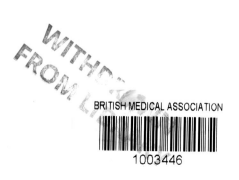

Videos associated with each of the chapters are online at MediaCenter.Thieme.com!

	WINDOWS & MAC	TABLET
Recommended Browser(s)	Recent browser versions on all major platforms and any mobile operating system that supports HTML5 video playback. *All browsers should have JavaScript enabled.*	
Flash Player Plug-in	Flash Player 9 or higher. *For Mac users, ATI Rage 128 GPU doesn't support full-screen mode with hardware scaling.*	Tablet PCs with Android OS support Flash 10.1.
Recommended for optimal usage experience	Monitor resolutions: • Normal (4:3) 1024×768 or higher • Widescreen (16:9) 1280×720 or higher • Widescreen (16:10) 1440×900 or higher A high-speed internet connection (minimum 384 Kps) is suggested.	WiFi or cellular data connection is required.

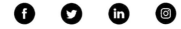

Connect with us on social media

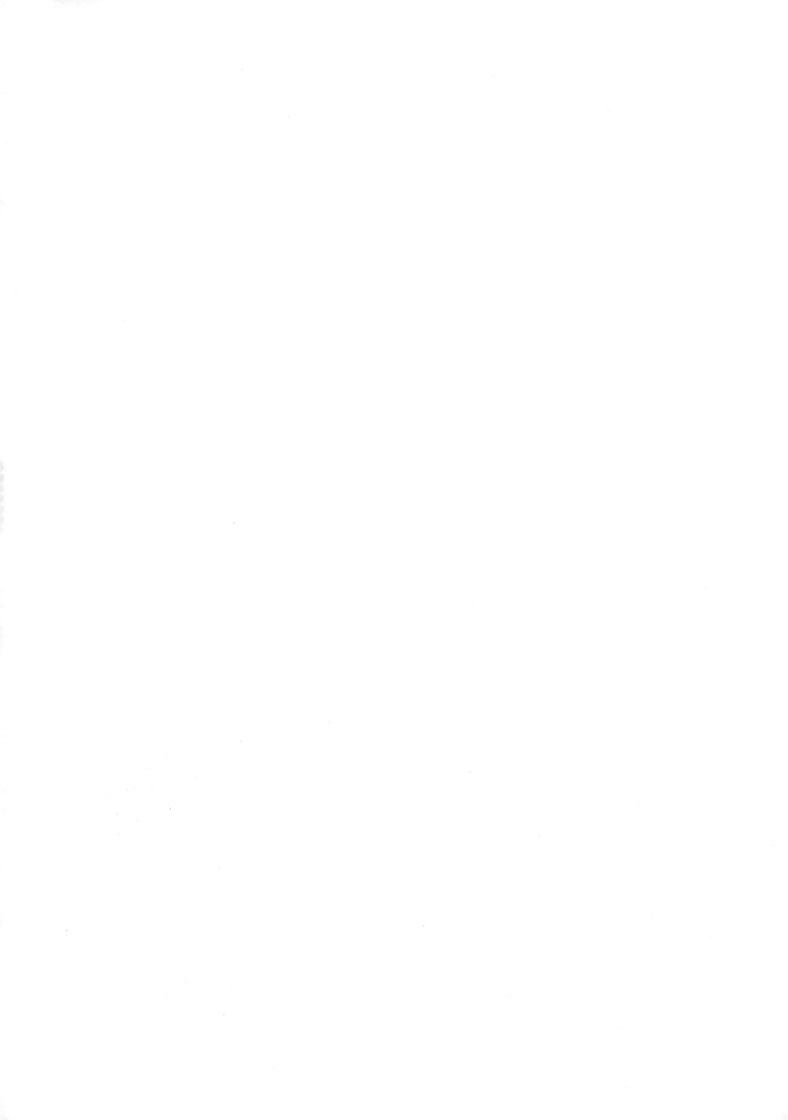

Gastroenterological Endoscopy

Michael B. Wallace, MD
Professor of Medicine
Division of Gastroenterology and Hepatology
Mayo Clinic
Jacksonville, FL, USA

Paul Fockens, MD
Professor and Chair
Department of Gastroenterology and Hepatology
Academic Medical Center
University of Amsterdam
Amsterdam, The Netherlands

Joseph Jao-Yiu Sung, MD, PhD
Mok Hing Yiu Professor of Medicine and Director
Institute of Digestive Diseases
The Chinese University of Hong Kong
Shatin, New Territories, Hong Kong

Associate Editors
Todd H. Baron, Nicholas J. Shaheen, Michael John Bourke,
D. Nageshwar Reddy, Lauren B. Gerson

Third edition

With contributions by:

Jürgen Hochberger, Juergen Maiss, Jonathan Cohen, Peter D. Siersema, Anthony T. R. Axon, Andrew Axon, Till Wehrmann, Hans-Dieter Allescher, Bret Petersen, Louis M. Wong Kee Song, Mouen Khashab, Matthew D. Rutter, Daniel Blero, Jacques Devière, Eduardo Rodrigues-Pinto, Philip Chiu, Rajvinder Singh, Yamamoto, Jamie Barkin, Jodie Barkin, John Chi To Wong, Christine Boumitri, Nikhil A. Kumta, Michel Kahaleh, David Lee, Juliana Yang, Ali A. Siddiqui, Ralf Kiesslich, Michael Vieth, Vanbiervliet, Rob Hawes, Hye Yeon Jhun, Prateek Sharma, Maximilien Barret, Roos E Pouw, Kamar Belghazi, Jacques JGM Bergman, David E. Fleischer, Hassan Siddiki, Albert J Bredenoord, Froukje van Hoeij, Douglas G. Adler, Moe Kyaw, James Lau, Takuji Gotoda, Chris Thompson, Andrew Storm, Steven A. Edmundowicz, Jonathan Leighton, Lucinda Harris, Greg Haber, Prashant Mudireddy, Joseph Murray, Alberto Rubio Tapia, Ibrahim Mostafa Ibrahim, Mostafa Ibrahim, Nancy N. Fanous, Doug Rex, David Tate, Evelien Dekker, Frank G.J. Kallenberg, Joep E.G. IJspeert, Barbara A.J. Bastiaansen, Geert D'Haens, Marjolijn Duijvestein, Helmut Messmann, Alexander Meier, Disaya Chavalitdhamrong, Rome Jutabha, Guido Costamagna, Pietro Familiari, Cristiano Spada, Marianna Arvanitakis, Omer Basar, William R. Brugge, Stavros Stavropoulos, Jennifer L. Maranki, Gregory G. Ginsberg, James H. Tabibian

787 illustrations

Thieme
Stuttgart • New York • Delhi • Rio De Janeiro

Library of Congress Cataloging-in-Publication Data
Names: Wallace, Michael B. (Michael Bradley), editor. |
    Fockens, Paul, editor. |
    Sung, Joseph J. Y. (Joseph Jao Yiu), 1959- editor.
Title: Gastroenterological endoscopy / [edited by] Michael B. Wallace,
    Paul Fockens, Joseph Jao Yiu Sung ; associate editors, Todd H. Baron,
    Nicholas J. Shaheen, Michael John Bourke, D. Nageshwar Reddy, Lauren B.
    Gerson; with contributions by Jhurgen Hochberger [and others].
Description: Third edition. | Stuttgart, Germany ; New York, NY : Georg
    Thieme Verlag, 2018. | Includes bibliographical references and index.
Identifiers: LCCN 2017059936 | ISBN 9783131258533
Subjects: | MESH: Endoscopy, Digestive System | Digestive System
    Diseases–diagnosis
Classification: LCC RC804.G3 | NLM WI 141 | DDC 616.3/307545--dc23 LC record
    available at https://lccn.loc.gov/2017059936

Important note: Medicine is an ever-changing science undergoing continual development. Research and clinical experience are continually expanding our knowledge, in particular our knowledge of proper treatment and drug therapy. Insofar as this book mentions any dosage or application, readers may rest assured that the authors, editors, and publishers have made every effort to ensure that such references are in accordance with **the state of knowledge at the time of production of the book**.

Nevertheless, this does not involve, imply, or express any guarantee or responsibility on the part of the publishers in respect to any dosage instructions and forms of applications stated in the book. **Every user is requested to examine carefully** the manufacturers' leaflets accompanying each drug and to check, if necessary in consultation with a physician or specialist, whether the dosage schedules mentioned therein or the contraindications stated by the manufacturers differ from the statements made in the present book. Such examination is particularly important with drugs that are either rarely used or have been newly released on the market. Every dosage schedule or every form of application used is entirely at the user's own risk and responsibility. The authors and publishers request every user to report to the publishers any discrepancies or inaccuracies noticed. If errors in this work are found after publication, errata will be posted at www.thieme.com on the product description page.

Some of the product names, patents, and registered designs referred to in this book are in fact registered trademarks or proprietary names even though specific reference to this fact is not always made in the text. Therefore, the appearance of a name without designation as proprietary is not to be construed as a representation by the publisher that it is in the public domain.

© 2018 by Georg Thieme Verlag KG

Thieme Publishers Stuttgart
Rüdigerstrasse 14, 70469 Stuttgart, Germany
+49 [0]711 8931 421, customerservice@thieme.de

Thieme Publishers New York
333 Seventh Avenue, New York, NY 10001 USA
+1 800 782 3488, customerservice@thieme.com

Thieme Publishers Delhi
A-12, Second Floor, Sector-2, Noida-201301
Uttar Pradesh, India
+91 120 45 566 00, customerservice@thieme.in

Thieme Publishers Rio, Thieme Publicações Ltda.
Edifício Rodolpho de Paoli, 25ª andar
Av. Nilo Peçanha, 50 – Sala 2508
Rio de Janeiro 20020-906 Brasil
+55 21 3172 2297 / +55 21 3172 1896

Cover design: Thieme Publishing Group
Typesetting by DiTech Process Solutions

Printed in Germany by CPI Books GmbH

5 4 3 2 1

ISBN 978-3-13-125853-3

Also available as an e-book:
eISBN 978-3-13-147013-3

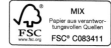

MIX
Papier aus verantwortungsvollen Quellen
FSC® C083411

Dedication

In Memory of Dr. Lauren Battat Gerson

We mourn the untimely demise of our colleague Dr. Lauren Battat Gerson, who passed away on July 21, 2017. Lauren contributed to the field of *gastrointestinal endoscopy* in so many ways, including as an associate editor for this book. She will be remembered for all the lives she touched and patients she cared for. A memorial article was published in *Gastrointestinal Endoscopy*, volume 86, issue 4, pages 579–80.

Preface

We proudly present the third edition of *Gastroenterological Endoscopy*, 15 years after the first and 8 years after the second edition. This book, founded by Professors Classen, Tytgat, and Lightdale, now passes the torch to a second generation of editors. It nonetheless continues the tradition of excellence, depth, and breadth that its founding editors started. We strive to continue publishing the leading reference in the field of gastrointestinal endoscopy. Professors Fockens, Sung, and Wallace have brought together an outstanding team of associate editors: Todd Baron, Michael Bourke, Nicholas Shaheen, Nageshwar (Nagy) Reddy, and Lauren Gerson. After completion of the book, but prior to its publication, we were tremendously saddened by the sudden passing of Dr. Gerson, whose contribution carries on with the book. A memoriam to Dr. Gerson appears in the opening pages of this book.

The list of contributing authors is a who's who of endoscopy. We are fortunate to have both, senior masters and new innovators. In the preface to the second edition, the "new" procedures of the day were NOTES, ESD, and advanced imaging. Much has passed since 2010. NOTES (natural orifice transluminal endoscopic surgery) has largely waned, but it led endoscopy into the "third space," the submucosa between the lumen and the outside (intra-abdominal) world. Submucosal endoscopy enabled POEMS (per-oral endoscopic myotomy surgery) for achalasia and its new variations, gastric-POEMS (for gastroparesis) and STER (submucosal tunnel endoscopic resection), for subepithelial tumors. New devices such as over-the-scope clips have enabled safe closure of full-thickness defects. Initially, these were applied to unplanned perforations and bleeding, but as we became increasingly confident of closure, they enabled planned full-thickness resection of tumors and even tissue sampling of the gastroenteric nervous system, which further opens new methods of research and treatment. Endoscopic resection by EMR and ESD is now practiced worldwide with refinements in devices and techniques to make it easier and safer while still preserving its efficacy. A major recent advancement in endoscopy was the development of lumen-apposing metal stents (LAMS), initially for drainage of pancreatic fluid collections. Like NOTES, LAMS have opened a new world of possibilities to endoscopists including EUS-guided biliary drainage directly from lumen to bile duct (not retrograde through the papilla). Lumen-to-lumen apposition has opened the way for gastroenteric bypass in duodenal obstruction (or double biliary and duodenal bypass in the case of double obstruction from pancreatic head tumors). Creative endoscopists, driven by patients' needs, developed methods of biliary access in patients with surgically altered anatomy through a variety of transluminal routes. It is remarkable to witness the impact of new technology (LAMS, clips) and techniques (POEMS, NOTES) on unanticipated downstream innovations. These are truly disruptive events, all captured in the third edition.

In addition to the editors and authors, we wish to thank the outstanding staff at Thieme for editorial assistance in producing this large volume of work. We hope that endoscopists throughout the world will engage this new knowledge and, most importantly, apply it to improve the care of patients with gastrointestinal and other relevant diseases.

The editors

List of Contributors

Associate Editors

Todd H. Baron, MD
Professor
Director of Advanced Therapeutic
Endoscopy
University of North Carolina
North Carolina, USA

Nicholas J. Shaheen, MD, MPH
Professor, Medicine and Epidemiology
Chief, Division of Gastroenterology and
Hepatology
University of North Carolina School of
Medicine
North Carolina, USA

Michael John Bourke, FRACP
Professor
Department of Gastroenterology and
Hepatology
Westmead Hospital
Sydney, Australia

D. Nageshwar Reddy, MD, DM, DSc, FAMS,
FRCP, FASGE, FACG, MWGO
Chairman and Chief of Gastroenterology
Asian Institute of Gastroenterology
Hyderabad, India

Lauren B. Gerson, MD, MSc
Associate Clinical Professor
University of California San Francisco
Director of Clinical Research
Gastroenterology Fellowship Program
California Pacific Medical Center
California, USA

Contributors

Douglas G. Adler MD, FACG, AGAF, FASGE
Professor
Director of Therapeutic Endoscopy
Director
GI Fellowship Program
Gastroenterology and Hepatology
University of Utah School of Medicine
Huntsman Cancer Center
Utah, USA

Hans-Dieter Allescher, MD, PhD
Professor
Center for Internal Medicine
Klinikum Garmisch-Partenkirchen
Garmisch-Partenkirchen, Germany

Marianna Arvanitakis, MD, PhD
Department of Gastroenterology
Erasme University Hospital ULB
Brussels, Belgium

Andrew Eliot Axon, BA (Hons), MA (Cantab)
Head
Parklane Plowden Barristers Chambers
Leeds and Newcastle, UK

Anthony T. R. Axon, MD, FRCP
Professor
University of Leeds
Leeds, UK

Jamie S. Barkin, MD, MACP, MACG, AGAF,
FASGE
Professor of Medicine
Miller School of Medicine
University of Miami
Florida, USA

Jodie A. Barkin, MD
Gastroenterology Fellow
Department of Medicine, Division of
Gastroenterology
Leonard M. Miller School of Medicine
University of Miami
Florida, USA

Maximilien Barret, MD
Department of Gastroenterology and
Hepatology
Academic Medical Center
Amsterdam, The Netherlands

Omer Basar, MD
Research Fellow
Pancreas Biliary Center
Gastrointestinal Unit
Massachusetts General Hospital
Boston, Massachusetts, USA
Professor
Hacettepe Medical School
Department of Gastroenterology
Ankara, Turkey

Barbara A.J. Bastiaansen, MD
Department of Gastroenterology and
Hepatology
Academical Medical Center
University of Amsterdam
Amsterdam, The Netherlands

Kamar Belghazi, MD
Department of Gastroenterology and
Hepatology
Academic Medical Center
Amsterdam, The Netherlands

J.J.G.H.M. Bergman, MD, PhD
Professor
Department of Gastroenterology &
Hepatology
Academic Medical Center
Amsterdam, The Netherlands

Daniel Blero, MD
Professor
Department of Gastroenterology
Hepatopancreatology, and Digestive
Oncology, Université Libre de Bruxelles
Hôpital Erasme
Brussels, Belgium

Christine Boumitri, MD
Gastroenterology Fellow
Department of Gastroenterology and
Hepatology
University of Missouri
Missouri, USA

Albert J. Bredenoord, MD
Department of Gastroenterology and
Hepatology
Academic Medical Centre
Amsterdam, The Netherlands

William R. Brugge, MD
Director, Pancreas-Biliary Center
Professor
Massachusetts General Hospital
Harvard Medical School
Massachusetts, USA

Disaya Chavalitdhamrong, MD
Division of Gastroenterology
Harbor-UCLA Medical Center
California, USA

Philip Wai Yan Chiu, MD (CUHK),
MBChB (CUHK), FRCSEd, FCSHK, FHKAM
(Surgery)
Professor
Department of Surgery, Institute of
Digestive Disease
The Chinese University of Hong Kong
New Territories, Hong Kong

Jonathan Cohen, MD, FASGE, FACG
Clinical Professor
New York University School of Medicine
New York, USA

Guido Costamagna, MD, FACG
Professor
Head of Department of Digestive and
Endocrine-Metabolic Diseases
Director of Digestive Endoscopy Unit
Catholic University of Rome
Rome, Italy
Chair of Excellence in Digestive Endoscopy
University of Strasbourg
Strasbourg, France

Geert R.A.M. D'Haens, MD, PhD
Professor
Department of Gastroenterology and
Hepatology
Academic Medical Center
Amsterdam, The Netherlands

Evelien Dekker, MD, PhD
Department of Gastroenterology &
Hepatology
Academic Medical Center
Amsterdam, The Netherlands

Jacques Deviere, MD, PhD
Professor
Director
Division of Gastroenterology
Hepatopancreatology and Digestive oncology
Erasme Hospital, ULB
Brussels, Belgium

Marjolijn Duijvestein, MD, PhD
Department of Gastroenterology and
Hepatology
Academic Medical Center
Amsterdam, The Netherlands

Steven A. Edmundowicz, MD, FASGE
Professor
Medical Director, Digestive Health Center
University of Colorado Anschutz Medical
Campus
University of Colorado Hospital
Colorado, USA

Pietro Familiari MD, PhD
Digestive Endoscopy Unit
Fondazione Policlinico Universitario A.
Gemelli
Rome, Italy

Nancy N. Fanous, MSc., MD
Consultant Gastroenterologist and
Hepatologist
Police Hospital
General Administration of Medical Services
at Ministry of Interior
Department of Gastroenterology,
Hepatology and Endoscopy
Cairo, Egypt

David E. Fleischer, MD
Professor
Mayo College of Medicine
Staff Physician
Mayo Clinic
Arizona, USA

Gregory G. Ginsberg, MD
Professor
University of Pennsylvania Perelman School
of Medicine
Penn Medicine
Abramson Cancer Center
Gastroenterology Division
Director of Endoscopic Services
Perelman Center for Advanced Medicine
Pennsylvania, USA

Takuji Gotoda, MD, PhD, FASGE, FACG, FRCP
Professor
Division of Gastroenterology and Hepatology
Department of Medicine
Nihon University School of Medicine
Tokyo, Japan

Gregory B. Haber, MD
Chief
Division of Gastroenterology
Lenox Hill Hospital
Northwell Health System
New York, USA

Lucinda A. Harris, MD
Associate Professor
Division of Gastroenterology and Hepatology
Mayo Clinic College of Medicine
Arizona, USA

Robert H. Hawes, MD
Professor
University of Central Florida College of
Medicine
Medical Director
Florida Hospital Institute for Minimally
Invasive Therapy
Florida, USA

Juergen Hochberger, MD, PhD, FASGE
Chairman
Department of Gastroenterology
Vivantes Friedrichshain Hospital
Teaching Hospital of Humboldt University
Charité
Berlin, Germany

Froukje B. van Hoeij, MD
Research fellow
Department of Gastroenterology and
Hepatology
Academic Medical Center
Amsterdam, The Netherlands

Mostafa Ibrahim, MD
Department of Gastroenterology, Hepatopa-
ncreatology and Digestive Oncology
Erasme Hospital
Université libre de Bruxelles
Brussels, Belgium

Ibrahim Mostafa Ibrahim, MD, PhD, FACG,
MWGO, FRCP (Glasg.)
Professor of Gastroenterology, Hepatology
and Liver Transplantation
Theodor Bilharz Research Institute, Ministry
of Scientific Research
Chair, Education Committee World Endosco-
py Organization
Vice President, Pan Arab Association of
Gastroenterology
Giza Governorate, Egypt

Joep Evert Godfried IJspeert, MD
Epidemiologist
Department of Gastroenterology and
Hepatology
Academic Medical Centre
University of Amsterdam
Amsterdam, The Netherlands

Hye Yeon Jhun, MD
Gastroenterology Fellow
University of Kansas Medical Center
Kansas, USA

Rome Jutabha, MD
Professor
Division of Digestive Diseases
David Geffen School of Medicine at UCLA
Director, UCLA Center for Small Bowel
Diseases
Ronald Reagan UCLA Medical Center
Advisory Board, UCLA Center for World
Health
California, USA

Michel Kahaleh, M.D., AGAF, FACG, FASGE
Professor
Medical Director Pancreas Program
Division of Gastroenterology and
Hepatology
Department of Medicine
Weill Cornell Medicine
New York, USA

Frank G.J. Kallenberg, MD
Department of Gastroenterology and
Hepatology
Academic Medical Center
University of Amsterdam
Amsterdam, The Netherlands

Mouen A. Khashab, MD
Associate Professor
Director
Therapeutic Endoscopy
Division
Gastroenterology and Hepatology
Johns Hopkins Hospital
Maryland, USA

Ralf Kiesslich, MD
Professor
Department of Gastroenterology and
Hepatology
Helios HSK Wiesbaden

Nikhil A. Kumta, MD, MS
Assistant Professor
Department of Medicine
Dr. Henry D. Janowitz Division of
Gastroenterology
Mount Sinai Hospital
New York, USA

Moe Kyaw, MRCP, MSc, MBA
Institute of Digestive Diseases
The Chinese University of Hong Kong
Prince of Wales Hospital
New Territories, Hong Kong

James YW Lau, FRCS
Department of Surgery
Prince of Wales Hospital
The Chinese University of Hong Kong
New Territories, Hong Kong

David Lee, MD
Gastroenterology Fellow
H.H. Chao Comprehensive Digestive Disease
Center
Division of Gastroenterology and
Hepatology
University of California Irvine Medical
Center
California, USA

Jonathan A. Leighton, MD, FACG, AGAF,
FASGE, FACP
Professor
Mayo Clinic
Arizona, USA

Juergen Maiss, MD, PhD
Kerzel and Maiss Gastroenterology
Associates
Forchheim, Germany

Jennifer L. Maranki, MD, MSc
Assistant Professor
Section of Gastroenterology and Hepatology
Temple University School of Medicine
Pennsylvania, USA

Alexander Meier, MD
III. Medical Clinic
Klinikum Augsburg
Augsburg, Germany

Helmut Messmann, MD
Professor
Director III. Med. Department
Klinikum, Augsburg

Prashant R. Mudireddy, MD
GI Fellow
Department of Gastroenterology
Lenox Hill Hospital
Northwell Health System
New York, USA

Joseph A. Murray, MD
Professor
Consultant
Department of Immunology
Division of Gastroenterology and
Hepatology
Mayo Clinic
Minnesota, USA

Bret T. Petersen, MD
Professor
Division of Gastroenterology
Mayo Clinic
Rochester, Minnesota, USA

Roos Elisabeth Pouw, MD, PhD
Department of Gastroenterology and
Hepatology
Academic Medical Center
Amsterdam, The Netherlands

Douglas Kevin Rex, MD
Distinguished Professor
Indiana University School of Medicine
Chancellor's Professor, Indiana University–
Purdue University Indianapolis
Director of Endoscopy, Indiana University
Hospital
Division of Gastroenterology/Hepatology
Indiana University Health
Indiana, USA

Eduardo Rodrigues-Pinto, MD
Department of Gastroenterology
Centro Hospitalar São João
Porto, Portugal

Alberto Rubio-Tapia, MD
Assistant Professor
Division of Gastroenterology and
Hepatology
Mayo Clinic
Minnesota, USA

Matthew D. Rutter, MD, FRCP
Professor
University Hospital of North Tees
Queen's Medical Campus, Durham
University
Cleveland, UK

Prateek Sharma, MD
Professor
University of Kansas School of Medicine
Department of Veterans Affairs Medical
Center
Missouri, USA

Hassan Siddiki, MD, MS
Clinical Fellow
Department of Gastroenterology and
Hepatology
Mayo Clinic
Arizona, USA

Ali Ahmed Siddiqui, MD
Professor
Division of Gastroenterology
Thomas Jefferson University Hospital
Pennsylvania, USA

Peter D. Siersema, MD, PhD, FASGE
Professor
Department of Gastroenterology and
Hepatology
Radboud University Medical Center
Nijmegen, The Netherlands

Rajvinder Singh, FRCP FRACP
Professor of Medicine and Director of
Gastroenterology
Department of Gastroenterology
Division of Medicine
University of Adelaide & the Lyell McEwin
Hospital
Adelaide, Australia

Louis M. Wong Kee Song, MD
Professor
Division of Gastroenterology and Hepatology
Mayo Clinic
Minnesota, USA

Cristiano Spada, MD, PhD
Digestive Endoscopy Unit
Fondazione Policlinico Universitario A.
Gemelli
Rome, Italy

Stavros N. Stavropoulos, MD, FASGE
Chief, GI Endoscopy
Director, Program in Advanced GI Endoscopy
Winthrop University Hospital
Mineola, New York, USA
Adjunct Professor
Columbia University
New York, New York, USA
Adjunct Clinical Professor of Medicine
Temple University
Pennsylvania, USA

Andrew C. Storm, MD
Therapeutic Endoscopy Fellow
Division of Gastroenterology and
Hepatology
Mayo Clinic
Minnesota, USA

James H. Tabibian, MD, PhD
Instructor
Division of Gastroenterology
Advanced Endoscopy Training Program
Hospital of the University of Pennsylvania
Pennsylvania, USA

David James Tate, MA (Cantab), MRCP
Department of Gastroenterology and
Hepatology
Westmead Hospital
Sydney, Australia

Christopher C. Thompson, MD, MSc, FACG,
FASGE
Director of Therapeutic Endoscopy
Associate Professor
Division of Gastroenterology, Hepatology
and Endoscopy
Brigham and Women's Hospital
Harvard Medical School
Massachusetts, USA

Geoffroy Vanbiervliet, MD, MSc
Hospital Practitioner
Endoscopie Digestive
Hôpital L'Archet, CHU Nice
Nice, France

Michael Vieth, MD
Klinikum Bayreuth
Institute of Pathology
Bayreuth, Germany

Till Wehrmann, MD, PhD
Head
Department of Gastroenterology
DKD Helios Klinik Wiesbaden
Wiesbaden, Germany

John Chi To Wong, MD, FRCPC, DABIM
Clinical Professional Consultant
Institute of Digestive Disease
The Chinese University of Hong Kong
Prince of Wales Hospital
New Territories, Hong Kong

Hironori Yamamoto, MD, PhD
Professor
Department of Medicine
Division of Gastroenterology
Jichi Medical University
Tochigi, Japan

Juliana Yang, MD
Gastroenterology Fellow
Division of Digestive and Liver Diseases
University of Texas Southwestern Medical
Center
Texas, USA

Contents

Contents

III General Diagnostic and Therapeutic Procedures and Techniques

Contents

IV Upper Gastrointestinal Tract Disease

Contents

VI Biliopancreatic, Hepatic, and Peritoneal Diseases

Index

Video Contents

Abbreviations

automated endoscope reprocessors	AER	fine-needle aspiration	FNA
argon plasma coagulation	APC	gastric antral vascular ectasia	GAVE
American Society for Gastrointestinal Endoscopy	ASGE	gastrointestinal	GI
adenosine triphosphate	ATP	high- level disinfection	HLD
complementary metal oxide semiconductor	CMOS	instructions for use	IFUs
carbapenem–resistant enterobacteriaceae	CRE	Japanese Gastroenterological Endoscopy Society	JGES
dual antiplatelet therapy	DAPT	liquid chemical germicide	LCG
esophagogastroduodenoscopy	EGD	multidrug-resistant organism	MDRO
endoscopic mucosal resection	EMR	Mallory–Weiss tear	MWT
endoscopic retrograde cholangiopancreatography	ERCP	not recommended	NR
endoscopic submucosal dissection	ESD	polymerase chain	PCR
European Society of Gastrointestinal Endoscopy	ESGE	percutaneous endoscopic gastrostomy/jejunostomy	PEG/PEJ
endoscopic ultrasound	EUS	peptic ulcer disease	PUD

Section I

Introduction to Endoscopy

1 Education and Training in Endoscopy

Jürgen Hochberger, Jürgen Maiss, and Jonathan Cohen

1.1 Introduction

Optimal patient care and quality outcomes are becoming increasingly important in clinical medicine. Specialist medical societies have produced guidelines and recommendations for minimum quality requirements for performance of endoscopic techniques (▶ Table 1.1).[1] However, in most of these guidelines, terms such as "self-reliance" and "under supervision" are not clearly defined. Optimal methods, duration, and proper endpoints of training are still topics of debate.[2] There has been a growing trend to de-emphasize the number or procedures performed in favor of demonstration of competent and independent performance.[3]

Recently, endoscopy simulators have rekindled debate on whether training in basic manual skills is better provided outside the patient.[4,5,6,7,8] Despite the growing availability of various training models, practical skills are still routinely acquired by performing actual procedures under the supervision of a senior endoscopist. This chapter presents an overview of training issues and the role of simulators in training.

1.2 Clinical Education

A few general principles can be applied to the entire field of endoscopic training:

- The endpoint of training is the acquisition of competency to perform the examinations without supervision at a level comparable to that achieved by practitioners in the community.
- While certain general endoscopic basic skills are crucial to many procedures, training must be procedure specific. Competency in one technique does not necessarily guarantee competency in another technique.
- Procedures performed for diagnostic purposes should also enable related tissue sampling or therapies associated with that procedure.

1.2.1 Clinical Training to Competency in Esophagogastroduodenoscopy and Colonoscopy: Studies, Guidelines, and Assessment

Since the early 1980s, trainees have been required to keep a record of all procedures performed,[1] in particular for colonoscopy.

The ability to reach the cecum is the most common criterion by which colonoscopies have been judged.[9] Data from early studies showed variable learning curves and led to the concept of minimal numbers of procedures required.[1] Sedlack et al presented in 2011 a new assessment tool, the so-called Mayo Colonoscopy Skills Assessment Tool (MCSAT), to describe learning curves for colonoscopy.[10] They evaluated forty-one GI fellows who performed 6,635 colonoscopies. Independent cecal intubation rates of 85% and cecal intubation times of 16 minutes or less were achieved at 275 procedures on average, which is more than previous gastroenterology training recommendations required.

In 2014, the Training Committee of the American Society for Gastrointestinal Endoscopy (ASGE) presented the "Assessment of Competency in Endoscopy" (ACE) tool as a refinement of the MCSAT.[9] The ACE tool added important quality parameters such as a metric assessment of fine-tip control and polyp detection rates. In 2016, a prospective, multicenter trial was published evaluating the ACE tool at 10 institutions across the United States including 93 gastrointestinal (GI) fellows.[11] A total of 184 senior endoscopists assessed 1,061 colonoscopies, which included 6 motor and 6 cognitive skills on a 4-point scale. The average fellow reached required cognitive and motor skills endpoints by 250 procedures, with over 90% of fellows surpassing these thresholds by 300 procedures.[11] Procedure times, polyp detection rates, and polyp miss rates with increasing experience are shown in ▶ Fig. 1.1 and ▶ Fig. 1.2.

Barton et al[12] described in 2012 the value of the Direct Observation of Procedural Skills (DOPS) method developed by an expert group of colonoscopists and clinical educators in the United Kingdom. Colonoscopists wishing to participate in the British National Health Service National Bowel Cancer Screening Programme (BCSP) were assessed. Assessments from 147 candidates and 28 assessors were analyzed. Candidates had to prove experience in a minimum of 500 colonoscopies with a self-reported cecal intubation rate of ≥ 90% and a polyp detection rate of ≥ 20%. The assessment had high reliability using generalizability theory (G) with G = 0.81 and correlated highly with a global expert assessment. Both, candidates and assessors, believed that the DOPS was a valid assessment of competence.

Anderson[13] recently described how DOPS evaluation has been successfully integrated for trainees as well as for independent endoscopists into the "UK National Bowel Cancer Screening Programme." The Joint Advisory Group (JAG) sets the standards for endoscopy training and the accreditation of endoscopy units as base training

Table 1.1 Recommendations regarding the minimum numbers of procedures required for competence.*

Organization	EGD	Colonoscopy	ERCP
American Society for Gastrointestinal Endoscopy	100	100	100
British Society of Gastroenterology	300	100	150
Conjoint Committee for the Recognition of Training in Gastrointestinal Endoscopy (Australia)	200	100	200
European Diploma of Gastroenterology	300	100	150

Abbreviations: EGD, esophagogastroduodenoscopy; ERCP, endoscopic retrograde cholangiopancreatography.

Source: Hochberger et al 2010.[1]

*Numbers often under debate.

units.[14,15] A Global Rating Scale web-based system is used for continuous assessment of performance and DOPS is regularly applied in order to monitor continuously individual performances. An individual web-based logbook and e-portfolio of each endoscopist is created via a national database system that is the base for credentialing and certification. Feedback of data to individuals helps in benchmarking and identification of those with suboptimal performance and a need for extra training and close audits. The system has recently been extended to upper GI endoscopy and other techniques.[16]

1.2.2 Training in Endoscopic Retrograde Cholangiopancreatography

Proficiency in all aspects of endoscopic retrograde cholangiopancreatography (ERCP) requires several years of practical training and continuous refinement of knowledge and skills.[8] With the advent of noninvasive tests such as magnetic resonance cholangiopancreatography (MRCP) and endoscopic ultrasonography (EUS), ERCP is an almost purely therapeutic procedure. This is creating a new challenge in the training of young endoscopists, as ERCP procedures are becoming more complex and are concentrated in large- or mid-volume endoscopy centers.[17,18]

In most fellowship training programs, traditional ERCP training follows education in diagnostic gastroscopy and colonoscopy and is often begun when the trainee has been introduced to polypectomy, hemostasis, or EUS training as part of a "learning pyramid" (▶Fig. 1.3).[1]

Jowell et al[19] found that a minimum of 180 to 200 ERCPs are needed to be performed before a trainee could attain competency in ERCP.[19] (▶Fig. 1.4) Approximately, 80 to 100 ERCPs per

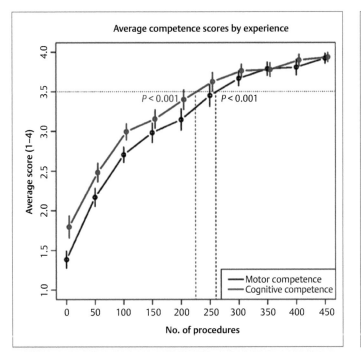

Fig. 1.1 Procedure time by experience. (Reproduced with permission from Sedlack et al 2016.[11])

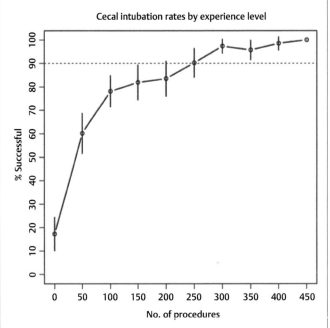

Fig. 1.2 Polyp detection and miss rates by experience. (Reproduced with permission from Sedlack et al 2016.[11])

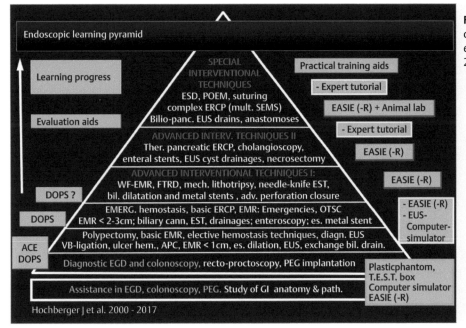

Fig. 1.3 The "learning pyramid" as an example of stepwise clinical training in interventional endoscopy. (Adapted from Hochberger et al 2010.[1])

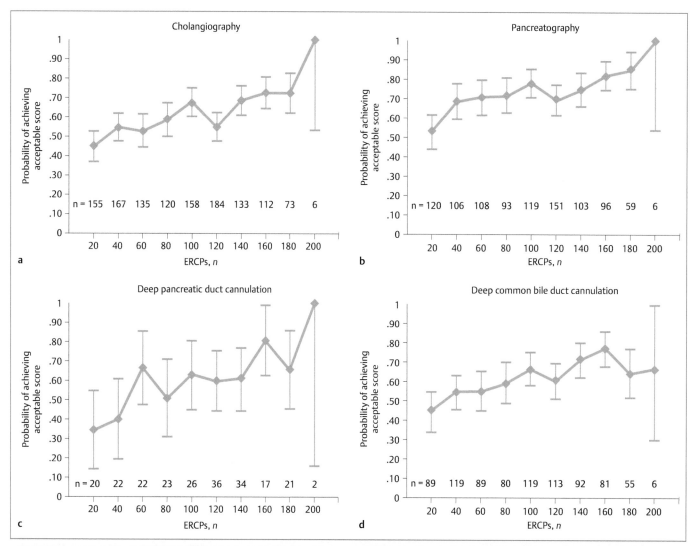

Fig. 1.4 The probability (with 95% confidence intervals) of achieving an acceptable score for cholangiography **(a)**, pancreatography **(b)**, deep pancreatic cannulation **(c)**, and deep biliary cannulation **(d)** during training of fellows in endoscopic retrograde cholangiopancreatography (ERCP), as reported by Jowell et al[19] for 17 gastroenterology fellows during 1,450 ERCP procedures.

endoscopist per year appear to be necessary to maintain adequate competence for biliary procedures and 250 ERCPs per endoscopist per year for complex therapeutic procedures in the pancreas.[20] The ERCP volume plays a role in complication rates. In various studies, a minimum of 40 to 50 endoscopic sphincterotomies (ESTs) per endoscopist per year was found to be associated with a lower complication rate in comparison to endoscopists with a lower EST frequency.[8,21] Rabenstein et al[22] showed that both prior experience and ongoing volume of ERCPs influence the success and complication rate.

Now that most ERCPs are performed for therapeutic purposes, it is a matter of controversy whether cannulation is the next technique for the trainee to learn after he or she is able to maneuver the duodenoscope competently to the papilla. For example, it is well known that for routine stent exchanges in the setting of a prior sphincterotomy, fewer procedures ($n = 60$) are needed to obtain competence than is the case with cannulation of a native papilla ($n = 180–200$), and it is also known that stent exchanges are associated with a lower risk profile compared to cannulation. Patients with benign biliary strictures, chronic obstructive pancreatitis, and recurrent bile duct stones in the setting of prior sphincterotomy are also associated with lower risk during training.

The ASGE published their latest core curriculum for training in ERCP in 2016.[8,23] Trainees who elect to perform ERCP should have completed at least 18 months of standard gastroenterology training, followed by at least 12 months of ERCP training.

Schutz and Abbott[24] developed an ERCP grading scale based on procedural difficulty using benchmarks such as cannulation rates to gauge competency. A modification of this score was adopted by the ASGE as part of their quality-assessment document. Absolute numbers of procedures partially performed by a fellow may not realistically reflect competence.[25] Where possible, trainee logbook records should specify particular skills completed by the fellow (cannulation, sphincterotomy, stent placement, tissue sampling), and should also indicate cases that the trainee completed without assistance. The ASGE guidelines state that most fellows require at least 180 ERCP cases before competency can be assessed, with at least half being therapeutic.[8] Although not all of the trainees may ultimately perform ERCP after the completion of their training, all fellows should at least develop an understanding of the diagnostic and therapeutic role of the procedure, including indications, contraindications, and possible complications.[26]

The decision by a program director as to whether to train one or more fellows each year to achieve sufficient competence will depend in some measure on the volume of ERCPs performed at the institution and the availability of experts in ERCP (▶ Fig. 1.4).[19] For example, with an annual volume of 400 cases and three fellows, it would be reasonable to have one fellow perform 300 or more cases and provide the other two with an exposure to ERCP, rather than have all three individuals equally share cases, with a low likelihood that any of the three would reach competence by the end of the fellowship.

1.2.3 Complementary E-learning and Video Courses

Live endoscopy courses, interactive teaching programs, and video materials can help trainees to recognize pathology better and to understand the appropriate application of therapeutic techniques.[27] However, such passive activities cannot replace the performance of the actual procedures.

1.3 Incorporation of Simulators in Training

The Gastroenterology Core Curriculum, Third Edition in May 2007 states in section IV.A.6.(b): "Fellows must participate in training using simulation."[23] To date, no simulator experience alone has been validated as sufficient to replace actual patient experience. To guide adoption of simulators for specific roles in training and assessing skill, the ASGE initiated a PIVI (*Preservation and Incorporation of Valuable Endoscopic Innovations*) task force in 2011.[28] This group set the following two thresholds for justifying adoption of a particular simulator:

- *Threshold for incorporation into training.* For an endoscopy simulator to be integrated into the standard instruction for a procedure, it must demonstrate a 25% or greater reduction in the median number of clinical cases required for the trainees to achieve the minimal competence parameters for that procedure.
- *Threshold for assessing skill.* Simulator-based assessment tools must be procedure-specific and predictive of independently defined minimal competence parameters from real procedures with a kappa value of at least 0.70 for high-stakes assessment.[28]

The logistic and cost issues for a particular simulator would need to be weighed. For example, a high-cost computer simulator that had a 25% reduction in a learning curve might not make any sense for a program in which trainees typically had sufficient actual case experience to develop competency. In contrast, a lower cost simulator in which a program typically had insufficient cases would be well worth the investment.

1.4 Endoscopy Simulators and Training Models

1.4.1 Plastic Phantoms and Other Static Models

The initial experimental models for endoscopy training were made of plastic and textile tissues.[1] In 1974, Classen and Ruppin[29] in Erlangen presented an anatomically shaped plastic phantom that allowed examination of the upper GI tract. Christopher Williams and his group in London have been working on the first semi-rigid colonoscopy phantoms. A robust further development represents the Kyoto Kagaku Colonoscope Training Model, which presents greater technical difficulty to reach the cecum and allows a more realistic loop reduction ▶ Fig. 1.6.[29] Grund and co-workers in Tübingen, Germany, developed a series of advanced static models for different training purposes.[32,33] They include artificial tissues for electrosurgical interventions and recently specific ERCP techniques. Unfortunately, those models are not commercially available so far and there are no published data validating their use in training.

In addition, a number of device manufacturers have produced their own models to facilitate training in the procedures in which their accessories are used. The Cook Medical ERCP Trainer recently developed by Costamagna et al[34] allows to practice cannulation and different ERCP techniques except sphincterotomy via a plastic papilla with varying ampullary anatomy, orientation, and cannulation difficulty.

Another promising simulator is the "T.E.S.T box simulator" (▶ Fig. 1.5).[35] The model, designed by Christopher Thompson has demonstrated an ability to distinguish skills levels with significant

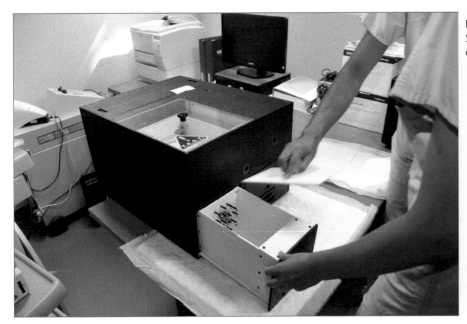

Fig. 1.5 The Thompson Endoscopic Part Task Simulator Training (T.E.S.T.) box containing five different training modules.[33]

1.4.2. Computer Simulators

Various computer simulation systems have been developed since the early 1980s.[1] Rapid progress in computer technology and electronics at the early 2000s allowed the development of commercially available systems. The first of these models was the Simbionix GI Mentor (3D Systems Healthcare, Littleton, CO,

United States, formerly Simbionix Corporation), at the time in the shape of a human torso mannequin.[34] The system creates a relatively realistic virtual endoscopy environment and allowed the simulation of various diagnostic and interventional procedures at different levels. During training, teaching modules with anatomy and pathology (▶Fig. 1.7) atlases are at the trainee's disposition. Beginners can train their dexterity in a "GI Fundamental Skills" module including navigation, targeting, retroflection, loop reduction, or in "Cyberscopy," a module to further enhance hand–eye coordination. Different modules such as upper and lower GI endoscopy, sigmoidoscopy, EUS, ERCP, and hemostasis training are available. EUS and ERCP modules allow parallel viewing of radiographic and endoscopic simulations. Virtual sphincterotomy, stone extraction, and other techniques have been implemented. In addition to the current GI Mentor model (3D Systems Healthcare), the EndoVR virtual reality endoscopy simulator (CAE Healthcare, Montreal, Canada, formerly "Accutouch" by Immersion Medical, Inc., Gaithersburg, MD, United States) has been used in multiple studies (see later). Recently, another system the so-called "Endo X" has been presented (Medical-X BV, EM Rotterdam, the Netherlands (▶Fig. 1.8). The system provides mainly upper and lower GI techniques, but also includes analyzing tools such as insufflation performance simulation and video recording of the procedure. All devices allow user-specific training curricula and reflect the user-specific learning curve. Modules are supervised by a virtual tutor and the whole system can be connected to a real supervisor via internet for additional personal feedback and to view learning curves of different trainees by the supervisor (▶Fig. 1.9). Various studies have demonstrated the benefits of additional computer simulator training in connection with colonoscopy.[1,28]

In a prospective simulation study, four fellows at the Mayo Clinic received 6 hours of simulator-based training, compared with four fellows without training. The simulator-trained fellows outperformed the traditionally trained fellows during their initial 15 to 30 colonoscopies in all performance aspects except for insertion time ($p < 0.05$). Beyond 30 procedures, there were no differences in performance between the two groups (evidence level B).

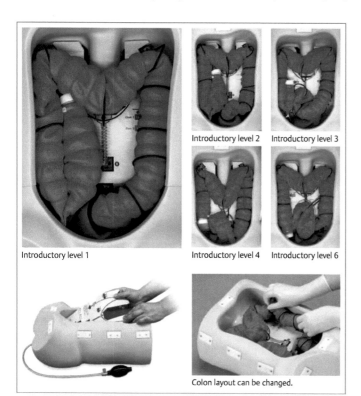

Introductory level 1
Introductory level 2
Introductory level 3
Introductory level 4
Introductory level 6
Colon layout can be changed.

Fig. 1.6 The Kyoto Kagaku colonoscopy training model with different possibilities to vary the difficulty of passage of the sigmoid (Level 1-6). (Images are provided courtesy of Kyoto Kagaku, Kyoto, Japan.)

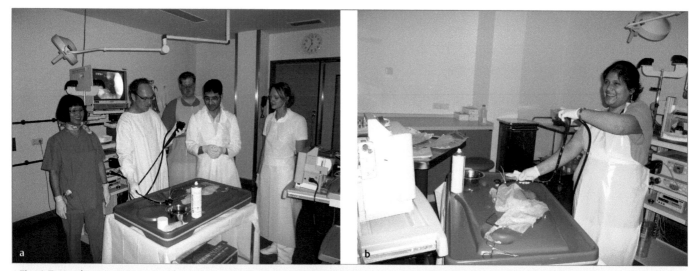

Fig. 1.7 Hands-on training using the compactEASIE simulator. (a) Groups of three or four fellows per simulator and teacher receiving instructions. (b) Individual practice, for example, for basic gastroscopy.[1]

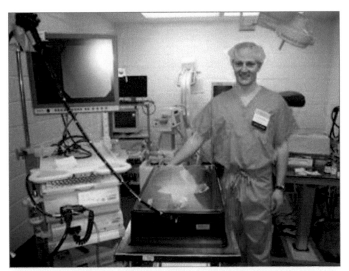

Fig. 1.8 The EASIE-R model designed by Kai Matthes and based on the compactEASIE simulator.[1]

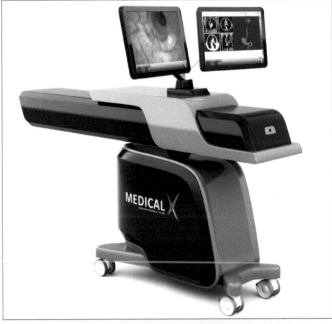

Fig. 1.9 A computer simulation model for gastroscopy and colonoscopy skills (Image is provided courtesy of Medical-X BV, EM Rotterdam, the Netherlands).

In a randomized controlled multicenter trial of 45 first-year GI fellows in New York comparing 10 independent hours of work on the Simbionix GI Mentor II versus no simulator training, trainees who worked on the simulator had significantly better objective technical and cognitive performance on their first 20 to 80 real supervised colonoscopy examinations but no difference in the time required to achieve competency nor in subjective proctor assessment of patient discomfort. These studies suggest that virtual reality simulator training prior to real cases accelerates early training, but improvement in final competency has not yet been established. Nor has there been any computer-based skills test that has been correlated with competent performance on actual endoscopic procedures.

1.4.3 Training Courses with Live Animals

Animal models offer a realistic learning environment; however, a substantial organizational, technical, and financial effort is required. Ethical considerations, animal welfare, and problems of hygiene, along with the need for dedicated endoscopes for animal use and substantial staff and financial expenditure, are major restrictions. Currently, training courses on live animals are performed for many different techniques including endoscopic submucosal dissection and peroral endoscopic myotomy.[36,37]

1.4.4 Ex Vivo Porcine Tissue Models (EASIE, Erlanger Endo-Trainer, EASIE-R)

Clean pig stomachs with a dedicated mold have been used for training in diagnostic gastroscopy for many years.[1] As in the pulsatile organ perfusion simulator described by Szinicz et al,[40] a roller pump can be used to simulate spurting arterial bleeding in hollow GI viscera.

The "compactEASIE" device is a simplified version of the original biosimulation model and was developed in 1998 (▶ Fig. 1.10**a-c**). For ERCP interventions such as sphincterotomy and stent placement the hepatobiliary system with the liver, extrahepatic bile ducts, and gallbladder is dissected and added to the upper GI tract. Bile duct stones can be simulated by inserting pieces of plastic stents into the bile duct. Matthes and Cohen have reported an interesting model called the "neopapilla."[41]

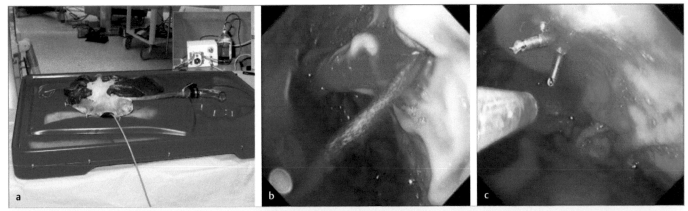

Fig. 1.10 (a) The compactEASIE model for hands-on training using specially prepared pig organs. **(b)** A roller pump drives artificial blood into vessels that have been sutured into a pig stomach, to provide training in hemostasis procedures in realistic conditions. **(c)** Practicing hemoclipping with the compactEASIE simulator.

Training in more than 30 interventional endoscopic techniques can be provided (▶Table 1.2). It is generally recommended to use special animal endoscopes for the training with isolated ("ex vivo") pig organs. Sedlack et al[42] compared computer simulator, harvested porcine organ, and live anesthetized pigs for ERCP training. The authors concluded the harvested porcine organ model to be the most realistic model for instruction in both basic and advanced ERCPs.

1.4.5 Training Courses

Ways of Integrating Educational Material, Demonstration, Practice, Feedback, and Evaluation into a Comprehensive Workshop

Regular training workshops on endoscopic hemostasis using the compactEASIE simulator have been available since 1997. EASIE team training comprises the simultaneous training of doctors and nurses in different interventional endoscopic techniques using this type of simulator and was first described in detail in 2001.[1]

Basic skills. To assess an individual's capacity for brain–hand coordination, a practical simulator test for manual skills was developed. For this hand–eye dexterity test performed before the training course, four 2- to 3-mm dots are created on the anterior wall of the ex vivo porcine simulator using a thermal device. The dots are arranged in the form of a square standing on one corner, with a diagonal length of 2 cm. Precision in the brain–hand coordination test can be evaluated by asking the trainee to touch each mark with the probe in a clockwise fashion. The time needed to complete the task is also measured. In this exercise, precision is weighted more heavily than speed.

Studies on training using ex vivo simulators (e.g., compactEASIE) for fellows and the EASIE team-training method

Since the introduction of the EASIE simulator, considerable efforts have been made to assess the value of additional simulator training using the EASIE model in endoscopic hemostasis. Several prospective trials have been conducted in recent years to provide objective evidence that participants benefit from simulator training. A prospective randomized study conducted in collaboration with the New York Society for Gastrointestinal Endoscopy (NSYGE) was undertaken.[6] The results provided the first evidence of benefit from simulator training in the treatment of upper GI bleeding. In this prospective training project, 37 gastroenterology fellows from nine hospitals in New York were first evaluated in five endoscopic techniques using the compactEASIE simulator. These included manual skills, ulcer hemostasis using injection, a coagulation probe and hemoclipping, as well as variceal band ligation. Twenty-eight fellows with comparable skills were then randomly assigned either to an intensive training group attending three 1-day simulator hands-on workshops over a period of 7 months or to a control group only receiving traditional clinical training in endoscopy in their home hospitals (▶Fig. 1.11). During the 7-month study period, it was demonstrated that the additional simulator training in four endoscopic hemostasis techniques significantly enhanced the participants' skills in comparison with the fellows who only

received a clinical training. In particular, the evaluation of clinical cases following the training period showed a higher initial hemostasis rate and a lower complication rate among simulator-trained fellows, although the difference in the complication rate was not significant. These results were confirmed in a national training

Table 1.2 Selection of endoscopic interventions for which training can be carried out using the compactEASIE simulator

Training goal	Technique
Ulcer hemostasis	Injection techniques
	Thermal probes
	Clip application
	Over-the-scope-clip (OTSC)
	others
Variceal treatment	Multiple band ligation Cyanoacrylate glue injection
	Sclerotherapy
Tissue resection techniques	Snare polypectomy, loop application Saline-assisted polypectomy/endoscopic mucosal resection (EMR) including piecemeal EMR, capEMR, "band and snare" technique Endoscopic submucosal dissection (ESD) Full-thickness resection (FTRD) Rotablation of tissue
Tissue coagulation and cryoablation	Argon plasma coagulation (APC) Radiofrequency ablation (RFA) Cryoablation, etc.
Stricture management and stenting	Balloon dilation, bougienage Stenting: esophageal, gastro-duodenal, enteral, colonic
ERCP	Cannulation techniques, sphincterotomy and precut techniques, (Over) Guidewire exchange techniques (long and short wire/Rx) Stone extraction (balloon, basket), mechanical lithotripsy, Dilatation and bougienage Stents, plastic, self-expanding metal stents (SEMS) Complex stenting techniques (multiple, bi-hilar stents) Fine caliber cholangioscopy
Complication management	Bleeding, perforation closure

project conducted in France on training in endoscopic hemostasis that started 1 year later, with a similar study design.[43] The efficacy of the EASIE simulator was also confirmed in another project including novice endoscopists, in which remarkable levels of skill in hemostatic techniques were achieved using intensified simulator training every second week.[7]

1.4.6 Incorporating Simulator Training into Educational Programs and Maintaining Skills in Complex Procedures

Simulator training in interventional endoscopy provides an effective opportunity for endoscopy trainees to gain considerable experience in ERCP techniques without time limitations and patient risk. In the New York study on EASIE simulator training in

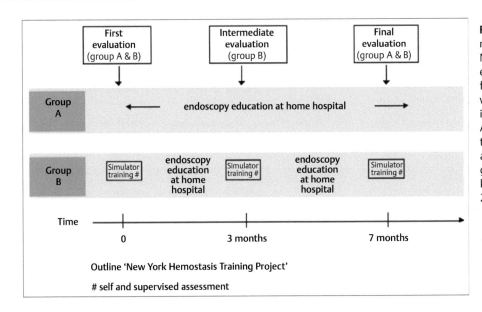

Fig. 1.11 Outline of a prospective and randomized study of training conducted in New York City, comparing conventional clinical education in endoscopic hemostasis provided for 14 gastroenterology fellows with 14 fellows who received additional hands-on training in simulators in three 1-day workshops. After a period of 7 months, the intensive training group had significantly improved in all disciplines, while the conventional clinical group had only improved in variceal band ligation. (Adapted from Hochberger et al 2005.[6])

hemostasis, the trainees achieved significant improvement in the performance of multiple skills on the simulator after only three workshops.[44] It appears that a structured educational program with access to simulator training, in addition to supervised real cases in the hospital plus DOPS evaluation, would increase the effectiveness of education in any interventional technique. The results of the real hemostasis cases performed in the New York study highlight this potential.[40] The analogous French training project confirmed that more complex techniques like clipping or injection/gold-probe application need repeat training courses to acquire and to maintain competence compared to easier techniques like band ligation.[39]

The role of simulators in training the proper application of new devices and new techniques is not really known. However, many manufacturers have already now made specific certified training and supervision of the first clinical cases obligatory for new suturing, closure, or resective devices.

There is little doubt that the knowledge and skills gained once may decline over time. Apart from sphincterotomy volume, little is known about deterioration of skill or outcome with infrequently practiced techniques. British experience with web-based e-portfolio of trainees and independent endoscopists highlights that central monitoring of practice may play a role in the future.

References

[1] Hochberger J, Maiss J, Matthes K, et al. Training and Education in Endoscopy. In: Classen M, Tytgat GNJ, Lightdale C, eds. Gastroenterological Endoscopy. Stuttgart: Georg Thieme Verlag, 2010:92–105

[2] Barrison IG, Jacques JP. Gastroenterology training in Europe-unmet educational needs beyond the machines: response from the European Section and Board of Gastroenterology. Gut. 2016; 65(1):187

[3] Forbes N, Mohamed R, Raman M. Learning curve for endoscopy training: is it all about numbers? Best Pract Res Clin Gastroenterol. 2016; 30(3):349–356

[4] Grover SC, Scaffidi MA, Khan R, et al. Progressive learning in endoscopy simulation training improves clinical performance: a blinded randomized trial. Gastrointest Endosc. 2017; 86(5):881–889

[5] Ekkelenkamp VE, Koch AD, de Man RA, Kuipers EJ. Training and competence assessment in GI endoscopy: a systematic review. Gut. 2016; 65(4):607–615

[6] Hochberger J, Matthes K, Maiss J, et al. Training with the compactEASIE biologic endoscopy simulator significantly improves hemostatic technical skill of gastroenterology fellows: a randomized controlled comparison with clinical endoscopy training alone. Gastrointest Endosc. 2005; 61(2):204–215

[7] Maiss J, Millermann L, Heinemann K, et al. The compactEASIE is a feasible training model for endoscopic novices: a prospective randomised trial. Dig Liver Dis. 2007; 39(1):70–78, discussion 79–80

[8] Jorgensen J, Kubiliun N, Law JK, et al; ASGE Training Committee. Endoscopic retrograde cholangiopancreatography (ERCP): core curriculum. Gastrointest Endosc. 2016; 83(2):279–289

[9] Sedlack RE, Coyle WJ, Obstein KL, et al; ASGE Training Committee. ASGE's assessment of competency in endoscopy evaluation tools for colonoscopy and EGD. Gastrointest Endosc. 2014; 79(1):1–7

[10] Sedlack RE. Training to competency in colonoscopy: assessing and defining competency standards. Gastrointest Endosc. 2011; 74(2):355–366.e1, 2

[11] Sedlack RE, Coyle WJ; ACE Research Group. Assessment of competency in endoscopy: establishing and validating generalizable competency benchmarks for colonoscopy. Gastrointest Endosc. 2016; 83(3):516–523.e1

[12] Barton JR, Corbett S, van der Vleuten CP; English Bowel Cancer Screening Programme. UK Joint Advisory Group for Gastrointestinal Endoscopy. The validity and reliability of a direct observation of procedural skills assessment tool: assessing colonoscopic skills of senior endoscopists. Gastrointest Endosc. 2012; 75(3):591–597

[13] Anderson JT. Assessments and skills improvement for endoscopists. Best Pract Res Clin Gastroenterol. 2016; 30(3):453–471

[14] Gavin DR, Valori RM, Anderson JT, et al. The national colonoscopy audit: a nationwide assessment of the quality and safety of colonoscopy in the UK. Gut. 2013; 62(2):242–249

[15] Rees CJ, Thomas Gibson S, Rutter MD, et al; on behalf of: the British Society of Gastroenterology, the Joint Advisory Group on GI Endoscopy, the Association of Coloproctology of Great Britain and . Ireland. UK key performance indicators and quality assurance standards for colonoscopy. Gut. 2016; 65(12):1923–1929

[16] Ward ST, Hancox A, Mohammed MA, et al. The learning curve to achieve satisfactory completion rates in upper GI endoscopy: an analysis of a national training database. Gut. 2017; 66(6):1022–1033

[17] Shahidi N, Ou G, Telford J, Enns R. When trainees reach competency in performing ERCP: a systematic review. Gastrointest Endosc. 2015; 81(6):1337–1342

[18] Hochberger J, Menke D, Maiss J. ERCP training. In: Baron TH, Kozarek R, Carr-Locke DL, eds. ERCP. Philadelphia, PA: Saunders - Elsevier, 2008:61–72

[19] Jowell PS, Baillie J, Branch MS, et al. Quantitative assessment of procedural competence. A prospective study of training in endoscopic retrograde cholangiopancreatography. Ann Intern Med. 1996; 125(12):983–989

[20] Freeman ML. Adverse outcomes of endoscopic retrograde cholangiopancreatography: avoidance and management. Gastrointest Endosc Clin N Am. 2003; 13(4):775–798, xi

[21] Freeman ML, Nelson DB, Sherman S, et al. Complications of endoscopic biliary sphincterotomy. N Engl J Med. 1996; 335(13):909–918

[22] Rabenstein T, Hahn EG. Post-ERCP pancreatitis: is the endoscopist's experience the major risk factor? JOP. 2002; 3(6):177–187

[23] American Association for the Study of Liver Diseases, American College of Gastroenterology, American Gastroenterological Association (AGA) Instutute, and American Society for Gastrointestinal Endoscopy (2007): The Gastroenterology Core Curriculum, Third Edition. Gastroenterology 132(5): 2012-8.

[24] Schutz SM, Abbott RM. Grading ERCPs by degree of difficulty: a new concept to produce more meaningful outcome data. Gastrointest Endosc. 2000; 51(5):535–539

[25] Wani S, Hall M, Wang AY, et al. Variation in learning curves and competence for ERCP among advanced endoscopy trainees by using cumulative sum analysis. Gastrointest Endosc. 2016 Apr; 83(4):711–9.e11

[26] Kowalski T, Kanchana T, Pungpapong S. Perceptions of gastroenterology fellows regarding ERCP competency and training. Gastrointest Endosc. 2003; 58(3):345–349

[27] Baumgart DC, Wende I, Grittner U. Tablet computer-based multimedia enhanced medical training improves performance in gastroenterology and endoscopy board style exam compared with traditional medical education. Gut. 2016; 65(3):535–536

[28] Cohen J, Bosworth BP, Chak A, et al. Preservation and Incorporation of Valuable Endoscopic Innovations (PIVI) on the use of endoscopy simulators for training and assessing skill. Gastrointest Endosc. 2012; 76(3):471–475

[29] Classen M. [Endoscopy of the digestive tract in the continuing education of internists and gastroenterologist]. Internist (Berl) 1982;23:243–244

[30] Williams CB. Fiberoptic colonoscopy: teaching. Dis Colon Rectum 1976;19:395–399

[31] Plooy AM, Hill A, Horswill MS, et al. Construct validation of a physical model colonoscopy simulator. Gastrointest Endosc. 2012; 76(1):144–150

[32] Grund KE, Schumpelick V. Competence: the way to surgical endoscopy Chirurg. 2002; 73(1):32–37

[33] Lange V, Grund KE. Chirurg. 2001; 72:164–165

[34] Costamagna G. Experience Cook Medical's collaborative approach to learning. Available at: https://www.cookmedical.eu/endoscopy/experience-cook-medicals-collaborative-approach-to-learning/

[35] Thompson CC, Jirapinyo P, Kumar N, et al. Development and initial validation of an endoscopic part-task training box. Endoscopy. 2014; 46(9):735–744

[36] Bar-Meir S. A new endoscopic simulator. Endoscopy. 2000; 32(11):898–900

[37] Sedlack RE. The state of simulation in endoscopy education: continuing to advance toward our goals. Gastroenterology. 2013; 144(1):9–12

[38] Berr F, Ponchon T, Neureiter D, et al. Experimental endoscopic submucosal dissection training in a porcine model: learning experience of skilled Western endoscopists. Dig Endosc. 2011; 23(4):281–289

[39] Hochberger J, Kruse E, Wedi E, et al. Training in endoscopic mucosal resection and endoscopic submucosal dissection. In: Cohen J, ed. Successful Gastrointestinal Endoscopy. Oxford, UK: Wiley-Blackwell, 2011:204–237

[40] Szinicz G, Beller S, Bodner W, Zerz A, Glaser K. Simulated operations by pulsatile organ-perfusion in minimally invasive surgery. Surg Laparosc Endosc 1993;3:315–317

[41] Matthes K, Cohen J. The Neo-Papilla: a new modification of porcine ex vivo simulators for ERCP training (with videos). Gastrointest Endosc 2006;64:570–576

[42] Sedlack R, Petersen B, Binmoeller K, Kolars J. A direct comparison of ERCP teaching models. Gastrointest Endosc. 2003; 57(7):886–890

[43] Maiss J, Prat F, Wiesnet J, et al. The complementary Erlangen active simulator for interventional endoscopy training is superior to solely clinical education in endoscopic hemostasis: the French training project: a prospective trial. Eur J Gastroenterol Hepatol. 2006; 18(11):1217–1225

[44] Matthes K, Cohen J, Kochman ML, et al. Efficacy and costs of a one-day hands-on EASIE endoscopy simulator train-the-trainer workshop. Gastrointest Endosc. 2005; 62(6):921–927

2 The Value of Clinical Research

Michael B. Wallace and Peter D. Siersema

2.1 Introduction

In this review, we will cover major topics relevant to the performance and communication of clinical research, including key issues such as the value to clinical care, keys to conducting research, and how to build teams of successful researchers within institutions and between institutions. We will provide a basic overview on how to design clinical trials, generate research ideas, write grants, and conduct day-to-day clinical research. We will provide valuable information on how to present at national and international meetings and write and publish manuscripts. Finally, we will cover issues such as ethics and the future of scientific publications.

Clinical research provides value through guiding physicians and other caregivers on how to choose the optimal method of diagnosing and treating diseases. It is fundamentally different from basic research, which focuses on mechanisms of diseases as well as normal and abnormal biological processes. Clinical research particularly focuses on the patient. In our daily practice, we struggle through decisions in virtually all patients including, which diagnostic tests to perform, what the optimal treatments are, and how to deal with the costs and adverse effects of our diagnostic and treatment approaches. It is widely acknowledged that there are major gaps in our knowledge. High-value clinical research should include several key elements including:
- Selecting clinically relevant interventions for comparison to current standards of care.
- Inclusion of relevant and diverse populations.
- Collection of health-related outcomes important to patients, physicians, and payers.

All clinical trials should be performed in a rigorous scientific manner that adheres to several key principles to provide accurate and reliable information.[1] Studies performed in a highly selected group of patients, who are fundamentally different from the patient we are currently caring for, do not provide reliable guidance. The value of clinical trials is only as great as the extent to which those results are communicated and made available to patients, colleagues, and providers. The process of scientific publication has long been the mechanism by which we communicate these results, although many other options are increasingly available; such as communication at scientific conferences, internet, and social-media based methods of data sharing.

2.2 Keys to Success

Clinical research is both tremendously rewarding and challenging. Over many years of conducting research we have defined four key elements to success:
- A tough skin.
- A team approach.
- Attention to detail and a questioning approach.
- Having long-term as well as short-term goals.

2.2.1 A Tough Skin

Even the most successful clinical investigators face many hurdles while conducting and publishing clinical research. Most competitive medical journals have acceptance rates of well under 20%. Large federal grants are even more competitive with funding rates now less than 10%. Thus, even excellent research proposals and papers may be rejected for funding and publication. To ultimately succeed, clinical investigators must be willing to accept the short-term failures and persist in conducting and publishing the research they believe in.

2.2.2 Building Teams

Building teams enables each member of the team to bring unique talents and ideas to a research project. Many of the best research projects occur at the boundary zones between different areas of expertise. A specific example of this is our research on the role of endoscopic ultrasound in lung cancer.[2,3] Both the field of endoscopic ultrasound and the field of lung cancer were represented by very different groups of physicians; however, working together identified unique contributions of each team. Beyond physicians, a successful team should include senior mentors, junior investigators, statisticians, experts in clinical trial design, study coordinators, and editorial assistants.

Fellows play one of the most important roles in the team. For the fellow, the goals are to perform the research and to learn the process. The only way to do this, is to practice. Most academic medical centers include research activities as a part of their core curriculum. In addition to clinical fellows, who spend part of their time doing research, many programs offer dedicated research fellowships in clinical investigation. These programs often include dedicated training in research methodologies and advanced degrees such as a Master or Doctoral degree. Such didactic training has been shown to increase the likelihood of long-term research success.[4]

Research collaboration, both within an area of interest and across disciplines, fosters long-term academic productivity. In addition, collaboration with colleague researchers in other centers, both on a national and international level, often increases the clinical value of observations. Developing a long-term plan to integrate with other colleagues is critical. Key elements of this include shared authorship and shared responsibilities, both of which are best outlined at the beginning of a study. A challenging issue for many large groups is authorship on manuscripts. Overall, it is best to acknowledge the contributions of each member either throughout authorship, if they meet guidelines, or through acknowledgment. It is important to recognize that it is not necessary to include a division chair on every manuscript. The International Committee of Medical Journal Editors (ICMJE) provides widely accepted definitions of authorship.[5]

Study coordinators do the majority of the day-to-day work of clinical trials. Clinical coordinator should be chosen based on the skills necessary for each trial. In some cases, a nurse is required when important clinical decisions need to be made. In other circumstances, data coordinators can collect clinical trial information in a reliable and efficient manner. Coordinators should be respected members of the team who are included in research planning discussions and acknowledged in manuscripts.

Statisticians play a key role in the design and analysis of studies. A common mistake is to involve statisticians only at the end of the study when analysis is needed. A much more effective strategy is to involve statisticians at the planning stages. In this way, variables can be carefully defined and chosen in a way that will optimize data analysis. Statisticians can also significantly improve the overall study design. For example, simple changes in study design can substantially alter the sample size needed.[6]

Finally, partnering with editorial assistants may be highly valuable for some investigators. The skill of writing manuscripts is very different than the skill of conducting research. Many large academic centers have medical editors who can facilitate how we communicate our scientific discovery with the broader community.

2.3 Designing Clinical Trials

The field of endoscopy has matured substantially over the past 20 to 30 years. From one where simply describing our observations and experience was enough to be published, to now where competitive journals typically only publish well-designed controlled clinical trials and cohort studies. In order to be published, such high-quality clinical studies should be carefully designed to achieve our primary goal of seeking scientific truth. Designing clinical trials follows a general pattern from generating ideas, to study design, to grant writing, and finally completion of the study. Each of these is discussed further.

2.3.1 Generating Ideas

Generating ideas should be the easiest of all research activities. All those involved in patient care know that many decisions we make, for both diagnosis and treatment, have only a limited amount of scientific evidence. Thus, in almost every patient encounter, we can identify opportunities for research.

2.3.2 Refining Ideas

Many studies can take months or even years to complete, so the long list of possible research topics needs to be refined based on several key factors:

- Is the topic of high interest to the investigator?
- Are the resources to study the question available to the investigator, including adequate numbers of patients, access to large databases, collaborators with sufficient expertise, and funding sources?

Research questions should be further defined based on a very detailed review of the current literature. Ultimately, research is aimed at extending the envelope of knowledge beyond what is currently known. Many resources are available (PubMed, Google Scholar, Medline, etc.) to identify current knowledge and its gaps including review of published research and consultation with other experts.

Almost all published studies end with a statement such as "further research is necessary to confirm/clarify…." These statements offer excellent clues on how to further refine a specific research question. Moreover, some outcomes need to be confirmed or even excluded because they seem clinically not rational.

2.3.3 Clinical Trial Design

Clinical trial design balances precision and accuracy of a particular research question with available resources. Theoretical and practical issues must be taken into consideration. For treatment trials, the definitive randomized control trial is often not feasible, cost-effective, or even ethical.

Studies of new diagnostic technologies, which are particularly common in the field of endoscopy, often begin with a pilot study assessing the general safety and efficacy of a new device such as a new endoscopic imaging technology. This should initially be compared to historical controls. If promising, further studies should then be performed comparing the new method to the current standard in a controlled cohort or randomized study. Many diagnostic trials follow a crossover design where each patient undergoes both procedures, either back-to-back or in a sequential crossover design. Such methods may reduce by 10- to 20-fold the number of patients needed compared with a simple randomized design since each patient serves as his/her own control, thus minimizing variability.[6] Nonetheless, particularly back-to-back studies are prone to bias if not well conducted, for example, when the same investigator performs both procedures in the same subject.

Treatment studies also began typically as an initial safety study. Ideally, these should be compared to historical controls and, if the data are promising, lead to prospective randomized controlled trials. The classic randomized controlled trial is well-suited in this area and can be done efficiently, particularly when there are significant improvements with a new technology compared to existing technology. Such studies have led to major landmark publications and have set new standards of care for endoscopy.[7]

Trials of causation and association, such as the link between *Helicobacter pylori* and gastric ulcers and gastric lymphoma,[8] often cannot be addressed through prospective clinical trials. In these cases, large cohort or case–control studies may be better suited. Cohort studies are valuable for common conditions such as the association between nonsteroidal anti-inflammatory drug use and peptic ulcer disease. However, for more rare conditions, case–control study design is more efficient. This includes studies such as the association between gastroesophageal reflux disease and esophageal adenocarcinoma.[9]

2.3.4 Grant Writing

The skill of grant writing is similar to the skill of publishing clinical trials. A well-written grant must convince the funding agency that:

- the question is important.
- your methods are well-suited.
- the question and approach is novel.
- your team is the best one to answer the question.

Most successful research teams build on a long arc of successful investigation in the specific area. Because of their established record, they can achieve each of the elements mentioned above and continue to push the frontier of knowledge forward. Having said this, it also means that the initial steps on the research path are often not easy!

2.3.5 Conducting Clinical Trials

Once the study is designed and funded, the day-to-day work of completing the study is often assigned to study coordinators, with oversight from the principal investigator. If the idea was well formed and refined, the trial carefully designed, and the team of collaborators well chosen, clinical trial conduct usually proceeds without difficulties. However, even in these circumstances, regular meetings to review enrollment and identify any problems with study data collection are very important. In some studies, where the outcomes are highly uncertain, a planned interim analysis should be considered to allow for appropriate adjustment.

2.3.6 Presentation and National Meetings

Once the study is complete, or during a planned interim analysis, the communication of study results is often done in a multifactorial way including presentation at national meetings. This is often the first opportunity to communicate important results to colleagues and to receive feedback. By their nature, presentations at national meetings are very short relative to the full publication. Most large meetings include options for either oral or poster presentation. Oral presentation typically involves a slide review of the study aims and hypothesis, and a short review of the background, followed by methods, results, and conclusions. This must be communicated in a short period of time, typically 8 to 12 minutes. The message should be kept relatively simple with two to three main points that are communicated. Fewer slides that are carefully worded and presented communicate much more than very densely written slides and rapid speech. The presenter should always be highly respectful of his or her time allocation and allow for a question and answer session.

2.3.7 Manuscript Writing

Many investigators fall short at the final stage of the scientific process. The classical writers' block has prevented many excellent studies from being fully published. Each investigator has his or her own style of writing and overcoming writers' block. One of the most valuable methods is to remind ourselves that the manuscript does not have to be perfect on the first draft. It is often easier to *edit* a manuscript than to *write* a manuscript. For this reason, simply getting the ideas down on paper can overcome the most challenging obstruction. With current voice recognition technology, this can be done simply by dictating a manuscript. Begin by assembling all the key elements of the study, such as tables, figures, and the previous grant submission. Large aspects of the manuscript may have been previously written, such as the background section of the grant, which should change little other than a timely update of the most recent literature. The methods section should largely be identical to the methods written in the original grant application. The results also should largely reflect the key data elements including figures and tables. The discussion is perhaps the most difficult to write. A discussion section should generally follow a general sequence as outlined in the following:

- Summarize your key findings.
- Discuss how your findings compared to literature that supports the results.
- Discuss how your findings extend knowledge compared to other studies.
- Discuss how your findings may conflict with other published results and explain why these differences exist.
- Discuss the strengths and limitations of your study.
- Discuss the implications and conclusions of your study.
- Discuss what future research should be done.

2.4 Ethics

Scientific exploration, particularly studies that involve commercial devices, has potential for conflicts of interest. Scientific misconduct occurs when we lose sight of our primary goal, to discover new knowledge, and instead focus on personal gains. We have recently published a summary of the key ethical issues in scientific publication and how to prevent them.[10,11] Common ethical problems include the following.

2.4.1 Conflict of Interest

Conflicts of interest should be clearly declared and should err on the side of overdisclosure even if the author feels there may not be a direct conflict of interest. It is better to allow the reader to decide if the conflict of interest is present and how it might influence the scientific study. Examples include consulting fees or equity interest in a commercial product or company related to the study.

2.4.2 Registration of Clinical Trials and Underreporting of Negative Trials

The ICMJE guidelines, to which many journals adhere, require clinical trials to be registered at the outset of the study.[12] According to the ICMJE, a clinical trial is defined as "any research study that prospectively assigns human participants or groups of humans to one or more health-related interventions to evaluate the effects on health outcomes."[12] Some studies, such as a retrospective chart review, do not require registration. All studies that meet this definition should be listed on one of the many acceptable registration sites such as:

- www.anzctr.org.au
- www.clinicaltrials.gov
- www.ISRCTN.org
- www.umin.ac.jp/ctr/index/htm
- www.trialregister.nl
- https://eudract.ema.europa.eu/

2.4.3 Falsification of Data

Although this is the most dangerous of all ethical issues, it is often very difficult to detect. Most issues of data falsification come to light through collaborators who have questions about the authenticity of data and raise these concerns to either institutional leadership or journal editors.

2.4.4 Plagiarism

The ability to copy and paste text material and the broadly available content throughout the World Wide Web have made plagiarism an increasingly common practice. On the other hand, software tools to search text within any manuscript and compare it to other published work have made it very easy to detect plagiarism.[10,11]

A more challenging issue is the reuse of text by the same author, so called "text recycling." Authors must remember that the copyright of published manuscript belongs to the journal and cannot be reused verbatim. Direct reuse should be quoted and referenced with permission from the original source or preferably rewritten in new words.

2.5 Manuscript Submission and Review Process

Most medical journals follow a standard process for submission and review, although new online open access journals are changing this process. For most journals, the approach is to submit a manuscript, typically through a website. The journal's managing editors and chief editor typically screen manuscripts to identify those that should be sent for full peer review. Many competitive journals may not send some manuscripts out for review.

Once an article clears the initial screening, it is typically sent for review to two or more independent experts in a field. They provide a critical review of the manuscript and often make a recommendation regarding whether manuscripts should be published and what improvements should be made. The decision on whether manuscripts should be published is ultimately made by the editorial team and chief editor. Most journals prioritize studies that are novel, well designed, well written, and appropriate for the audience of the journal. For this reason, the authors should carefully select the most appropriate journal. It is a common mistake to choose a journal simply based on the reported impact factors. Ultimately, the goal of publishing manuscripts is to communicate the new knowledge with the audience that is most likely to benefit, as opposed to the most widely read or cited journals.

2.5.1 Expanding the Reach

Many journals now expand their reach beyond just the print publication including online publication and even online-only publication. Professional and public social media sites, such as such as Facebook, Twitter, WeChat, ResearchGate, Doximity, and LinkedIn, allow peer-to-peer and journal-to-peer sharing of articles and online discussion and will likely continue and gain more popularity.

2.5.2 The Future of Scientific Publications

Publication through printed journals, which are distributed to individuals and libraries in monthly issues, has been the preferred method of scientific publication for more than a century. Scientific publication is rapidly evolving and includes open access journals, with or without peer review. While some well-respected open access journals (e.g., F1000, PLoS) publish high-quality scientific articles,[13,14] others are fraught with opportunities to publish poorly designed or even plagiarized material.

The mechanism of editorial review is changing toward a more open and peer-to-peer communication. While anyone can post their scientific discovery online, the role of journals and editors will continue to be valuable. For many busy scientists and physicians, it will remain valuable to have an expert editor identify the most important new studies relevant to their needs among rapid explosion of studies being performed and published. The journal itself will likely evolve into a refined portal of information linking each study with the physicians and scientist who can most apply that new knowledge. Despite these very rapid and uncertain changes, there is no doubt that clinical research and the communication will be valuable to physicians, scientists, and patients alike, with the role of editors to ensure that knowledge is effectively and accurately conveyed.

References

[1] Tunis SR, Stryer DB, Clancy CM. Practical clinical trials: increasing the value of clinical research for decision making in clinical and health policy. JAMA. 2003; 290(12):1624–1632

[2] Wallace MB, Pascual JM, Raimondo M, et al. Minimally invasive endoscopic staging of suspected lung cancer. JAMA. 2008; 299(5):540–546

[3] Wallace MB. Endoscopic ultrasound staging of lung cancer. Am J Respir Crit Care Med. 2005; 172(3):400–401, author reply 401

[4] Kapoor K, Wu BU, Banks PA. The value of formal clinical research training in initiating a career as a clinical investigator. Gastroenterol Hepatol (N Y). 2011; 7(12):810–813

[5] ICMJE. Defining the role of authors and contributors. 2016. Available at: http://www.icmje.org/recommendations/browse/roles-and-responsibilities/defining-the-role-of-authors-and-contributors.html. Accessed February 16, 2016

[6] van den Broek FJ, Kuiper T, et al. Study designs to compare new colonoscopic techniques: clinical considerations, data analysis, and sample size calculations. Endoscopy. 2013; 45(11):922–927

[7] Lau JY, Leung WK, Wu JCY, et al. Omeprazole before endoscopy in patients with gastrointestinal bleeding. N Engl J Med. 2007; 356(16):1631–1640

[8] Parsonnet J, Hansen S, Rodriguez L, et al. Helicobacter pylori infection and gastric lymphoma. N Engl J Med. 1994; 330(18):1267–1271

[9] Lagergren J, Bergström R, Lindgren A, Nyrén O. Symptomatic gastroesophageal reflux as a risk factor for esophageal adenocarcinoma. N Engl J Med. 1999; 340(11):825–831

[10] Wallace MB, Siersema PD. Ethics in publication. Gastrointest Endosc. 2015; 82(3):439–442

[11] Wallace MB, Siersema PD. Ethics in publication. Endoscopy. 2015; 47(7):575–578

[12] ICMJE. Clinical trials registration. 2015. Available at: http://www.icmje.org/about-icmje/faqs/clinical-trials-registration/. Accessed April 3, 2015

[13] Björk B-C, Solomon D. Open access versus subscription journals: a comparison of scientific impact. BMC Med. 2012; 10(1):73

[14] Gargouri Y, Hajjem C, Larivière V, et al. Self-selected or mandated, open access increases citation impact for higher quality research. PLoS One. 2010; 5(10): e13636

Section II

The Patient and Endoscopy

3 Informed Consent for Gastrointestinal Endoscopy

Andrew E. Axon and Anthony T. R. Axon

3.1 Introduction

Informed consent for gastrointestinal endoscopy is an essential part of a quality endoscopy service. It empowers patients to determine their own medical management based on an understanding of their clinical condition and the potential risks, benefits, and alternatives to the proposed intervention. It also protects the endoscopist and the clinical institution providing the service from liability for complications arising outside their control. It therefore benefits all parties. This chapter considers the principles underlying informed consent in digestive endoscopy. It draws attention to the rights of the patient giving consent and discusses when and how consent should be taken and by whom. It sets out what information should be disclosed and considers those cases where consent may not be required or is undesirable. In particular, the chapter addresses the medicolegal issues that are evolving with the increasing burden of litigation that is influencing medical management in the 21st century.

Historically, the medical profession has adopted a paternalistic approach to patient management. Hippocrates said "... sometimes you will have to deftly comfort [your patient] without revealing the true progress of his illness because many patients take a turn for the worse when they find out about their condition and the prognosis."[1] A prototype of informed consent operated as long ago as the 14th century, but it was employed more to protect the doctor than to enable patient autonomy.[2] Since the beginning of the 20th century, patients have been able to sue their surgeon successfully if their expressed wishes concerning an operation had been ignored, but there was no requirement for "informed consent" until late in that century.[2] Following the Nuremberg trials, ethics relating to medical research came under scrutiny, but this did not have a major impact on medical practice in the United Kingdom. In 1967, Pappworth controversially published *"Human guinea pigs"—a history*.[3,4] This led to the adoption of local ethics committees and requirement of informed consent from patients recruited for research.

In 1994, the World Health Organization published a declaration of patients' rights in Europe.[5] It stated:

Patients have the right to be fully informed about their health status, including the medical facts about their condition; about the proposed medical procedures, together with the potential risks and benefits of each procedure; about alternatives to the proposed procedures, including the effect of non-treatment; and about the diagnosis, prognosis and progress of treatment. The informed consent of the patient is a prerequisite for any medical intervention. A patient has the right to refuse or to halt a medical intervention. The implications of refusing or halting such an intervention must be carefully explained to the patient.

These are the principles that today underlie the concept of informed consent, but their application varies according to the legislation in individual countries. However, in spite of the general acceptance that informed consent in endoscopy is important, studies suggest that it is often poorly done and is sometimes neglected altogether.[6,7] This chapter is based on recent guidelines produced by National endoscopy societies,[8,9] and on case law.

3.2 What Is "Informed Consent"?

It is legally defined as follows:

... An adult person of sound mind is entitled to decide which, if any, of the available forms of treatment to undergo, and his or her consent must be obtained before treatment interfering with that person's bodily integrity is undertaken. The doctor is therefore under a duty to take reasonable care to ensure that the patient is aware of any material risks involved in any treatment, and of any reasonable alternative or variant treatments ....[10]

The concept of informed consent requires the sharing of sufficient information between doctor and patient so as to protect the patient's right of autonomy. Whether or not this duty is met will depend on: what information is provided; how it is provided; and where and when it is provided.

3.3 Clinician and Patient Relationship

The relationship between providers and recipients of clinical care lies at the heart of understanding the modern concept of informed consent. The starting point is a recognition that the relationship between the doctor and the patient is a partnership, involving a mutual understanding that medical treatment is uncertain of success and may involve risks. It is then that the patient is able to make decisions concerning their treatment and accept responsibility for taking those risks and living with their consequences.

Historically, the doctor/patient relationship was characterized very differently, one in which "the doctor knows best" and the patient is a passive and potentially reluctant recipient of medical care. This was the default position in the United Kingdom during the 1960s, when to tell a patient he or she had cancer was usually a sentence of death, and medical students were taught not to use the "C" word. Most therapy was ineffective and public understanding of medical matters was limited. To deprive a patient of all hope offended the first Hippocratic principal "Do no harm." Furthermore, many patients preferred the doctor to do his/her best without wanting to know the details. Until the late 20th century, the common law accepted that the nature and extent of information to be provided by a doctor to a patient was primarily a matter of clinical judgment:

... a decision what degree of disclosure of risks is best calculated to assist a particular patient to make a rationale choice as to whether or not to undergo a particular treatment must primarily be a matter of clinical judgment.[11]

More recently, there has been a fundamental shift away from this paternalistic approach. Today, the internet generation is well-educated about medical matters and is aware that effective treatments are available for most conditions, that medicine has subspecialized, and that certain doctors and hospitals are better qualified to treat them than others. Patients and their relatives are also aware that if the advice given is inappropriate or if procedures go wrong, they have recourse to the court for compensation.

3.4 What Information Is Required?

For the reasons stated above, this is not simply a clinical question gauged by risk versus benefit. It includes an assessment of what information the patient might attach significance to, be it the risk of complications, alternative treatment, or the consequences of not providing treatment. The significance of a given risk to a patient (as opposed to the clinician), will reflect a variety of personal factors besides its magnitude: for example, its nature, his/her attitude to health and wellbeing, and the importance that the patient attaches to the benefits the treatment might bring. The information given should enable patients to make a decision based on what is important to them, which is not the same as a clinical judgment as to the benefits or otherwise of an intended procedure.

In endoscopy, the procedure will have been advised to establish or exclude a specific diagnosis, provide therapy, prevent an illness from arising, or undertake research, or it may be a combination of these. For screening or research, the patient will usually have already received an explanatory invitation; for diagnosis, therapy, or surveillance, an explanation will have been given by the referring clinician. However, it is the endoscopist's responsibility to ensure that the patient is aware of his or her clinical condition, the reasons for the endoscopy, the potential complications and any alternative options that are available. Information must be provided indicating what the specific procedure will entail, and includes details of any preparation, dietary measures, or medication changes needed before the procedure. Sedation options should be included with an explanation of their advantages and disadvantages. The risk of complications must be clearly set out based preferably on local data. The written information should list possible side effects that might arise following the procedure and indicate any restrictions in activity or medication following the procedure.

Depending on local and regional customs and laws, the consent form should state who will perform the endoscopy, whether trainees will be involved, the cost, and whether tissue will be retrieved and stored and for what purpose, indicating specifically whether it might be used for research. If images or other recordings are to be made, it should state whether they might be used for teaching or publication.

If the patient is to be involved in a clinical trial, the consent protocol approved by an appropriate ethics committee must be used. If the endoscopy is to be part of a live teaching demonstration, it should conform to advice published by national or international endoscopy organizations.[12]

A consent form should be completed and signed by the patient. The person taking the consent should indicate that the above issues had been addressed and that the patient had given consent.

3.5 How Should the Information Be Provided?

Informed consent will be adequately obtained only if the information provided is comprehensible. The duty is not fulfilled by bombarding the patient with technical information, which they cannot reasonably be expected to grasp. If possible, patients should be provided with written information expressed in layman's terms, and confirmation should be obtained that it has been read and understood by the patient. The process may involve other professionals such as trainee endoscopists or nursing staff but the principles remain the same. Those engaged in the consent procedure will require a full understanding of the patient's medical condition, the intended procedure, its benefits, and the risks associated with treatment. This is because questions may well be asked which require an accurate and complete response. It is important that all of those involved in the consent process have received training and are aware of the medical and legal implications.

3.6 Where and When Should the Consent Be Taken?

Provided that the situation is not an emergency, patients should be given time to consider the implications of the endoscopic procedure so that they can discuss it with their primary health doctor, friends, or relatives if they choose to do so. Written information is therefore most important. Patients should not be coerced, so it is undesirable for decision making to take place in the endoscopy room just before the procedure. Under certain circumstances, such as open access digestive endoscopy or screening colonoscopy, postal consent may be appropriate in relatively fit individuals and protocols are accessible in the literature that address this[13]; even so, an opportunity for further discussion should be offered, and confirmation of consent must be recorded, before the procedure begins.

3.7 Withdrawal of Consent

Withdrawal of consent during an endoscopy is not uncommon.[8,9,14] It is not always clear whether this is an effect of sedation-induced confusion or because the patient has genuinely withdrawn consent. If it is clear that consent has been withdrawn, the procedure should be abandoned. However, if it seems to be an effect of confusion, it is reasonable to temporarily desist and re-review after reassurance. If there is a serious risk involved in stopping the procedure, for example, major bleeding occurring during polypectomy, clinical judgment must be used. All endoscopy units should possess a written protocol prepared with input from the nursing staff who are the professionals mainly responsible for patient comfort and welfare during the procedure. This protocol should be followed in the event that consent is withdrawn.

3.8 Exceptions to the Requirement of Consent

Firstly, a doctor is not required to make disclosures to a patient if, in the reasonable exercise of medical judgment, he/she considers that it would be detrimental to the health of the patient. This is what is known as the "therapeutic exception." However, this is a limited exception to the general principle and should not be used to enable a doctor to prevent a patient from making an informed choice which the doctor considers to be contrary to the patient's best interests. Such would subvert the concept of patient autonomy which informed consent is intended to protect.

Secondly, a situation can arise in which the patient would rather trust their doctor to make treatment choices for them and in so doing request not to be informed of the risks arising from a recommended procedure. Under these circumstances, a doctor is not obliged to provide the information that would otherwise be required to obtain informed consent. It should be stressed that whether or not a patient falls into this category is a matter of judgment and one that should be approached with caution.

Thirdly, a doctor is excused from conferring with a patient in circumstances of necessity, for example, where the patient requires treatment urgently but the patient is unconscious or otherwise unable to make a decision. Clinical staff are often confronted by patients who may lack the capacity to make decisions. In these circumstances and in absence of preexisting consent from the patient, the approach to informed consent remains the same, although the individuals involved in deciding the course of treatment may differ, whether it is a relative with power of attorney or a court-appointed representative.

References

[1] Dunkas N. Works of Hippocrates. Paper presented at: Second European Symposium on Ethics in Gastroenterology and Digestive Endoscopy; 2006; Kos Greece

[2] Leclercq WK, Keulers BJ, Scheltinga MR, et al. A review of surgical informed consent: past, present, and future. A quest to help patients make better decisions. World J Surg. 2010; 34(7):1406–1415

[3] Pappworth MH. "Human guinea pigs"--a history. BMJ. 1990; 301(6766):1456–1460

[4] Pappworth MH. Human Guinea Pigs: Experimentation on Man. London: Routledge; 1967

[5] World Health Organization. A Declaration on the Promotion of Patients' rights in Europe: European Consultation on the Rights of Patients Amsterdam, 28 -30 March 1994. Copenhagen: World Health Organization; 1994

[6] Triantafyllou K, Stanciu C, Kruse A, et al; European Society of Gastrointestinal Endoscopy. Informed consent for gastrointestinal endoscopy: a 2002 ESGE survey. Dig Dis. 2002; 20(3–4):280–283

[7] Kopacova M, Bures J. Informed consent for digestive endoscopy. World J Gastrointest Endosc. 2012; 4(6):227–230

[8] Everett SM, Griffiths H, Nandasoma U, et al; Guideline for obtaining valid consent for gastrointestinal endoscopy procedures. British Society of Gastroenterology Gut. 2016; 65(10):1585-1601

[9] Zuckerman MJ, Shen B, Harrison ME, III, et al; Standards of Practice Committee. Informed consent for GI endoscopy. Gastrointest Endosc. 2007; 66(2):213–218

[10] Montgomery v Lanarkshire Health Board [2015] UKSC 11

[11] Sidaway v Board of Governors of the Bethlem Royal Hospital and Maudsley Hospital [1985] AC 871

[12] Dinis-Ribeiro M, Hassan C, Meining A,, et al. European Society of Gastrointestinal Endoscopy. Live endoscopy events (LEEs): European Society of Gastrointestinal Endoscopy Position Statement - Update 2014. Endoscopy. 2015; 47(1):80–86

[13] Shepherd H, Hewitt D. Guidelines for Postal Consenting for Outpatient Endoscopic Procedures. British Society of Gastroenterology; 2009

[14] Ward B, Shah S, Kirwan P, Mayberry JF. Issues of consent in colonoscopy: if a patient says 'stop' should we continue? J R Soc Med. 1999; 92(3):132–133

4 Patient Preparation and Sedation for Endoscopy

T. Wehrmann

4.1 Introduction

Sedation in endoscopy is drug-induced reduction of the patients' consciousness. The aim of sedation in endoscopic procedures is to increase the patient's comfort and to improve endoscopic performance, especially during therapeutic procedures. Traditionally, the sedation regimen most commonly used for conscious sedation during gastrointestinal endoscopy was a combination of benzodiazepines and opioids. However, the use of propofol has enormously increased during the last two decades, and several studies showed advantages of propofol over the traditional regimens in terms of faster recovery time. Conversely, one must be aware that the complication rates of endoscopic procedures might increase when using propofol sedation. Therefore, a thorough risk evaluation before the procedure and monitoring during the procedure are paramount. In addition, properly trained staff and emergency equipment are essential. Sedation can be provided by anesthesiologists, nonanesthesiologist physicians (i.e., gastroenterologists or surgeons), or a well-trained nursing staff, depending on institutional and regional restrictions. Nurse-administered sedation for low-risk endoscopic procedures and low-risk patients has become accepted in some European countries. Ideally, a sedation regimen is tailored to the individual patient after assessment of clinical risk and patient anxiety level, as well as to the complexity of planned endoscopic procedure.

Analgesia is the elimination of pain by analgesic agents. The combination of sedation and analgesia is used to achieve optimal patient tolerance during diagnostic and therapeutic endoscopic procedures. Patient tolerance, in turn, is important for successful completion and safety, which leads to better patient compliance with subsequent endoscopies.[1] Procedural sedation provokes a high level of physician and patient satisfaction, and may improve the quality of an endoscopic examination.[2,3] Although it is feasible to perform routine endoscopies without sedation in selected patients, for complex endoscopic procedures sedation is required.[4,5,6] The sedation frequency for endoscopic procedures has risen significantly during the last two decades.[7,8,9,10] As a consequence, several guidelines have been published regarding endoscopic sedation.[4,5,6,11,12,13,14,15,16,17]

4.2 Presedation Assessment

Before choosing a sedation strategy, an appropriate risk assessment is necessary. Cardiorespiratory problems, which could occur during endoscopy, should be carefully evaluated for each patient. A detailed past medical history and a focused physical examination should be conducted. This includes at least vital signs and weight measurement, heart and lung auscultation, blood pressure measurement, and an airway assessment using the Mallampati classification (▶ Table 4.1).

Patients should then be classified using the criteria of the American Society of Anesthesiologists (ASA) (▶ Table 4.2), and the respective ASA score should be documented. Patients with an ASA class ≥ III are at an increased risk for sedation-related complications.[18] Morphologic characteristics that may make airway management more difficult, such as a reduced ability to open the mouth (Mallampati III or IV),[19] a short neck (chin-hyoid distance < 4 cm), and history of difficult endotracheal intubation, should be considered. Further risk factors to be aware of are a history of sleep apnea, alcohol or substance abuse, adverse reaction to sedation, and anticipated prolonged procedure duration; such patients are not suitable for nurse-administered sedation, and sedation must be performed by a second physician who is not directly involved in the endoscopic procedure. Otherwise, the assistance of an anesthesiologist should be considered.[1,3,4,5,6]

Pregnancy testing is recommended for women of childbearing age who may be pregnant. In general, endoscopy during pregnancy is not recommended unless there is a strong indication, and, if possible, should be postponed until the second trimester.[20]

A presedation visit is important for the evaluation of possible risk factors and for planning of the individualized sedation regimen. Furthermore, informed written consent should be obtained for both the endoscopy and the sedation plans, including possible adverse events. Recommendations regarding fasting before elective procedures vary. According to ASA recommendations, patients should fast a minimum of 2 hours prior to a procedure following clear liquid ingestion and 6 hours for a light meal.[21]

Requirements regarding airway management and cardiac life support must be available, and endoscopic sedation should only be provided by properly trained staff. Maintenance of personal qualification of the endoscopy team through repeated participation in dedicated training courses is recommended.[4,5,6]

Table 4.1 Mallampati classification system for difficult laryngoscopy and intubation

Class I	Class II	Class III	Class IV
Soft palate, uvula, and pillars are visible	Soft palate and base of the uvula are visible	Only soft palate is visible	Only hard palate is visible

Table 4.2 Physical status classification system of the American Society of Anesthesiologists (ASA)

ASA class	Definition
I	*Healthy; no risk*
II	Mild to moderate systemic disease, with no functional limitation; *minimal risk*
III	Severe systemic disease, but not incapacitating; *moderate risk*
IV	Severe incapacitating disease that is a constant threat to life; *high risk*
V	Moribund, patient is not expected to survive 24 hours irrespective of procedure/operation; *very high risk*

Source: Adapted from the ASA task force.[13]

4.3 Monitoring during Endoscopic Sedation

4.3.1 Introduction

Changes of the patient's level of consciousness during endoscopic sedation occur along a continuum. Although most endoscopic (diagnostic) procedures are performed under moderate sedation, a prediction of patient response to sedation is not always possible, and some patients may move past moderate sedation levels into deep sedation.[3] Therefore, clinical monitoring of the patient's level of consciousness is important and requires the full attention of qualified staff (nurse or physician certified in cardiac life support) who are not involved in the endoscopic procedure, especially in difficult therapeutic procedures and/or when deep sedation is planned.

Observation of patient awareness, compliance with the procedure, pain reactions, and reflex status is difficult to assess in a darkened procedure room and during the performance of endoscopic interventions. Therefore, adequate monitoring of cardiorespiratory parameters is mandatory to allow for detection of early signs of patient distress; clinical assessment should be supported by objective data through technical monitoring.

4.3.2 Hemodynamic Monitoring

Heart rate and blood pressure should be determined before sedation is initiated, and should be monitored every 3 to 5 minutes during the procedure, depending on clinical requirements, and especially during propofol administration.[4,5,6,11,12,13,14,15,16,17] Hemodynamic parameters may be affected not only by the sedative agents but also by the endoscopic procedure. For example, tachycardia and hypertension may be indicative of inadequate depth of sedation, whereas bradycardia and hypotension may be caused by oversedation.

Electrocardiography

Electrocardiography (ECG) is only recommended in patients with significant cardiovascular disease to detect and analyze cardiac arrhythmia during endoscopy.[4,5,6] ECG is not required for low-risk patients (ASA I or II).[4,5,6] Other patients in whom ECG monitoring should be considered are elderly patients and those in whom prolonged procedures are anticipated. However, the precise value of ECG monitoring in these groups of patients has not been established.

Pulse Oximetry

This noninvasive method, used to monitor hemoglobin oxygenation, is recommended for all patients, irrespective of the sedation regimen or type of endoscopic procedure.[3,4,5,6,11,12,13,14,15,16,17] Although oxygen desaturation can be readily assessed, it is relatively insensitive for detecting hypoventilation, because oxygen desaturation is a late sign of depressed ventilation. Typically, hypoxemia occurs within 5 minutes of medication administration or intubation of the endoscope.[22] Patients with a baseline oxygen saturation of less than 95% are at risk for respiratory

complications during sedation, and require close monitoring.[22] Limitations of pulse oximetry include the inability to detect an adequate signal as a consequence of hypothermia, low cardiac output, or motion artifacts.

Capnography

The noninvasive monitoring of carbon dioxide in exhaled breath is more sensitive in detecting hypoventilation than direct visual observation or pulse oximetry.[23] Pulse oximetry is less sensitive when apnea occurs, because 60 to 120 seconds may elapse before arterial oxygen saturation begins to fall. Data from two randomized controlled studies show that episodes of apnea or disordered respiration can be detected significantly more frequently when using capnography as compared to pulse oximetry, but no difference in clinically relevant outcomes was seen.[24,25] Therefore, most guidelines do not recommend routine use of capnography for monitoring during endoscopic sedation.[4,5,6] However, the use of capnography is reasonable for patients with a high risk for respiratory depression.[6]

Documentation of the Sedation Procedure and Administration of Supplemental Oxygen

Most guidelines recommend that monitoring data (clinical and technical parameters), as well as drug administration, should be routinely documented.[4,5,6,11,12,13,14,15,16,17]

Oxygen supplementation has been shown to significantly reduce the frequency of severe hypoxemia.[26,27] However, oxygen supplementation can decrease respiratory drive in patients with pronounced hypercapnia due to chronic obstructive pulmonary disease. Additionally, preventive oxygen supplementation might cause a delay in detection of hypoventilation.[28] However, most guidelines recommend the use of oxygen supplementation during endoscopic sedation.[3,4,5,6]

4.4 Pharmacology

4.4.1 Introduction

The most commonly used drugs for sedation in gastrointestinal endoscopy are benzodiazepines, opioids, and propofol. Propofol use has increased enormously in the last decade after several studies demonstrated advantages over traditional benzodiazepine/opioid combinations, including faster recovery, and with the same safety profile.[29,30,31] The pharmacologic profiles of the drugs most commonly used for sedation in endoscopy are listed in ▶ Table 4.3.

4.4.2 Benzodiazepines

Benzodiazepines enhance the effect of the neurotransmitter gamma-aminobutyric acid (GABA), which results in sedative, hypnotic, anxiolytic, anticonvulsant, and amnesic action.[32] The benzodiazepines diazepam and midazolam are the most commonly used sedatives in gastrointestinal endoscopy, and have comparable efficacy and safety.[32,33] Because benzodiazepines do not have an analgesic effect, addition of an opioid is often

Table 4.3 Pharmacological characteristics of intravenous medications used for sedation and analgesia in endoscopy

Agent	Effects	Dose	Onset	Duration	Side effects
Diazepam	Sedative, anxiolytic, amnesic	0.03–0.1 mg/kg over 2 to 3 min (maximum 2–10 mg)	1–5 min	15–60 min Half-life 20–100 h (36–200 h for main active metabolite)	Cardiorespiratory depression, prolonged effect or delayed recovery in elderly, obese, or impaired hepatic function
Midazolam	Sedative, anxiolytic, amnesic, nonanalgesic	0.015–0.03 mg/kg (1–2 mg) over 2 to 3 min May repeat after 2–5 min, to a maximum of 0.1 mg/kg (in elderly, initial dose 1–1.5 mg decrease maximum to 0.07 mg/kg)	1–2 min	15–30 min Half-life 1.8–3 h (up to 21 h for active metabolite)	Cardiorespiratory depression; prolonged effect or delayed recovery in elderly, obese, or impaired hepatic function; dose reduction in combination with other agents
Meperidine	Analgesic, sedative, nonamnesic	25–50 mg over 3 to 5 min May repeat after 5–10 min	3–5 min	60–150 min Half-life 3–8 h	Hypotension, prolonged duration and recovery. Interaction with MAO inhibitors
Fentanyl	Analgesic, sedative, nonamnesic	0.5–1 µg/kg over 3 or more min May repeat after 5–10 min (maximum 50–100 µg)	2–3 min	20–30 min Half-life 25–100 min	Respiratory depression, dose reduction in combination with benzodiazepines
Ketamine	Dissociative, sedative, analgesic, hallucinogen	0.5–1 mg/kg over 1 to 2 min (25–50 mg)	30–50 s	5–20 min Half-life 2–4 h	Minimal cardiorespiratory depression, preserved protective reflexes
Propofol	Sedative, amnesic, nonanalgesic	0.5–1 mg/kg (initial dose > 70kg 40mg, >70 kg 60 mg, elderly dose reduction by 20%) Repeat every 2–5 min, 10–20 mg	30–45 s	7–8 min	Respiratory depression, hypotension, seldom bradycardia, painful injection

necessary. Midazolam is frequently the drug of choice over diazepam for endoscopic procedures because of its rapid onset, short duration of action, 1.5 to 3.5 times higher sedation potency, and lack of associated phlebitis.[34] In addition, midazolam has less respiratory depression and superior patient satisfaction compared to diazepam.[34,35] However, the potency of midazolam increases in patients older than 60 years, with an increased potential for causing respiratory depression. Therefore, the dose of midazolam should be decreased and the intervals between administrations should be longer in such patients.[35]

An advantage of benzodiazepines is temporary reversibility through the antagonist flumazenil (0.1–0.3 mg intravenous bolus). Because the half-life of action of flumazenil is shorter than that of midazolam/diazepam, resedation may occur after flumazenil reversal.[3]

4.4.3 Opioids

Introduction

Opioids have a high analgesic effect, in addition to a mild sedative effect. The two most commonly used opiates for gastrointestinal endoscopy are meperidine/pethidine and fentanyl.[9,10] They are often used in combination with benzodiazepines during endoscopic procedures, which is important as the sedation effect is quite pronounced. Because of the increased central nervous system depression, the opioid dose should be reduced when combination therapy is used, especially in the elderly and in patients with significant renal or liver dysfunction. Moderate sedation with a benzodiazepine/opioid combination results in high levels of physician and patient satisfaction, with a low risk of serious adverse events.[3,29]

Pethidine Hydrochloride (Meperidine)

Pethidine hydrochloride (meperidine) should be used primarily in procedures lasting longer than 30 minutes, because of its half-life of 3 to 4 hours. It is metabolized in the liver to normeperidine, an active metabolite with a half-life of 15 to 20 hours. Therefore, the clearance of meperidine may be significantly prolonged in patients with renal and hepatic insufficiency.[3] In addition, the combination of meperidine with monoamine oxidase inhibitors is contraindicated due to the potential for life-threatening complications.[36]

Fentanyl

Because of its high degree of fat solubility fentanyl has a rapid onset and brief duration of action. In addition, it reduces the incidence of nausea as compared to meperidine and has analgesic properties approximately 100 times more potent than morphine, with relatively little effect on the cardiovascular system. Fentanyl has a shorter overall procedure duration during upper endoscopy and colonoscopy due to faster recovery.

A dose reduction of 50% or more is recommended in the elderly.[3] Fentanyl has a narrow therapeutic range with a high risk of respiratory depression, which may persist longer than the analgesic effect.[3] In addition, it must be injected slowly to avoid chest-wall rigidity associated with rapid administration.[3]

The central nervous effects of all described opioids can be reversed by intravenous administration of naloxone. The onset of action is only 1 to 2 minutes but its half-life is 30 to 45 minutes, and patients receiving naloxone should be monitored for at least 2 hours.[3]

4.4.4 Propofol

Pharmacology

Propofol, a phenol derivate, is a short-acting hypnotic agent. It has a rapid onset of action and a rapid elimination, which leads to significantly faster time to sedation and shorter recovery times compared to other agents.[3,29,37] Propofol is significantly more efficacious than the combination of midazolam and meperidine for therapeutic endoscopies.[31,37,38]

Propofol has a weaker amnesic effect than midazolam, and has virtually no analgesic effects. However, the lack of analgesia is somewhat compensated when deeper sedation is reached. Dose reduction is not necessary for patients with moderately severe liver disease or renal failure, whereas a dose reduction is mandatory in patients with cardiac dysfunction and in the elderly.[3] For interventional endoscopic procedures, propofol has been shown to be at least as safe as midazolam/pethidine, even when used in high-risk octogenarians.[39] Furthermore, previously published randomized controlled studies demonstrate that propofol does not cause acute or transient deterioration of minimal encephalopathy in patients with liver cirrhosis and is associated with an improved recovery in those patients.[40,41,42] Therefore, propofol is preferred instead of midazolam for sedation in patients with hepatic cirrhosis.[3,4,5,6]

While propofol can induce and maintain all levels of sedation, ranging from moderate sedation to general anesthesia, it has a narrow therapeutic window, so that sedation might become more deeply than intended, and reversal agent exists.[3] However, data from the world-wide safety registry of 646,080 patients who received propofol sedation administered by gastroenterologists showed a mortality rate of 1 per 161,515, lower than that seen when standard sedation (opioids and benzodiazepines) is used (1 per 10,000),[43,44] and comparable to published data on general anesthesia administered by anesthesiologists (1 per 10,000–50,000).[44,45] The most common severe complications are dose-dependent hypotension, particularly in volume-depleted patients, and transient apnea following induction doses.

The wide variability in patient response to propofol should be considered. In some patients, only small doses of propofol induce deep sedation or even anesthesia. Because it is lipophilic, it should be handled in an aseptic fashion and measures should be taken to minimize the risk of bacterial contamination. Propofol contains soybean and egg lecithin and is therefore contradicted in patients with egg or soybean allergy.[3]

Administration Techniques

Propofol might be administered intravenously as repeated bolus injection, continuous infusion, or a combination. For gastrointestinal endoscopy sedation, propofol is most commonly administered by an initial bolus, adapted to patient's weight, age, and comorbidities, followed by repeated boluses (10–20 mg), or by a continuous propofol infusion adapted to the desired sedation and patient conditions. The latter technique of continuous infusion is most commonly used by anesthesiologists, whereas the bolus application is currently used when nonanesthesiologist-administered propofol (NAAP) sedation is used. Another mode for the administration of propofol is the so-called balanced propofol sedation (BPS). This is achieved by a small induction dose of a benzodiazepine and/or an opioid, followed by small incremental doses of propofol. BPS might provide the benefits of propofol sedation, with a reduced risk of dose-related adverse reactions.[13,46,47] However, most guidelines recommend the use of propofol monosedation.[4,5,6,11,12,13,14,15,16,17]

4.4.5 Who Should Perform Endoscopic Sedation?

This question is still a matter of debate within the medical community.[3,47] Some anesthesiologists believe that only those trained in the administration of general anesthesia should administer propofol, and that the use of propofol by nonanesthesiologists is unsafe. While the package insert of propofol restricts its use to anesthesiologists, this insert was created in the late 1980s before evidence accumulated that nonanesthesiologists can safely administer propofol for endoscopic procedures. Of course, it is necessary for endoscopists and nursing staff to be able to manage the typical adverse effects of propofol and be trained in life support techniques.[3,47] All currently available guidelines state that the endoscopist is not permitted to administer propofol and to monitor the patient. This task must be done by an additional person, who has the sole responsibility to administer the sedative and to monitor the patient.[4,5,6,11,12,13,14,15,16,17] This person can be an anesthesiologist (monitored anesthesia care [MAC]), a specially trained nonanesthesiologist physician (NAAP sedation), or a dedicated nurse (nurse-administered propofol sedation, NAPS). The mode of propofol application is, in most countries, regulated by law, for example, in most states of the United States and in France, the use of propofol is restricted to anesthesiologists; therefore, the only mode of propofol sedation is MAC in these countries. However, there is no proven clinical benefit of providing MAC for low-risk patients (ASA I–II) undergoing routine endoscopic procedures, and it is suggested that MAC should be reserved for patients with an increased risk of sedation-related complications.[6,47] Recently, it was shown that NAAP is safe in patients with obstructive sleep apnea, and that the use of MAC in ASA I and II patients for upper endoscopy and colonoscopy is not cost-effective.[48] The use of NAAP or even NAPS is now recommended by most international guidelines for patients with a lower risk profile (excluding ASA class IV–V and those with expected difficult airway management).[3,4,5,6] Furthermore, NAAP and NAPS should only be performed where appropriately trained staff and facilities for monitoring and providing proper airway management, including availability of supplemental oxygen and equipment for advanced cardiac life support, are available. To optimize patient safety, many guidelines recommend regular participation in structured education curricula for teams involved in NAAP/NAPS.[4,5,6]

4.5 Postprocedure Care

4.5.1 Monitoring during Recovery

Following conclusion of the procedure the patient remains at risk for cardiopulmonary complications because the sedation/anesthesia medications have not been completely metabolized, while at the same time the procedure stimulation is gone. Therefore, postprocedural monitoring of the cardiopulmonary system by qualified staff is necessary. This monitoring should take place in a separate recovery room/area with equipment for appropriate cardiopulmonary monitoring and resuscitation.[3] No defined recommendations regarding postprocedure monitoring exist. Because most of the serious adverse effects of sedation occur within 30 minutes after the last administration of benzodiazepines and opioids,[49] patients should be monitored for at least 30 minutes in a recovery room. Furthermore, patients who have obstructive sleep apnea and patients who have received reversal agents need special postsedation management based on ASA guidelines, because prolonged recovery times or rebound may occur in these patients.[3]

4.5.2 Discharge

There is no consensus on the duration of postprocedure monitoring, because it varies widely based on the individual patient, type of sedation, and procedure performed. Some authors recommend patients can be safely discharged approximately 30 minutes after the last application of sedation/analgesia/anesthesia agents if no adverse effects have occurred.[49] Others would discharge the patient once vital signs are stable and the patient has reached an appropriate level of consciousness.[17] Therefore, defined discharge criteria might be useful for objective guidance. Various scoring systems exist, of which the Aldrete score is the most commonly used.[50] It evaluates respiration, oxygen saturation, blood pressure, consciousness, and activity. Irrespective of which scoring system is used, a checklist to assess discharge criteria (suggested minimum criteria are shown in ▶ Table 4.4) is recommended. The results should be documented before the patient is allowed to leave the endoscopy unit, and with an accompanying adult.[3,4,5,6] In general, patients should have sufficient return of their motor skills, with the ability to walk, tolerate liquids, and dress themselves. The patient should be strongly advised not to drive a car

Table 4.4 Criteria for home discharge after endoscopic sedation

- Stable vital signs for at least 1 h
- Ability to dress, walk, and micturate without difficulty
- No excessive pain or nausea
- Intake of oral fluids without difficulty
- Adult escort
- Postsedation care at home available
- Written and verbal instructions outlining possible complications
- Phone number to be called in case of emergency

or operate machinery until full recovery can safely be expected. The exact time until the patient will regain the ability to drive or work depends on the half-life of the drugs administered, the patient's comorbidity, and intended activities (e.g., employment as a traffic pilot, heavy equipment operator, etc.). Time to full recovery using psychomotor tests is significantly less after monosedation with propofol as compared to midazolam monotherapy or midazolam/opioid sedation.[3] Driving skills return to baseline levels within 2 hours after last propofol administration.[51,52,53] However, whether patients should be allowed to drive after propofol monosedation remains uncertain.[3] Patients should be able to drive, work, and engage in legally binding decisions the day after the procedure (current European guidelines recommend an interval of 6–12 hours).[4,5,6] Furthermore, patients should be provided written instructions because of amnesic effects of the procedural sedation.[4,5,6]

References

[1] Cohen LB, Ladas SD, Vargo JJ, et al. Sedation in digestive endoscopy: the Athens international position statements. Aliment Pharmacol Ther. 2010; 32(3):425–442

[2] Abraham NS, Fallone CA, Mayrand S, et al. Sedation versus no sedation in the performance of diagnostic upper gastrointestinal endoscopy: a Canadian randomized controlled cost-outcome study. Am J Gastroenterol. 2004; 99(9):1692–1699

[3] Müller M, Wehrmann T. How best to approach endoscopic sedation? Nat Rev Gastroenterol Hepatol. 2011; 8(9):481–490

[4] Riphaus A, Wehrmann T, Weber B, et al. S3 Guideline: sedation for gastrointestinal endoscopy. Endoscopy. 2009; 41:787–815

[5] Riphaus A, Wehrmann T, Hausmann J, et al; German Society of General and Visceral Surgery. German Crohn's disease / ulcerative colitis Association e. V. German Society of Anaesthesiology and Intensive Care Medicine e. V. (DGAI). Gesellschaft Politics and Law in Health Care (GPRG). S3-guidelines "sedation in gastrointestinal endoscopy" 2014 (AWMF register no. 021/014) [in German] Z Gastroenterol. 2015; 53(8):802–842

[6] Dumonceau JM, Riphaus A, Aparicio JR, et al; NAAP Task Force Members. European Society of Gastrointestinal Endoscopy, European Society of Gastroenterology and Endoscopy Nurses and Associates, and the European Society of Anaesthesiology Guideline: Non-anesthesiologist administration of propofol for GI endoscopy. Endoscopy. 2010; 42(11):960–974

[7] Ladas SD, Aabakken L, Rey JF, et al; European Society of Gastrointestinal Endoscopy Survey of National Endoscopy Society Members. Use of sedation for routine diagnostic upper gastrointestinal endoscopy: a European Society of Gastrointestinal Endoscopy Survey of National Endoscopy Society Members. Digestion. 2006; 74(2):69–77

[8] Baudet JS, Borque P, Borja E, et al. Use of sedation in gastrointestinal endoscopy: a nationwide survey in Spain. Eur J Gastroenterol Hepatol. 2009; 21(8):882–888

[9] Riphaus A, Rabofski M, Wehrmann T. Endoscopic sedation and monitoring practice in Germany: results from the first nationwide survey. Z Gastroenterol. 2010; 48(3):392–397

[10] Riphaus A, Geist F, Wehrmann T. Endoscopic sedation and monitoring practice in Germany: re-evaluation from the first nationwide survey 3 years after the implementation of an evidence and consent based national guideline. Z Gastroenterol. 2013; 51(9):1082–1088

[11] Byrne MF, Chiba N, Singh H, Sadowski DC; Clinical Affairs Committee of the Canadian Association of Gastroenterology. Propofol use for sedation during endoscopy in adults: a Canadian Association of Gastroenterology position statement. Can J Gastroenterol. 2008; 22(5):457–459

[12] Cohen LB, Delegge MH, Aisenberg J, et al; AGA Institute. AGA Institute review of endoscopic sedation. Gastroenterology. 2007; 133(2):675–701

[13] American Society of Anesthesiologists Task Force on Sedation and Analgesia by Non-Anesthesiologists. Practice guidelines for sedation and analgesia by non-anesthesiologists. Anesthesiology. 2002; 96(4):1004–1017

[14] Heneghan S, Myers J, Fanelli R, Richardson W; Society of American Gastrointestinal Endoscopic Surgeons. Society of American Gastrointestinal Endoscopic Surgeons (SAGES) guidelines for office endoscopic services. Surg Endosc. 2009; 23(5):1125–1129

[15] Lichtenstein DR, Jagannath S, Baron TH, et al; Standards of Practice Committee of the American Society for Gastrointestinal Endoscopy. Sedation and anesthesia in GI endoscopy. Gastrointest Endosc. 2008; 68(5):815–826

[16] López Rosés L; Subcomité de Protocolos Of The Spanish Society Of Gastrointestinal Endoscopy Seed. Sedation/analgesia guidelines for endoscopy. Rev Esp Enferm Dig. 2006; 98(9):685–692

[17] Waring JP, Baron TH, Hirota WK, et al; American Society for Gastrointestinal Endoscopy, Standards of Practice Committee. Guidelines for conscious sedation and monitoring during gastrointestinal endoscopy. Gastrointest Endosc. 2003; 58(3):317–322

[18] Miller MA, Levy P, Patel MM. Procedural sedation and analgesia in the emergency department: what are the risks? Emerg Med Clin North Am. 2005; 23(2):551–572

[19] Mallampati SR, Gatt SP, Gugino LD, et al. A clinical sign to predict difficult tracheal intubation: a prospective study. Can Anaesth Soc J. 1985; 32(4):429–434

[20] Qureshi WA, Rajan E, Adler DG, et al; American Society for Gastrointestinal Endoscopy. ASGE Guideline: Guidelines for endoscopy in pregnant and lactating women. Gastrointest Endosc. 2005; 61(3):357–362

[21] American Society of Anesthesiologists committee. Practice guidelines for preoperative fasting and the use of pharmacologic agents to reduce the risk of pulmonary aspiration: application to healthy patients undergoing elective procedures: a report by the American Society of Anesthesiologist Task Force on Preoperative Fasting. Anesthesiology. 1999; 90(3):896–905

[22] Qadeer MA, Lopez AR, Dumot JA, Vargo JJ. Hypoxemia during moderate sedation for gastrointestinal endoscopy: causes and associations. Digestion. 2011; 84(1):37–45

[23] Vargo JJ, Zuccaro G, Jr, Dumot JA, et al. Automated graphic assessment of respiratory activity is superior to pulse oximetry and visual assessment for the detection of early respiratory depression during therapeutic upper endoscopy. Gastrointest Endosc. 2002; 55(7):826–831

[24] Qadeer MA, Vargo JJ, Dumont JA, et al. Capnographic monitoring of respiratory activity improves safety of sedation for endoscopic cholangiopancreatography and ultrasonography. Gastroenterology. 2009; 136:1568–1576

[25] Beitz A, Riphaus A, Meining A, et al. Capnographic monitoring reduces the incidence of arterial oxygen desaturation and hypoxemia during propofol sedation for colonoscopy: a randomized, controlled study (ColoCap Study). Am J Gastroenterol. 2012; 107(8):1205–1212

[26] Wang CY, Ling LC, Cardosa MS, et al. Hypoxia during upper gastrointestinal endoscopy with and without sedation and the effect of pre-oxygenation on oxygen saturation. Anaesthesia. 2000; 55(7):654–658

[27] Bell GD, Bown S, Morden A, et al. Prevention of hypoxaemia during upper-gastrointestinal endoscopy by means of oxygen via nasal cannulae. Lancet. 1987; 1(8540):1022–1024

[28] Fu ES, Downs JB, Schweiger JW, et al. Supplemental oxygen impairs detection of hypoventilation by pulse oximetry. Chest. 2004; 126(5):1552–1558

[29] McQuaid KR, Laine L. A systematic review and meta-analysis of randomized, controlled trials of moderate sedation for routine endoscopic procedures. Gastrointest Endosc. 2008; 67(6):910–923

[30] Koshy G, Nair S, Norkus EP, et al. Propofol versus midazolam and meperidine for conscious sedation in GI endoscopy. Am J Gastroenterol. 2000; 95(6):1476–1479

[31] Wehrmann T, Kokabpick S, Lembcke B, et al. Efficacy and safety of intravenous propofol sedation during routine ERCP: a prospective, controlled study. Gastrointest Endosc. 1999; 49(6):677–683

[32] Horn E, Nesbit SA. Pharmacology and pharmacokinetics of sedatives and analgesics. Gastrointest Endosc Clin N Am. 2004; 14(2):247–268

[33] Zakko SF, Seifert HA, Gross JB. A comparison of midazolam and diazepam for conscious sedation during colonoscopy in a prospective double-blind study. Gastrointest Endosc. 1999; 49(6):684–689

[34] Cole SG, Brozinsky S, Isenberg JI. Midazolam, a new more potent benzodiazepine, compared with diazepam: a randomized, double-blind study of preendoscopic sedatives. Gastrointest Endosc. 1983; 29(3):219–222

[35] Christe C, Janssens JP, Armenian B, et al. Midazolam sedation for upper gastrointestinal endoscopy in older persons: a randomized, double-blind, placebo-controlled study. J Am Geriatr Soc. 2000; 48(11):1398–1403

[36] Stack CG, Rogers P, Linter SP. Monoamine oxidase inhibitors and anaesthesia. A review. Br J Anaesth. 1988; 60(2):222–227

[37] Singh H, Poluha W, Cheung M, et al. Propofol for sedation during colonoscopy. Cochrane Database Syst Rev. 2008(4):CD006268

[38] Jung M, Hofmann C, Kiesslich R, Brackertz A. Improved sedation in diagnostic and therapeutic ERCP: propofol is an alternative to midazolam. Endoscopy. 2000; 32(3):233–238

[39] Riphaus A, Stergiou N, Wehrmann T. Sedation with propofol for routine ERCP in high-risk octogenarians: a randomized, controlled study. Am J Gastroenterol. 2005; 100(9):1957–1963

[40] Amorós A, Aparicio JR, Garmendia M, et al. Deep sedation with propofol does not precipitate hepatic encephalopathy during elective upper endoscopy. Gastrointest Endosc. 2009; 70(2):262–268

[41] Riphaus A, Lechowicz I, Frenz MB, Wehrmann T. Propofol sedation for upper gastrointestinal endoscopy in patients with liver cirrhosis as an alternative to midazolam to avoid acute deterioration of minimal encephalopathy: a randomized, controlled study. Scand J Gastroenterol. 2009; 44(10):1244–1251

[42] Bamji N, Cohen LB. Endoscopic sedation of patients with chronic liver disease. Clin Liver Dis. 2010; 14(2):185–194

[43] Sharma VK, Nguyen CC, Crowell MD. A national study of cardiopulmonary unplanned events after GI endoscopy. Gastrointest Endosc. 2007; 66(1):27–34

[44] Rex DK, Deenadayalu VP, Eid E, et al. Endoscopist-directed administration of propofol: a worldwide safety experience. Gastroenterology. 2009; 137(4):1229–1237, quiz 1518–1519

[45] Lagasse RS. Anesthesia safety: model or myth? A review of the published literature and analysis of current original data. Anesthesiology. 2002; 97(6):1609–1617

[46] Lee CK, Lee SH, Chung IK, et al. Balanced propofol sedation for therapeutic GI endoscopic procedures: a prospective, randomized study. Gastrointest Endosc. 2011; 73(2):206–214

[47] Vargo JJ, Cohen LB, Rex DK, Kwo PY. Position statement: nonanesthesiologist administration of propofol for GI endoscopy. Gastrointest Endosc. 2009; 70(6):1053–1059

[48] Vargo JJ. Procedural sedation. Curr Opin Gastroenterol. 2010; 26(5):421–424

[49] Newman DH, Azer MM, Pitetti RD, Singh S. When is a patient safe for discharge after procedural sedation? The timing of adverse effect events in 1367 pediatric procedural sedations. Ann Emerg Med. 2003; 42(5):627–635

[50] Aldrete JA. Modifications to the postanesthesia score for use in ambulatory surgery. J Perianesth Nurs. 1998; 13(3):148–155

[51] Horiuchi A, Nakayama Y, Katsuyama Y. Safety and driving ability following low-dose propofol sedation. Digestion. 2008; 78(4):190–194

[52] Riphaus A, Gstettenbauer T, Frenz MB, Wehrmann T. Quality of psychomotor recovery after propofol sedation for routine endoscopy: a randomized and controlled study. Endoscopy. 2006; 38(7):677–683

[53] Vargo JJ. Doc, can I drive home? Am J Gastroenterol. 2009; 104(7):1656–1657

5 Design of the Endoscopy Suite

Hans-Dieter Allescher

5.1 Introduction

Endoscopic techniques continue to develop rapidly, and a myriad of other diagnostic imaging modalities have become more and more important and clinically relevant. When planning and designing a new endoscopic suite, these changing demands of technical equipment and information technologies have to be considered. Former guidelines can only be partially adapted to these recent changes. New demands to imaging, flexibility, and connectivity have to be defined. In general, the space and facilities required in endoscopic units depend on the spectrum and quantity of the procedure performed and the staff available. Additionally, it is important to predefine which endoscopic techniques should be performed or subsequently introduced. When required, the facilities should be sufficiently versatile and flexible to allow handling of emergency cases without disrupting routine procedures.

There are some general questions and considerations which should be answered in a checklist before planning and building an endoscopic suite.

5.2 General Questions and Considerations

1. For what purposes are the endoscopy suite used?
   a) Only elective/planned procedures?
   b) Only outpatient or ambulatory patients or also inpatients?
   c) Estimated number of procedures and procedure types per day/week?
   d) Number and frequency of complex procedures (e.g., endoscopic submucosal dissection [ESD], peroral endoscopic myotomy [POEM], double-balloon endoscopy, cholangioscopy)?
   e) What types of therapeutic and invasive procedures are performed?
   f) Are special patient groups treated (e.g., pediatric patients, bariatric patients)?
2. What types of complex procedures are performed?
   a) Frequency of X-ray and radiological demands?
   b) Need for navigated work or procedures?
   c) Need for combined imaging (e.g. endoscopic ultrasound [EUS] plus radiology)?
   d) Are there plans for NOTES (natural orifice transluminal endoscopic surgery) procedures (POEM, peroral endoscopic tumor resection [POET], ESD)?
   e) Are other procedures and tests (manometry, capsule endoscopy, function tests) performed within the unit?
3. What are the streams of material/patients/doctors/nurses?
   a) What is the most effective way for patients to navigate from the time of admission until the end of recovery?
   b) Which pathway is most effective for endoscopic staff and nurses?
   c) How can the time and efficiency of physicians be optimized?
   d) How can the endoscopic equipment be used most effectively?

   e) How and when is the endoscopic report generated and given/explained to the patient?
4. Which reprocessing concept is planned?
   a) Processing of endoscopes within the unit or in central facility?
   b) Reprocessing of material or exclusive single use?
   c) What concept of reprocessing the endoscopes is carried out (separation of unclean and clean area), and what type of reprocessing machines will be used?
   d) What room concept (ceiling supplies or trollies) is planned?
5. How is sedation performed in the endoscopic suite?
   a) Percentage of procedures with sedation.
   b) What type of sedation is used and what is the process for patient monitoring during and after the procedure?
   c) Need for and frequency of general anesthesia.
   d) How is general anesthesia performed?
   e) Does the endoscopy suite provide care to children of all ages?

5.3 Guidelines for Planning an Endoscopy Suite

The space concept of an endoscopic suite is influenced by many factors. If the endoscopy suite is planned de novo or in a new building, an ideal room concept can be realized. However, if the unit is built into an existing building, there is always a compromise between demands and technical feasibility. The number of endoscopy rooms within the endoscopy suite depends on several factors such as the estimated number of endoscopic procedures and the breakdown by type, complexity, and need for fluoroscopy or radiography. Precise updated numbers and a development plan for the upcoming years should be made available for planning, as these statistics are often outdated.[1]

Furthermore, transport and waiting times as well as the management of patients outside of the procedure rooms are relevant. A clearly defined and structured monitoring of sedated patients is mandatory, and sufficient space, monitors, and staff personal for this need to be considered. Some units have individual preprocedural rooms for each patient, to assess, undress, recover, dress, and review patients before discharge. In some countries, the requirements for the postprocedural recovery are clearly regulated and need to be considered before planning.[2] When there is limited recovery space and when more than one patient shares a room, there should be one or two interview rooms available for postprocedure consultation (▶Fig. 5.1, ▶Fig. 5.2).

5.4 Pathways for Patients, Staff, and Material

When planning a new unit, it is advisable to first plan the pathways of individual patient populations (inpatients, outpatients), endoscopes, doctors, and nursing staff. Questions to be addressed include: where does the patient (outpatient or bedbound) enter

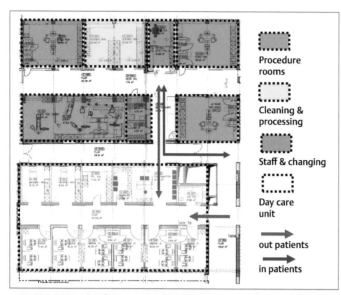

Fig. 5.1 Example of a concept of an endoscopy unit with adjacent daycare unit. It is important to visualize pathways of patents, doctors, and staff for optimizing work flow.

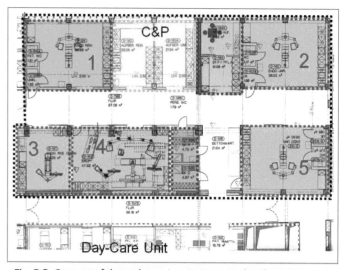

Fig. 5.2 Concept of the endoscopic suite in more detail consisting of procedure rooms (*red*), area for cleaning and processing of endoscopes (*green*), area for staff base, and changing of staff personnel (*blue*).

the endoscopy unit, where do the preparation, undressing, and preprocedural assessment take place, and how and where does the patient leave the unit. If possible, preparation and recovery of the patients should be carried out independently of the procedure rooms, as this increases flexibility and productivity of the unit. On the other hand, separated recovery areas require additional staff and space. Furthermore, it is advisable to separate patients waiting for procedures from those recovering. Additionally, the number and timing of outpatient procedures performed without sedation have to be estimated, as these patients require less infrastructure and nearby changing rooms eventually with direct access to the procedure room.

For the endoscopists, it is important to define the endoscopic workflow beforehand. Who performs sedation (specialized staff, Nurse Administered Propofol Sedation [NAPS] nurses, anesthetist, second physician)? When and how is the procedure report created? Will there be a report given to the patient prior to leaving the unit, or will it be finalized after the patient leaves? According to the answers, the pathways (computer-based report generation location, printout, and signature) have to be developed. Similar pathways should be defined for equipment and material including endoscopes and working/break areas for the endoscopy staff. A close proximity between procedure rooms and cleaning and disinfection area is desirable. In this context, it is important to define how the contaminated endoscopes are transported back to the unclean area of the cleaning facilities and how the cleaned endoscopes are transported back into the procedure room. In many modern endoscopy units, a special closed trolley system is used for this purpose.

5.5 Location of the Unit

The strategic location of the unit is crucial and should be based on the number of inpatient and/or outpatient procedures. If the majority of endoscopic examinations are outpatient procedures, a location next to the outpatient department or day care unit is desirable (▶Fig. 5.1, ▶Fig. 5.2), unless daycare facilities are fully provided for within the unit itself.[1,3] At many units, the majority

of patients are ambulatory, with a significant minority arriving in wheelchairs or trolleys, or even on hospital beds. A suitable reception area is needed, as well as an area for patients to await endoscopy on trolleys, on which they will be transported directly into the endoscopy room. Changing facilities in or near this waiting area must be provided. The waiting area can also serve as the recovery area to which patients are returned after endoscopy, though it is advisable to have separate waiting and recovery areas. Waiting and recovery areas must also be provided with toilet facilities. After full recovery, ambulatory patients should await discharge in the reception area, which can also be occupied by relatives and friends. Waiting-room space can be calculated on the basis of eight chairs for each endoscopy procedure room. This is based on two or three seats for the waiting patient and family members, and two each for family members of the two patients in recovery and the patient undergoing the procedure.

If outpatients and inpatients are treated, then simultaneous but separate patient flow pathways should be created (▶Fig. 5.1). There should be an interview room where the details of the procedure prior to endoscopy and the results of endoscopy and further arrangements can be discussed in privacy with the patients and/or their relatives, as appropriate.

5.6 Number of Rooms

In general, upper and lower gastrointestinal (GI) tract endoscopies are separated, and thus there is a minimum of two endoscopy rooms even for a small unit. For larger units, approximately one endoscopy room per 1,000 examinations (diagnostic and low-scale therapeutic) annually is a rough estimate for capacity planning. The British Society of Gastroenterology recommends a minimum of 2 + 1 endoscopy rooms for 3,000 endoscopies per year.[3,4]

In larger units, the concept should also include a radiography unit and a multipurpose room for various procedures such as laser therapy, EUS, and emergency cases.[5] Providing care for emergency cases has to be standardized and separated into those suitable for the endoscopy unit and those who should be treated in the intensive care unit or operating room. If a high volume of emergency and unscheduled cases are seen, then it is important to have at least one additional room for flexibility without interrupting the routine scheduled endoscopic program.[3]

When additional techniques such as video capsule endoscopy and functional GI tests (manometry, breath test, absorptive tests) are planned and performed by the same staff, additional rooms for these tests and for reviewing capsule endoscopy should be planned for. In larger units or specialized centers performing 6,000 procedures (the 4 + 2 room model), a dedicated room for EUS, laser therapy, and photodynamic therapy should also be present.[6,7,8,9,10,11,12,13,14,15,16]

Therapeutic endoscopic procedures are increasingly time-consuming and result in lower productivity per room. Such interventional techniques as ESD, POEM, and double-balloon enteroscopy, which have longer procedure times, should be taken into account for workflow. There are recent reviews and published overviews on the time demands of the various endoscopic procedures, which have been validated.[8,9,17]

The amount of teaching that takes place in the endoscopy unit also has considerable impact on procedure performance time and can amount to as much as an additional 30% of time per procedure.

Furthermore, the concept of report generation has to be considered (see below). If the report is generated immediately after the procedure with a computer-based documentation system, the time can be utilized for patient and room turnover. Thus, a single endoscopist could continuously work in one room. However, often the concept of switching rooms between procedures is applied. This increases the productivity of the individual endoscopist, but report writing and documentation might be less accurate. Capacity planning is important, and all calculations for procedure room capacity have to incorporate a realistic period (e.g., 10–15 minutes) for cleaning and setting up the room for the next procedure.[6-16] However, capacity and productivity planning is often greatly affected by local characteristics (waiting time, in-house transportation, recovery facilities). Room productivity is a valuable quality measure for organization of the unit. However, productivity of a procedure room is also influenced by the availability of instruments (endoscopes) and the cleaning preparation cycles.

5.7 X-Ray Requirements

Besides ERCP and percutaneous transhepatic procedures, which depend on optimal X-ray imaging, several therapeutic endoscopic interventions such as dilation, placement of stents and probes, and double-balloon enteroscopy require radiographic guidance. If a unit requires more than 200 to 500 radiographic examinations per year, then a dedicated radiography room is recommended. In this case, either the third room in the 2 + 1 model should have such facilities or it should be possible in a separate additional room. Sharing X-ray facilities with other departments is possible, but there is a considerable loss of effective procedure time. Interventional ERCP strongly depends on the technical demands and optimal conditions of the procedure room. Movement of the endoscopy equipment to radiology should be minimized, and precautions are needed that when the equipment is moved it does not adversely affect the safety and performance.

In most modern hospitals, a picture archiving and central storage system (PACS) is available, which allows digital archiving and distribution of X-rays. As PACS provides digital X-rays, high-quality monitors are needed to display the digital pictures in the various procedure rooms.

5.8 The Endoscopic Examination Room

5.8.1 Size of the Rooms

A continuous point of discussion is the minimum size of an endoscopic procedure room. A general or multipurpose endoscopy room, primarily intended for GI endoscopy, should have a floor surface area of not less than 30 m². For rooms with X-ray facilities, a minimum room size of 36 m² is recommended (▶ Fig. 5.3).[17] The requirements of recommended procedure room size have changed over the last years. According to the British Society of Gastroenterology, from 1990 a room measuring 25 to 30 m² was considered adequate if there was sufficient storage space outside the room for endoscopes and additional equipment.[4] The corresponding American recommendation was an area of approximately 6.25 × 4.75 m or 30 m² in size, as appropriate.[7] In a 2015 consensus statement of the German digestive society, a minimum room size of 30 m² is recommended. For rooms with X-ray, the minimum size is 36 m².

In addition to the size of the procedure room, other general requirements should be met. The width of the entrance and corridors should be sufficient to allow for the transportation of beds, stretchers, and wheelchairs. It must be possible to turn beds around in the corridor. The standard door width should be 1.28 m, and the opening should have sliding doors. An "engaged" or "in use" sign as well as signs for "Laser" or "X-ray" should be

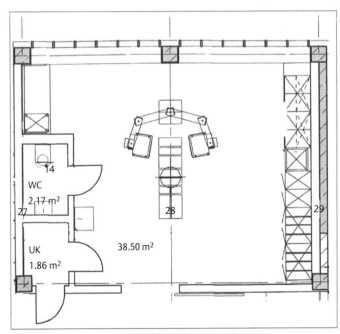

Fig. 5.3 Concept of a procedure room in more detail. The ground floor size is 38.5 m². In addition to a ceiling supply unit with two monitor systems, fitted cupboards (right side), a computer documentation area (upper left corner), changing room (UK) and toilet (WC) are integrated.

present on the entrance doors to endoscopy rooms, where appropriate. The floor material in the procedure room must be fluid resistant and easy to clean and must conform to anesthetic and high-frequency electrical requirements (e.g., nonconducting).

5.8.2 Equipment

The endoscopy room should contain a mobile examination table with adjustable height and positioning, a desk and chair, radiography viewing space, a work surface with a sink and cupboards, and waste containers for the various types of waste. There should be facilities for proper hand disinfection and storage of protective clothing and equipment. Storage space for accessories should be available in the endoscopy room or in an adjacent storage area.[14]

There should be fitted cupboards for endoscopes and ancillary equipment, and washing facilities for staff and equipment. The procedure rooms should be equipped with high-quality video screens for viewing digital images.

It is essential to have piped oxygen gas and suction facilities as well as pressured air. Insufflation using CO_2 is becoming routine for interventional endoscopic procedures and is increasingly used also during routine endoscopy. Thus, CO_2 outlets positioned close to the endoscopic processor should be considered in order to avoid CO_2 supply via gas cylinders. Placement of oxygen and suction outlets has to be well considered as the lines to the patient or the endoscope should not cross the working area or the floor. Thus, suction should be close to the endoscopic processor and oxygen close to the patient's head.

Sufficient power outlets are necessary in the procedure room to ensure flexible working conditions and so that auxiliary equipment can be used safely. The electric sockets can be either wall-mounted or attached to the ceiling supply units. The electric sockets should be connected to various circuits. Some power outlets should also be connected to the hospital's emergency energy supply. Sockets used for endoscopic light sources and the video processor as well as the surveillance monitors should have an uninterrupted emergency power supply. The compressed air supply, intravenous fluids hooks, suction lines, and connections for closed circuit television should preferably be fixed to the ceiling, to prevent cables crossing the floor.

Within the endoscopy room, air conditioning and temperature control must be optimal. If there are outside windows, then blinds or blackout facilities are needed. Ceiling lighting should be bright, but easily dimmed. There is a new trend to use colored lights such as blue or green light for procedure rooms, as blue light increases the contrast and facilitates viewing of the monitor image while still having enough surrounding light for handling and controlling the patient. Various functions of the endoscopic procedure room (room light, video recording, picture documentation, video switching and video streaming, video sources for the monitor, communication) can be handled with touch screen–based devices. There are several commercial systems which offer such functionality as complete room service package (e.g., Endo-Alpha by Olympus, OR1 by Storz). Other optional features such as writing surfaces and dictation facilities depend on the report generation management (see documentation).

Cubicles, or at least curtained-off partitions and washing facilities, should be available for patients who have undergone sigmoidoscopy or colonoscopy.

5.8.3 Monitor Systems and Anesthesia

Surveillance monitors are mandatory in each procedure room for optimal patient safety during the procedure, as well as during the recovery period. The monitor display should be positioned in such way that it can be easily viewed and controlled. The monitor system should consist of a noninvasive blood pressure measurement, a pulse oximeter, and an ECG. There is some debate as to whether CO_2 monitoring should be performed during endoscopic procedures.[17] Due to the high rates of artifacts of current systems, no specific recommendations for the use of CO_2 monitoring can be given. The positioning of the monitor should also consider that cables and lines connect to the patients, and these should not cross the working areas of the endoscopist. A positioning of the monitor system opposite to the endoscopist near the video monitor is a possible solution, which avoids these problems (▶ Fig. 5.4). The suction equipment may be either free-standing or placed on a trolley or incorporated in a ceiling supply unit (▶ Fig. 5.4). As in most operating rooms, documentation of the vital parameters (respiratory rate, heart rate, blood pressure, medication administration) is increasingly carried out via digital online recording of the respective parameters. The implementation of an IT-based documentation of monitoring data has to be taken into account and a separate computer workplace in the procedure room close to the patient has to be planned for the anesthetist or personnel performing sedation and monitoring.

In addition, there should be a resuscitation equipment within the unit. A resuscitation trolley should be in the endoscopy room or easily available. In some units, it has been found convenient to place markers on the floor so that mobile equipment is placed correctly.

As general anesthesia has changed mostly to intravenous agents, the installation requirements for general anesthesia have decreased. However, the needs of the anesthesiologist should be considered during the primary planning. There should be anesthesiology trolleys or equipment and infrastructure (pressure

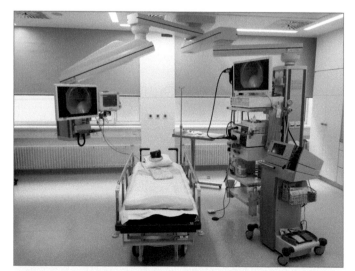

Fig. 5.4 Example of an endoscopic room for upper GI endoscopy with optimized positioning of video monitors and surveillance monitors.

air and oxygen sockets, IT connections) to accommodate the needs of the anesthetist. Preferentially, the X-ray room should be equipped with such facilities.

5.8.4 Video Integration and PC-Based Documentation

Modern GI endoscopy uses digital video endoscopy almost exclusively. While the analogue video signal (SVHS, RGB) is still available, most newly designed units use the digital high-definition video technique. Whether videos are stored centrally or in the local endoscopic documentation system depends on the video concept of the unit or the hospital. Increasingly, the Digital Imaging and Communications in Medicine (DICOM) standard is used to store endoscopic pictures in the PACS. This offers the advantage that all images are stored with the respective patient case in a central system which is generally accessible. A corresponding video standard is yet to be developed.

As IT-based documentation of endoscopic procedures is standard, a specialized area for documentation within the procedure room has to be planned. This area should be located outside either the sterile or contaminated procedure area but should be close enough to access written or PC-documented information (Clinical Information System [KIS] or PACS information). In the radiographic procedure room, this documentation area must be located outside the radiation area.

Various commercial endoscopic documentation systems with integrated report generation are available. As endoscopic terminology has been widely standardized, reports can be generated with these systems. Integrated systems also allow video streaming and video switching. For the integration of additional equipment, additional video inputs and video lines have to be planned and installed. It is advisable to have a separate video planning concept for a new unit. In most larger units, it is advisable to centralize video information to a central video switchboard which allows central video streaming or storage. Most integrated systems (EndoAlpha, OR-1) are based on such a concept.

As already mentioned, IT documentation is also standard for sedation as well as for documentation of procedure parameters (endoscope and equipment and material used). Thus, in addition to the IT working place for the endoscopists, additional areas have to be planned for anesthetists and nursing staff. Recently, there have been attempts to switch the documentation process to handheld devices, which will then decrease space requirements. However, this emphasizes the need for high-speed WLAN connectivity in the endoscopic suite.

5.8.5 Endoscopes and Endoscopic Equipment

Sufficient endoscopes must be available within a endoscopic unit to allow a smooth sequence of the endoscopic procedures and to allow for optimal work efficiency of the endoscopists and endoscopic staff.

The number of endoscopes needed is dependent on the reprocessing cycles, the number of procedures and rooms active in parallel, and the amount of specialized procedures that require specialized endoscopes and equipment (e.g., therapeutic endoscopes, large working channel, pediatric scopes).

In addition to the equipment within the procedure room, a mobile endoscopy trolley carrying all essential instruments and endoscopic processors should always be on standby, as occasionally an endoscopic procedure has to be carried out in other parts of the hospital, such as the intensive care unit or the surgical or radiological department.

5.9 Endoscopic Ultrasound and Laser Treatment Room, Radiography Room

Large endoscopy units, from the so-called 4 + 2 room model and upward, should have a room dedicated to EUS, laser, or photodynamic therapy. Since such procedures tend to be time consuming, they should be scheduled and planned carefully so as to not interfere with general routine endoscopic activities. Radiographic facilities should be available when required during ERCP, dilation procedures, insertion of stents, etc. Such facilities avoid the inconvenience and waste of time involved in transporting patients and fragile equipment to and from the radiology department. An alternative for smaller endoscopy units is to modify one of the rooms in the radiography department to accommodate endoscopy.

The choice of radiography system should consider the special needs of the endoscopist. In most modern units, a C-arm system with flexible X-ray planes is used. Digital X-ray with a pulse radiographic beam is preferable due to high image quality and low radiation exposure. A solid phase X-ray detector is a new X-ray standard which offers less respiration and movement artifacts, which is helpful especially for ERCP and percutaneous interventions (▶Fig. 5.5). New technologies allow 3D imaging and image fusion of the ultrasound with DICOM CT and MR data. This technology involves magnetic field tracking, and prerequisites for such procedures can be planned in new procedure rooms.

The radiographic procedure room is often used with additional imaging modalities such as endosonography and cholangiography. Therefore, the display capacity of this room must be versatile

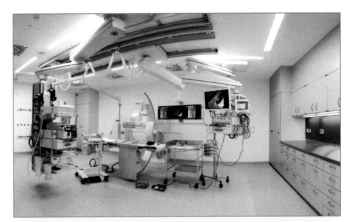

Fig. 5.5 Modern multifunctional intervention room with X-ray and operative hygiene standard. Technical installations (e.g. for X-ray Siemens artis Zee with solid state detector) are in a separate room to gain space for anesthesiology and additional equipment. Modern video switching (Olympus Exera III with switching tool) allows versatile combination of video sources and distribution on the various procedure monitors. Ceiling supplies (Trumpf Medical) allow optimal hygiene standard and flexibility.

and flexible (see later). A "2 and 2" or "3 and 2" monitor system is recommended with flexible inputs to the various monitors, for example, by the use of a special switching device. The radiography monitor and the videoendoscopic monitor should be mounted together and positioned in such a way that the endoscopist and assistant personnel have a direct, unobstructed view. Preferentially, the main monitor system is composed of a radiographic and one endoscopic monitor, whereas the third monitor should be used for reference (X-ray) or additional imaging modalities (EUS, cholangiography, mother–baby endoscopy) (► Fig. 5.5). The second monitor system for the assistant personnel should be composed of one X-ray and one endoscopic monitor.

The radiographic room should have enough space for the X-ray protection and shielding system and should be especially equipped for procedures performed under general anesthesia.

5.10 Preparation and Recovery Room

Preparation and recovery rooms should be located close to the endoscopy unit. In general, three beds per endoscopy room are required.[7,10] Seven square meters per bed is standard. The use of sedatives such as midazolam and/or propofol during upper or lower tract endoscopy requires recovery facilities (with nursing supervision), since it may be as long as an hour before these patients are able to leave the endoscopy unit. Oxygen and suction devices are essential in addition to pulse oximeters, electrocardiography monitoring, and resuscitation equipment.

5.11 Cleaning and Disinfection Area

Disinfection is a central problem in the endoscopic unit. Thus, the concepts for cleaning and reprocessing the endoscopes is of utmost importance and should be handled with local disinfection experts. Processing of the endoscopes can be done in a centralized area for the entire hospital, but requires elaborate logistics for transport to and from the unit. More commonly, a disinfection and reprocessing area is located within the endoscopic unit. When planning a new unit, there are two different concepts for the cleaning area. In one concept, the cleaning area is accessible directly from the procedure room. This is only practical in smaller units with few procedure rooms. In larger units with more than three procedure rooms, the cleaning area is best located centrally. For optimal hygiene, a one-way system for endoscope transport and processing has to be established. The cleaning and reprocessing area has to be divided into separate unclean and clean areas. These two areas should be completely separated by a separating wall and best by double side or load through washing and reprocessing machines, which act as separator for the two rooms.[17,18] This completely avoids mixing of used and unused endoscopes and eliminates possible endoscope contamination. Cleaning of endoscopes should be carried out by fully-automated washing and disinfection machines by skilled personal. The unclean areas should contain stainless-steel work surfaces, with a double sink and an ultrasonic bath for initial cleaning. There should

be 1.5 m on either side of the sink to position endoscopes. There should be enough room for brushing, ultrasonic cleaner, tightness control, and a compressed-air system for mechanical cleaning. After cleaning and disinfection of the endoscopes, they should be stored either hanging in a closed storage cabinet or in specially designed venting cabinets. There are various venting cabinets that are commercially available.

The entire cleaning process should be controlled by RFID chip or bar code–mediated control of the endoscopes, processing machines, and the venting cabinet. This allows generation of an endoscope "history" where all relevant data from the endoscope are collected in a central data file. These data include time and use of the endoscopes in the individual patients, time and responsible person who cleaned and processed the endoscope, processing protocol, time and success of the disinfection process, and time during transfer of the endoscope to the venting cabinet. With this log file, continuous monitoring of the endoscope use as well as cleaning and processing can be established. These data can be used to define interval for service and evaluation of endoscopes, hygiene controls, and mandatory service procedures.

The capacity of the disinfection equipment and washing machines needed for a given unit depends on the number of examinations, the time planned per examination, and the time needed to clean, disinfect, and dry (cleaning cycle) the endoscope. As vapors from disinfectants need to be removed from the room, a powerful ventilation system has to be in place for the cleaning and processing area to exclude the possibility of inhalation of toxic or allergenic vapors. There should be separate containers for waste, dirty linen, etc. There should be at least one dirty sink.

5.12 Staffing

Assistance for GI endoscopy is a task for fully-trained professional nurses and technicians.[12,13,19] The nursing staff carries a major responsibility for patient safety. In some countries, nursing staff can be trained and specialized for administration of sedation and monitoring of the patient during the endoscopic procedure (NAPS nurses).[2] In other countries, for example, France, the sedation and administration of sedatives are required to be performed by anesthetists.[20]

Per European guidelines, there must be one properly trained nurse assistant in each procedure room, and two for any complex endoscopies such as ERCP and sophisticated therapy. One head nurse should be in charge of the unit for the day, and at least one other handling the recovery area. Lower level staff can be trained to perform cleaning and disinfection effectively, and to assist with recovery duties. However, the procedure-related nurses should maintain their skills in handling those functions and may occasionally rotate through these areas. Since emergency procedures performed outside of regular hours are often the most difficult and dangerous ones, it is essential to have GI nursing staff on 24-hour call. This also ensures a more consistent approach to cleaning and disinfection of endoscopic equipment for patient safety. The extent to which the nurse manager is involved in actual procedures will depend on the size of the unit. In a department with four or five procedure rooms, the nurse manager should allocate at least half of his or her time for office and managerial activities. The amount of secretarial assistance will depend on the methods used for scheduling and reporting. An appropriate technician must be available if radiography equipment is in use—not only to assist with the procedures, but also to help in maintaining and monitoring radiation safety standards.

References

[1] Mulder CJJ. The endoscopy unit. In: Tytgat GNJ, Mulder CJJ, eds. Procedures in Hepatogastroenterology. 2nd ed. Dordrecht: Kluwer Academic; 1997:345–53

[2] Riphaus A, Wehrmann T, Weber B, et al; Sektion Enoskopie im Auftrag der Deutschen Gesellschaft für Verdauungs- und Stoffwechselerkrankungen e.V. (DGVS). Bundesverband Niedergelassener Gastroenterologen Deuschlands e. V. (Bng). Chirurgische Arbeitsgemeinschaft für Endoskopie und Sonographie der Deutschen Gesellschaft für Allgemein- und Viszeralchirurgie (DGAV). Deutsche Morbus Crohn/Colitis ulcerosa Vereinigung e. V. (DCCV). Deutsche Gesellschaft für Endoskopie-Assistenzpersonal (DEGEA). Deutsche Gesellschaft für Anästhesie und Intensivmedizin (DGAI). Gesellschaft für Recht und Politik im Gesundheitswesen (GPRG). S3-Guidelines–Sedation in endoscopy. Z Gastroenterol. 2008; 46(11):1298–1330

[3] Working Party of the Clinical Services Committee of the British Society of Gastroenterology. Provision of gastrointestinal endoscopy and related services for a district general hospital. Gut. 1991; 32(1):95–105

[4] Lennard-Jones JE, Williams CB, Axon A. Provision of Gastrointestinal Endoscopy and Related Services for a District General Hospital: Report of the British Society of Gastroenterology. London: British Society of Gastroenterology; 1990

[5] Mulder CJJ, Tan AC, Huibregeste K. Guidelines for designing an endoscopy unit: report of the Dutch Society of Gastroenterologists. Endoscopy. 1997; 29(1):I–VI

[6] Phillip J, Allescher H.D., Hohner R. Endoskopie: Struktur und Ökonomie. Bad Homburg, Eaglewood, NJ: Normed Verlag, International Medical Publishers; 1998

[7] Waye JD, Rich ME. Planning an Endoscopy Suite for Office and Hospital. Tokyo: Igaku-Shoin Medical; 1990

[8] Staritz M, Alkier R, Krzoska B. et al Zeitbedarf für endoskopische Diagnostik und Therapie: Ergebnisse einer Multicenterstudie. Z Gastroenterol 1992; 30(8):509–518

[9] Phillip J, Sahl RJ, Ruus P. Zeitaufwand für endoskopische Untersuchungen. Z Gastroenterol. 1990; 28(1):1–9

[10] Burton D, Ott BJ, Gostout CJ, DiMagno EP. Approach to designing a gastrointestinal endoscopy unit. Gastrointest Endosc Clin N Am. 1993; 3:525–540

[11] Sivak MV, Senick JM. The endoscopy unit. In: Sivak MV, ed. Gastroenterologic Endoscopy. Philadelphia, PA: Saunders; 1987:42–66

[12] Axon ATR. Staffing of endoscopy units. Acta Endosc. 1989; 19:213–216

[13] Lennard-Jones JE, Slade GE. Report of a working party on the staffing of endoscopy units. Gut. 1987; 28(12):1682–1685

[14] Marmarinou J. The autonomous endoscopy unit. Designing it for maximum efficiency. AORN J. 1990; 51(3):764–773, 766, 768–769 passim

[15] Marasco JA, Marasco RF. Designing the ambulatory endoscopy center. Gastrointest Endosc Clin N Am. 2002; 12(2):185–204, v

[16] Seifert E, Weismüller J. How to run an endoscopy unit? Experience in the Federal Republic of Germany. Results of a survey of 31 centers. Endoscopy. 1986; 18(1):20–24

[17] Denzer U, Beilenhoff U, Eickhoff A, et al; Deutsche Gesellschaft für Gastroenterologie, Verdauungs-und Stoffwechselkrankheiten. S2k guideline: quality requirements for gastrointestinal endoscopy, AWMF registry no. 021–022 [in German] Z Gastroenterol. 2015; 53(12):1496–1530

[18] Beilenhoff U, Neumann CS, Rey JF, et al; ESGE Guidelines Committee. European Society of Gastrointestinal Endoscopy. European Society of Gastroenterology and Endoscopy Nurses and Associates. ESGE-ESGENA Guideline: cleaning and disinfection in gastrointestinal endoscopy. Endoscopy. 2008; 40(11):939–957

[19] Neumann CS, the members of the ESGENA Education. Working Group ESGENA Statement: Staffing in endoscopy. 2008. Available at: www.esgena.org/statements-curricula

[20] Dumonceau JM, Riphaus A, Aparicio JR, et al. ESGE-ESGEGA-ESA guideline: non-anesthesiologist administration or propofol for GI endoscopy. Endoscopy. 2010; 42:960–974

6 Cleaning and Disinfection in Endoscopy

Bret T. Petersen

6.1 Introduction

Cleaning and disinfection of endoscopes are critical safety and quality tasks that all gastrointestinal endoscopy departments must be attentive to. The soiled environment in which endoscopes are used yields a significant bioburden for cleaning and eradication before their reuse in subsequent patients. The complexity of endoscope design further challenges the task of producing a microbe-free instrument. Our recognition of reprocessing requirements and adoption of standardized approaches to reprocessing developed slowly over several decades.[1] The Spaulding criteria for critical instruments, which are those that contact intact but contaminated mucosal membranes, stipulate that reprocessing should achieve, at a minimum, high-level disinfection (HLD). This level of reprocessing eradicates all living bacteria, viruses, and most spores, unless present in high numbers. Current international guidelines for HLD all espouse stepwise processes, which include precleaning at the bedside, thorough submersion and manual cleaning, standardized disinfection by exposure to approved liquid chemical germicides (LCGs) at specific parameters, and followed by rinsing, drying, and appropriate storage. Recent outbreaks of infections subsequent to endoscopic retrograde cholangiopancreatography (ERCP) have been attributed to persistent contamination at the elevator mechanisms, despite appropriate reprocessing. This has prompted interim advice to ensure optimal training and oversight of cleaning staff while intensifying attention to all standard steps of HLD, plus consideration of local benefit of use of double reprocessing cycles, ethylene oxide sterilization after each procedure, adenosine triphosphate (ATP) testing to assay the adequacy of the cleaning phase of reprocessing, and intermittent or per procedure endoscope cultures after full HLD.

Recurring clusters of infections, primarily related to lapses in standard reprocessing steps, have repeatedly focused the attention of the medical community and the broader regulatory and patient communities on the issue of reprocessing. This has culminated in the development of multiple national and international standards and guidelines for reprocessing, from many affiliated medical and technical specialty groups. Despite differences in detail and specificity, most existing guidelines are highly uniform in their requirements.[2,3,4,5,6,7]

6.2 Principles of Disinfection

6.2.1 Definitions

The language of reprocessing employs numerous terms with varied derivations from both regulatory and scientific origins. *Reprocessing* refers to a validated process that is used to render a used or soiled medical device fit for a subsequent single use.[8] It typically includes steps to remove gross soil by cleaning (or washing), and disinfection or sterilization to inactivate microorganisms. *Cleaning* is the physical removal of soil and contaminants to minimize transfer from one patient to another or between uses in a single patient. It should enable successful subsequent disinfection or sterilization and prevent accumulation of residual soil throughout the useful life of the product.[9] *Disinfection* is the process that employs physical or chemical means to destroy pathogenic and nonpathogenic microorganisms present on inanimate objects, such as medical devices. Hence, *disinfectants* are the agents used to destroy the microorganisms. Individual agents are sometimes referred to as germicides, fungicides, sporicides, etc., based on the microorganisms they are designed to inactivate. In contrast, *antiseptics* are agents that reduce or eliminate microorganisms on skin or in living tissues.

Disinfection is commonly categorized by the degree of clearance of microorganisms: HLD eradicates all bacteria, viruses, and most but not all spores when present in high numbers; *intermediate-level disinfection* inactivates all bacteria, mycobacteria, and most viruses but not bacterial spores; *low-level disinfection* destroys most bacteria, viruses, and fungal spores, but some mycobacteria, nonlipid viruses, and bacterial spores remain viable.

Sterilization achieves 100% eradication of all forms of life or infectious agents. This degree of certainty cannot be measured or accurately achieved; hence, sterility is often equated to a very low probability of less than 10^{-6} ($< 1/10^6$ = less than one in a million) of a nonsterile unit following sterilization. This "sterility assurance level" (SAL) is required for injectable medications and medical devices by the Food and Drug Administration (FDA) in the United States.[10] HLD is also intended to reduce microbial load to a SAL of 10^{-6}, with the exception that some resistant spore forms are not eradicated.

The intensity of reprocessing for all medical devices is based on the *Spaulding classification*, which stipulates that the degree of disinfection or sterilization should be based on the risk of transmission, as related to the nature of contact with the patient (▶ Table 6.1).[11] Those instruments that enter the bloodstream or other sterile environments require sterilization between uses. Those that contact intact mucous membranes and do not normally penetrate sterile tissue require HLD, and those that contact intact skin require low-level disinfection.

6.2.2 Application to Gastrointestinal Endoscopes

By the Spaulding criteria, gastrointestinal endoscopes require HLD, in accord with their routine exposure to nonsterile mucous membranes. Endoscopes or devices that are used in sterile environments, such as percutaneous laparoscopic passage and insertion via an enterotomy during a laparotomy, are deemed to require sterilization. Devices breaking the mucosal surface, such as needles and biopsy cables, and those entering sterile systems such as the biliary tree or pancreatic ducts, must be sterilized between uses. Many busy endoscopy departments opt for use of sterile single-use accessories such as biopsy cables,

Table 6.1 Spaulding criteria for intensity of reprocessing of medical devices based on exposure risk[11]

Category	Definition	Reprocessing	Examples
Critical	Contact sterile tissue, including the vascular system	Sterilization	• Surgical instruments • Vascular and urinary catheters • Endoscopic biopsy cables • EUS needles, ERCP devices • Endoscopes for intraoperative or transabdominal use
Semicritical	Contact intact mucous membranes or nonintact skin	High-level disinfection	• GI endoscopes • Respiratory therapy and anesthesia equipment • Laryngoscope blades
Noncritical	Contact only intact skin	Low-level disinfection	• Beds and rails • Bedpans

Abbreviations: GI, gastrointestinal; ERCP, endoscopic retrograde cholangiopancreatography; EUS, endoscopic ultrasound.

Table 6.2 Steps in reprocessing of flexible endoscopes

Bedside (point-of-use) precleaning	• Prior to transport to reprocessing room • Manually wipe exterior surfaces with water and enzymatic detergent • Aspirate or flush detergent through air/water and biopsy channels until clear	• Removes visible soil and blood before drying and adherence • Optimally reduces bioburden by 10^3
Manual washing	• Disassembly, followed by leak testing • Full submersion of entire endoscope • Manual washing and brushing of exterior with enzymatic solution • Brushing and flushing of accessible channels • Thorough water rinse	• Optimally reduces bioburden by 10^6
High-level disinfection	• Automated preferable to manual • Multiple machines and agents—require compatibility per IFUs • Adhere to IFUs for minimum concentration and contact times	• Optimally reduces bioburden by 10^6 • Narrow margin of safety primarily in complex instruments with elevators
Alcohol flushing	• Usually an AER cycle • Rinse of all LCG • Alcohol flush to facilitate removal of water and full drying	• Reduces risk of patient or personnel exposure • Facilitates complete removal of water
Forced air drying	• Filtered or "medical" air • Often heated • No fixed time/temperature parameters	• Enhances microbial kill • Prevents moist environment for proliferation of residual organisms during storage
Appropriate storage	• Upright, dry, ventilated without exposure to ambient soiled atmosphere	• Ensures clean, patient-ready endoscope at start of next procedure, calendar

Abbreviations: AER, automated endoscope reprocessors; IFUs, instructions for use; LCG, liquid chemical germicide.

sphincterotomes, and biliary guidewires to avoid the expense and organizational processes required for sterilizing inexpensive high-volume devices.

The most uniformly adopted approach to reprocessing of endoscopes employs several standardized steps (▶Table 6.2),[2,3,4,5,6,7] including:

1. *Bedside precleaning* (or "point-of-use processing") using water and detergent to wipe the endoscope exterior and flushing or aspirating it through the air and water channels to remove grossly visible blood and soil before they have an opportunity to dry and more tightly adhere to the instrument. After this gross cleaning, disassembly of all valves and parts is performed, followed by leak testing.
2. *Manual mechanical cleaning*, distant from the bedside, with full submersion in water and detergent while physically wiping all exterior surfaces and brushing the accessible inner channels. This requires flushing and aspiration of large volumes of water and detergent followed by a thorough rinse. Detergents facilitate disaggregation and removal of debris but are not efficient microbicides. Some automated endoscope reprocessors (AERs) employ a validated "brushless" cleaning process prior to disinfection cycles.
3. HLD of all exposed surfaces via full submersion and perfusion through all lumens using an approved LCG and appropriate parameters for concentration, temperature, and duration of contact. HLD can be achieved with prolonged passive soaking in appropriate LCG solutions; however, data suggest greater shortfalls in meeting requisite parameters and greater risk of inadequate bacterial clearance.[12]
4. *Rinse* with sterile or filtered water or tap water, followed by *alcohol flush* of all accessible channels (umbilical cord, biopsy, elevator cables) to evacuate residual LCG and water, thereby facilitating complete drying. This step is usually automated and accomplished by most AER machines.
5. *Forced air drying* to ensure complete removal of moisture from the endoscope channels.
6. *Upright storage* in clean, dry cabinets away from flow of ambient microorganisms. Straight upright storage theoretically facilitates drainage of any potentially retained liquids. Varieties of specialty cabinets with filtered or heated air flow, and some with flat storage, are marketed for this purpose.

HLD performed with careful adherence to validated manufacturers' instructions for use (IFUs) results in clean endoscopes with remarkably low risk of residual clinically important contaminants. Adequate reprocessing of gastrointestinal endoscopes, however, is hampered by several specific challenges, including: (1) the immense bioburden they acquire during use, (2) the relatively narrow margin of safety achieved when all reprocessing steps are appropriately performed, (3) the risk for development of intractable biofilm when cleaning steps are insufficiently performed, (4) the lack of rapid and accurate bioindicators of the process end points, (5) training, support, and ongoing supervision for staff who performs the repetitive tasks, and (6) the need for efficient turnaround of instruments in busy clinical environments.

Following use, endoscopes commonly harbor 10^6 to 10^9 microorganisms. Following combined precleaning and manual cleaning, endoscopes enter HLD with a bioburden of about 10^1 to 10^5 microorganisms.[13,14] HLD achieves a further 6 log (10^6) reduction, culminating in a theoretical terminal bioburden of 10^{-6} to 10^1 organisms per instrument.[15] While this is generally well below the inoculum required for detrimental clinical effects, any shortcoming or hindrance to optimal performance clearly risks shortcomings in the terminal cleanliness and safety of the instrument. Failure of the initial precleaning and cleaning steps risks the development of adherent biofilm, which cannot be reliably removed or sterilized with repeated optimal performance of standard HLD. Reliable, inexpensive, rapid biomarkers to assess adequacy of reprocessing by assaying for residual contamination would clearly improve performance and cleaning outcomes. No such indicators exist, however. A variety of indicators for residual blood, protein, and other components of living tissue have been evaluated, but none appear reliable for assessment of the fully reprocessed instrument.[16] Testing for ATP, which is present in all living cells, is widely used in food preparation and cleaning industries, but ATP results obtained from reprocessed endoscopes do not correlate with terminal culture results.[17] Gross differences in ATP levels are evident between well-cleaned and poorly cleaned instruments, prior to HLD, so it may prove useful as a check on training and monitoring of performance by cleaning personnel.[18]

6.2.3 Liquid Chemical Germicides and Automated Endoscope Reprocessors

Multiple LCGs are available for reprocessing of flexible endoscopes (▶ Table 6.3).[19] Initially, several LCGs were labelled as both disinfectant and sterilant, with the difference based primarily on parameters of temperature and duration of contact. Others, including many widely employed today, serve as disinfectants but do not have regulatory clearance as sterilizing agents.[20] The available agents differ in their required contact times, endoscope and reprocessing machine compatibilities, potential toxicities, and expense.

Some LCGs are consumed with each reprocessing cycle, but many are labelled for reuse, defined by time intervals or cycles of use in automated reprocessing machines. Repeated reprocessing cycles dilute the LCG, eventually risking decline in concentration below their minimum effective concentration. Agent-specific test strips should be employed to monitor LCG concentration over time. Manufacturers' IFUs should be followed regarding frequency of testing, generally per procedure.

AERs are designed to automate a variety of tasks formerly done manually during HLD. They enhance consistency in many parameters of reprocessing cycles (time, volume, temperature, pressure, concentration, etc.) and enclose LCGs and contain their fumes, thus limiting exposure of staff to potential irritants. Several are labelled to accomplish washing by vigorous perfusion of detergents prior to HLD.[21] The FDA and manufacturers have advised that this function does not replace manual washing for duodenoscopes and echoendoscopes. All AERs provide HLD, generally by complete submersion and vigorous channel flushing of appropriately-timed cycles of LCG followed by thorough rinsing. Most proceed with automated alcohol flushing and at least initial air flushing. Many AERs record and document the endoscope, LCG, and cycle parameters during performance. Compatibility between endoscopes, LCGs, and AERs should be ensured and the IFU should be closely followed to avoid risk of insufficient HLD

Table 6.3 Liquid chemical germicides commonly employed in gastrointestinal endoscope reprocessing as high-level disinfectants or chemical sterilants

Agent	Advantages	Disadvantages
Glutaraldehyde	• Long experience, numerous studies • Inexpensive • Good materials compatibility	• Respiratory irritation • Pungent and irritating odor • Slow mycobactericidal activity as sole agent • Coagulates blood and fixes tissue to surfaces • Allergic contact dermatitis
Hydrogen peroxide	• No activation required • Does not coagulate blood or fix biomaterial to surfaces—may enhance removal of organic matter • No disposal issues • Inactivates cryptosporidium	• Material compatibility concerns • Serious eye damage with contact
Ortho-phthalaldehyde (OPA)	• Fast—shorter reprocessing cycles • No activation required • Odor not significant • Excellent materials compatibility claimed • Does not coagulate blood or fix biomaterial to surfaces	• Stains protein gray (skin, membranes, clothing, etc.) • Higher expense than glut • Eye irritation with contact • Slow sporicidal activity • Anaphylactic reactions to OPA in bladder cancer with repeated exposure during cystoscopy
Peracetic acid	• Low-temperature liquid chemical sterilization	• Potential material incompatibility
Peracetic acid–hydrogen peroxide	• No activation required	

Source: Data from Rutala and Weber.[20]

cycles, chronic microbial contamination of machines, and staff exposure to reprocessing agents.

6.3 Transmission of Infection by Gastrointestinal Endoscopy

A 2013 compilation of known outbreaks of infection attributed to interpatient transmission during gastrointestinal endoscopy in the United States and Europe identified 47 clusters of cases involving 235 patients, including 19 outbreaks in upper endoscopy (56 patients), 5 outbreaks during lower endoscopy (6 patients) and 23 outbreaks during ERCP (89 patients).[22] Most identified outbreaks, involving 85% or more of patient cases, were attributed to deficiencies in cleaning and disinfection of endoscopes or water bottles, or contaminated AERs.[15] The predominant organisms involved were *Helicobacter pylori*, *Salmonella*, hepatitis C virus, and *Pseudomonas aeruginosa*. Undoubtedly, publication and other public reporting mechanisms significantly underrepresent the likely occurrences of disease transmission during endoscopy. More recently, numerous outbreaks involving patient-to-patient transmission of multidrug-resistant organisms (MDROs) have been reported to occur following ERCP, as discussed in the following.

6.3.1 Transmission by Endoscopes with Elevators

Multiple cases of *P. aeruginosa* cholangitis after ERCP were recognized many years ago.[23] They were attributed to insufficient drying of the endoscope at the end of the procedure day, and largely eradicated by use of an alcohol flush and forced air drying between procedures. Multiple episodes of duodenoscope transmission of carbapenem-resistant enterobacteriaceae (CRE) or other MDROs were published or publicly acknowledged in the 2013–2015 time frame, some having occurred up to 5 years earlier.[24,25,26,27,28,29] As of early 2016, approximately 25 outbreaks have infected at least 250 patients, with at least 20 deaths.[30] When closely evaluated, most centers appear to have been adhering to HLD guidelines, without shortfalls in practice or equipment. The risk appears to be related to the challenge of cleaning and disinfection in tight crevices surrounding the elevator mechanism and its actuation cable. Several studies suggest further risk from wear and degradation with routine use.[29,31] The U.S. FDA and others have provided a series of mandatory, advisable, and future interventions to prevent such episodes in the future (▶ Table 6.4).[15,23,32,33] The role of routine servicing based on time or procedure numbers remains unknown. Limited case reports and culture studies suggest similar risk of persistent contamination after reprocessing of echoendoscopes.[34,35]

6.3.2 Failure or Breach in Reprocessing

On occasion, endoscopy unit staff identify inappropriate or incomplete reprocessing for one or more endoscopes. Breaches in reprocessing are not uncommon; however, transmission of an infectious agent is far less so, due to variations in prevalence and infectivity

Table 6.4 Means toward reducing risk in complex instruments

1. Ensuring quality of endoscope reprocessing

- Optimal training, oversight, and competency evaluation of existing processes
- Endoscope culture after HLD and quarantine until return of negative cultures
- Selective endoscope culture following use in MDRO (+) patient and quarantine until return of negative cultures
- Surveillance culture of endoscopes intermittently for quality assurance of HLD process
- Routine or intermittent surveillance testing of bioburden (e.g., ATP) for QA of washing processes before HLD

2. Enhanced or alternative approaches to reprocessing

- Routine per procedure ETO sterilization following HLD
- Selective or intermittent ETO sterilization, for suspicion of biofilm (culture positivity) or following use in patient carrying MDRO
- Routine use of double cycles of washing + HLD after each procedure (wash→ HLD→ wash→ HLD)
- "Liquid sterilization" using peracetic acid

3. Identification of high-risk patients to guide use of alternative endoscope reprocessing

- Routine surveillance for CRE and/or other MDROs (via PCR or culture and sensitivity) by anal swab in all patients undergoing ERCP → with subsequent intensified/alternative reprocessing if positive

4. Potential new technologies

- Alternative designs for endoscopes that harbor elevators or other complex functions:
- Enhanced access for cleaning—removable tips
- Tolerance to high-temperature autoclaving
- Single-use disposable components
- New modalities for precleaning and/or washing
- New low-temperature sterilization technologies

Abbreviations: ATP, adenosine triphosphate; CRE, carbapenem-resistant enterobacteriaceae; ERCP, endoscopic retrograde cholangiopancreatography; ETO, ethylene oxide; HLD, high- level disinfection; MDRO, multidrug-resistant organism; PCR, polymerase chain reaction; QA, quality assurance.

Source: Adapted from Petersen,[23] Rutala and Weber,[15] and FDA.[32,33]

of significant organisms, immune clearance of the gut, and the degree to which the lapse in reprocessing reduced the likely clearance of pathogens. An organized approach is useful for addressing the shortfall in reprocessing. Steps include investigating the risk to patients, communicating with appropriate local and regulatory groups, and potentially undertaking a notification and call-back program for exposed patients. Several algorithms have been described to accomplish the necessary elements.[36,37] Both the scope of breaches in reprocessing and nuance regarding the nature of the breach may influence the institutions' decisions regarding patient notification. In the current era, most guidance advises informing patients and serologic or culture testing are selectively based on the perceived risk.

6.3.3 Unusual Organisms

Almost all contaminating organisms are efficiently eradicated if they can be adequately exposed to standard means of cleaning (by mechanical action and detergents) and HLD employing appropriate germicides. In contrast, prions are transmissible infectious agents that are highly resistant to commonly employed methods of HLD and sterilization. They are the etiologic agent of a variety of extremely rare, and lethal, spongiform encephalopathies, which predominantly infect tissues of the central nervous system, such as Creutzfeldt–Jacob disease (CJD), kuru, and others. While prions can be inactivated by more intense application of nonstandard cleaning agents and sterilization parameters, many guidelines advise against reuse of medical devices that are exposed to nervous system tissues of patients with CJD.[38]

6.4 Design and Oversight of Reprocessing Facilities

The recent clusters of infection attributed to persistent contamination despite apparent adherence to current reprocessing guidelines have prompted renewed emphasis on reprocessing facility design, unit leadership, and training and supervision of reprocessing staff. All of these issues are assessed during accreditation evaluation. Facility design is more standardized than in the past. Designs routinely incorporate expectations for sufficient air exchanges to avoid exposure of staff to reprocessing fumes and chemicals, and floor plans that enable instrument flow from dirty to clean, with avoidance of crossover to dirty areas often carefully evaluated.

Quality performance in most settings is highly dependent on the tenor and expectations set by the leadership and administrative staff of the organization. Recent infection outbreaks have prompted the U.S. FDA and accreditation agencies to further emphasize these issues. Training, competency testing, repeated continuing oversight of performance, and documentation of both administrative and technical steps are all highlighted in recent FDA and Centers for Disease Control and Prevention (CDC) guidance.[7,39]

References

[1] Petersen BT. Gaining perspective on reprocessing of GI endoscopes. Gastrointest Endosc. 1999; 50(2):287–291

[2] Petersen BT, Chennat J, Cohen J, et al. Multisociety guideline on reprocessing flexible GI endoscopes: 2016 update. Gastrointest Endosc. 2017; 85(2):282–294

[3] Gastroenterologic Society of Australia. Clinical Update: Infection Control in Clinical Endoscopy. 3rd ed. Melbourne: Gastroenterologic Society of Australia; 2010

[4] Beilenhoff U, Neumann CS, Rey JF, et al; ESGE Guidelines Committee. European Society of . Gastrointestinal Endoscopy. European Society of Gastroenterology and Endoscopy Nurses and Associates. ESGE-ESGENA Guideline: cleaning and disinfection in gastrointestinal endoscopy. Endoscopy. 2008; 40(11):939–957

[5] The British Society of Gastroenterology Endoscopy Committee. Guidelines for decontamination of equipment for gastrointestinal endoscopy. 2014. Available at: http://www.bsg.org.uk/clinical-guidance/general/guidelines-for-decontamination-of-equipment-for-gastrointestinal-endoscopy.html. Accessed October 12, 2015

[6] Rutala WA, Weber DJ; Healthcare Infection Control Practices Advisory Committee (HICPAC). Guideline for disinfection and sterilization in healthcare facilities, 2008. Available at: http://www.cdc.gov/hicpac/Disinfection_Sterilization/3_0disinfectEquipment.html. Accessed August 15, 2016

[7] Hospital Infection Control Professional Advisory Committee (HICPAC), Centers for Disease Control and Prevention (CDC). Essential elements of a reprocessing program for flexible endoscopes – Recommendations of the Healthcare Infection Control Practices Advisory Committee. 2016. Available at: https://www.cdc.gov/hicpac/pdf/Flexible-Endoscope-Reprocessing.pdf. Accessed September 1, 2017

[8] Reprocessing Medical Devices in Health Care Settings: Validation Methods and Labeling Guidance for Industry and Food and Drug Administration Staff, Appendix A - Definitions. https://www.fda.gov/ucm/groups/fdagov-public/@fdagov-meddev-gen/documents/document/ucm253010.pdf. Accessed Sept 1, 2017.

[9] Food and Drug Administration. Reprocessing medical devices in health care settings: validation methods and labeling—guidance for industry and food and drug administration staff. March 17, 2015. Available at: http://www.fda.gov/downloads/MedicalDevices/DeviceRegulationandGuidance/GuidanceDocuments/UCM253010.pdf. Accessed August 10, 2016

[10] Food and Drug Administration. Guidance for industry: sterile drug products produced by aseptic processing– current good manufacturing practice. 2004. Available at: https://webcache.googleusercontent.com/search?q=cache:XRs-8gHSVGKYJ:https://www.fda.gov/downloads/Drugs/Guidances/ucm070342.pdf+&cd=1&hl=en&ct=clnk&gl=us. Accessed September 1, 2017.

[11] Spaulding EH. Chemical disinfection and antisepsis in the hospital. J Hosp Res. 1972; 9:5–31

[12] Funk SE, Reaven NL. High-level endoscope disinfection processes in emerging economies: financial impact of manual process versus automated endoscope reprocessing. J Hosp Infect. 2014; 86(4):250–254

[13] Alfa MJ, Degagne P, Olson N. Worst-case soiling levels for patient-used flexible endoscopes before and after cleaning. Am J Infect Control. 1999; 27(5):392–401

[14] Chu NS, McAlister D, Antonoplos PA. Natural bioburden levels detected on flexible gastrointestinal endoscopes after clinical use and manual cleaning. Gastrointest Endosc. 1998; 48(2):137–142

[15] Rutala WA, Weber DJ. ERCP scopes: what can we do to prevent infections? Infect Control Hosp Epidemiol. 2015; 36(6):643–648

[16] Komanduri S, Abu Dayyeh BK, Bhat YM, et al; ASGE Technology Committee. Technologies for monitoring the quality of endoscope reprocessing. Gastrointest Endosc. 2014; 80(3):369–373

[17] Visrodia K, Hanada Y, Pennington KM, et al. Duodenoscope reprocessing surveillance with adenosine triphosphate testing and terminal cultures: a clinical pilot study. Gastrointest Endosc. 2017;S0016–5107(17)31782–0

[18] Alfa MJ, Olson N, Murray BL. Comparison of clinically relevant benchmarks and channel sampling methods used to assess manual cleaning compliance for flexible gastrointestinal endoscopes Am J Infect Control. 2014; 42(1):e1–e5

[19] Food and Drug Administration. FDA-cleared sterilants and high level disinfectants with general claims for processing reusable medical and dental devices - March 2015. Available at: https://www.fda.gov/MedicalDevices/DeviceRegulationandGuidance/ReprocessingofReusableMedicalDevices/ucm437347.htm. Accessed August 28, 2016

[20] Rutala WA, Weber DJ. Disinfection, sterilization, and antisepsis: an overview. Am J Infect Control. 2016; 44(5, Suppl):e1–e6

[21] Desilets D, Kaul V, Tierney WM, et al; ASGE Technology Committee. Automated endoscope reprocessors. Gastrointest Endosc. 2010; 72(4):675–680

[22] Kovaleva J, Peters FT, van der Mei HC, Degener JE. Transmission of infection by flexible gastrointestinal endoscopy and bronchoscopy. Clin Microbiol Rev. 2013; 26(2):231–254

[23] Petersen BT. Duodenoscope reprocessing: risk and options coming into view. Gastrointest Endosc. 2015; 82(3):484–487

[24] Petersen BT, Ginsburg GG, Koch J. Infection using ERCP endoscopes. Gastroenterology. 2016; 151(1):46–50

[25] Epstein L, Hunter JC, Arwady MA, et al. New Delhi metallo-β-lactamase-producing carbapenem-resistant Escherichia coli associated with exposure to duodenoscopes. JAMA. 2014; 312(14):1447–1455

[26] Wendorf KA, Kay M, Baliga C, et al. Endoscopic retrograde cholangiopancreatography-associated AmpC Escherichia coli outbreak. Infect Control Hosp Epidemiol. 2015; 36(6):634–642

[27] Alrabaa SF, Nguyen P, Sanderson R, et al. Early identification and control of carbapenemase-producing Klebsiella pneumoniae, originating from contaminated endoscopic equipment. Am J Infect Control. 2013; 41(6):562–564

[28] Gastmeier P, Vonberg RP. Klebsiella spp. in endoscopy-associated infections: we may only be seeing the tip of the iceberg. Infection. 2014; 42(1):15–21

[29] Verfaillie CJ, Bruno MJ, Voor in 't Holt AF, et al. Withdrawal of a novel-design duodenoscope ends outbreak of a VIM-2-producing Pseudomonas aeruginosa. Endoscopy. 2015; 47(6):493–502

[30] United States Senate. Preventable tragedies: superbugs and how ineffective monitoring of medical device safety fails patients. Available at: http://www.help.senate.gov/imo/media/doc/Duodenoscope%20Investigation%20FINAL%20Report.pdf. Accessed February 16, 2016

[31] Ross AS, Baliga C, Verma P. A quarantine process for the resolution of duodenoscope-associated transmission of multidrug-resistant Escherichia coli. Gastrointest Endosc. 2015; 82(3):477–483

[32] US Food and Drug Administration. Design of endoscopic retrograde cholangiopancreatography (ERCP) duodenoscopes may impede effective cleaning: FDA safety communication. Available at: http://www.fda.gov/MedicalDevices/Safety/AlertsandNotices/ucm434871.htm. Accessed August 30, 2016

[33] US Food and Drug Administration (FDA). Supplemental measures to enhance reprocessing: FDA safety communication. Available at: www.fda.gov/MedicalDevices/Safety/AlertsandNotices/ucm454766.htm. Accessed August 30, 2016

[34] Chapman CG, Siddiqui UD, Manzano M, et al. Risk of infection transmission in curvilinear array echoendoscopes: results of a prospective reprocessing and culture registry. Gastrointest Endosc. 2017; 85(2):390–397.e1

[35] Visrodia K, Petersen BT. Echoing concerns related to endoscope reprocessing. Gastrointest Endosc. 2017; 85(2):398–400

[36] Weber DJ, Rutala WA. Assessing the risk of disease transmission to patients when there is a failure to follow recommended disinfection and sterilization guidelines. Am J Infect Control. 2013; 41(5, Suppl):S67–S71

[37] Banerjee S, Nelson DB, Dominitz JA, et al; Standards of Practice Committee. Reprocessing failure. Gastrointest Endosc. 2007; 66(5):869–871

[38] Rutala WA, Weber DJ; Society for Healthcare Epidemiology of America. Guideline for disinfection and sterilization of prion-contaminated medical instruments. Infect Control Hosp Epidemiol. 2010; 31(2):107–117

[39] Hospital Infection Control Professional Advisory Committee. United States Centers for Disease Control and Prevention. Atlanta, GA, 2016

7 Electrosurgical Principles for Endoscopy

Louis M. Wong Kee Song and Michael B. Wallace

7.1 Introduction

Electrosurgery is an integral part of many therapeutic applications in gastrointestinal endoscopy. Electrosurgical units generate high-frequency alternating current (AC), which connects to accessories, such as polypectomy snares and sphincterotomes, for the purpose of cutting and/or coagulation.[1] An electrosurgical unit (ESU) converts low-frequency AC from a household electrical outlet (60 Hz in North America; 1 hertz [Hz] = 1 cycle per second) to > 300 KHz (▶ Fig. 7.1). At these higher frequencies, there is insufficient time for cellular depolarization to occur before the current alternates again and undesirable neuromuscular stimulation (electric shock) is therefore avoided. Since the frequencies employed in electrosurgery are in the range of amplitude-modulated radio broadcasts, the term radiofrequency (RF) current is also used.

The amount and rate of heat produced at the cellular level through passage of RF current through tissue determine the end result. A high current concentration or density (measure of current applied per unit area) delivered by an electrosurgical knife or wire rapidly boils and vaporizes cells along the cleavage line, resulting in electrosurgical cutting. At low current density, tissue coagulation occurs since cells are heated more slowly and desiccate without any cutting. Several variables affect the current density and, consequently, the final tissue outcome (▶ Fig. 7.2). Many of these variables are operator-dependent, such as selection of the ESU settings, type of accessory utilized, and technique and duration of application, so that the proportion of cells cut to those coagulated can be controlled to achieve the desired tissue effect.[2,3] An understanding of the basic electrosurgical properties and the interplay of these variables on the final tissue outcome are paramount for the safe and effective use of electrosurgery during endoscopy. Herein, the fundamental principles of electrosurgery

and practical recommendations regarding utilization of electrosurgical devices for commonly performed procedures, such as polypectomy, sphincterotomy, and hemostasis, are highlighted.

The term *cautery* is often erroneously used during electrosurgery.[4,5] An example of a cautery device is the Heat Probe Unit (HPU-20, Olympus Corp., Tokyo, Japan), which uses an electrically heated probe that is then applied to tissue for coagulation (hemostasis) without any cutting (**Video 7.1**). The procedure is similar to hot iron branding and, unlike electrosurgery, there is no passage of electrical current through tissue.

7.2 Electrosurgical Principles

7.2.1 Electrical and Tissue Variables

The three interacting electrical properties of current (I), voltage (V), and resistance or impedance (R) affect temperature rise in tissue and are governed by Ohm's law (▶ Table 7.1). The terms resistance and impedance are applicable to direct current and AC, respectively.

Impedance is influenced by the water and electrolyte content of tissue. Tissues with high water content, such as blood vessels, pose less resistance to current flow than dehydrated tissues, such as bone and fat. Consequently, a lipomatous lesion is more difficult to transect with a snare relative to a nonfatty polyp at similar electrosurgical settings. Fibrosis and scarring also increase tissue impedance, which may necessitate adjustments in power and/or current waveform to achieve the desired effect. The buildup of charred tissue at the tip of a hemostatic probe or RF ablation catheter impedes current flow, hence the need to clean the electrodes intermittently during the procedure for efficient contact coagulation.

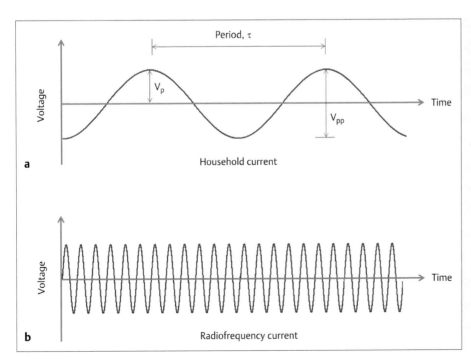

Fig. 7.1 (a) Household alternating current versus **(b)** high-frequency (radiofrequency) alternating current. Vp is peak voltage amplitude. Vpp is peak-to-peak voltage amplitude.

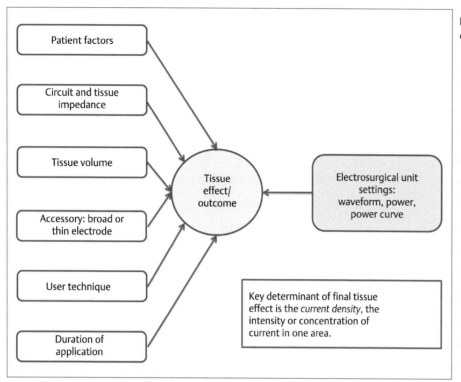

Fig. 7.2 Factors that impact the current density and final tissue outcome.

Table 7.1 Electrosurgical variables and equations

		Variables
Variable	Unit	Definition
Current (I)	Ampere (A)	Flow of electric charge (electrons) in a circuit per unit time
Voltage (V)	Volt (V)	Force that pushes an electric charge through resistance along the circuit
Resistance or impedance (R)	Ohm (Ω)	Measure of impediment to current flow
Power (P)	Watt (W)	Work, or amount of energy per unit time
Energy (Q)	Joule (J)	Capacity to do work
		Equations
Ohm's law	$I = V / R$ $V = I \times R$ $R = V / I$	
Power	$P = V \times I$ $P = V^2 / R$ $P = I^2 \times R$	
Energy	$P \times t$ (s)	

Voltage is the force that drives current through tissue. Voltage spikes must be greater than 200 peak volts (Vp) in order to generate adequate current density for electrosurgical cutting. Below 200 Vp, only tissue coagulation occurs regardless of the power setting. ESU outputs that maintain voltage constantly below the 200-Vp threshold are typical of bipolar applications for hemostasis, as well as the monopolar soft coagulation mode found in certain ESUs.

Current density ultimately determines the end result at the treated site and impacts the design or selection of the active electrode to suit a specific clinical purpose. Current density is lower when the RF energy extends over a greater volume of tissue, resulting in slower heating. Hence, the energy spread over the jaws of a flat hemostatic forceps (e.g., Coagrasper, Olympus Corp.,

Tokyo, Japan) or probe (e.g., TouchSoft, Genii Inc., St. Paul, MN) promotes coagulation as opposed to the high current density delivered along the thin wire of a sphincterotome that promotes cutting. Moreover, the operator can affect the current density by controlling the contact area between tissue and the active electrode.

Another operator-dependent variable is the power setting, which in turn impacts current density. As tissue heats, impedance rises, which decreases current flow and, consequently, power (▶Table 7.1). Through feedback tissue sensing, modern ESUs have outputs that are able to maintain power relatively constant over a range of measured impedances during current activation. These outputs with broad power-to-impedance curves are useful during certain procedures, such as polypectomy, where automatic sensing and power regulation reduce the potential for snare entrapment by providing adequate power during the entire resection process (▶Fig. 7.3). On the other hand, narrow power-to-impedance curves are characteristic of bipolar or monopolar outputs designed for contact hemostasis, with peak power delivered between 30 and 250 ohms (Ω) (▶Fig. 7.4). Tissues with resistances within this range, such as blood vessels, are targeted to receive the maximum power output that optimizes coagulation and, as tissue impedance increases with ongoing heating, the power output falls significantly so that the tissue does not overly desiccate and cause the accessory to stick. Although the manufacturer's suggested power settings for specific procedures are a good starting point for a particular ESU, adjustments can be made based on the operator's preference, technique, and desired outcome.

One variable that is entirely under the control of the operator is duration (time) of current application, which can impact the final outcome to a large degree. Taking into consideration that the total amount of energy (J) delivered equals power (W) ×time (s), how fast or slow the power is being deposited becomes important. The outcome of delivering 50 W of power

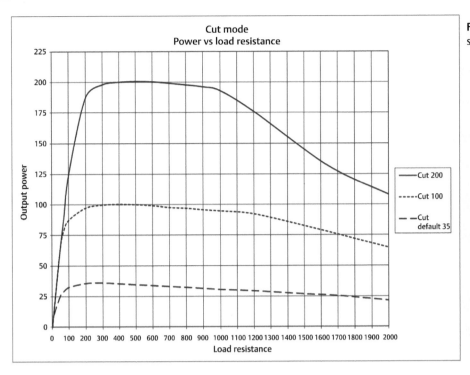

Fig. 7.3 Broad power-to-resistance curves suitable for snare polypectomy.

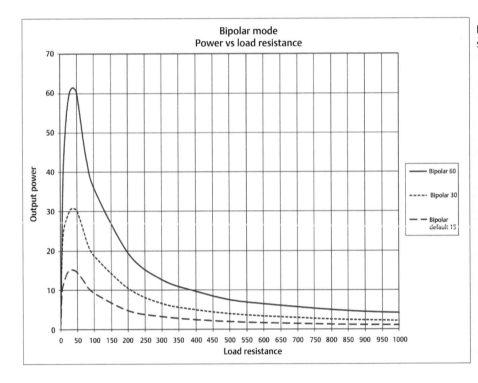

Fig. 7.4 Narrow power-to-resistance curves suitable for bipolar hemostasis.

for 2 seconds is quite different than that of delivering 20 W for 5 seconds, even though the total amount of heat energy delivered (100 J) is the same. Furthermore, if the time of application and power settings remain the same, either a continuous or modulated waveform will deliver an identical amount of total energy but with a very different outcome (see the section Electrosurgical Units and Waveforms).

7.2.2 Monopolar versus Bipolar Circuit

The terms monopolar and bipolar refer to the manner in which the electrosurgical circuit is completed. In a monopolar circuit, RF current oscillates from the active electrode (e.g., polypectomy snare) through the patient's body via the path of least resistance

to the inactive or dispersive electrode (electrosurgical pad), and returns to the ESU to complete the circuit (▶ Fig. 7.5). The term *dispersive* electrode conveys an understanding that the energy exiting the patient through the pad is so much less concentrated that the risk of a burn injury at the pad site is reduced. Placement of the dispersive electrode close to the target site is recommended to keep the circuit as short as possible.

In a bipolar circuit, the active and return electrodes are in close proximity to each other, as illustrated by the bipolar hemostatic probe (e.g., Gold Probe, Boston Scientific Inc., Natick, MA) (▶ Fig. 7.6). Current travels from the active to return electrodes through only a small volume of tissue in contact with the tip of the probe. An electrosurgical pad is not required for bipolar accessories. Except for hemostasis applications, bipolar devices

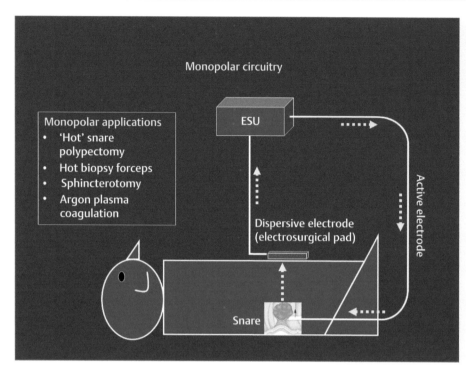

Fig. 7.5 Schematic of monopolar circuit. Current flows from the active electrode (e.g., snare) through the patient's body to the dispersive electrode (pad) placed on the patient's skin.

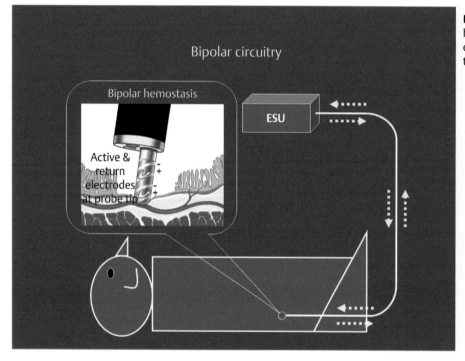

Fig. 7.6 Schematic of bipolar circuit. Bipolar hemostasis probe with active and return electrodes closely spaced at the probe's tip (inset).

are far less commercially available for endoscopic use than their monopolar counterparts.

7.3 Electrosurgical Units and Waveforms

ESUs enable the user to select from a menu of current waveforms a particular output, such as "Cut," "Coag," and "Blend." An understanding of the waveform selected for a given ESU is important since manufacturer's labeling of the outputs is not standardized and can be misleading (▶Table 7.2). For instance, an output labeled "Coag" with voltage spikes above 200 V is quite capable of electrosurgical cutting.

ESUs produce current outputs ranging from low-voltage, continuous sinusoidal waves to interrupted (modulated) waveforms with much higher voltages (▶Fig. 7.7). When voltage is maintained below 200 Vp, continuous waveforms produce superficial contact coagulation without electrosurgical cutting. These coagulation current outputs can be recognized by particular labels, such as "Soft Coag" or "TouchSoft" when used with monopolar devices and "BiCap" or "Bipolar" when used with bipolar accessories. With voltages between 200 and 600 Vp, continuous waveforms promote maximum cutting effects since they can rapidly produce high current densities along the active electrode to vaporize (cut) cells. Cells that are situated further away from the active electrode do not heat fast enough to vaporize, so they coagulate. Thus, even if a waveform is named "Pure Cut," some

Table 7.2 Output Terminology for Commonly Used Electrosurgical Units in Gastrointestinal Endoscopy

ConMed BiCap® III	ConMed Beamer™ Mate	ERBE VIO 300 D	ERBE VIO 200 S	ERBE ICC 200	ERBE VIO 100 C	Genii gi4000	Olympus ESG-100
		Soft Coag®	Soft Coag®	Soft Coag®	Soft Coag®	TouchSoft®	Soft Coag®
Coag	Coag (Hot Biopsy & Pure Coag)	Forced Coag	Forced Coag	Forced Coag	Forced Coag	Coag	Forced Coag 1 and 2
		Swift Coag®				Blend Coag	
Pulse Blend						Pulse Blend Cut	
Blend	Blend Cuts 1 and 2	Dry Cut			Dry Cut	Blend Cut	
Pulse Cut	Pulse Cut (Polyp and Papilla)	Endo Cut I or Q®	Endo Cut I or Q®	Endo Cut®		Pulse Cut	Pulse Cut Slow/Fast
Pure Cut	Pure Cut	Auto Cut®	Auto Cut®	Auto Cut®	Auto Cut®	Cut	Cut 1, 2, 3
Bipolar	BiCap® & Cut	Bipolar	Bipolar	Bipolar	Bipolar	Bipolar	Bipolar
		Spray Coag*					
Argon-assisted Coagulation*	Beamer Plus: Argon Steady, Slow, Fast, Super [amplified beam] (additional unit required)	APC 2 Forced, Pulse 1 & 2, Precise [amplified beam] (additional unit required)	APC 2 Forced [amplified beam] (additional unit required)	APC300 Forced [standard beam] (additional unit required)		ArC Smart Beam™ [linear beam] (included in unit)	

*non-contact coagulation modes

Genii and TouchSoft are US Registered Trademarks of Genii, Inc.; VIO, Endo Cut, Swift Coag and Soft Coag are Trademarks of Erbe Electromedizin; BiCap and Beamer are Trademarks of ConMed Corp. All information taken from Operator's Manuals. Table is provided courtesy of Marcia Morris, MS, with modification.

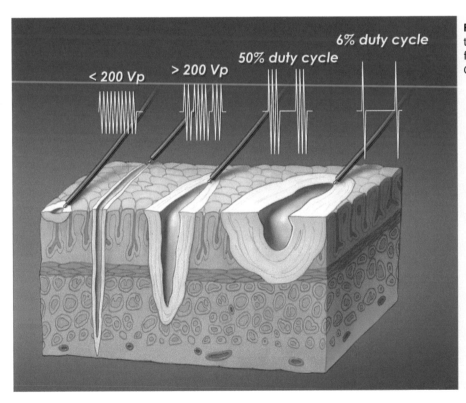

Fig. 7.7 Schematic of current waveforms (see text for details). (Repoduced with permission from Macmillan publishers Ltd: Am J Gastroenterol, copyright 2009.[3])

coagulation will always be present along the margins of the cut. Although higher voltages deepen the coagulation spread along the cut margin, tissue charring becomes problematic when voltage is increased above 600 Vp for these continuous waves.

Modulated or interrupted waveforms heat tissue more slowly than continuous waves and are designed for outputs intended to produce varying amounts of coagulation, ablation, and hemostasis. By interrupting the current flow, tissue has a chance to cool, and the proportion of cells that desiccate without bursting increases. These modulated waveforms are recognized by particular labels, such as "Blend," "Forced Coag," and "Coag." Peak voltages for modulated waveforms range from well over 200 Vp to 4,500 Vp, and even higher for noncontact fulguration modes.

High-voltage modulated waveforms are used to ionize argon gas during noncontact argon plasma coagulation (APC).

One should not assume that a specific label, such as "Blend," from one ESU corresponds to the same waveform output from another ESU with the same name. When reporting ESU settings in research studies and publications, quantitative descriptions of the waveforms based on the *duty cycle* and/or *crest factor* should be used to enable comparison and categorization of the qualitative waveform labels from different ESUs (▶ Table 7.3). The duty cycle relates the percentage of time that the current is actually on during the activation period. For example, an output that is supplying current half the time and remains off the rest of the time has a 50% duty cycle. Continuous sine waves, often labeled as

Table 7.3 Monopolar output features for selected electrosurgical units

Peak volts	Duty cycle	Crest factor	Conmed Beamer	BSC EndoStat	BSC EndoStat III	ERBE ICC 200	ERBE VIO 300	Genii gi4000	Meditron 3000B/ Pentax	Olympus ESG-100	Valleylab Force 2
< 200	100%	1.4				Soft Coag	Soft Coag	TouchSoft		Soft Coag	
> 200	100%	1.4	Pure Cut, Pulse Cut 1, 2*	Cut	Cut, Control Cut	Autocut, Endo Cut	Autocut, Endo Cut I, Q	Cut, Pulse Cut	Cut	Cut 1, 2, 3 Pulse Cut Slow, Fast	Cut
	70%	1.8	Blend Cut		Blend						
	50%			Blend				Blend Cut, Pulse Blend Cut	Blend 1		Blend 1 (CF 3.4)
	50%	2.5	Super Blend								
	37%										Blend 2
	30%	2.7			Coag						
		3.0	Pure Coag				Dry Cut Effect 1–4				
		3.2					Dry Cut Effect 5–6				
		3.7	Hot Bx								
		3.8					Dry Cut Effect 7–8				
	25%								Blend 2		Blend 3
	12%			Coag				Blend Coag (CF 6.3)	Blend 3		
	8%	5.0								Forced 1, 2	
		5.4					Swift Coag				
		6.0					Forced Coag	Coag			
	6%									Coag	
	4%				Forced Coag						
		7.4					Spray Coag				
		8.5									Coag

Increasing voltage (arrow, left margin)

*ConMed Beamer Polyp Pulse Cut 1, 2 and Papilla Pulse Cut 1, 2 crest factor (CF) not available.

Source: Data from Morris M et al[3] and Tokar et al.[7] Additional data published or provided by the electrosurgical generator manufacturers: Conmed Corp., Utica, New York, United States; EndoStat distributed by Boston Scientific Inc., Natick, Massachusetts, United States; ERBE USA Inc., Marietta, Georgia, United States; Genii Inc., St. Paul, Minnesota, United States; Meditron, a division of Cooper Surgical, Trumbull, Connecticut, United States; Valleylab, Medtronic, Dublin, Ireland. Not all ESUs listed may be currently marketed.

"Cut," have a 100% duty cycle, whereas waveforms with duty cycles ranging from 20 to 80% often have labels such as "Swift Coag," "Blend," and "Blend Cut." Waveforms named "Coag" typically have duty cycles of 6 to 12%, and although current is not flowing during much of the activation period, voltage spikes are well above 1,500 Vp when current does flow and therefore some electrosurgical cutting occurs especially with wire electrodes, such as polypectomy snares. Operators who utilize the "Coag" output and smoothly close a snare through polyp tissue are taking advantage of this cutting action along the snare wire, coupled with marked hemostasis promoted by the long rest periods in the cycle and the high voltage peaks that drive coagulation into tissue.

As an alternative to duty cycle, the crest factor can also be used to quantify waveforms. Crest factor takes into consideration average and peak voltages, as well as the frequency of the modulation, and becomes a better indicator of the expected depth and intensity of coagulation relative to the duty cycle for modulated waveforms. Continuous sinusoidal waveforms have a constant crest factor of 1.4 and in this instance the maximum peak voltage should also be stated. Highly modulated, high-voltage waveforms typical of "Coag" types (6% duty cycle) have crest factors in the range of 5 to 7. In general, high duty cycles correlate with low crest factors indicative of waveforms designed to produce more cutting with limited coagulation, whereas low duty cycles correlate with higher crest factors that predict increasing depth of coagulation and hemostasis (▶ Table 7.3).

Specialized proprietary microprocessor outputs are available in some ESUs. For example, the "ENDO CUT" (Erbe Electromedizin, Tubingen, Germany) mode fractionates (pulses) the current output to promote controlled cutting of tissue and provide a well-defined and constant zone of coagulation during the entire cutting process. The "ENDO CUT" mode consists of an initial incision (cut) phase followed by phases of alternating cutting and coagulation current (▶ Fig. 7.8), with the capability to adjust the duration (speed) of the cutting phase, the interval duration between cutting cycles, and the intensity of the coagulation

effect.[6,7] Most of the ESUs listed in ▶ Table 7.2 also have similar controlled pulse modes and all have various options for providing more or less coagulation along the cut zones.

7.4 Practical Applications

7.4.1 Snare Polypectomy

The optimal electrosurgical settings for "hot" snare polypectomy that maximizes resection efficiency and minimizes adverse events, such as bleeding and transmural burn syndrome, have not been established. Comparisons among available studies are hampered by the qualitative labels of the current waveforms used during polypectomy. Polypectomy practice and the electrosurgical method utilized vary among endoscopists. According to a U.S. survey, most endoscopists use "Pure Coagulation" (46%) or "Blend" (46%) current and a minority utilize "Pure Cut" (3%) or modify the current waveform (4%) during polypectomy.[8]

Although the risk of transmural burn syndrome might, in theory, be increased with a "Pure Coagulation" current as it drives coagulation deeper into tissue, that type of current has been used in a relatively safe manner for resecting large colon polyps (> 2 cm).[9,10] A comparative study of "Blend" versus "Continuous Coagulation" current showed similar rates of adverse events overall, but timing of postpolypectomy hemorrhage was related to the current waveform utilized. All immediate or very early (< 12 hours) bleeds occurred when blended current was utilized, and all delayed bleeds (2–8 days) occurred when coagulation current was used.[11] In one study, the postpolypectomy bleeding rate was relatively low at 1.1% when "Pure Current" was applied, although prophylactic endoscopic loop or endoscopic clip placement was undertaken in 12% of the polypectomy defects to minimize the risk of bleeding.[12] The use of "Pure Cut" current as opposed to "Blend" or "ENDO CUT" current was found to be a risk factor for immediate postpolypectomy bleeding in a large, prospective, multicenter study.[13] The use of proprietary current outputs, such

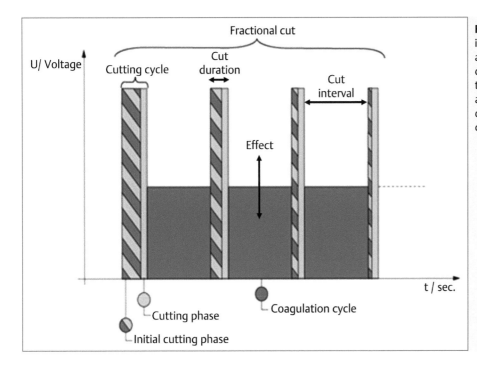

Fig. 7.8 ENDO CUT mode. After an initial incision (cut) phase, bursts of cutting alternating with coagulation current are delivered. The duration of the cutting cycle, the interval duration between cutting cycles, and the intensity (effect) of the coagulation cycle can be adjusted. (This figure is provided courtesy of ERBE Inc., Marietta, GA.)

as "ENDO CUT," is promoted by some experts in the field of endoscopic resection.[14] The use of "ENDO CUT" resulted in significantly less deep thermal ulceration, necrosis, and acute inflammation relative to a low-power coagulation current in an animal model,[15] as well as in better assessment of the resection margins and histologic quality of the specimens relative to a blended current.[16]

Findings from the above-mentioned studies are consistent with predicted outcomes based on the principles of electrosurgery. In general, a "Pure Cut" current leads to increased immediate bleeding, whereas overuse of a "Pure Coagulation" current increases the risk of delayed postpolypectomy hemorrhage and transmural burn syndrome. In addition to the current waveform, the speed of snare closure and type of snare utilized will influence the polypectomy process. A thin (monofilament) snare will deposit a higher current density than a thick snare wire, resulting in faster transection. ESU settings or operator technique may need to be adjusted accordingly based on the selected snare.

From a practical perspective, a reasonable approach for all polyp types is to constrict the polyp without overtightening, begin current application, and then smoothly close the wire using a low duty cycle waveform that enables cutting and coagulation at the same time (**Video 7.2**). For standard polypectomy, interrupted waveforms with duty cycles of 4 to 12% and broad power-to-impedance curves are suitable, with power outputs averaging 20 W. These waveforms have high-voltage peaks that allow some electrosurgical cutting along the wire, while at the same time driving coagulation adequately through snared tissue. Tenting of the polyp away from the wall prior to current activation may decrease the risk of perforation, and moving the ensnared polyp back and forth during transection will minimize contact between the polyp surface and intestinal wall, hence decreasing the risk of contralateral burn injury (**Video 7.2**). The use of submucosal fluid injection to provide a safety cushion against deeper tissue heating is also reasonable, particularly during resection of large sessile polyps. Snare entrapment in desiccated tissue can be minimized by avoiding excessive snare strangulation or by resecting a thick stalk polyp with too low a power setting. If entrapment occurs, the snare should be loosened and a pause taken prior to resuming the transection process, with stepwise adjustments in power setting or electrosurgical waveform toward mostly a cutting current.

7.4.2 Hot Biopsy

The use of monopolar hot biopsy forceps (**Video 7.3**) is discouraged due to the 15% rate of residual polyp tissue, thermal artifact interfering with histopathological evaluation, and risk of delayed bleeding and perforation due to deep thermal damage attributed to the large cups of the forceps, particularly in the thin-walled right colon.[6] However, the reported experience with the hot biopsy forceps utilized predominantly coagulation current. The use of a soft coagulation or "Cut" current is more appropriate since both waveforms have lower peak voltages, resulting in less intense coagulation and overall thermal injury. Moreover, utilization of the hot biopsy forceps with "Soft Coag" or "ENDO CUT" current was found useful for the removal of scarred, nonlifting, residual polyp tissue (so-called hot biopsy

avulsion) (**Video 7.4**) without adverse events in a small study of 20 patients.[17]

If utilized, the hot biopsy forceps technique should be restricted to the removal of polyps < 5 mm in size, with grasping and tenting of the polyp away from the bowel wall to limit thermal injury to the submucosa. The use of a fractionated cutting current or low-voltage soft coagulation current waveform set at low power (10–15 W) is suggested, with pedal activation of 1 to 2 seconds.

7.4.3 Sphincterotomy

Factors that affect the performance of sphincterotomy include the selected waveform, power setting, length of wire in contact with tissue, and force of the sphincterotome applied onto tissue. From an electrosurgical standpoint, only "Coag"-type waveforms with duty cycles lower than 37% have been associated with a significant increase in postsphincterotomy pancreatitis due to wider thermal spread, local edema, and restricted pancreatic outflow.[3] Thus, endoscopists who perform sphincterotomy generally select waveforms that promote more cutting and less coagulation, such as low-voltage, 100% duty cycle, "Pure Cut" outputs or modulated waveforms with duty cycles > 40%. The power settings also tend to be higher (30–60 W) relative to polypectomy settings since cutting efficiency increases with rising power. Proprietary microprocessor-controlled outputs, such as "ENDO CUT I" or "Pulse Cut," are increasingly being used for sphincterotomy. The use of such outputs that can "pulse" or "fractionate" the cut is useful in reducing the risk of an uncontrolled zipper cut, particularly in the hands of less experienced endoscopists.[3,6]

A meta-analysis of four prospective randomized trials (804 patients) comparing "Pure Cut" to "mixed" current, which included blended current and "ENDO CUT," showed a higher rate of minor postbiliary sphincterotomy bleeding in the "Pure Cut" group, but no significant differences in the rates of pancreatitis or major bleeding between the two groups.[18]

7.4.4 Hemostasis

Contact Bipolar

Bipolar applications in gastrointestinal endoscopy are mostly limited to the use of bipolar coagulation probes for hemostasis since the development of bipolar accessories for polypectomy and sphincterotomy is technically complex and expensive. Bipolar outputs designed for use with bipolar probes combine a low-voltage, continuous waveform with a narrow power-to-impedance curve. A power setting of 15 to 20 W is generally sufficient for endoscopic hemostasis (▶ Table 7.4). For larger caliber vessels, such as those found in peptic ulcers and Dieulafoy's lesions, the bipolar probe should be applied for a longer time interval with firm contact pressure to promote deeper coagulation (**Video 7.5**). Shorter contact duration with light to moderate pressure is recommended in the small intestine and colon (**Video 7.6**).

Contact Monopolar

Dedicated monopolar hemostatic forceps (e.g., Coagrasper) and probes (e.g., TouchSoft Coagulator, Genii Inc., St. Paul, MN) for endoscopic use are available, which are particularly suitable for

Table 7.4 Suggested settings for hemostasis of nonvariceal bleeding lesions

Thermal modalities	Upper GI lesions				Lower GI lesions				
	PUD	*Dieulafoy*	*MWT*	*GAVE*	*Diverticular bleeding*	*Postpolypectomy bleeding*	*Angioectasia*	*Focal ulcer*	*Cancer*
Bipolar									
Probe size (large [10 Fr] or small [7 Fr])	Large	Large	Large or small	Large	Large > small	Large > small	Large > small	Large > small	Large > small
Power (W)	15–20	15–20	12–15	15	12–15	12–15	12–15	12–15	12–15
Application duration (s)	7–10	7–10	3–5	3–5	2–4	2–4	2–4	2–4	2–4
No. of applications (range)	Variable (1–5)	Variable (1–5)	Variable (1–5)	Multiple	Variable (1–5)	Variable (1–5)	Variable (1–5)	Variable (1–5)	Variable (1–5)
Probe–tissue contact pressure	Firm	Firm	Moderate	Moderate	Light-moderate	Light-moderate	Light-moderate	Moderate	Moderate
End point	Bleed stops; white coagulum; cavitation	Bleed stops; white coagulum; cavitation	Bleed stops; white coagulum	Bleed stops; white coagulum	Bleed stops; white coagulum	Bleed stops	Bleed stops; white coagulum	Bleed stops	Bleed stops
APC[a]									
Power (W)	NR	NR	30–45	35–60	30–45	30–45	30–45	30–45	30–45
Argon gas flow rate (L/min)			1	1	1	1	1	1	1
Probe-to-tissue distance (mm)			1–2	1–2	1–2	1–2	1–2	1–2	1–2
End point			Bleed stops; coagulum	White coagulum	Bleed stops; white coagulum	Bleed stops	Bleed stops; coagulum	Bleed stops	Bleed stops

Abbreviations: APC, argon plasma coagulation; GAVE, gastric antral vascular ectasia; MWT, Mallory–Weiss tear; NR, not recommended; PUD, peptic ulcer disease.

[a]Non-amplified APC generators

hemostasis of actively bleeding as well as nonbleeding vessels during procedures such as endoscopic mucosal resection (EMR) and endoscopic submucosal dissection (ESD). Low-voltage (< 200 Vp), continuous waveforms (e.g., "Soft Coag" or "TouchSoft") are utilized with these devices to optimize coagulation of blood vessels, with manufacturer's suggested power settings ranging from 50 W (colon) to 80 W (stomach). The application of brief (1–2 s) pulses of coagulation current, in addition to vascular coaptation by the closed jaws of the Coagrasper forceps, results in effective sealing of the blood vessel (**Video 7.7**). The Coagrasper device may also be suitable for other nonvariceal bleeding lesions, although care regarding its use for the treatment of a visible vessel in an ulcer is warranted, since grasping and tenting the vessel from an indurated base may result in vascular tearing and bleeding.

Argon-Assisted Coagulation

Argon-assisted or argon plasma coagulation (APC) is a noncontact monopolar method used primarily for coagulation of superficial vascular lesions, such as gastric antral vascular ectasia (**Video 7.8**) and angiodysplasias, and for tissue ablation, such as residual Barrett's epithelium and polyp tissue (**Video 7.9**). APC works through delivery of RF energy to the target tissue via electrically conductive ionized argon gas (plasma). Nonionized gas outside of the argon beam does not conduct energy to the tissue.

Some APC-enabled ESUs (e.g., ERBE VIO/APC2 and ConMed Beamer Mate) are equipped with amplified power profiles such that lower power settings produce similar tissue effects relative to nonamplified APC generators.[7] A good starting point is to select the manufacturer's recommended power setting in the lower range for a particular indication and increase power output until the desired tissue effect is achieved.

In general, power settings of 40 to 60 W are adequate for hemostasis and superficial tissue ablation, with the argon flow rate maintained at 1 L/minute. For high-power amplified ESUs, the settings are typically about half that of nonamplified APC generators. Ideally, the APC probe should be maintained at a distance of 1 to 2 mm from the target site, as ionization will not begin if the probe is too far from tissue. If the ideal distance cannot be maintained and the probe is further away from tissue, it is best to augment the power setting rather than the argon flow rate since increasing the latter only serves to further dilute the ionized particles in the stream. Inadvertent probe–tissue contact may result in localized pneumatosis from dissection of tissue layers by argon gas, an often benign event. APC-induced perforations, however, have occurred and likely correlate with tissue contact with the probe tip, power setting, and duration of application.

7.4.5 Miscellaneous

Electrosurgery figures prominently in various other procedures, including EMR, ESD, peroral endoscopic myotomy (POEM), and radiofrequency ablation (RFA) of Barrett's esophagus (BE). Dedicated generators and RFA catheters (BARRX, Covidien, Sunnyvale, CA) are commercially available for BE,[19] as well as a variety of electrosurgical knives for ESD[20] and POEM.[21] For the latter, the selected current waveforms and power settings are influenced by the type of knives used for incision and dissection, lesion characteristics and location, and operator preference. A review of these techniques and available electrosurgical accessories is beyond the scope of this chapter.

7.5 Electrosurgical Hazards and Safety

7.5.1 Unintended Burn Injury

Older ground-referenced ESUs are outdated, since current seeking the path of least resistance could travel through electrically conductive grounded materials, causing thermal injury at alternate sites. Modern ESUs have isolated outputs such that the system is disabled if there is any break in the return circuit or when excessive leakage is detected, thus greatly minimizing the risk of alternate site thermal injury through other ground paths. Return electrode contact quality monitoring (RECQM) is a standard feature in most ESUs and, combined with dual-foil dispersive electrodes ("split" pads), RECQM-equipped units will not activate if a hazardous concentration of current is detected at the interface between the electrosurgical pad and the patient. These units have virtually eliminated the incidence of a skin burn at the pad site. Proper placement of the electrosurgical pad is nevertheless important. Flank or upper thigh placement is common in gastrointestinal endoscopy, and high-resistance areas, such as bony prominences, hair, scars, and prosthetic joints, should be avoided. The avoidance of the term "grounding pad" conveys an understanding that ESUs that were ground-referenced are obsolete.

Alternate site burns can occur via current division or diversion through processes such as capacitive coupling, direct coupling, and insulation defects. Capacitive coupling is the phenomenon by which current appears to leak across insulation to a second electrically conductive structure, potentially causing inadvertent thermal injury away from the target site. These electrical discharges are uncommon with current endoscopic technology. Direct connection between the active electrode and another electrically conductive accessory can lead to serious alternate site burns, such as thermal injury to the biliary tree as a result of current conduction between a sphincterotome wire and a frayed guidewire. Endoscopic insulation failure occurs when the instrument's shaft is compromised due to wear and tear or poor handling. Small cracks are more hazardous than easily detectable ones

because they concentrate current and are more likely to cause injury. Thus, careful inspection of all accessories prior to use is mandatory.

7.5.2 Implanted Electromagnetic Devices

The electrical current produced by ESUs can interfere with implanted electromagnetic devices, including permanent pacemakers (PPMs), implantable cardioverter-defibrillators (ICDs), and medication pumps, resulting in undesirable effects, such as device reprogramming, pacemaker inhibition, and ICD-induced shocks.

For PPMs, no reprogramming is needed if the patient is not dependent on the pacemaker. If the patient is pacemaker-dependent and prolonged use of electrosurgery is anticipated, the PPM should be synchronized to the asynchronous mode (VOO or DOO). For a patient with an ICD, a cardiology team or a team dedicated in the management of implantable cardiac devices should be consulted. The ICD should be reprogrammed to inactivate tachyarrhythmia detection before the use of electrosurgery. Alternatively, a magnet can be used if it can be secured over the pulse generator of the ICD. Continuous cardiopulmonary monitoring during the procedure is mandatory, with cardioversion–defibrillation equipment on standby. When feasible, the bipolar mode should be used over monopolar applications. If a monopolar output is required, the dispersive electrode (pad) should be placed away from the leads of the implanted device, with judicious use of current application. Postprocedure, the PPM or ICD should be reprogrammed to restore baseline function of the device.[22,23]

7.5.3 Bowel Explosion

Explosion has occurred in poorly prepped or unprepped colons exposed to electrosurgery. Polyethylene glycol or sodium phosphate cleansing preparations render the bowel safe for electrosurgery by decreasing the concentrations of combustible gases, mainly hydrogen, methane, and oxygen. The use of carbon dioxide for insufflation may also reduce the risk of explosion. Mannitol- or sorbitol-based preparations are contraindicated due to hydrogen gas production from these sugars by colonic bacterial fermentation. Enema preparations are insufficient for the safe performance of electrosurgery during flexible sigmoidoscopy, and explosion has been documented during unprepped proctoileoscopy and APC in a patient with subtotal colectomy.[24]

7.6 Conclusion

ESUs and electrosurgical devices are widely utilized during therapeutic endoscopy, yet remain a poorly understood technology among users, regardless of years of experience.[25] A key understanding of the fundamental properties of electrosurgery aids in the educated selection of ESU settings and devices for a particular indication and desired tissue effect, and enhances the safety and performance of commonly performed procedures, such as snare polypectomy, hot biopsy, sphincterotomy, hemostasis, and APC.

References

[1] Tucker RD, Sievert CE, Kramolowsky EV, et al. The interaction between electrosurgical generators, endoscopic electrodes, and tissue. Gastrointest Endosc. 1992; 38(2):118–122

[2] Morris ML. Electrosurgery in the gastroenterology suite: principles, practice, and safety. Gastroenterol Nurs. 2006; 29(2):126–132, quiz 132–134

[3] Morris ML, Tucker RD, Baron TH, Wong Kee Song LM. Electrosurgery in gastrointestinal endoscopy: principles to practice. Am J Gastroenterol. 2009; 104(6):1563–1574

[4] Munro MG, Abbott JA, Vilos GA, Brill AI. Radiofrequency electrical energy guidelines for authors: what's in a name? J Minim Invasive Gynecol. 2015; 22(1):1–2

[5] Wong Kee Song LM, Gostout CJ, Tucker RD, et al. Electrosurgery in gastrointestinal endoscopy: terminology matters. Gastrointest Endosc. 2016; 83(1):271–273

[6] Rey JF, Beilenhoff U, Neumann CS, Dumonceau JM; European Society of Gastrointestinal Endoscopy (ESGE). European Society of Gastrointestinal Endoscopy (ESGE) guideline: the use of electrosurgical units. Endoscopy. 2010; 42(9):764–772

[7] Tokar JL, Barth BA, Banerjee S, et al; ASGE Technology Committee. Electrosurgical generators. Gastrointest Endosc. 2013; 78(2):197–208

[8] Singh N, Harrison M, Rex DK. A survey of colonoscopic polypectomy practices among clinical gastroenterologists. Gastrointest Endosc. 2004; 60(3):414–418

[9] Binmoeller KF, Bohnacker S, Seifert H, et al. Endoscopic snare excision of "giant" colorectal polyps. Gastrointest Endosc. 1996; 43(3):183–188

[10] Brooker JC, Saunders BP, Shah SG, Williams CB. Endoscopic resection of large sessile colonic polyps by specialist and non-specialist endoscopists. Br J Surg. 2002; 89(8):1020–1024

[11] Van Gossum A, Cozzoli A, Adler M, et al. Colonoscopic snare polypectomy: analysis of 1485 resections comparing two types of current. Gastrointest Endosc. 1992; 38(4):472–475

[12] Parra-Blanco A, Kaminaga N, Kojima T, et al. Colonoscopic polypectomy with cutting current: is it safe? Gastrointest Endosc. 2000; 51(6):676–681

[13] Kim HS, Kim TI, Kim WH, et al. Risk factors for immediate postpolypectomy bleeding of the colon: a multicenter study. Am J Gastroenterol. 2006; 101(6):1333–1341

[14] Burgess NG, Bahin FF, Bourke MJ. Colonic polypectomy (with videos). Gastrointest Endosc. 2015; 81(4):813–835

[15] Bahin FF, Burgess NG, Kabir S, et al. Comparison of the histopathological effects of two electrosurgical currents in an in vivo porcine model of esophageal endoscopic mucosal resection. Endoscopy. 2016; 48(2):117–122

[16] Fry LC, Lazenby AJ, Mikolaenko I, et al. Diagnostic quality of: polyps resected by snare polypectomy: does the type of electrosurgical current used matter? Am J Gastroenterol. 2006; 101(9):2123–2127

[17] Veerappan SG, Ormonde D, Yusoff IF, Raftopoulos SC. Hot avulsion: a modification of an existing technique for management of nonlifting areas of a polyp (with video). Gastrointest Endosc. 2014; 80(5):884–888

[18] Verma D, Kapadia A, Adler DG. Pure versus mixed electrosurgical current for endoscopic biliary sphincterotomy: a meta-analysis of adverse outcomes. Gastrointest Endosc. 2007; 66(2):283–290

[19] American Society for Gastrointestinal Endoscopy Technology Committee. Mucosal ablation devices. Gastrointest Endosc. 2008; 68(6):1031–1042

[20] Maple JT, Abu Dayyeh BK, Chauhan SS, et al; ASGE Technology Committee. Endoscopic submucosal dissection. Gastrointest Endosc. 2015; 81(6):1311–1325

[21] Pannala R, Abu Dayyeh BK, Aslanian HR, et al; ASGE Technology Committee. Per-oral endoscopic myotomy (with video). Gastrointest Endosc. 2016; 83(6):1051–1060

[22] Parekh PJ, Buerlein RC, Shams R, et al. An update on the management of implanted cardiac devices during electrosurgical procedures. Gastrointest Endosc. 2013; 78(6):836–841

[23] Nelson G, Morris ML. Electrosurgery in the gastrointestinal suite: knowledge is power. Gastroenterol Nurs. 2015; 38(6):430–439

[24] Lin OS, Biehl T, Jiranek GC, Kozarek RA. Explosion from argon cautery during proctoileoscopy of a patient with a colectomy. Clin Gastroenterol Hepatol. 2012; 10(10):1176–1178.e2

[25] Watanabe Y, Kurashima Y, Madani A, et al. Surgeons have knowledge gaps in the safe use of energy devices: a multicenter cross-sectional study. Surg Endosc. 2016; 30(2):588–592

8 Antibiotic Prophylaxis in Endoscopy

Mouen A. Khashab and Brooks D. Cash

8.1 Introduction

Antibiotic prophylaxis in endoscopy plays a critical role in minimization of infectious complications associated with endoscopic procedures. Although bacteremia is relatively common after both diagnostic and therapeutic procedures, the incidence of infectious endocarditis is very low. Therefore, administration of prophylactic antibiotics solely for the prevention of infectious endocarditis is not recommended for patients undergoing endoscopic procedures. Antibiotic prophylaxis may have an important role in the prevention of infectious complications resulting from certain endoscopic procedures and in specific clinical settings. These include endoscopic retrograde cholangiopancreatography (ERCP) in patients with biliary obstruction and incomplete ductal drainage, ERCP in liver transplant patients, endoscopic ultrasound (EUS)-guided fine needle aspiration (FNA) of cystic lesions, percutaneous endoscopic gastrostomy (PEG), and endoscopy in cirrhotic patients presenting with gastrointestinal (GI) bleeding, among others.

Bacterial translocation of GI microbial flora into the bloodstream may occur during endoscopy due to procedure-related trauma. Resulting bacteremia carries a minor risk of localization of infection in distant tissues. In addition, endoscopy may also result in local infections where a typically sterile space or tissue is breached and contaminated by an endoscopic accessory or by contrast injection. In this chapter, infectious complications related to endoscopy and the role of periprocedural antibiotic prophylaxis for the prevention of these complications are presented.

8.2 Bacteremia Related to Endoscopic Procedures

Bacteremia can arise following endoscopic procedures and is considered a surrogate marker for infective endocarditis (IE) risk. However, clinically important infections arising from GI endoscopy are uncommon, with only 25 cases of IE reported with temporal association to an endoscopic procedure.[1,2,3] Additionally, no data exist that validate a causal association between endoscopic procedures and IE. Likewise, there are no data indicating that antibiotic prophylaxis preceding endoscopic procedures prevents the occurrence of IE.

8.2.1 Procedures Associated with Low Risk of Bacteremia

Bacteremia after gastroscopy and colonoscopy occurs in approximately 4% of patients and is not associated with infectious complications.[4,5,6] Bacteremia is even uncommon (6.3%) with therapeutic colonic procedures such as colonic stent insertion for colonic obstruction.[7]

The frequency of bacteremia after EUS, with or without FNA, is similar to that of upper endoscopy. Prospective studies in patients undergoing EUS-FNA of cystic or solid lesions along the upper GI indicate a bacteremia rate of 4.0 to 5.8%.[8,9,10,11] Likewise, EUS-FNA of solid rectal and perirectal lesions is associated with a low risk of bacteremia, with one study reporting a risk of 2%.[12]

8.2.2 Procedures Associated with High Risk of Bacteremia

The highest rates of bacteremia have been reported with esophageal dilation, sclerotherapy of esophageal varices, and ERCP in patients with biliary obstruction. The rate of bacteremia following esophageal dilation ranged between 12 and 22% in three prospective trials,[13,14,15] and may be higher with dilation of malignant strictures[14] and with passage of multiple dilators.[14] The cultured organisms are typically commensal to the mouth. In one study, viridans streptococci was the organism isolated in 79% of cases.[13]

The rate of bacteremia associated with variceal sclerotherapy is approximately 15%,[16,17,18,19] while that associated with endoscopic variceal ligation is about 9%.[20,21,22]

ERCP in patients with a nonobstructed biliary tree is associated with a relatively low rate of bacteremia of 6%, rising to 18% in the setting of biliary obstruction due to stones or tumors.[23]

8.3 Antibiotic Prophylaxis for the Prevention of Infective Endocarditis

The American Heart Association (AHA) recommends that administration of prophylactic antibiotics merely for the prevention of IE is not recommended for patients undergoing GI endoscopic procedures.[24] This recommendation is due to the absence of data demonstrating a conclusive link between endoscopic procedures and the development of IE, in addition to a lack of evidence that antibiotic prophylaxis prevents IE following endoscopy.[24] Similarly, the American Society for Gastrointestinal Endoscopy (ASGE) recommends against the routine administration of antibiotic prophylaxis solely for prevention of IE.[25]

The AHA specifically recognized cardiac conditions associated with the highest risk of poor clinical outcome from IE, including: (1) prosthetic (mechanical or bioprosthetic) cardiac valve; (2) history of previous IE; (3) cardiac transplant recipients who develop cardiac valvulopathy; and (4) patients with congenital heart disease (CHD), including (a) those with unrepaired cyanotic CHD including palliative shunts and conduits, (b) those with completely repaired CHD with prosthetic material or devices, placed surgically or by catheter, for the first 6 months after the procedure, and (c) those with repaired CHD with residual defects at the site or adjacent to the site of a prosthetic patch or device.[24] The AHA suggests administration of antibiotics with coverage of enterococci in patients with these specific cardiac conditions who also have established infections of the GI tract where enterococci may be part of the infecting bacterial flora (such as cholangitis).[24] Although resulting infections are likely to be polymicrobial, coverage for enterococci is recommended because only enterococci are likely to result in IE.

8.3.1 Antibiotic Prophylaxis for the Prevention of Procedural-Related Infections (Other Than IE)

Antibiotic prophylaxis may have an important role in the prevention of infectious complications resulting from certain endoscopic procedures and in specific clinical settings.

ERCP

Patients with acute cholangitis are typically treated with antibiotics and biliary drainage via ERCP.[26] Additional antibiotic administration for procedural prophylaxis is not recommended. Cholangitis and sepsis are known complications of ERCP, occurring in up to 3% of patients.[27,28,29,30,31,32,33,34] Antibiotic prophylaxis has been shown to reduce the incidence of bacteremia associated with ERCP,[35,36] but this does not clearly translate into a reduction in the incidence of cholangitis. A recent Cochrane systematic review that comprised 9 randomized clinical trials and 1,573 patients established that prophylactic antibiotics reduced bacteremia and seemed to prevent cholangitis and septicemia in patients undergoing elective ERCP.[37] However, in the subgroup of patients with uncomplicated ERCP, the effect of antibiotics was less prominent.[37] In one study, incomplete biliary drainage was predictive of 91% of all cases of sepsis.[38] Antibiotic therapy may therefore have particular value where drainage achieved at ERCP is incomplete or achieved with difficulty, such as with hilar cholangiocarcinoma and primary sclerosing cholangitis.[38,39,40] In one of the few trials that indicated a benefit of antibiotics in patients undergoing ERCP for biliary obstruction, prophylactic antibiotics were continued postprocedurally for several days.[41] The ASGE recommends against antibiotic prophylaxis prior to ERCP where obstructive biliary tract disease is not suspected or when complete biliary drainage is expected.[25] On the other hand, the ASGE recommends that antibiotic prophylaxis be administered prior to ERCP in patients following liver transplantation and/or known or suspected biliary obstruction, where there is a possibility that complete biliary drainage may not be achieved.[25] Antibiotics should also be continued postprocedure when biliary drainage is incomplete.

There are no studies that have assessed the value of antibiotic prophylaxis in patients undergoing ERCP who have pancreatic cystic lesions that communicate with the main pancreatic duct. However, the incidence of infectious complications in this setting seems to be uncommon given that ERCP is commonly performed in patients with such cystic lesions (e.g., intraductal papillary mucinous neoplasms, pseudocysts) without reports of cyst infections.

Acute cholecystitis may result from placement of biliary self-expandable metallic stents (SEMSs) and is believed to be due to cystic duct obstruction. This occurs in 2 to 12% of cases.[42] In two meta-analyses, the incidence of cholecystitis was similar between covered and uncovered SEMSs.[43,44] The majority of reported cases of cholecystitis after biliary SMES placement occurred in patients with malignant biliary obstruction,[42] and tumor involvement of the cystic duct orifice is an independent risk factor for acute cholecystitis after SEMS insertion.[45] The role of prophylactic antibiotics has not been studied, but may help prevent this complication, especially since surgery is frequently needed to manage this untoward event.

8.4 EUS-FNA

Two large series encompassing 672 patients undergoing EUS-FNA of a variety of solid lesions reported sepsis as a complication in only 3 patients.[46,47] Therefore, prophylactic antibiotics are not recommended prior to EUS-FNA of solid lesions.[25]

Periprocedural administration of antibiotics has been recommended for EUS-FNA of cystic lesions in order to prevent cyst infection.[29] The benefit of this practice has not been evaluated in prospective randomized studies. Reports of infected cystic lesions following FNA are scarce. One comparative retrospective trial that included 253 patients studied the effect of prophylactic antibiotics during EUS-FNA of pancreatic cysts.[48] The incidence of infectious complications was very low (one cyst infection in the antibiotic group and one fever episode in the nonantibiotic group), and antibiotics did not confer a protective effect against infections. Infections and antibiotic-related complications occurred more commonly in the group of patients who received prophylactic antibiotics (4.4 vs. 0.6%, $p = 0.04$).[48] Infectious complications after EUS-FNA of mediastinal cysts seem to occur more commonly. Multiple case reports and case series with limited numbers of patients reported infection of mediastinal cysts and mediastinitis following EUS-FNA, some occurring despite the use of appropriate intravenous antibiotic prophylaxis.[49,50] The ASGE suggests administration of prophylactic antibiotics in patients undergoing EUS-FNA of cystic lesions, although the benefit of this practice has not been proven.[25]

The risk of bacteremia and infectious complications after EUS-FNA in the lower GI was studied in one prospective trial which assessed complications of EUS-FNA of solid rectal and perirectal lesions in 100 patients.[12] Two patients developed bacteremia, but without signs or symptoms of infection. Based on these findings, the ASGE recommends against antibiotic prophylaxis prior to diagnostic EUS or EUS-FNA of solid lesions in the lower GI tract.[25]

The role of prophylactic antibiotics in patients undergoing interventional EUS procedures (e.g., pseudocyst drainage, biliary drainage, fine needle injection of cysts/tumors, fiducial placement) has not been studied. Most interventional EUS studies have included patients who received periprocedural antibiotics and a short course of antibiotics thereafter,[51,52,53,54,55,56] and postprocedural infections are infrequent using this practice.

8.5 Percutaneous Endoscopic Gastrostomy/Jejunostomy

Patients undergoing placement of PEG tubes are frequently susceptible to infectious complications because of age, compromised nutritional intake, immunosuppression, and comorbid conditions. A systematic review of randomized studies evaluating the use of prophylactic antibiotics for PEG placement included

12 trials and 1,271 patients.[57] A pooled analysis demonstrated that administration of prophylactic antibiotics resulted in a statistically significant reduction in the incidence of peristomal infection (odds ratio [OR], 0.36; 95% confidence interval [CI], 0.26–0.50).[57] An antibiotic that provides adequate coverage of cutaneous organisms such as cefazolin 1 g intravenously should be given 30 minutes prior to the procedure.[25,58]

The role of prophylactic antibiotics before percutaneous endoscopic jejunostomy (PEJ) placement has not been studied. However, administration of antibiotics should offer similar protection against peristomal infections observed in patients who undergo PEG placement, especially when it is considered that complications, including local infections, seem to be more common with PEJ.[59,60]

8.6 Cirrhosis with GI Bleeding

A Cochrane meta-analysis of 12 randomized controlled trials that comprised 1,241 patients showed that antibiotic administration in cirrhotic patients with GI bleeding was associated with significantly lower overall mortality, mortality from bacterial infections, incidence of bacterial infections, rebleeding, and length of hospital stay.[61] Antibiotic therapy should therefore be commenced at presentation in such patients. Intravenous ceftriaxone seems to be the optimal choice and has been shown to be superior to oral norfloxacin in one randomized controlled trial.[62]

8.7 Synthetic Vascular Grafts and Other Nonvalvular Cardiovascular Devices

There are no reported cases of vascular graft infection related to GI endoscopic procedures. The AHA does not recommend antibiotic prophylaxis following vascular graft or other nonvalvular cardiovascular device (pacemakers, defibrillators, coronary artery stents, peripheral vascular stents, and vena cava filters) in patients undergoing endoscopy.[63]

8.8 Orthopaedic Prostheses

There exist scant case reports of pyogenic arthritis which followed endoscopic procedures, and thus it is believed that infection of prosthetic joints related to endoscopy is exceptionally rare.[64] Although the American Association of Orthopedic Surgeons (AAOS) initially recommended antibiotic prophylaxis for patients with total joint replacement before invasive procedure that may cause bacteremia, this recommendation was subsequently withdrawn since it was not based on clinical evidence.

8.9 Patients Receiving Peritoneal Dialysis

Patients on continuous ambulatory peritoneal dialysis can develop peritonitis due to translocation of microorganisms across the bowel wall.[65] Endoscopic procedures in these patients can result in peritonitis. A retrospective study found that peritonitis developed in 6.3% of patients after colonoscopy without antibiotic

prophylaxis and did not occur in patients who received prophylactic antibiotics.[66] The International Society for Peritoneal Dialysis (ISPD) recommended administration of antibiotics such as ampicillin (1 g) plus a single dose of an aminoglycoside, with or without metronidazole, given intravenously immediately before endoscopic procedures.[67] An alternative suitable strategy is the administration of prophylactic antibiotics by the intraperitoneal route the night before the endoscopic procedure. The ISPD recommended that the abdomen be emptied of fluid prior to the procedure.[67]

References

[1] Sekino Y, Fujisawa N, Suzuki K, et al. A case of recurrent infective endocarditis following colonoscopy. Endoscopy. 2010; 42(Suppl 2):E217

[2] Yu-Hsien L, Te-Li C, Chien-Pei C, Chen-Chi T. Nosocomial acinetobacter genomic species 13 TU endocarditis following an endoscopic procedure. Intern Med. 2008; 47(8):799–802

[3] Malani AN, Aronoff DM, Bradley SF, Kauffman CA. Cardiobacterium hominis endocarditis: Two cases and a review of the literature. Eur J Clin Microbiol Infect Dis. 2006; 25(9):587–595

[4] Liebermann TR. Bacteremia and fiberoptic endoscopy. Gastrointest Endosc. 1976; 23(1):36–37

[5] Norfleet RG, Mitchell PD, Mulholland DD, Philo J. Does bacteremia follow upper gastrointestinal endoscopy? Am J Gastroenterol. 1981; 76(5):420–422

[6] O'Connor HJ, Hamilton I, Lincoln C. et al. Bacteraemia with upper gastrointestinal endoscopy--a reappraisal. Endoscopy. 1983; 15(1):21–23

[7] Chun YJ, Yoon NR, Park JM, et al. Prospective assessment of risk of bacteremia following colorectal stent placement. Dig Dis Sci. 2012; 57(4):1045–1049

[8] Barawi M, Gottlieb K, Cunha B, et al. A prospective evaluation of the incidence of bacteremia associated with EUS-guided fine-needle aspiration. Gastrointest Endosc. 2001; 53(2):189–192

[9] Levy MJ, Norton ID, Wiersema MJ, et al. Prospective risk assessment of bacteremia and other infectious complications in patients undergoing EUS-guided FNA. Gastrointest Endosc. 2003; 57(6):672–678

[10] Janssen J, König K, Knop-Hammad V, et al. Frequency of bacteremia after linear EUS of the upper GI tract with and without FNA. Gastrointest Endosc. 2004; 59(3):339–344

[11] Early DS, Acosta RD, Chandrasekhara V, et al; ASGE Standards of Practice Committee. Adverse events associated with EUS and EUS with FNA. Gastrointest Endosc. 2013; 77(6):839–843

[12] Levy MJ, Norton ID, Clain JE, et al. Prospective study of bacteremia and complications With EUS FNA of rectal and perirectal lesions. Clin Gastroenterol Hepatol. 2007; 5(6):684–689

[13] Zuccaro G, Jr, Richter JE, Rice TW, et al. Viridans streptococcal bacteremia after esophageal stricture dilation. Gastrointest Endosc. 1998; 48(6):568–573

[14] Nelson DB, Sanderson SJ, Azar MM. Bacteremia with esophageal dilation. Gastrointest Endosc. 1998; 48(6):563–567

[15] Hirota WK, Wortmann GW, Maydonovitch CL, et al. The effect of oral decontamination with clindamycin palmitate on the incidence of bacteremia after esophageal dilation: a prospective trial. Gastrointest Endosc. 1999; 50(4):475–479

[16] Camara DS, Gruber M, Barde CJ. et al. Transient bacteremia following endoscopic injection sclerotherapy of esophageal varices. Arch Intern Med. 1983; 143(7):1350–1352

[17] Cohen LB, Korsten MA, Scherl EJ. et al. Bacteremia after endoscopic injection sclerosis. Gastrointest Endosc. 1983; 29(3):198–200

[18] Brayko CM, Kozarek RA, Sanowski RA, Testa AW. Bacteremia during esophageal variceal sclerotherapy: its cause and prevention. Gastrointest Endosc. 1985; 31(1):10–12

[19] Snady H, Korsten MA, Waye JD. The relationship of bacteremia to the length of injection needle in endoscopic variceal sclerotherapy. Gastrointest Endosc. 1985; 31(4):243–246

[20] Lin OS, Wu SS, Chen YY, Soon MS. Bacterial peritonitis after elective endoscopic variceal ligation: a prospective study. Am J Gastroenterol. 2000; 95(1):214–217

[21] Berner JS, Gaing AA, Sharma R. et al. Sequelae after esophageal variceal ligation and sclerotherapy: a prospective randomized study. Am J Gastroenterol. 1994; 89(6):852–858

[22] da Silveira Rohr MR, Siqueira ES, Brant CQ, et al. Prospective study of bacteremia rate after elastic band ligation and sclerotherapy of esophageal varices in patients with hepatosplenic schistosomiasis. Gastrointest Endosc. 1997; 46(4):321–323

[23] Nelson DB. Infectious disease complications of GI endoscopy: Part I, endogenous infections. Gastrointest Endosc. 2003; 57(4):546–556

[24] Wilson W, Taubert KA, Gewitz M, et al; American Heart Association Rheumatic Fever, Endocarditis, and Kawasaki Disease Committee. American Heart Association Council on Cardiovascular Disease in the Young. American Heart Association Council on Clinical Cardiology. American Heart Association Council on Cardiovascular Surgery and Anesthesia. Quality of Care and Outcomes Research Interdisciplinary Working Group. Prevention of infective endocarditis: guidelines from the American Heart Association: a guideline from the American Heart Association

Rheumatic Fever, Endocarditis, and Kawasaki Disease Committee, Council on Cardiovascular Disease in the Young, and the Council on Clinical Cardiology, Council on Cardiovascular Surgery and Anesthesia, and the Quality of Care and Outcomes Research Interdisciplinary Working Group. Circulation. 2007; 116(15):1736–1754

[25] Khashab MA, Chithadi KV, Acosta RD, et al; ASGE Standards of Practice Committee. Antibiotic prophylaxis for GI endoscopy. Gastrointest Endosc. 2015; 81(1):81–89

[26] Khashab MA, Tariq A, Tariq U, et al. Delayed and unsuccessful endoscopic retrograde cholangiopancreatography are associated with worse outcomes in patients with acute cholangitis. Clin Gastroenterol Hepatol. 2012; 10(10):1157–1161

[27] Kapral C, Mühlberger A, Wewalka F, et al. Working Groups Quality Assurance and Endoscopy of Austrian Society of Gastroenterology and Hepatology (OeGGH). Quality assessment of endoscopic retrograde cholangiopancreatography: results of a running nationwide Austrian benchmarking project after 5 years of implementation. Eur J Gastroenterol Hepatol. 2012; 24(12):1447–1454

[28] Andriulli A, Loperfido S, Napolitano G, et al. Incidence rates of post-ERCP complications: a systematic survey of prospective studies. Am J Gastroenterol. 2007; 102(8):1781–1788

[29] Barkay O, Khashab M, Al-Haddad M, Fogel EL. Minimizing complications in pancreaticobiliary endoscopy. Curr Gastroenterol Rep. 2009; 11(2):134–141

[30] Colton JB, Curran CC. Quality indicators, including complications, of ERCP in a community setting: a prospective study. Gastrointest Endosc. 2009; 70(3):457–467

[31] Masci E, Toti G, Mariani A, et al. Complications of diagnostic and therapeutic ERCP: a prospective multicenter study. Am J Gastroenterol. 2001; 96(2):417–423

[32] Ismail S, Kylänpää L, Mustonen H, et al. Risk factors for complications of ERCP in primary sclerosing cholangitis. Endoscopy. 2012; 44(12):1133–1138

[33] Loperfido S, Angelini G, Benedetti G, et al. Major early complications from diagnostic and therapeutic ERCP: a prospective multicenter study. Gastrointest Endosc. 1998; 48(1):1–10

[34] Bilbao MK, Dotter CT, Lee TG, Katon RM. Complications of endoscopic retrograde cholangiopancreatography (ERCP). A study of 10,000 cases. Gastroenterology. 1976; 70(3):314–320

[35] Sauter G, Grabein B, Huber G. et al. Antibiotic prophylaxis of infectious complications with endoscopic retrograde cholangiopancreatography. A randomized controlled study. Endoscopy. 1990; 22(4):164–167

[36] Niederau C, Pohlmann U, Lübke H, Thomas L. Prophylactic antibiotic treatment in therapeutic or complicated diagnostic ERCP: results of a randomized controlled clinical study. Gastrointest Endosc. 1994; 40(5):533–537

[37] Brand M, Bizos D, O'Farrell P, Jr. Antibiotic prophylaxis for patients undergoing elective endoscopic retrograde cholangiopancreatography. Cochrane Database Syst Rev. 2010(10):CD007345

[38] Motte S, Deviere J, Dumonceau JM. et al. Risk factors for septicemia following endoscopic biliary stenting. Gastroenterology. 1991; 101(5):1374–1381

[39] De Palma GD, Galloro G, Siciliano S. et al. Unilateral versus bilateral endoscopic hepatic duct drainage in patients with malignant hilar biliary obstruction: results of a prospective, randomized, and controlled study. Gastrointest Endosc. 2001; 53(6):547–553

[40] Bangarulingam SY, Gossard AA, Petersen BT. et al. Complications of endoscopic retrograde cholangiopancreatography in primary sclerosing cholangitis. Am J Gastroenterol. 2009; 104(4):855–860

[41] Byl B, Devière J, Struelens MJ, et al. Antibiotic prophylaxis for infectious complications after therapeutic endoscopic retrograde cholangiopancreatography: a randomized, double-blind, placebo-controlled study. Clin Infect Dis. 1995; 20(5):1236–1240

[42] Saxena P, Singh VK, Lennon AM. et al. Endoscopic management of acute cholecystitis after metal stent placement in patients with malignant biliary obstruction: a case series. Gastrointest Endosc. 2013; 78(1):175–178

[43] Saleem A, Leggett CL, Murad MH, Baron TH. Meta-analysis of randomized trials comparing the patency of covered and uncovered self-expandable metal stents for palliation of distal malignant bile duct obstruction. Gastrointest Endosc. 2011; 74(2):321–327.e1, 3

[44] Almadi MA, Barkun AN, Martel M. No benefit of covered vs uncovered self-expandable metal stents in patients with malignant distal biliary obstruction: a meta-analysis. Clin Gastroenterol Hepatol. 2013; 11(1):27–37.e1

[45] Isayama H, Kawabe T, Nakai Y, et al. Cholecystitis after metallic stent placement in patients with malignant distal biliary obstruction. Clin Gastroenterol Hepatol. 2006; 4(9):1148–1153

[46] Williams DB, Sahai AV, Aabakken L, et al. Endoscopic ultrasound guided fine needle aspiration biopsy: a large single centre experience. Gut. 1999; 44(5):720–726

[47] Eloubeidi MA, Tamhane A, Varadarajulu S, Wilcox CM. Frequency of major complications after EUS-guided FNA of solid pancreatic masses: a prospective evaluation. Gastrointest Endosc. 2006; 63(4):622–629

[48] Guarner-Argente C, Shah P, Buchner A. et al. Use of antimicrobials for EUS-guided FNA of pancreatic cysts: a retrospective, comparative analysis. Gastrointest Endosc. 2011; 74(1):81–86

[49] Diehl DL, Cheruvattath R, Facktor MA, Go BD. Infection after endoscopic ultrasound-guided aspiration of mediastinal cysts. Interact Cardiovasc Thorac Surg. 2010; 10(2):338–340

[50] Annema JT, Veseliç M, Versteegh MI, Rabe KF. Mediastinitis caused by EUS-FNA of a bronchogenic cyst. Endoscopy. 2003; 35(9):791–793

[51] Khashab MA, Dewitt J. EUS-guided biliary drainage: is it ready for prime time? Yes! Gastrointest Endosc. 2013; 78(1):102–105

[52] Khashab MA, Fujii LL, Baron TH, et al. EUS-guided biliary drainage for patients with malignant biliary obstruction with an indwelling duodenal stent (with videos). Gastrointest Endosc. 2012; 76(1):209–213

[53] Khashab MA, Kim KJ, Tryggestad EJ, et al. Comparative analysis of traditional and coiled fiducials implanted during EUS for pancreatic cancer patients receiving stereotactic body radiation therapy. Gastrointest Endosc. 2012; 76(5):962–971

[54] Shah JN, Marson F, Weilert F, et al. Single-operator, single-session EUS-guided anterograde cholangiopancreatography in failed ERCP or inaccessible papilla. Gastrointest Endosc. 2012; 75(1):56–64

[55] Khashab MA, Valeshabad AK, Modayil R, et al. EUS-guided biliary drainage by using a standardized approach for malignant biliary obstruction: rendezvous versus direct transluminal techniques (with videos). Gastrointest Endosc. 2013; 78(5):734–741

[56] Khashab MA, Varadarajulu S. Endoscopic ultrasonography as a therapeutic modality. Curr Opin Gastroenterol. 2012; 28(5):467–476

[57] Lipp A, Lusardi G. Systemic antimicrobial prophylaxis for percutaneous endoscopic gastrostomy. Cochrane Database Syst Rev. 2006(4):CD005571

[58] Jain NK, Larson DE, Schroeder KW, et al. Antibiotic prophylaxis for percutaneous endoscopic gastrostomy. A prospective, randomized, double-blind clinical trial. Ann Intern Med. 1987; 107(6):824–828

[59] Maple JT, Petersen BT, Baron TH. et al. Direct percutaneous endoscopic jejunostomy: outcomes in 307 consecutive attempts. Am J Gastroenterol. 2005; 100(12):2681–2688

[60] Maple JT. Direct percutaneous endoscopic jejunostomy in the obese: proceed with caution. Gastrointest Endosc. 2008; 67(2):270–272

[61] Chavez-Tapia NC, Barrientos-Gutierrez T, Tellez-Avila F, et al. Meta-analysis: antibiotic prophylaxis for cirrhotic patients with upper gastrointestinal bleeding - an updated Cochrane review. Aliment Pharmacol Ther. 2011; 34(5):509–518

[62] Fernández J, Ruiz del Arbol L, Gómez C, et al. Norfloxacin vs ceftriaxone in the prophylaxis of infections in patients with advanced cirrhosis and hemorrhage. Gastroenterology. 2006; 131(4):1049–1056, quiz 1285

[63] Baddour LM, Epstein AE, Erickson CC, et al; American Heart Association Rheumatic Fever, Endocarditis, and Kawasaki Disease Committee of the Council on Cardiovascular Disease in the Young. Council on Cardiovascular Surgery and Anesthesia. Council on Cardiovascular Nursing. Council on Clinical Cardiology. Interdisciplinary Council on Quality of Care and Outcomes Research. A summary of the update on cardiovascular implantable electronic device infections and their management: a scientific statement from the American Heart Association. J Am Dent Assoc. 2011; 142(2):159–165

[64] Zimmerli W, Trampuz A, Ochsner PE. Prosthetic-joint infections. N Engl J Med. 2004; 351(16):1645–1654

[65] Piraino B, Bernardini J, Brown E, et al. ISPD position statement on reducing the risks of peritoneal dialysis-related infections. Perit Dial Int. 2011; 31(6):614–630

[66] Yip T, Tse KC, Lam MF, et al. Risks and outcomes of peritonitis after flexible colonoscopy in CAPD patients. Perit Dial Int. 2007; 27(5):560–564

[67] Piraino B, Bernardini J, Brown E, et al. ISPD position statement on reducing the risks of peritoneal dialysis-related infections. Perit Dial Int. 2011; 31(6):614–630

9 Quality Assurance in Endoscopy

Matthew D. Rutter

9.1 The Importance of Quality

In recent years, the publication of several key studies has brought the importance of quality in health care services into sharp focus. For example, a study from the United States in 2000 indicated that as many as 98,000 people were dying each year as a result of medical errors.[1] In endoscopy, which is a pivotal investigation in the diagnosis and management of gastrointestinal (GI) pathology, the quality agenda has been advanced further by the introduction of organized colorectal cancer screening programs. High-quality endoscopy delivers better health outcomes and better patient experience,[2] yet it is widely recognized that significant variation exists in the performance of endoscopists and of endoscopy units,[3,4,5,6,7] and as tens of millions endoscopic procedures are performed every year across the world, the potential health impact of suboptimal endoscopic quality is large.

The current variation in endoscopic quality between services and between individuals is best evidenced in colonoscopy. For example, a recent United Kingdom study demonstrated a four-fold variation in postcolonoscopy colorectal cancer (PCCRC) rates between hospitals.[8] It is known that the majority of PCCRCs arise from missed cancers, missed premalignant polyps, or incomplete polypectomy.[9,10] Back-to-back colonoscopy studies show that there is a three- to sixfold variation in adenoma detection rates (ADRs) between endoscopists, and even greater variation in serrated polyp detection rates.[11,12] Even when polyps are found, removal may be incomplete: the CARE study concluded that 10% of nonpedunculated polyps of 5 to 20 mm, 23% of nonpedunculated polyps of 15 to 20 mm, and 48% of serrated polyps of 10 to 20 mm were incompletely resected.[13]

Quality variation is not limited to colonoscopy. In endoscopic retrograde cholangiopancreatography (ERCP), which is one of the most complex and high-risk commonly performed endoscopic procedure, a wide variation is seen in procedure completion and in complication rates.[14,15,16,17,18,19,20,21] Gastric cancers and precursor lesions are also frequently missed in the upper GI tract—in one series, 7.2% of patients diagnosed with gastric cancer had had a negative gastroscopy within the preceding year, of which around three-quarters were due to endoscopist error.[22]

9.2 Performance Measures

Differences in endoscopic quality will only come to light if performance is measured. Services and individuals are unlikely to improve, nor can support be provided, unless they are aware of their performance and how it compares with benchmark standards. Such comparison can be a powerful motivator for individuals and services to improve, diminishing the variation in quality between endoscopists and services. It is also well-recognized that by simply monitoring a service, performance will improve—this is the Hawthorne effect, and it is essentially a free means to improve the quality of patient care.

Performance measures (PMs; also known as quality measures, quality indicators, key performance indicators, or clinical quality measures) are criteria that are used to assess the performance of a service or a component of the service. The provision of high-quality, patient-centered endoscopic care is complex, involving a multidisciplinary team, many detailed processes, and an array of specialist equipment to investigate and treat a wide range of people of differing age and comorbidity with differing levels of urgency. PMs can be used to measure all aspects (often called "domains") of the endoscopic service, from preprocedure, through the procedure itself, and in the postprocedural period. Examples of domains include timeliness, completeness of procedure, identification of pathology, management of pathology, complications, and patient experience. Ideally, a small number of PMs should be used to assess each domain: used together, they provide a global overview of the quality of the service. A good example of this process is the Endoscopy Global Rating Scale (GRS) used in the United Kingdom, which is now adopted in many other nations (▶ Fig. 9.1).

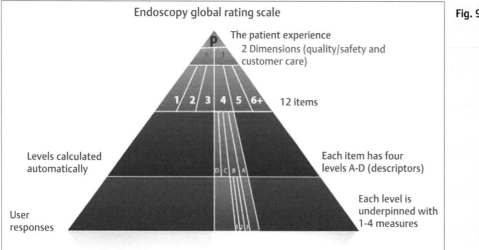

Fig. 9.1 The Endoscopy Global Rating Scale.

Endoscopy global rating scale

The patient experience
2 Dimensions (quality/safety and customer care)

12 items

Each item has four levels A–D (descriptors)

Levels calculated automatically

Each level is underpinned with 1-4 measures

User responses

ENDOSCOPY SAFETY CHECKLIST

☑ Affix patient ID label

Time Out — Before scope insertion		
Team introduction	☐ Yes
Patient ID	☐ Yes
Correct screen on reporting software	☐ Yes
Correct procedure	☐ Yes
Indication	☐ Yes
Consent	☐ Yes
Monitoring (IV access / O_2 sats)	☐ Yes
Allergies	☐ Yes ☐ No
Comorbidity	☐ Yes ☐ No
Anticoagulants	☐ Yes ☐ No
Correct scope & kit	☐ Yes
Sign Out — End of procedure Samples & labelling	☐ Yes ☐ N/A
Accurate report	☐ Yes
Follow-Up	☐ Yes

Name (Dr / Nurse)...............................Date & Time....................Signature................................

St MARK'S HOSPITAL

Wolfson Unit for Endoscopy

Fig. 9.2 An example of an endoscopy checklist.[33]

PMs can be categorized as outcome measures, structural measures, or process measures. Outcome measures assess the results of clinically meaningful aspects of care directly, and are usually considered the most important measures—for example, the pancreatitis rate following ERCP. However, it may not always be feasible to measure such outcomes—the data may be too difficult to capture, the event may be rare and therefore difficult to analyze with statistical certainty, or the timeframe to capture such data may be too long for it to be a useful measure of current performance (e.g., PCCRC rates, where several years need to pass before the true figure can be calculated). In these situations, the use of surrogate PMs may be required. These may also be outcome measures—for example, ADR is used as a surrogate for PCCRC rate. Where surrogate measures are used, it is desirable that there is evidence of a correlation between these measures and an important health outcome—reassuringly, in this example, there is increasingly compelling evidence demonstrating a strong correlation between an individual endoscopist's ADR and its PCCRC rate.[23,24] Surrogate measures may also be structural measures, which look at aspects of health care infrastructure (e.g., information about staffing levels or whether a provider has an electronic endoscopy reporting system), or process measures, which measure whether specific quality actions are being implemented (e.g., the proportion of patients that have had a preprocedure

endoscopy checklist completed; ▶Fig. 9.2—there is compelling evidence from surgery that the introduction of the WHO surgical checklist can result in a reduction of complications by a third and mortality by almost half).[25,26]

Colorectal cancer screening has facilitated the implementation of PMs for diagnostic colonoscopy. However, measures for therapeutic colonoscopy and for most other aspects of GI endoscopy are either nonexistent or very much in their infancy.

It is usually desirable to identify a minimum standard and a target standard for each PM. Although PMs will remain relatively static over time, quality improvement is a dynamic process and as such the standards within such measures will usually increase over time as techniques and technologies improve. The standards may also vary according to the specific procedure—for example, the minimum standard for ADR will be higher for fecal occult blood diagnostic colonoscopy compared to screening colonoscopy. At present, there are many PMs where no evidence-based minimum standard has been defined. With time, further research can help determine what the appropriate standards should be; nevertheless, in the interim it may still be useful to measure and benchmark performance against other similar services.

An example of endoscopic PMs is given in ▶Fig. 9.3.

TABLE 4. Summary of proposed quality indicators for ERCP

Quality indicator	Grade of recommendation	Measure type	Performance target (%)
Preprocedure			
1. Frequency with which ERCP is performed for an indication that is included in a published standard list of appropriate indications and the indication is documented (priority indicator)	1C+	Process	> 90
2. Frequency with which informed consent is obtained, including specific discussions of risks associated with ERCP, and fully documented	1C	Process	> 98
3. Frequency with which appropriate antibiotics for ERCP are administered for settings in which they are indicated	2B	Process	> 98
4. Frequency with which ERCP is performed by an endoscopist who is fully trained and credentialed to perform ERCP	3	Process	> 98
5. Frequency with which the volume of ERCPs performed per year is recorded per endoscopist	1C	Process	> 98
Intraprocedure			
6a. Frequency with which deep cannulation of the ducts of interest is documented	1C	Process	> 98
6b. Frequency with which deep cannulation of the ducts of interest in patients with native papillae without surgically altered anatomy is achieved and documented (priority indicator)	1C	Process	> 90
7. Frequency with which fluoroscopy time and radiation dose are measured and documented	2C	Process	> 98
8. Frequency with which common bile duct stones < 1 cm in patients with normal bile duct anatomy are extracted successfully and documented (priority indicator)	1C	Outcome	≥ 90
9. Frequency with which stent placement for biliary obstruction in patients with normal anatomy whose obstruction is below the bifurcation is successfully achieved and documented (priority indicator)	1C	Outcome	≥ 90
Postprocedure			
10. Frequency with which a complete ERCP report that details the specific techniques performed, particular accessories used, and all intended outcomes is prepared	3	Process	> 98
11. Frequency with which acute adverse events and hospital transfers are documented	3	Process	> 98
12. Rate of post-ERCP pancreatitis (priority indicator)	1C	Outcome	N/A
13. Rate and type of perforation	2C	Outcome	≤ 0.2
14. Rate of clinically significant hemorrhage after sphincterotomy or sphincteroplasty in patients undergoing ERCP	1C	Outcome	≤ 1
15. Frequency with which patients are contacted at or greater than 14 days to detect and record the occurrence of delayed adverse events after ERCP	3	Process	> 90

Fig. 9.3 American Society for Gastrointestinal Endoscopy (ASGE) performance measures for ERCP.[34]

9.3 Practicalities of Measurement

PMs should enable assessors to identify specific deficits in the service, permitting them to be addressed and thus resulting in better patient outcomes. Several different attributes should be considered when constructing PMs:

9.3.1 Clinical Importance

As described earlier, PMs should correlate with important health outcomes. Measures should be as evidence-based as possible. However, current evidence for most endoscopic PMs (and particularly for minimum standards) is low—further research is required, but in the meantime, expert consensus opinion is an appropriate interim approach to ensure that PMs are clinically meaningful for their target audience.

9.3.2 Standardization

The standardization of PM definitions and methodology of measurement is important to permit meaningful comparison between individuals and services. PMs should be as objective (such as using an *unadjusted* cecal intubation rate—unadjusted for

strictures or poor bowel preparation) and reproducible as possible. Current endoscopic PM definitions and methodology calculations are poorly described and inconsistent, although there is welcome movement to correct this by producing international standards.[27] Another component that requires standardization is in the robustness of the methodology for capturing complications—otherwise, a perverse situation arises where poor services may appear to perform better, simply because they have not identified the complications that have occurred.

Different PMs lend themselves to different methodologies. PMs based on common events such as cannulation of the intended duct at ERCP, or adenoma detection at colonoscopy, are suited to quantitative analysis. However, rarer events, such as missed cancer or endoscopic perforation, may be best examined by qualitative review of each adverse event (root cause analysis). Rarer events can also be examined at an endoscopy unit level rather than endoscopist level, although this methodology can sometimes overlook poorly performing individuals.

9.3.3 Practicality

The trade-off of all PMs is the practicality of capturing and analyzing the data. While a multitude of highly complex PMs may be justifiable on quality grounds, it may be unrealistic or impossible to implement such measures in a busy service. Considerations include the number of PMs, the number of data sources required to calculate the PM (e.g., ADR requires both pathology and endoscopy data, whereas polypectomy rate does not), and whether data are stored electronically or not—electronic endoscopy reporting systems are an important component in allowing timely data collection and automated, standardized PM reporting.

9.3.4 Governance Infrastructure

The practicality and objectivity of quality assurance (QA) is influenced greatly by the governance infrastructure. QA requires political will and strong leadership at all levels. For programs to succeed, they need to be organized and embedded in the routine activities of an endoscopy service. Locally, support is required from hospital management. However, commitment from regional or national authorities is also desirable—the best current QA systems have arisen from colorectal cancer screening programs, where instituted (▶ Fig. 9.4). These modestly funding schemes adopt a centralized approach to QA using automatic (electronic) capture of data and calculation of PMs. This ensures an objective, standardized approach to PM calculation, while the centralized nature saves time and money.

The best programs are those where the QA process is mandatory and are overseen by those who have authority to act on the findings. If a scheme is voluntary, those whose performance is suboptimal may simply not participate to the ongoing detriment of patient care. Where it is not possible to mandate participation, some success has been achieved with schemes that incentivize participation—this has happened in both the United Kingdom and the United States, where participation or nonparticipation may result in financial reward or penalty.[28]

9.3.5 Negative Aspects

PMs are designed to measure and improve quality. However, there can be unintended consequences. Perhaps, the best described is the concept of "gaming"—that is, the endoscopist may either inappropriately adjust his/her practice simply to chase the PM target, or may adjust his/her reporting to make his/her figures appear better than they actually are (e.g., claiming that a failed colonoscopy was actually a flexible sigmoidoscopy so that it does not count against their cecal intubation rate). Clearly, this is an issue of integrity. Centralizing the process and using robust and objective measures less susceptible to gaming helps mitigate this risk, although it does not remove the risk altogether.

Another potential negative aspect of PMs relates to how data are published. Open publication of PMs, either among the wider health care service or to the public, permits users and commissioners of the service to assess quality for themselves. This can be very powerful in incentivizing improvements in quality. However, it can also have unintended consequences if data are open to misinterpretation or inappropriate comparison.

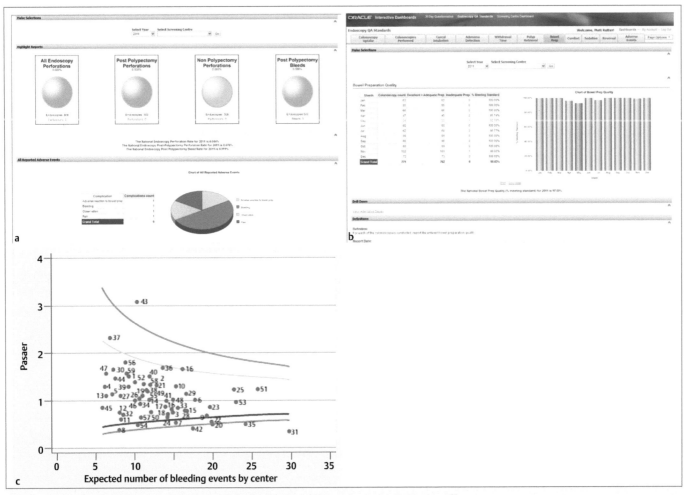

Fig. 9.4 An example of automated output from the English Bowel Cancer Screening Programme.[35]

This may lead to a defensive endoscopic culture, where endoscopists are unwilling to take on more complex cases where outcomes are likely to be worse. Strategies to address these issues include clear descriptions about the limitations of each PM, using procedure complexity adjustment, and carefully defining exclusions when calculating PMs. The pros and cons both of open publication of data and of using named or anonymized reporting of PM data should also be considered, particularly when programs are being investigated—the initial use of a degree of data anonymity can give individuals greater confidence that the process is a supportive one.

9.4 Quality Improvement

Measuring quality is only one component of the broader concept of quality improvement. Quality improvement also requires the creation of a supportive culture within endoscopic services, including training, accreditation, and management of underperformance.

In recent years, the quality of endoscopy training has become increasingly sophisticated and structured, incorporating virtual reality simulators, cadaveric models (particularly for therapeutic procedures) and programs involving evidence-based one-to-one training, bespoke courses with trainers with expertise not only in endoscopy but also in teaching methodology, and formative training assessments (▶Fig. 9.5).

Formal accreditation (credentialing) of endoscopy trainees prior to independent practice is increasingly common and undoubtedly adds a level of protection for patients from inexperienced and incompetent endoscopists. Nevertheless, its global introduction, particularly for endoscopists who are currently practicing independently, is controversial. Many services have compromised by introducing accreditation only for newly-trained endoscopists, anticipating that, within a generation, all independently practicing endoscopists will have been accredited at inception.

When potential underperformance is identified by measuring PMs, it is important that further analysis and action is handled in a supportive and constructive manner. Many organizations have developed well-defined, open, structured processes for managing underperformance,[29] and when handled sensitively, experience shows that most endoscopists embrace such support. However, this is not universal and on occasions there may be resistance to engagement with such processes from individuals or even from services. This may be driven by embarrassment or fear that one's abilities might be demonstrated to be suboptimal, and may be pronounced if there are financial or service drivers to continue with the status quo. Nevertheless, it is essential for high-quality patient care that these barriers are overcome.

Unfortunately, trials of initiatives to improve specific aspects of endoscopic quality have not been universally successful. For example, evidence reveals that endoscopists who spend more time inspecting the colonic mucosa find more pathology[11]; however, initiatives to mandate a minimum withdrawal time have produced mixed results.[30,31,32] We should not use this as evidence to give up on quality improvement though—these studies further our understanding of the techniques that underpin high-quality endoscopy, allowing us to refine training methodology. Moreover, such direct interventions are only one component of quality improvement—more global quality improvement initiatives have been highly successful: for example, in the United Kingdom, introducing PMs along with additional measures such as structured training programs resulted in significant improvement in endoscopy quality, where cecal intubation rate improved from 76.9 to 92.3%.[18]

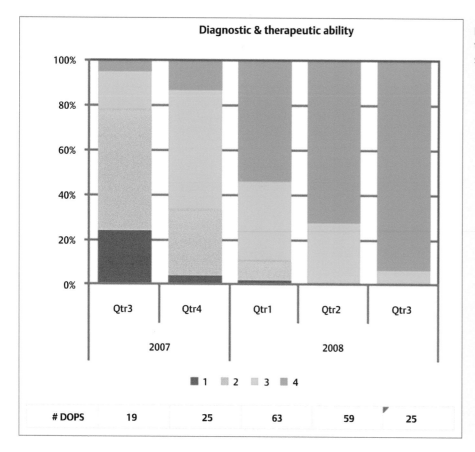

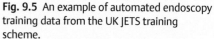

Fig. 9.5 An example of automated endoscopy training data from the UK JETS training scheme.

9.5 Summary

Quality in endoscopy is essential to maximize the benefit and minimize potential harm from these common, invasive procedures. The potential benefit to public health from improving endoscopy quality is large. Despite half a century having passed since the advent of flexible endoscopy, embedding QA and quality improvement into everyday endoscopic practice remains very much in its infancy. PMs are being developed for all aspects of clinical care. The importance of objective, standardized, and automated processes, mandated and coordinated at a regional or national level, is increasingly recognized. There remains, however, a need to prioritize research to strengthen the evidence base for quality metrics and effective quality improvement initiatives.

References

[1] Kohn LT, Corrigan JM, Donaldson MS. To Err Is Human: Building a Safer Health System. Washington, DC: Committee on Quality of Health Care in America, Institute of Medicine; 2000

[2] Rutter MD, Rees CJ. Quality in gastrointestinal endoscopy. Endoscopy. 2014; 46(6):526–528

[3] Rajasekhar PT, Rutter MD, Bramble MG, et al. Achieving high quality colonoscopy: using graphical representation to measure performance and reset standards. Colorectal Dis. 2012; 14(12):1538–1545

[4] Baillie J, Testoni PA. Are we meeting the standards set for ERCP? Gut. 2007; 56(6):744–746

[5] Cotton PB. Are low-volume ERCPists a problem in the United States? A plea to examine and improve ERCP practice-NOW. Gastrointest Endosc. 2011; 74(1):161–166

[6] Williams EJ, Taylor S, Fairclough P, et al. Risk factors for complication following ERCP; results of a large-scale, prospective multicenter study. Endoscopy. 2007; 39(9):793–801

[7] Williams EJ, Taylor S, Fairclough P, et al; BSG Audit of ERCP. Are we meeting the standards set for endoscopy? Results of a large-scale prospective survey of endoscopic retrograde cholangio-pancreatograph practice. Gut. 2007; 56(6):821–829

[8] Valori R, Morris E, Rutter MD. Rates of Post Colonoscopy Colorectal Cancer (PC-CRC) Are Significantly Affected by Methodology, but Are Nevertheless Declining in the NHS. UEG Week; 2014; Vienna

[9] Pabby A, Schoen RE, Weissfeld JL, et al. Analysis of colorectal cancer occurrence during surveillance colonoscopy in the dietary Polyp Prevention Trial. Gastrointest Endosc. 2005; 61(3):385–391

[10] Robertson DJ, Lieberman DA, Winawer SJ, et al. Colorectal cancers soon after colonoscopy: a pooled multicohort analysis. Gut. 2014; 63(6):949–956

[11] Barclay RL, Vicari JJ, Doughty AS. et al. Colonoscopic withdrawal times and adenoma detection during screening colonoscopy. N Engl J Med. 2006; 355(24):2533–2541

[12] Chen SC, Rex DK. Endoscopist can be more powerful than age and male gender in predicting adenoma detection at colonoscopy. Am J Gastroenterol. 2007; 102(4):856–861

[13] Pohl H, Srivastava A, Bensen SP, et al. Incomplete polyp resection during colonoscopy-results of the complete adenoma resection (CARE) study. Gastroenterology. 2013; 144(1):74–80.e1

[14] Raftopoulos SC, Segarajasingam DS, Burke V. et al A cohort study of missed and new cancers after esophagogastroduodenoscopy. Am J Gastroenterol. 2010; 105(6):1292–1297

[15] Cohen J, Safdi MA, Deal SE, et al; ASGE/ACG Taskforce on Quality in Endoscopy. Quality indicators for esophagogastroduodenoscopy. Am J Gastroenterol. 2006; 101(4):886–891

[16] Faigel DO, Pike IM, Baron TH, et al; ASGE/ACG Taskforce on Quality in Endoscopy. Quality indicators for gastrointestinal endoscopic procedures: an introduction. Am J Gastroenterol. 2006; 101(4):866–872

[17] Park WG, Cohen J. Quality measurement and improvement in upper endoscopy. Tech Gastrointest Endosc. 2012; 14(1):13–20

[18] Gavin DR, Valori RM, Anderson JT. et al. The national colonoscopy audit: a nationwide assessment of the quality and safety of colonoscopy in the UK. Gut. 2013; 62(2):242–249

[19] Enochsson L, Swahn F, Arnelo U. Nationwide, population-based data from 11,074 ERCP procedures from the Swedish Registry for Gallstone Surgery and ERCP. Gastrointest Endosc. 2010; 72(6):1175–1184, 1184.e1–1184.e3

[20] Baron TH, Petersen BT, Mergener K, et al; ASGE/ACG Taskforce on Quality in Endoscopy. Quality indicators for endoscopic retrograde cholangiopancreatography. Am J Gastroenterol. 2006; 101(4):892–897

[21] Cotton PB, Garrow DA, Gallagher J, Romagnuolo J. Risk factors for complications after ERCP: a multivariate analysis of 11,497 procedures over 12 years. Gastrointest Endosc. 2009; 70(1):80–88

[22] Yalamarthi S, Witherspoon P, McCole D, Auld CD. Missed diagnoses in patients with upper gastrointestinal cancers. Endoscopy. 2004; 36(10):874–879

[23] Corley DA, Jensen CD, Marks AR, et al. Adenoma detection rate and risk of colorectal cancer and death. N Engl J Med. 2014; 370(14):1298–1306

[24] Kaminski MF, Regula J, Kraszewska E, et al. Quality indicators for colonoscopy and the risk of interval cancer. N Engl J Med. 2010; 362(19):1795–1803

[25] Haynes AB, Weiser TG, Berry WR, et al; Safe Surgery Saves Lives Study Group. A surgical safety checklist to reduce morbidity and mortality in a global population. N Engl J Med. 2009; 360(5):491–499

[26] de Vries EN, Prins HA, Crolla RM, et al; SURPASS Collaborative Group. Effect of a comprehensive surgical safety system on patient outcomes. N Engl J Med. 2010; 363(20):1928–1937

[27] Rutter MD, Senore C, Bisschops R, et al. The European Society of Gastrointestinal Endoscopy Quality Improvement Initiative: developing performance measures. Endoscopy. 2016; 48(1):81–89

[28] Calderwood AH, Jacobson BC. Colonoscopy quality: metrics and implementation. Gastroenterol Clin North Am. 2013; 42(3):599–618

[29] Thomas-Gibson S, Barton JR, Green J, et al. Mentoring and Quality Assurance of Screening Endoscopists in the NHS Bowel Cancer Screening Programme. NHS BCSP Publication; 2013

[30] Barclay RL, Vicari JJ, Greenlaw RL. Effect of a time-dependent colonoscopic withdrawal protocol on adenoma detection during screening colonoscopy. Clin Gastroenterol Hepatol. 2008; 6(10):1091–1098

[31] Lin OS, Kozarek RA, Arai A, et al. The effect of periodic monitoring and feedback on screening colonoscopy withdrawal times, polyp detection rates, and patient satisfaction scores. Gastrointest Endosc. 2010; 71(7):1253–1259

[32] Sawhney MS, Cury MS, Neeman N, et al. Effect of institution-wide policy of colonoscopy withdrawal time> or =7 minutes on polyp detection. Gastroenterology. 2008; 135(6):1892–1898

[33] Matharoo M, Thomas-Gibson S, Haycock A, Sevdalis N. Implementation of an endoscopy safety checklist. Frontline Gastroenterol. 2014; 5(4):260–265

[34] Adler DG, Lieb JG, II, Cohen J, et al. Quality indicators for ERCP. Gastrointest Endosc. 2015; 81(1):54–66

[35] Blanks RG, Nickerson C, Patnick J. et al. Evaluation of colonoscopy performance based on post-procedure bleeding complications: application of procedure complexity-adjusted model. Endoscopy. 2015; 47(10):910–916

10 Endoscopic Complications

Daniel Blero and Jacques Devière

10.1 Introduction

An endoscopic complication can be defined as an adverse event that requires a deviation from the initial plan for diagnosis and/or treatment, and this adverse event can be qualified as severe when it prolongs hospitalization and/or results in an unscheduled hospital admission.[1] The frequency of endoscopic complications is likely to increase in proportion to the indications and complexity of therapeutic procedures. The best way to prevent complication is to carefully analyze procedural indications and avoid unnecessary invasive examinations. Gastrointestinal (GI) endoscopy is a discipline evolving quickly within a multidisciplinary environment with paradigm changes such as the development of alternative, noninvasive diagnostic techniques, for example, magnetic resonance cholangiopancreatography (MRCP), which has entirely replaced diagnostic endoscopic retrograde cholangiopancreatography (ERCP) for imaging the biliopancreatic tract. With an increasing complexity of endoscopic procedures, the need for extensive knowledge of techniques and accessories has become paramount, and it is now clear that many of these procedures must be concentrated in specialized referral centers. Acquiring and maintaining experience in a multidisciplinary environment is essential to select the best procedure for a specific indication and to consequently reduce the risk of adverse events. Now that therapeutic endoscopy offers even more alternatives to open surgery, it is also important to disseminate information about the outcomes of these procedures in order to avoid inappropriate therapeutic approaches to manage known or suspected complications. For example, postprocedural management following submucosal and transmural endotherapy may result in imaging findings of incidental free air that may be inappropriately managed with aggressive surgery.[2]

Preprocedural patient education and informed consent (see Chapter 3) are paramount. Standardization of treatment, organization of the therapeutic endoscopy team and its training, and adherence to guidelines are also essential in order to minimize, prevent, and adequately manage adverse events. The most frequent complications of diagnostic and therapeutic endoscopy are reviewed in this chapter. Different modalities of medical, endoscopic, and surgical management are also considered.

10.2 General Considerations

10.2.1 Cardiopulmonary and Sedation-Related Events

A cornerstone for proper performance of endoscopy is that the selection, and the monitoring of sedation should commensurate with the planned procedure. Cardiopulmonary adverse events account for up to 50% of severe morbidity and mortality related to GI endoscopy.[3,4] These adverse events range from clinically insignificant oxygen desaturation to clinical dysrhythmias, oversedation, aspiration pneumonia, respiratory failure, myocardial infarction, and shock. Many of these adverse events are linked to inappropriate sedation levels considering the type of procedure and the status of the patient, but they may also be associated with other adverse events such as bleeding, sepsis, and perforation.

Before undertaking moderate sedation (see Chapter 4), the patient's medical and surgical history, baseline medications with a particular focus on antithrombotic agents, and drug allergies must be assessed. The American Society of Anesthesiologists (ASA) score is a useful predictor of procedural sedation risk. Other risk factors include age, type of anesthesia, inpatient status, emergency procedure, and trainee involvement. Patients should not temporarily discontinue their cardiovascular medications except for antithrombotic agents when high-risk bleeding procedure is performed (see ▶ Table 10.1),[5] and this decision should be undertaken with advice from other specialists (cardiology, neurology, etc.) in patients at high risk for thrombosis.

Pharyngeal anesthesia is usually recommended when no or minimal sedation is administered. It should be used with caution or avoided in nonintubated patients with suspected gastric outlet obstruction or gastroparesis, and in the presence of active upper GI bleeding as it increases the risk of aspiration pneumonia.[3] Preoxygenation of patients with ischemic cardiovascular disease, as well as administration of supplemental oxygen during the procedure to avoid ischemic events, is recommended. All patients must be monitored using pulse oximetry before, during, and after the examination and continued until full recovery. Managing and avoiding cardiopulmonary adverse events requires competency in basic life support, knowledge of the patient's underlying medical status, and pharmacological properties of the drugs used and their reversal agents.

10.2.2 Infection

Although rare,[6] infections can result from the transmission of microorganisms through the endoscope from one patient to another or (even more rarely) through reprocessed devices, from the translocation of bacteria from the endogenous digestive flora through a tear or perforation in the mucosa, from contamination of a sterile compartment by patient's GI flora (i.e., typically during ERCP in the presence of obstructed ducts and inadequate drainage), or by the transmission of microorganisms from patients to personnel of the endoscopy unit (and vice versa).

All reported cases of patient-to-patient transmitted infections were due to failure to properly follow multisociety guidelines for disinfecting and reprocessing flexible endoscopes,[7,8] first published in 2003. It must be noted, however, that this type of infection remains of major importance as recently illustrated when contamination of duodenoscopes not adequately designed to allow proper disinfection resulted in severe iatrogenic infections.[9]

Regarding prevention of bacterial translocation during endoscopy, prophylactic antimicrobial regimens are recommended in cases of suspected incomplete biliary drainage, puncture of

Table 10.1 Bleeding risk of endoscopic procedures

Bleeding risk	Endoscopic procedure	Continuation of aspirin?	Continuation of clopidogrel or prasugrel?
Low risk	EGD and colonoscopy +/- biopsy	Yes	Yes
	EUS without FNA	Yes	Yes
	Colonic polypectomy < 1 cm	Yes	No
	Dilation of digestive stenosis	Yes	No
	EUS FNA of solid mass	Yes	No
	Digestive stenting	Yes	No
	ERCP stent placement or papillary balloon dilation without endoscopic sphincterotomy	Yes	Yes
	Argon plasma coagulation for angiodysplasia	Yes	Yes
High risk	EMR, ESD, and ampullary resection	No	No
	Endoscopic sphincterotomy	Yes	No
	Endoscopic sphincterotomy +/- large balloon papillary dilation	No	No
	Colonic polypectomy > 1 cm	Yes	No
	EUS FNA of cystic lesions	No	No
	Percutaneous endoscopic gastrostomy	Yes	N.A.
	Esophageal variceal band ligation	Yes	No

Abbreviations: EGD, esophagogastroduodenoscopy; EMR, endoscopic mucosal resection; ERCP, endoscopic retrograde cholangiopancreatography; ESD, endoscopic submucosal dissection; EUS, endoscopic ultrasound; FNA, fine-needle aspiration.

Source: Reproduced with permission from Boustière C, Veitch A, Vanbiervliet G, et al; European Society of Gastrointestinal Endoscopy. Endoscopy and antiplatelet agents. European Society of Gastrointestinal Endoscopy (ESGE) Guideline. Endoscopy 2011;43(5):445–461.

fluid collections or cysts, percutaneous endoscopic gastrostomy placement, and in patients with variceal bleeding. In some cases, prophylaxis entails single-dose administration before treatment, while in others it may need to be continued, such as in patients with inadequately drained bile ducts or those with variceal bleeding. New techniques involving transmural access, such as endoscopic ultrasound (EUS)-guided biliary drainage, peroral endoscopic myotomy (POEM), and gastric transmural therapy, also require antibiotic prophylaxis with or without continued treatment. Unfortunately, prospective evidence for these indications is lacking.

The protection of endoscopy personnel from infection/contamination by patient body fluids should be instituted and followed according to institutional universal exposure educational guidelines and postexposure management.[10]

10.3 Upper Gastrointestinal Endoscopy

10.3.1 Diagnostic Upper Gastrointestinal Endoscopy

Diagnostic upper GI endoscopy is usually considered to be a safe procedure, with overall complication and mortality rates at 0.13 and 0.004%, respectively.[11] Procedure-induced Mallory–Weiss tear occurs in < 0.5% of diagnostic endoscopies and is generally not associated with significant bleeding.[12] Bleeding after mucosal biopsy is rare in the absence of thrombocytopenia, coagulopathy, or portal hypertension. Biopsies can be safely performed in patients with a platelet count > 20,000/mm.[3,13] Perforation secondary to diagnostic upper GI endoscopy is extremely rare, with an estimated frequency of < 0.03%.[3] Risk factors for perforation include endoscopist inexperience, presence of cervical osteophytes, Zenker's diverticulum, pharyngeal pouches, and esophageal stricture. Eosinophilic esophagitis is a recognized risk for mucosal tearing and perforation during diagnostic procedures.[14,]

10.3.2 Therapeutic Upper Gastrointestinal Endoscopy

Therapeutic upper GI endoscopy has dramatically increased over the last 10 years and is associated with a much higher rate (approximately 10 times) of adverse events than diagnostic procedures.[15]

Stricture and Achalasia Dilation

Dilation of esophageal strictures and achalasia pneumatic dilation are associated with specific complications including perforation, bleeding, and bronchial aspiration. Bronchial aspiration can be prevented by endotracheal intubation, which is recommended in patients with comorbidities, although it is also associated with specific adverse events.[16] Perforation risk varies with indication and technique used. Up to 4% risk has been described for pneumatic dilation of achalasia.[17] It can be reduced by starting with a balloon diameter of 30 mm and not dilating greater than 35 mm.[17] With the advent of POEM, the use of pneumatic dilation is likely to decrease.[18] The risk of perforation when dilating malignant and caustic strictures is twofold compared with benign (peptic) strictures.[19] Complex strictures (defined as an asymmetry, < 12 mm in diameter, or endoscopically impassable) are also associated with increased rates of complications.[19] Another established risk factor for perforation is the level of operator experience. The risk of perforation during dilation is four times higher for trainees who have performed fewer than 500 upper GI endoscopies.[3] Most perforations occur at the first session of dilation.[20] Three separate studies failed to show that bougie dilators are safer than balloon dilators in patients with benign strictures.[21]

Stent Insertion

Self-expandable metal stent (SEMS) placement is a method for palliating malignant dysphagia and malignant tracheoesophageal fistula.[22,23] SEMS can also be used to close upper GI fistulas in benign conditions.[24,25] Unfortunately, complications are frequent (20–40%).[26] Thoracic or epigastric pain is common after SEMS placement but is usually transient. Acute perforation is rare unless prior dilation was required. The risk of late perforation and bleeding seems to be higher with larger stents, and particular caution should be taken when stenting the gastroesophageal junction where asymmetrical pressure against the esophageal wall may precipitate ulceration, perforation, and/or bleeding. The use of larger stents, however, does decrease the rate of other adverse events, such as stent migration and tumor ingrowth.[26] After placement of a stent across the gastroesophageal junction, proton pump inhibitor (PPI) use and postural precautions are mandatory. The efficacy of antireflux stents has not been established.[27]

Late complications of stenting also include relapsing stenosis due to tissue hyperplasia (in the uncovered parts of partially covered stents) and tumor overgrowth. If the stent is placed for a benign indication, tissue hyperplasia may be treated by temporary placement of a second fully covered stent inside the first one, which will pressure necrose the inflammatory tissue and allow stent removal.[24,25,26] Following SEMS removal, secondary fibrotic strictures at the proximal or distal ends may occur, and are usually easily managed with dilation.

Polypectomy, Endoscopic Mucosal Resection, and Endoscopic Submucosal Dissection

Polypectomy, endoscopic mucosal resection (EMR), and endoscopic submucosal dissection (ESD) are commonly associated with bleeding, although most bleeding is intraprocedural, controlled endoscopically, and is not clinically relevant. Perforation occurs in 3% of esophageal resections and in 1% of gastric resections.[28,29,30] Cicatricial strictures are a late complication that mainly occur after circumferential esophageal resection.[31] Delayed bleeding after esophageal or gastric EMR/ESD is uncommon (< 5%).[28,30] To prevent delayed bleeding, some authors recommend coagulation of all visible submucosal vessels during the procedure for gastric resections, but this and second-look endoscopy are not routinely recommended.[32] PPI therapy is usually prescribed after the procedure. Delayed bleeding occurs more frequently after duodenal mucosal resection compared with esophageal and gastric resection, with bleeding rates ranging from 4 to 33%. Some authors suggest closure of the mucosa after resection with placement of multiple clips.[33]

In the last two decades, ablative therapies (such as argon plasma coagulation, photodynamic therapy, and mainly radiofrequency ablation) have emerged for the treatment of premalignant or early superficial malignant lesions, and as palliative therapy for some advanced tumors. Photosensitivity is a specific complication associated with the use of photodynamic therapy, but can also result in the development of strictures, especially when applied in the esophagus.[34,35] Stricture formation as a late complication can occur after circumferential radiofrequency ablation for treatment of dysplastic Barrett's esophagus.

Hemostasis of Nonvariceal Bleeding

Hemostasis of nonvariceal bleeding includes a combination of injection therapy and thermal or mechanical therapy. Although adrenaline injection (0.1 mg/mL) does not result in complications, injection of sclerosants (such as polidocanol, ethanolamine, or absolute alcohol) should be avoided as they do not control bleeding[36] and could lead to life-threatening tissue necrosis.[37] Coaptive coagulation can be obtained by the use of bipolar coagulation or heater probes. Perforation rates with these devices range from 0 to 2%, and are increased when treatment is repeated.[38,39] Monopolar probes have higher rates of perforation and have largely been abandoned.

Endoscopic tools available to treat esophageal variceal bleeding include band ligation, variceal obliteration, and sclerotherapy. Endoscopic band ligation is as effective as sclerotherapy with fewer and less severe complications (perforation rates: < 0.7 vs. 2–5%; superficial ulceration rates: 5–15 vs. 70–90%, respectively) and a major impact on overall mortality. It has become the preferred technique for acute bleeding, and primary and secondary prophylaxis of variceal bleeding.[40,41,42] Injection of cyanoacrylate is more effective than endoscopic band ligation for gastric variceal bleeding but is not without risks, such as embolization, which occurs in 2 to 5% of cases.[43] Pulmonary embolism is usually limited and with marginal clinical consequences. Paradoxical embolism may occur (especially in unsedated patients who have transient opening of the foramen ovale) with lethal outcome.

Removal of Foreign Bodies

Adverse event rates encountered during the removal of foreign bodies can reach 8%.[44] The most common complication is aspiration pneumonia, which can be prevented by endotracheal intubation, sometimes difficult in an emergency situation. Another major complication is mucosal tearing, which occurs during retrieval of sharp objects through the esophagus. Tearing can be prevented by using a protector hood at the distal extremity of the scope or by the use of an overtube. However, an overtube itself can induce mucosal tearing and perforation of the esophagus. Its use should be restricted to patients placed in the left lateral decubitus position in order to ensure neck overextension during overtube insertion.

10.3.3 Management of Upper Gastrointestinal Perforation

While perforation is a feared and well-known complication of upper GI endoscopy, its management has evolved and is no longer considered an absolute indication for surgery. Endoscopic closure of small perforations (< 2 cm) recognized during the procedure can be achieved using through-the-scope (TTS) clips. Larger over-the-scope closing devices may be useful in selected situations.[45,46] SEMSs (partially or fully covered) have also been used to treat large perforations, especially those occurring after dilatation.[24,26] An algorithm for the management of upper GI perforation is presented in ▶ Fig. 10.1.[27,45,47] Since prompt recognition and management of perforations is paramount, a careful examination at the end of a procedure in high-risk situations can be performed with injection of water-soluble contrast agents under fluoroscopy, if possible.

In the case of suspected delayed esophageal perforation (characterized by persistent or increasing pain, fever, respiratory distress, and hemodynamic instability), a water-soluble contrast radiographic study is the examination of choice. Alternatively, computed tomography (CT) scan of the neck and chest can be used. Endoscopic closure can be performed in concert with drainage of any fluid visualized collection, when possible.[24]

In the case of gastric or duodenal perforation, the same principles are applicable, but endoscopic closure mainly relies on the use of clips combined with gastric aspiration.[45]

10.3.4 Management of Upper GI Bleeding

Bleeding during therapeutic endoscopy is part of the procedure especially during polypectomy, EMR, or ESD. Immediate and late bleeding can be managed using coagulation forceps (preferred during EMR or ESD) or clips. Bleeding occurring after esophageal stenting, especially when occurring late after the initial procedure, should always be evaluated by proper imaging, given the potential risk of esophago-aortic fistulas.[48]

10.4 Small Bowel Endoscopy

Various endoscopic techniques can be used to explore the small intestine. These include push enteroscopy, single and double-balloon enteroscopy (SBE and DBE, respectively), spiral enteroscopy, and video capsule endoscopy. The most widely available published data concern DBE and video capsule endoscopy. The most common adverse events associated with DBE include perforation, bleeding, pancreatitis, and adverse events related to sedation. The rate of adverse events associated with DBE ranges from 0.4 to 0.8% for diagnostic procedures and 3 to 4% for therapeutic procedures.[49,50] The rate of pancreatitis associated with the antegrade DBE is consistently reported to be around 0.3%. The mechanisms of pancreatitis remain poorly understood. Pancreatitis may be prevented by avoiding inflation of the balloon at the duodenal level.[51] Management of perforation following enteroscopy usually requires prompt surgical intervention.

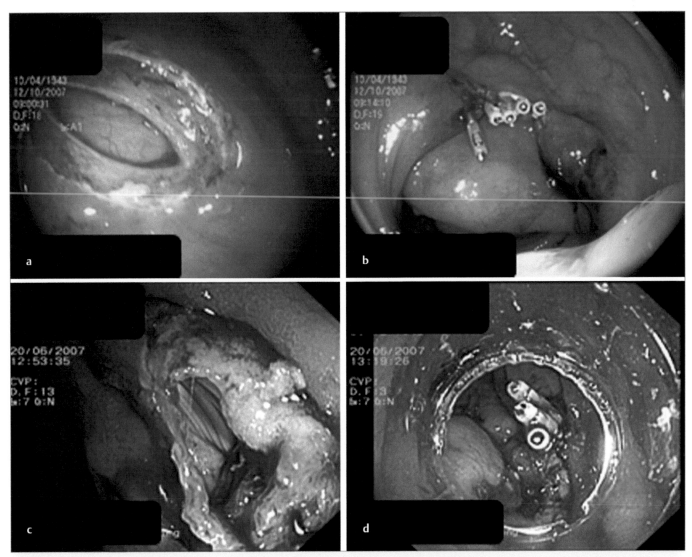

Fig. 10.1 Perforation during colonoscopy may occur after polypectomy (**a, c**) or may be due to direct trauma of the endoscope (**b, d**). When limited in size, most are amenable to immediate treatment with endoscopic clip placement.

The main complication of video capsule endoscopy is capsule retention (frequency 1–2%).[52] Retention is more common in cases of stenosis, especially those associated with Crohn's disease. The identification of a radiological abnormality of the small bowel is associated with a risk of capsule retention of 15.4%, usually requiring surgical or DBE exploration for retrieval.[53]

10.5 Colonoscopy

Colonoscopy is the gold standard for diagnosis of colorectal cancer and treatment of colorectal polyps. The rate of significant adverse events for diagnostic colonoscopy ranges from 0.02 to 0.07%.[54] The bowel preparation itself, if performed with sodium phosphate, may be associated with hypovolemia, hyperphosphatemia, and eventually death. Age, preexisting renal failure, and the use of nonsteroidal anti-inflammatory drugs (NSAIDs) are risks factors for this complication.[55]

10.5.1 Perforation

The reported frequency of this most feared complication varies in the literature. In a multicenter, prospective survey of 9,223 colonoscopies performed in England, the perforation rate was 0.11% for diagnostic and 0.21% for therapeutic colonoscopy.[54]

Three different mechanisms exist by which colonic perforation might occur during endoscopy: pneumatic perforation of an already weakened colonic wall; mechanical perforation owing to excessive pressure by the scope against the colonic wall; and posttherapeutic colonoscopy perforation, which can occur when the colonic wall has been made fragile by polypectomy, EMR, ESD, and/or coagulation during therapeutic colonoscopy. Following the results of a report of 183 colonic perforations, the most predominant site of perforation was the sigmoid colon (72%), followed by the ascending and descending colon (8.6% each), the rectum (6.9%), and the transverse colon (3.4%).[56] Risks factors for perforation during colonoscopy include the following: therapeutic colonoscopy (polypectomy, EMR, stricture dilation, and argon plasma coagulation use), age > 75 years, diverticular disease, previous intra-abdominal surgery, colonic obstruction, and female gender.[57]

Intraprocedural perforations occurring during EMR or ESD (the latter in approximately 30% of cases)[58] are frequently recognized immediately, with the "target sign" on the resection specimen useful. EMR perforation risk factors include transverse or right colon location, en-bloc resection, and presence of high-grade

dysplasia or submucosal cancer in the resected specimen.[59] In most situations, the recognition of peritoneal structures is obvious, but a sudden lack of insufflation and/or acute pain are signs that perforation has occurred.[56] In half of cases, perforations are < 2 cm in length and are not easily recognized. This is why, the diagnosis is often delayed (from 1 hour to weeks after the procedure).[56] An overt perforation with associated peritonitis is easy to diagnose, while patients having localized peritoneal signs due to minimal perforation, sometimes delayed and known as "the postpolypectomy syndrome" or "transmural burn syndrome," may be more challenging to diagnose. The clinical outcome of postpolypectomy syndrome is usually favorable with conservative treatment.[58] In any case of suspected perforation, an abdominal CT scan is the preferred examination for differentiating colonic perforation from postpolypectomy syndrome, which is characterized by the absence of diffuse air leak.

10.5.2 Management of Colonic Perforation

Owing to the frequency and diversity of perforation types (mechanisms, size, and location), management remains controversial (▶ Fig. 10.2).[60,61,62,63,64] Endoscopic techniques that have been used to close GI perforations in the setting of natural orifice translumenal endoscopic surgery (NOTES) and submucosal dissection have resulted in enhanced management strategies for perforations and are expected to evolve.

Although most patients with colonic perforation require surgical intervention, some can be effectively managed conservatively, especially if the endoscopist is able to close the perforation endoscopically.[65,66] The efficacy of clipping, in terms of intention to treat, is not fully determined; a review of 75 cases revealed a success rate ranging from 69 to 93%, without mortality in patients in whom endoscopic closure was achieved,[66] but these values are probably overestimates. Key factors for endoscopic success are small perforations (<2 cm), early recognition, a clean bowel, and prompt and complete closure.[67] Over-the-scope clips, such as the OVESCO (Ovesco Endoscopy, Germany), are being used with favorable results. A recent systematic review of all iatrogenic GI perforations reported clinically successful endoscopic closure in 90% using standard clips and 88% using over-the-scope clips.[45] Although this likely does not represent a true comparison, it stresses the fact that, at least in the colon, standard TTS clips remain the first choice.[59] Prospective randomized studies are needed to define the role of

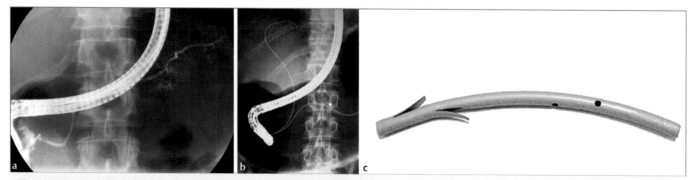

Fig. 10.2 Intrarectal indometacin must be administered before any procedure performed on an intact papilla. High-risk patients (acinarization **[a]**, multiple manipulations on a normal pancreas) may benefit from additional prevention of pancreatitis with PPS. If a guidewire is inserted into the pancreas, it can be left in place and may facilitate further biliary cannulation **(b)**. At the end of the procedure, it is used to insert a PPS (5Fr, without proximal flaps) **(c)**.

various techniques of endoscopic closures. When endoscopic treatment of a perforation is foreseen, CO_2 insufflation (if not already used) should be immediately instituted and special attention given to a possible drop in blood pressure related to a decreased cardiac preload induced by intraperitoneal hypertension. Prompt peritoneal decompression should be performed by needle puncture. Conservative treatment consists of bowel rest, intravenous hydration, administration of broad-spectrum antibiotics, and close clinical monitoring. Successful closure is noted by clinical improvement within the first 48 hours. Such an approach can be considered for all patients who are in good clinical condition with localized symptoms of peritonitis and in whom the perforation is contained, either by endoscopic closure or by spontaneous sealing.[67,68]

Surgical treatment is standard for patients with generalized peritonitis and/or objective failure of endoscopic closure, in patients who deteriorate under conservative treatment, and finally in patients presenting with colonic disease that otherwise requires surgery (such as colon cancer). Simple closure of the perforation is often possible in the absence of intraperitoneal fecal contamination; resection with immediate intestinal anastomosis and colectomy with temporary colostomy are alternatives.

The outcomes of patients with colonic perforation requiring surgery are associated with morbidity and mortality rates of 21 to 53% and 0 to 26%, respectively.[57,58,68] Surgical site infection is frequent, and leading causes of death are cardiopulmonary complications and multiple organ failure.[57,58]

10.5.3 Bleeding

Bleeding is the most frequent complication after polypectomy (incidence: 0.3–6.1%).[69,70] There is no evidence that aspirin or NSAID use increases the risk of bleeding after mucosal biopsy or polypectomy.[71] However, the reader is referred to national societal guidelines concerning the management of anticoagulation and antiplatelet agents during endoscopy.[5] The risk of bleeding depends on the type and size of the polyp and the technique of polypectomy.

Immediate bleeding occurring during endoscopy (1.5% of cases) must be differentiated from delayed bleeding occurring from a few hours to 1 month after polypectomy (2% of cases). In most cases, persistent active bleeding can be managed endoscopically using endoscopic hemostatic tools, such as snaring of residual stalks for compression, epinephrine injection, electrocautery (coagulation forceps or tip of the snare), endoloop, and clips. The use of cautery should be performed with caution owing to the thinness of the colonic wall. Immediate bleeding may be prevented by the use of pure coagulation for pedunculated polyps,[72] epinephrine injection, clipping, or closing the stalk with an endoloop. No prophylactic measures have proved to be efficient in preventing delayed bleeding.[73] Bleeding occurring during EMR or ESD is preferably managed by coagulation.[74]

10.5.4 Unusual Complications

Very rare adverse events associated with colonoscopy include glutaraldehyde-induced colitis (probably due to endoscope mishandling during reprocessing) and extracolonic trauma such as splenic rupture and liver hematoma due to excessive abdominal pressure exerted during difficult insertion.[75,76]

10.6 ERCP

ERCP has changed the paradigm of management of biliopancreatic diseases but is also one of the most demanding endoscopic procedures. In addition to adverse events common with upper GI endoscopic procedures, specific adverse events related to biliopancreatic manipulations include bleeding, perforation, infection, and pancreatitis[77] (see ▶Table 10.2). According to a retrospective review of 21 studies, including 16,855 patients, the incidence rate of ERCP-related complications was 6.85% (1.67% were severe complications), with a mortality rate of 0.33%.[78] These findings were confirmed in two prospective studies, including 7,252 patients, with an overall complication rate of 5.3% and mortality rate of 0.34%.[79,80] Important factors modulating the risk of complications are the indication for ERCP and the case volume of the operator, which could be responsible for a two- to threefold increase in the rate of severe complications.[81] For these reasons, the need for concentrating these procedures in high-volume centers has become more and more obvious over the last two decades.

Table 10.2 ERCP complications classification

	Mild	Moderate	Severe
Bleeding	Hemoglobin drop < 3 g/dL and no need for transfusion	Transfusion of ≤ 4 units and no angiographic or surgical intervention	Transfusion of ≥ 5 units or surgical/radiological intervention
Perforation	Possible or only a very slight leak of fluid or contrast agent, treatable by fluid and suction for 3 days or less	Any definite perforation treated medically for 4–10 days	Medical treatment for more than 10 days or intervention (percutaneous, endoscopic, or surgical)
Infection (cholangitis)	More than 38°C for 24–48 hours	Febrile or septic illness requiring >3 days of hospital treatment or endoscopic or percutaneous intervention	Septic shock or surgery
Post-ERCP pancreatitis	Clinical pancreatitis, amylase levels at least three times normal at more than 24 hours after the procedure, requiring admission or prolongation of planned hospitalization	Pancreatitis requiring hospitalization of 4–10 days	Hospitalization for >10 days, or hemorrhagic pancreatitis, phlegmon or pseudocyst, or intervention (percutaneous drainage or surgery)

Source: Adapted with permission from Cotton PB et al, Gastrointest Endosc 1991; 37(3): 383–393.

10.6.1 Bleeding

Bleeding is often associated with sphincterotomy, and occurs in 1.3% of ERCPs with a reported mortality rate of 0.05%.[78] Half are recognized during the procedure.[81,82] Most bleeding is mild to moderate in severity. Risk factors are related to: the patient's condition, such as cholangitis before the procedure; coagulopathy, liver cirrhosis, or chronic renal failure; anatomical variants (peripapillary diverticulum, stone impaction, papillary stenosis, and Billroth II gastrectomy); or the technique used and the operator (low case volume of the unit or operator, needle knife sphincterotomy, sphincterotomy length, and "recut" of a previous sphincterotomy).[77,81,82,83]

Most patients can be managed by medical and endoscopic treatment.[77] Treatment of postsphincterotomy bleeding includes the use of epinephrine injection (0.1 mg/mL) for oozing-type bleeding.[84] Additional thermal methods, such as sphincterotome wire and electrocautery/heater probe use, can be used in the management of a visible vessel or a bleeding point.[85] Mechanical devices, such as TTS clips, although difficult to manipulate with a side-viewing scope, can be used as second-line treatment to control bleeding at the level of the sphincterotomy, avoiding its placement on the pancreatic orifice.[86] Balloon tamponade at the site of sphincterotomy has been described but its efficacy has not been established.[87]

The use of the Endocut Mode (Erbe, Inc., Germany), an automatically controlled cut/coagulation system, has become widely adopted and reduces the rate of minor bleeding.[88,89] Finally, for patients with altered anatomy or with coagulation disorders, balloon sphincteroplasty (endoscopic papillary balloon dilation) could be used since it reduces the risk of bleeding (but unfortunately increases the risk of pancreatitis when performed on an intact papilla).[77]

10.6.2 Perforation

Perforation, although rare, is one of the most feared adverse events of ERCP, occurring in 0.6% of the procedures.[77,78] The most frequent is retroperitoneal duodenal perforation occurring at the site of sphincterotomy. Free peritoneal perforation of the duodenum or jejunum is rare and often associated with altered anatomy (Billroth II gastrectomy, duodenal stricture, or peridiverticular papilla). Perforation of the bile duct itself usually follows stricture dilation or traumatic wire insertion through a stricture.[90] Most patients with free peritoneal perforation will require surgery, whilst most patients with retroperitoneal duodenal perforation can be initially managed conservatively with nasogastric suction, hydration, and administration of broad-spectrum antibiotics. If possible, a nasobiliary catheter should be placed to ensure external biliary or pancreatic drainage. When retroperitoneal perforation is recognized during the procedure, this placement should be immediately attempted. Surgical or radiological drainage of retroperitoneal collections should be considered on a case-by-case basis, keeping in mind the severity of this complication with a reported mortality around 5%.[78,81,91,92]

ERCP-related perforation can largely be prevented by using a finely-tuned technique of sphincterotomy, always performed over a guidewire, ensuring correct orientation of the cutting wire during the course of the sphincterotomy. Incision should be performed step by step, avoiding a zipper cut, recognizing the anatomy of the papilla, and tailoring the size of the sphincterotomy to the size of distal common bile duct. In difficult cases or for removal of large stones, endoscopic balloon dilation of the papilla after a small or incomplete sphincterotomy is now a valid option.[93,94]

10.6.3 Infections

Post-ERCP infections include cholangitis, cholecystitis, and "pancreatic sepsis" (which may refer to severe necrotic pancreatitis and/or infection of a pseudocyst). Cholangitis and sepsis occur in more than 85% of patients whose opacified bile ducts drain incompletely.[95] Post-ERCP acute cholecystitis has an incidence rate of < 0.5% and may be related to the injection of contrast medium into a poorly emptying gallbladder or to the occlusion of the cystic duct by a tumor, a stone, and/or a covered self-expandable stent.[77]

Properly disinfected endoscopes and use of sterile accessories are paramount in prevention. Drainage of any opacified obstructed structure is recommended and "diagnostic" opacification of an obstructed duct is strictly contraindicated. Antibiotic prophylaxis has proven effective in patients at risk of infective endocarditis, in patients known to have a pancreatic pseudocyst, or in patients displaying cholestasis or jaundice with enlarged bile ducts.[96,97] This prophylaxis should be prolonged if drainage is incomplete.

10.6.4 Post-ERCP Pancreatitis

Post-ERCP pancreatitis (PEP) remains the most prevalent cause of morbidity and mortality after ERCP. Although its incidence has decreased with improved techniques and indications as well as with prophylactic measures, it remains above 2% in large cohorts.[98,99] It is a clinical situation in which new postprocedural pancreatic pain is associated with at least a threefold increase in serum levels of amylase or lipase.[100] The severity of PEP is defined on the basis of the additional length of hospital stay needed to manage the condition (▶ Table 10.2). Different risk factors related to the operator case volume, to the procedure itself, and to patient susceptibility have been recognized in large prospective studies (▶ Box 10.1).[78,81] Severe PEP accounts for less than 10% of PEP cases[100]; although risk factors for PEP have been identified, predictors of severity are lacking. The only drug prophylaxis for PEP that has proven efficient is intrarectal administration of 100 mg of diclofenac or indomethacin, and this has been adopted as standard therapy to be given for any ERCP performed on an intact papilla (or involving manipulations on the pancreatic duct).[98,101] In addition, it was recently shown that such prophylaxis should be given systematically before the procedure and not "on demand" according to the per-procedures findings or events.[102] Over the past 20 years, two major endoscopic techniques for preventing PEP in high-risk patients have been developed: guidewire-directed biliary cannulation[103] and prophylactic pancreatic stent (PPS) insertion. Four meta-analyses of prospective, randomized trials comparing PEP rates with and without PPS insertion conclude that PPS not only reduces PEP rates but also decreases the rate of severe cases of PEP in high-risk patients.[104,105,106] This finding was confirmed in the intention-to-treat analysis of studies investigating the risk of PEP development, which included patients in whom PPS insertion failed.[107] Nevertheless, PPS placement is associated with an adverse event rate of 4%,[107] mainly related to guidewire- or stent-induced pancreatic duct injuries. The additional benefit of PPS in average-risk ERCPs when NSAIDs are administered is unclear, and its use should be limited to higher risk cases, mainly when a manipulation of the pancreatic duct is performed, in case of precut or papillectomy or when acinarization is observed. Three- or five-centimeter-long 5 French PPS without internal (proximal) flange but with external (distal) flaps are considered the best choice.[108,109] PPS insertion is strongly recommended, despite the recognized complications, in patients who are at high risk of PEP (▶ Box 10.2).[98,110,111] Finally, the best way to prevent complications is not to perform the procedure, and recently, one of the most controversial indications, sphincter of Oddi dysfunction type III, associated with highest risk of PEP has been shown to be ineffectively treated with biliary sphincterotomy.[112]

Box 10.1 Patient- and procedure-related risk factors of Post-ERCP pancreatitis (PEP)

Patient-related factors
- Female gender
- Young age
- History of suspected sphincter of Oddi dysfunction
- History of pancreatitis, recurrent or post-ERCP pancreatitis

Procedure-related factors
- Difficult or multiple cannulation attempts
- Multiple pancreatic contrast injections
- Pancreatic acinarization
- Precut sphincterotomy
- Endoscopic papillary balloon dilation
- Sphincter of Oddi manometry
- Distal common bile duct diameter ≤ 10 mm
- Procedures not involving stone removal

Source: Adapted with permission from Woods KE, Willingham FF. World J Gastrointest Endosc. 2010; 2(5): 165–78.

Box 10.2 Indications for prophylactic pancreatic stent placement during ERCP

Definitive
- Pancreatic sphincterotomy for sphincter of Oddi dysfunction/acute recurrent pancreatitis
- Ampullectomy

Highly recommended
- Difficult biliary cannulation, involving instrumentation or injection of the pancreatic duct
- Pancreatic sphincterotomy (major and minor)
- Aggressive instrumentation of the pancreatic duct (cytology brushing, biopsies)
- Balloon dilatation of an intact biliary sphincter (balloon sphincteroplasty)
- Prior PEP
- Precut sphincterotomy starting at the papillary orifice

Source: Adapted with permission from Devière J. Gastrointest Endosc Clin N Am. 2011; 21(3): 499–510.

PEP is mild to moderate in >90% of the cases.[98,100] PEP is managed as with pancreatitis from other etiologies.

10.7 Other Techniques

Over the last 10 years, the therapeutic capabilities of endoscopy have been extended to techniques involving the passage of instruments through the GI tract or of endoscopes into the submucosal space. Most of these techniques are still in development, and all of these should be done in high-volume centers with extensive technical experience. Some of these procedures, however, have become part of the routine armamentarium in large endoscopy units, such as EUS-guided celiac block/neurolysis for refractory pancreatic pain, EUS-guided cyst drainages, and POEM for achalasia. The major potential complications associated with these techniques are summarized.

10.7.1 EUS-Guided Celiac Block/Neurolysis

This technique used for managing pain related to pancreatic cancer or chronic pancreatitis is usually used in cases not manageable with usual drug therapy. It consists of injecting absolute ethanol or corticoids at the bifurcation between the aorta and the celiac trunk. Usually, the needle is flushed with local anesthetic, which is injected initially. This reduces the transient exacerbation of pain (reported in up to 30% of cases) but also confirms the injection takes place outside the stomach and is not intravascular. Indeed, intramural injection may lead to necrosis of the gastric wall and abscess formation (especially when neurolysis is performed), while damage to a vessel can induce bleeding or rare spinal cord injury. Another delayed complication, almost unpreventable, is diarrhea. This occurs in 3 to 5% of the cases, and is often transient and managed symptomatically.[113,114]

10.7.2 EUS-Guided Drainage of Pancreatic Fluid Collections

Endotherapy has become accepted as a gold standard for management of symptomatic pancreatic pseudocysts and acute fluid collections.[115] Complications related with this technique may occur during the procedure or delayed. Periprocedural complications include bleeding, of which the incidence has been dramatically reduced with the use of linear EUS endoscopes to perform the procedure, and leakage of the pseudocyst contents. If a bleeding occurs during the procedure, it is most often due to puncture of a vessel. A coagulation device (Cystotome, Cook Endoscopy, Winston-Salem, North Carolina, United States; Endoflex, Voerde, Germany) can be used and the procedure completed by the placement plastic stents or SEMSs, which will also has a tamponade effect.[116] However, there are no established indications for SEMS placement for pseudocyst drainage. Recently developed short, biflanged stents (Axios, Boston Scientific, Marlborough, Massachusetts, United States; Nagi stent, Taewoong, Seoul, Korea; Spaxus stent, Taewoong, Seoul, Korea) are useful for drainage of pseudocysts and necrosis and facilitating access to pancreatic necrosis for direct necrosectomy. They may be associated with severe complications, mainly vascular injuries.[117] Leakage following placement usually occurs either by loss of guidewire access after puncture or by misdeployment or slippage into the peritoneal cavity when the collection is not bulging into the GI tract. If such a leak occurs, the first priority is to regain access to the residual cavity and provide adequate decompression.

Delayed bleeding may also occur within a few days after the procedure. In this case, it is most often due to a pseudoaneurysm, and the initial therapeutic approach should be an interventional angiography.

Finally, a late complication is recurrence of the collection after stent removal. It is most often due to the presence of a disconnected pancreatic duct.[118] Magnetic resonance pancreatography (if possible with secretin) is recommended before any decision to remove the transmural stents. If ductal disconnection is present, stents (exclusively plastic, not SEMS) should remain in place indefinitely.

10.7.3 Peroral Endoscopic Myotomy

POEM, and more largely any intervention requiring access to the submucosal space (also called third space endoscopy to differentiate it from the luminal and extraluminal cavities), including esophageal or pyloric myotomies but also resection of submucosal tumors, has become a standard procedure in tertiary specialized centers. These techniques offer new possibilities of treatment, potentially more effective than surgery in selected cases. They are, however, associated with specific complications. In one of the largest series to date,[119] (1,680 patients treated with POEM), major complications occurred in 55 (3.3%) patients, including 13 (0.8%) postoperative mucosa breach, 3 (0.2%) delayed bleeding, 8 (0.5%) hydrothorax, 25 (1.5%) pneumothorax that required thoracic tube placement, and 6 (0.4%) other complications. Four patients required ICU admission and 14 (0.8%) stayed more than 10 days in the hospital. The rate of major complications decreased over time and reached a plateau of 1% after 3.5 years. Multivariate analysis identified experience < 1 year (odds ratio [OR], 3.00; 95% confidence interval [CI], 1.12–8.06), air insufflation (OR, 2.78; 95% CI, 1.03–7.52), and mucosal edema (OR 1.92; 95% CI, 1.05–3.49) as risk factors. Other than the need for case volume and experience, it is clear that CO_2 insufflation is essential when performing such procedures.

When performed by experienced physicians, these techniques are very safe, but one must be aware about incidental imaging findings such as pneumomediastinum, pneumothorax, and pneumoperitoneum, which are not as common with other endoscopic techniques. When pneumoperitoneum occurs during the procedure, it must be relieved when associated with hemodynamic disturbances. The presence of free air must only be considered when associated with clinical symptoms and one should understand this to avoid unnecessary interventions.[120]

10.8 Conclusion

Therapeutic endoscopy continues to progress and therefore potential complications need to be recognized and properly prevented and treated. Prevention of complications relies on a fine knowledge of the patient's condition and procedural indications. Scheduling must consider the available resources, evaluate if proper experience is available, and draw different strategies for managing complications. Early diagnosis of complications and multidisciplinary approach are paramount. The best approach will, in most cases, be dictated by local expertise. Concentration of cases will become necessary with the sophistication of techniques, which will require more resources and experience and patient education about the risks. Local expertise will remain a cornerstone in management.

10.9 Key Points

- Avoidance of unnecessary invasive examinations is the best way to prevent adverse events.
- Preprocedural patient information and informed consent are paramount.
- Acquiring and maintaining experience and competency in specific procedures is essential to reduce the risk of adverse events. Inexperienced and/or undertrained endoscopists should avoid performing advanced complex, therapeutic endoscopic procedures.
- Standardization of training and adherence to guidelines are required in order to prevent and manage adverse events.
- Assessing center- and operator-specific complication rates are important issues leading to improved quality and safety.

References

[1] Cotton PB, Eisen GM, Aabakken L, et al. A lexicon for endoscopic adverse events: report of an ASGE workshop. Gastrointest Endosc. 2010; 71(3):446–454

[2] Cai MY, Zhou PH, Yao LQ, et al. Thoracic CT after peroral endoscopic myotomy for the treatment of achalasia. Gastrointest Endosc. 2014; 80(6):1046–1055

[3] Quine MA, Bell GD, McCloy RF, et al. Prospective audit of upper gastrointestinal endoscopy in two regions of England: safety, staffing, and sedation methods. Gut. 1995; 36(3):462–467

[4] Vargo JJ, Niklewski PJ, Williams JL, et al. Patient safety during sedation by anesthesia professionals during routine upper endoscopy and colonoscopy: an analysis of 1.38 million procedures. Gastrointest Endosc. 2017; 85(1):101–108

[5] Veitch AM, Vanbiervliet G, Gershlick AH, et al. Endoscopy in patients on antiplatelet or anticoagulant therapy, including direct oral anticoagulants: British Society of Gastroenterology (BSG) and European Society of Gastrointestinal Endoscopy (ESGE) guidelines. Endoscopy. 2016; 48(4):c1

[6] Kimmey MB, Burnett DA, Carr-Locke DL, et al. Technology assessment position paper: transmission of infection by gastrointestinal endoscopy. Gastrointest Endosc. 1993; 39:885–888

[7] Petersen BT, Chennat J, Cohen J, et al; ASGE Quality Assurance In Endoscopy Committee. Society for Healthcare Epidemiology of America. Multisociety guideline on reprocessing flexible gastrointestinal endoscopes: 2011. Gastrointest Endosc. 2011; 73(6):1075–1084

[8] Beilenhoff U, Neumann CS, Biering H, et al; ESGE. ESGENA. ESGE/ESGENA guideline for process validation and routine testing for reprocessing endoscopes in washer-disinfectors, according to the European Standard prEN ISO 15883 parts 1, 4 and 5. Endoscopy. 2007; 39(1):85–94

[9] Rubin ZA, Murthy RK. Outbreaks associated with duodenoscopes: new challenges and controversies. Curr Opin Infect Dis. 2016; 29(4):407–414

[10] U.S. Public Health Service. Updated U.S. Public Health Service guidelines for the management of occupational exposures to HBV, HCV and HIV and recommandations for post-exposure prophylaxis. MMWR. 2001; 50:1–42

[11] Silvis SE, Nebel O, Rogers G, et al. Endoscopic complications. Results of the 1974 American Society for Gastrointestinal Endoscopy Survey. JAMA. 1976; 235(9):928–930

[12] Montalvo RD, Lee M. Retrospective analysis of iatrogenic Mallory-Weiss tears occurring during upper gastrointestinal endoscopy. Hepatogastroenterology. 1996; 43(7):174–177

[13] Van Os EC, Kamath PS, Gostout CJ, Heit JA. Gastroenterological procedures among patients with disorders of hemostasis: evaluation and management recommendations. Gastrointest Endosc. 1999; 50(4):536–543

[14] Straumann A, Bussmann C, Zuber M, et al. Eosinophilic esophagitis: analysis of food impaction and perforation in 251 adolescent and adult patients. Clin Gastroenterol Hepatol. 2008; 6(5):598–600

[15] Green J. BSG guidelines: complications of gastrointestinal endoscopy. 2006. Available at: www.bsg.org.uk

[16] Siddiqui N, Katznelson R, Friedman Z. Heart rate/blood pressure response and airway morbidity following tracheal intubation with direct laryngoscopy, GlideScope and Trachlight: a randomized control trial. Eur J Anaesthesiol. 2009; 26(9):740–745

[17] Boeckxstaens GE, Annese V, des Varannes SB, et al; European Achalasia Trial Investigators. Pneumatic dilation versus laparoscopic Heller's myotomy for idiopathic achalasia. N Engl J Med. 2011; 364(19):1807–1816

[18] Bechara R, Ikeda H, Inoue H. Peroral endoscopic myotomy: an evolving treatment for achalasia. Nat Rev Gastroenterol Hepatol. 2015; 12(7):410–426

[19] Hernandez LV, Jacobson JW, Harris MS. Comparison among the perforation rates of Maloney, balloon, and savary dilation of esophageal strictures. Gastrointest Endosc. 2000; 51(4 Pt 1):460–462

[20] Metman EH, Lagasse JP, d'Alteroche L, et al. Risk factors for immediate complications after progressive pneumatic dilation for achalasia. Am J Gastroenterol. 1999; 94(5):1179–1185

[21] Saeed ZA, Winchester CB, Ferro PS, et al. Prospective randomized comparison of polyvinyl bougies and through-the-scope balloons for dilation of peptic strictures of the esophagus. Gastrointest Endosc. 1995; 41(3):189–195

[22] Nicholson DA, Haycox A, Kay CL, et al. The cost effectiveness of metal oesophageal stenting in malignant disease compared with conventional therapy. Clin Radiol. 1999; 54(4):212–215

[23] Dumonceau JM, Cremer M, Lalmand B, Devière J. Esophageal fistula sealing: choice of stent, practical management, and cost. Gastrointest Endosc. 1999; 49(1):70–78

[24] Swinnen J, Eisendrath P, Rigaux J, et al. Self-expandable metal stents for the treatment of benign upper GI leaks and perforations. Gastrointest Endosc. 2011; 73(5):890–899

[25] Murino A, Arvanitakis M, Le Moine O, et al. Effectiveness of Endoscopic Management Using Self-Expandable Metal Stents in a Large Cohort of Patients with Post-bariatric Leaks. Obes Surg. 2015; 25(9):1569–1576

[26] Spaander MC, Baron TH, Siersema PD, et al. Esophageal stenting for benign and malignant disease: European Society of Gastrointestinal Endoscopy (ESGE) Clinical Guideline. Endoscopy. 2016; 48(10):939–948

[27] Sgourakis G, Gockel I, Radtke A, et al. The use of self-expanding stents in esophageal and gastroesophageal junction cancer palliation: a meta-analysis and meta-regression analysis of outcomes. Dig Dis Sci. 2010; 55(11):3018–3030

[28] May A, Gossner L, Behrens A, et al. A prospective randomized trial of two different endoscopic resection techniques for early stage cancer of the esophagus. Gastrointest Endosc. 2003; 58(2):167–175

[29] Okano A, Hajiro K, Takakuwa H, et al. Predictors of bleeding after endoscopic mucosal resection of gastric tumors. Gastrointest Endosc. 2003; 57(6):687–690

[30] Ahmad NA, Kochman ML, Long WB, et al. Efficacy, safety, and clinical outcomes of endoscopic mucosal resection: a study of 101 cases. Gastrointest Endosc. 2002; 55(3):390–396

[31] Katada C, Muto M, Manabe T, et al. Esophageal stenosis after endoscopic mucosal resection of superficial esophageal lesions. Gastrointest Endosc. 2003; 57(2):165–169

[32] Kim EH, Park SW, Nam E, et al. The role of second-look endoscopy and prophylactic hemostasis after gastric endoscopic submucosal dissection: A systematic review and meta-analysis. J Gastroenterol Hepatol. 2017; 32(4):756–768

[33] Apel D, Jakobs R, Spiethoff A, Riemann JF. Follow-up after endoscopic snare resection of duodenal adenomas. Endoscopy. 2005; 37(5):444–448

[34] Dumot JA, Greenwald BD. Argon plasma coagulation, bipolar cautery, and cryotherapy: ABC's of ablative techniques. Endoscopy. 2008; 40(12):1026–1032

[35] Pouw RE, Sharma VK, Bergman JJ, Fleischer DE. Radiofrequency ablation for total Barrett's eradication: a description of the endoscopic technique, its clinical results and future prospects. Endoscopy. 2008; 40(12):1033–1040

[36] Marmo R, Rotondano G, Piscopo R, et al. Dual therapy versus monotherapy in the endoscopic treatment of high-risk bleeding ulcers: a meta-analysis of controlled trials. Am J Gastroenterol. 2007; 102(2):279–289, quiz 469

[37] Lazo MD, Andrade R, Medina MC, et al. Effect of injection sclerosis with alcohol on the rebleeding rate of gastroduodenal peptic ulcers with nonbleeding visible vessels: a prospective, controlled trial. Am J Gastroenterol. 1992; 87(7):843–846

[38] Rutgeerts P, Vantrappen G, Van Hootegem P, et al. Neodymium-YAG laser photocoagulation versus multipolar electrocoagulation for the treatment of severely bleeding ulcers: a randomized comparison. Gastrointest Endosc. 1987; 33(3):199–202

[39] Lau JYW, Sung JJ, Lam YH, et al. Endoscopic retreatment compared with surgery in patients with recurrent bleeding after initial endoscopic control of bleeding ulcers. N Engl J Med. 1999; 340(10):751–756

[40] Lo GH, Lai KH, Cheng JS, et al. Emergency banding ligation versus sclerotherapy for the control of active bleeding from esophageal varices. Hepatology. 1997; 25(5):1101–1104

[41] Stiegmann GV, Goff JS, Michaletz-Onody PA, et al. Endoscopic sclerotherapy as compared with endoscopic ligation for bleeding esophageal varices. N Engl J Med. 1992; 326(23):1527–1532

[42] de Franchis R. Updating consensus in portal hypertension: report of the Baveno III Consensus Workshop on definitions, methodology and therapeutic strategies in portal hypertension. J Hepatol. 2000; 33(5):846–852

[43] Binmoeller KF. Glue for gastric varices: some sticky issues. Gastrointest Endosc. 2000; 52(2):298–301

[44] Ikenberry SO, Jue TL, Anderson MA, et al; ASGE Standards of Practice Committee. Management of ingested foreign bodies and food impactions. Gastrointest Endosc. 2011; 73(6):1085–1091

[45] Verlaan T, Voermans RP, van Berge Henegouwen MI, et al. Endoscopic closure of acute perforations of the GI tract: a systematic review of the literature. Gastrointest Endosc. 2015; 82(4):618–28.e5

[46] Voermans RP, Le Moine O, von Renteln D, et al; CLIPPER Study Group. Efficacy of endoscopic closure of acute perforations of the gastrointestinal tract. Clin Gastroenterol Hepatol. 2012; 10(6):603–608

[47] Kowalczyk L, Forsmark CE, Ben-David K, et al. Algorithm for the management of endoscopic perforations: a quality improvement project. Am J Gastroenterol. 2011; 106(6):1022–1027

[48] Lindenmann J, Maier A, Fink-Neuboeck N, et al. Fatal aortic hemorrhage after OTSC and subsequent esophageal stenting for sealing of iatrogenic esophageal perforation. Endoscopy. 2015; 47:E-280–E-281

[49] Mensink PB, Haringsma J, Kucharzik T, et al. Complications of double balloon enteroscopy: a multicenter survey. Endoscopy. 2007; 39(7):613–615

[50] Möschler O, May A, Müller MK, Ell C; German DBE Study Group. Complications in and performance of double-balloon enteroscopy (DBE): results from a large prospective DBE database in Germany. Endoscopy. 2011; 43(6):484–489

[51] Kopacova M, Tacheci I, Rejchrt S, et al. Double balloon enteroscopy and acute pancreatitis. World J Gastroenterol. 2010; 16(19):2331–2340

[52] Karagiannis S, Faiss S, Mavrogiannis C. Capsule retention: a feared complication of wireless capsule endoscopy. Scand J Gastroenterol. 2009; 44(10):1158–1165

[53] Atay O, Mahajan L, Kay M, et al. Risk of capsule endoscope retention in pediatric patients: a large single-center experience and review of the literature. J Pediatr Gastroenterol Nutr. 2009; 49(2):196–201

[54] Bowles CJ, Leicester R, Romaya C, et al. A prospective study of colonoscopy practice in the UK today: are we adequately prepared for national colorectal cancer screening tomorrow? Gut. 2004; 53(2):277–283

[55] Thomson A, Naidoo P, Crotty B. Bowel preparation for colonoscopy: a randomized prospective trail comparing sodium phosphate and polyethylene glycol in a predominantly elderly population. J Gastroenterol Hepatol. 1996; 11(2):103–107

[56] Garbay JR, Suc B, Rotman N, et al. Multicentre study of surgical complications of colonoscopy. Br J Surg. 1996; 83(1):42–44

[57] Lohsiriwat V. Colonoscopic perforation: incidence, risk factors, management and outcome. World J Gastroenterol. 2010; 16(4):425–430

[58] Repici A, Tricerri R. Endoscopic polypectomy: techniques, complications and follow-up. Tech Coloproctol. 2004; 8(Suppl 2):s283–s290

[59] Burgess NG, Bassan MS, Mc Leod D, et al. Deep mural injury and perforation after colonic endoscopic mucosal resection: a new classification and analysis of risk factors. Gut. 2016:(e-pub ahead of print)

[60] Agresta F, Michelet I, Mainente P, Bedin N. Laparoscopic management of colonoscopic perforations. Surg Endosc. 2000; 14(6):592–593

[61] Hansen AJ, Tessier DJ, Anderson ML, Schlinkert RT. Laparoscopic repair of colonoscopic perforations: indications and guidelines. J Gastrointest Surg. 2007; 11(5):655–659

[62] Kilic A, Kavic SM. Laparoscopic colotomy repair following colonoscopic polypectomy. JSLS. 2008; 12(1):93–96

[63] Makharia GK, Madan K, Garg PK, Tandon RK. Colonoscopic barotrauma treated by conservative management: role of high-flow oxygen inhalation. Endoscopy. 2002; 34(12):1010–1013

[64] Donckier V, André R. Treatment of colon endoscopic perforations. Acta Chir Belg. 1993; 93(2):60–62

[65] Avgerinos DV, Llaguna OH, Lo AY, Leitman IM. Evolving management of colonoscopic perforations. J Gastrointest Surg. 2008; 12(10):1783–1789

[66] Parodi A, Repici A, Pedroni A, et al. Endoscopic management of GI perforations with a new over-the-scope clip device (with videos). Gastrointest Endosc. 2010; 72(4):881–886

[67] Cobb WS, Heniford BT, Sigmon LB, et al. Colonoscopic perforations: incidence, management, and outcomes. Am Surg. 2004; 70(9):750–757, discussion 757–758

[68] Iqbal CW, Cullinane DC, Schiller HJ, et al. Surgical management and outcomes of 165 colonoscopic perforations from a single institution. Arch Surg. 2008; 143(7):701–706, discussion 706–707

[69] Gibbs DH, Opelka FG, Beck DE, et al. Postpolypectomy colonic hemorrhage. Dis Colon Rectum. 1996; 39(7):806–810

[70] Sorbi D, Norton I, Conio M, et al. Postpolypectomy lower GI bleeding: descriptive analysis. Gastrointest Endosc. 2000; 51(6):690–696

[71] Hui AJ, Wong RM, Ching JY, et al. Risk of colonoscopic polypectomy bleeding with anticoagulants and antiplatelet agents: analysis of 1657 cases. Gastrointest Endosc. 2004; 59(1):44–48

[72] Van Gossum A, Cozzoli A, Adler M, et al. Colonoscopic snare polypectomy: analysis of 1485 resections comparing two types of current. Gastrointest Endosc. 1992; 38(4):472–475

[73] Lee CK, Lee SH, Park JY, et al. Prophylactic argon plasma coagulation ablation does not decrease delayed postpolypectomy bleeding. Gastrointest Endosc. 2009; 70(2):353–361

[74] Neuhaus H. ESD around the world: Europe. Gastrointest Endosc Clin N Am. 2014; 24(2):295–311

[75] Ahishali E, Uygur-Bayramiçli O, Dolapçioğlu C, et al. Chemical colitis due to glutaraldehyde: case series and review of the literature. Dig Dis Sci. 2009; 54(12):2541–2545

[76] Michetti CP, Smeltzer E, Fakhry SM. Splenic injury due to colonoscopy: analysis of the world literature, a new case report, and recommendations for management. Am Surg. 2010; 76(11):1198–1204

[77] Chandrasekhara V, Khashab MA, Muthusamy VR, et al; ASGE Standards of Practice Committee. Adverse events associated with ERCP. Gastrointest Endosc. 2017; 85(1):32–47

[78] Andriulli A, Loperfido S, Napolitano G, et al. Incidence rates of post-ERCP complications: a systematic survey of prospective studies. Am J Gastroenterol. 2007; 102(8):1781–1788

[79] Williams EJ, Taylor S, Fairclough P, et al. Risk factors for complication following ERCP; results of a large-scale, prospective multicenter study. Endoscopy. 2007; 39(9):793–801

[80] Wang P, Li ZS, Liu F, et al. Risk factors for ERCP-related complications: a prospective multicenter study. Am J Gastroenterol. 2009; 104(1):31–40

[81] Freeman ML, Nelson DB, Sherman S, et al. Complications of endoscopic biliary sphincterotomy. N Engl J Med. 1996; 335(13):909–918

[82] Ferreira LE, Fatima J, Baron TH. Clinically significant delayed postsphincterotomy bleeding: a twelve year single center experience. Minerva Gastroenterol Dietol. 2007; 53(3):215–223

[83] Vandervoort J, Soetikno RM, Tham TC, et al. Risk factors for complications after performance of ERCP. Gastrointest Endosc. 2002; 56(5):652–656

[84] Vásconez C, Llach J, Bordas JM, et al. Injection treatment of hemorrhage induced by endoscopic sphincterotomy. Endoscopy. 1998; 30(1):37–39

[85] Kuran S, Parlak E, Oguz D, et al. Endoscopic sphincterotomy-induced hemorrhage: treatment with heat probe. Gastrointest Endosc. 2006; 63(3):506–511

[86] Baron TH, Norton ID, Herman L. Endoscopic hemoclip placement for post-sphincterotomy bleeding. Gastrointest Endosc. 2000; 52(5):662

[87] Mosca S, Galasso G. Immediate and late bleeding after endoscopic sphincterotomy. Endoscopy. 1999; 31(3):278–279

[88] Kohler A, Maier M, Benz C, et al. A new HF current generator with automatically controlled system (Endocut mode) for endoscopic sphincterotomy--preliminary experience. Endoscopy. 1998; 30(4):351–355

[89] Norton ID, Petersen BT, Bosco J, et al. A randomized trial of endoscopic biliary sphincterotomy using pure-cut versus combined cut and coagulation waveforms. Clin Gastroenterol Hepatol. 2005; 3(10):1029–1033

[90] Stapfer M, Selby RR, Stain SC, et al. Management of duodenal perforation after endoscopic retrograde cholangiopancreatography and sphincterotomy. Ann Surg. 2000; 232(2):191–198

[91] Christensen M, Matzen P, Schulze S, Rosenberg J. Complications of ERCP: a prospective study. Gastrointest Endosc. 2004; 60(5):721–731

[92] Avgerinos DV, Llaguna OH, Lo AY, Voli J, Leitman IM. Management of endoscopic retrograde cholangiopancreatography: related duodenal perforations. Surg Endosc. 2009; 23(4):833–838

[93] Liao WC, Lee CT, Chang CY, et al. Randomized trial of 1-minute versus 5-minute endoscopic balloon dilation for extraction of bile duct stones. Gastrointest Endosc. 2010; 72(6):1154–1162

[94] Heo JH, Kang DH, Jung HJ, et al. Endoscopic sphincterotomy plus large-balloon dilation versus endoscopic sphincterotomy for removal of bile-duct stones. Gastrointest Endosc. 2007; 66(4):720–726, quiz 768, 771

[95] Motte S, Deviere J, Dumonceau JM, et al. Risk factors for septicemia following endoscopic biliary stenting. Gastroenterology. 1991; 101(5):1374–1381

[96] Byl B, Devière J, Struelens MJ, et al. Antibiotic prophylaxis for infectious complications after therapeutic endoscopic retrograde cholangiopancreatography: a randomized, double-blind, placebo-controlled study. Clin Infect Dis. 1995; 20(5):1236–1240

[97] Harris A, Chan AC, Torres-Viera C, et al. Meta-analysis of antibiotic prophylaxis in endoscopic retrograde cholangiopancreatography (ERCP). Endoscopy. 1999; 31(9):718–724

[98] Dumonceau JM, Andriulli A, Elmunzer BJ, et al; European Society of Gastrointestinal Endoscopy. Prophylaxis of post-ERCP pancreatitis: European Society of Gastrointestinal Endoscopy (ESGE) Guideline - updated June 2014. Endoscopy. 2014; 46:799–815

[99] Testoni PA, Mariani A, Aabakken L, et al. Papillary cannulation and sphincterotomy techniques at ERCP: European Society of Gastrointestinal Endoscopy (ESGE) Clinical Guideline. Endoscopy. 2016; 48:657–683

[100] Cotton PB, Garrow DA, Gallagher J, Romagnuolo J. Risk factors for complications after ERCP: a multivariate analysis of 11,497 procedures over 12 years. Gastrointest Endosc. 2009; 70(1):80–88

[101] Elmunzer BJ, Waljee AK, Elta GH, et al. A meta-analysis of rectal NSAIDs in the prevention of post-ERCP pancreatitis. Gut. 2008; 57(9):1262–1267

[102] Luo H, Zhao L, Leung J, et al. Routine pre-procedural rectal indometacin versus selective post-procedural rectal indometacin to prevent pancreatitis in patients undergoing endoscopic retrograde cholangiopancreatography: a multicentre, single-blinded, randomised controlled trial . Lancet. 2016; 387(10035):2293–2301

[103] Cheung J, Tsoi KK, Quan WL, et al. Guidewire versus conventional contrast cannulation of the common bile duct for the prevention of post-ERCP pancreatitis: a systematic review and meta-analysis. Gastrointest Endosc. 2009; 70(6):1211–1219

[104] Masci E, Mariani A, Curioni S, Testoni PA. Risk factors for pancreatitis following endoscopic retrograde cholangiopancreatography: a meta-analysis. Endoscopy. 2003; 35(10):830–834

[105] Singh P, Das A, Isenberg G, et al. Does prophylactic pancreatic stent placement reduce the risk of post-ERCP acute pancreatitis? A meta-analysis of controlled trials. Gastrointest Endosc. 2004; 60(4):544–550

[106] Mazaki T, Masuda H, Takayama T. Prophylactic pancreatic stent placement and post-ERCP pancreatitis: a systematic review and meta-analysis. Endoscopy. 2010; 42(10):842–853

[107] Freeman ML, Overby C, Qi D. Pancreatic stent insertion: consequences of failure and results of a modified technique to maximize success. Gastrointest Endosc. 2004; 59(1):8–14

[108] Chahal P, Tarnasky PR, Petersen BT, et al. Short 5Fr vs long 3Fr pancreatic stents in patients at risk for post-endoscopic retrograde cholangiopancreatography pancreatitis. Clin Gastroenterol Hepatol. 2009; 7(8):834–839

[109] Zolotarevsky E, Fehmi SM, Anderson MA, et al. Prophylactic 5-Fr pancreatic duct stents are superior to 3-Fr stents: a randomized controlled trial. Endoscopy. 2011; 43(4):325–330

[110] Tarnasky PR, Palesch YY, Cunningham JT, et al. Pancreatic stenting prevents pancreatitis after biliary sphincterotomy in patients with sphincter of Oddi dysfunction. Gastroenterology. 1998; 115(6):1518–1524

[111] Harewood GC, Pochron NL, Gostout CJ. Prospective, randomized, controlled trial of prophylactic pancreatic stent placement for endoscopic snare excision of the duodenal ampulla. Gastrointest Endosc. 2005; 62(3):367–370

[112] Yaghoobi M, Pauls Q, Durkalski V, et al. Incidence and predictors of post-ERCP pancreatitis in patients with suspected sphincter of Oddi dysfunction undergoing biliary or dual sphincterotomy: results from the EPISOD prospective multicenter randomized sham-controlled study. Endoscopy. 2015; 47(10):884–890

[113] Alvarez-Sánchez MV, Jenssen C, Faiss S, Napoléon B. Interventional endoscopic ultrasonography: an overview of safety and complications. Surg Endosc. 2014; 28(3):712–734

[114] Chantarojanasiri T, Aswakul P, Prachayakul V. Uncommon complications of therapeutic endoscopic ultrasonography: What, why, and how to prevent. World J Gastrointest Endosc. 2015; 7(10):960–968

[115] Varadarajulu S, Bang JY, Sutton BS, et al. Equal efficacy of endoscopic and surgical cystogastrostomy for pancreatic pseudocyst drainage in a randomized trial. Gastroenterology. 2013; 145(3):583–90.e1

[116] Hookey LC, Debroux S, Delhaye M, et al. Endoscopic drainage of pancreatic-fluid collections in 116 patients: a comparison of etiologies, drainage techniques, and outcomes. Gastrointest Endosc. 2006; 63(4):635–643

[117] Bang JY, Hasan M, Navaneethan U, et al. Lumen-apposing metal stents (LAMS) for pancreatic fluid collection (PFC) drainage: may not be business as usual. Gut. 2016; 0:1–3. doi:10.1136/gutjnl-2016-312812

[118] Arvanitakis M, Delhaye M, Bali MA, et al. Pancreatic-fluid collections: a randomized controlled trial regarding stent removal after endoscopic transmural drainage. Gastrointest Endosc. 2007; 65(4):609–619

[119] Zhang X-C, Zhou P-H. Major perioperative complications of POEM: experience based on 1680 patients. Gastrointest Endosc. 2016; 83:1000

[120] Bechara R, Onimaru M, Ikeda H, Inoue H. Per-oral endoscopic myotomy, 1000 cases later: pearls, pitfalls, and practical considerations. Gastrointest Endosc. 2016; 84:330–338

11 Anticoagulation and Endoscopy

Eduardo Rodrigues-Pinto and Todd H. Baron

11.1 Introduction

Anticoagulation and endoscopy often go hand in hand, and management of antithrombotic therapy in patients undergoing endoscopic procedures can be challenging. The risk of endoscopy in patients on antithrombotics depends on the risks of procedural hemorrhage and thrombosis due to discontinuation of therapy. The decision-making process is challenging when moderate-to high-risk patients, for thrombosis off anticoagulation, undergo high-risk bleeding procedures. Management also differs between elective and emergency procedures. Appropriate decision making requires knowledge of thrombotic risk, procedure-related bleeding risk, concepts of bridging anticoagulation, and timing of cessation and reinitiation of antithrombotic agents. A discussion between clinicians specializing in preoperative management of antithrombotic agents and coagulation disorders, primary providers prescribing these agents, and the proceduralist is essential. Ideally, this communication should occur well in advance of the procedure to increase patient safety and facilitate patient education. In this chapter, we review antiplatelet agents, anticoagulants, procedure risks, assessment of thrombotic risk, antithrombotic management, postprocedure care, and endoscopy procedures in the actively bleeding patient on antithrombotic therapy.

A large number of patients require long-term treatment with anticoagulant and antiplatelet agents (APAs), collectively known as antithrombotic agents. Antithrombotics are prescribed to reduce the risk of thromboembolic complications in patients with certain cardiovascular and thromboembolic conditions.[1] In addition, dual antiplatelet therapy (DAPT; combination treatment with aspirin and a thienopyridine) after coronary-artery stent placement has dramatically increased.[2]

In patients undergoing elective endoscopic procedures in whom the decision is made to discontinue these agents, familiarity with these medications is required to optimize the timing of cessation before, and reinitiation after procedures. The absolute risk of an embolic event in patients whose anticoagulation is interrupted for 4 to 7 days is approximately 1%.[3] In addition to drug cessation, the risk of thromboembolism might be increased by dehydration caused by preparation for endoscopic examinations.[4] Similarly, in those patients for whom the decision is made to continue antithrombotic agents for elective procedures, the clinician must understand the risk that these agents impart on procedural-induced bleeding. Finally, it is important to understand how to manage these agents in the setting of urgent/emergent endoscopic procedures and in the presence of acute gastrointestinal bleeding (GIB).

The goal is to minimize thromboembolic events and major hemorrhage in the periprocedural period. For patients taking antithrombotics who require endoscopy, the urgency of the procedure, its bleeding risks, the effect of the antithrombotic drug(s) on the bleeding risk, and the risk of a thromboembolic event related to periprocedural interruption of antithrombotic agents must be considered.[5]

Although guidelines from major Gastroenterological societies provide a framework for management of antithrombotics, the decision-making process may not always be straightforward.[6,7,8]

11.2 Antithrombotics

11.2.1 Antiplatelet Agents

APAs decrease platelet aggregation, thus preventing thrombus formation. APAs are usually used in patients with ischemic heart disease, coronary stents, and cerebrovascular disease. Aspirin causes irreversible inhibition of the cyclooxygenase 1 and 2 enzyme systems; after cessation of aspirin, 7 to 9 days are required to regain full platelet function.[9] Clopidogrel (Plavix, Bristol-Myers Squibb/Sanofi Pharmaceuticals Partnership, Bridgewater, New Jersey, United States), prasugrel (Effient, Eli Lilly and Company, Indianapolis, Indiana, United States), ticlopidine (Ticlid, Roche Pharmaceuticals, Nutley, New Jersey, United States), and ticagrelor (Brilinta, AstraZeneca, Wilmington, Delaware, United States) are thienopyridines, which inhibit the P2Y12 component of the adenosine diphosphate (ADP) receptors, preventing activation of the glycoprotein IIb/IIIa (GPIIb/IIIa) receptor complex.[10,11] Restoration of normal platelet aggregation requires 5 to 7 days for clopidogrel and prasugrel and 3 to 5 days for ticagrelor. Dipyridamole (Persantine, Teva Pharmaceuticals USA, Sellersville, Pennsylvania, United States) reversibly inhibits platelet aggregation; its duration of action is about 2 days after discontinuation. Abciximab (ReoPro, Eli Lilly and Company, Indianapolis, Indiana, United States), eptifibatide (Integrilin, Merck Sharp & Dohme Corp, Whitehouse Station, New Jersey, United States), and tirofiban (Aggrastat, Medicure Pharma, Inc, Somerset, New Jersey, United States) are GPIIb/IIIa receptor inhibitors that limit platelet aggregation, respectively, for 24 hours, 4 hours, and 1 to 2 seconds after discontinuation.[10,11]

11.2.2 Anticoagulants Agents

Anticoagulants prevent the clotting of blood by interfering with the native clotting cascade. Warfarin (Coumadin, Bristol-Myers Squibb Company, Princeton, New Jersey, United States) is an oral anticoagulant that inhibits the vitamin K–dependent clotting factors II, VII, IX, and X and proteins C and S.[10,11] Heparin derivatives (unfractionated heparin [UFH] and low-molecular-weight heparin [LMWH]) are administered intravenously and should be administered 4 to 6 hours and 24 hours, respectively, before high-risk procedures.[10,11] Fondaparinux (Arixtra, GlaxoSmithKline, Research Triangle Park, North Carolina, United States) is a specific inhibitor of factor Xa, with anticoagulant effects lasting for at least 36 hours.[10,11] Rivaroxaban (Xarelto, Janssen Pharmaceuticals, Inc, Raritan, New Jersey, United States), apixaban (Eliquis, Bristol-Myers Squibb Company, Princeton, New Jersey, United States), and edoxaban (Savaysa,

Daiichi Sankyo Co, LTD, Tokyo, Japan) are direct factor Xa inhibitors, while dabigatran (Pradaxa, Boehringer Ingelheim Pharmaceuticals Inc, Ridgefield, Connecticut, United States), hirudins, and argatroban (Acova, Abbott Laboratories, North Chicago, Illinois, United States) are direct thrombin inhibitors.[10,11] Direct oral anticoagulants (DOACs) reach a maximum effect 1.25 to 3 hours after ingestion and should be discontinued ≥ 48 hours before a high-risk procedure.[11] These agents overcome some of the vitamin K antagonists (VKAs) pitfalls such as their narrow therapeutic window, the need for frequent monitoring, and dose adjustments as well as the interaction with foods and/or other drugs. However, specific antidotes are limited, with only idarucizumab (Praxbind, Boehringer Ingelheim, Inc, Ridgefield, Connecticut, United States) approved for use in cases of life-threatening uncontrolled bleeding or prior to emergency surgery in patients on dabigatran.[12] Prothrombin time and activated partial thromboplastin time are poor measures of drug effect and are insensitive and often minimally prolonged or normal in spite of therapeutic drug levels.[13]

Procedure Risks

There is an intrinsic risk of hemorrhage associated with endoscopic procedures. Hemorrhage may be immediately apparent at the time of endoscopy or may be delayed for up to 2 weeks following the procedure.

In general, a patient undergoing a procedure associated with low risk of bleeding (low-risk procedure) can (and should) safely continue antithrombotic therapy, particularly if the patient is at high risk for a thromboembolic event (high-risk patient).[1] Conversely, a patient undergoing a high-risk procedure can temporarily discontinue antithrombotic agents safely if the patient is at low risk for a thromboembolic event (low-risk patient).[1] The decision-making process is challenging when patients at moderate-to-high risk for thromboembolic events undergo high-risk procedures. Management also differs between elective and emergency procedures.[1] Elective endoscopic procedures should be deferred until short-term anticoagulation therapy is completed.

Common endoscopic procedures vary in their potential to induce bleeding (▶ Table 11.1).[4,11,14] Studies on postprocedural bleeding risks have been conducted in patients who are not on antithrombotic regimens and thus may not accurately reflect the bleeding risk of patients using antithrombotic therapies.

Assessment of Thrombotic Risk

The probability of a thromboembolic event related to the temporary interruption of antithrombotic therapy for an endoscopic procedure depends on the indication for antithrombotic therapy and individual patient characteristics (▶ Table 11.2).[4,11,14]

Antiplatelet Agents Management

While the American Society for Gastrointestinal Endoscopy (ASGE) recommends continuation of low-dose aspirin and nonsteroidal anti-inflammatory drugs in the periendoscopic period,[11] the European Society for Gastrointestinal Endoscopy (ESGE) recommends continuing aspirin for all endoscopic procedures, with the exception of endoscopic submucosal dissection, large colonic endoscopic mucosal resection (EMR) (>2 cm), upper GI EMR, and ampullectomy (▶ Table 11.3).[14] In the latter cases, aspirin discontinuation should be considered on an individual-patient basis depending on thrombosis and hemorrhage risks.[14] Japanese guidelines consider withdrawal of aspirin monotherapy in high-risk endoscopic procedures for 3 to 5 days in patients at low risk of thromboembolism; aspirin monotherapy should be continued in patients at high risk of thromboembolism.[4] In patients on long-term low-dose aspirin

Table 11.1 Risk stratification of endoscopic procedures based on the risk of hemorrhage

Low risk	High risk
Diagnostic procedures including mucosal biopsy	Endoscopic polypectomy
ERCP with stent placement or papillary balloon dilation without sphincterotomy	ERCP with sphincterotomy or large balloon papillary dilation
Device-assisted enteroscopy without polypectomy	Endoscopic hemostasis
Capsule endoscopy	Ampullectomy
Enteral stent deployment[a] (controversial)	EMR or ESD
EUS without FNA	Endoscopic dilatation of strictures
Argon plasma coagulation	Endoscopic therapy of varices
Barrett's ablation	PEG[b]/PEJ
	EUS with FNA[c]
	EUS-guided biliary drainage
	Transmural drainage procedures (e.g., pancreatic fluid collections, gallbladder drainage)
	Tumor ablation

Abbreviations: EMR, endoscopic mucosal resection; ERCP, endoscopic retrograde cholangiopancreatography; ESD, endoscopic submucosal dissection; EUS, endoscopic ultrasound; FNA, fine-needle aspiration; PEG/PEJ: percutaneous endoscopic gastrostomy/jejunostomy

[a]Enteral stent deployment risk is controversial for American Society for Gastrointestinal Endoscopy (ASGE), low risk for Japanese guidelines, and high risk for European Society for Gastrointestinal Endoscopy (ESGE).

[b]PEG on aspirin or clopidogrel therapy is low risk for ASGE, but high risk for ESGE and Japanese guidelines; does not apply to dual antiplatelet therapy.

[c]EUS-FNA of solid masses on acetylsalicylic acid/nonsteroidal anti-inflammatory drugs is low risk.

Table 11.2 Risk stratification for discontinuation of clopidogrel, prasugrel, or ticagrelor, and warfarin therapy based on risk of thrombosis and consideration of need for bridge therapy

Low risk	High risk
Clopidogrel, prasugrel, or ticagrelor	
Ischemic heart disease without coronary stents	Drug-eluting coronary artery stents within 12 months of placement
Cerebrovascular disease	Bare metal coronary artery stents within 1 month of placement
Peripheral vascular disease	
Warfarin	
Prosthetic metal heart valve in aortic position	Prosthetic metal heart valve in mitral position
Xenograft heart valve	Prosthetic heart valve and atrial fibrillation
Atrial fibrillation without valvular disease	Atrial fibrillation and mitral stenosis[a]
> 3 months after venous thromboembolism	< 3 months after venous thromboembolism
Thrombophilia syndromes	

[a]Uncertainty exists regarding the thrombotic risk of temporarily discontinuing warfarin in patients with atrial fibrillation and mitral stenosis, but there is insufficient evidence at present to alter the risk category

Table 11.3 Summary of societal guidelines for management of antithrombotic therapy

			Procedures with low bleeding risk				Procedures with high bleeding risk
Conditions with low thromboembolic risk	Aspirin/thienopyridines	ESGE ASGE	Continue	Aspirin	ESGE ASGE	Case by case	
		JGES	• Continue when patient on antithrombotic monotherapy • Consider withdrawal case by case when DAPT or triple therapy	Thienopyridines	ESGE ASGE JGES	Discontinue ± substitution with aspirin during procedure	
	Anticoagulants	ESGE ASGE	Continue	Anticoagulants	ESGE ASGE	Discontinue	
		JGES	Continue in diagnostic procedures without biopsy		JGES	Discontinue with heparin-bridging therapy[a]	
Conditions with high thromboembolic risk	Aspirin/thienopyridines/DAPT	ESGE ASGE	Continue	Aspirin	ESGE ASGE	Continue	
		JGES	• Continue when patient on antithrombotic monotherapy • Consider withdrawal case by case when DAPT or triple therapy		JGES	Case by case	
				Thienopyridines	ESGE ASGE JGES	Delay procedures if possible. If not possible, discontinue and substitute with aspirin	
				DAPT	ESGE ASGE JGES	Delay procedures if possible. If not possible, discontinue and substitute with aspirin	
	Anticoagulants	ESGE ASGE	Continue	Anticoagulants	ESGE ASGE JGES	Discontinue ± heparin-bridging therapy[a]	
		JGES	Continue in diagnostic procedures without biopsy				

Abbreviations: ASGE, American Society for Gastrointestinal Endoscopy; DAPT, dual antiplatelet therapy; ESGE, European Society of Gastrointestinal Endoscopy; JGES, Japanese Gastroenterological Endoscopy Society.

[a]Caution should be used in patients undergoing complex therapeutic procedures.

for secondary prevention, aspirin interruption was associated with a three times increased risk of cardiovascular or cerebrovascular events, and 70% of these events occurred ≤ 7 to 10 days after interruption.[15] For low-risk endoscopic procedures, thienopyridines should be continued, as single or DAPT.[11,14] For high-risk endoscopic procedures in patients at low thrombotic risk, thienopyridines should be discontinued 5 days (if taken as monotherapy) to 7 days (if taken as DAPT) before the procedure.[4] In patients on DAPT, aspirin should be continued.[11,14] For high-risk endoscopic procedures in patients at high thrombotic risk, when it is not feasible to withdraw thienopyridines, replacement with aspirin should be performed after consultation with the prescribing doctor.[4,11,14]

Anticoagulants Agents Management

Warfarin should be continued for low-risk endoscopic procedures (▶Table 11.3); however the international normalized ratio (INR) should not exceed the therapeutic range measured in the week before the procedure.[11,14] For low-risk endoscopic procedures, the morning dose of DOACs should be omitted on the day of the procedure.[11,14] For high-risk endoscopic procedures in patients at low thrombotic risk, warfarin should be discontinued 5 days before the procedure.[11,14] For high-risk endoscopic procedures in patients at high thrombotic risk, warfarin should be discontinued 5 days prior to the procedure, with bridging therapy with LMWH.[11,14] For high-risk endoscopic procedures in patients on DOACs, the last dose of DOACs should be taken at least 48 hours before the procedure (72 hours prior for patients on dabigatran with a creatinine clearance of 30–50 mL/min).[11,14]

Although all guidelines recommend bridging therapy for patients with high thromboembolic risk requiring temporary withdrawal of anticoagulants, a recent meta-analysis of 35 studies found an increased risk of overall and major bleeding but a similar thromboembolic risk in patients receiving periprocedural heparin-bridging therapy.[16,17] Thus, caution should be taken to balance the benefits of bridging therapy and the risks of bleeding in patients needing temporary discontinuation of anticoagulant. All patients on warfarin should be advised that there is an increased risk of postprocedure bleeding compared to nonanticoagulated patients, even when temporarily discontinued.[11,14] In a multivariate analysis, however, most bleeding was immediate and successfully treated endoscopically without significant consequence.[18] Hemorrhage secondary to high-risk endoscopic procedures can often be controlled by further endoscopic therapeutic measures, and is rarely fatal. Thrombotic adverse events such as stroke from interruption of anticoagulation can be catastrophic.[19]

Postendoscopic Procedure

If APAs or anticoagulants are discontinued, there is consensus that antithrombotic therapy should be resumed upon completion of the procedure. Warfarin should be restarted within 24 hours of the procedure in patients with valvular heart disease and a low risk for thromboembolism; in patients at high risk for thromboembolism, UFH or LMWH should be restarted as soon as "bleeding stability allows" and continued until the INR reaches an appropriate therapeutic level.[20] UFH may be restarted 2 to 6 hours after a therapeutic procedure. The optimal time to restart LMWH after endoscopy has not been determined. Delaying reinitiation of LMWH 48 to 72 hours after surgery should be considered in patients believed to be at high risk for bleeding adverse events.[2] There are no data regarding optimal timing of resumption of DOACs after endoscopic procedures. If they cannot be restarted within 24 hours after a high-risk procedure, then bridge therapy should be considered for patients at high risk for thromboembolism.[21,22] Reinitiation of DOACs should be delayed for at least 48 hours after high-risk procedures because full anticoagulation occurs shortly after administration; for patients in whom biliary sphincterotomy is performed, resumption of these agents should be delayed for at least 72 hours; for patients who are at high risk of delayed bleeding and who are at low risk for antithrombotic events, it would be reasonable to hold anticoagulation for 7 days.[23] APAs should be resumed once hemostasis has been achieved. Clopidogrel administered at maintenance doses has delayed onset and can be reinitiated within 24 hours; clopidogrel loading results in rapid onset of action and should be considered among patients at risk for thrombosis with a lower risk of bleeding than anticipated; other APAs, including aspirin, can be reinitiated within 24 hours.

Endoscopy Procedures in the Actively Bleeding Patient on Antithrombotic Therapy

Endoscopic evaluation and therapy in patients using antithrombotics with active GIB is both warranted and safe.[5] The decision to stop, reduce, and/or reverse antithrombotic therapy (and thereby risking thromboembolic consequences) must be weighed against the risk of continued bleeding. Reversal of anticoagulation with four-factor prothrombin complex concentrate (PCC) rather than fresh-frozen plasma should be used for patients with VKA-associated major bleeding, in addition to intravenous vitamin K.[24] Vitamin K should not be given routinely in patients with mechanical valves because this may create a hypercoagulable condition.[25] However, endoscopic hemostatic therapy is very effective even in patients with moderately elevated INR, and it should not be postponed to correct coagulopathy in patients with an INR < 2.5, as normalizing the INR does not reduce rebleeding. Patients who require anticoagulation after endoscopic therapy receive UFH because of its relatively shorter half-life after successful endoscopic hemostasis for high-risk stigmata.

Regarding the new DOACs in patients with severe GIB, hemodialysis can be used in patients receiving dabigatran but not for rivaroxaban, edoxaban, and apixaban because of their decreased renal excretion and because they are highly protein bound. Charcoal hemoperfusion also may be effective.[25] Although factor VIIa and four-factor PCC have been used in these situations, their value in reversing the clinical anticoagulant effects and controlling clinical hemorrhage is uncertain.[26]

For patients on APAs with life-threatening or serious bleeding, options include stopping these agents and/or administration of platelets. Consultation with the prescribing specialist should occur in situations of significant GIB in patients with high risk for thrombosis. The risk of an adverse cardiac event associated with cessation of the APA therapy likely exceeds the benefit of decreasing postendoscopic bleeding.

References

[1]   Baron TH, Kamath PS, McBane RD. Management of antithrombotic therapy in patients undergoing invasive procedures. N Engl J Med. 2013; 368(22):2113–2124

[2]   Douketis JD, Spyropoulos AC, Spencer FA, et al; American College of Chest Physicians. Perioperative management of antithrombotic therapy: Antithrombotic Therapy and Prevention of Thrombosis, 9th ed: American College of Chest Physicians Evidence-Based Clinical Practice Guidelines. Chest. 2012; 141(2, Suppl):e326S–e350S

[3]   Garcia DA, Regan S, Henault LE, et al. Risk of thromboembolism with short-term interruption of warfarin therapy. Arch Intern Med. 2008; 168(1):63–69

[4]   Fujimoto K, Fujishiro M, Kato M, et al; Japan Gastroenterological Endoscopy Society. Guidelines for gastroenterological endoscopy in patients undergoing antithrombotic treatment. Dig Endosc. 2014; 26(1):1–14

[5]   Abraham NS, Castillo DL. Novel anticoagulants: bleeding risk and management strategies. Curr Opin Gastroenterol. 2013; 29(6):676–683

[6]   Tang RS, Chan FK. Prevention of gastrointestinal events in patients on antithrombotic therapy in the peri-endoscopy period: review of new evidence and recommendations from recent guidelines. Dig Endosc. 2015; 27(5):562–571

[7]   Anderson MA, Ben-Menachem T, Gan SI, et al; ASGE Standards of Practice Committee. Management of antithrombotic agents for endoscopic procedures. Gastrointest Endosc. 2009; 70(6):1060–1070

[8]   Boustière C, Veitch A, Vanbiervliet G, et al; European Society of Gastrointestinal Endoscopy. Endoscopy and antiplatelet agents. Endoscopy. 2011; 43(5):445–461

[9]   Patrono C, Ciabattoni G, Patrignani P, et al. Clinical pharmacology of platelet cyclo-oxygenase inhibition. Circulation. 1985; 72(6):1177–1184

[10] Di Minno A, Spadarella G, Prisco D. et al. Antithrombotic drugs, patient characteristics, and gastrointestinal bleeding: clinical translation and areas of research. Blood Rev. 2015; 29(5):335–343

[11] Acosta RD, Abraham NS, Chandrasekhara V, et al; ASGE Standards of Practice Committee. The management of antithrombotic agents for patients undergoing GI endoscopy. Gastrointest Endosc. 2016; 83(1):3–16

[12] Vanden Daelen S, Peetermans M, Vanassche T. et al. Monitoring and reversal strategies for new oral anticoagulants. Expert Rev Cardiovasc Ther. 2015; 13(1):95–103

[13] Cuker A, Siegal DM, Crowther MA, Garcia DA. Laboratory measurement of the anticoagulant activity of the non-vitamin K oral anticoagulants. J Am Coll Cardiol. 2014; 64(11):1128–1139

[14] Veitch AM, Vanbiervliet G, Gershlick AH, et al. Endoscopy in patients on antiplatelet or anticoagulant therapy, including direct oral anticoagulants: British Society of Gastroenterology (BSG) and European Society of Gastrointestinal Endoscopy (ESGE) guidelines. Endoscopy. 2016; 48(4):385–402

[15] Biondi-Zoccai GG, Lotrionte M, Agostoni P, et al. A systematic review and meta-analysis on the hazards of discontinuing or not adhering to aspirin among 50,279 patients at risk for coronary artery disease. Eur Heart J. 2006; 27(22):2667–2674

[16] Siegal D, Yudin J, Kaatz S. Periprocedural heparin bridging in patients receiving vitamin K antagonists: systematic review and meta-analysis of bleeding and thromboembolic rates. Circulation. 2012; 126(13):1630–1639

[17] Hui AJ, Wong RM, Ching JY. et al. Risk of colonoscopic polypectomy bleeding with anticoagulants and antiplatelet agents: analysis of 1657 cases. Gastrointest Endosc. 2004; 59(1):44–48

[18] Kim HG, Friedland S. Safe and effective colon polypectomy in patients receiving uninterrupted anticoagulation: can we do it? Gastrointest Endosc. 2014; 79(3):424–426

[19] Nishimura RA, Otto CM, Bonow RO, et al; ACC/AHA Task Force Members. 2014 AHA/ACC Guideline for the Management of Patients With Valvular Heart Disease: a report of the American College of Cardiology/American Heart Association Task Force on Practice Guidelines. Circulation. 2014; 129(23):e521–e643

[20] Weitz JI, Quinlan DJ, Eikelboom JW. Periprocedural management and approach to bleeding in patients taking dabigatran. Circulation. 2012; 126(20):2428–2432

[21] Dzik WS. Reversal of drug-induced anticoagulation: old solutions and new problems. Transfusion. 2012; 52(Suppl 1):45S–55S

[22] Baron TH, Kamath PS, McBane RD. New anticoagulant and antiplatelet agents: a primer for the gastroenterologist. Clin Gastroenterol Hepatol. 2014; 12(2):187–195

[23] Holbrook A, Schulman S, Witt DM, et al; American College of Chest Physicians. Evidence-based management of anticoagulant therapy: Antithrombotic Therapy and Prevention of Thrombosis, 9th ed: American College of Chest Physicians Evidence-Based Clinical Practice Guidelines. Chest. 2012; 141(2, Suppl):e152S–e184S

[24] Tripodi A. The laboratory and the new oral anticoagulants. Clin Chem. 2013; 59(2):353–362

[25] Kaatz S, Kouides PA, Garcia DA, et al. Guidance on the emergent reversal of oral thrombin and factor Xa inhibitors. Am J Hematol. 2012; 87(Suppl 1):S141–S145

[26] Siegal DM, Cuker A. Reversal of novel oral anticoagulants in patients with major bleeding. J Thromb Thrombolysis. 2013; 35(3):391–398

Section III

General Diagnostic and Therapeutic Procedures and Techniques

12 Upper Gastrointestinal Endoscopy

Philip W.Y. Chiu and Rajvinder Singh

12.1 History of Upper Gastrointestinal Endoscopy

The development of endoscopy can be traced back to the ancient Roman time where archeologists discovered the vaginal speculum at the ruins of Pompeii.[1] In 1853, Desormeaux first proposed the concept of endoscope and its essential components, including optical body and light source. In 1868, Kussmaul first performed upper endoscopy through a rigid tube, but the examination was far from satisfactory because of the poor light illumination.[2] Johann Mikulicz, being the first surgeon to perform suture repair of perforated gastric ulcer, developed improved models and performed the first esophagogastroscopy in 1881. His modifications included mirrors to produce 30-degree-angled field of vision and a miniature version of Thomas Edison's electric incandescent globe as the light source. He was first to describe the endoscopic observation of gastric carcinoma. The concept of flexible endoscope was introduced by Henry Elsner in 1911 where the endoscope was created with both rigid and flexible parts. Rudolph Schindler, a gastroenterologist, modified the Elsner two-part gastroscope to include a separate channel for flushing of lens and developed the Wolf–Schindler gastroscope in the 1930s. This scope consisted of multiple prisms for transmission of images and a bending angle of 30 to 34 degrees. This scope became widely adopted due to the safety and efficacy. Diagnostic endoscopy was enhanced by the developments in flexible fiberoptics in 1954 by Harold Hopkins at the Imperial College of London.[3] The Hopkins system consisted of glass rods coated in reflective cladding, permitting high-intensity light transmission and image transmission. Dr. Basil Hirschowitz from University of Michigan produced a prototype flexible gastroscope based on these fiberoptic bundles and performed the first gastroscopy on himself and subsequently on a patient in 1957.[4] The enhancement of optical fibers further enhanced the development of endoscope. The introduction of videoendoscopy further revolutionized the performance of endoscopic examination. In 1983, charge-coupled device (CCD) was used to replace coherent fiberoptic image bundle by the Welch Allyn Company to capture images focused by a small lens. The image was converted to display on a TV monitor.[5,6] This allowed the endoscopist, trainees, and nurses to appreciate the endoscopic examination together and unleash the possibility of therapeutic endoscopy.[7]

The modern gastroscopes are forward-viewing endoscopes with a short insertion shaft dedicated for examination of the esophagus, stomach, and duodenum (▶Table 12.1).[8] The length of the insertion tube varies between 925 and 1,100 mm, and the diameter varies from 4.9 to 12.8 mm depending on the functionality and indications. A typical gastroscope has one working channel and the size varies from 2 to 3.8 mm, and a dual-channel gastroscope is available for specific therapeutic purpose. An ultrathin endoscopy is also available with a diameter between 4.9 and 6 mm and a working channel of 1.5 to 2 mm.[9] This can be used for transnasal or transoral upper endoscopic examination

to alleviate patients discomfort without sedation, as well as negotiation through tight constrictive upper gastrointestinal (GI) tumors.

12.2 General Diagnostic Techniques

12.2.1 Indications

Generally, upper GI endoscopy is indicated as an investigation for patients who have symptoms relating to upper GI diseases. The American Society for Gastrointestinal Endoscopy (ASGE) guidelines for appropriate use of GI endoscopy described indications for esophagogastroduodenoscopy (EGD).[10] For patients with symptoms of upper GI diseases, endoscopists should be alerted of the differential diagnosis related to these symptoms and search for those diseases during upper endoscopy. Patients with upper abdominal symptoms associated with alarm signs and symptoms, and those with new-onset dyspepsia who are older than 50 years should receive early EGD. For patients with symptoms of upper GI hemorrhage, the most common pathologies include bleeding peptic ulcers, variceal bleeding, bleeding from upper GI malignancies, and hemorrhagic gastritis. For patients with dysphagia, upper endoscopy is indicated to examine for presence of esophageal cancer and cancer at the cardia of the stomach. However, as upper endoscopy is not the most appropriate investigation for functional diseases, patients with dysphagia and a normal endoscopy should be further investigated with high-resolution manometry to rule out esophageal dysmotility disorders including achalasia, and 24-hour pH study for chronic gastroesophageal reflux disease (GERD). Patients with symptoms of gastroesophageal reflux which persist despite appropriate treatment should be investigated with an EGD. For patients with clinical suspicion of coeliac disease or a positive serological test, routine biopsy of the duodenum is important to rule out villous atrophy.

Axon et al reported the guidelines on indications for performance of upper GI endoscopy.[11] The guidelines were set for referral of EGD based on appropriate symptoms and indications from evaluation of systematic reviews of published data and recommendations from expert panels. The appropriate indications for EGD are summarized in ▶Table 12.2.

Indications—For Screening of Upper Gastrointestinal Cancers

There is an increase in acceptance of performing upper GI endoscopy as a screening procedure, especially in countries with high incidence of gastric cancer. Meanwhile, the cost and effectiveness of such screening program should be cautiously introduced as the prevalence of upper GI cancers varies among different countries worldwide.[12] In countries such as Japan with high prevalence of gastric cancers, national screening program started as

Table 12.1 Technological specifications for various gastroscopes used for upper gastrointestinal endoscopy[8]

Manufacturer	Model	Insertion tube length/ diameter (mm)	Image type	Image characteristic	Compatible processor	Biopsy channel	Special features
Olympus Excera III	GIF H190	1,030/9.2	Video	Color CCD	CV190	1/2.8	HD with waterjet
Olympus Excera	GIF H180J	1,030/9.9	Video	Color CCD	CV180/160/140/92	1/2.8	Standard with waterjet
	GIF H180	1,030/9.8	Video	Color CCD	CV180/160/140/93	1/2.8	HD
	GIF Q180	**1,030/8.8**	Video	Color CCD	CV180/160/140/94	1/2.8	Standard (high resolution)
	GIF N180	1,100/4.9	Video	Color CCD	CV180/160/140/95	1/2.0	Ultrathin
	GIF XP180N	1,100/5.5	Video	Color CCD	CV180/160/140/96	1/2.0	Ultrathin
	GIF 2TH180	1,030/12.6	Video	Color CCD	CV180/160/140/97	2/2.8,3.7	Dual channel
	GIF 1TQ160	1,030/11.3	Video	Color CCD	CV180/160/140/98	1/3.7	Therapeutic
	GIF XTQ160	1,030/12.9	Video	Color CCD	CV180/160/140/99	1/6.0	Therapeutic
	GIF Q160Z	1,030/10.9	Zoom video	Color CCD	CV180/160/140/100	1/2.8	Optical zoom 115×
Olympus Lucera Elite	GIF HQ290	1,030/9.9	Video	Color CCD	CV290	1/2.8	HD with waterjet and dual focus
Olympus Lucera	GIF H260	1,030/9.8	Video	Color CCD	CV260/260SL	1/2.8	Standard
	GIF H260Z	1,030/10.5	Video	Color CCD	CV260SL	1/2.8	Optical zoom 80×
	GIF N260	1,100/5.2	Video	Color CCD	CV 260/260SL/240	1/2.0	Ultrathin
	GIF XP260	1,100/5.5	Video	Color CCD	CV260/260SL/240	1/2.0	Ultrathin
Fujinon	EG 530WR	1,100/9.3	Video	HD	EPX4400HD/EPX2500	1/2.8	Standard
	EG 450PE5	1,100/8.1	Video	HD	EPX4400HD	1/2.2	Slim
	EG 530N	1,100/5.9	Video	HD	EPX4400HD/EPX2500	1/2.0	Ultra slim
	EG530NP	1,100/4.9	Video	HD	EPX4400HD/EPX2500	1/2.0	Ultra slim
	EG450CT5	1,100/10.8	Video	HD	EPX4400HD	1/3.8	Therapeutic
	EG 450D5	1,090/11.5	Video	HD	EPX4400HD	2/3.8,2.8	Dual channel
	EG 590WR	1,100/9.6	Video	HD (SuperCCD)	EPX4400HD	1/2.8	Standard
	EG 590ZW	1,100/9.8	Video	HD (SuperCCD)	EPX4400HD	1/2.8	Optical magnification
Pentax	EG29-i10	1,050/9.8	Video	HD+	EPK-i5010	1/3.2	Close focus with waterjet
	EG27-i10	1,050/9.0	Video	HD+	EPK-i5010	1/2.8	Close focus
	EG 2790i	1,050/9.0	Video	HD	EPK-i5010	1/2.8	
	EG 2990i	1,050/9.8	Video	Standard (SD)	EPK-i5010	1/2.8	Waterjet
	EG 1690K	1,100/5.4	Video	Standard (SD)	EPK-I, EPK1000	1/2.0	
	EG 2490K	1,050/8.0	Video	Standard (SD)	EPK-I, EPK1000	1/2.4	
	EG 2790K	1,050/9.0	Video	Standard (SD)	EPK-I, EPK1000	1/2.8	
	EG 2990K	1,050/9.8	Video	Standard (SD)	EPK-I, EPK1000	1/2.8	
	EG 3490K	1,050/11.6	Video	Standard (SD)	EPK-I, EPK1000	1/3.8	Waterjet
	EG 3470ZK	1,050/11.6	Video	Standard (SD)	EPK-I, EPK1000	1/2.8	
	EG 3890TK	1,050/12.8	Video	Standard (SD)	EPK-I, EPK1000	2/3.8, 2.8	Dual channel

early as the 1960s.[13] Photofluorography (or barium radiography) was employed as the screening method, and in 1983 all residents older than 40 years were recommended to receive gastric cancer screening. Five case–control studies demonstrated that screening by photofluorography in Japan significantly decreases gastric cancer mortality by 40 to 60%. Recently, gastroscopy is increasingly performed for screening of gastric cancer in Japan,[14] and studies suggested that most of the gastric cancers were diagnosed by EGD rather than photofluorography. Currently, more than 60% of gastric cancers are diagnosed at an early stage in Japan,[15] while technological advances in endoscopy and imaging will further improve the diagnosis and management.[16]

Indications—Therapeutic Procedures

The therapeutic procedures for upper GI endoscopy have been increasing over the past decades. Currently, upper GI endoscopy is indicated as primary treatment for upper GI hemorrhage.[17] Endoscopic resection with techniques such as endoscopic mucosal resection (EMR) and endoscopic submucosal dissection (ESD) is the standard treatment for early-stage upper GI neoplasia.[18,19] Palliative endoscopic stenting is the optimal treatment for advanced or metastatic carcinoma of esophagus, stomach, and pancreas, which causes obstruction.[20] Upper GI endoscopy is indicated for removal of foreign bodies. Various interventions can be achieved

Table 12.2 Appropriate indications for performance of upper gastrointestinal endoscopy[11]

Upper gastrointestinal symptoms/signs	Significant upper abdominal pain
	Dyspepsia (especially new onset at the age of 40)
	Significant heartburn not responsive to PPI therapy
	Dysphagia
	Odynophagia
	Recurrent vomiting
	Palpable epigastric mass
Upper gastrointestinal hemorrhage	Passage of tarry stool
	Hematemesis
	Coffee ground vomiting
	Positive occult blood test
	Anemia
General symptoms	Unexplained weight loss
	Malaise/anorexia
Abnormal investigation(s)	Abnormal barium meal/swallow results
	Hypochromic microcytic anemia (low hemoglobin)

through EGD for management of complications after upper GI and bariatric surgeries, including balloon dilatation for anastomotic strictures and stenting for leakage.[21]

Indications—Intraoperative Upper Endoscopy

Recently, with the concept of endolaparoscopic approach for treatment of upper GI diseases, there is an increase in use of upper endoscopy during laparoscopic surgery.[22,23] The objectives for intraoperative upper endoscopy usually include the following: (1) localization of the disease/neoplasia; (2) providing endoluminal guidance to assess adequacy of the resection margins; and (3) as a combined endolaparoscopic approach for resection of early gastric neoplasia or GI stromal tumor. As gaseous insufflation is necessary to achieve good endoscopic visualization, the use of CO_2 insufflation is recommended during intraoperative upper GI endoscopy to avoid overdistension of the GI tract, which may hinder further laparoscopic surgical procedures.

12.2.2 Contraindications

Upper GI endoscopy is generally contraindicated when patients are suspected to have upper GI perforations including perforated peptic ulcers. Cohort studies demonstrated therapeutic procedures, such as clipping and stenting, may be successful in the management of upper GI perforations including Boerhaave's disease and anastomotic leakage.[21] These exceptional conditions will require careful clinical planning and availability of expertise. The other contraindication for upper GI endoscopy is an inadequate timing of fasting before the procedure, for patients with symptoms of gastric outlet obstruction and achalasia. These patients will have either food residue in the esophagus or large amount of undigested food in stomach. Performing upper GI endoscopy during these clinical conditions may induce significant regurgitation, leading to aspiration pneumonia.

In the guidelines by ASGE and guidelines published by the joint working party in England, patients with symptoms that are considered functional in origin are generally not indicated for EGD.[10,11] However, EGD should still be indicated to exclude mechanical causes when these symptoms persist.[24] In countries with moderate to high incidence of gastric cancers, patients with upper abdominal symptoms should receive a diagnostic EGD—"a scope and treat strategy" rather than the test and eradicate *Helicobacter pylori* without endoscopy, i.e., "test and treat strategy," which is more commonly advocated in low-prevalence populations.[25]

12.3 Preparation of the Patient

For a typical diagnostic upper GI endoscopy, the patient is usually fasted for 6 hours for food and 4 hours for fluid before the procedure. The patient should arrive at the endoscopy unit as an outpatient if he/she is physically fit or be admitted to the daycare center of the hospital if he/she requires a prolonged recovery time after the endoscopy. An informed consent should be obtained from the patient, including the indication and risks of the procedure. The risks of upper GI endoscopy generally include bleeding, perforation of 1:10,000, and aspiration pneumonia.

Before EGD, a "time-out" procedure will be carried out according to local recommendations. Local anesthesia to the throat may help to reduce and prevent gag reflux during insertion of the endoscope through the hypopharynx and reduce patients' discomfort.[26] The patient is placed in a left lateral position facing the endoscopist to facilitate insertion of the endoscope and prevent aspiration. A mouthpiece will be placed between the teeth to protect the endoscope during the examination.

12.4 Sedation

The aim of sedation for upper GI endoscopy is to reduce the anxiety during the procedure, relief of the discomfort and pain induced, and provide a safe and stable condition for endoscopists to perform a good high-quality diagnostic and therapeutic procedure.[27]

Diagnostic upper GI endoscopy can be performed without sedation, but patients may experience significant discomfort during the procedure and may be hesitant to commit to future screening endoscopy. The prescription of sedation for diagnostic upper GI endoscopy is thus optional depending on patients' acceptance, availability of recovery areas, decision of endoscopists, and location of the endoscopy suite.[28] In Germany, 74% of the upper GI endoscopies were performed under sedation.[29] In Switzerland, the use of sedation for upper GI endoscopy has markedly increased from 60% in 1990 to 78% in 2003.[30] However, only 20% of the upper GI endoscopies were performed under sedation in Spain.[31] The level of sedation is defined by American Society of Anesthesiologists (ASA) as illustrated in ▶ Table 12.3. Generally, sedation during diagnostic upper GI endoscopy should achieve minimal to moderate sedative effects, which correspond to Ramsay sedation score 3 and 4 (▶ Table 12.4).

Table 12.3 American Society of Anesthesiologists (ASA) level of sedation[27]

Sedation level	Minimal sedation (anxiolysis)	Moderate sedation	Deep sedation	General anesthesia
Responsiveness	Normal	Verbal or tactile stimuli	Repeated painful stimuli	Unresponsive to painful stimuli
Airway	Normal	No intervention required	Intervention may be required	Intervention usually required
Spontaneous ventilation	Normal	Adequate	May be inadequate	Usually inadequate
Cardiovascular function	Normal	Normal	Usually maintained	May be impaired

Table 12.4 Ramsay sedation score[27]

Ramsay score	Response
1	The patient is anxious and agitated or restless or both
2	The patient is cooperative, orientated, and tranquil
3	The patient responds to commands only
4	Drowsiness: The patient exhibits brisk response to light glabellar tap or loud auditory stimulus
5	Drowsiness: The patient exhibits a sluggish response to light glabellar tap or loud auditory stimulus
6	The patient exhibits no response

Patients are more "settled" during therapeutic upper GI endoscopy when intravenous sedation is administered. The commonly used agents for sedation in upper GI endoscopy include intravenous benzodiazepines, propofol, and fentanyl. Intravenous midazolam was demonstrated to be more effective than diazepam with higher patients' satisfaction.[32] Moreover, intravenous midazolam has an "amnesic effect," which possibly contributed to higher satisfaction. However, major decisions concerning patients on the endoscopic findings should not be conducted immediately after the procedure because of this effect. Barriga et al evaluated the adequacy of conscious sedation during upper endoscopy using midazolam alone compared with midazolam and fentanyl.[33] Although, from the endoscopists' perspective, patients in the combination group had better tolerance, no significant differences were found in the patient assessments. These results suggest that an adequate level of sedation can be obtained safely by either midazolam or midazolam and fentanyl. In a double-blind, placebo-controlled trial, 130 patients were randomly assigned to receive either 7.5 mg of midazolam orally or a placebo as premedication.[34] The results demonstrated that median anxiety score during upper endoscopy was significantly lower in the midazolam group than that in control. A significantly larger number of patients in the midazolam group reported partial or complete amnesia. Patients were more willing to receive repeat endoscopy in the midazolam group. However, the median recovery time was significantly longer in the midazolam group than control, with no differences in the satisfaction score and hemodynamic changes. Recently, propofol is increasingly used for sedation during advanced and prolonged therapeutic upper endoscopy with excellent sedative effect and high patients' satisfaction. Although propofol is generally safe with good hemodynamic stability, it is associated with a dose-dependent effect on blood pressure and heart rate. Moreover, there is no pharmacological antagonist, and monitored anesthesia care is the preferred approach.[28]

12.5 Use of Antifoaming Agents and Antispasmotics

In ideal setting, the use of antifoaming agents will help to clear the mucus and froth to enhance observation of any luminal pathology.[35] A mixture of mucolytic and defoaming agent can be given 30 minutes before the procedure. In Japan, the formula recommended includes 100-mL water with 20,000-U pronase (Kaken Pharmaceutical, Tokyo, Japan), 1 g of sodium bicarbonate, and 10 mL of dimethylpolysiloxane.[35] Pronase is not available worldwide; an alternative mixture will be 100-mL water mixed with 2 mL of acetylcysteine (200 mg/mL Parvolex, Celltech, United Kingdom; or Mucomyst, Bristo-Myers Squibb, United States) and 0.5 mL (40 mg/mL) activated dimethicone (Infacol, Forest Laboratories, United Kingdom; or Gascon, Kissei Pharmacuetical, Japan).[36]

Antispasmotics may be indicated for detail endoscopic examination of stomach, as peristalsis may obscure minute lesions and early gastric cancers. The most common agent used as antispasmodics is intravenous bolus of butylscopolamine bromide (Buscopan).[37] Peppermint oil solution administered intraluminally was reported to achieve similar effect of reducing gastric motility when compared to Buscopan, while it has less side effects of dry mouth and blurred vision.[38]

12.6 Procedural Steps for Upper Gastrointestinal Endoscopy

12.6.1 Insertion and Observation

After checking of the functionality of gastroscope, it is first inserted under direct visualization through the mouth into the oral cavity. After passing through the oral cavity into the hypopharynx, the larynx and the vocal cords will be observed for any abnormality. The endoscope will pass posterior to the larynx over the pyriform fossa through the cricopharyngeus. The patient will be asked to swallow in order to relax the cricopharyngeus for passage of the endoscope. The endoscopic view should be maintained during passage through the cricopharyngeus for observation of Zenker's diverticulum especially in elderly.

12.6.2 Esophagus

The gastroscope will then be passed into esophagus (▶ Fig. 12.1a). Abnormal esophageal pathology will be observed reaching the squamocolumnar junction (SCJ: Z-line) (▶ Fig. 12.1). The esophagus can be divided according to the anatomical region into three parts:
- *Cervical esophagus.* The cervical part of esophagus starts from cricopharyngeus, which usually is located at approximately 15 cm from the incisors to thoracic inlet where the esophagus enters the thorax posterior to the trachea.
- *Thoracic esophagus.* The thoracic esophagus starts from thoracic inlet, which is around 20 cm from the incisors and ends when esophagus enters into the abdominal cavity through the esophageal hiatus at the diaphragm at around 38 to 40 cm from incisor.

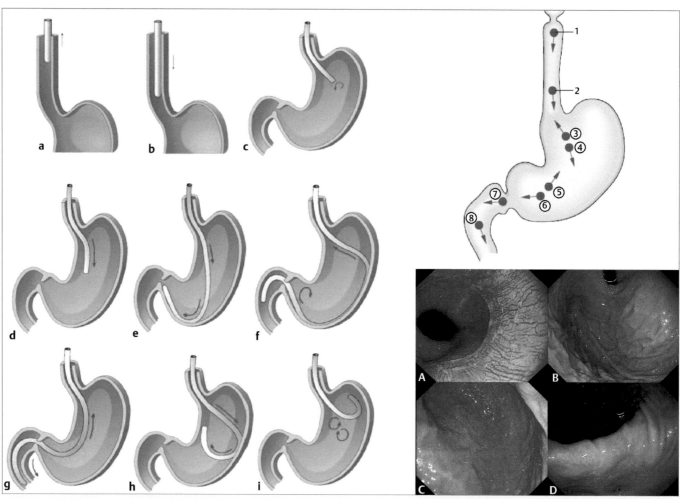

Fig. 12.1 ESGE quality control recommendations for an illustrated report on upper gastrointestinal endoscopy. **1(a)**, upper esophagus image taken 20 cm from incisor. **2(b)**, 2 cm above the squamocolumnar junction. **3(h)**, cardia in retroversion. **4(d)**, upper part of lesser curvature. **5(e)**, angular incisura. **6(e)**, antrum. **7(f)**, duodenal bulb. **8(g)**, second part of duodenum. **(A)**, gastroesophageal junction. **(B)**, retroflexed view of the gastric cardia. **(C)**, body of stomach. **(D)**, angular incisura.[42]

- *Abdominal esophagus.* The abdominal esophagus starts from the esophageal hiatus and ends at the esophagogastric junction (EGJ). It is generally less than 5 cm in length and it is where the lower esophageal sphincter is located. The level of the Z-line will be noted, and any abnormality or irregularity of the Z-line will be observed.

12.6.3 Esophagogastric Junction

EGJ is defined as the level of proximal gastric rugae fold according to the American Gastroenterology Association guidelines.[39] Meanwhile, the level of SCJ is defined as the distal end of esophageal palisading vessels as defined by Japanese Society of Esophageal Disease in 2000 (▶Fig. 12.1).[40] In healthy people, SCJ and EGJ should coincide at the same level. A sliding hiatal hernia is endoscopically defined as more than 2 cm separation of the caudally displaced EGJ and diaphragmatic impression.[41]

12.6.4 Stomach and Duodenum

The stomach is divided into the cardia, fundus, body, greater and lesser curvature, angular incisura, antrum, prepyloric canal, and pylorus. After passage through the gastroesophageal junction, the stomach should be examined systematically for

various pathologies over all the regions. In order to avoid prolonged gaseous distension, the stomach is examined after duodenal examination (▶Fig. 12.1d–f). The gastroscope should be passed through the pylorus entering into the first part of duodenum. Usually passage of the gastroscope through the pylorus requires targeting in close proximity, as the antral-pyloric region is a moving target upon active peristalsis (▶Fig. 12.1f, g). Intubation of second part of duodenum requires consecutive steps of manipulation of gastroscope, as the junction between first and second part of duodenum is an oblique uprising turn. After examination of the duodenal bulb, the tip of the scope is placed at the end of bulb pushing forward with the tip bending upward to the right. The left hand holding the shaft should also turn right when advancing the scope through the junction. The passage through the genu superius is usually blind, and the second part of duodenum will come to view after this passage with the gastroscope blending left and down. The endoscopist should then pull back the scope to reduce the loop formed in the stomach and the ampulla of Vater will be observed at superior wall of the second part of the duodenum. The scope shall be slowly withdrawn for observation of pathologies over the junction, especially as peptic ulcers at the inferior wall can be missed. For patients with upper GI bleeding where the source of bleeding cannot be identified, the duodenum should be intubated as far as possible to examine the third and fourth parts. After examination of the duodenum, the endoscopy is withdrawn back to stomach and rotated counterclockwise in 180-degree turn into a retroflexed position—the "J" maneuver for examination of the fundus, cardia, and proximal body of stomach.

Upper GI endoscopic examination should be conducted in a systematic manner. The European Society of Gastrointestinal Endoscopy (ESGE) recommended a minimal checklist of eight images should be taken during upper GI endoscopy[42] (▶Fig. 12.1). The anatomic locations recommended by ESGE included: image 1, upper esophagus at 20 cm from incisor; image 2, 2 cm above SCJ; image 3, cardia in retroversion; image 4, upper part of lesser curvature; image 5, angulus in partial inversion; image 6, antrum; image 7, duodenal bulb; and image 8, second part of duodenum.

The systematic screening protocol for stomach (SSS) provides a basis for standardized endoscopic examination of stomach to avoid missing lesions at blind spots[43,44] (▶Fig. 12.2). Firstly, after withdrawal from the duodenum, the stomach should be adequately distended to avoid missing lesions between folds and rugae. The gastric luminal wall should be adequately irrigated to remove mucus and secretions. With the gastroscope in antegrade manner, we first examine the four quadrants of the antrum (anterior, posterior, lesser curvature, and greater curvature). Next, the four quadrants of the lower body will be examined. Afterward, the four quadrants of the midupper body will be examined (▶Fig. 12.2). We then retroflex the gastroscope and examine the four quadrants of the gastric fundus-cardia region over anterior, posterior, lesser curvature, and greater curvature. While keeping the gastroscope in the retroflex position, further examination will be conducted at middle-upper body over lesser curve, anterior and posterior part. Finally, the angular incisura will be examined over lesser curve, anterior and posterior sides.

12.6.5 Transnasal Upper Endoscopy

Recently, the development of transnasal endoscopy allowed diagnostic upper endoscopy to be performed with scopes of much reduced caliber. The diameter of transnasal endoscope ranged from 4.9 to 5.9 mm (▶Table 12.1). This ultrathin endoscope is usually passed through one of the nostrils under local anesthesia with xylocaine spray, through the nasal cavity between middle and inferior turbinates into the nasopharynx. Through the nasopharynx, the larynx and the hypopharynx will be observed. The remaining procedure will be similar to those of ordinary upper endoscopy. Clinical studies confirmed a high success rate in endoscopic examination using transnasal endoscope, as well as excellent patients' satisfaction. The working channel allowed biopsy to be taken during transnasal endoscopy. However, the adoption of transnasal endoscopy is not high worldwide, probably related to the limitation in maneuverability of ultrathin endoscope as well as lower image quality.[45]

12.7 Common Pathologies for Upper Gastrointestinal Endoscopy

The pathological findings during upper GI endoscopy can be classified into benign or neoplastic diseases. These pathologies can be incidentally detected when patients do not have symptoms.

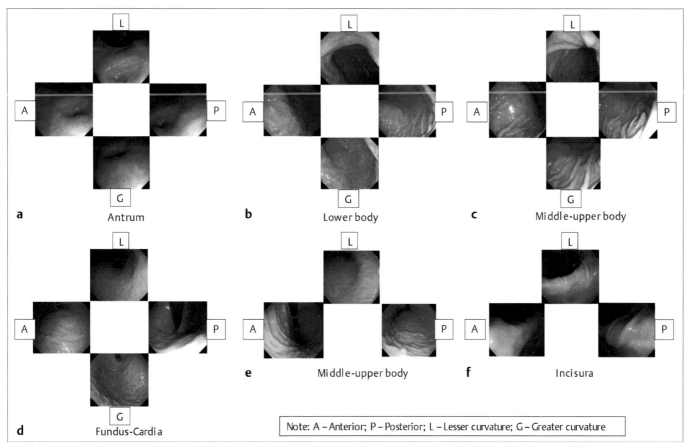

Note: A – Anterior; P – Posterior; L – Lesser curvature; G – Greater curvature

Fig. 12.2 Systematic screening protocol for stomach in upper gastrointestinal endoscopy.[44] The photos represented standard locations for examination and documentation in stomach.

While for those who present with symptoms or having complications including upper GI hemorrhage and obstruction, endoscopists should focus on identifying the relevant pathologies.

12.7.1 I: Upper Gastrointestinal Cancers

Cancer of the Stomach

Adenocarcinomas (ACs) of stomach are classified into intestinal and diffuse type according to the Lauren classification.[46] Borrmann et al described the macroscopic appearance of gastric cancer in four types which correlates with clinical prognosis.[47] Recently, type 0 was added into this classification to represent superficial and early-stage carcinoma (▶Table 12.5).[48] Type I describes protruding-type tumors, type II represents ulcerative and localized growth, type III are infiltrative and ulcerative tumors, and type IV represents diffusely infiltrative type or linitis plastica. Early gastric cancer is defined as carcinoma involving the mucosa or submucosal irrespective of the lymph node status (▶Table 12.6).[48] The macroscopic appearance of early gastric cancer can be classified into type 0 I (polypoid), which can be subclassified into type 0 Ip (pedunculated) and type 0 Is (sessile); type 0 II represents nonpolypoid type, which can be subclassified into type 0 IIa (elevated), IIb (flat), and IIc (depressed), and type 0 III represents excavated tumors, which carries higher risks of submucosal invasion.

Endoscopic characterization of early gastric cancer depends on changes in microvascular (MV) and microstructural (MS) patterns, as well as the presence of demarcation line. Yao et al reported the VS classification (V, vascular; S, surface) for diagnosis of early gastric cancer under magnifying endoscopy.[43,49] The changes in MS and MV pattern can be described as regular, irregular, or absence, as shown in ▶Fig. 12.3. The observation of these changes should be conducted using gastroscopes with either the mechanical zoom or dual-focus function (▶Table 12.1). For the MS pattern, the microanatomical changes include changes in the marginal crypt epithelium (MCE) and crypt openings. Intramucosal early gastric cancers demonstrate irregular MS pattern as evidence by irregular linear, curved, or polygonal pattern of MCE. The direction of arrangements of MCE will also be irregular, and length and width will not be uniform (▶Fig. 12.3). For MV pattern, we will observe changes in capillaries, collecting venules, and microvessels. Early gastric neoplasia usually demonstrate irregular vascular pattern including nonuniform microvessels with irregular sizes and shapes (▶Fig. 12.3). The presence of a demarcation line is an important distinguishing feature between chronic gastritis and early gastric cancers. The diagnosis of early gastric cancer is based on the presence of (1) irregular MV pattern with demarcation line and/or (2) irregular MS pattern with demarcation line.

Carcinoma of the Esophagus

Carcinoma of esophagus is generally primary in origin. The most common histological types of esophageal carcinoma include squamous cell carcinoma and AC. Superficial esophageal carcinoma are carcinomas limited to the submucosa (T1a and T1b), while early-stage esophageal cancers are carcinomas with invasion limited to the mucosa without metastasis (T1aN0M0). Superficial esophageal carcinoma is difficult to diagnose as it has only slight changes in MV and MS patterns.

For advance esophageal carcinoma, the following features should be documented during endoscopy: (1) location of the tumor in relation to the circumference; (2) proximal and distal extend of the tumor; (3) anatomical location as defined by the region of esophagus and relevant distance from incisor; and (4) macroscopic classification of the tumor. The macroscopic classification is according to type 0 to 5 as shown in ▶Table 12.5. Superficial esophageal carcinoma can be further classified according to the Paris classification into Type 0 Ip (protruded), Is (sessile), IIa (elevated), IIb (flat), IIc (depressed), and III (excavated) (▶Table 12.6). Superficial esophageal neoplasia is difficult to recognize upon white light endoscopy

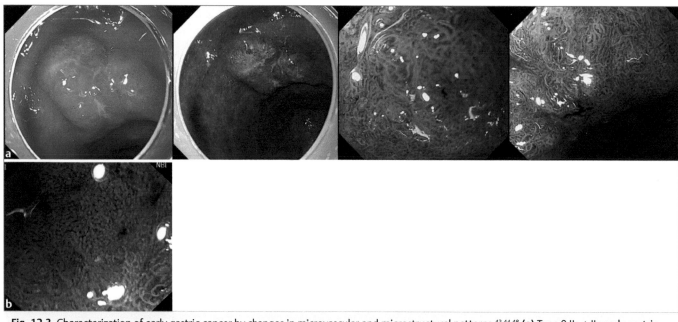

Fig. 12.3 Characterization of early gastric cancer by changes in microvascular and microstructural patterns.[43,44,48] (a) Type 0 IIa + IIc early gastric cancer with presence of irregular microsurface (MS) pattern under narrow-band imaging (NBI) magnifying endoscopy. (b) Early gastric cancer with irregular microvascular (MV) pattern and demarcation line (DL) under NBI magnifying endoscopy.

Table 12.5 Macroscopic classification of esophageal and gastric carcinoma[46]

Type	Japan Gastric Cancer Association classification	Borrmann's classification	Endoscopic appearance (esophagus)	Endoscopic appearance (stomach)
Type 0	Superficial type	NA		
Type 1	Protruding type	Protruding type		
Type 2	Ulcerative and localized type	Superficial growth		
Type 3	Ulcerative and infiltrative type	Excavating growth		
Type 4	Diffusely infiltrative type	Infiltrating growth with lateral spreading		

as there are only subtle changes in MV patterns. Inoue et al reported the changes in patterns of intrapapillary capillary loops (IPCLs) for superficial squamous esophageal neoplasia and correlation between dilatation of IPCL to depth to tumor invasion (▶Fig. 12.4). Kumagai et al first correlated the changes of MV pattern under magnifying endoscopy with the diagnosis of superficial esophageal neoplasia.[50] The caliber of IPCL was found to be significantly larger for M1 cancers when compared to normal esophageal mucosa under observation with stereoscopic microscopy and Microfil injection on surgical specimens, as well as magnifying endoscopy in 82 patients with superficial esophageal neoplasia. The original classification by Inoue et al classified IPCL into five types: type I

Table 12.6 Paris classification of superficial esophageal and gastric neoplasia[47]

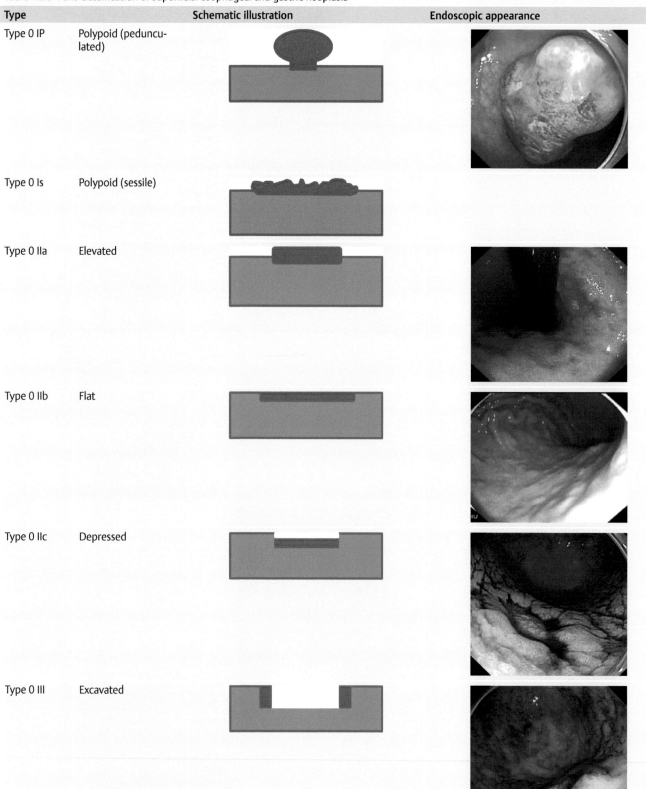

Type		Schematic illustration	Endoscopic appearance
Type 0 IP	Polypoid (pedunculated)		
Type 0 Is	Polypoid (sessile)		
Type 0 IIa	Elevated		
Type 0 IIb	Flat		
Type 0 IIc	Depressed		
Type 0 III	Excavated		

represents normal nondilated IPCL; type II represents elongated IPCL corresponding to inflammation; type III IPCLs are borderline lesions which potentially include esophagitis and low-grade intraepithelial neoplasia; type IV IPCLs are dilated loops representing high-grade intraepithelial neoplasia; type V IPCL patterns represent carcinoma of esophagus, while type V1 and V2 patterns are dilated loops, while type V1 and V2 patterns are dilated loops of IPCL with tortuosity, and neoplasia with these patterns indicate M1 or M2 invasion; type V3 patterns are dilated, torturous loops with elongated tail representing M3 invasion; and type Vn pattern corresponds to neovascularization and indicates submucosal invasion.[51,52]

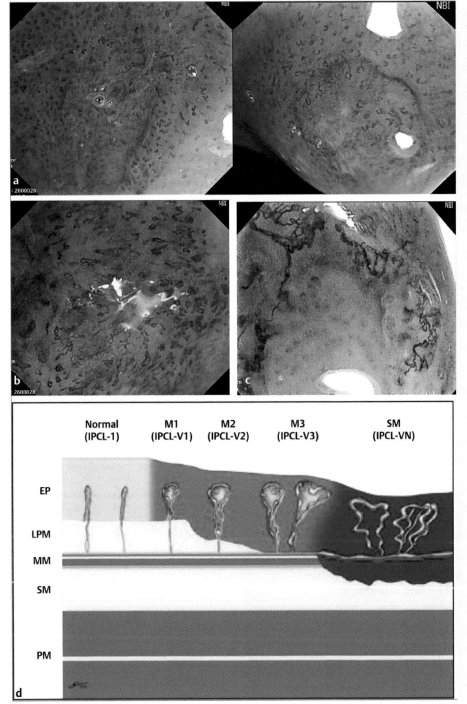

Fig. 12.4 Superficial esophageal neoplasia with irregular intrapapillary capillary loops (IPCL).[49,50] **(a)** IPCL type V1 pattern showing dilated loops, representing intramucosal esophageal carcinoma or severe dysplasia; A demarcation line is identified between normal and abnormal IPCL. **(b)** IPCL type V3 pattern: dilated torturous loops with elongated tail, representing superficial esophageal neoplasia with M3 or SM1 invasion. **(c)** IPCL type Vn pattern—neovascularization with no recognizable pattern of IPCL, representing esophageal cancer with submucosal invasion. **(d)** Intrapapillary capillary loop (IPCL) changes and the correlation with depth of invasion.[51]

12.7.2 II: Upper Gastrointestinal Hemorrhage

Upper GI hemorrhage is one of the most common emergency diseases requiring hospitalization worldwide. Upper endoscopy is the current standard for diagnosis and treatment of upper GI hemorrhage. The most common causes include bleeding peptic ulcers, esophageal and gastric variceal bleeding, bleeding from gastric, and esophageal cancers.[53] The less common causes included Dieulafoy's lesions, hemorrhagic gastritis, and gastric antral vascular ectasia (GAVE). Forest et al classified bleeding peptic ulcers into three types: Forest type I represents actively bleeding ulcers, which can be subclassified into spurting (Ia) and oozing (Ib) ulcers. Forest type II represents ulcers with endoscopic

stigmata of recent hemorrhage, including ulcers with a visible vessel (IIa), adherent clot (IIb), and red or black dot (IIc) at base of the ulcer. Endoscopic therapy should be applied for treatment for Forest Ia, Ib, IIa, and IIb ulcers.[54]

Esophageal and gastric variceal bleeding should be suspected when patients with a background history of liver cirrhosis present with an upper GI bleed. During diagnostic endoscopy, active bleeding can be sometimes observed. Bleeding from esophageal varices can be evidenced by presence of a small white clot as stigmata of recent hemorrhage. Retroflexion of the endoscope is essential to confirm presence of gastric varices. Patients with GAVE has bleeding from dilated small superficial vessels located over the antrum, while those with bleeding from Dieulafoy's lesions are related to erosion over small arterioles of the gastric wall.

12.7.3 III: GERD and Barrett's Esophagus

GERD is present in about 10 to 20% of the general population. About 40% of patients with GERD will go on to develop erosive esophagitis, out of which 10 to 15% will have Barrett's esophagus (BE). These patients can subsequently develop AC with an incidence of 0.3% per year.[55] Lately, larger population-based studies have reduced this figure further to less than 0.2% per year. GERD is a known risk factor for developing AC presumably due to ongoing active and chronic inflammatory process. A case–control study performed by Lagergren et al revealed that the odds of developing AC increased by 7.7 times in patients with GERD.[56] However, the prevalence of BE in patients without reflux symptoms ranges from 6 to 10% (note: prevalence in the GERD group which is 10 to 15%). The majority of patients with BE are not diagnosed because they are asymptomatic.[57]

BE is defined as an endoscopically apparent area of columnar-lined epithelium above the esophagogastric junction (▶ Fig. 12.5). Controversies with regard to the ideal definition still persist despite recognition of the presence of the condition more than 60 years ago. Intestinal metaplasia (IM) is required for the diagnosis in the United States, Continental Europe, and Australia but not in Britain and Japan.[58,59] It is important for the endoscopist to identify BE and its associated landmarks: the diaphragmatic pinch, the gastroesophageal junction, and SCJ.[55] The description of metaplastic change should be standardized according to Prague's classification, which includes the circumferential and maximal length of the Barrett's segment.[60] According to recent guidelines of American College of Gastroenterology (ACG),[55] in patients with suspected BE, at least eight random biopsies should be obtained to maximize the yield of IM. For patients with short (1–2 cm) segments of suspected BE where eight biopsies may not be possible, at least four biopsies per centimeter of circumferential BE should be taken.

12.8 Screening for BE

Screening is done to identify individuals with cancer or those with high risk of developing cancer. However, almost 40% of patients with esophageal adenocarcinoma (EAC) do not have reflux symptoms,[61] and these patients would certainly be missed if patients with chronic GERD are screened. Cost issues and the invasiveness of the current screening tool have also limited the effectiveness of an "endoscopic" screening strategy. Until better criteria are established for more targeted screening and perhaps newer methods introduced (including biomarkers or less invasive methods, e.g., the "cytosponge"), screening for BE in general population is still largely contentious. The recent guidelines of ACG recommended screening for BE may be considered in men

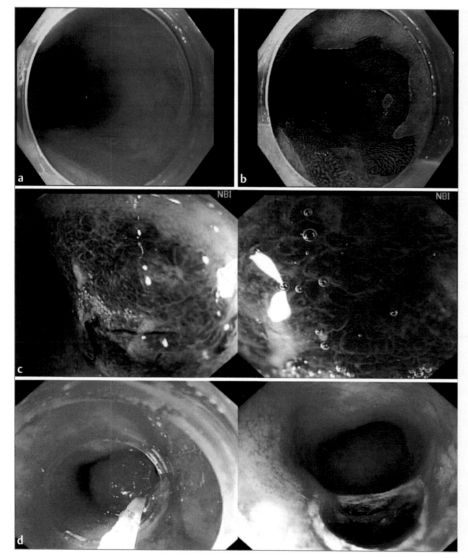

Fig. 12.5 Endoscopic diagnosis of Barrett's esophagus. (a) Barrett's esophagus on standard white light imaging. (b) Barrett's esophagus on narrow-band imaging. (c) Irregular microsurface pattern signifying high-grade dysplasia in BE. (d) High-grade dysplasia in BE treated by endoscopic mucosal resection.

with chronic (>5 years) and/or frequent symptoms of GERD with two or more risk factors for BE or EAC.[55] These risk factors included: (1) age > 50 years; (2) Caucasian race; (3) presence of central obesity; (4) current or past history of smoking; and (5) family history of BE or EAC in first-degree relative.

12.9 Surveillance for BE

It is hoped that for surveillance to succeed, any evidence of dysplasia and early carcinoma can be detected and treated promptly generally by less invasive endoscopic means.[62,63] Surveillance endoscopy is only appropriate for patients without significant comorbidities and fit to undergo therapy, be it surgery or endoscopic resection/ablation. When BE is identified, multiple systematic biopsy specimens should be obtained after any macroscopic lesion is sampled. The present recommended approach is to obtain four-quadrant biopsy specimens every 2-cm interval in patients without dysplasia, and 1-cm intervals in patients with prior dysplasia.[55] Recently, the development of WATS biopsy technique allowed better and deeper sampling, and improved the detection of esophageal dysplasia by 40%.[64] For patients with established BE of any length and with no dysplasia, an acceptable interval for surveillance is every 3 to 5 years. For patients with indefinite dysplasia, a repeat endoscopy after acid-suppression therapy for 3 to 6 months is recommended, while surveillance endoscopy should be performed at an interval of 12 months if indefinite dysplasia is confirmed. For patients with low-grade dysplasia (LGD), endoscopy therapy should be preferred, although surveillance every 12 months is an acceptable alternative.[55]

12.10 Barrett's Esophagus–Related Dysplasia

If dysplasia is indeterminate and/or if there is evidence of acute inflammation due to GERD, repeat biopsies should be performed after 8 weeks of effective acid-suppression therapy. Compliance with therapy is paramount. LGD should be managed by extensive rebiopsy after intensive acid suppression for 8 to 12 weeks. Lately, it has been recommended that a diagnosis of LGD in the community should prompt further confirmation by an expert GI pathologist. If persisting, surveillance should be 6 monthly for as long as it remains stable. If apparent regression occurs on two consecutive examinations, surveillance intervals may be increased to annually. Some centers advocate treating "confirmed" LGD with radiofrequency ablation. High-grade dysplasia is associated with a focus of invasive AC in 30 to 40% of patients (▶ Fig. 12.5c). Endoscopic therapy has superseded esophagectomy and is now considered the mainstay of treatment for these patients (▶ Fig. 12.5d).

12.11 Complications of Upper Gastrointestinal Endoscopy

The procedure-related mortality of EGD was reported to be 1 in 9,000, while the risk of complication in gastroscopy ranged from 0.01 to 0.1%.[65,66] The risk of mortality from EGD is generally higher among patients who presented with upper GI hemorrhage and variceal bleeding. Reiertsen et al reported the mortality of diagnostic EGD to be 0.04%, while nonfatal complications occurred in 0.14% of the 7,314 procedures.[67] The most common complaints after EGD are sore throat and abdominal discomfort.[68] The general risk of perforation is reported to be around 0.01%, while therapeutic EGD had significantly higher risks of perforation. Niv et al reported the risk of perforation as 1 in 31,480 EGD procedures.[69] The common causes of perforation after EGD are mostly related to therapeutic procedures, including EMR and ESD, endoscopic dilatation, and removal of foreign body. The rate of cardiopulmonary unplanned events was 0.6% and the risk correlated to ASA class.[67] Aspiration pneumonia is one of the important risks for EGD, and patients are usually instructed to keep nil per oral for at least 6 hours before the procedure. However, patients with undiagnosed achalasia and gastric outlet obstruction will have increased risks of aspiration, and diagnostic EGD should be performed with extra caution and prolonged fasting for these cases.

References

[1] Kravetz RE. Vaginal speculum. Am J Gastroenterol. 2006; 101(11):2456

[2] Kluge F, Seidler E. Zur Erstanwendung der Osophago- und Gastroskopie: Briefe von Adolf Kussmaul und seinen Mitarbeitern. Medizinhist J. 1986; 21(3–4):288–307

[3] Hopkins HH, Kapany NS. A flexible fiberscope, using static scanning. Nature. 1954; 173:39–41

[4] Hirschowitz BI, Curtiss LE, Peters CW, Pollard HM. Demonstration of a new gastroscope, the fiberscope. Gastroenterology. 1958; 35(1):50–53, discussion 51–53

[5] Sivak MV. Gastrointestinal endoscopy: past and future. Gut. 2006; 55(8):1061–1064

[6] Classen M, Phillip J. Electronic endoscopy of the gastrointestinal tract. Initial experience with a new type of endoscope that has no fiberoptic bundle for imaging. Endoscopy. 1984; 16(1):16–19

[7] Niwa H, Kawaguchi A, Miyahara T, Koyama H. Clinical use of new video-endoscopes (EVIS 100 and 200). Endoscopy. 1992; 24(3):222–224

[8] Varadarajulu S, Banerjee S, Barth BA, et al; ASGE Technology Committee. GI endoscopes. Gastrointest Endosc. 2011; 74(1):1–6.e6

[9] Rodriguez SA, Banerjee S, Desilets D, et al; ASGE Technology Committee. Ultrathin endoscopes. Gastrointest Endosc. 2010; 71(6):893–898

[10] Early DS, Ben-Menachem T, Decker GA, et al; ASGE Standards of Practice Committee. Appropriate use of GI endoscopy. Gastrointest Endosc. 2012; 75(6):1127–1131

[11] Axon AT, Bell GD, Jones RH, et al. Guidelines on appropriate indications for upper gastrointestinal endoscopy. Working Party of the Joint Committee of the Royal College of Physicians of London, Royal College of Surgeons of England, Royal College of Anaesthetists, Association of Surgeons, the British Society of Gastroenterology, and the Thoracic Society of Great Britain. BMJ. 1995; 310(6983):853–856

[12] Leung WK, Wu MS, Kakugawa Y, et al; Asia Pacific Working Group on Gastric Cancer. Screening for gastric cancer in Asia: current evidence and practice. Lancet Oncol. 2008; 9(3):279–287

[13] Hamashima C, Shibuya D, Yamazaki H, et al. The Japanese guidelines for gastric cancer screening. Jpn J Clin Oncol. 2008; 38(4):259–267

[14] Suzuki H, Gotoda T, Sasako M, Saito D. Detection of early gastric cancer: misunderstanding the role of mass screening. Gastric Cancer. 2006; 9(4):315–319

[15] Hisamichi S. Screening for gastric cancer. World J Surg. 1989; 13(1):31–37

[16] ASGE Technology Committee. High-definition and high-magnification endoscopes. Gastrointest Endosc. 2014; 80(6):919–927

[17] Lau JY, Barkun A, Fan DM, et al. Challenges in the management of acute peptic ulcer bleeding. Lancet. 2013; 381(9882):2033–2043

[18] Gotoda T, Ho KY, Soetikno R, et al. Gastric ESD: current status and future directions of devices and training. Gastrointest Endosc Clin N Am. 2014; 24(2):213–233

[19] Wani S, Sharma P. Challenges with endoscopic therapy for Barrett's esophagus. Gastroenterol Clin North Am. 2015; 44(2):355–372

[20] Costamagna G, Marchese M, Iacopini F. Self-expanding stents in oesophageal cancer. Eur J Gastroenterol Hepatol. 2006; 18(11):1177–1180

[21] Fernández-Esparrach G, Córdova H, Bordas JM, et al. Endoscopic management of the complications of bariatric surgery. Experience of more than 400 interventions [in Spanish] Gastroenterol Hepatol. 2011; 34(3):131–136

[22] Teoh AY, Chiu PW. Collaboration between laparoscopic surgery and endoscopic resection: an evidence-based review. Dig Endosc. 2014; 26(Suppl 1):12–19

[23] Kato M, Uraoka T, Isobe Y, et al. A case of gastric adenocarcinoma of fundic gland type resected by combination of laparoscopic and endoscopic approaches to neoplasia with non-exposure technique (CLEAN-NET). Clin J Gastroenterol. 2015; 8(6):393–399

[24] Cooper GS. Indications and contraindications for upper gastrointestinal endoscopy. Gastrointest Endosc Clin N Am. 1994; 4(3):439–454

[25] Wu JC, Chan FK, Ching JY, et al. Empirical treatment based on "typical" reflux symptoms is inappropriate in a population with a high prevalence of Helicobacter pylori infection. Gastrointest Endosc. 2002; 55(4):461–465

[26] Campo R, Brullet E, Montserrat A, et al, . Topical pharyngeal anesthesia improves tolerance of upper gastrointestinal endoscopy: a randomized double-blind study. Endoscopy. 1995; 27(9):659–664

[27] Igea F, Casellas JA, González-Huix F, et al; Spanish Society of Digestive Endoscopy. Sedation for gastrointestinal endoscopy. Endoscopy. 2014; 46(8):720–731

[28] Triantafillidis JK, Merikas E, Nikolakis D, Papalois AE. Sedation in gastrointestinal endoscopy: current issues. World J Gastroenterol. 2013; 19(4):463–481

[29] Riphaus A, Rabofski M, Wehrmann T. Endoscopic sedation and monitoring practice in Germany: results from the first nationwide survey. Z Gastroenterol. 2010; 48(3):392–397

[30] Heuss LT, Froehlich F, Beglinger C. Changing patterns of sedation and monitoring practice during endoscopy: results of a nationwide survey in Switzerland. Endoscopy. 2005; 37(2):161–166

[31] Baudet JS, Borque P, Borja E, et al. Use of sedation in gastrointestinal endoscopy: a nationwide survey in Spain. Eur J Gastroenterol Hepatol. 2009; 21(8):882–888

[32] Lee MG, Hanna W, Harding H. Sedation for upper gastrointestinal endoscopy: a comparative study of midazolam and diazepam. Gastrointest Endosc. 1989; 35(2):82–84

[33] Barriga J, Sachdev MS, Royall L, et al, . Sedation for upper endoscopy: comparison of midazolam versus fentanyl plus midazolam. South Med J. 2008; 101(4):362–366

[34] Mui LM, Teoh AY, Ng EK, et al. Premedication with orally administered midazolam in adults undergoing diagnostic upper endoscopy: a double-blind placebo-controlled randomized trial. Gastrointest Endosc. 2005; 61(2):195–200

[35] Bhandari P, Green S, Hamanaka H, et al. Use of Gascon and Pronase either as a pre-endoscopic drink or as targeted endoscopic flushes to improve visibility during gastroscopy: a prospective, randomized, controlled, blinded trial. Scand J Gastroenterol. 2010; 45(3):357–361

[36] Chang CC, Chen SH, Lin CP, et al. Premedication with pronase or N-acetylcysteine improves visibility during gastroendoscopy: an endoscopist-blinded, prospective, randomized study. World J Gastroenterol. 2007; 13(3):444–447

[37] Gotoda T, Uedo N, Yoshinaga S, et al. Basic principles and practice of gastric cancer screening using high-definition white-light gastroscopy: Eyes can only see what the brain knows. Dig Endosc. 2016; 28(Suppl 1):2–15

[38] Imagawa A, Hata H, Nakatsu M, et al. Peppermint oil solution is useful as an antispasmodic drug for esophagogastroduodenoscopy, especially for elderly patients. Dig Dis Sci. 2012; 57(9):2379–2384

[39] Sharma P, McQuaid K, Dent J, et al; AGA Chicago Workshop. A critical review of the diagnosis and management of Barrett's esophagus: the AGA Chicago Workshop. Gastroenterology. 2004; 127(1):310–330

[40] Takubo K, Aida J, Sawabe M, et al. The normal anatomy around the oesophagogastric junction: a histopathologic view and its correlation with endoscopy. Best Pract Res Clin Gastroenterol. 2008; 22(4):569–583

[41] Huang Q. Definition of the esophagogastric junction: a critical mini review. Arch Pathol Lab Med. 2011; 135(3):384–389

[42] Rey JF, Lambert R; ESGE Quality Assurance Committee. ESGE recommendations for quality control in gastrointestinal endoscopy: guidelines for image documentation in upper and lower GI endoscopy. Endoscopy. 2001; 33(10):901–903

[43] Yao K. The endoscopic diagnosis of early gastric cancer. Ann Gastroenterol. 2013; 26(1):11–22

[44] Veitch AM, Uedo N, Yao K, East JE. Optimizing early upper gastrointestinal cancer detection at endoscopy. Nat Rev Gastroenterol Hepatol. 2015; 12(11):660–667

[45] Tanuma T, Morita Y, Doyama H. Current status of transnasal endoscopy worldwide using ultrathin videoscope for upper gastrointestinal tract. Dig Endosc. 2016; 28(Suppl 1):25–31

[46] Hu B, El Hajj N, Sittler S, et al. Gastric cancer: Classification, histology and application of molecular pathology. J Gastrointest Oncol. 2012; 3(3):251–261

[47] Li C, Oh SJ, Kim S, et al. Macroscopic Borrmann type as a simple prognostic indicator in patients with advanced gastric cancer. Oncology. 2009; 77(3–4):197–204

[48] The Paris endoscopic classification of superficial neoplastic lesions: esophagus, stomach, and colon: November 30 to December 1, 2002. Gastrointest Endosc. 2003; 58(6, Suppl):S3–S43

[49] Yao K, Anagnostopoulos GK, Ragunath K. Magnifying endoscopy for diagnosing and delineating early gastric cancer. Endoscopy. 2009; 41(5):462–467

[50] Kumagai Y, Inoue H, Nagai K, et al. Magnifying endoscopy, stereoscopic microscopy, and the microvascular architecture of superficial esophageal carcinoma. Endoscopy. 2002; 34(5):369–375

[51] Inoue H, Kaga M, Ikeda H, et al. Magnification endoscopy in esophageal squamous cell carcinoma: a review of the intrapapillary capillary loop classification. Ann Gastroenterol. 2015; 28(1):41–48 Review

[52] Sato H, Inoue H, Ikeda H, et al. Utility of intrapapillary capillary loops seen on magnifying narrow-band imaging in estimating invasive depth of esophageal squamous cell carcinoma. Endoscopy. 2015; 47(2):122–128

[53] Sung JJ, Kuipers E, Barkun A. Gastrointestinal Bleeding. 2nd ed. Hoboken, NJ: Wiley-Blackwell; 2012

[54] Forrest JA, Finlayson ND, Shearman DJ. Endoscopy in Gastrointestinal Bleeding. Lancet 1974; 304(7877):394–397

[55] Shaheen NJ, Falk GW, Iyer PG, Gerson LB; American College of Gastroenterology. ACG Clinical Guideline: diagnosis and management of Barrett's esophagus. Am J Gastroenterol. 2016; 111(1):30–50, quiz 51

[56] Lagergren J, Bergström R, Lindgren A, Nyrén O. Symptomatic gastroesophageal reflux as a risk factor for esophageal adenocarcinoma. N Engl J Med. 1999; 340(11):825–831

[57] Cameron AJ, Zinsmeister AR, Ballard DJ, Carney JA. Prevalence of columnar-lined (Barrett's) esophagus. Comparison of population-based clinical and autopsy findings. Gastroenterology. 1990; 99(4):918–922

[58] Playford RJ. New British Society of Gastroenterology (BSG) guidelines for the diagnosis and management of Barrett's oesophagus. Gut. 2006; 55(4):442–443

[59] Sampliner RE; The Practice Parameters Committee of the American College of Gastroenterology. Practice guidelines on the diagnosis, surveillance, and therapy of Barrett's esophagus. Am J Gastroenterol. 1998; 93(7):1028–1032

[60] Sharma P, Dent J, Armstrong D, et al. The development and validation of an endoscopic grading system for Barrett's esophagus: the Prague C & M criteria. Gastroenterology. 2006; 131(5):1392–1399

[61] Devesa SS, Blot WJ, Fraumeni JF, Jr. Changing patterns in the incidence of esophageal and gastric carcinoma in the United States. Cancer. 1998; 83(10):2049–2053

[62] Sampliner RE; Practice Parameters Committee of the American College of Gastroenterology. Updated guidelines for the diagnosis, surveillance, and therapy of Barrett's esophagus. Am J Gastroenterol. 2002; 97(8):1888–1895

[63] Wang KK, Wongkeesong M, Buttar NS; American Gastroenterological Association. American Gastroenterological Association medical position statement: role of the gastroenterologist in the management of esophageal carcinoma. Gastroenterology. 2005; 128(5):1468–1470

[64] Anandasabapathy S, Sontag S, Graham DY, et al. Computer-assisted brush-biopsy analysis for the detection of dysplasia in a high-risk Barrett's esophagus surveillance population. Dig Dis Sci. 2011; 56(3):761–766

[65] McLernon DJ, Donnan PT, Crozier A, et al, . A study of the safety of current gastrointestinal endoscopy (EGD). Endoscopy. 2007; 39(8):692–700

[66] Sharma VK, Nguyen CC, Crowell MD, et al. A national study of cardiopulmonary unplanned events after GI endoscopy. Gastrointest Endosc. 2007; 66(1):27–34

[67] Reiertsen O, Skjøtø J, Jacobsen CD, Rosseland AR. Complications of fiberoptic gastrointestinal endoscopy--five years' experience in a central hospital. Endoscopy. 1987; 19(1):1–6

[68] Abbas SZ, Shaw S, Campbell D, et al. Outpatient upper gastrointestinal endoscopy: large prospective study of the morbidity and mortality rate at a single endoscopy unit in England. Dig Endosc. 2004; 16:1443–1661

[69] Niv Y, Gershtansky Y, Tal Y, et al. Analysis of 7-year physician-reported adverse events in esophagogastroduodenoscopy. J Patient Saf. 2012; 8(2):65–68

13 Enteroscopy Techniques

Tomonori Yano, Satoshi Shinozaki, Alan Kawarai Lefor, and Hironori Yamamoto

13.1 Introduction

Enteroscopy techniques are utilized worldwide because of the widespread availability of device-assisted enteroscopy and capsule endoscopy. The anatomical state of the small intestine precluded conventional endoscopy from deep insertion in the 20th century. The emergence of device-assisted enteroscopy at the beginning of 21st century has revolutionized the paradigm for the diagnosis and management of small intestinal diseases. The insertion mechanism in all device-assisted enteroscopy is straightforward, utilizing wedged overtube folding and shortening redundant loops so that endoscopist's maneuver is directly transferred to the tip of endoscope. Device-assisted enteroscopy includes double-balloon endoscopy (DBE), single-balloon endoscopy (SBE), and spiral endoscopy. All device-assisted enteroscopy can reach the deep small intestine, enabling detailed visualization, endoscopic ultrasound, biopsy, hemostasis, balloon dilation, polypectomy, and foreign body retrieval. Indications for device-assisted enteroscopy include diagnosis, observation, and therapeutic interventions for a wide range of small intestinal diseases, and is also useful for total colonoscopy in patients who underwent failed cecal intubation by conventional colonoscopy and for biliary interventions in patients with surgically altered anatomy. Total enteroscopy is usually accomplished by using both upper and lower endoscopic insertion. Although the rate of total enteroscopy varies among the kinds of device-assisted enteroscopy procedures and patients, DBE is superior to SBE or spiral endoscopy. Device-assisted enteroscopy will continue to have a major impact on the diagnosis and treatment of small intestinal diseases throughout the 21st century.

13.2 Overview of Enteroscopy Procedures

13.2.1 Anatomical Characteristics of the Small Intestine

The small intestine includes the duodenum, jejunum, and ileum, between the stomach and colon. It is located far from the mouth and anus, and is not fixed by peritoneal attachments with multiple complicated flexion points. This anatomical state makes it difficult to visualize the entire small intestine with conventional endoscopy.

13.2.2 Classification and Principles of Device-Assisted Enteroscopy

At the beginning of 21st century, the development and availability of device-assisted enteroscopy provided full access to the entire small intestine, for both diagnostic and thera-

peutic interventions. Device-assisted enteroscopy includes DBE (▶Fig. 13.1), SBE (▶Fig. 13.2), and spiral endoscopy (▶Fig. 13.3). Double- and single-balloon endoscopy are collectively known as balloon-assisted endoscopy. Although various devices are used, the mechanism is the same involving "folding redundant loops of the small intestine" (▶Fig. 13.4). This allows direct transmission of manipulation from the hand to the tip of endoscope even in the deep small intestine. Further, the working length of the endoscope does not have to be as long as the length of the intestine because device-assisted enteroscopy effectively shortens the intestine by repeat folding ("pleating") of redundant loops. The endoscopes also have a working channel which enables biopsies, marking, endoscopic ultrasonography, and various therapeutic interventions such as balloon dilation and hemostasis.

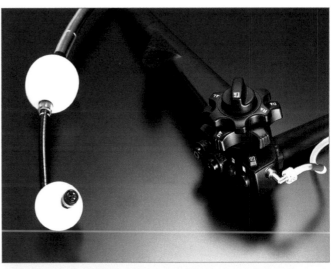

Fig. 13.1 Double-balloon endoscopy (DBE).

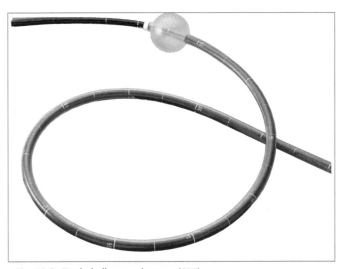

Fig. 13.2 Single-balloon endoscopy (SBE).

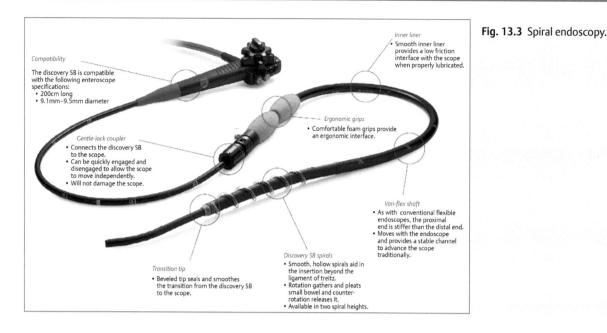

Fig. 13.3 Spiral endoscopy.

Compatibility

The discovery SB is compatible with the following enteroscope specifications:
• 200cm long
• 9.1mm–9.5mm diameter

Inner liner
• Smooth inner liner provides a low friction interface with the scope when properly lubricated.

Gentle-lock coupler
• Connects the discovery SB to the scope.
• Can be quickly engaged and disengaged to allow the scope to move independently.
• Will not damage the scope.

Ergonomic grips
• Comfortable foam grips provide an ergonomic interface.

Vari-flex shaft
• As with conventional flexible endoscopes, the proximal end is stiffer than the distal end.
• Moves with the endoscope and provides a stable channel to advance the scope traditionally.

Transition tip
• Beveled tip seals and smoothes the transition from the discovery SB to the scope.

Discovery SB spirals
• Smooth, hollow spirals aid in the insertion beyond the ligament of treitz.
• Rotation gathers and pleats small bowel and counter-rotation releases it.
• Available in two spiral heights.

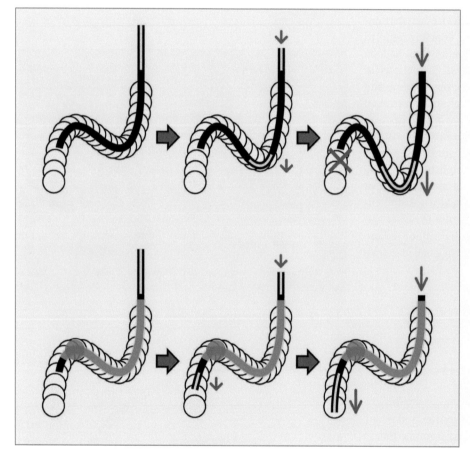

Fig. 13.4 Principle of device-assisted enteroscopy.

13.2.3 Balloon-Assisted Enteroscopy (Double-Balloon Endoscopy/Single-Balloon Endoscopy)

Balloon-assisted endoscopy uses a soft overtube with a balloon at the tip. The overtube fully accommodates the working length of the endoscope. The balloon of the overtube wedges against the intestinal wall so that it can fold the small intestine enabling direct transfer of the endoscopic manipulation from the shaft to the tip of the endoscope. Balloon-assisted endoscopy includes DBE and SBE. DBE has two balloons, one at the tip of the endoscope and the other at the tip of the overtube, and SBE has a balloon only at the tip of the overtube. Yamamoto et al first developed and reported DBE in 2001,[1] which was then released in 2003 by Fujifilm Corp. (Tokyo, Japan). At about the same time, capsule endoscopy was also reported and made available.[2] In 2007, SBE was released by Olympus Corp. (Tokyo, Japan). The development and worldwide availability of balloon-assisted endoscopy has revolutionized the diagnosis and treatment of small intestinal diseases.

13.2.4 Spiral Endoscopy

Spiral endoscopy (Spiral Medical, LLC, Massachusetts, United States) utilizes a helical overtube that accommodates an endoscope (inner diameter is 9.8 mm and full length is 118 cm). The rotating overtube with protrusions hooks the fold, and the redundant small intestine is folded and fixed on the overtube.[3] Once the tip of the overtube passes the ligament of Treitz, the tip of endoscope passively moves forward by rotating the overtube without pushing the endoscope.

13.3 General Diagnostic Techniques

The insertion route is determined by symptoms and findings of prior studies, including computed tomography (CT) scan, esophagogastroduodenoscopy, and colonoscopy. Preparation before upper and lower balloon-assisted enteroscopy is the same as that used for esophagogastroduodenoscopy and colonoscopy, respectively. Upper device-assisted enteroscopy only requires fasting from the night before the procedure, and lower balloon-assisted enteroscopy requires preparation with 2 to 4 L of polyethylene glycol and/or laxative. Because of the longer examination time compared with conventional endoscopy, deep sedation is recommended for upper balloon-assisted enteroscopy and conscious sedation for lower balloon-assisted enteroscopy.

Generally, balloon-assisted enteroscopy is performed with one endoscopic operator and one assistant who handles the overtube. However, it can also be performed by only one person with or without an apparatus to assist.[4,5] Balloon-assisted endoscopy is performed as follows: (1) the operator places an overtube on the proximal side of the endoscope and inserts the endoscope in the mouth or anus; (2) the operator inserts the endoscope using the "hooking the fold" technique as long as possible, and then proceeds with the overtube along the endoscope. At this time, the balloon at the tip of the endoscope is inflated so that the endoscope is not pulled proximally by interfering with overtube insertion. With SBE, the operator has to hook the endoscope to the fold by flexing the endoscope tip upward/downward; (3) the operator inflates the balloon at the tip of the overtube, and then pulls both the overtube and endoscope so that the redundant loop is shortened on the overtube. (4) the operator deflates the balloon at the tip of the endoscope in DBE, and then releases upward/downward on the endoscope in SBE. The operator then passes the endoscope deeper into the small intestine. By repeating steps (2) to (4) above, deep enteroscopy is accomplished (**Video 13.1**, **Video 13.2**).

In upper enteroscopy, balloon inflation is not needed in the stomach. In lower enteroscopy, balloon inflation is used, even in the colon.

13.4 General Therapeutic Techniques

13.4.1 Hemostasis

Device-assisted enteroscopy enables endoscopic hemostasis in the distal small intestine, as far as the endoscope reaches. The most important and difficult issue is to identify the bleeding source distally in the small intestine. If a patient presents with obscure gastrointestinal bleeding, the examination of choice is probably a dynamic CT scan with contrast because of its low invasiveness and short procedure time. Based on the results of the CT scan, clinical manifestations, and conventional endoscopy, the appropriate device (capsule endoscope or device-assisted enteroscopy) is selected. If the CT scan shows extravasation, a mass lesion, wall thickening, or stricture, device-assisted enteroscopy is selected rather than capsule endoscopy. However, capsule endoscopy is used in patients with a negative CT scan. In case of overt obscure gastrointestinal bleeding, upper device-assisted enteroscopy is recommended. During upper enteroscopy, the appearance of bloody enteric contents indicates that the bleeding source is near because retrograde flow of intestinal contents usually does not occur in the small intestine. Therefore, a marking clip should be placed as a landmark where the bloody fluid is first seen. The operator can easily lose orientation in the distal small intestine without a landmark. The operator should then try to find the bleeding source around the area of the marking clip. If there is massive bleeding obscuring the visual field, use of the "gel immersion method" should be considered to obtain clear visualization and enable precise hemostasis.[6] When we investigate a patient with mid-gastrointestinal bleeding, the lumen of the small bowel is narrow and may be filled with blood. It is difficult to secure the visual field during enteroscopy for massive bleeding, because the injected water is rapidly mixed with fresh blood. Clear gel of an appropriate viscosity to prevent rapid mixing is injected through the accessory channel, instead of water. After gel injection, the bleeding source is clearly observed in the space occupied by the gel.

Bleeding sources in the small intestine are divided into three groups: vascular lesions, tumors/polyps, and ulcers/erosions.[7] Tumors/polyps and ulcers/erosions are usually treated by surgical or medical management after confirming the diagnosis by device-assisted enteroscopy. However, the mainstay of treatment for vascular lesions in the small intestine is endoscopic hemostasis using device-assisted enteroscopy.[8] Small intestinal vascular lesions are endoscopically classified by the Yano–Yamamoto classification based on the size and pulsatile nature of the lesion.[9] A lesion that is not pulsatile is considered to be a venous/capillary lesion, and is usually treated by argon plasma coagulation. Pulsatile vascular lesions are considered to be arterial in origin, and are usually treated by clip application.

13.4.2 Balloon Dilation

There are a number of diseases that cause small intestinal strictures including Crohn's disease, Behcet's disease, nonspecific multiple small intestinal ulcerous disease, nonsteroidal anti-inflammatory drug–induced enteritis, ischemic enteritis, traumatic delayed-onset stricture, postoperative stricture, and scar formation after chemotherapy or radiotherapy. In these situations, device-assisted enteroscopy usually enables endoscopic balloon dilation as far as the endoscope reaches. Indications for balloon dilation include (1) fibrotic strictures with obstructive symptoms after medical treatment, (2) asymptomatic strictures with proximal bowel dilation shown by diagnostic imaging (fluoroscopic examination, computed tomography, and magnetic resonance imaging). Factors precluding balloon dilation include (1) a stricture that exceeds 50 mm in length, (2) a stricture with severe angulation, (3) a stricture with an active ulcer that seems to involve the muscularis layer, (4) a stricture with abscess formation, and (5) a stricture with a malignant appearance.[10]

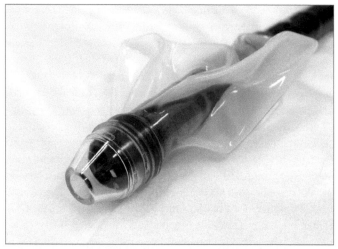

Fig. 13.5 Calibrated small-caliber-tip transparent hood.

Endoscopic balloon dilation requires real-time fluoroscopic guidance. After reaching the stricture using device-assisted enteroscopy, endoscopic observation of the stricture and selective contrast studies are necessary to ascertain the indication for dilation. Using DBE, wedging, or inflating, the balloon at the tip of the endoscope prevents reflux of contrast media, resulting in clear visualization of the stricture. Next, the operator passes a soft guidewire through the stricture, and then introduces a through-the-scope dilation balloon. The location of the balloon is adjusted referring to real-time fluoroscopic images. The dilation time is usually about 1 minute.

Determining the correct balloon size is always difficult because the precise diameter of the stricture is difficult to estimate based on endoscopic imaging and selective contrast studies. The use of a transparent hood with calibration lines marked along the side may be used (▶Fig. 13.5).[11] By wedging the stricture, one can measure the actual diameter. We recommend stepwise dilation to prevent iatrogenic perforation. Although 12-mm dilation is a typical goal for balloon dilation during the first session, 8- to 10-mm dilation may be appropriate in patients with severe strictures (< 6 mm in diameter before dilation). After the first session, additional repeat dilations are sometimes performed at 3- to 6-month intervals to attain 15-mm dilation as the final goal.

13.4.3 Polypectomy/Endoscopic Mucosal Resection

Using device-assisted enteroscopy, small intestinal polyps can be treated endoscopically, in the same manner as resecting a colon polyp. The small intestinal wall is thinner than that of the stomach or colon. Therefore, a submucosal saline injection prior to polypectomy is recommended to avoid perforation.

13.4.4 Retrieval of Foreign Bodies

Device-assisted enteroscopy enables retrieval of intraluminal foreign bodies or a trapped capsule endoscope. The optimal hood and retrieval tool to be used for retrieval is based on the size and shape of the foreign body.

Table 13.1 Commercially available endoscopes for balloon-assisted endoscopy in 2016.

	Working length	Outer diameter	Diameter of the working channel
Double-balloon endoscopes			
• EN-580XP	2,000	7.5	2.2
• EN-580T	2,000	9.4	3.2
• EI-580BT	1,550	**9.4**	3.2
Single-balloon endoscope			
• SIF-Q260	2,000	9.2	2.8

13.5 Accessory Devices and Techniques

Since the endoscopes used in device-assisted enteroscopy have a long working length and a small working channel, the tools which can be used are limited. ▶Table 13.1 shows the specifications of commercially available endoscopes for device-assisted enteroscopy as of 2016. For diagnostic DBE, a 2.2-mm working channel accommodates biopsy forceps, an injection needle, a snare, or an argon plasma coagulation probe. However, clip application devices and dilation balloons cannot be used. A DBE or SBE with a 2.8-mm or larger working channel can accommodate clip application devices and dilation balloons as well. Although most conventional biliary tract devices cannot be used in device-assisted enteroscopy as long as 2,000 mm, short DBE can accommodate these devices. Short DBE enables biliary interventions via a wide working channel in patients with surgically altered anatomy.

13.6 Indications for the Use of Device-Assisted Enteroscopy

13.6.1 Indications for Diagnostic Use

Investigation of obscure gastrointestinal bleeding, small intestinal tumors, small intestinal strictures, and inflammatory bowel disease is the main indications for the diagnostic use of device-assisted enteroscopy.

13.6.2 Indications for Follow-Up of Small Intestinal Lesions

Device-assisted enteroscopy is useful to follow up small intestinal lesions due to previously diagnosed Crohn's disease or Behcet's disease. The degree of inflammatory change can be easily determined by direct observation of the small intestinal mucosa using device-assisted enteroscopy.

13.6.3 Therapeutic Indications for Device-Assisted Enteroscopy

Therapeutic interventions using device-assisted enteroscopy include endoscopic hemostasis, endoscopic polypectomy, balloon dilation of small intestinal strictures, and retrieval of foreign bodies such as a capsule endoscope.

13.6.4 Miscellaneous Indications for Device-Assisted Enteroscopy

Balloon-assisted endoscopy enables total colonoscopy after failure of cecal intubation with conventional colonoscopy. Balloon-assisted endoscopy also enables endoscopic retrograde cholangiopancreatography in patients with surgically altered anatomy, such as a Roux-en-Y anastomosis.

13.7 Procedure-Specific Quality Measures

Accomplishing total enteroscopy is important for a high-quality examination. When we attempt total enteroscopy using balloon-assisted endoscopy, we try to insert the balloon-assisted endoscope (upper or lower) as far as possible and mark the most distal site of insertion with a tattoo or clip. Balloon-assisted endoscopy is then performed from the other side (lower or upper), and we try to reach the marking point to confirm total enteroscopy.

Based on a systematic review, the rate of total enteroscopy using DBE combining oral and anal routes is 44% (569/1143), and using upper balloon-assisted enteroscopy alone, total enteroscopy is accomplished in 1.6% (9/569).[12] Takano et al reported that the rate of total enteroscopy using SBE is 16.7% (20/120).[13] Takenaka et al reported that the rate of total enteroscopy in patients with Crohn's disease using upper enteroscopy only is 12.2% (11/90).[14]

Since SBE does not use a balloon on the endoscope, preparation is simple and fast. However, when using DBE, the balloon at the tip of endoscope is wedged against and fixed on the small intestine to prevent slipping of the endoscope. When performing SBE, slipping of the endoscope is more frequent than with DBE because there is no balloon at the tip of the endoscope. The rate of total enteroscopy using DBE is significantly higher than that of SBE.[13,15] Japanese and German randomized-controlled trials reported a rate of total enteroscopy of 0 and 22% using SBE and 57 and 66% using DBE, respectively.[13,15]

The rate of total enteroscopy using DBE was different in Japan and other countries, just after its release. However, this difference is getting smaller recently. A recent prospective study reported that the rate of total enteroscopy was 71% (34/48) in Japan[16] and 71% (45/63) in Europe.[15,17] We suggest two possible explanations for the recent improvement in the rate of total enteroscopy. One is the introduction of carbon dioxide for endoscopic insufflation, and the other is improvement in the insertion technique, especially for retrograde insertion, as shown by studies from Europe.

There are few direct comparisons between balloon-assisted endoscopy and spiral endoscopy.[17,18,19] Deep enteroscopy is superior when performing DBE and procedure times are shorter when performing spiral endoscopy. There is no significant difference in diagnostic and therapeutic yield. However, a randomized-controlled study regarding the rate of total enteroscopy, comparing DBE and spiral endoscopy concludes 92% (12/13) for DBE and 8% (1/13) for spiral endoscopy.[17] The mean maximal insertion depth for upper enteroscopy was 346 cm for DBE and 268 cm for spiral endoscopy ($p < 0.001$), and for lower enteroscopy was 209 cm for DBE and 78 cm for spiral endoscopy ($p < 0.001$). Although spiral endoscopy has some advantages

compared with DBE, it needs further development to be more clinically useful.

Introduction of device-assisted enteroscopy-assisted endoscopic retrograde cholangiopancreatography (ERCP) enables an approach to the biliary tract even in patients with surgically altered anatomy such as a Roux-en-Y reconstruction or Billroth-II reconstruction. A recent review reported an overall success rate of device-assisted enteroscopy-assisted ERCP of 48 to 94%.[20] A Japanese multicenter study using a short-type double-balloon endoscope reported a 98% (304/311) success rate for reaching the target site, a 96% (293/304) success rate of biliary cannulation, and a 98% (277/283) success rate of treatment.[21] Device-assisted enteroscopy-assisted ERCP is undoubtedly a useful procedure in patients with surgically altered anatomy. A short device-assisted enteroscope with a wide working channel use is especially recommended to enable successful biliary interventions.

13.8 Procedure-Specific Training Requirements

13.8.1 Minimizing Air Insufflation for Deep Intubation

Excessive air insufflation diminishes the efficacy of deep endoscope insertion because of poor folding of redundant loops. Carbon dioxide insufflation is useful for device-assisted enteroscopy just as it is in conventional colonoscopy. Since carbon dioxide is absorbed more rapidly by intestinal mucosa than air by 100-fold or more, the use of carbon dioxide insufflation facilitates total enteroscopy[22] and deep intubation,[23] and it also diminishes discomfort after enteroscopy.[24,25] Despite the usefulness of carbon dioxide insufflation, excessive carbon dioxide in the intestinal lumen decreases insertion efficacy. Minimum insufflation is important for efficient intubation as well as the patient's comfort.

13.8.2 Necessity of X-Ray Fluoroscopy during Device-Assisted Enteroscopy

For less experienced practitioners of device-assisted enteroscopy, fluoroscopy is frequently used to confirm the shape of the endoscope during insertion. However, advancements in the technique of device-assisted enteroscopy have decreased the use of fluoroscopy.[26] For the proficient endoscopist performing device-assisted enteroscopy, fluoroscopy is usually not necessary except patients with severe peritoneal adhesions, strictures, or masses requiring indirect visualization using contrast media.

13.9 Minimizing Procedure-Specific Complications

13.9.1 Complications of Balloon-Assisted Endoscopy

Complications of balloon-assisted endoscopy include perforation, bleeding, aspiration pneumonia, infection, and mucosal injury. While these events occur even when performing conventional endoscopy, acute pancreatitis is a balloon-assisted endoscopy-specific complication. A systematic review of 9047 DBE procedures reported 61 major complications (0.72%) including 20 perforations (0.2%), 17 patients with acute pancreatitis (0.2%), 8 patients with aspiration pneumonia (0.09%), 6 patients with bleeding (0.07%), and 10 patients with miscellaneous (1.1%).[12] There is only one study of complications after SBE with a small number of patients.[27]

The rate of acute pancreatitis after upper DBE is 0.3 to 0.5% from large retrospective studies.[12,28] However, in a prospective study, hyperamylasemia occurs in 25 to 50% of patients after upper DBE and acute pancreatitis occurred in 3 to 12% of patients.[29,30] Long procedure time and insertion depth were significant predictive factors for the development of hyperamylasemia.[29]

Since the main locus of pancreatitis after balloon-assisted endoscopy is the body and tail of the pancreas, mechanical torque of the pancreas by balloon-assisted endoscopy during insertion is a possible cause. Although pancreatitis after device-assisted enteroscopy is predominantly reported after the upper DBE, it has been reported after upper SBE,[31] lower DBE,[32] and lower SBE.[33] In upper DBE, pancreatitis is probably caused by compression and deviation of the pancreas by straightening the duodenum. Both the duodenum and pancreas are fixed in the retroperitoneum. To avoid iatrogenic pancreatitis, "pulling" movements should be slow and gentle, and the procedure time for DBE be less than 2 hours. When strong compression of the pancreas occurs during "pulling," both the endoscope and overtube should be pushed together, minimizing compression of the pancreas.

A recent Japanese prospective multicenter study reported a 10.6% (33/311) rate of complications with the short-type double-balloon endoscope-assisted ERCP in patients with surgically altered anatomy.[21] In 311 patients, pancreatitis occurred in 11 patients (3.5%) and perforation in 6 patients (1.9%).[21] These patients were treated nonoperatively except for one patient with a perforation requiring emergency operative repair.[21] Device-assisted enteroscopy-assisted ERCP is safe and is the first choice for interventions in patients with surgically altered anatomy.

13.9.2 Complications of Spiral Endoscopy

The main complications of spiral endoscopy are mucosal injury and perforation. The use of a thick overtube, 17.5 mm outer diameter, and spiral protrusions on the overtube may damage the small intestinal mucosa. Actually, in an animal study, laparoscopic imaging showed ecchymosis and peritoneal tearing during spiral endoscopy insertion due to torsion on the mesenteric root.[34] Careful insertion of the overtube during spiral endoscopy may be important to avoid complications. Further, special attention should be paid to patients with adhesions due to previous laparotomy.

13.10 Conclusions

The development of device-assisted enteroscopy has revolutionized the diagnosis and treatment of small intestinal disorders for the last decade. Device-assisted enteroscopy will continue to have a major impact on the diagnosis and treatment of small intestinal diseases throughout the 21st century.

References

[1] Yamamoto H, Sekine Y, Sato Y, et al. Total enteroscopy with a nonsurgical steerable double-balloon method. Gastrointest Endosc. 2001; 53(2):216–220

[2] Iddan G, Meron G, Glukhovsky A, Swain P. Wireless capsule endoscopy. Nature. 2000; 405(6785):417

[3] Akerman PA, Agrawal D, Cantero D, Pangtay J. Spiral enteroscopy with the new DSB overtube: a novel technique for deep peroral small-bowel intubation. Endoscopy. 2008; 40(12):974–978

[4] Araki A, Tsuchiya K, Okada E, et al. Single-operator method for double-balloon endoscopy: a pilot study. Endoscopy. 2008; 40(11):936–938

[5] Ohtsuka K, Kashida H, Kodama K, et al. Diagnosis and treatment of small bowel diseases with a newly developed single balloon endoscope. Dig Liver Dis. 2008; 20:134–137

[6] Yano T, Nemoto D, Ono K, et al. Gel immersion endoscopy: a novel method to secure the visual field during endoscopy in bleeding patients (with videos). Gastrointest Endosc. 2016; 83(4):809–811

[7] Shinozaki S, Yamamoto H, Yano T, et al. Long-term outcome of patients with obscure gastrointestinal bleeding investigated by double-balloon endoscopy. Clin Gastroenterol Hepatol. 2010; 8(2):151–158

[8] Shinozaki S, Yamamoto H, Yano T, et al. Favorable long-term outcomes of repeat endotherapy for small-intestine vascular lesions by double-balloon endoscopy. Gastrointest Endosc. 2014; 80(1):112–117

[9] Yano T, Yamamoto H, Sunada K, et al. Endoscopic classification of vascular lesions of the small intestine (with videos). Gastrointest Endosc. 2008; 67(1):169–172

[10] Sunada K, Shinozaki S, Nagayama M, et al. Long-term outcomes in patients with small intestinal strictures secondary to Crohn's disease after double-balloon endoscopy-assisted balloon dilation. Inflamm Bowel Dis. 2016; 22(2):380–386

[11] Hayashi Y, Yamamoto H, Yano T, et al. A calibrated, small-caliber tip, transparent hood to aid endoscopic balloon dilation of intestinal strictures in Crohn's disease: successful use of prototype. Endoscopy. 2013; 45(Suppl 2 UCTN):E373–E374

[12] Xin L, Liao Z, Jiang YP, Li ZS. Indications, detectability, positive findings, total enteroscopy, and complications of diagnostic double-balloon endoscopy: a systematic review of data over the first decade of use. Gastrointest Endosc. 2011; 74(3):563–570

[13] Takano N, Yamada A, Watabe H, et al. Single-balloon versus double-balloon endoscopy for achieving total enteroscopy: a randomized, controlled trial. Gastrointest Endosc. 2011; 73(4):734–739

[14] Takenaka K, Ohtsuka K, Kitazume Y, et al. Comparison of magnetic resonance and balloon enteroscopic examination of the small intestine in patients with Crohn's disease. Gastroenterology. 2014; 147(2):334–342.e3

[15] May A, Färber M, Aschmoneit I, et al. Prospective multicenter trial comparing push-and-pull enteroscopy with the single- and double-balloon techniques in patients with small-bowel disorders. Am J Gastroenterol. 2010; 105(3):575–581

[16] Yamamoto H, Yano T, Ohmiya N, et al. Double-balloon endoscopy is safe and effective for the diagnosis and treatment of small-bowel disorders: prospective multicenter study carried out by expert and non-expert endoscopists in Japan. Dig Endosc. 2015; 27(3):331–337

[17] Messer I, May A, Manner H, Ell C. Prospective, randomized, single-center trial comparing double-balloon enteroscopy and spiral enteroscopy in patients with suspected small-bowel disorders. Gastrointest Endosc. 2013; 77(2):241–249

[18] Frieling T, Heise J, Sassenrath W, et al. Prospective comparison between double-balloon enteroscopy and spiral enteroscopy. Endoscopy. 2010; 42(11):885–888

[19] May A, Manner H, Aschmoneit I, Ell C. Prospective, cross-over, single-center trial comparing oral double-balloon enteroscopy and oral spiral enteroscopy in patients with suspected small-bowel vascular malformations. Endoscopy. 2011; 43(6):477–483

[20] Shimatani M, Takaoka M, Tokuhara M, et al. Review of diagnostic and therapeutic endoscopic retrograde cholangiopancreatography using several endoscopic methods in patients with surgically altered gastrointestinal anatomy. World J Gastrointest Endosc. 2015; 7(6):617–627

[21] Shimatani M, Hatanaka H, Kogure H, et al; Japanese DB-ERC Study Group. Diagnostic and therapeutic endoscopic retrograde cholangiography using a short-type double-balloon endoscope in patients with altered gastrointestinal anatomy: a multicenter prospective study in japan. Am J Gastroenterol. 2016; 111(12):1750–1758

[22] Li X, Zhao YJ, Dai J, et al. Carbon dioxide insufflation improves the intubation depth and total enteroscopy rate in single-balloon enteroscopy: a randomised, controlled, double-blind trial. Gut. 2014; 63(10):1560–1565

[23] Domagk D, Bretthauer M, Lenz P, et al. Carbon dioxide insufflation improves intubation depth in double-balloon enteroscopy: a randomized, controlled, double-blind trial. Endoscopy. 2007; 39(12):1064–1067

[24] Hirai F, Beppu T, Nishimura T, et al. Carbon dioxide insufflation compared with air insufflation in double-balloon endoscopy: a prospective, randomized, double-blind trial. Gastrointest Endosc. 2011; 73(4):743–749

[25] Lenz P, Meister T, Manno M, et al. CO2 insufflation during single-balloon enteroscopy: a multicenter randomized controlled trial. Endoscopy. 2014; 46(1):53–58

[26] Mehdizadeh S, Ross A, Gerson L, et al. What is the learning curve associated with double-balloon enteroscopy? Technical details and early experience in 6 U.S. tertiary care centers. Gastrointest Endosc. 2006; 64(5):740–750

[27] Aktas H, de Ridder L, Haringsma J, et al . Complications of single-balloon enteroscopy: a prospective evaluation of 166 procedures. Endoscopy. 2010; 42(5):365–368

[28] Mensink PB, Haringsma J, Kucharzik T, et al. Complications of double balloon enteroscopy: a multicenter survey. Endoscopy. 2007; 39(7):613–615

[29] Zepeda-Gómez S, Barreto-Zuñiga R, Ponce-de-León S, et al. Risk of hyperamylasemia and acute pancreatitis after double-balloon enteroscopy: a prospective study. Endoscopy. 2011; 43(9):766–770

[30] Kopácová M, Rejchrt S, Tachecí I, Bures J. Hyperamylasemia of uncertain significance associated with oral double-balloon enteroscopy. Gastrointest Endosc. 2007; 66(6):1133–1138

[31] Sharma MK, Sharma P, Garg H, et al. Clinical acute pancreatitis following antegrade single balloon enteroscopy. Endoscopy. 2011; 43(Suppl 2 UCTN):E20–E21

[32] Gerson LB, Tokar J, Chiorean M, et al. Complications associated with double balloon enteroscopy at nine US centers. Clin Gastroenterol Hepatol. 2009; 7(11):1177–1182, 1182.e1–1182.e3

[33] Yip WM, Lok KH, Lai L, et al. Acute pancreatitis: rare complication of retrograde single-balloon enteroscopy. Endoscopy. 2009; 41(Suppl 2):E324

[34] Soria F, Lopez-Albors O, Morcillo E, et al. Experimental laparoscopic evaluation of double balloon versus spiral enteroscopy in an animal model. Dig Endosc. 2011; 23(1):98

14 Wireless Video Capsule Endoscopy

Jodie A. Barkin, Lauren B. Gerson, and Jamie S. Barkin

14.1 Introduction

Video capsule endoscopy (VCE), introduced globally in 2000 and in the United States in 2001, has enabled the gastroenterologist to view the small intestine from the pylorus to the ileocecal valve, territory that usually spans 16 to 20 feet (400–800 cm) in most humans. VCE can be done in the inpatient or outpatient setting. VCE can be swallowed by the patient or, if need be, endoscopically deployed into the duodenum. Small bowel preparation prior to VCE has been shown to improve visualization and diagnostic yield. Previously classified as obscure gastrointestinal bleeding and recently renamed as small bowel bleeding, suspected small bowel bleeding is the most common indication for VCE. VCE is indicated after the patient has undergone adequate esophago-gastroduodenoscopy and colonoscopy. VCE may find lesions in up to 60% of patients with obscure gastrointestinal bleeding, and should be performed as close as possible to an obscure overt bleeding event to increase diagnostic yield. Suspicion of small bowel Crohn's disease or assessment of Crohn's disease activity is a frequent indication for VCE; however, VCE's role in patients with stable active Crohn's disease is unclear. While VCE administration is considered to be generally safe, there is a potential risk of capsule retention, defined as nonpassage of VCE into the cecum within a 2-week period. In patients with suspected small bowel bleeding, retention rates are approximately 1 to 2%, whereas the risk of VCE retention in patients with inflammatory bowel disease may range from 2 to 13%. This chapter will discuss preparation and indications for VCE, available technology, reading techniques, and management of findings.

14.2 Technology

VCE was approved by the Food and Drug Administration (FDA) in 2001 as an adjunctive aid for diagnosis of small intestinal disorders, and in 2003 as a first-line modality for this indication. Initial VCE devices required the patient to wear aerials secured to the chest and abdomen in order to transmit images by radiofrequency telemetry to a data recorder. While initial capsule technology captured 8 hours of data (approximately 70,000 images), newer batteries now allow for 12 hours of data gathering, ensuring greater completion rates to the cecum. While initial capsules featured a field of view of 140 degrees and now feature mainly 160 degrees, newer capsules are in development that allow for a 360-degree field of view, as it has four cameras located around the center of the capsule (CapsoCam, CapsoVision Inc, Saratoga, California, United States). Whether increased field of view translates to increased diagnostic yield is currently under investigation. All VCE capsules contain light-emitting diodes (LEDs) that allow for emission of light in the otherwise dark small intestine, and feature chips with complementary metal-oxide-semiconductor technology. A newer generation VCE from Korea (MiroCam, IntroMedic, Seoul, Korea) uses the body rather than telemetry to conduct the signal, increasing the operating time (capture rate three frames per second as opposed to two frames per second). An esophageal capsule that is a "double-header" with 2 cameras is able to capture 14 frames per second. Current commercially available VCE systems are compared in ▶ Table 14.1. To date, comparative studies between capsule brands have not shown significant differences in diagnostic yields. Use of a second VCE compared to one has been associated with increased rates of small bowel pathologic findings.

The current generation of VCEs has only demonstrated visualization of the papilla in 10% of cases or less. However, a new VCE under development with a 360-degree field of view has increased the ampulla detection rate to approximately 70%.[6] As expected in an exclusively diagnostic modality, VCE is limited by an inability to provide therapeutic capabilities, lack of external control of capsule movement, and potential difficulty in localizing the exact site of a lesion.[7] Newer generations of VCE with possible external control of capsule movement through the small bowel are in development but are not commercially available at this time.[8]

Table 14.1 Comparison of video capsule endoscopes for small bowel imaging.[1,2,3,4,5]

	PillCam SB3	EndoCapsule 10	CapsoCam SV1	MiroCam	OMOM
Manufacturer	Given Imaging	Olympus	CapsoVision	IntroMedic	Chongqing Jinshan
Length (mm)	26	26	31	24.5	28
Diameter (mm)	11	11	11	10.8	13
Weight (g)	1.9	3.3	4	3.25	
Type of image sensor	CMOS	CMOS	CMOS	CMOS	CMOS
Frame rate (per second)	2 to 6 (adaptive frame rate)	2	20	3	2
Number of cameras	1	1	4	1	1
Field of view (degrees)	156	160	360	170	140
Battery life (h)	12	12	15	12	8

Abbreviation: CMOS, complementary metal oxide semiconductor.

14.3 Setting and Preparation for Video Capsule Endoscopy

VCE can be done in the inpatient or outpatient setting, although the latter is generally preferred as gastric and small bowel transit times are improved when patients are ambulatory. In the inpatient setting, particularly if patients are receiving narcotics or other motility-altering medications and are bedridden, placement of the capsule endoscope into the duodenum is recommended using a through-the-scope capsule-loading device that is advanced into the duodenum, and the capsule is released into the second portion of the duodenum, bypassing the stomach. In addition, a vigorous preparation and use of promotility drugs may be beneficial.

Many studies, including a 2009 meta-analysis, have demonstrated that small bowel preparation improves small bowel visualization and diagnostic yield of VCE.[9] The patient should be on a clear liquid diet the day prior to capsule administration. Administration of 2 or 4 L of polyethylene glycol solution on the night prior to testing was shown to increase visualization quality. In patients taking narcotic medications or other medications, i.e., anticholinergics and antihistamines, which are associated with gastroparesis, cessation of these medications 2 to 3 days prior to VCE administration is recommended. An alternative is that the patient can receive either metoclopramide 10 mg three times daily before meals or erythromycin 250 mg every 8 hours for 2 to 3 days prior to VCE administration. However, given the high rate of gastric retention in patients with gastroparesis or narcotic-induced gastroparesis, endoscopic placement is highly recommended.

In patients taking anticoagulants, including warfarin or the novel anticoagulants, no adjustment in dosage of medication is recommended prior to VCE administration; in fact, studying patients on these medications may help to increase diagnostic yield given the potentially increased risk for bleeding.[10,11]

14.4 VCE Administration

The approximate VCE dimensions are 11 mm × 26 mm or the size of a "large jelly bean," and most subjects do not have issues swallowing the capsule. In patients who express concern, having the patient to swallow, and not chew, a jellybean can serve as a test of tolerability, particularly in children or adolescents. Albeit rare, if a patient aspirates a capsule, urgent bronchoscopy should be performed for removal. Once successfully administered, some gastroenterology units will keep the patient in observation for an hour with application of the real-time viewer, in order to assure gastric passage. Should the VCE remain in the stomach after 1 hour, prokinetic agents such as metoclopramide 10 mg can be administered prior to discharge. Patients are allowed to ingest clear liquids 2 hours after VCE administration and a light meal 4 hours after administration. Depending on capsule technology, the study is completed within 8 to 12 hours and the data recorder returned and uploaded. Patients are not instructed to watch for signs of capsule passage in the stool, as this is often not reliable. However, in the case of newer capsules (CapsoCam), patients are provided with a hat and wand in order to collect the capsule, which is then sent back to the company for uploading.[1,12] Should the VCE appear to not have passed during reading of the video, an abdominal X-ray can be considered within 2 weeks postingestion to assure passage, or sooner if the patient reports abdominal pain.

14.5 Indications for VCE

Previously classified as obscure gastrointestinal (GI) bleeding and recently renamed as small bowel bleeding, suspected small bowel bleeding is the most common indication for VCE. It is divided into overt (melena or bright red blood) and occult (iron-deficiency anemia and heme-positive stool). VCE is indicated after the patient has undergone adequate esophagogastroduodenoscopy and colonoscopy[7,13] (▶ Fig. 14.1). Some studies suggest a "second-look" endoscopy with duodenal biopsies to exclude celiac disease and possibly a second colonoscopy, as occult lesions in the esophagus, stomach (Dieulafoy's lesion, Cameron's ulcers, gastric antral vascular ectasia), and colon (arteriovenous malformations [AVMs]) may be discovered on second endoscopy. The most common lesion found depends on the age of the patient. In those older than 40 years, vascular lesions including AVMs are most frequently found. Predisposing conditions to AVMs in addition to age include chronic kidney disease, aortic stenosis, and patients with left ventricular assist devices (Heyde's syndrome), hereditary hemorrhagic telangiectasias, and radiation. Additionally, in those older than 40 years, causative etiologies include drug effects including nonsteroidal anti-inflammatory drugs (NSAIDs) causing erosions, ulcers, and diaphragms; Dieulafoy's lesions; and benign and malignant neoplasms including metastases. In those younger than 40 years, inflammatory bowel disease (IBD), Dieulafoy's lesions, Meckel's diverticulum, and polyposis syndromes are the most common.[7] Images of characteristic VCE findings are shown in ▶ Fig. 14.2.

Neoplasms may occur in those younger than 40 years but are more common in those older than 40 years. Malignant neoplasms include primary small bowel adenocarcinomas, neuroendocrine tumors, and metastatic implants primarily from melanomas, renal cell carcinoma, and lung and breast malignancies. The appearance of small bowel neoplasms varies based on histologic type. Lesions arising from the mucosa may be flat or raised, and may have surface ulceration. Submucosal lesions may protrude into the lumen and have either a normal or ulcerated surface. Neoplasms may also have an associated stricture. In the case of adenocarcinomas, lesions may be either infiltrative or exophytic, and may be ulcerated, strictured, or bloody. Metastatic melanomas classically appear pigmented.[14]

VCE may find lesions in up to 60% of patients with obscure GI bleeding.[15] VCE should be performed as close as possible to an obscure overt bleeding event to increase diagnostic yield, with one report of a VCE sensitivity of 92% in patients with ongoing overt small bowel bleeding at the time of VCE.[16,17] A false-negative rate for VCE of 10% has been reported in a pooled study of VCE performed for both bleeding and nonbleeding.[18] VCE has improved diagnostic accuracy compared to computed tomography (CT) or magnetic resonance (MR) enterography for visualization of flat mucosal lesions such as AVMs, small bowel diaphragms, and erosions. CT/MR enterography has improved accuracy for mass lesions, and VCE and enterography should be viewed as complementary.[13]

Suspicion of small bowel Crohn's disease or assessment of Crohn's disease activity is a frequent indication for VCE. These patients should, first, have an unrevealing CT/MR enterography, prior to VCE administration. If they have symptoms compatible

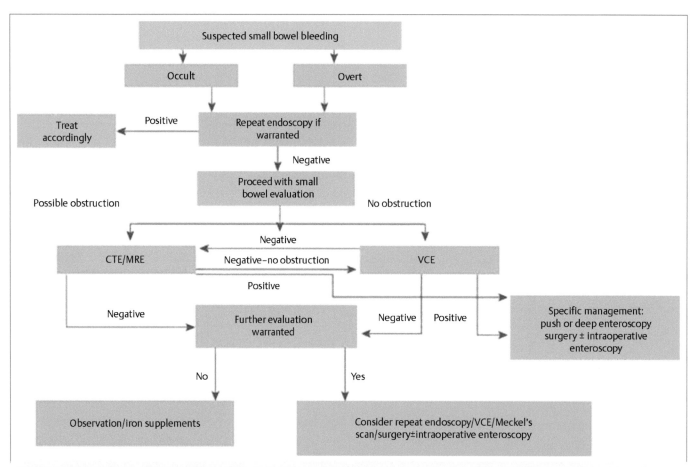

Fig. 14.1 Algorithm for suspected small bowel bleeding. CTE, computed tomography enterography; MRE, magnetic resonance enterography; VCE, video capsule endoscopy. (Reproduced with permission from Gerson et al.[7])

with a partial small bowel obstruction or have had prior intestinal resection, they should be considered for a patency capsule prior to VCE. Similar to patients with obscure GI bleeding, VCE is better for diagnosis of flat mucosal lesions, whereas CT/MR enterography is better for transmural disease, again providing complementary information. VCE's role in patients with stable active Crohn's disease is unclear as the risk of retention in patients with known Crohn's disease can be as high as 13%.[19,20] Small bowel ulcers are not pathognomonic for Crohn's disease as they can be caused by medications (i.e., NSAIDs), ischemia and vasculitis, and infections (i.e., tuberculosis and *Cytomegalovirus*).

In patients with unexplained diarrhea, VCE may be diagnostic for parasitic infectious causes, Whipple's disease, or suspected celiac disease. VCE, however, is not regularly used as first-line evaluation for celiac disease, but may be useful as an adjunctive modality in patients with an equivocal diagnosis or in patients unable or unwilling to undergo conventional endoscopy.[13] VCE may rarely be employed to elucidate the causes of unexplained abdominal pain, providing a valid explanation in only up to about 20% of patients, and should not be routinely used in this subgroup of patients.[16]

14.6 Contraindications to VCE

Relative contraindications to VCE administration are predisposition to capsule retention and inability to swallow the capsule, which can be overcome by endoscopic deployment. The only absolute contraindication to capsule administration is known symptomatic luminal obstruction.

14.7 Risk of VCE Retention

While VCE administration is considered to be generally safe, the potential risk of retention deserves additional discussion. VCE retention is defined as nonpassage of VCE into the cecum within a 2-week period.[19] VCE retention has only been documented in patients with an anatomical cause, and has not been reported in normal subjects. In patients with suspected small bowel bleeding, retention rates are approximately 1 to 2%, with most common causes including small bowel neoplasms, strictures due to usage of NSAIDs, radiation enteritis, prior surgical anastomoses, or IBD.[15,21,22,23,24,25] It should be noted that the risk of VCE retention in patients with IBD is not insignificant, with rates ranging from 2 to 13% in some series.[13,15,22,25]

In patients with the potential for VCE retention, evaluation prior to VCE administration is advised. In most cases, conduction of a CT or MR enterography examination is advised in patients with known Crohn's disease or indeterminate IBD or abdominal pain potentially related to a small bowel stricturing process. Unfortunately, a normal examination does not entirely exclude the possibility of retention, as it misses lesions, i.e., diaphragms of NSAIDs and localized strictures in IBD patients. Administration of a swallowed PillCam patency capsule (Given Imaging Ltd, Yoqneam, Israel) can be performed prior to VCE. The patency capsule features a dissolvable lactose body and a radiofrequency identification (RFID) tag. Approximately 30 hours after administration, the patient can be scanned to determine whether the RFID tag is present, indicating the potential for retention with administration of a VCE.[26]

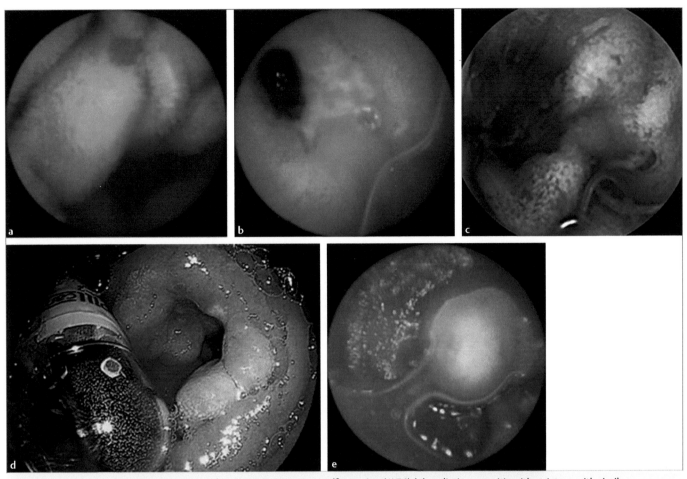

Fig. 14.2 Video capsule endoscopy images showing arteriovenous malformation (AVM) **(a)**; radiation enteritis with stricture with similar appearance to Crohn's disease **(b)**; small bowel hookworm with bleeding **(c)**; jejunal adenocarcinoma with capsule retention **(d)**; and small bowel carcinoid tumor **(e)**.

In patients with VCE retention, management depends on the etiology and symptoms from capsule retention. Small bowel neoplasms are usually resected. In patients with IBD, administration of anti-inflammatory agents often can be associated with passage of the capsule, although this process may require weeks to months. However, small bowel perforation from VCE has been reported in patients with active IBD. Usage of deep enteroscopy has been successful in the removal of retained VCE in many cases.[25,27] If patients have new abdominal symptoms associated with capsule retention, intervention for capsule removal is indicated.

14.8 Reading a VCE Study

While there are no formal guidelines in place for training, it has been recommended that gastroenterology fellows wishing to undergo training in VCE read at least 50 studies with attendings in order to become certified. Reading should include identification of important landmarks, including the esophagogastric junction, duodenal bulb, ileocecal valve, first cecal image, and ampulla if visualized. Capsule reading software systems feature the ability to change reading speed (in terms of frame rates), number of frames visualized (from one to four at a time), light intensity, and many feature quadrant locators. The current software programs feature the ability to blend like images in order to reduce the number of frames presented to the reader. Studies have shown that reading rates exceeding 15 to 20 frames per second are associated with

higher miss rates.[28] Additional features vary based on the specific reading software used. Some software may automatically flag images for the reader with possible presence of blood, such as the Suspected Blood Indicator feature (Given Imaging Ltd, Yoqneam, Israel). Other software features may provide image enhancement or superimpose identical images or images filled with bubbles and debris to optimize reading speeds, such as the Endocapsule EC-10 software (Olympus America Inc., Center Valley, Pennsylvania, United States).

VCE reading accuracy depends on the reader, capsule preparation, and the rapidity of capsule passage. VCE reading features multiple images, rapidly passing through the visual field, which may cause reader fatigue, exacerbated by reading multiple studies sequentially. Similar to a radiologist's interpretation, providing clinical information by the ordering physician is vital to an accurate reading.

It is recommended that the reader inspects the esophagus and stomach, as missed lesions have been reported in up to 25% of patients with suspected small bowel bleeding.[7,29,30] Next, the reader should identify the first duodenal image and first cecal image, in order to calculate total small bowel transit time. Findings should be classified as being in the proximal two-thirds or distal one-third of the small bowel, as these locations will determine subsequent approach for deep enteroscopy as anterograde or retrograde. The quality of the preparation should be assessed for each segment, based on the ability to visualize the entire lumen which is not obscured by bubbles or other debris. Lesions should be classified using the Saurin classification system, where P2 denotes a definite lesion (angiodysplastic lesion, ulceration, or neoplasm) and P1 a finding of unclear certainty (red spot or erosion).[31] The colonic mucosa should also be examined if possible to assess for the presence of findings in the colon, including missed polyps.

14.9 Conclusion

VCE has completed a fantastic journey, allowing direct visualization of the entire small bowel. As with any diagnostic modality, VCE is not 100% accurate but has contributed significant information regarding causes of obscure GI bleeding, diarrhea, and, on occasion, abdominal pain. Advances in VCE technology have improved diagnostic ability, and we are looking forward to 360-degree visualization and steerable VCE in the future, with continued optimism for improved diagnostic accuracy and patient outcomes.

References

[1] CapsoVision. CapsoCam. February 17, 2016. Available at: http://www.capsovision.com/index.php/capsocam.html

[2] PillCam SB. Given Imaging. March 1, 2016. Available at: http://www.capsovision.com/

[3] ENDOCAPSULE 10 System. Olympus America – Medical. March 1, 2016. Available at: http://medical.olympusamerica.com/products/endocapsule-10-system

[4] IntroMedic. March 1, 2016. Available at: http://intromedic.com/eng/item/item_010100_view.asp?search_kind=&gotopage=1&no=3

[5] OMOM Capsule Endoscopy System Manufacturer from Chongqing China. March 1, 2016. Available at: http://jinshangroup.gmc.globalmarket.com/products/details/omom-capsule-endoscopy-system-4543846.html

[6] Pioche M, Vanbiervliet G, Jacob P, et al; French Society of Digestive Endoscopy (SFED). Prospective randomized comparison between axial- and lateral-viewing capsule endoscopy systems in patients with obscure digestive bleeding. Endoscopy. 2014; 46(6):479–484

[7] Gerson LB, Fidler JL, Cave DR, Leighton JA. ACG Clinical Guideline: diagnosis and management of small bowel bleeding. Am J Gastroenterol. 2015; 110(9):1265–1287, quiz 1288

[8] Keller J, Fibbe C, Volke F, et al. Inspection of the human stomach using remote-controlled capsule endoscopy: a feasibility study in healthy volunteers (with videos). Gastrointest Endosc. 2011; 73(1):22–28

[9] Rokkas T, Papaxoinis K, Triantafyllou K, et al. Does purgative preparation influence the diagnostic yield of small bowel video capsule endoscopy?: A meta-analysis. Am J Gastroenterol. 2009; 104(1):219–227

[10] Boal Carvalho P, Rosa B, Moreira MJ, Cotter J. New evidence on the impact of antithrombotics in patients submitted to small bowel capsule endoscopy for the evaluation of obscure gastrointestinal bleeding. Gastroenterol Res Pract. 2014; 2014:709217

[11] Van Weyenberg SJ, Van Turenhout ST, Jacobs MA, et al. Video capsule endoscopy for previous overt obscure gastrointestinal bleeding in patients using anti-thrombotic drugs. Dig Endosc. 2012; 24(4):247–254

[12] Friedrich K, Gehrke S, Stremmel W, Sieg A. First clinical trial of a newly developed capsule endoscope with panoramic side view for small bowel: a pilot study. J Gastroenterol Hepatol. 2013; 28(9):1496–1501

[13] Pennazio M, Spada C, Eliakim R, et al. Small-bowel capsule endoscopy and device-assisted enteroscopy for diagnosis and treatment of small-bowel disorders: European Society of Gastrointestinal Endoscopy (ESGE) Clinical Guideline. Endoscopy. 2015; 47(4):352–376

[14] Lewis BS, Keuchel M, Wiedbrauck F, et al. Malignant tumors. In: Keuchel M, Hagenmüller F, Tajiri H, eds. Video Capsule Endoscopy. Heidelberg: Springer-Verlag; 2014:337–358

[15] Liao Z, Gao R, Xu C, Li ZS. Indications and detection, completion, and retention rates of small-bowel capsule endoscopy: a systematic review. Gastrointest Endosc. 2010; 71(2):280–286

[16] Katsinelos P, Fasoulas K, Beltsis A, et al. Diagnostic yield and clinical impact of wireless capsule endoscopy in patients with chronic abdominal pain with or without diarrhea: a Greek multicenter study. Eur J Intern Med. 2011; 22(5):e63–e66

[17] Pennazio M, Santucci R, Rondonotti E, et al. Outcome of patients with obscure gastrointestinal bleeding after capsule endoscopy: report of 100 consecutive cases. Gastroenterology. 2004; 126(3):643–653

[18] Lewis BS, Eisen GM, Friedman S. A pooled analysis to evaluate results of capsule endoscopy trials. Endoscopy. 2005; 37(10):960–965

[19] Cave D, Legnani P, de Franchis R, Lewis BS; ICCE. ICCE consensus for capsule retention. Endoscopy. 2005; 37(10):1065–1067

[20] Barkin JS, Friedman S. Wireless capsule endoscopy requiring surgical intervention: the world's experience. Am J Gastroenterol. 2002; 97(9):S298

[21] Li F, Gurudu SR, De Petris G, et al. Retention of the capsule endoscope: a single-center experience of 1000 capsule endoscopy procedures. Gastrointest Endosc. 2008; 68(1):174–180

[22] Cheifetz AS, Kornbluth AA, Legnani P, et al. The risk of retention of the capsule endoscope in patients with known or suspected Crohn's disease. Am J Gastroenterol. 2006; 101(10):2218–2222

[23] Rondonotti E, Pennazio M, Toth E, et al; European Capsule Endoscopy Group. Italian Club for Capsule Endoscopy (CICE). Iberian Group for Capsule Endoscopy. Small-bowel neoplasms in patients undergoing video capsule endoscopy: a multicenter European study. Endoscopy. 2008; 40(6):488–495

[24] Höög CM, Bark LÅ, Arkani J, et al. Capsule retentions and incomplete capsule endoscopy examinations: an analysis of 2300 examinations. Gastroenterol Res Pract. 2012; 2012:518718

[25] Cheon JH, Kim YS, Lee IS, et al; Korean Gut Image Study Group. Can we predict spontaneous capsule passage after retention? A nationwide study to evaluate the incidence and clinical outcomes of capsule retention. Endoscopy. 2007; 39(12):1046–1052

[26] Caunedo-Alvarez A, Romero-Vazquez J, Herrerias-Gutierrez JM. Patency and Agile capsules. World J Gastroenterol. 2008; 14(34):5269–5273

[27] Baichi MM, Arifuddin RM, Mantry PS. What we have learned from 5 cases of permanent capsule retention. Gastrointest Endosc. 2006; 64(2):283–287

[28] Zheng Y, Hawkins L, Wolff J, et al. Detection of lesions during capsule endoscopy: physician performance is disappointing. Am J Gastroenterol. 2012; 107(4):554–560

[29] Lepileur L, Dray X, Antonietti M, et al. Factors associated with diagnosis of obscure gastrointestinal bleeding by video capsule enteroscopy. Clin Gastroenterol Hepatol. 2012; 10(12):1376–1380

[30] Gerson LB. Outcomes associated with deep enteroscopy. Gastrointest Endosc Clin N Am. 2009; 19(3):481–496

[31] Saurin JC, Delvaux M, Gaudin JL, et al. Diagnostic value of endoscopic capsule in patients with obscure digestive bleeding: blinded comparison with video push-enteroscopy. Endoscopy. 2003; 35(7):576–584

15 Colonoscopy: Preparation, Instrumentation, and Technique

John C. T. Wong and Joseph J. Y. Sung

15.1 Introduction

Since the development of colonoscopy over a quarter of a century ago, technological developments and evidence-based medicine have evolved, expanding colonoscopy's role in the screening, diagnosis, prognosis, and treatment of wide-ranging gastrointestinal conditions. Colonoscopy requires astute hand–eye coordination and manual dexterity, but extends beyond technical skills, to demand patience and thoughtfulness to factors such as sedation and quality assurance. This chapter provides an overview of established and novel literature related to the preparation, instrumentation, techniques, and quality measure for colonoscopy, an increasingly utilized and rewarding procedure.

15.2 Preparation

15.2.1 Indications and Contraindications

An appropriate indication for colonoscopy is the first step in ensuring a quality examination. ▶ Table 15.1 lists current diagnostic and therapeutic colonoscopy indications as recommended by the American Society of Gastrointestinal Endoscopy (ASGE).[1] As our understanding of disease pathology grows, and the capabilities of devices and accessories become more sophisticated, these indications will continue to evolve. Despite these guidelines, whether the investigation will alter an individual's overall disease or treatment course must be considered. Also, contraindications to colonoscopy, such as suspected or known colonic perforation, fulminant colitis, and acute diverticulitis, should be acknowledged to minimize harm in an otherwise safe procedure. Colonoscopy during pregnancy or soon after an acute and severe medical event like a myocardial infarction should weigh the benefits and risks.

15.2.2 Patient Preparation

The contribution of precolonoscopy patient preparation to procedural success should not be underestimated, as the most proficient endoscopic skills may be futile in the face of a poor bowel preparation, which has been associated with longer procedural time, more incomplete procedures, reduced polyp and adenoma detection, increased procedure-related adverse events, variable adherence to surveillance intervals, and higher medical costs.[2,3,4,5,6,7] Endoscopy centers should have a systematic and clear approach to dietary modification, bowel preparation, and use of medications prior to colonoscopy, with the aim of achieving a bowel preparation adequate for the detection of polyps greater than 5 mm in size permitting compliance with surveillance interval guidelines in over 85% of colonoscopies performed per endoscopist.[8] Patients with the following risk factors for poor bowel preparation: advancing age, obesity, stroke, dementia, diabetes, prior colorectal resection, inpatient colonoscopy, prior inadequate preparation, non-English speakers (in English-dominant societies), lower socioeconomic status, lower health literacy, and long interval to colonoscopy should receive additional attention, such as oral and written instructions, assistance from patient navigators or more extensive dietary and preparation protocols.[9,10,11,12] Otherwise, in a patient without such risk factors, a low-residue diet has been shown in randomized-controlled trials to be comparable in bowel preparation quality, but better tolerated than a clear liquid diet on the day prior to a colonoscopy.[13,14] Bowel preparation regimes can be categorized based on osmolarity and volume. Iso-osmotic regimes largely rely on a cathartic effect for bowel cleansing, and include 4 L of polyethylene glycol electrolyte lavage solution (PEG-ELS) and 2 L of PEG-ELS with ascorbic acid (Moviprep). Four liters of PEG-ELS is now recommended by multiple guidelines to be administered in a split fashion, with the latter half taken on the day of the colonoscopy due to higher patient satisfaction and superior adenoma detection rates as shown by meta-analysis and systematic reviews.[15,16,17,18] For an afternoon colonoscopy, 2 L of PEG-ELS with ascorbic acid on the morning of the procedure can achieve comparable bowel cleansing, greater patient preference, and less impact of daily activities and sleep compared to a 2-day protocol.[19,20] Hyperosmolar regimes include sodium sulfate, sodium phosphate, magnesium citrate, and sodium picosulfate/magnesium citrate, and although their lower volume appears attractive, their use should be avoided in patients with renal insufficiency. Hypo-osmotic regimes are primarily low-volume PEG paired with sports drink, but a recent meta-analysis demonstrated fewer satisfactory bowel preparations were achieved compared to

Table 15.1 Diagnostic, screening/surveillance, and therapeutic indications for colonoscopy as recommended by the American Society of Gastrointestinal Endoscopy [Early]

Diagnostic indications	Investigation for unexplained gastrointestinal (GI) bleeding (e.g., positive fecal occult blood, hematochezia, melena after exclusion of an upper GI source); unexplained chronic diarrhea; unexplained iron deficiency anemia; colonic abnormalities on barium enema or other imaging (e.g., filling defect or stricture); localization of neoplasia for marking
Screening/surveillance indications	Sporadic, familial (e.g., familial adenomatous polyposis, hereditary nonpolyposis colorectal cancer), synchronous and metachronous colorectal cancer screening; surveillance after polypectomy; surveillance of dysplasia in inflammatory bowel disease
Therapeutic indications	Polypectomy; endoscopic mucosal resection; endoscopic submucosal dissection; hemostasis for lower gastrointestinal bleeding (e.g., from neoplasia, angiodysplasia, radiation proctitis, postpolypectomy); palliative colonic stenting; dilation of anastomotic or Crohn's related stricture; removal of foreign body; decompression of sigmoid volvulus or colonic pseudo obstruction

traditional PEG.[21] Preparations currently commercially available in the United States were recently summarized.[22] Regardless of the regime used, the optimal interval between prep completion and colonoscopy commencement should be 4 to 6 hours, as longer duration correlates to worst proximal colon cleansing due to chyme from the small intestine.[23] However, completing preparation by 2 hours before commencement of sedation will minimize gastric residue.[24]

Aspirin users need not withhold treatment, as a case–control study showed it is not a risk factor for postpolypectomy bleeding.[25] However, patients on antiplatelet like clopidogrel, traditional anticoagulant like warfarin, and/or novel oral anticoagulants (factor Xa inhibitors like rivaroxaban, and direct thrombin inhibitors like dabigatran) deserve heightened attention, and their modification must take into account indication for use, medication half-life, creatinine clearance, onset of action, time to peak effect, and the colonoscopy's urgency and bleeding risk, among other factors. In general, if their use is for a defined period of time, and the indication is not urgent, colonoscopy can be performed after completion of treatment course. If their use is indefinite, joint discussion with the prescribing clinician and patient is recommended. Reviews by the European Society of Gastrointestinal Endoscopy (ESGE) in 2011 and the ASGE from 2016 summarized the key pharmacokinetic properties and recommendations prior to colonoscopy for some of these medications.[26,27] Finally, constipating medications such as iron tablets and narcotics should also be discontinued at least 3 to 5 days before the procedure.

15.3 Basic Instrumentation

15.3.1 Sedation

Colonoscopy is an invasive procedure that can invoke anxiety. Patients have come to expect sedation for a pain-free examination, but comfort must be balanced with safety to achieve the optimal procedure. The elderly, the obese, patients with chronic cardiopulmonary conditions, such as chronic obstructive pulmonary disease, obstructive sleep apnea, and cirrhosis are more sensitive to sedation effects, either due to altered drug metabolism or decreased baseline function, and deserve careful titration of medications. The use, type, and administrator of sedation during colonoscopy vary worldwide. Endoscopist-administered intravenous benzodiazepine and opiate for moderate sedation is an established regime worldwide. Midazolam acts on the γ-aminobutyric acid (GABA) receptor to achieve antegrade amnestic, anxiolytic, and sedative effects, and is metabolized by the liver. Used at doses of approximately 2.5 to 5 mg, it has an onset of action within 1 to 2 minutes, and a duration of action of approximately 1 hour. Of note is that midazolam can induce paradoxical reaction including disorientation, agitation, and aggression in approximately 1% of patients, though this can be reversed with flumazenil.[28]

Intravenous propofol (2,6-diisopropofol), alone or in combination with an opiate, has been advocated as a superior choice for sedation due to both its rapid onset of action and distribution into peripheral tissues, resulting in a short duration of action and faster patient recovery. Meta-analysis of randomized-controlled trials have shown propofol use has a similar or lower risk of hypoxia or hypotension, shorter recovery time, and higher patient satisfaction compared to traditional sedation with midazolam,

meperidine, and/or fentanyl.[29,30,31] Controversy, however, surrounds who are qualified to administer the drug because of a potential for deep sedation without the availability of a reversal agent. Nonanesthesiologist administration of propofol (NAAP) is prevalent in European countries like Germany, Switzerland, and Denmark, whereas anesthetic support predominates in France and the United States.[32,33,34] Current literature have not shown an increase in adverse events among NAAP, and the differences in practice are more likely related to medical training, reimbursement, and societal lobbying.[35] Regardless of the type of sedation used, the endoscopy team should have fundamental knowledge in emergency airway and resuscitation management, and multiple national societies have developed endoscopy sedation curriculums.[36,37]

15.3.2 Colonoscope

A colonoscope consists of three sections: the insertion tube, the control handle, and the connection port (▶Fig. 15.1a). Depending on manufacturer and model, the flexible insertion tube is of variable length (1,330–1,700 mm) and diameter (11.1–15 mm), and can have variable stiffness, controlled by a clockwise/counterclockwise turn dial at the base of the control handle, which in turn differentially tightens or relaxes a tension coil along the length of the tube.[38] The insertion tube also houses the light and image bundles, and the working channel for passage of accessories and suction. At the tip of the tube are the light illumination system, charged couple device for color image generation, forward-viewing lens, air/water channel, and opening of the working channel, which is at the 5 to 6 o'clock position (▶Fig. 15.1b, c). The control handle has two stacked turn dials for up/down and left/right tip deflection, each of which can be locked into place (▶Fig. 15.1d, e). Also, there are standard push buttons for image freeze, suction, and air and water insufflation. Additional programmable buttons can activate image enhancements such as narrow-band imaging (NBI) (Olympus Medical Systems), i-Scan (Pentax), FICE (Fujinon), and magnification. NBI filters white light leaving light of 415 nm (blue) and 540 nm (green) wavelengths to be absorbed by hemoglobin. Color, vessel, and epithelial surface patterns are enhanced, permitting characterization of colorectal polyp type by the NICE classification.[39] At the base of the handle near the variable stiffness controller is the entry port for the working channel (2.8–4.2 mm in diameter).[38] The connection port attaches to the image processor, and sources of electricity, light, water, and air or carbon dioxide, the use of which is associated with less abdominal pain postprocedure.[40] All equipment can be pendant mounted to reduce electrical wiring on the floor. High-definition colonoscopes are now standard of care, providing up to 1-million pixel resolution, which are displayed on high-definition monitors. Image-recording equipment for endoscopic photos or videos are also important as part of documentation.

15.3.3 Accessories

The basic accessories accompanying colonoscopy include the biopsy forceps, injection needle, polypectomy snare, and hemoclips (▶Fig. 15.1f). The biopsy forceps can be used for tissue sampling or removal of diminutive polyps. It consists of a flexible metal sheath with/without an overlying polymer housing a

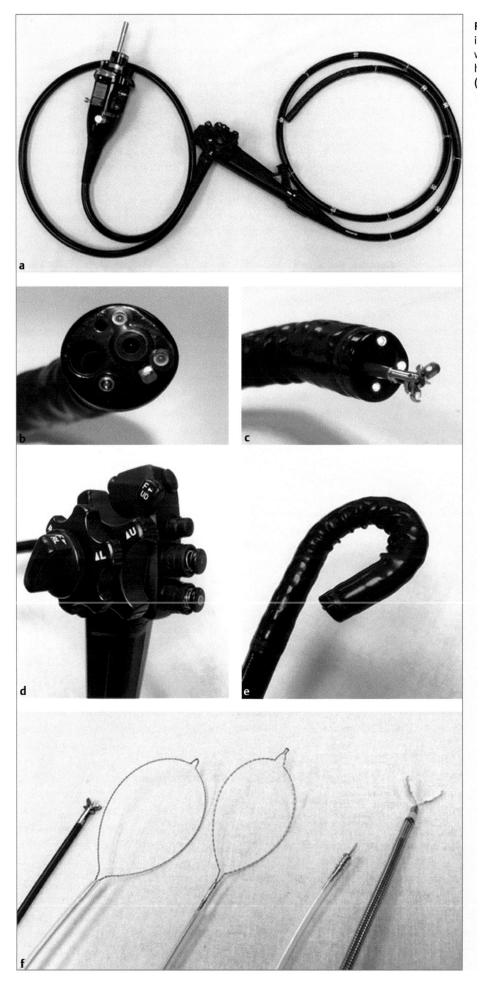

Fig. 15.1 **(a)** Adult colonoscope, **(b)** tip of insertion tube, **(c)** biopsy forceps exiting working channel of insertion tube, **(d)** control handle, **(e)** insertion tube tip deflection, **(f)** basic colonoscopy accessories.

cable connecting a two-piece plastic handle at one end to opposing biopsy cups at the other end. Forceps differ by number and size of biopsy cups, surface (smooth/alligator jaws/rat tooth), fenestration, rotatability, and presence of a central needle spike, which can minimize slippage, and facilitate double-bite biopsies. The injection needle consists of an outer sheath with an inner hollow beveled-tip needle approximately 4 to 8 mm long, which can be advanced and retracted by a plastic handle, and is used for submucosal lifting prior to polyp removal, adrenaline injection for hemostasis, or tattooing. Central to colonoscopy's role in reducing colorectal cancer (CRC) incidence and mortality is the polypectomy snare. Endoscopist should be aware of the varying designs available and the situations most suited for his or her use. In addition to differences in shape (crescent/hexagonal/oval), the opened diameter (15–25 mm), wire diameter, and wire design (straight/twisted/spiked to prevent slippage) should be appreciated. Polypectomy may be complicated by bleeding or perforation, which can be managed by clip devices by experienced endoscopists. Depending on patient's clinical response after clipping, small perforations can be successfully managed without surgery. Beyond these basic accessories is the rapid development of tools to enhance mucosal exposure such as Endocuff, Endorings, and the 330-degree wide-angle full-spectrum endoscope (FUSE), which have all been shown to increase adenoma detection rates.[41,42,43]

15.4 Technique

15.4.1 Scope Insertion

Prior to scope insertion, an anorectal examination should be performed. Often underappreciated, visual evaluation for hemorrhoids, anal fissures, fistula openings, neurologic examination of the sacral nerve, manual assessment of sphincter tone, squeeze pressure, pelvic floor function, anorectal masses, and prostatic hypertrophy or nodules are all possible.[44]

The general principles to technical success in diagnostic colonoscopy include coordinated movement between the left and right hands, preferential use of tip steering and clockwise/anticlockwise shaft torquing over vigorous pushing for scope advancement, recognition and algorithmic resolution of loop formation, use of abdominal pressure, patient position change and alternate equipment as rescue maneuvers, patience on the part of the endoscopist, and dutiful attention to sensory feedback from the colonoscope and patient comfort. On insertion of the colonoscope through the anus and on air insufflation, the rectum is visualized as a large reservoir extending approximately 15 cm proximal from the anal verge, occasionally with some residual effluent. If the bowel preparation in the rectosigmoid is clearly

insufficient to detect polyps greater than 5 mm, a colonoscopy performed for screening or surveillance should be terminated and rescheduled with more intensive preparation.[8] Scope retroflexion to examine the distal rectum can be performed by distending the rectum by insufflation, then applying upward tip deflection while pushing in the scope (**Video 15.1**). Once retroflexed views are achieved, sideways tip deflection or shaft torquing can provide circumferential views of the rectum. Retroflexion may also be performed at the end of the colonoscopy on scope withdrawal. However, in cases of active proctitis or narrowed scarred rectum, retroflexion should not be performed due to perforation risk. Scope advancement across the sigmoid colon is often the most challenging part of the procedure, but can be achieved by careful tip deflection, shaft manipulation, and minimal pushing to simulate a corkscrew motion to traverse sequential folds. However, as the rectum is at the back of the pelvis, then courses anteriorly to the sigmoid colon, then spirals to the retroperitoneum where the descending colon is fixed, formation of an alpha loop with the loop apex directed toward the diaphragm is not uncommon (▶Fig. 15.2a). Formation of an N-shaped loop due to sigmoid mesentery hypermobility should be suspected when an excessive length of instrument can be introduced relatively resistance free along a featureless colon, until loss of 1:1 progression along the descending colon and patient discomfort occurs (▶Fig. 15.2b). Loop formation can stretch the sigmoid colon like an accordion from a length of approximately 30 cm up to approximately 70 cm, which can be taken advantage for polyp detection. Removal of small sigmoid polyps detected on scope insertion should be considered as use of distance and clock-face position to find them again on scope withdrawal may be unreliable, unless nearby suction marking is performed. To minimize loop formation, suprapubic abdominal pressure toward the left lower abdominal quadrant at the apex of the sigmoid colon, or moving the patient from the left lateral to the supine position can be tried. To straighten a formed loop, 90- to 180-degree clockwise torque steering while scope withdrawal and deflation should be performed. The water immersion technique, which involves scope insertion "underwater," has been shown in randomized controlled trials to reduce sigmoid loop formation as evidenced by a magnetic endoscope imaging device, and achieves faster cecal intubation with less patient discomfort compared to air insufflation among minimally sedated procedures.[45,46] A straightened colonoscope should be floppy at the level of the anus, and easily rests on the patient bed, while a looped device will feel stiff. Stenosing sigmoid diverticular disease from hypertrophied circular muscles, or adhesions from prior lower intra-abdominal/pelvic surgery can represent a challenge even for experienced physicians, and require the scope to adapt to a fixed bend. Changing to a thinner pediatric colonoscope (~ 11 mm in diameter), a gastroscope (~ 9 mm in

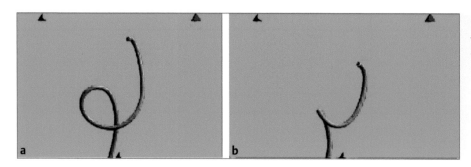

Fig. 15.2 (a) Alpha loop, (b) N-loop as visualized by magnetic endoscope imaging device.[83]

diameter), a different endoscopist, or even an alternate method of investigation like computed tomography (CT) colonography may be warranted. Starting with a pediatric colonoscope can also be considered in thinner women, and depending on prior colonoscopy difficulties and findings. After negotiating the sigmoid colon, advancement across the approximately 20-cm-long descending colon is usually straightforward, but the splenic flexure may appear acutely angulated due to the patient's left lateral position, which can be changed to the supine position to facilitate passage. Once beyond the splenic flexure, all loops should be straightened by a hooking maneuver so the colonoscope should at most be 40 to 50 cm from the anal verge with a straight scope. The transverse colon can be recognized by the typical air-filled triangular lumen, and use of clockwise torque, gentle scope advancement/withdrawal, and suctioning can be used to reach the hepatic flexure. For assistance, applying variable shaft stiffness to prevent recurrent sigmoid looping, changing the patient from left lateral to supine position (if not done already) to negate an antigravity effect, and left iliac fossa abdominal pressure directed toward the epigastrium to minimize inferior stretching of the transverse mesocolon can all assist with scope advancement. The hepatic flexure can sometimes be recognized by the bluish hue of the liver, but can be mistaken for the cecum, due to acute angulation as the anterior proximal transverse colon transitions to the posterior distal ascending colon, but the hepatic flexure will be clean compared to an often fluid-filled cecum. If the patient is in the left lateral position, the hepatic flexure can be exposed by rotating the patient's right shoulder toward the bed. Deep inspiration by the patient will cause diaphragmatic descent, which along with suctioning, and if necessary, position change to the right lateral decubitus, can propel the scope along the ascending colon to the base of the cecum, where the appendiceal orifice and convergence of the three teniae coli must be clearly visualized. In case of semisolid or solid debris that cannot be suctioned away, patient position change can expose the obscured underlying mucosa. A blind spot to carefully evaluate is between the appendiceal orifice and the ileocecal valve, which can vary in appearance from a subtle slit to a lipomatous bulge on the first fold distal to the cecal pole. The orifice to the ileum can be on the proximal side of the fold, and visualization may require scope retroflexion in the cecum. To facilitate valve intubation, which should be attempted in all cases, air should be aspirated from the cecum to reduce tension across the fold lips, which can also be oriented by use of biopsy forceps. The distal ileum has a distinctive appearance with lymphoid hyperplasia and finger-like projections can be seen on air and water insufflation, respectively.

15.4.2 Scope Withdrawal

On successful intubation of the cecum or terminal ileum, focus should then turn to performing a thorough high-quality examination during withdrawal of the colonoscope, when most polyps are detected and removed if feasible (▶Fig. 15.3a, ▶Fig. 15.3b). Miss rates for adenomas greater than 1 cm, 6 to 9 mm, and less than or equal to 5 mm have been reported to be between 2 and 6%, 13%, and approximately 27%, respectively, on tandem colonoscopy studies, and is the most significant contributor (between 50 and 60%) to postcolonoscopy colorectal cancer (PCCRC).[47,48,49] General principles of scope withdrawal

include meticulous cleansing of the mucosa, adequate luminal distension, intentional and patient inspection of the interhaustral space, careful attention to subtle changes in color, surface, and vascular pattern, and standardized description of endoscopic appearances. Scope withdrawal along the ascending colon requires particular attention, as polyps can be subtly flat, likely contributing to the lack of colonoscopy's efficacy in decreasing right-sided CRC mortality.[50,51] Polyps with a mucus cap should raise suspicion for a serrated lesion, like a sessile serrated adenoma. Performing a second examination of the ascending colon is particularly important when polyps were detected during the first examination (odds ratio [OR] = 2.8, 95% confidence interval [CI] = 1.7–4.7) and when the endoscopist's confidence in the quality of the first examination is low (OR = 4.8, 95% CI = 1.9–12.1), as these are risk factors for finding additional lesions on a second inspection.[52] The second examination can be either by retroflexed view or forward view, as these views produced a similar increase in adenoma detection rate in a recent study.[52] To retroflex in the cecum, first ensure the endoscope is free of any loops, then maximal tip deflection on the up/down control is performed. The scope is then advanced, and with torque and/or left/right tip deflection, the retroflexed view can be obtained. This view will move paradoxically to the colonoscope's advance/withdrawal movements, similar to the retroflex view during gastroscopy. During withdrawal on forward view, by using a combination of tip deflection and shaft torquing to "work" and flatten the haustral folds like the hands of a clock, circumferential and proximal fold evaluation can be systematically achieved (**Video 15.2**). Repeated scope advancement and withdrawal are also integral to a careful examination, especially when a segment of colon "flies by." Between the transverse colon, the inner aspects of the hepatic and splenic flexures are also potential blind spots that deserve added attention (▶Fig. 15.3c, d). At the sigmoid, interhaustral spaces should be exposed by the tip of the scope or by irrigation. Finally, at the rectum, the proximal sides of the semilunar transverse folds of Houston should be carefully examined for lesions, after which rectal retroflexion should be performed, if not already done, to rule out lower rectal pathology (▶Fig. 15.3e, f). If air insufflation was used, suctioning should be performed throughout the withdrawal phase to minimize postprocedural discomfort. Overall, a withdrawal time of 6 minutes is considered minimal standard of care during a screening colonoscopy.[7] On completion of the procedure, the quality of bowel preparation after intraprocedural clearance of residual debris should be rated using a standardized scale such as the Boston Bowel Preparation Scale, which has moderate-to-high intra- (k = 0.77) and interobserver reliability (k = 0.74). Higher scores (greater than or equal to 5), have been associated with better polyp detection.[53,54] In cases of poor bowel preparation, a future procedure within 1 year with more comprehensive education and intensive preparation is recommended.

15.4.3 Polypectomy

All colorectal polyps visualized should be characterized by size (relative to open biopsy forceps or snare), location, and morphology by the Paris endoscopic classification.[55] Image enhancements like NBI and the NICE classification for optical diagnosis

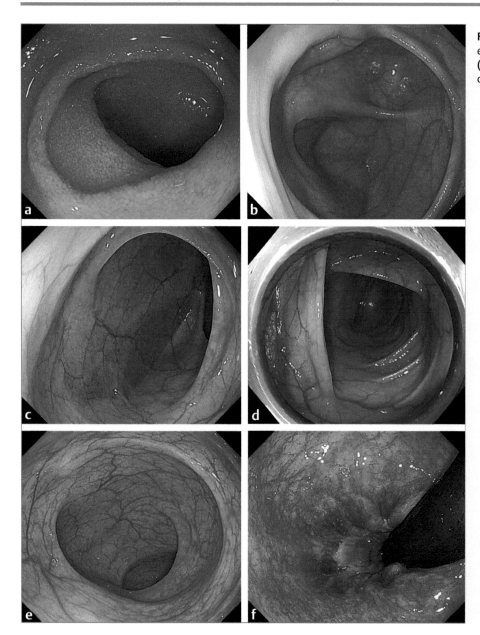

Fig. 15.3 High-definition white light endoscopic images of **(a)** terminal ileum, **(b)** cecum, **(c)** hepatic flexure, **(d)** transverse colon, **(e)** rectum, **(f)** rectal retroflexion.

are increasingly used, with some advocating a "predict, resect, discard" approach to diminutive (≤ 5 mm) lesions (▶ Fig. 15.4).[39,56] A complete discussion of polypectomy techniques is beyond the scope of this chapter, but endoscopists should appreciate up to approximately 20% of PCCRC are estimated to be from incomplete polypectomy.[49] Diminutive polyps are now increasingly recommended to be removed by cold (i.e., without electrocautery) snaring, due to higher rates of residual tissue from cold biopsy.[57,58] Hot (i.e., with electrocautery) snare polypectomy is applied for pedunculated lesions, and large sessile or flat polyps which may first be lifted with saline, methylene blue, and/or epinephrine. The technique is similar to cold snare polypectomy except that after the polyp is captured with a snare, it should be tented away from the mucosal plane during cautery to minimize postpolypectomy electrocoagulation syndrome (**Video 15.3**).

15.4.4 Complications

The main complications of colonoscopy relate to the cardiopulmonary effects of sedation, and polypectomy, specifically bleeding,

perforation, postpolypectomy electrocoagulation syndrome, and death. Sedation-related adverse events make up the majority of endoscopic complications. Depending on the type of sedation used, and the level achieved, cardiopulmonary effects range from transient fluctuations in blood pressure, heart rate, respiratory rate, and oxygen desaturation to shock, cardiac arrhythmias, cardiac arrest, aspiration pneumonia, respiratory suppression, and death. Higher American Society of Anesthesiologists (ASA) class, older patients, underlying cardiopulmonary disease, obesity, inpatients, and trainee procedural involvement are risk factors for sedation-related adverse events.[59,60] Standardized preprocedural assessment, careful titration of sedatives, along with physiologic monitoring during colonoscopy are crucial to a safe procedure. Postpolypectomy bleed may be immediate or delayed by several days up to 4 weeks, occurring with an incidence of approximately 1% in a contemporary series.[61] Risk factors for immediate bleeding identified from a 2010 literature review by the ASGE included age greater than 65, cardiovascular or chronic renal disease, anticoagulation use, poor bowel preparation, polyp greater than 1 cm, cutting mode electrosurgical current, or inadvertent cold

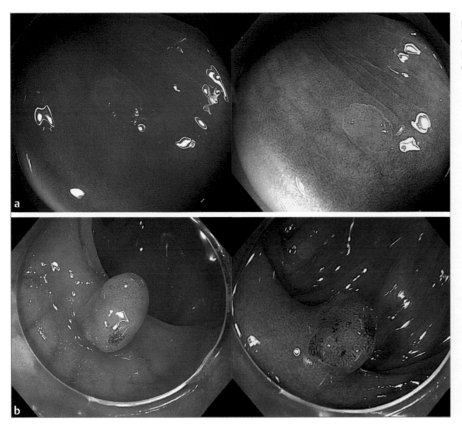

Fig. 15.4 Paired high-definition white light and narrow-band images of **(a)** hyperplastic polyp (NICE class I), **(b)** tubular adenoma (NICE class II).

cutting.[60,62] Bleeding from the residual stalk of a pedunculated lesion can be initially controlled by regrasping it with a snare for approximately 5 minutes. More definitive therapy by hemoclips, epinephrine injection or cautery by thermal probes, biopsy forceps, or snare tip can then be applied (**Video 15.3**). Delayed postpolypectomy bleeding may be due to sloughing of eschar that was covering a vessel. Right-sided polypectomy of lesions greater than 1 cm by low-volume colonoscopists (< 300 total procedures) complicated by immediate postpolypectomy bleeding is at the highest risk for delayed bleeding.[63,64] Patients with signs of active bleeding should undergo therapeutic colonoscopy for hemostasis, while those whose bleeding gradually subsides, may be observed expectantly. Perforation may be due to mechanical forces exerted on the bowel wall, particularly when obstruction is the procedural indication, barotrauma from excessive air insufflation, or polypectomy. Multiple studies have shown a perforation rate of approximately 0.1%, with the sigmoid and ascending colon as the most common affected sites.[65,66] If detected during the procedure, CO_2 insufflation should be switched to (if not already used), the site of perforation turned to a nondependent position, and hemoclips be used to tightly close the defect if amenable. Surgical consultation should be sought in case of clinical deterioration. Postpolypectomy electrocoagulation syndrome usually presents within 5 days of colonoscopy, manifested by abdominal pain, fever, leukocytosis without radiographic evidence of perforation. This rare transmural injury and localized peritonitis are due to electrocoagulation, and can usually be managed by analgesia and antibiotics. Postcolonoscopy splenic injury occurs predominantly in women, presenting with abdominal pain, drop in hemoglobin, and splenic laceration with/without hemoperitoneum on CT. Surgical intervention is usually required.[67] Overall, colonoscopy-specific related mortality is exceedingly rare.[61]

15.5 Quality Measures

Over the past decade, there have been increasing efforts to evaluate quality in medicine, so to reduce variations in practice, and to improve clinical outcomes. This is likewise the case in gastroenterology and screening colonoscopy which have been shown to reduce CRC incidence and mortality, provided the examination is of high quality.[50,68,69,70] The most recent society guidelines from Europe and the United States on quality colonoscopy were developed to provide evidence-based principles to standardize procedural and institutional practice with the goals of enhancing performance characteristics and patient outcomes.[71,72] A summary of pre-, intra-, and postprocedure-related quality indicators for colonoscopy, along with expected performance targets, proposed jointly by the American College of Gastroenterology and the ASGE are listed in ▶ Table 15.2.[72] European guidelines were more expansive to discuss quality in organization and implementation of a screening program, professional requirements and training, and pathology reporting standards.[73] Currently, the most important quality indicator is the adenoma detection rate (ADR), which is the proportion of screening colonoscopies in which one or more adenoma is detected. Endoscopists with an ADR less than 20% have an interval cancer risk 10 times higher than physicians with a higher ADR.[74] More specifically, a population-based study from the United States found for every 1% increase in ADR, there was a 3 to 4% decrease in patient CRC risk and mortality.[75] Currently, the target ADR for men and women on screening colonoscopies are greater than 30% and greater than 20%, respectively, with recent results suggesting a higher ADR benchmark for high-risk individuals such as those with prior adenomas, and a separate target for sessile serrated adenomas.[72,76,77] To determine ADR and other quality indicators by manual reviews of colonoscopy

Table 15.2 List of colonoscopy quality indicators proposed by the American Society of Gastrointestinal Endoscopy[72]

Quality indicators	Performance targets
Preprocedure	
Frequency with which endoscopy is performed for an indication that is included in a published standard list of appropriate indications, and the indication is documented	> 80%
Frequency with which informed consent is obtained and fully documented	> 98%
Frequency with which colonoscopies follow recommended postpolypectomy and postcancer resection surveillance intervals and 10-year intervals between screening colonoscopies in average-risk patients who have negative examination results and adequate bowel cleansing	> 90%
Frequency with which ulcerative colitis and Crohn's colitis surveillance is recommended within proper intervals	> 90%
Intraprocedure	
Frequency with which the procedure note documents the quality of preparation	> 98%
Frequency with which the bowel preparation is adequate to allow the use of recommended surveillance or screening intervals	> 85%
Frequency with which visualization of the cecum by notation of landmarks and photodocumentation of landmarks is documented in every screening procedure	> 95%
Frequency with which adenomas are detected in asymptomatic, average-risk individuals (screening)	≥ 30% for men, ≥ 20% for women
Frequency with which withdrawal time is measured	> 98%
Average withdrawal time in negative-result screening colonoscopies	≥ 6 min average
Frequency of recommended tissue sampling when colonoscopy is performed for surveillance in ulcerative colitis and Crohn's colitis	> 98%
Frequency with which endoscopic removal of pedunculated polyps and sessile polyps < 2 cm is attempted before surgical referral	> 98%
Postprocedure	
Incidence of perforation and postpolypectomy bleeding	< 1:500 for perforation, < 1% for postpolypectomy bleeding
Frequency with which postpolypectomy bleeding is managed without surgery	> 90%
Frequency with which appropriate recommendation for timing of repeat colonoscopy is documented and provided to the patient after histologic findings are reviewed	> 90%

and pathology reports can be a time- and resource-intensive process. Several groups have used natural language processing to extract information from text reports in an automated fashion, and showed results such as accurate identification of screening procedures, and ADR determination were comparable to manual chart review.[78,79] Physician performance can now be submitted to data registries like the GI Quality Improvement Consortium in the United States or the Endoscopy Global Rating Scale in the United Kingdom, for comparison against recognized standards. Identifying suboptimal adherence to current quality benchmarks provides opportunities for quality improvement, such as endoscopy training programs which have been shown to increase ADR by greater than 10%, with a durable effect of up to 5 months.[80,81] Finally, as physician awareness for quality colonoscopy increases, public reporting of endoscopist performance may become more widespread and expected, which itself has the benefit of increasing ADR by approximately 5%.[82]

References

[1] Early DS, Ben-Menachem T, Decker GA, et al; ASGE Standards of Practice Committee. Appropriate use of GI endoscopy. Gastrointest Endosc. 2012; 75(6):1127–1131

[2] Harewood GC, Sharma VK, de Garmo P. Impact of colonoscopy preparation quality on detection of suspected colonic neoplasia. Gastrointest Endosc. 2003; 58(1):76–79

[3] Froehlich F, Wietlisbach V, Gonvers JJ, et al. Impact of colonic cleansing on quality and diagnostic yield of colonoscopy: the European Panel of Appropriateness of Gastrointestinal Endoscopy European multicenter study. Gastrointest Endosc. 2005; 61(3):378–384

[4] Sherer EA, Imler TD, Imperiale TF. The effect of colonoscopy preparation quality on adenoma detection rates. Gastrointest Endosc. 2012; 75(3):545–553

[5] Lebwohl B, Kastrinos F, Glick M, et al. The impact of suboptimal bowel preparation on adenoma miss rates and the factors associated with early repeat colonoscopy. Gastrointest Endosc. 2011; 73(6):1207–1214

[6] Ben-Horin S, Bar-Meir S, Avidan B. The impact of colon cleanliness assessment on endoscopists' recommendations for follow-up colonoscopy. Am J Gastroenterol. 2007; 102(12):2680–2685

[7] Rex DK, Imperiale TF, Latinovich DR, Bratcher LL. Impact of bowel preparation on efficiency and cost of colonoscopy. Am J Gastroenterol. 2002; 97(7):1696–1700

[8] Johnson DA, Barkun AN, Cohen LB, et al; US Multi-Society Task Force on Colorectal Cancer. Optimizing adequacy of bowel cleansing for colonoscopy: recommendations from the US multi-society task force on colorectal cancer. Gastroenterology. 2014; 147(4):903–924

[9] Ness RM, Manam R, Hoen H, Chalasani N. Predictors of inadequate bowel preparation for colonoscopy. Am J Gastroenterol. 2001; 96(6):1797–1802

[10] Chung YW, Han DS, Park KH, et al. Patient factors predictive of inadequate bowel preparation using polyethylene glycol: a prospective study in Korea. J Clin Gastroenterol. 2009; 43(5):448–452

[11] Nguyen DL, Wieland M. Risk factors predictive of poor quality preparation during average risk colonoscopy screening: the importance of health literacy. J Gastrointestin Liver Dis. 2010; 19(4):369–372

[12] Chan WK, Saravanan A, Manikam J, et al. Appointment waiting times and education level influence the quality of bowel preparation in adult patients undergoing colonoscopy. BMC Gastroenterol. 2011; 11:86

[13] Melicharkova A, Flemming J, Vanner S, Hookey L. A low-residue breakfast improves patient tolerance without impacting quality of low-volume colon cleansing prior to colonoscopy: a randomized trial. Am J Gastroenterol. 2013; 108(10):1551–1555

[14] Sipe BW, Fischer M, Baluyut AR, et al. A low-residue diet improved patient satisfaction with split-dose oral sulfate solution without impairing colonic preparation. Gastrointest Endosc. 2013; 77(6):932–936

[15] Kilgore TW, Abdinoor AA, Szary NM, et al. Bowel preparation with split-dose polyethylene glycol before colonoscopy: a meta-analysis of randomized controlled trials. Gastrointest Endosc. 2011; 73(6):1240–1245

[16] Enestvedt BK, Tofani C, Laine LA, et al. 4-Liter split-dose polyethylene glycol is superior to other bowel preparations, based on systematic review and meta-analysis. Clin Gastroenterol Hepatol. 2012; 10(11):1225–1231

[17] Lieberman DA, Rex DK, Winawer SJ, et al; United States Multi-Society Task Force on Colorectal Cancer. Guidelines for colonoscopy surveillance after screening and polypectomy: a consensus update by the US Multi-Society Task Force on Colorectal Cancer. Gastroenterology. 2012; 143(3):844–857

[18] Hassan C, Bretthauer M, Kaminski MF, et al; European Society of Gastrointestinal Endoscopy. Bowel preparation for colonoscopy: European Society of Gastrointestinal Endoscopy (ESGE) guideline. Endoscopy. 2013; 45(2):142–150

[19] Matro R, Shnitser A, Spodik M, et al. Efficacy of morning-only compared with split-dose polyethylene glycol electrolyte solution for afternoon colonoscopy: a randomized controlled single-blind study. Am J Gastroenterol. 2010; 105(9):1954–1961

[20] Longcroft-Wheaton G, Bhandari P. Same-day bowel cleansing regimen is superior to a split-dose regimen over 2 days for afternoon colonoscopy: results from a large prospective series. J Clin Gastroenterol. 2012; 46(1):57–61

[21] Siddique S, Lopez KT, Hinds AM, et al. Miralax with gatorade for bowel preparation: a meta-analysis of randomized controlled trials. Am J Gastroenterol. 2014; 109(10):1566–1574

[22] Saltzman JR, Cash BD, Pasha SF, et al; ASGE Standards of Practice Committee. Bowel preparation before colonoscopy. Gastrointest Endosc. 2015; 81(4):781–794

[23] Siddiqui AA, Yang K, Spechler SJ, et al. Duration of the interval between the completion of bowel preparation and the start of colonoscopy predicts bowel-preparation quality. Gastrointest Endosc. 2009; 69(3 Pt 2):700–706

[24] American Society of Anesthesiologists Committee. Practice guidelines for preoperative fasting and the use of pharmacologic agents to reduce the risk of pulmonary aspiration: application to healthy patients undergoing elective procedures: an updated report by the American Society of Anesthesiologists Committee on Standards and Practice Parameters. Anesthesiology. 2011; 114(3):495–511

[25] Yousfi M, Gostout CJ, Baron TH, et al. Postpolypectomy lower gastrointestinal bleeding: potential role of aspirin. Am J Gastroenterol. 2004; 99(9):1785–1789

[26] Boustière C, Veitch A, Vanbiervliet G, et al; European Society of Gastrointestinal Endoscopy. Endoscopy and antiplatelet agents. Endoscopy. 2011; 43(5):445–461

[27] Acosta RD, Abraham NS, Chandrasekhara V, et al; ASGE Standards of Practice Committee. The management of antithrombotic agents for patients undergoing GI endoscopy. Gastrointest Endosc. 2016; 83(1):3–16

[28] Tae CH, Kang KJ, Min BH, et al. Paradoxical reaction to midazolam in patients undergoing endoscopy under sedation: incidence, risk factors and the effect of flumazenil. Dig Liver Dis. 2014; 46(8):710–715

[29] Singh H, Poluha W, Cheung M, et al. Propofol for sedation during colonoscopy. Cochrane Database Syst Rev. 2008(4):CD006268

[30] Qadeer MA, Vargo JJ, Khandwala F, et al. Propofol versus traditional sedative agents for gastrointestinal endoscopy: a meta-analysis. Clin Gastroenterol Hepatol. 2005; 3(11):1049–1056

[31] McQuaid KR, Laine L. A systematic review and meta-analysis of randomized, controlled trials of moderate sedation for routine endoscopic procedures. Gastrointest Endosc. 2008; 67(6):910–923

[32] Heuss LT, Froehlich F, Beglinger C. Nonanesthesiologist-administered propofol sedation: from the exception to standard practice. Sedation and monitoring trends over 20 years. Endoscopy. 2012; 44(5):504–511

[33] Slagelse C, Vilmann P, Hornslet P. et al. Nurse-administered propofol sedation for gastrointestinal endoscopic procedures: first Nordic results from implementation of a structured training program. Scand J Gastroenterol. 2011; 46(12):1503–1509

[34] Inadomi JM, Gunnarsson CL, Rizzo JA, Fang H. Projected increased growth rate of anesthesia professional-delivered sedation in the United States: 2009 to 2015. Gastrointest Endosc. 2010; 72(3):580–586

[35] Rex DK, Deenadayalu VP, Eid E, et al. Endoscopist-directed administration of propofol: a worldwide safety experience. Gastroenterology. 2009; 137(4):1229–1237, quiz 1518–1519

[36] Dumonceau JM, Riphaus A, Aparicio JR, et al; NAAP Task Force Members. European Society of Gastrointestinal Endoscopy, European Society of Gastroenterology and Endoscopy Nurses and Associates, and the European Society of Anaesthesiology Guideline: non-anesthesiologist administration of propofol for GI endoscopy. Endoscopy. 2010; 42(11):960–974

[37] Vargo JJ, DeLegge MH, Feld AD, et al; American Association for the Study of Liver Diseases. American College of Gastroenterology. American Gastroenterological Association Institute. American Society for Gastrointestinal Endoscopy. Society for Gastroenterology Nurses and Associates. Multisociety sedation curriculum for gastrointestinal endoscopy. Gastroenterology. 2012; 143(1):e18–e41

[38] Varadarajulu S, Banerjee S, Barth BA, et al; ASGE Technology Committee. GI endoscopes. Gastrointest Endosc. 2011; 74(1):1–6.e6

[39] Hewett DG, Kaltenbach T, Sano Y, et al. Validation of a simple classification system for endoscopic diagnosis of small colorectal polyps using narrow-band imaging. Gastroenterology. 2012; 143(3):599–607.e1

[40] Wu J, Hu B. The role of carbon dioxide insufflation in colonoscopy: a systematic review and meta-analysis. Endoscopy. 2012; 44(2):128–136

[41] van Doorn SC, van der Vlugt M, Depla A, et al. Adenoma detection with Endocuff colonoscopy versus conventional colonoscopy: a multicentre randomised controlled trial. Gut 2015 Dec 16. pii: gutjnl-2015-310097

[42] Dik VK, Gralnek IM, Segol O, et al. Multicenter, randomized, tandem evaluation of EndoRings colonoscopy—results of the CLEVER study. Endoscopy. 2015; 47(12):1151–1158

[43] Gralnek IM, Siersema PD, Halpern Z, et al. Standard forward-viewing colonoscopy versus full-spectrum endoscopy: an international, multicentre, randomised, tandem colonoscopy trial. Lancet Oncol. 2014; 15(3):353–360

[44] Talley NJ. How to do and interpret a rectal examination in gastroenterology. Am J Gastroenterol. 2008; 103(4):820–822

[45] Asai S, Fujimoto N, Tanoue K, et al. Water immersion colonoscopy facilitates straight passage of the colonoscope through the sigmoid colon without loop formation: randomized controlled trial. Dig Endosc. 2015; 27(3):345–353

[46] Leung CW, Kaltenbach T, Soetikno R, et al, Water immersion versus standard colonoscopy insertion technique: randomized trial shows promise for minimal sedation. Endoscopy. 2010; 42(7):557–563

[47] Rex DK, Cutler CS, Lemmel GT, et al. Colonoscopic miss rates of adenomas determined by back-to-back colonoscopies. Gastroenterology. 1997; 112(1):24–28

[48] van Rijn JC, Reitsma JB, Stoker J, et al, Polyp miss rate determined by tandem colonoscopy: a systematic review. Am J Gastroenterol. 2006; 101(2):343–350

[49] Adler J, Robertson DJ. Interval colorectal cancer after colonoscopy: exploring explanations and solutions. Am J Gastroenterol. 2015; 110(12):1657–1664, quiz 1665

[50] Baxter NN, Goldwasser MA, Paszat LF, et al. Association of colonoscopy and death from colorectal cancer. Ann Intern Med. 2009; 150(1):1–8

[51] Singh H, Nugent Z, Demers AA, et al. The reduction in colorectal cancer mortality after colonoscopy varies by site of the cancer. Gastroenterology. 2010; 139(4):1128–1137

[52] Kushnir VM, Oh YS, Hollander T, et al. Impact of retroflexion vs. second forward view examination of the right colon on adenoma detection: a comparison study. Am J Gastroenterol. 2015; 110(3):415–422

[53] Lai EJ, Calderwood AH, Doros G, et al, The Boston bowel preparation scale: a valid and reliable instrument for colonoscopy-oriented research. Gastrointest Endosc. 2009; 69(3 Pt 2):620–625

[54] Clark BT, Protiva P, Nagar A, et al. Quantification of adequate bowel preparation for screening or surveillance colonoscopy in men. Gastroenterology. 2016; 150(2):396–405, quiz e14–e15

[55] The Paris endoscopic classification of superficial neoplastic lesions: esophagus, stomach, and colon: November 30 to December 1, 2002. Gastrointest Endosc. 2003; 58(Suppl 6):S3–S43

[56] Lieberman D, Brill J, Canto M, et al. Management of diminutive colon polyps based on endoluminal imaging. Clin Gastroenterol Hepatol. 2015; 13(11):1860–1866, quiz e168–e169

[57] Lee CK, Shim JJ, Jang JY. Cold snare polypectomy vs. cold forceps polypectomy using double-biopsy technique for removal of diminutive colorectal polyps: a prospective randomized study. Am J Gastroenterol. 2013; 108(10):1593–1600

[58] Raad D, Tripathi P, Cooper G, Falck-Ytter Y. Role of the cold biopsy technique in diminutive and small colonic polyp removal: a systematic review and meta-analysis. Gastrointest Endosc. 2015 Nov 9. pii: S0016–5107(15)03054–0

[59] Sharma VK, Nguyen CC, Crowell MD, et al. A national study of cardiopulmonary unplanned events after GI endoscopy. Gastrointest Endosc. 2007; 66(1):27–34

[60] Romagnuolo J, Cotton PB, Eisen G, Identifying and reporting risk factors for adverse events in endoscopy. Part I: cardiopulmonary events. Gastrointest Endosc. 2011; 73(3):579–585

[61] Levin TR, Zhao W, Conell C, et al. Complications of colonoscopy in an integrated health care delivery system. Ann Intern Med. 2006; 145(12):880–886

[62] Kim HS, Kim TI, Kim WH, et al. Risk factors for immediate postpolypectomy bleeding of the colon: a multicenter study. Am J Gastroenterol. 2006; 101(6):1333–1341

[63] Choung BS, Kim SH, Ahn DS, et al. Incidence and risk factors of delayed postpolypectomy bleeding: a retrospective cohort study. J Clin Gastroenterol. 2014; 48(9):784–789

[64] Zhang Q, An SI, Chen Zy, et al. Assessment of risk factors for delayed colonic post-polypectomy hemorrhage: a study of 15553 polypectomies from 2005 to 2013. PLoS One. 2014; 9(10):e108290

[65] Korman LY, Overholt BF, Box T, Winker CK. Perforation during colonoscopy in endoscopic ambulatory surgical centers. Gastrointest Endosc. 2003; 58(4):554–557

[66] Arora G, Mannalithara A, Singh G. et al. Risk of perforation from a colonoscopy in adults: a large population-based study. Gastrointest Endosc. 2009; 69 (3 Pt 2):654–664

[67] Saad A, Rex DK. Colonoscopy-induced splenic injury: report of 3 cases and literature review. Dig Dis Sci. 2008; 53(4):892–898

[68] Winawer SJ, Zauber AG, Ho MN, et al; The National Polyp Study Workgroup. Prevention of colorectal cancer by colonoscopic polypectomy. N Engl J Med. 1993; 329(27):1977–1981

[69] Zauber AG, Winawer SJ, O'Brien MJ, et al. Colonoscopic polypectomy and long-term prevention of colorectal-cancer deaths. N Engl J Med. 2012; 366(8):687–696

[70] Nishihara R, Wu K, Lochhead P, et al. Long-term colorectal-cancer incidence and mortality after lower endoscopy. N Engl J Med. 2013; 369(12):1095–1105

[71] Rembacken B, Hassan C, Riemann JF, et al. Quality in screening colonoscopy: position statement of the European Society of Gastrointestinal Endoscopy (ESGE). Endoscopy. 2012; 44(10):957–968

[72] Rex DK, Schoenfeld PS, Cohen J, et al. Quality indicators for colonoscopy. Am J Gastroenterol. 2015; 110(1):72–90

[73] von Karsa L, Patnick J, Segnan N, et al; European Colorectal Cancer Screening Guidelines Working Group. European guidelines for quality assurance in colorectal cancer screening and diagnosis: overview and introduction to the full supplement publication. Endoscopy. 2013; 45(1):51–59

[74] Kaminski MF, Regula J, Kraszewska E, et al. Quality indicators for colonoscopy and the risk of interval cancer. N Engl J Med. 2010; 362(19):1795–1803

[75] Corley DA, Jensen CD, Marks AR, et al. Adenoma detection rate and risk of colorectal cancer and death. N Engl J Med. 2014; 370(14):1298–1306

[76] Sanaka MR, Rai T, Navaneethan U, et al. Adenoma detection rate in high-risk patients differs from that in average-risk patients. Gastrointest Endosc. 2016; 83(1):172–178

[77] Ross WA, Thirumurthi S, Lynch PM, et al. Detection rates of premalignant polyps during screening colonoscopy: time to revise quality standards? Gastrointest Endosc. 2015; 81(3):567–574

[78] Raju GS, Lum PJ, Slack RS, et al. Natural language processing as an alternative to manual reporting of colonoscopy quality metrics. Gastrointest Endosc. 2015; 82(3):512–519

[79] Imler TD, Morea J, Kahi C, et al. Multi-center colonoscopy quality measurement utilizing natural language processing. Am J Gastroenterol. 2015; 110(4):543–552

[80] Coe SG, Crook JE, Diehl NN, Wallace MB. An endoscopic quality improvement program improves detection of colorectal adenomas. Am J Gastroenterol. 2013; 108(2):219–226, quiz 227

[81] Ussui V, Coe S, Rizk C, et al. Stability of increased adenoma detection at colonoscopy. Follow-up of an endoscopic quality improvement program-EQUIP-II. Am J Gastroenterol. 2015; 110(4):489–496

[82] Abdul-Baki H, Schoen RE, Dean K, et al. Public reporting of colonoscopy quality is associated with an increase in endoscopist adenoma detection rate. Gastrointest Endosc. 2015; 82(4):676–682

[83] Classen M, Tytgat GN, Lightdale CJ, eds. Gastroenterlogical Endoscopy. New York, NY: Thieme; 2010

16 Endoscopic Retrograde Cholangiopancreatography

Christine Boumitri, Nikhil A. Kumta, and Michel Kahaleh

16.1 Introduction

Endoscopic retrograde cholangiopancreatography (ERCP) has re-shaped the management of biliary and pancreatic disease since its introduction in 1968. From a diagnostic tool to a therapeutic tool with expanding use and indications, ERCP continues to be an innovative and exceptional technique with continuous improvements to provide the safest and most effective procedures. While its use as a diagnostic tool is falling out of favor with advances in noninvasive imaging, its therapeutic applications continue to expand for biliary and pancreatic strictures management, stone extraction, and biliary leaks. This procedure has proven to be safe in the pediatric and pregnant population. Performance in high-volume centers by experienced endoscopists is essential with increasing demand for complex cases, which raises the question of training and credentialing.

16.2 Overview of Procedure

The first attempt to cannulate the ampulla of Vater was in 1968 by a group of surgeons in the United States.[1] In 1969, Dr. Itaru Oi presented the first endoscopic cholangiopancreatography (ECPG) at an international meeting and was considered one of the pioneers along with Dr. Kazuei Ogoshi from Japan.[2,3] ERCP started to gain success in the early 1970s. Soon after, therapeutic applications of ERCP were developed starting with the first reported sphincterotomy in 1974 by Dr. Kawai in Japan and Dr. Classen in Germany followed by the first biliary stenting in 1979 by Dr. Soehendra.[4,5,6] Over the last four decades ERCP has shifted from being a diagnostic tool to being used almost exclusively as a therapeutic tool especially with the presence of other diagnostic tools such as magnetic resonance cholangiopancreatography (MRCP), and endoscopic ultrasound (EUS).

16.3 General Diagnostic Techniques

With advances in imaging modalities of the biliary tree and pancreas including computed tomography (CT) scan and magnetic resonance imaging (MRI), the use of ERCP as a diagnostic tool has significantly decreased except for certain instances such as sphincter of Oddi manometry. Regardless of the final intent of the procedure, biliary cannulation remains the first and most important step of all ERCPs.

16.3.1 Biliary Cannulation

The first step starts by establishing the duodenal position to achieve an "en face" position with the major papilla. This can be achieved by advancing the endoscope 2 to 3 cm after reaching the second part of the duodenum with counterclockwise torque. The right left wheel is then turned right and locked

followed by clockwise rotation of the shaft with upper deflection of the big wheel. Another technique is to advance the tip of the endoscope to the distal second part of the duodenum and then repeat the same steps mentioned above.[7] Once the duodenal position is achieved, biliary cannulation is attempted. Selective biliary cannulation remains one of the most difficult aspects of the procedure with failed cannulation occurring in up to 20% of cases outside of high-volume expert centers.[8] It is important to know that repetitive and prolonged cannulation increase the risk of post-ERCP pancreatitis (PEP). Cannulation can be achieved with either catheters or sphincterotomes. Most endoscopists use sphincterotomes for biliary cannulation since diagnostic ERCP has fallen out of favor and most procedures are performed with a therapeutic intent. Contrast opacification of the biliary tree is a long-established technique but is being used less due to the increased risk of PEP with inadvertent contrast filling of the pancreatic duct (PD). Wire-guided cannulation is becoming the preferred method of cannulation. This could be achieved by either direct access with the sphincterotome (ST) or by advancing the ST 2 to 3 mm beyond the luminal aspect of the papilla, then gently advancing the guidewire, or the "wire lead" technique where the wire acts as an introducer especially in situation where the papilla is small. Cannulation can fail in certain instances and is considered difficult after 5 minutes of attempting common bile duct (CBD) cannulation, five failed attempts or after more than two inadvertent pancreatic duct cannulation.[9,10] Multiple risk factors have been associated with failed cannulation such as Billroth I and II surgeries, Roux-en-Y gastrojejunostomy, hepaticojejunostomy, Whipple surgery, gastric outlet obstruction, or duodenal narrowing and malignant biliary tract obstructions such as periampullary tumors distorting the ampulla of Vater.[11,12,13,14,15,16] The literature is not clear whether periampullary diverticulum is a risk for failed cannulation or not. Boix et al reported that cannulation is more difficult in type 1 diverticula (where the papilla is inside the diverticulum).[12,17,18,19]

In the instance of failed or difficult access, the endoscopist should consider alternative ways of cannulation. If repetitive attempts of biliary cannulation result in access to PD, a PD stent can be placed thus decreasing the chance of PEP and facilitating access into the bile duct. Another option would be to use the dual-wire technique in which case the wire is left in the PD and sphincterotome is withdrawn from the papilla and loaded with a second guidewire for biliary cannulation. This technique can be used in patients with pancreas divisum. Access sphincterotomy describes techniques where cutting is performed prior to cannulation in order to facilitate access into the bile duct, another term is needle–knife sphincterotomy or precut sphincterotomy.

16.3.2 Sphincter of Oddi Manometry

Sphincter of Oddi manometry (SOM) is the gold standard to study pressure dynamics of the sphincter of Oddi in patients with high clinical suspicion for sphincter of Oddi dysfunction (SOD). According to the Milwaukee classification, there are three types of SOD. A recent update of Rome criteria (Rome IV) for sphincter of Oddi disorders considered that the classification of SOD into three types no longer applies since patients with SOD type I (dilated bile duct and elevated liver enzymes) have organic stenosis and benefit from sphicterotomy.[20] On the other hand, patients with SOD type II (dilated bile duct or elevated liver enzymes) should be labeled as *suspected functional biliary sphincter disorder* (FBSD).[20] SOM can be especially helpful in establishing the diagnosis of patients with type II and III SOD and sphincterotomy should be considered based on manometry results.[21,22] However, the EPISOD trial revealed that patients with SOD type III do not respond to sphincter ablation better than sham intervention and only patients with type II SOD would benefit from manometry directed sphincterotomy.[23,24,25] This procedure is technically challenging and requires high expertise in a center that is known to provide it. There is variation in pressure measurements depending on catheter size, probe position, and point of time when spasm is captured.[26] It is also associated with high risk of pancreatitis up to 9%.[27] The patient should be well sedated during the procedure and any drugs that might stimulate (narcotics, cholinergics) or relax (nitrates, calcium channel blockers, glucagon) the sphincter should be avoided 8 to 12 hours before the procedure and intraprocedure. Opioids should be avoided due to risk of inducing SO spasms.[28,29,30,31] Meperidine at a dose less than or equal to ≤ 1 mg/kg, ketamine, droperidol (discontinued in the united states), and propofol use have not been shown to significantly affect the basal pressure of the sphincter.[32,33,34,35,36] Two types of catheters are available for SOM: water perfused and solid state.[37] The procedure starts by passing the catheter along the working channel of the duodenoscope; once the duodenum is reached, a baseline or zero duodenal pressure is measured and recorded before cannulation.[22] This is followed by cannulation of the biliary or pancreatic duct. The need to measure both pancreatic and biliary sphincter remains controversial.[38] Cannulation can be achieved with the manometry catheter or with the aid of a 0.018 guidewire. It is reasonable to perform ERCP prior to manometry to make sure that there is no stone or obstruction that might obviate manometry. Contrast injection has not been shown to affect manometry results.[39] Once cannulation is obtained, measurement of ductal pressure is noted. This is obtained by the slow flow of pressurized water from an external pump to the sphincter of Oddi through the catheter. The catheter is then withdrawn at 1 to 2-mm intervals by station pull-through technique pausing for 60 to 90 seconds once the area of the sphincter is reached.[40] A basal sphincter pressure of greater than 40 mm Hg is used to diagnose SOD.[41,42,43] This is the calculated mean pressure readings from three pull-throughs.[44] Patients with SOD type I (evidence of SO obstruction) are treated with sphincterotomy without manometry.[43] Patients with type II SOD may benefit from sphincterotomy if manometry reveals increased basal pressure. This was the case in three small-randomized studies, which showed that sphincterotomy was more effective than a sham procedure in these patients.[24,25,45]

16.4 General Therapeutic Techniques

The innovations in technologies and equipment led to the expansion of the therapeutic applications of ERCP. A brief review of the most common therapeutic techniques is described below. Among others, sphincterotomy, endoscopic papillary balloon dilation, stone extraction, and stent insertion are considered an integral part of therapeutic ERCP that advanced endoscopists should master.

16.4.1 Biliary Sphincterotomy

Having the ampulla between the 11 and 1 o'clock positions facilitates deep cannulation, after which, the sphincterotome can be withdrawn to the desired incision length. The sphincterotomy should be performed in the longitudinal axis and never be continued beyond the junction of the intramural segment of the CBD and the duodenal wall. There is significant variation in choice of electrosurgical current used (cutting current, blended current, "ENDO CUT" mode). Possible complications include bleeding, pancreatitis, as well as retroperitoneal perforation resulting from a fast and uncontrolled "zipper" cut.[46,47] The most common indications for biliary sphincterotomy are CBD stones with or without cholangitis, facilitation of biliary stent placement for malignant or benign biliary obstruction, benign papillary stenosis, SOD types I and II when manometry reveals high basal pressure, biliary leaks, and others.[48] Pancreatic sphincterotomy (PS) is usually performed for pancreatic SOD, biliary SOD that does not respond to treatment with biliary sphincterotomy, chronic pancreatitis with papillary stenosis or stricture, and pancreas divisum. PS can also be used to facilitate other biliary pancreatic intervention such as transpapillary drainage of pancreatic pseudocysts, chronic pancreatitis with ductal stones treated with pancreatic stents, and/or stone removal and malignant strictures.[49]

16.4.2 Endoscopic Papillary Balloon Dilation

Endoscopic papillary balloon dilation (EPBD) is an alternative to sphincterotomy, first introduced in 1983.[50] It carries less risk of perforation and bleeding compared with sphincterotomy. Reports of increased risk of PEP with the use of EPBD led to a decrease in use, though in the 1990s it regained popularity with multiple reports showing its safety and noninferiority to sphincterotomy.[51,52,53] Ideal patients to be selected for EPBD as a substitute to sphincterotomy are those with fewer than or equal to three stones, stone less than 10 mm in diameter, age less than 50, impaired hemostasis, CBD less than 12 mm, no previous or ongoing pancreatitis.[54,55,56] Endoscopic papillary large balloon dilation can also be used as adjunctive tool with sphincterotomy for large complicated CBD stones, where a small endoscopic sphincterotomy (ES) can help direct the direction of sphincter of Oddi dilation and prevent postprocedure pancreatitis by decreasing periampullary edema. In addition, the combination of a small ES with EPBD reduces the need for mechanical lithotripsy when compared to ES alone.[57] After cannulation, a 0.025- or 0.035-in guidewire is inserted into the bile duct followed by removal of the cannula and insertion of a balloon-tipped catheter (CRE Wire-Guided Balloon, Boston Scientific, Natick, Massachusetts) over the guidewire. Usually, two-thirds of the balloon is inside the distal CBD and one-third is outside the papillary orifice. The balloon is then inflated with diluted contrast until the waist disappears. The dilation is maintained for 15 to 30 seconds. Different dilator balloons sizes are also available depending on the size of the bile duct. When dilating strictures, the endoscopist should be cautious for an increased risk of perforation.

16.4.3 Stone Extraction

Stones that are less than 1 cm will pass spontaneously after performing sphincterotomy and stones larger than 2 cm will most likely require additional fragmentation either mechanically using baskets or with intraductal electrohydraulic or laser lithotripsy and, rarely, extracorporeal shock wave lithotripsy (ESWL).[58] Sphincterotomy should be large enough to allow passage of the stone, otherwise impacted stones may result. Extraction can be achieved using retrieval balloon catheter or Dormia basket to sweep out the stone; mechanical lithotripsy (BML-V237QR-30 or BML-V242 QR-30, Olympus Medical Systems, Tokyo) can be used to fragment large stones. In complicated cases where stone extraction cannot be achieved, temporary biliary stenting to achieve biliary drainage and prevent sepsis and cholangitis should be performed while medical therapy with oral dissolution agents are used to decrease stone size and facilitate endoscopic extraction.[59,60] If stones are unable to be visualized, then the endoscopist has to change scope position to the long position to make sure no stones are hidden behind the endoscope. Small stones can be missed when a large amount of dense contrast is injected into a dilated duct.[61]

16.4.4 Biliary Stenting

Indications for biliary stenting include treatment of obstructive jaundice from benign causes, such as biliary stones or bile leaks, and malignant etiologies. Both plastic and metallic stents can be used. Plastic stents are more commonly used for benign strictures. With the emergence of metallic stents, their use for malignant strictures has decreased but are still considered and used for palliation in patients with distal malignant biliary tumors when the expected survival is 3 to 6 months.[62] They are usually formed of Teflon, polyethylene, or polyurethane, and come in different configurations (straight, single pigtail, or double pigtails), lengths, and width. They tend to be obstructed by food debris and biofilm and usually require exchange within 3 to 6 months. Stents less than 8.5 F are usually advanced over the guidewire using a pushing catheter. Stents greater than 8.5 F have an inner guiding catheter that passes over the guidewire. When stenting a distal malignant biliary stricture, a 10-F plastic stent is preferable to a 7 F due to prolonged patency. Sphincterotomy or balloon dilation of the stricture is not necessary; however, this is not the case when dealing with hilar strictures or when placing more than one biliary stent.

Self-expandable metallic stents (SEMS) can be uncovered (uSEMS), partially covered (pcSEMS), or totally covered (cSEMS). These were introduced after plastic stents and are primarily used for palliation and drainage of malignant obstruction secondary to surgically unresectable tumors. These offer longer patency due to a larger diameter.[63,64,65,66] uSEMS are associated with higher occlusion rate due to tumor ingrowth, this problem is surpassed by using cSEMS, however, the latter is associated with higher migration rate. pcSEMS were created to overcome the issues faced with uncovered and fully covered metallic stents. No benefit to survival or morbidity was observed when comparing uSEMS to cSEMS.[67,68] Innovative mechanisms to decrease the rate of duodenal biliary reflux and metallic stent obstruction has led to the creation of antireflux valve metal stent (ARVMS) with preliminary results revealing superior duration of patency compared to cSEMS.[69] There is an increased use of SEMS for benign biliary conditions such as strictures, leaks, and postsphincterotomy bleeding.[70,71,72] While placing SEMS, it is crucial to obtain an adequate cholangiogram prior to deploying the stent that will help the endoscopist in assessing the location and length of the stricture and guide on the choice of stent to be used. Once the endoscopist has made the decision with the type of stent to be used, deployment of the stent should be performed under endoscopic and fluoroscopic guidance. The stent is passed over the guidewire and advanced to the stricture level; the introducer catheter is passed over it. Fluoroscopic images are obtained to give an approximation of the postdeployment proximal and distal ends of the SEMS.

16.5 Accessory Devices and Techniques

16.5.1 Endoscopes

Duodenoscopes

Duodenovideoscopes are side-viewing endoscopes that are designed for both diagnostic and therapeutic ERCP. They are equipped with an elevator that allows the manipulation of the accessories introduced in the working channel. The side-viewing endoscopes are available for the pediatric and adult populations. The adult duodenoscope is available from three different manufacturers (Olympus, Pentax, and Fujinon) (▶ Fig. 16.1). The insertion tube diameter can range between 10.8- and 12.1-mm diameter with a biopsy channel diameter between 3.2 and 4.8 mm according to the manufacturer.[73] The pediatric duodenoscopes have an outer diameter of 7.5 mm and an accessory channel of 2 mm. The use of the latter is limited though due to the paucity of accessories available for the smaller working channel especially when performing therapeutic ERCPs. In a recent review, Troendle et al suggested that pediatric duodenoscope should be the instrument of choice in patients less than 10 kg (22 lb), whereas adult duodenoscope could be safely used in patients greater than 10 kg.[74] We suggest that the use of the duodenoscope be at the discretion of the endoscopist based on a case-by-case basis and taking into account the patient's age and weight, nature of the ERCP procedure, and anticipated accessory channel equipment to be used.

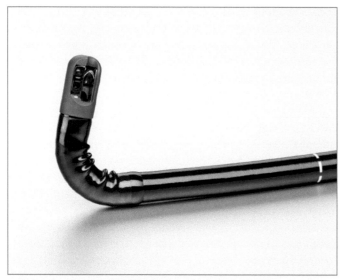

Fig. 16.1 ED34-i10T video duodenoscope with 4.2-mm working channel. (Image is provided courtesy of Pentax Medical, Montvale, NJ.)

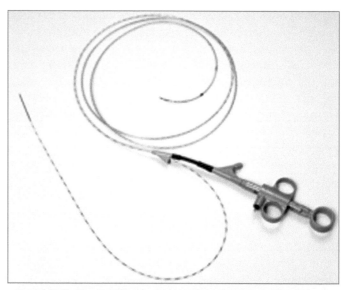

Fig. 16.2 Hydratome RX cannulating sphincterotome: preloaded with a Hydra Jagwire. (Image is provided courtesy of Boston Scientific. ©2016 Boston Scientific Corporation or its affiliates. All rights reserved.)

Forward-Viewing Endoscopes and Echoendoscopes

Forward-viewing endoscopes are used in patients with altered surgical anatomy where direct forward visualization will make it easier to reach the ampulla and the use of duodenoscope can entail a higher perforation risk, such as Billroth II, Roux-en-Y gastrectomy or gastric bypass, and hepaticojejunostomy. Accurate knowledge of the surgery that was performed is crucial such as the type and the length of anastomoses, the timing of the surgery, and, if possible, the surgeon who performed it. The endoscopes that can be used are enteroscopes, pediatric colonoscopes, or gastroscopes. With the emergence of device-assisted enteroscopy (DAE) such as double-balloon enteroscopy, single-balloon enteroscopy, and spiral enteroscopy, DAE-ERCP in patients with Roux-en-Y reconstruction has been reported in multiple case series.[75] Single-balloon enteroscopes can allow access to previously inaccessible anatomy. These scopes do not have elevators and thus the manipulation of the accessories may be challenging. Novel techniques to access the biliary tract using endoscopic ultrasound have been rising in patients with altered anatomy.[76] The therapeutic curvilinear echoendoscope has a 3.8-mm working channel and allows passage of standard ERCP accessories as well as placement of stents with large diameter (10F).

16.5.2 Equipment

Cannulation Catheters

Cannulation catheters are devices that are used to gain access to the ducts. There are more than 20 standard cannulation catheters from different providers with variable size, length, tip configurations, and number of lumens. These are generally made of Teflon (Dupont, Wilmington, Delaware), the size can range between 5 and 7 F, and can accommodate a 0.035-in guidewire, however, some can only accommodate a 0.025-in

guidewire such as the ultratapered catheter that can be alternatively used for minor papilla cannulation due to smaller tip size.[73,77] Another catheter that can facilitate minor papilla cannulation is the Cremer needle tip (Cook Endoscopy, Winston-Salem, North Carolina). The catheter tip can be either straight, tapered, or rounded. Tapered catheters can allow better duct access but carries an increased risk of submucosal injection. Another catheter that allows the endoscopist to control the tip and angulate it up to 90 degrees is the swing-tip catheter (Olympus America Inc., Center Valley, Pennsylvania) and this can facilitate insertion into bile ducts in challenging cases.

Sphincterotomes

Sphincterotomes are catheters that have the advantage of both performing a sphincterotomy and biliary cannulation. These consist of Teflon with a continuous wire with a distal 2 to 3 cm exposed wire that can exit at variable distance from the tip. The other end of the wire is connected to an electrosurgical unit that provides current for sphincterotomy (▶ Fig. 16.2). There are several types of sphincterotomes, with the earliest precut sphincterotomy being the pull type where the wire extends to the tip. With the rising use of sphincterotomes for cannulation, there have been different types of devices manufactured to overcome difficulties encountered. S-shaped tips are available for patient with altered anatomy, sphincterotome with a cutting wire directed at the opposite direction of the standard sphincterotome for patients with Billroth II, as well as rotatable sphincterotome. These catheters are available in single, double, and triple lumens. Double-lumen sphincterotomes allow for either injection of contrast or introduction of a guidewire. Triple-lumen sphincterotomes allow injection of contrast through the additional port without the need to remove the wire. A small syringe is used to facilitate injection

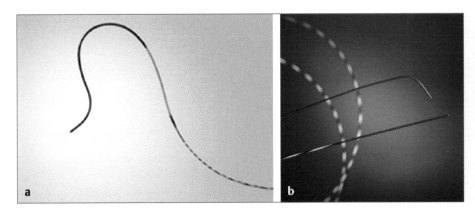

Fig. 16.3 (a) VisiGlide 2 guidewires (Image is provided courtesy of Olympus, all rights reserved). **(b)** Hydra Jagwire guidewire with straight or angled tip. (Image is provided courtesy of Boston Scientific. © 2016 Boston Scientific Corporation or its affiliates. All rights reserved.)

and overcome resistance that can be encountered by the assistant due to smaller lumen. A sphincterotome with ability for stone extraction is also available (Stonetome, Boston Scientific, Natick, Massachusetts); this can render cannulation harder because of increased catheter diameter. Current that can be applied while performing sphincterotomy includes cutting, auto-cut, coagulation, or blended. Cutting is associated with a higher chance of bleeding when compared with others and decreased risk of developing PEP when performing pancreatic sphincterotomy. Needle–knife and precut sphincterotomes are used when conventional methods to cannulate the bile ducts have failed.

Guidewires

Guidewires are used to cannulate the bile or pancreatic ducts. They are available in different diameters and lengths ranging from 0.018 to 0.035 in and from 260 to 480 cm.[78] Different types of guidewires are available for different indication and are beyond the scope of this chapter, however, we mention conventional, hydrophilic, and *hybrid*, guidewires. Those used for electrocautery applications should be coated. Hydrophilic wires are mostly used in difficult papillae or strictures; however, these can be slippery leading to loss of position during exchange. Thus, newer combination (hybrid) wires such as Jagwire, Hydra Jagwire (Boston Scientific); FX, X (ConMed, Utica, New York); VisiGlide (Olympus America Inc.); and Metro (Cook Endoscopy) are available and provide a stiffer shaft (▶ Fig. 16.3). A full report and detailed review of different guidewires are available in the American Society for Gastrointestinal Endoscopy (ASGE) technology assessment report.[79]

16.6 Accepted Indications

The ASGE has set practice guidelines for the role of ERCP in diseases of the biliary tree and pancreas. These guidelines are available online with the most detailed document dating back to 2005.[80] A list of acceptable indications were published in the guidelines of appropriate use of gastrointestinal (GI) endoscopy in 2012.[81] More recently, the ASGE has released an update of the role of ERCP in benign biliary disease.[82] A summary of acceptable indications based on these guidelines are listed in ▶ Box 16.1.

Box 16.1 ERCP indications

1. **Biliary Tract Diseases:**
   - Biliary obstruction
     - Choledocholithiasis
     - Malignant biliary strictures
     - Benign biliary strictures (PSC, postoperative, chronic pancreatitis)
     - Biliary SOD
     - Sump syndrome
     - Choledochocele
   - Sphincter of Oddi manometry
   - Bile leak
2. **Pancreatic Diseases:**
   - Pancreatic cancer and other pancreatic malignancies with brushing and biopsy
   - Recurrent acute pancreatitis
   - Chronic pancreatitis: treatment of symptomatic stones, strictures, and pseudocysts
   - Pancreatic duct leaks
   - Pancreatic fluid collections (PFC)
   - Pancreatic SOD
3. **Ampullary Diseases:**
   - Ampullary carcinoma in poor surgical candidate to relieve obstruction
   - Papillary stenosis
4. **Therapeutic ERCP:**
   - Tissue sampling
   - Balloon dilation of strictures
   - Stone extraction
   - Endoscopic sphincterotomy
   - Stent placement
   - Nasobiliary or nasopancreatic drain placement
   - Cholangioscopy and pancreatoscopy
   - Drainage of PFC
   - Ampullectomy of adenomatous neoplasms of the major papilla

PSC: Primary Sclerosing Cholangitis
SOD: Sphincter of Oddi Dysfunction

It is important to emphasize that the endoscopist should be competent in performing ERCPs regardless of the indications. This should be considered a quality measure in addition to following the guidelines. According to the ASGE guidelines, ERCP should not be performed if the patient refuses the procedure, the endoscopist lacks adequate training in ERCP, or there is lack of equipment and accessories. In addition, ERCP should not be performed for the evaluation of abdominal pain when a pancreatic or biliary etiology is not suspected or in the evaluation of gallbladder disease without bile duct disease. Endoscopists should avoid ERCP when the anatomy limits access to papilla, when patient is in the midst of an acute episode of pancreatitis, and should reconsider options in high-risk procedure.

The indications of ERCP in the pediatric population mirror that of the adults. In pregnant patients, ERCP is now considered a safe and effective procedure when performed by a competent endoscopist and for the appropriate indications. Pregnant women are at higher risk of developing cholelithiasis since the hormonal changes associated with pregnancy increase bile lithogenicity and causes bile stasis.[83,84] ERCP for diagnostic purpose is not an accepted indication for ERCP in a pregnant patient. The most common indication for ERCP in this patient group is biliary pancreatitis, cholangitis, and bile duct injury. Other indications should be approached on a case-by-case basis and risk of serious adverse event should be discussed with the patient.[85,86,87] The best time to perform ERCP is the second trimester where the risk of ionizing radiation on fetal development is diminished compared to the first trimester.[88] According to American Congress of Obstetricians and Gynecologists, "exposure to less than 5 rad (50 mGy) has not been associated with an increase in fetal anomalies or pregnancy loss."[89] Kahaleh et al reported a mean fetal radiation exposure of 40 mrad (range 1–180 mrad) in 15 pregnant women undergoing ERCP and concluded that ERCP during pregnancy is efficacious and safe when performed for the right indications and when adequate measures are taken to minimize exposure of the fetus to ionizing radiation such as limiting fluoroscopy time and applying external lead shielding to the lower abdomen/pelvis.[90]

16.7 Procedure-Specific Quality Measures

Procedure-specific quality measures can now be monitored by standardization of reports. Preprocedure, intraprocedure, and postprocedure indicators common to all endoscopy reports are specified in ▶ Box 16.2.[91] This standardization is also extended to more complex procedure such as ERCP. A summary of the proposed quality indicators for ERCP is available online from the ASGE.[92] For ERCP, the recommended priority indicators are appropriate indication, cannulation rate, stone extraction success rate, stent insertion success rate, and frequency of PEP.[92]

Box 16.2 Essential Data to be included in endoscopy reports

- Date of procedure
- Patient identification data
- Endoscopist(s)
- Nurses and assistant(s)
- Documentation of relevant patient history and physical examination
- Documentation of informed consent
- Procedure indication(s)
- Type of endoscopic instrument used
- Medications administered (type of sedation, antibiotics, antispasmodics)
- Anatomic extent of examination
- Limitation(s) of examination, if any
- Tissue or fluid samples obtained
- Findings
- Diagnostic impression
- Types of therapeutic intervention and results
- Adverse events, if any
- Disposition
- Recommendations for subsequent care

16.8 Procedure-Specific Training Requirements

ERCP is an advanced therapeutic procedure and an additional year of training has become the standard in the United States beyond the 3-year gastroenterology training program. Advanced endoscopy is currently blossoming and innovations in techniques and devices are happening every day. There is a high demand among graduating gastroenterology fellows for advanced training with 58 fellowship programs participating in the ASGE advanced endoscopy fellowship throughout the United States. An additional year of training in advanced endoscopy not only allows fellows to have dedicated training from experts, but also accelerates their professional development by performing research in advanced endoscopy, gaining leadership skills, and refining their endoscopy skills. Most trainees start by observing their mentors doing the procedures, assisting the endoscopist while learning how to handle the catheters, guidewires, and other equipment. Once they are at the hands-on stage, they will first learn how to use the side-viewing scope with esophageal intubation, passing the pylorus, and how to achieve the short position at the papilla level. Most trainees keep a logbook of their achievements as they progress in their training. According to the ASGE guidelines for advanced endoscopy and the American Gastroenterological Association (AGA) gastroenterology core curriculum, the number of ERCPs needed before trainees' competency can be assessed is 200.[93,94,95]

16.9 Procedure-Specific Complications

ERCP remains a complex procedure that is technically demanding. Adequate training and experience are needed to ensure quality and minimize adverse events. Among endoscopic procedures, ERCP has the highest rate of complications ranging between 5 and 10%.[47] The most common complications of ERCP are bleeding, infection, PEP, and perforation. These are mentioned in details in ▶ Table 16.1 with predisposing factors, how to manage and prevent these complications.[46,47] In managing PEP, it is important to mention that rectal administration of indomethacin/nonsteroidal anti-inflammatory drugs (NSAIDs) pre- or post-ERCP can decrease the severity and incidence of PEP.[96,97,98,99,100] One of the largest trials published in the New England Journal of Medicine in 2012 showed that PEP developed in 9.2% of the indomethacin group compared to 16.9% of the placebo group ($p = 0.005$).[97] The European Society for Gastrointestinal Endoscopy guidelines recommends prophylactic rectal indomethacin for all patients undergoing ERCP, including those at average risk for pancreatitis, however, a recent randomized-controlled trial revealed no benefit of prophylactic administration of rectal indomethacin in decreasing the incidence or severity of PEP in all patients undergoing ERCP.[9,101] Thus, we need further trials to clarify the role of indomethacin in preventing PEP. In addition, cardiopulmonary adverse events related to sedation are also common and could be prevented by adequately risk assessing each patient prior to the procedure, avoiding unnecessary procedures, and using endotracheal intubation with general anesthesia when needed.

Table 16.1 Procedure-related complications: incidence, risk factors, treatment, and prevention

Complication	Incidence	Risk factors	Treatment	Prevention

Post-ERCP pancreatitis	Adult: 5–7%
	Pediatric: 3–11%
		1. Patient related:
		  a) Young age
		  b) Female sex
		  c) History of previous post-ERCP pancreatitis
		  d) Nondilated ducts
		  e) Normal bilirubin
		  f) Suspected SOD
		2. Procedure related:
		  a) Difficult cannulation
		  b) Pancreatic sphincterotomy
		  c) Precut sphincterotomy
		  d) Pancreatic sampling
		  e) Multiple pancreatic injections
			Similar to acute pancreatitis:
			1. Nil per mouth
			2. Intravenous hydration with lactate ringer
			3. Pain control
			4. Enteral feeding
			5. Close monitoring
				1. Perform ERCP only when clinically indicated
				2. Prophylactic pancreatic duct stenting in high-risk cases
				3. Rectal administration of indomethacin
				4. Guidewire cannulation technique
				5. Early precut sphincterotomy
				6. Aggressive hydration

Bleeding	Adult
	Immediate: 10–30%
	Severe (melena, hematemesis, > 2 g/dL drop in Hgb level, requirement of secondary intervention endoscopy, transfusion): 0.1–2%
	Pediatrics: 1–2%
		1. Presence of coagulopathy or thrombocytopenia
		2. Initiation of anticoagulation within 3 days of sphincterotomy
		3. Cholangitis
		4. Low-volume case of endoscopist
		5. Ampullary stone impaction
		6. Periampullary diverticula
		7. Zipper cut
		8. Needle–knife sphincterotomy
			1. Endoscopic therapy:
			  a) Dilute epinephrine injection 1: 10,000
			  b) Coagulation
			  c) Combination therapy (epinephrine and coagulation)
			  d) Clip placement
			  e) fcSEMS
			  f) Catheter-delivered hemostatic powder
			2. Angiographic embolization
			3. Surgery
				1. Correct coagulopathy (platelet count > 50,000, INR < 1.5–2)
				2. Blended current
				3. Hold anticoagulation for 3 days after procedure
				4. Prophylactic epinephrine injection (Role not clear)

Perforation	Adult: 0.3–0.6%
	Pediatrics: < 1%
		1. Free wall perforation:
		  a) Force and angle related
		  b) Diverticulum
		  c) Esophageal stricture
		  d) Altered anatomy (Billroth II, Roux-en-Y)
		  e) Gastric outlet obstruction from pancreatic tumor
		2. Retroperitoneal perforation:
		  a) Needle–knife precut access
		  b) Suspected SOD
		3. Bile and pancreatic ducts perforation:
		  a) Wire-related manipulation
		  b) Stricture dilation
			1. Endoscopic treatment:
			  a) Through the scope clips
			  b) OTSC
			  c) Endoscopic Suturing
			  d) fcSEMS
			  e) Plastic or fcSEM stents for ductal injury
			2. Percutaneous drainage of collection if needed
			3. Surgery
			  a) In addition to above always:
			  b) Admit patient
			  c) Keep nil per mouth
			  d) Obtain imaging as needed
			  e) Surgical consult for backup
			  f) Intravenous (IV) hydration
			  g) IV antibiotics
			  h) Proton pump inhibitors
				1. Know altered anatomy and use forward-viewing scope if needed
				2. Avoid pushing against resistance
				3. Use floppy-tipped hydrophilic wires

Infection	Adult: < 2%
	Pediatrics: < 1%
		1. Cholangitis
		  a) Failed or incomplete biliary drainage
		  b) Jaundice
		  c) PSC
		  d) Rendezvous technique
		  e) Lack of endoscopists' experience
		2. Cholecystitis
		  a) fcSEMS across cystic duct
		  b) Tumor-involving cyst duct
			1. Endoscopic drainage
			2. Percutaneous drainage
			3. Surgery
				1. Antibiotics prophylaxis if incomplete drainage
				2. Aspiration and lavage of infected bile from obstruction prior to contrast injection
				3. Minimize contrast injection in bile ducts
				4. Obtain complete drainage

ERCP, endoscopic retrograde cholangiopancreatography; fcSEMS, self-expandable metallic stents; INR, international normalized ratio; OTSC, over-the-scope clip; PSC, primary sclerosing cholangitis; SOD, sphincter of Oddi dysfunction.

Recent outbreaks of infections caused by drug-resistant bacteria, specifically carbapenem-resistant enterobacteriaceae (CRE) associated with the use duodenoscopes for ERCP have raised major concerns worldwide. Multiple incidents of duodenoscope-associated infection have been reported in the United States.[102] On February 19, 2015, the United States Food and Drug Administration (FDA) issued a safety communication on duodenoscope cleaning and urged all health care professionals to strictly follow the cleaning instructions provided by the duodenoscope manufacturer to prevent duodenoscope-associated infection. In January of 2016, Olympus America announced initiation for arrangements for return of TJF-Q180V duodenoscopes for the forceps elevator replacement to ensure that the devices are consistent with the new parameters cleared by the FDA.

References

[1] McCune WS, Shorb PE, Moscovitz H. Endoscopic cannulation of the ampulla of vater: a preliminary report. Ann Surg. 1968; 167(5):752–756

[2] Oi I, Takemoto T, Kondo T. Fiberduodenoscope: direct observation of the papilla of Vater. Endoscopy. 1969; 1(3):101–103

[3] Cotton PB. Cannulation of the papilla of Vater by endoscopy and retrograde cholangiopancreatography (ERCP). Gut. 1972; 13(12):1014–1025

[4] McHenry L, Lehman GA. Four decades. In: Todd H. Baron RAK, David L. Carr-Locke eds. ERCP. 2nd ed. New York, NY: Elsevier, 2013: Chapter 1, 2-9

[5] Burcharth F, Jensen LI, Olesen K. Endoprosthesis for internal drainage of the biliary tract. Technique and results in 48 cases. Gastroenterology. 1979; 77(1):133–137

[6] Soehendra N, Reynders-Frederix V. Palliative bile duct drainage—a new endoscopic method of introducing a transpapillary drain. Endoscopy. 1980; 12(1):8–11

[7] Bourke MJ. Cannulation of the major papilla. In: Baron TH, Kozarek RA, Carr-Locke DL, eds. ERCP. 2nd ed. New York, NY: Elsevier, 2013; 104–115

[8] Williams EJ, Taylor S, Fairclough P, et al; BSG Audit of ERCP. Are we meeting the standards set for endoscopy? Results of a large-scale prospective survey of endoscopic retrograde cholangio-pancreatograph practice. Gut. 2007; 56(6):821–829

[9] Dumonceau JM, Andriulli A, Elmunzer BJ, et al; European Society of Gastrointestinal Endoscopy. Prophylaxis of post-ERCP pancreatitis: European Society of Gastrointestinal Endoscopy (ESGE) Guideline—updated June 2014. Endoscopy. 2014; 46(9):799–815

[10] Wang P, Li ZS, Liu F, et al. Risk factors for ERCP-related complications: a prospective multicenter study. Am J Gastroenterol. 2009; 104(1):31–40

[11] Baron TH, Petersen BT, Mergener K, et al. Quality indicators for endoscopic retrograde cholangiopancreatography. Gastrointest Endosc. 2006; 63(4, Suppl):S29–S34

[12] Fukatsu H, Kawamoto H, Kato H, et al. Evaluation of needle-knife precut papillotomy after unsuccessful biliary cannulation, especially with regard to postoperative anatomic factors. Surg Endosc. 2008; 22(3):717–723

[13] Choudari CP, Sherman S, Fogel EL, et al. Success of ERCP at a referral center after a previously unsuccessful attempt. Gastrointest Endosc. 2000; 52(4):478–483

[14] Nordback I, Airo I. Endoscopic retrograde cholangiopancreatography (ERCP) and sphincterotomy (EST) after BII resection. Ann Chir Gynaecol. 1988; 77(2):64–69

[15] Freeman ML, Guda NM. ERCP cannulation: a review of reported techniques. Gastrointest Endosc. 2005; 61(1):112–125

[16] Faylona JM, Qadir A, Chan AC, et al. Small-bowel perforations related to endoscopic retrograde cholangiopancreatography (ERCP) in patients with Billroth II gastrectomy. Endoscopy. 1999; 31(7):546–549

[17] Boix J, Lorenzo-Zúñiga V, Añaños F, et al. Impact of periampullary duodenal diverticula at endoscopic retrograde cholangiopancreatography: a proposed classification of periampullary duodenal diverticula. Surg Laparosc Endosc Percutan Tech. 2006; 16(4):208–211

[18] Lobo DN, Balfour TW, Iftikhar SY. Periampullary diverticula: consequences of failed ERCP. Ann R Coll Surg Engl. 1998; 80(5):326–331

[19] Balik E, Eren T, Keskin M, et al. Parameters that may be used for predicting failure during endoscopic retrograde cholangiopancreatography. J Oncol. 2013; 2013:201681

[20] Cotton PB, Elta GH, Carter CR, et al. Gallbladder and sphincter of Oddi disorders. Gastroenterology 2016

[21] Cohen S, Bacon BR, Berlin JA, et al. National Institutes of Health State-of-the-Science Conference Statement: ERCP for diagnosis and therapy, January 14–16, 2002. Gastrointest Endosc. 2002; 56(6):803–809

[22] Pfau PR, Banerjee S, Barth BA, et al. Sphincter of Oddi manometry. Gastrointest Endosc. 2011; 74(6):1175–1180

[23] Cotton PB, Durkalski V, Romagnuolo J, et al. Effect of endoscopic sphincterotomy for suspected sphincter of Oddi dysfunction on pain-related disability following cholecystectomy: the EPISOD randomized clinical trial. JAMA. 2014; 311(20):2101–2109

[24] Toouli J, Roberts-Thomson IC, Kellow J, et al. Manometry based randomised trial of endoscopic sphincterotomy for sphincter of Oddi dysfunction. Gut. 2000; 46(1):98–102

[25] Geenen JE, Hogan WJ, Dodds WJ, et al. The efficacy of endoscopic sphincterotomy after cholecystectomy in patients with sphincter-of-Oddi dysfunction. N Engl J Med. 1989; 320(2):82–87

[26] Small AJ, Kozarek RA. Sphincter of Oddi dysfunction. Gastrointest Endosc Clin N Am. 2015; 25(4):749–763

[27] Wong GS, Teoh N, Dowsett JD, et al. Complications of sphincter of Oddi manometry: biliary-like pain versus acute pancreatitis. Scand J Gastroenterol. 2005; 40(2):147–153

[28] Economou G, Ward-McQuaid JN. A cross-over comparison of the effect of morphine, pethidine, pentazocine, and phenazocine on biliary pressure. Gut. 1971; 12(3):218–221

[29] Greenstein AJ, Kaynan A, Singer A, Dreiling DA. A comparative study of pentazocine and meperidine on the biliary passage pressure. Am J Gastroenterol. 1972; 58(4):417–427

[30] Radnay PA, Brodman E, Mankikar D, Duncalf D. The effect of equi-analgesic doses of fentanyl, morphine, meperidine and pentazocine on common bile duct pressure. Anaesthesist. 1980; 29(1):26–29

[31] Joehl RJ, Koch KL, Nahrwold DL. Opioid drugs cause bile duct obstruction during hepatobiliary scans. Am J Surg. 1984; 147(1):134–138

[32] Fogel EL, Sherman S, Bucksot L, et al. Effects of droperidol on the pancreatic and biliary sphincters. Gastrointest Endosc. 2003; 58(4):488–492

[33] Wilcox CM, Linder J. Prospective evaluation of droperidol on sphincter of Oddi motility. Gastrointest Endosc. 2003; 58(4):483–487

[34] Varadarajulu S, Tamhane A, Wilcox CM. Prospective evaluation of adjunctive ketamine on sphincter of Oddi motility in humans. J Gastroenterol Hepatol. 2008; 23(8 Pt 2):e405–e409

[35] Goff JS. Effect of propofol on human sphincter of Oddi. Dig Dis Sci. 1995; 40(11):2364–2367

[36] Schmitt T, Seifert H, Dietrich CF, et al. Propofol sedation in endoscopic manometry of Oddi's sphincter Z Gastroenterol. 1999; 37(3):219–227

[37] Petersen BT. An evidence-based review of sphincter of Oddi dysfunction: part I, presentations with "objective" biliary findings (types I and II). Gastrointest Endosc. 2004; 59(4):525–534

[38] Raddawi HM, Geenen JE, Hogan WJ, et al. Pressure measurements from biliary and pancreatic segments of sphincter of Oddi. Comparison between patients with functional abdominal pain, biliary, or pancreatic disease. Dig Dis Sci. 1991; 36(1):71–74

[39] Blaut U, Sherman S, Fogel E, Lehman GA. Influence of cholangiography on biliary sphincter of Oddi manometric parameters. Gastrointest Endosc. 2000; 52(5):624–629

[40] Geenen JE, Hogan WJ, Dodds WJ, et al. Intraluminal pressure recording from the human sphincter of Oddi. Gastroenterology. 1980; 78(2):317–324

[41] Guelrud M, Mendoza S, Rossiter G, Villegas MI. Sphincter of Oddi manometry in healthy volunteers. Dig Dis Sci. 1990; 35(1):38–46

[42] Corazziari E, Shaffer EA, Hogan WJ, et al. Functional disorders of the biliary tract and pancreas. Gut. 1999; 45(Suppl 2):II48–II54

[43] Behar J, Corazziari E, Guelrud M, et al. Functional gallbladder and sphincter of oddi disorders. Gastroenterology. 2006; 130(5):1498–1509

[44] Eversman D, Fogel EL, Rusche M, et al. Frequency of abnormal pancreatic and biliary sphincter manometry compared with clinical suspicion of sphincter of Oddi dysfunction. Gastrointest Endosc. 1999; 50(5):637–641

[45] Sherman S, Lehman G, Jamidar P, et al. Efficacy of endoscopic sphincterotomy and surgical sphincteroplasty for patients with sphincter of Oddi dysfunction (SOD): randomized, controlled study. Gastrointest Endosc. 1994; 40:A125

[46] Rustagi T, Jamidar PA. Endoscopic retrograde cholangiopancreatography-related adverse events: general overview. Gastrointest Endosc Clin N Am. 2015; 25(1):97–106

[47] Rustagi T, Jamidar PA. Endoscopic retrograde cholangiopancreatography (ERCP)-related adverse events: post-ERCP pancreatitis. Gastrointest Endosc Clin N Am. 2015; 25(1):107–121

[48] Neuhaus H. Biliary sphincterotomy. In: Baron TH, Kozarek RA, Carr-Locke DL, eds. ERCP. 2nd ed. Saunders; 2013:129–138

[49] Jonathan M. Buscaglia ANK. Pancreatic sphincterotomy. In: Baron TH, Kozarek RA, Carr-Locke DL, eds. ERCP. 2nd ed. New York, NY: Saunders; 2013:166–77

[50] Staritz M, Ewe K, Meyer zum Büschenfelde KH. Endoscopic papillary dilation (EPD) for the treatment of common bile duct stones and papillary stenosis. Endoscopy. 1983; 15(Suppl 1):197–198

[51] Minami A, Nakatsu T, Uchida N, et al. Papillary dilation vs sphincterotomy in endoscopic removal of bile duct stones. A randomized trial with manometric function. Dig Dis Sci. 1995; 40(12):2550–2554

[52] Mathuna PM, White P, Clarke E, et al. Endoscopic balloon sphincteroplasty (papillary dilation) for bile duct stones: efficacy, safety, and follow-up in 100 patients. Gastrointest Endosc. 1995; 42(5):468–474

[53] Xu L, Kyaw MH, Tse YK, Lau JY. Endoscopic sphincterotomy with large balloon dilation versus endoscopic sphincterotomy for bile duct stones: a systematic review and meta-analysis. BioMed Res Int. 2015; 2015:673103

[54] Vlavianos P, Chopra K, Mandalia S, et al. Endoscopic balloon dilatation versus endoscopic sphincterotomy for the removal of bile duct stones: a prospective randomised trial. Gut. 2003; 52(8):1165–1169

[55] Sugiyama M, Izumisato Y, Abe N, et al. Predictive factors for acute pancreatitis and hyperamylasemia after endoscopic papillary balloon dilation. Gastrointest Endosc. 2003; 57(4):531–535

[56] Shim C-S. Balloon dilation of the native and postsphincterotomy papilla. In: Baron TH, Kozarek RA, Carr-Locke DL, eds. ERCP. 2nd ed. New York, NY: Elsevier, 2013; 139–151

[57] Teoh AY, Cheung FK, Hu B, et al. Randomized trial of endoscopic sphincterotomy with balloon dilation versus endoscopic sphincterotomy alone for removal of bile duct stones. Gastroenterology. 2013; 144(2):341–345.e1

[58] Lauri A, Horton RC, Davidson BR, et al. Endoscopic extraction of bile duct stones: management related to stone size. Gut. 1993; 34(12):1718–1721

[59] Lee TH, Han JH, Kim HJ, et al. Is the addition of choleretic agents in multiple double-pigtail biliary stents effective for difficult common bile duct stones in elderly patients? A prospective, multicenter study. Gastrointest Endosc. 2011; 74(1):96–102

[60] Han J, Moon JH, Koo HC, et al. Effect of biliary stenting combined with ursodeoxycholic acid and terpene treatment on retained common bile duct stones in elderly patients: a multicenter study. Am J Gastroenterol. 2009; 104(10):2418–2421

[61] Mishkin D, Carpenter S, Croffie J, et al; Technology Assessment Committee, American Society for Gastrointestinal Endoscopy. ASGE Technology Status Evaluation Report: radiographic contrast media used in ERCP. Gastrointest Endosc. 2005; 62(4):480–484

[62] Wilcox CM, Kim H, Seay T, Varadarajulu S. Choice of plastic or metal stent for patients with jaundice with pancreaticobiliary malignancy using simple clinical tools: a prospective evaluation. BMJ Open Gastroenterol. 2015; 2(1):e000014

[63] Kaassis M, Boyer J, Dumas R, et al. Plastic or metal stents for malignant stricture of the common bile duct?Results of a randomized prospective study. Gastrointest Endosc. 2003; 57(2):178–182

[64]   Prat F, Chapat O, Ducot B, et al. A randomized trial of endoscopic drainage methods for inoperable malignant strictures of the common bile duct. Gastrointest Endosc. 1998; 47(1):1–7

[65]   Mukai T, Yasuda I, Nakashima M, et al. Metallic stents are more efficacious than plastic stents in unresectable malignant hilar biliary strictures: a randomized controlled trial. J Hepatobiliary Pancreat Sci. 2013; 20(2):214–222

[66]   Zorrón Pu L, de Moura EG, Bernardo WM, et al. Endoscopic stenting for inoperable malignant biliary obstruction: a systematic review and meta-analysis. World J Gastroenterol. 2015; 21(47):13374–13385

[67]   Moole H, Dhillon S, Volmar F-H, et al. Is there a survival and morbidity benefit of covered over uncovered metal stents in malignant biliary strictures? A meta-analysis and systematic review. Gastrointest Endosc. 2015; 81(5):AB399

[68]   Yang Z, Wu Q, Wang F, et al. A systematic review and meta-analysis of randomized trials and prospective studies comparing covered and bare self-expandable metal stents for the treatment of malignant obstruction in the digestive tract. Int J Med Sci. 2013; 10(7):825–835

[69]   Lee YN, Moon JH, Choi HJ, et al. Effectiveness of a newly designed antireflux valve metal stent to reduce duodenobiliary reflux in patients with unresectable distal malignant biliary obstruction: a randomized, controlled pilot study (with videos). Gastrointest Endosc. 2016; 83(2):404–412

[70]   Poley JW, van Tilburg AJ, Kuipers EJ, Bruno MJ. Breaking the barrier: using extractable fully covered metal stents to treat benign biliary hilar strictures. Gastrointest Endosc. 2011; 74(4):916–920

[71]   Irani S, Baron TH, Akbar A, et al. Endoscopic treatment of benign biliary strictures using covered self-expandable metal stents (CSEMS). Dig Dis Sci. 2014; 59(1):152–160

[72]   Bakhru MR, Kahaleh M. Expandable metal stents for benign biliary disease. Gastrointest Endosc Clin N Am. 2011; 21(3):447–462, viii

[73]   Varadarajulu S, Banerjee S, Barth BA, et al; ASGE Technology Committee. GI endoscopes. Gastrointest Endosc. 2011; 74(1):1–6.e6

[74]   Troendle DM, Barth BA. Pediatric considerations in endoscopic retrograde cholangiopancreatography. Gastrointest Endosc Clin N Am. 2016; 26(1):119–136

[75]   Moreels TG. Altered anatomy: enteroscopy and ERCP procedure. Best Pract Res Clin Gastroenterol. 2012; 26(3):347–357

[76]   Carmona YF, Tyberg A, Zerbo S, et al. Transgastric biliary brushing: a novel endoscopic technique. Gastrointest Endosc. 2016; 83(1):257–258

[77]   Kethu SR, Adler DG, Conway JD, et al; ASGE Technology Committee. ERCP cannulation and sphincterotomy devices. Gastrointest Endosc. 2010; 71(3):435–445

[78]   Jacob L, Geenen JE. ERCP guide wires. Gastrointest Endosc. 1996; 43(1):57–60

[79]   Somogyi L, Chuttani R, Croffie J, et al; Technology Assessment Committee. Guidewires for use in GI endoscopy. Gastrointest Endosc. 2007; 65(4):571–576

[80]   Adler DG, Baron TH, Davila RE, et al; Standards of Practice Committee of American Society for Gastrointestinal Endoscopy. ASGE guideline: the role of ERCP in diseases of the biliary tract and the pancreas. Gastrointest Endosc. 2005; 62(1):1–8

[81]   Early DS, Ben-Menachem T, Decker GA, et al; ASGE Standards of Practice Committee. Appropriate use of GI endoscopy. Gastrointest Endosc. 2012; 75(6):1127–1131

[82]   Chathadi KV, Chandrasekhara V, Acosta RD, et al; ASGE Standards of Practice Committee. The role of ERCP in benign diseases of the biliary tract. Gastrointest Endosc. 2015; 81(4):795–803

[83]   Everson GT, McKinley C, Kern F, Jr. Mechanisms of gallstone formation in women. Effects of exogenous estrogen (Premarin) and dietary cholesterol on hepatic lipid metabolism. J Clin Invest. 1991; 87(1):237–246

[84]   Marzio L. Factors affecting gallbladder motility: drugs. Dig Liver Dis. 2003; 35(Suppl 3):S17–S19

[85]   Shelton J, Linder JD, Rivera-Alsina ME, Tarnasky PR. Commitment, confirmation, and clearance: new techniques for nonradiation ERCP during pregnancy (with videos). Gastrointest Endosc. 2008; 67(2):364–368

[86]   McGrath BA, Singh M, Singh T, Maguire S. Spontaneous common bile duct rupture in pregnancy. Int J Obstet Anesth. 2005; 14(2):172–174

[87]   Cappell MS. Risks versus benefits of gastrointestinal endoscopy during pregnancy. Nat Rev Gastroenterol Hepatol. 2011; 8(11):610–634

[88]   Ara B, Sahakian PAJ. ERCP in pregnancy. In: Baron TH, Kozarek RA, Carr-Locke DL, eds. ERCP. 2nd ed. New York, NY: Elsevier, 2013; 264–9

[89]   ACOG Committee on Obstetric Practice. ACOG Committee Opinion. Number 299, September 2004 (replaces No. 158, September 1995). Guidelines for diagnostic imaging during pregnancy. Obstet Gynecol. 2004; 104(3):647–651

[90]   Kahaleh M, Hartwell GD, Arseneau KO, et al. Safety and efficacy of ERCP in pregnancy. Gastrointest Endosc. 2004; 60(2):287–292

[91]   Rizk MK, Sawhney MS, Cohen J, et al. Quality indicators common to all GI endoscopic procedures. Gastrointest Endosc. 2015; 81(1):3–16

[92]   Adler DG, Lieb JG, II, Cohen J, et al. Quality indicators for ERCP. Gastrointest Endosc. 2015; 81(1):54–66

[93]   Verma D, Gostout CJ, Petersen BT, et al. Establishing a true assessment of endoscopic competence in ERCP during training and beyond: a single-operator learning curve for deep biliary cannulation in patients with native papillary anatomy. Gastrointest Endosc. 2007; 65(3):394–400

[94]   Jowell PS, Baillie J, Branch MS, et al. Quantitative assessment of procedural competence. A prospective study of training in endoscopic retrograde cholangiopancreatography. Ann Intern Med. 1996; 125(12):983–989

[95]   American Association for the Study of Liver Diseases; American College of Gastroenterology; AGA Institute; American Society for Gastrointestinal Endoscopy. A journey toward excellence: training future gastroenterologists—the gastroenterology core curriculum, third edition. Am J Gastroenterol 2007;102:921–927

[96]   Sotoudehmanesh R, Khatibian M, Kolahdoozan S, et al. Indomethacin may reduce the incidence and severity of acute pancreatitis after ERCP. Am J Gastroenterol. 2007; 102(5):978–983

[97]   Elmunzer BJ, Scheiman JM, Lehman GA, et al; U.S. Cooperative for Outcomes Research in Endoscopy (USCORE). A randomized trial of rectal indomethacin to prevent post-ERCP pancreatitis. N Engl J Med. 2012; 366(15):1414–1422

[98]   Ding X, Chen M, Huang S, et al. Nonsteroidal anti-inflammatory drugs for prevention of post-ERCP pancreatitis: a meta-analysis. Gastrointest Endosc. 2012; 76(6):1152–1159

[99]   Otsuka T, Kawazoe S, Nakashita S, et al. Low-dose rectal diclofenac for prevention of post-endoscopic retrograde cholangiopancreatography pancreatitis: a randomized controlled trial. J Gastroenterol. 2012; 47(8):912–917

[100]   Luo H, Zhao L, Leung J, et al. Routine pre-procedural rectal indometacin versus selective post-procedural rectal indometacin to prevent pancreatitis in patients undergoing endoscopic retrograde cholangiopancreatography: a multicentre, single-blinded, randomised controlled trial. Lancet. 2016; 387(10035):2293–2301

[101]   Levenick JM, Gordon SR, Fadden LL, et al. Rectal indomethacin does not prevent post-ERCP pancreatitis in consecutive patients. Gastroenterology. 2016; 150(4):911–917, quiz e19

[102]   Ha J, Son BK. Current issues in duodenoscope-associated infections: now is the time to take action. Clin Endosc. 2015; 48(5):361–363

17 Cholangioscopy

David Lee, Juliana Yang, and Ali A. Siddiqui

17.1 Introduction

The direct visualization of the biliary tree has long been out of reach for endoscopists. However, with recent advances in technique and equipment, cholangioscopy is gaining increased adoption for a wider variety of indications. From the direct visualization of benign versus malignant strictures to the removal of large or complicated biliary stones, cholangioscopy has become an essential tool in the toolkits of many endoscopists. In this chapter, we describe the recent advances which have led to the modern cholangioscope, as well as its most utilized indications. We also describe the variety of instruments available for use in conjunction with the cholangioscope, as well as the potential complications which can arise in cholangioscopy.

17.2 Overview of Cholangioscopy

In the modern era of endoscopy, the management of pancreaticobiliary ductal diseases utilizes multiple modalities, including endoscopic retrograde cholangiopancreatography (ERCP), endoscopic ultrasound (EUS), intraductal ultrasound (IDUS), and magnetic resonance cholangiopancreatography (MRCP).[1,2,3] These modalities are vital to the delineation of anatomy and evaluation of pancreaticobiliary ductal disease.[4] However, such imaging modalities are indirect methods and therefore suffer from the common problem of not allowing for direct visualization of biliary mucosal abnormalities.[1,5]

Peroral cholangioscopy is a noninvasive endoscopic method that is increasingly being utilized as a tool for the diagnosis and treatment of various biliary disorders.[6,7,8] Peroral cholangioscopy is performed by using a cholangioscope that is advanced through the duodenoscope accessory channel, or by direct insertion of a small endoscope into the bile duct. With the introduction of the SpyGlass direct visualization system, peroral cholangioscopy has now become universally adopted for the diagnosis and therapy of biliary tract disease. Studies have demonstrated the improved clinical efficacy of peroral cholangioscopy in characterizing benign versus malignant natures of biliary strictures, diagnosing intraductal tumors, better defining unknown biliary pathologies, and treating difficult to remove biliary stones.[9,10,11]

17.3 General Diagnostic Techniques

17.3.1 Two-Operator Systems: Mother-Baby Scopes

The first cholangioscope was described in 1941 and was used to exclude choledocholithiasis after cholecystectomy.[1] Twenty years later, this equipment was refined into a flexible choledochoscope that would gain access via a percutaneous, transhepatic approach. The peroral approach was introduced in the early 1970s,[12,13,14] utilizing a "mother-baby" system which required two endoscopists and a cumbersome operating system.[4,15,16,17] The "mother-baby" system (Olympus America, Center Valley, Pennsylvania, and Pentax, Montvale, New Jersey) was developed by Takekoshi et al, Nakajima et al, and Rosch, and had a smaller cholangioscope ("baby") that passed through the instrument channel of a larger duodenoscope ("mother").[18] This technology allowed for direct visualization of the pancreaticobiliary system, but was plagued by poor image acquisition, high cost, and lengthy procedures. These procedures were notorious for being very labor intensive and technically challenging (▶ Table 17.1).

17.3.2 Single-Operator System: SpyGlass Cholangiopancreatoscopy

Peroral cholangioscopy became more widespread following the introduction of the SpyGlass direct visualization system (Boston Scientific, Natick, Massachusetts, United States) in 2006, which improved the prior two-person ("mother-baby") operating system into a single-operator system.[18] The design of the system involves a SpyScope access and delivery catheter which is a single-operator, disposable catheter controlled by two dials allowing for four-way steer. It is 230 cm in length and has four channels: one 1.2-mm instrument channel, two 0.6-mm air and irrigation channels, and a 0.9-mm channel for fiberoptic probes.[8,16,19,20] These channels allow for simultaneous air insufflation and irrigation. The SpyGlass access catheter measures 10 F (3.3 mm) in outer diameter, and is a multiple-use device which conducts light to biliary ducts and transmits fiberoptic endoscopic images. It has a lens connected at the distal end of the image bundle that visualizes a 70-degree field of view.

In 2014, the new SpyGlass DS direct visualization system (Boston Scientific, Natick, Massachusetts, United States) was launched.

Table 17.1 Comparison of different peroral cholangioscopic equipment

	Fiberoptic "mother-baby scope"	SpyGlass direct visualization system	Direct cholangioscopy using ultraslim upper endoscope
Number of operators	Two	One	One
Tip deflection	Two way (up-down)	Four way (up-down, left-right)	Four way (up-down, left-right)
Separate irrigation channel	No	Yes	No
Exchangeable optics	No	Yes	No
Image quality	Moderate to good	Moderate to good	Excellent
Fragility	Yes	No	No

Adapted from J Interv Gastroenterol 2011;1(2):70–77.[71]

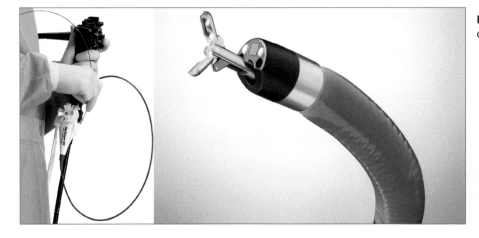

Fig. 17.1 Demonstration of the SpyGlass DS direct visualization system.

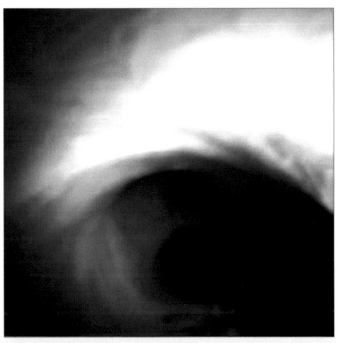

Fig. 17.2 Normal common hepatic duct as seen by the cholangioscopy.

This system consists of a fully integrated SpyScope DS access and delivery catheter, a single-use scope to eliminate probe reprocessing and image degradation (▶Fig. 17.1). It also has an integrated digital sensor that now allows for superior imaging, improved resolution, and a 60% wider field of view as compared to the first-generation system. At the time of this writing, there are only limited case reports published using the SpyGlass DS system, but the body of available literature is expected to expand greatly as this second-generation system gains adoption over the first-generation SpyGlass system (**Video 17.1**, **Video 17.2**).

17.3.3 Direct Cholangioscopy

With direct peroral cholangioscope (DPOC), an ultraslim (5–6 mm) upper endoscope is inserted via the mouth, advanced to the duodenum, and then manipulated across the major papilla and into the bile duct for evaluation of the mucosa and the lumen of the biliary tract (▶Fig. 17.2).[21] It requires the presence of biliary sphincterotomy and/or sphincteroplasty (papillary balloon dilation) in order to maneuver the scope into the bile duct. Upon initial insertion, there is often a significant amount of looping of the endoscope, especially in the gastric fundus and the duodenum,[21] and insertion of a guidewire into the bile duct is often required prior to introducing the scope so as to give the endoscope traction. Because of the difficulty in performing DPOC, this technique is rarely utilized outside of specialized or academic settings (**Video 17.3**).

An anchoring balloon has been trialed previously which would fix inside the intrahepatic duct branch to facilitate the advancement of the ultraslim scope.[20,21] Preliminary data indicated positive results, increasing the success rate from 45 to 95%. However, this device was voluntarily withdrawn from the market by the manufacturer due to concerns of increased risk of fatal air embolism.[21,22]

17.4 Accessory Devices and Techniques

17.4.1 Confocal Microscopy

The most recent development in cholangioscopy is probe-based confocal laser endomicroscopy (pCLE). This technology uses a flexible probe-based confocal aperture to focus light on a single spot. High contrast imaging is obtained by injecting a volatile organic compound, such as fluorescein, which in turn stains the extracellular matrix of the bile duct epithelium and allows for real-time microscopic images of the bile duct mucosa to be obtained. Abnormalities of the biliary epithelium, such as vascular congestion, dark granular patterns, thickened reticular structures, increased interglandular space, as well as blood flow and contrast uptake, can be directly visualized with this technique. This technique has been shown to be more sensitive and accurate at diagnosing cholangiocarcinoma in patients with indeterminate biliary strictures than conventional ERCP with tissue sampling (▶Fig. 17.3).[23] The pCLE technique is currently cited in the American Society of Gastrointestinal Endoscopy (ASGE) guidelines as a useful option in the work-up of biliary malignancy.[24]

17.4.2 Lithotripsy Probes

One of the most useful aspects of cholangioscopy is the ability to directly visualize and break up large bile duct stones.

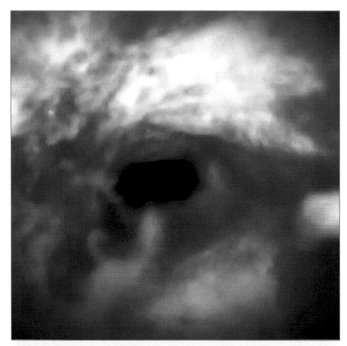

Fig. 17.3 Common hepatic duct stricture that is sclerotic and has abnormal vascular pattern. Biopsies demonstrated invasive cholangiocarcinoma.

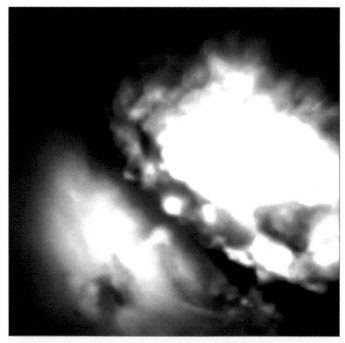

Fig. 17.4 Cholangioscopy demonstrating bile duct stone.

Several accessory devices are available from which the endoscopist may select for this purpose, including laser lithotripsy (LL) and electrohydraulic lithotripsy (EHL) systems. These accessories may be passed through the working channels of a cholangioscope (▶Fig. 17.4).

Several laser lithotripsy systems have been approved by the Food and Drug Administration (FDA) in the United States for biliary and pancreatic ductal indications. These probes focus a high-density laser light on the surface of a stone, locally creating a plasma bubble that propagates as compressive shock waves, shattering the adjacent stone.[25]

Holmium: yttrium aluminum garnet (YAG) lasers focus light in the near-infrared spectrum (2,100 nm), with pulses in the range of 500 to 1,000 mJ.[25,26] Typical power settings range from 0.6 to 1 J at 6 to 10 Hz, with a typical lithotripsy procedure using total laser energy of around 12 kJ.[25,27,28] Direct visualization is usually recommended to prevent inadvertent ductal damage. Holmium:YAG lasers have shown good efficacy in clearance of both biliary and pancreatic stones.[29]

Another popular system for laser lithotripsy is the so-called frequency-doubled, double-pulse neodymium:YAG (FREDDY) system. The FREDDY system uses a dual laser pulse. The recommended initial settings are 120 mJ single pulse at 3 to 5 Hz, increasing up to 160 mJ and 10 Hz if needed. The major purported advantage of the FREDDY system is that the green laser is absorbed by bile stones and not surrounding tissue, thereby minimizing the potential for ductal damage.[25]

EHL systems are comprised of a charge generator unit and a bipolar probe. A charge is released across the two electrodes of the probe, resulting in a spark and a hydraulic shock wave which propagates to shatter the adjacent stone. Optimal positioning of the probe tip is about 1 to 2 mm from the stone, about 5 mm from the tip of the endoscope, and aimed directly at the stone.[25] EHL does require the use of continuous saline irrigation to provide a medium for shock wave propagation, as well as to clear debris.[25] EHL systems too have shown good effect in stone clearance.[6]

17.4.3 Intraductal Biopsy Forceps

Cholangioscopy-directed biopsy to target indeterminate strictures of the biliary tract can be performed by passing a miniature Spybite biopsy forceps through the working channel under direct endoscopic visualization. The instrument is 270 cm in length, and has an outer diameter of 1 mm. The forceps' jaw can open to a 4.1-mm diameter at a 55-degree angle, and has a central spike which allows for targeted biopsies under direct visualization.

Another technique entails cholangioscopy-assisted biopsy by which the target biopsy site is first localized using cholangioscopic visualization, after which a conventional biopsy forceps is then passed through the working channel of the duodenoscope in order to obtain tissue samples under fluoroscopic guidance (▶Fig. 17.5).

17.5 Accepted Indications

17.5.1 Evaluation of Indeterminate and Malignant Biliary Strictures

The initial approach to obtain tissue confirmation in addressing a suspicious biliary stricture has traditionally been ERCP with brush cytology.[24] Unfortunately, the detection rate of brush cytology for cholangiocarcinoma (CCA) has been estimated at only 44 to 80%.[30,31,32,33,34,35] Negative or nondiagnostic findings on cytology usually necessitate referral to a more specialized center for cholangioscopy (▶Table 17.2).

Cholangioscopy with directed biopsies has arisen as a viable option to be offered under these circumstances. The ability to directly visualize a suspicious lesion and obtain biopsies under

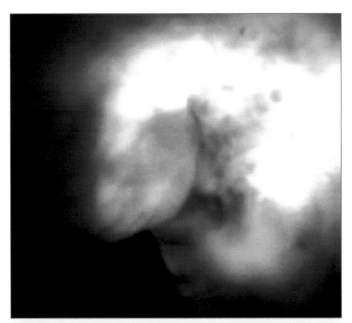

Fig. 17.5 A left hepatic stricture that is focally nodular and friable. Biopsies demonstrated invasive cholangiocarcinoma.

direct visualization is proving to be a powerful tool for interventional endoscopists. Visual findings on cholangioscopy that are concerning of a malignant biliary stricture include the presence of ulceration, intraductal masses or lesions, papillary or villous mucosal projections, or the presence of strictures with dilated, tortuous vessels ("tumor vessels").[8,36,37,38] Such findings have been shown to have greater sensitivity (92 vs. 66%) and specificity (93 vs. 51%) for malignancy compared to ERCP alone, even prior to obtaining targeted biopsy specimens (▶Fig. 17.6).[39]

There have been several studies validating the role of the Spy-Glass cholangioscopy system with directed biopsies in the diagnosis of malignancy in patients with otherwise indeterminate biliary strictures. Generally, studies have demonstrated a sensitivity and specificity of 49 to 89% and 96 to 100%, respectively, for the diagnosis of malignant strictures.[7,40,41,42,43] One study has demonstrated an accuracy of 77% in the diagnosis of malignancies that had been inconclusive from ERCP-guided brushings or EUS–fine-needle aspiration (EUS-FNA).[36]

The data have been more conflicting for the utility of cholangioscopy over other available modalities in the evaluation of whether primary sclerosing cholangitis (PSC)-related strictures were benign or malignant. In one study,[39] cholangioscopy was demonstrated to be superior to ERCP brush cytology in the diagnosis of CCA in PSC, quoting a sensitivity of 92% (vs. 66% for brush cytology), and specificity of 93% (vs. 51% for brush cytology). However, subsequent studies[44,45] have demonstrated sensitivities of only 33 to 50% for the detection of CCA via cholangioscopy in the setting of PSC, though specificity in these studies were similar at 100%. Some of this discrepancy may be related to user experience, though more studies are needed to better elucidate the proper role of cholangioscopy in CCA screening for patients with PSC. Currently, there is limited long-term data on whether cholangioscopy with directed biopsies of dominant strictures in patients with PSC increases CCA detection.[39,46] ▶Table 17.3 demonstrates the comparison of cholangioscopy to different advanced endoscopic imaging modalities for the evaluation of indeterminate biliary strictures.

Table 17.2 Indications for cholangioscopy

Diagnostic indications

Biopsy of indeterminate biliary strictures

Evaluation for malignant stricture in patients with primary sclerosing cholangitis

Diagnosing cholangiocarcinoma

Evaluation of indeterminate filling defect of bile ducts seen as seen on imaging or ERCP

Preoperative location of biliary intraductal tumors

Therapeutic indications

Photodynamic therapy of cholangiocarcinoma

Electrohydraulic lithotripsy (EHL) or laser lithotripsy (LL) for biliary duct stone dissolution and extraction

Electrohydraulic lithotripsy (EHL) or laser lithotripsy (LL) for biliary duct stone dissolution and extraction in patients with Mirizzi's syndrome type II

ERCP, endoscopic retrograde cholangiopancreatography.

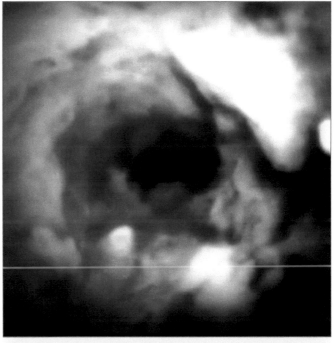

Fig. 17.6 Common hepatic duct stricture that has irregular villous tissue present circumferentially compatible with cholangiocarcinoma.

17.5.2 Diagnosis and Management of Choledocholithiasis

For conventional common bile duct (CBD) stones, ERCP extraction involves enlarging the papillary orifice by endoscopic biliary sphincterotomy (EBS) or by endoscopic papillary biliary dilation (EPBD).[47,48] The combination of these techniques is effective in clearing the majority of CBD stones, up to 85 to 95%.[43] However, approximately 5 to 15% of stones cannot be removed with conventional extraction methods, especially in cases of large stones (> 10–15 mm) or in cases with altered anatomy, biliary strictures, or periampullary diverticula.[47,48] In such cases, cholangioscopy-guided lithotripsy is a feasible alternative. Furthermore, impacted CBD stones larger than 20 mm in diameter often require fragmentation prior to retrieval.[47,49] Currently two

Table 17.3 Comparison of advanced endoscopic imaging modalities for the evaluation of indeterminate biliary strictures

	Advantages	Disadvantages
ERCP	Widely available	Procedural risks
	Workhorse technique with numerous accessories	Fluoroscopic (and endoscopic) images only
	Facilitates other diagnostic modalities (e.g., biliary brushing, biopsy, endomicroscopy) as well as therapy	Low sensitivity of conventional cytology and intra-ductal biopsies
EUS	Provides staging information	Limited views of the intrahepatic biliary tree (and nonvisualization of the right intrahepatic ductal system)
	Permits FNA	Generally, nondiagnostic in and of itself without FNA
	Can facilitate difficult biliary cannulation	Risk of tumor seeding if FNA primary tumor
Intraductal ultrasound	Can help direct ERCP-guided tissue acquisition	Limited depth of imaging
		Infrequently used in routine practice
Cholangioscopy	Excellent visualization of the biliary mucosa (with digital cholangioscopes)	High cost (disposable system $2,000 per case)
	May improve sensitivity, specificity, and overall accuracy compared to ERCP alone	Likely higher rates of pancreatitis, cholangitis, and perforation compared to ERCP alone
		Time-consuming
		Not widely available
Confocal laser endomicroscopy	Excellent sensitivity and negative predictive value	Marginal interobserver agreement
	Provides imaging at a cellular and subcellular level (lateral resolution of 3.5 µm)	Contact imaging of a very limited regional surface
		Time-consuming
		Not widely available
Optical coherence tomography	High resolution	Suboptimal sensitivity
	Improved sensitivity compared to ERCP-guided tissue acquisition	Resolution not as high as CLE
	Highly specific	Not widely available
	Permits larger surface areas to be examined compared to CLE	Not well-validated

CLE, confocal laser endomicroscopy; ERCP, endoscopic retrograde cholangiopancreatography; EUS, endoscopic ultrasound; FNA, fine-needle aspiration.

Adapted from World J Gastrointest Endosc. 2015;7(18):1268–1278.[72]

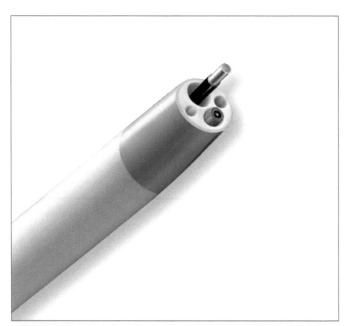

Fig. 17.7 EHL probe used through the SpyGlass DS direct visualization system.

modalities of lithotripsy are available for use with the cholangioscope: EHL and LL (▶Fig. 17.7).

EHL utilizes a bipolar probe that is capable of producing high-frequency hydraulic shock waves that can break up bile stones. It is vital to have a clear view of the bile duct, as the hydraulic shock wave can result in ductal injury or even perforation when misdirected. The overall complication rate is between 7 and 9%,[43,50] with the most common complications being cholangitis and hemobilia.[48] LL uses a pulsed laser that generates a plasma bubble, resulting in wave fracture of the CBD stone.[48,51] The clearance rate using LL has been reported to be between 64 and 97%.[52,53] As with EHL, LL also requires direct visualization with cholangioscopy in order to prevent inadvertent application to the bile duct wall.[48,54] These modern techniques are very useful in extracting large stones, residual stones, stones in atypical locations (i.e., Mirizzi's syndrome), stones with atypical shapes (i.e., barrel-shaped), and in altered anatomy.[8,55] The incidence of serious adverse events was 6.1% in direct stone fragmentation.[6]

Additionally, cholangioscopy-guided lithotripsy may find utility in type II Mirizzi's syndrome. Mirizzi's syndrome can be classified as type I and type II. The classic type I is when the impacted stone is in the cystic duct, causing extrinsic compression of the extrahepatic duct. In type II, however, the stone produces a cholecystocholedochal fistula and migrates to the common hepatic duct (CHD).[56] Extraction of the impacted stone from the CHD is technically challenging, and has often defaulted to extracorporeal shock wave lithotripsy (ESWL). However, complete ductal clearance for CHD stones using ESWL can be achieved in only 56 to 90% of cases.[48,57,58] The success rate of cholangioscopy-guided EHL and LL for difficult bile duct stones reported by Tsuyuguchi et al in 122 patients (53 with Mirizzi's syndrome) was around 96% for type II Mirizzi's syndrome, 0% for type I Mirizzi's syndrome, and 100% for impacted large stones.[59] A more recent series[60] indicated a 94% success rate of stone clearance using cholangioscopy-guided LL in patients with either Mirizzi's syndrome or cystic duct stones, including in those patients in whom surgical extraction had failed.

In hepatolithiasis, also known as intrahepatic choledocholithiasis, surgical resection of the lobe affected by the stone is the main treatment option. In untreated patients, hepatolithiasis can result in cholangitis, liver abscesses, cholangiocarcinoma, and biliary cirrhosis.[61] However, surgery carries risk, and patients are often not optimal surgical candidates, owing to their age or medical comorbidities. Conventional stone extraction is not always an option due to frequent biliary strictures associated with hepatolithiasis and the acute angulations of the hilar and intrahepatic ducts.[62] DPOC lithotripsy has been reported as a treatment option with a reported clearance rate of 64% and recurrence rate of 21.7%.[48,63] Another option is percutaneous transhepatic cholangioscopic lithotripsy. A transhepatic percutaneous drainage tract is created and allowed to mature for around 4 weeks.[64] The tract is then dilated and a video endoscopy is inserted into the intrahepatic duct. The clearance rate using LL and EHL is between 80 and 85%.[64,65,66] Major complications include liver laceration, hemobilia, shock, and intra-abdominal abscesses.[67] A novel variation of this, utilizing a modified triple-lumen catheter and proceeding without the need for tract maturation or extensive tract dilation, has been successfully performed.[68]

17.5.3 Photodynamic Therapy of Cholangiocarcinoma

Several studies have now suggested that the use of photodynamic therapy (PDT) can improve quality of life and perhaps survival in patients with unresectable hilar cholangiocarcinoma. With cholangioscopy-guided PDT, it is possible to identify tumor margins, determine the appropriate location for placement of the PDT diffuser catheter, allow for targeted therapy during PDT, and evaluate response to therapy.[69]

17.6 Complications of Cholangioscopy

The incidence of significant adverse events is similar to that of ERCP alone, with the caveat that cholangiopancreatoscopy showed higher rates of postcholangioscopy cholangitis (1%) compared to ERCP alone (0.2%). This was thought mainly to be related to intraprocedure saline irrigation and underlying pathology such as complex strictures. The risk of cholangitis seems to increase if

therapeutic interventions are undertaken during cholangioscopy, and has been reported upward of 7 to 10%, thought to be related to intraductal irrigation.[1] Prophylactic antibiotics are imperative and biliary drain and stents should also be considered postprocedure as well. Air embolism is another complication, and the use of carbon dioxide has been advocated instead of air in effort to avoid this. Other complications attributed to cholangioscopy include bile duct leak (1%) and hemobilia (0–3%) which have been attributed to intraductal lithotripsy.[8,43,70]

References

[1] Gabbert C, Warndorf M, Easler J, Chennat J. Advanced techniques for endoscopic biliary imaging: cholangioscopy, endoscopic ultrasonography, confocal, and beyond. Gastrointest Endosc Clin N Am. 2013; 23(3):625–646

[2] Yeh BM, Breiman RS, Taouli B, et al. Biliary tract depiction in living potential liver donors: comparison of conventional MR, mangafodipir trisodium-enhanced excretory MR, and multi-detector row CT cholangiography—initial experience. Radiology. 2004; 230(3):645–651

[3] Devereaux CE, Binmoeller KF. Endoscopic retrograde cholangiopancreatography in the next millennium. Gastrointest Endosc Clin N Am. 2000; 10(1):117–133, vii

[4] Nguyen NQ. Application of per oral cholangiopancreatoscopy in pancreatobiliary diseases. J Gastroenterol Hepatol. 2009; 24(6):962–969

[5] Yeh BM, Liu PS, Soto JA, et al. MR imaging and CT of the biliary tract. Radiographics. 2009; 29(6):1669–1688

[6] Chen YK, Parsi MA, Binmoeller KF, et al. Single-operator cholangioscopy in patients requiring evaluation of bile duct disease or therapy of biliary stones (with videos). Gastrointest Endosc. 2011; 74(4):805–814

[7] Chen YK, Pleskow DK. SpyGlass single-operator peroral cholangiopancreatoscopy system for the diagnosis and therapy of bile-duct disorders: a clinical feasibility study (with video). Gastrointest Endosc. 2007; 65(6):832–841

[8] Shah RJ, Adler DG, Conway JD, et al; ASGE Technology Committee. Cholangiopancreatoscopy. Gastrointest Endosc. 2008; 68(3):411–421

[9] de Bellis M, Fogel EL, Sherman S, et al. Influence of stricture dilation and repeat brushing on the cancer detection rate of brush cytology in the evaluation of malignant biliary obstruction. Gastrointest Endosc. 2003; 58(2):176–182

[10] Kitajima Y, Ohara H, Nakazawa T, et al. Usefulness of transpapillary bile duct brushing cytology and forceps biopsy for improved diagnosis in patients with biliary strictures. J Gastroenterol Hepatol. 2007; 22(10):1615–1620

[11] McGuire DE, Venu RP, Brown RD, et al. Brush cytology for pancreatic carcinoma: an analysis of factors influencing results. Gastrointest Endosc. 1996; 44(3):300–304

[12] Shore JM, Shore E. Operative biliary endoscopy: experience with the flexible choledochoscope in 100 consecutive choledocholithotomies. Ann Surg. 1970; 171(2):269–278

[13] Shore J, Lippman HN. A flexible choledochoscope. Lancet. 1965; 1(7397):1200–1201

[14] Takada T, Hanyu F, Kobayashi S, Uchida Y. Percutaneous transhepatic cholangial drainage: direct approach under fluoroscopic control. J Surg Oncol. 1976; 8(1):83–97

[15] Williamson JB, Judah JR, Gaidos JK, et al. Prospective evaluation of the long-term outcomes after deep small-bowel spiral enteroscopy in patients with obscure GI bleeding. Gastrointest Endosc. 2012; 76(4):771–778

[16] Kozarek RA. Direct cholangioscopy and pancreatoscopy at time of endoscopic retrograde cholangiopancreatography. Am J Gastroenterol. 1988; 83(1):55–57

[17] Kawakubo K, Isayama H, Sasahira N, et al. Clinical utility of single-operator cholangiopancreatoscopy using a SpyGlass probe through an endoscopic retrograde cholangiopancreatography catheter. J Gastroenterol Hepatol. 2012; 27(8):1371–1376

[18] Bogardus ST, Hanan I, Ruchim M, Goldberg MJ. "Mother-baby" biliary endoscopy: the University of Chicago experience. Am J Gastroenterol. 1996; 91(1):105–110

[19] Ramchandani M, Reddy DN, Lakhtakia S, et al. Per oral cholangiopancreatoscopy in pancreatico biliary diseases—expert consensus statements. World J Gastroenterol. 2015; 21(15):4722–4734

[20] Moon JH, Ko BM, Choi HJ, et al. Intraductal balloon-guided direct peroral cholangioscopy with an ultraslim upper endoscope (with videos). Gastrointest Endosc. 2009; 70(2):297–302

[21] Ghersi S, Fuccio L, Bassi M, et al. Current status of peroral cholangioscopy in biliary tract diseases. World J Gastrointest Endosc. 2015; 7(5):510–517

[22] Efthymiou M, Raftopoulos S, Antonio Chirinos J, May GR. Air embolism complicated by left hemiparesis after direct cholangioscopy with an intraductal balloon anchoring system. Gastrointest Endosc. 2012; 75(1):221–223

[23] Slivka A, Gan I, Jamidar P, et al. Validation of the diagnostic accuracy of probe-based confocal laser endomicroscopy for the characterization of indeterminate biliary strictures: results of a prospective multicenter international study. Gastrointest Endosc. 2015; 81(2):282–290

[24] Anderson MA, Appalaneni V, Ben-Menachem T, et al; American Society for Gastrointestinal Endoscopy (ASGE) Standards of Practice Committee. The role of

endoscopy in the evaluation and treatment of patients with biliary neoplasia. Gastrointest Endosc. 2013; 77(2):167–174

[25] DiSario J, Chuttani R, Croffie J, et al. Biliary and pancreatic lithotripsy devices. Gastrointest Endosc. 2007; 65(6):750–756

[26] Hochberger J, Tex S, Maiss J, Hahn EG. Management of difficult common bile duct stones. Gastrointest Endosc Clin N Am. 2003; 13(4):623–634

[27] Teichman JM, Schwesinger WH, Lackner J, Cossman RM. Holmium: YAG laser lithotripsy for gallstones. A preliminary report. Surg Endosc. 2001; 15(9):1034–1037

[28] Das AK, Chiura A, Conlin MJ, et al. Treatment of biliary calculi using holmium: yttrium aluminum garnet laser. Gastrointest Endosc. 1998; 48(2):207–209

[29] Maydeo A, Kwek BE, Bhandari S, et al. Single-operator cholangioscopy-guided laser lithotripsy in patients with difficult biliary and pancreatic ductal stones (with videos). Gastrointest Endosc. 2011; 74(6):1308–1314

[30] Pugliese V, Conio M, Nicolò G, et al. Endoscopic retrograde forceps biopsy and brush cytology of biliary strictures: a prospective study. Gastrointest Endosc. 1995; 42(6):520–526

[31] Farrell RJ, Jain AK, Brandwein SL, et al. The combination of stricture dilation, endoscopic needle aspiration, and biliary brushings significantly improves diagnostic yield from malignant bile duct strictures. Gastrointest Endosc. 2001; 54(5):587–594

[32] Park MS, Kim TK, Kim KW, et al. Differentiation of extrahepatic bile duct cholangiocarcinoma from benign stricture: findings at MRCP versus ERCP. Radiology. 2004; 233(1):234–240

[33] Ponchon T, Gagnon P, Berger F, et al. Value of endobiliary brush cytology and biopsies for the diagnosis of malignant bile duct stenosis: results of a prospective study. Gastrointest Endosc. 1995; 42(6):565–572

[34] Glasbrenner B, Ardan M, Boeck W, et al. Prospective evaluation of brush cytology of biliary strictures during endoscopic retrograde cholangiopancreatography. Endoscopy. 1999; 31(9):712–717

[35] Nakeeb A, Pitt HA, Sohn TA, et al. Cholangiocarcinoma. A spectrum of intrahepatic, perihilar, and distal tumors. Ann Surg. 1996; 224(4):463–473, discussion 473–475

[36] Siddiqui AA, Mehendiratta V, Jackson W, et al. Identification of cholangiocarcinoma by using the Spyglass Spyscope system for peroral cholangioscopy and biopsy collection. Clin Gastroenterol Hepatol. 2012; 10(5):466–471, quiz e48

[37] Seo DW, Lee SK, Yoo KS, et al. Cholangioscopic findings in bile duct tumors. Gastrointest Endosc. 2000; 52(5):630–634

[38] Tamada K, Ueno N, Tomiyama T, et al. Characterization of biliary strictures using intraductal ultrasonography: comparison with percutaneous cholangioscopic biopsy. Gastrointest Endosc. 1998; 47(5):341–349

[39] Tischendorf JJ, Krüger M, Trautwein C, et al. Cholangioscopic characterization of dominant bile duct stenoses in patients with primary sclerosing cholangitis. Endoscopy. 2006; 38(7):665–669

[40] Navaneethan U, Hasan MK, Lourdusamy V, et al. Single-operator cholangioscopy and targeted biopsies in the diagnosis of indeterminate biliary strictures: a systematic review. Gastrointest Endosc. 2015; 82(4):608–14.e2

[41] Shah RJ, Langer DA, Antillon MR, Chen YK. Cholangioscopy and cholangioscopic forceps biopsy in patients with indeterminate pancreaticobiliary pathology. Clin Gastroenterol Hepatol. 2006; 4(2):219–225

[42] Khan AH, Austin GL, Fukami N, et al. Cholangiopancreatoscopy and endoscopic ultrasound for indeterminate pancreaticobiliary pathology. Dig Dis Sci. 2013; 58(4):1110–1115

[43] Arya N, Nelles SE, Haber GB, et al. Electrohydraulic lithotripsy in 111 patients: a safe and effective therapy for difficult bile duct stones. Am J Gastroenterol. 2004; 99(12):2330–2334

[44] Arnelo U, von Seth E, Bergquist A. Prospective evaluation of the clinical utility of single-operator peroral cholangioscopy in patients with primary sclerosing cholangitis. Endoscopy. 2015; 47(8):696–702

[45] Kalaitzakis E, Sturgess R, Kaltsidis H, et al. Diagnostic utility of single-user peroral cholangioscopy in sclerosing cholangitis. Scand J Gastroenterol. 2014; 49(10):1237–1244

[46] Awadallah NS, Chen YK, Piraka C, et al. Is there a role for cholangioscopy in patients with primary sclerosing cholangitis? Am J Gastroenterol. 2006; 101(2):284–291

[47] Lauri A, Horton RC, Davidson BR, et al. Endoscopic extraction of bile duct stones: management related to stone size. Gut. 1993; 34(12):1718–1721

[48] Trikudanathan G, Navaneethan U, Parsi MA. Endoscopic management of difficult common bile duct stones. World J Gastroenterol. 2013; 19(2):165–173

[49] Yasuda I, Itoi T. Recent advances in endoscopic management of difficult bile duct stones. Dig Endosc. 2013; 25(4):376–385

[50] Blind PJ, Lundmark M. Management of bile duct stones: lithotripsy by laser, electrohydraulic, and ultrasonic techniques. Report of a series and clinical review. Eur J Surg. 1998; 164(6):403–409

[51] Lux G, Ell C, Hochberger J, et al. The first successful endoscopic retrograde laser lithotripsy of common bile duct stones in man using a pulsed neodymium-YAG laser. Endoscopy. 1986; 18(4):144–145

[52] McHenry L, Lehman G. Difficult bile duct stones. Curr Treat Options Gastroenterol. 2006; 9(2):123–132

[53] Hochberger J, Bayer J, May A, et al. Laser lithotripsy of difficult bile duct stones: results in 60 patients using a rhodamine 6G dye laser with optical stone tissue detection system. Gut. 1998; 43(6):823–829

[54] Parsi MA. Peroral cholangioscopy in the new millennium. World J Gastroenterol. 2011; 17(1):1–6

[55] Brauer BC, Chen YK, Shah RJ. Single-step direct cholangioscopy by freehand intubation using standard endoscopes for diagnosis and therapy of biliary diseases. Am J Gastroenterol. 2012; 107(7):1030–1035

[56] Corlette MB, Bismuth H. Biliobiliary fistula. A trap in the surgery of cholelithiasis. Arch Surg. 1975; 110(4):377–383

[57] Tandan M, Reddy DN, Santosh D, et al. Extracorporeal shock wave lithotripsy of large difficult common bile duct stones: efficacy and analysis of factors that favor stone fragmentation. J Gastroenterol Hepatol. 2009; 24(8):1370–1374

[58] Sauerbruch T, Stern M. Fragmentation of bile duct stones by extracorporeal shock waves. A new approach to biliary calculi after failure of routine endoscopic measures. Gastroenterology. 1989; 96(1):146–152

[59] Tsuyuguchi T, Sakai Y, Sugiyama H, et al. Long-term follow-up after peroral cholangioscopy-directed lithotripsy in patients with difficult bile duct stones, including Mirizzi syndrome: an analysis of risk factors predicting stone recurrence. Surg Endosc. 2011; 25(7):2179–2185

[60] Bhandari S, Bathini R, Sharma A, Maydeo A. Usefulness of single-operator cholangioscopy-guided laser lithotripsy in patients with Mirizzi syndrome and cystic duct stones: experience at a tertiary care center. Gastrointest Endosc. 2016; 84(1):56–61

[61] Plentz RR, Malek NP. Clinical presentation, risk factors and staging systems of cholangiocarcinoma. Best Pract Res Clin Gastroenterol. 2015; 29(2):245–252

[62] Katanuma A, Maguchi H, Osanai M, Takahashi K. Endoscopic treatment of difficult common bile duct stones. Dig Endosc. 2010; 22(Suppl 1):S90–S97

[63] Okugawa T, Tsuyuguchi T, K C S, et al. Peroral cholangioscopic treatment of hepatolithiasis: long-term results. Gastrointest Endosc. 2002; 56(3):366–371

[64] Neuhaus H. Endoscopic and percutaneous treatment of difficult bile duct stones. Endoscopy. 2003; 35(8):S31–S34

[65] Jan YY, Chen MF. Percutaneous trans-hepatic cholangioscopic lithotomy for hepatolithiasis: long-term results. Gastrointest Endosc. 1995; 42(1):1–5

[66] Lee SK, Seo DW, Myung SJ, et al. Percutaneous transhepatic cholangioscopic treatment for hepatolithiasis: an evaluation of long-term results and risk factors for recurrence. Gastrointest Endosc. 2001; 53(3):318–323

[67] Park JS, Jeong S, Lee DH, et al. Risk factors for long-term outcomes after initial treatment in hepatolithiasis. J Korean Med Sci. 2013; 28(11):1627–1631

[68] Wong JC, Lam SF, Lau JY. Novel use of an optical fiber in triple-lumen catheter for percutaneous choledochoscopy and holmium: yttrium aluminum garnet laser lithotripsy of intrahepatic bile duct stones. Gastrointest Endosc. 2015; 82(1):171

[69] Choi HJ, Moon JH, Ko BM, et al. Clinical feasibility of direct peroral cholangioscopy-guided photodynamic therapy for inoperable cholangiocarcinoma performed by using an ultra-slim upper endoscope (with videos). Gastrointest Endosc. 2011; 73(4):808–813

[70] Farrell JJ, Bounds BC, Al-Shalabi S, et al. Single-operator duodenoscope-assisted cholangioscopy is an effective alternative in the management of choledocholithiasis not removed by conventional methods, including mechanical lithotripsy. Endoscopy. 2005; 37(6):542–547

[71] Monga A, Ramchandani M, Reddy DN. Per-oral cholangioscopy. Journal of Interventional Gastroenterology. 2011; 1(2):70–77

[72] Tabibian JH, Visrodia KH, Levy MJ, Gostout CJ. Advanced endoscopic imaging of indeterminate biliary strictures. World Journal of Gastrointestinal Endoscopy. 2015; 7(18):1268–1278

18 Advanced Imaging Methods

Ralf Kiesslich and Arthur Hoffman

18.1 Introduction

Advanced imaging methods in gastrointestinal endoscopy are additional technological tools or endoscopic techniques, which should help refining in vivo diagnosis during ongoing endoscopy.

The aim of advanced imaging is to improve single or all parts of the diagnostic workflow of endoscopic procedures. Three steps are important: *recognition*, *characterization*, and *confirmation*. Recognition involves identification of all relevant lesions or changes of the inspected mucosa. Characterization is defined as differentiation of neoplastic from nonneoplastic changes and to decide whether an endoscopic treatment is possible or not (prediction of submucosal involvement in neoplastic changes). Confirmation is characterized by establishment of a definite diagnosis, which is mainly based on histologic evaluation of removed specimens. However, advanced imaging methods can correlate closely with final histology or display in vivo histology and can be used as reliable techniques for in vivo diagnosis (▶Fig. 18.1).

18.2 High-Definition Endoscopes

The development of advanced imaging technologies occurred in parallel with innovations of information technologies. Most important is the development of high-definition (HD) endoscopes (with and without optical zoom function) that has enabled to clearer identify vessel and mucosal surface architecture.

The chips used in current HD endoscopes produce signal images with resolutions that range from 850,000 pixels to more than 1 million pixels. HD video imaging can be displayed in a 16:9 aspect ratio. However, the 16:9 aspect ratio is not useful for display of images originating from round endoscopic lenses.

Thus, HD endoscopic video chips display images in either 4:3 or 5:4 aspect ratios.[1]

18.3 Virtual Chromoendoscopy

Virtual or electronic chromoendoscopy can be switched on and switched off during endoscopy by pushing a button at the hand piece of the endoscope. The emitted light to the mucosa or the reflecting light from the mucosa is altered using narrow band or postprocessing filters (▶Fig. 18.2). Virtual chromoendoscopy technologies include narrow-band imaging (NBI) (Olympus Medical Systems Tokyo, Japan), flexible spectral imaging color enhancement (FICE) (Fujinon, Fujifilm Medical Co, Saitama, Japan), and i-Scan (Pentax Endoscopy, Tokyo, Japan).[2]

The goal of virtual chromoendoscopy is to highlight vessel structures or surface architecture.

18.4 Narrow-Band Imaging

NBI is an endoscopic optical image enhancement technology, proprietary of Olympus Medical Systems. NBI is based on the penetration properties of light, which is directly proportional to wavelength. Short wavelengths penetrate only superficially into the mucosa, whereas longer wavelengths are capable of penetrating more deeply into tissue. Two narrow bands of light are emitted and centered at the specific wavelengths of 415 and 540 nm. The specific wavelengths correspond to light absorption peaks of hemoglobin. Because most of the NBI light is absorbed by the blood vessels in the mucosa, the resulting images emphasize the blood vessels in sharp contrast with the nonvascular structures in the mucosa.[2]

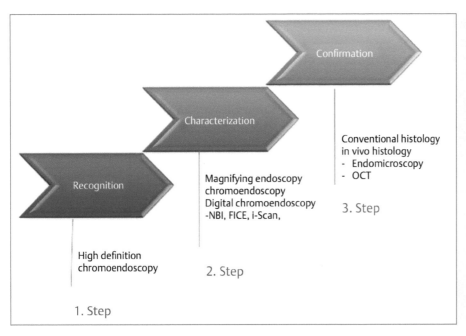

Fig. 18.1 Diagnostic steps in gastrointestinal endoscopy using advanced imaging techniques.

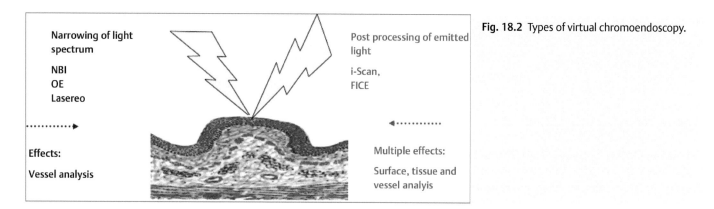

Fig. 18.2 Types of virtual chromoendoscopy.

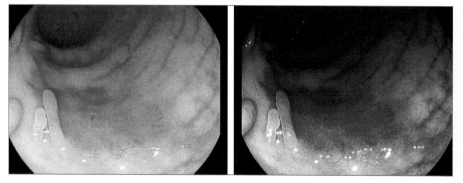

Fig. 18.3 Virtual chromoendoscopy using i-Scan.

18.5 Flexible Spectral Imaging Color Enhancement

FICE is a proprietary digital imaging postprocessing system of Fujinon. FICE takes white-light endoscopic images from the video processor and mathematically processes the image by emphasizing certain ranges of wavelengths. Three single-wavelength images can be selected and assigned to the red, green, and blue monitor inputs, respectively, to display a composite color-enhanced image in real time.[2]

Fujifilm has recently developed a new technique of virtual chromoendoscopy. The so-called Lasero system uses laser for its illumination. The laser is used as a function for narrow-band light that utilizes the characteristics of laser light as standard. Lasero has four observational modes and employs three kinds of illumination with different spectral distributions.[3]

18.6 i-Scan and Optical Enhancement

i-SCAN is a software-based digital, postprocessing image enhancement technology from Pentax Endoscopy that provides digital contrast to endoscopic images. Similar to FICE, i-Scan provides enhanced images of the mucosal surface and the blood vessels through postimage processing. There are three i-Scan modes: i-Scan 1, i-Scan 2, and i-Scan 3. Touching a button on the endoscope can access these modes. The switch from WLE to i-Scan occurs almost instantaneously.

i-Scan 1 is a surface-enhancement (SE) and contrast-enhancement (CE) mode that enhances contrast and thereby mucosal surface detail including enhanced mucosal surface texture and sharpened views of surface vessels. The image remains as bright as conventional WLE. i-Scan 2 increases the contrast between the mucosa and blood vessels, thereby improving the visibility of blood vessels and tissue architecture. i-Scan 3 differs from i-Scan 2 primarily in its ability to illuminate more distant regions better[2] (▶Fig. 18.3).

Most recently Pentax has introduced optical enhancement (OE) filtering, which uses similar technology as NBI. OE was developed to further highlight superficial vessel architecture in conjunction with bright illumination.[4]

Flat lesion (Paris classification type IIa) is visible within the colonic mucosa. i-Scan imaging is displayed on the right simultaneously (twin-mode). The lesion is highlighted and the border can be clearly delineated.

18.7 Clinical Application of Virtual Chromoendoscopy

Virtual chromoendoscopy can be used in upper and lower endoscopy. Areas of interest are gastroesophageal reflux disease with special focus on Barrett's esophagus, squamous cell cancer, gastric cancer colonic polyps, and inflammatory bowel diseases.

In Barrett's esophagus, virtual chromoendoscopy is able to achieve the so-called PIVI guidelines. The goals for Barrett's esophagus were to develop an imaging technology with targeted biopsies that should have a per-patient sensitivity of greater than or equal to 90% and a negative predictive value (NPV) of greater than or equal to 98% for detecting high-grade dysplasia or early cancer, compared with the current standard protocol, and the imaging technology should have a specificity that is sufficiently high (80%) to allow a reduction in the number of biopsies (compared with random biopsies). A recent meta-analysis concluded that the pooled sensitivity, NPV, and specificity for electronic chromoendoscopy by using NBI for detecting Barrett's associated dysplasia were 94.2% (95% confidence interval [CI], 82.6–98.2), 97.5% (95% CI, 95.1–98.7), and 94.4% (95% CI, 80.5–98.6), respectively.[5]

Virtual chromoendoscopy was also shown to be effective in characterizing small polyps in the colon and the so-called NICE classification was established using NBI technology. Virtual chromoendoscopy in expert hands can be used to guide the decision to leave suspected rectosigmoid hyperplastic polyps 5 mm or smaller in place (without resection), virtual chromoendoscopy provides a 90% or greater NPV (when used with high confidence) for adenomatous histology.[6]

Virtual chromoendoscopy seems not to be effective enough identifying colitis-associated dysplasia. Here, standard chromoendoscopy using intravital dyes remains standard of care for surveillance in ulcerative colitis.[2,7]

18.8 Chromoendoscopy

Chromoendoscopy, which is a well-known technique in gastrointestinal endoscopy since decades, refers to the topical application of stains or dyes at the time of endoscopy in an effort to enhance tissue characterization, differentiation, or diagnosis.

Commonly used stains for chromoendoscopy are classified as absorptive (Lugol's solution and methylene blue) or contrast dyes (indigo carmine and acetic acid) (▶ Table 18.1).[8]

Chromoendoscopy requires a spraying catheter for homogenous application of the different stains. Chromoendoscopy can be performed in a targeted fashion (staining of areas of interest, e.g., colonic polyps) or untargeted fashion (e.g., pan-chromoendoscopy in ulcerative colitis). The use of chromoendoscopy has never evolved as a mainstream diagnostic tool, because of the additional time, which is required. Furthermore, the concentration of the dyes is not well standardized. However, there is clear clinical evidence

that several clinical conditions benefit from chromoendoscopic diagnosis.[8,9]

18.9 Clinical Application of Chromoendoscopy

Lugol's solution is a prerequisite for diagnosing squamous cell cancer because it can highlight clearly the borders of the neoplastic changes. In Barrett's esophagus, acetic acid is commonly used in expert centers to unmask subtle mucosal irregularities. The pooled sensitivity, NPV, and specificity for acetic acid chromoendoscopy for the detection of dysplasia or early cancer in Barrett's were 96.6% (95% CI, 95–98), 98.3% (95% CI, 94.8–99.4), and 84.6% (95% CI, 68.5–93.2), respectively.[2]

Chromoendoscopy has been recommended for surveillance in patients with ulcerative colitis although the studies supporting its usage have been nonrandomized and of low quality. The SCENIC international guidelines[7] clearly state the following:

1. When performing surveillance with white-light colonoscopy, HD is recommended rather than standard definition.
2. When performing surveillance with standard-definition colonoscopy, chromoendoscopy is recommended rather than white-light colonoscopy.
3. When performing surveillance with HD colonoscopy, chromoendoscopy is suggested rather than white-light colonoscopy.

The use of pan-chromoendoscopy for colon cancer screening in sporadic cancer has also been shown to be effective in terms of improving of adenoma detection rate. However, other technologies also have shown similar benefits. Thus, pan-chromoendoscopy in screening colonoscopy is not recommended as a standard screening routine.[10]

18.10 Confocal Laser Endomicroscopy

Confocal laser endomicroscopy (CLE) is an endoscopic modality developed to obtain very high magnification and resolution images of the mucosal layer of the gastrointestinal (GI) tract. CLE is based on tissue illumination with a low-power laser with subsequent detection of the fluorescence of light reflected from the tissue through a pinhole. The term confocal refers to the alignment of both illumination and collection systems in the same focal plane. The laser light is focused at a selected depth in the tissue of interest and reflected light is then refocused onto the detection system by the same lens. Only returning light refocused through the pinhole is detected. The light reflected and scattered at other geometric angles from the illuminated object or refocused out of plane with the pinhole is excluded from detection. This dramatically increases the spatial resolution of CLE allowing cellular imaging and evaluation of tissue architecture at the focal plane during endoscopy.[11]

18.11 Probe-Based CLE

The probe-based CLE (pCLE) system comprises a fiberoptic bundle with an integrated distal lens that is connected to a laser scanning unit. The probe-based system to date has a fixed focal

Table 18.1 Commonly used stains for chromoendoscopy[8]

Stains	Mechanism of action	Main applications
Absorptive stains		
Lugol's solution	Glycogen-containing normal squamous epithelium is stained dark brown; inflammation, columnar mucosa, dysplasia, and cancer remain unstained	Esophageal squamous cell cancer and dysplasia
Methylene blue	Absorptive epithelial cells of the small bowel, colon, and intestinal metaplasia at any site are stained blue; dysplasia and cancer are variably stained or unstained	Ulcerative colitis
Contrast stains		
Indigo carmine	Nonabsorbed dark bluish dye highlighting mucosal topography	Colonic polyps Ulcerative colitis
Acetic acid	Interaction with protein of superficial cells leading to highlighting of surface architecture	Barrett's esophagus

length and so it can only scan in a single plane unlike current microscope systems that can create cross-sectional images at different depths. In pCLE systems, the individual optical fibers function as the pinhole. Cellvizio confocal miniprobes (Mauna Kea Technologies, Paris, France) created for GI tract applications include CholangioFlex, GastroFlex UHD, and ColoFlex UHD.[11] All probes generate dynamic (9–12 frames/s) images. The depth of imaging from the surface of the confocal lens is 40 to 70 mm for CholangioFlex probes and 55 to 65 mm for both GastroFlex UHD and ColoFlex UHD probes. The maximal field of view for CholangioFlex probes is 325 mm and 240 mm for GastroFlex UHD and ColoFlex UHD probes. The resolution of the CholangioFlex probe is 3.5 mm, whereas for GastroFlex UHD and ColoFlex UHD probes, it is 1 mm (Mauna Kea Technologies).

18.12 Endoscope-Based CLE

Endoscope-based CLE (eCLE) uses a confocal microscope (Optiscan, Victoria, Australia) integrated into the distal tip of a conventional endoscope (Pentax, Tokyo, Japan). The diameter of the eCLE endoscope is 12.8 mm, and the tip length is increased to accommodate the laser microscope so that there is a 5-cm rigid portion. It can be used for upper and lower GI tract examinations. With this setup, white-light endoscopy and eCLE can be performed simultaneously with images displayed on dual monitors. Images are collected at a scan rate of 1.6 frames/s (1024 × 512 pixels) or 0.8 frames/s (1024 × 1024 pixels) with an adjustable depth of scanning ranging from 0 to 250 μm, a field of view of 475 × 475 μm. The lateral resolution is 0.7 μm, and the axial resolution is 7 μm[11] (▶ Fig. 18.4).

18.13 Clinical Application

Endomicroscopy enables in vivo histology during ongoing endoscopy. Cellular and subcellular structures can be seen. Prerequisite for endomicroscopic imaging with the above-mentioned systems is the use of fluorescein intravenously as contrast agent. The use of fluorescein is safe and well tolerable. However, patients will develop a short-lasting discoloration of the skin.[12]

Endomicroscopy was extensively studied in different diseases. There is clear evidence that endomicroscopy is clinically effective in reducing the number of biopsies and to immediately diagnose GI cancers. This has been shown in Barrett's esophagus, gastric cancer, and colitis-associated dysplasia.[12]

However, the endoscope-based system is no longer commercially available. The probe-based system can still be used. However, it is expensive, has a distinct learning curve, and the resolution of the current systems can almost be achieved by using HD endoscopes with magnifying capabilities. However, the probe-based system has the advantage entering the biliary system and can differentiate biliary strictures.

In my opinion, endomicroscopy will further evolve in the field of functional and molecular imaging. Here, endomicroscopy is the only technology, which can define mucosal barrier function and molecular characteristics of different diseases.[13,14]

18.14 Optical Coherence Tomography

Optical coherence tomography (OCT) is a technology that obtains cross-sectional images of target tissue with high resolution on the order of a low-power microscope. Interferometry is the technique used in OCT that measures the path length of reflected light and processes the information for image generation. OCT is similar to ultrasound but uses light as the signal instead of an acoustic signal. Compared with endosonography, OCT offers a higher spatial resolution on the order of 1 to 15 μm, but less depth of penetration. OCT can operate with air or water interface. The images generated by OCT correlate with the subsurface of tissue. The original iteration of OCT was conventional time domain OCT. Frequency domain OCT has been developed to provide faster real-time imaging with high resolution. Volumetric laser

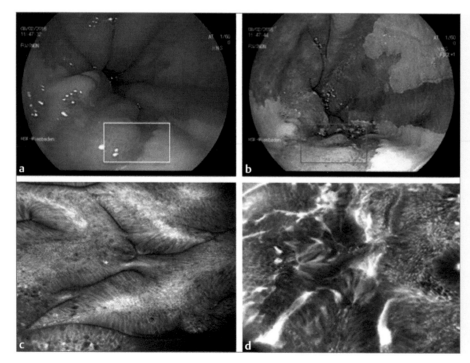

Fig. 18.4 Virtual chromoendoscopy and endomicroscopy of Barrett's associated neoplasia. **(a)** Short segment Barrett's esophagus is visible on white-light endoscopy. **(b)** Virtual chromoendoscopy using FICE highlights a depressed area. **(c)** Endomicroscopy of normal Barrett's epithelium. **(d)** Barrett's associated dysplasia can be identified within the depressed area (dark and irregular cells are visible).

endomicroscopy provides resolution to 10 µm and imaging depth down to 3 mm scanning over a 6-cm length of esophagus over a period of 90 seconds.[15]

Optical frequency domain imaging (OFDI) uses the same image interpretation technology as OCT, but by using a rotating scanning laser, it is able to assess several areas of the mucosa simultaneously. This allows for rapid assessment of a large field of mucosa and shortening scanning time to several minutes.[16]

Although spectrally encoded confocal microscopy has better transverse resolution than OFDI, OFDI can penetrate deeper into tissues, which potentially enables the visualization of different morphologic features.

The first comprehensive volumetric microscopy of the human distal esophagus was successfully demonstrated with OFDI and a balloon-centering catheter, providing a wealth of detailed information about the structure of the esophageal wall.[17] Today the microscopic imaging technology can also be integrated into a tethered capsule that can be swallowed. This new method is less invasive than traditional endoscopy and might help screening large groups of patients for specific disorders and provides microscopic information from the entire esophagus as the pill passes through the GI tract.

18.15 Conclusions

Advanced imaging techniques are techniques for improved endoscopic diagnosis. Chromoendoscopy and especially virtual chromoendoscopy has evolved in conjunction with HD endoscopes as techniques for daily use. These techniques facilitate detection and characterization of GI lesions. Neoplastic areas can be differentiated from nonneoplastic changes with high confidence, which leads to more targeted biopsies and more accurate prediction of final histology.

Optical coherence tomography and endomicroscopy are techniques exploring histologic details, which enables in vivo histology. Specific histologic features can be recognized and functional and molecular imaging becomes possible.

However, endoscopic imaging technologies are continuously and rapidly evolving and will alter the way in which we perform GI endoscopy and how we manage GI diseases in the future. Accurate image interpretation is key for these advanced imaging techniques, and for these technologies to be widely adopted, nonexperts must also be able to perform such interpretations.

References

[1] Bhat YM, Dayyeh BK, Chauhan SS, et al; ASGE Technology Committee. High-definition and high-magnification endoscopes. Gastrointest Endosc. 2014; 80(6):919–927
[2] Manfredi MA, Abu Dayyeh BK, Bhat YM, et al; ASGE Technology Committee. Electronic chromoendoscopy. Gastrointest Endosc. 2015; 81(2):249–261
[3] Morimoto Y, Kubo M, Kuramoto M et al. Development of a new generation endoscope system with Lasers, Lasereo Fujifilm Research and Development 2013;58:1–6
[4] Press release HOYA, Pentax, May, 2016. https://www.ncbi.nlm.nih.gov/pubmed/?term=Thosani+N%2C+Abu+Dayyeh+BK%2C+Sharma+P%2C+et+al%3B+ASGE+Technology+Committee.+ASGE. Accessed October 12, 2017.
[5] Thosani N, Abu Dayyeh BK, Sharma P, et al; ASGE Technology Committee. ASGE Technology Committee systematic review and meta-analysis assessing the ASGE Preservation and Incorporation of Valuable Endoscopic Innovations thresholds for adopting real-time imaging-assisted endoscopic targeted biopsy during endoscopic surveillance of Barrett's esophagus. Gastrointest Endosc. 2016; 83(4):684–6–98.e7
[6] Abu Dayyeh BK, Thosani N, Konda V, et al; ASGE Technology Committee. ASGE Technology Committee systematic review and meta-analysis assessing the ASGE PIVI thresholds for adopting real-time endoscopic assessment of the histology of diminutive colorectal polyps. Gastrointest Endosc. 2015; 81(3):502.e1–502.e16
[7] Laine L, Kaltenbach T, Barkun A, et al; SCENIC Guideline Development Panel. SCENIC international consensus statement on surveillance and management of dysplasia in inflammatory bowel disease. Gastroenterology. 2015; 148(3):639–651.e28
[8] Wong Kee Song LM, Adler DG, Chand B, et al; ASGE Technology Committee. Chromoendoscopy. Gastrointest Endosc. 2007; 66(4):639–649
[9] Rey JW, Kiesslich R, Hoffman A. New aspects of modern endoscopy. World J Gastrointest Endosc. 2014; 6(8):334–344
[10] Konda V, Chauhan SS, Abu Dayyeh BK, et al; ASGE Technology Committee. Endoscopes and devices to improve colon polyp detection. Gastrointest Endosc. 2015; 81(5):1122–1129
[11] Chauhan SS, Dayyeh BK, Bhat YM, et al; ASGE Technology Committee. Confocal laser endomicroscopy. Gastrointest Endosc. 2014; 80(6):928–938
[12] Teubner D, Kiesslich R, Matsumoto T, et al. Beyond standard image-enhanced endoscopy confocal endomicroscopy. Gastrointest Endosc Clin N Am. 2014; 24(3):427–434
[13] Atreya R, Neumann H, Neufert C, et al. In vivo imaging using fluorescent antibodies to tumor necrosis factor predicts therapeutic response in Crohn's disease. Nat Med. 2014; 20(3):313–318
[14] Goetz M, Malek NP, Kiesslich R. Microscopic imaging in endoscopy: endomicroscopy and endocytoscopy. Nat Rev Gastroenterol Hepatol. 2014; 11(1):11–18
[15] Konda V, Banerjee S, Barth BA, et al; ASGE Technology Committee. Enhanced imaging in the GI tract: spectroscopy and optical coherence tomography. Gastrointest Endosc. 2013; 78(4):568–573
[16] Potsaid B, Baumann B, Huang D, et al. Ultrahigh speed 1050nm swept source/Fourier domain OCT retinal and anterior segment imaging at 100,000 to 400,000 axial scans per second. Opt Express. 2010; 18(19):20029–20048
[17] Gora MJ, Sauk JS, Carruth RW, et al. Imaging the upper gastrointestinal tract in unsedated patients using tethered capsule endomicroscopy. Gastroenterology. 2013; 145(4):723–725

19 The Contribution of Histopathology to Endoscopy

Michael Vieth

According to Rudolf Virchow (1858), the etiology of all diseases can be boiled down to alterations of single cells.[1] Thus morphology and visualization is the basis by which diseases can be identified. It all began in about 1595 with Hans Janssen, who probably built the first microscope. Janssen's creation was nearly 45 cm in length and could magnify objects three- to ninefold.[2] During the 17th century, scientists in The Netherlands, England, and Italy began to dissect insects and plants and thus the microscope became the foundation for the natural sciences. At the end of the 18th century, Bichat was regarded as the founder of histology with his descriptions of 21 different tissues.[3] The first professional histologic laboratory was opened midway through the 19th century in Prague (1851) followed by one in Leipzig (1875).[4,5] Prerequisites were not only the optics but also the development of specimen fixation, embedding and preparing paraffin blocks, cutting with a microtome, and, last but not least, histochemical staining. The majority of histologic staining methods were described until the 1930s. Immunohistochemical methods were introduced in the 1980s, from 1990 on in situ hybridization, and from 2000 on, molecular pathology became more and more sophisticated and relevant for treatment and diagnosis.

Parallel to these developments, optical endoscopic visualization improved markedly in the last few decades. Endoscopy and histopathology share the morphologic analysis as their basis and these share the characterization of epithelia, vessels, infections, and neoplasia, among others. Whereas identification of color and pit pattern is the domain of endoscopy, histopathology can deliver risk factors and precise analysis of cells and tissue and depth of infiltration to build the basis for modern diagnosis (▶Fig. 19.1) and treatment options (▶Fig. 19.2).

Endoscopy and histopathology are interrelated. Sampling without prior precise surface analysis will not lead to representative biopsy material whereas histopathology allows more exact analysis of inflammation, possible infection, and better classification of tumors. Finally, by demonstration of mutations such as RAS in colorectal carcinoma, histopathology at the subcellular level has a direct consequence for therapy. The main contribution of histopathology has to be seen in the fact that histopathology delivers the precise etiology of changes seen endoscopically or by other methods. Therefore, it is essential that pathologists always report cause and etiology of their findings in their histopathologic diagnosis. Histopathology is important for screening for neoplasia, confirmation of clinical diagnosis, early diagnosis of neoplasia, differential diagnosis between benign and malignant, diagnosis of metabolic disease drug-induced changes, parasitic, bacterial, viral infections, inflammatory diseases, detection of immunopathologic diseases, intraoperative consultation for further treatment, and, last but not least, science.

19.1 Prerequisites

Close collaborations is warranted between endoscopists and pathologists for a precise diagnosis. For colorectal biopsies, the benefits of such a collaboration have been clearly demonstrated

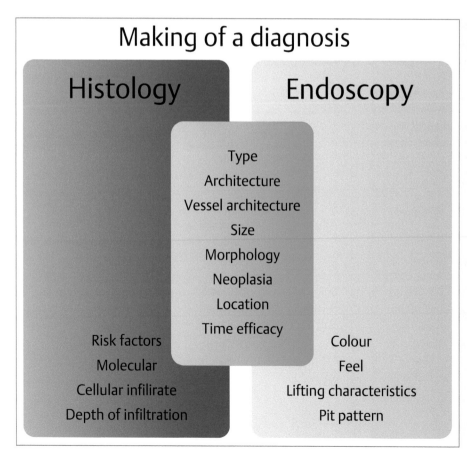

Fig. 19.1 Making of a diagnosis in endoscopy and histology with a considerable overlap but some features addressed by endoscopy or histology, only.

Operation
Robot assisted operation
Endoscopic intervention
Endoscopic operation
Snare biopsy
Endoscopic resection (EMR; ESD, etc...)
Diagnostic endoscopic resection for clarifying the diagnosis and planning of therapy
Endoscopic ablation (thermal, RFA, Argon-Plasma, etc...)

Fig. 19.2 Steadily growing list of interventional treatment options in the GI tract. Medications such as chemotherapy or biologics, etc. do not belong to this list.

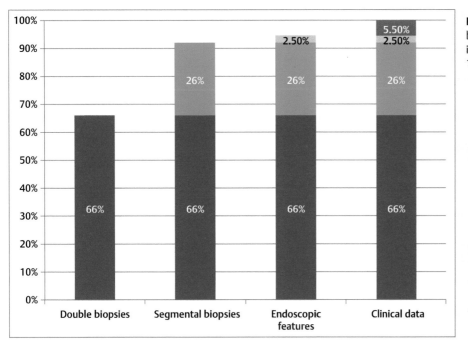

Fig. 19.3 Improvement of colitis diagnostics by change of biopsy technique and clinical information from 66% correctness to almost 100% (modified after Dejaco et al).

(▶Fig. 19.3).[6] It makes no sense at all to hide key information from the pathologist with the misguided notion of introducing objectivity to histologic diagnosis.[7] The endoscopist should provide the pathologists with a copy of the endoscopic report (optimum) but at least with the endoscopic diagnosis (minimum), preferably with images (in case of unexpected or unusual findings). In the United States this is currently not the case; pathologists rarely receive any endoscopic images. Pertinent clinical data include duration of symptoms, previous medications, and general clinical information such as prior diagnoses.

On receipt of a sample, standard protocol is for the pathologist to describe the received material. In the case of biopsies, the number of biopsy fragments received is recorded, but more detailed descriptions of the fragments are usually not necessary. The size of the fragments is mentioned. In all other cases, a gross examination is performed to ensure precise information of the resection margin status. In specimens removed for neoplasia, measurements of the tumor and its relationship to the specimen's margins are recorded to ensure proper future therapeutic steps and allow proper staging. For cases for which clarification about the sample is required, the pathologists need to contact the clinician. Regularly scheduled clincopathologic conferences ensure proper flow of information, specimens, and diagnoses. Endoscopists and pathologists need to understand the requirements of the other part and certainty of diagnostics (▶Fig. 19.1, ▶Fig. 19.4).

Proper orientation is important to avoid artefacts that can interfere with the pathologist's ability to interpret the histopathologic findings. Endoscopic resections should be carefully oriented in the endoscopy suite to ensure proper analysis of the resection margins. Specimens can be orientated by thread marks or latex colors or even India ink. Pinning these samples on thick paper or cork helps as well. Stretching a specimen prior to fixation should be definitively avoided. Specimens should be loosely pinned on paper or cork. The reasoning is that specimens can shrink up to 50% during fixation with formalin and this may cause artefacts that hamper the histologic diagnosis. Pinning through the lesion itself and close to the edges of the lesion should be avoided as well.

In addition, it should be noted that adequate fixation also is essential for all samples, including those obtained for cytologic evaluation (endoscopic ultrasound–fine-needle aspiration [EUS-FNA]). Some methods, such as electron microscopy, require special fixatives, whereas frozen sections and some molecular analyses require fresh nonfixated material. Immunohistochemical analyses can deliver false results if the incorrect fixative was used. If the endoscopist is unclear about the fixative, the pathologist's office should be contacted for clarification.

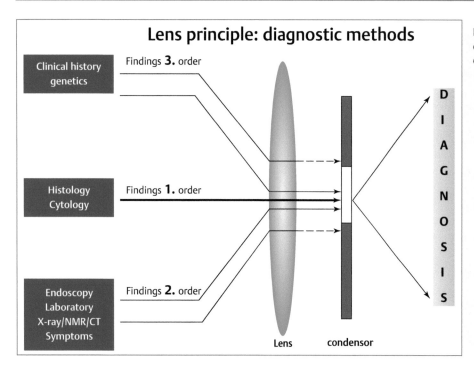

Fig. 19.4 Lens principle of diagnosis comparing different diagnostic methods and certainty of results.

19.2 Clinical Impact of Histopathology by Segment within the Gastrointestinal Tract

19.2.1 Esophagus

The most frequent indication for taking esophageal biopsies is refractory gastroesophageal reflux disease (GERD).

However, there are some limitations to the clinical impact of such biopsies: first, there are no clear recommendations where exactly to take them and how many biopsies should be obtained. Secondly, using biopsy protocols and clear histopathologic grading schemes increases the utility of such samples. It has been shown that when clear recommendations are introduced, histopathologic results correlate with endoscopic findings in GERD.[8,][9] However, such protocols have not been widely introduced and thus, in classical reflux disease with no suspicion for mimickers or neoplasia, biopsy results do not deliver information beyond the endoscopic diagnosis since the treatment and dosage of drugs are based on the combination of typical symptoms and lesions for prescribing the full dosage of proton pump inhibitors (PPIs) compared to cases with no mucosal breaks (nonerosive reflux disease [NERD]) for which patients are prescribed half the standard dosage of PPI. It is noteworthy that the vast majority of patients with GERD present with endoscopically negative reflux disease rather than with mucosal breaks.

It should be noted that in addition to GERD, esophageal inflammatory conditions also include various infections, drug-associated injury, neoplastic lesions, and even esophageal involvement in chronic inflammatory bowel disease (IBD). In such cases, histology has a clinical impact since the etiology of the inflammation can often be given and thus sufficient treatment options discussed. Biopsies in patients in whom there is a clinical suspicion for GERD should be taken (if at all) within a range of 0.5 cm above the Z-line and preferably in line with the lesser curvature of the stomach since histologic changes are known to be more striking there than elsewhere.

Cases suspicious for Barrett's esophagus (BE) should be biopsied according to the Seattle protocol, namely with four biopsies in every 2 cm. Unfortunately, this protocol is rarely followed in routine cases, but, when strictly adhered to, the Seattle protocol ensures a high probability of detecting dysplasia, if any. No biopsies should be taken from a straight, normal-appearing Z-line. Definitions of BE differ worldwide. In the United States, biopsies from columnar tongues longer than 1 cm are recommended. If goblet cells (intestinal metaplasia) are detected histopathologically, the diagnosis of BE is proven. However, there are variable different definitions worldwide with and without goblet cells with and without columnar metaplasia identified endoscopically (e.g., British Barrett's guidelines, German Barrett's guidelines, Japanese Barrett's guidelines, European Barrett's guidelines, Czech Barrett's guidelines). Pathologists are generally unaware of the endoscopic appearance and may state that the specimen is "suggestive of BE" when goblet cells are present. However, if there are tongues less than 5 mm or an irregular Z-line, the patient likely has "intestinal metaplasia of the Z-line." It is important that gastroenterologists correctly convey this information to their patients.

In patients for whom there is a clinical suspicion for eosinophilic esophagitis (EOE), biopsies should be taken from the distal, middle, and upper esophagus (two each in different containers) to allow differentiation of eosinophils in GERD within the distal esophagus from eosinophilic esophagitis, in which more proximal eosinophils are expected. The eosinophilic infiltrates in EOE can be rather discontinuous, focal, and sometimes even very sparse (< the requested 20/mm^2) especially in patients taking PPI or partially treated with steroids and thus multiple samples are ideal.

In patient in whom there is a suspicion of moniliasis/candidiasis, biopsies are recommended from the whitish sloughed material with and without mucosal breaks; in other words, from the edge or erosions/ulcers that encompass both the exudate/granulation tissue as well as the intact epithelium. The same applies to cases with suspicion for viral infections such as herpes simplex virus (HSV, which is detected in the edges of a necrosis of an ulcer) and cytomegalovirus (CMV, which is principally detected in the endothelial cells in granulation tissue or the center of an ulceration).

19.2.2 Stomach

Limiting the value of histopathology to the *Helicobacter* status of the stomach has little clinical impact when gastric biopsies can yield a wealth of other information. The histopathologic interpretation of gastric inflammatory lesions is well harmonized worldwide by the means of the updated Sydney system that allows a semiquantitative grading of various inflammatory infiltrates, intestinal metaplasia, and atrophy.[10] Additionally, pathologists add the etiology of the gastritis in the report. Biopsies should be taken 3 cm above the pylorus, from the lesser and greater curvature in the antrum, and form the middle of the body (two biopsies) according to the updated Sydney system. A biopsy from the incisura is considered optional (▶Fig. 19.5). This sampling allows detection of gastritis associated with *H. pylori* as well as the autoimmune/pernicious anemia type.

Gastric polyps can be biopsied first prior to deciding what to do next since more than 80% of all gastric polyps are nonneoplastic tumor–like lesions rather than neoplasms. This situation is completely different from that of the colorectum where adenomas are common. Gastric erosions and ulcerations should always be biopsied as here also, the pathologist can frequently determine the etiology of the lesion.[11,12] Routine biopsies from the antrum and corpus (two each) should never be forgotten even in cases endoscopically suspicious for carcinoma since the gastritis status may ensure the correctness of the diagnosis (e.g., a gastric carcinoma in an otherwise normal stomach would rather be unusual and should prompt the pathologist to question the diagnosis once more).[13] Ulcerations should be resampled during the healing phase since almost 20% of gastric carcinomas are not diagnosed at the first endoscopy but are diagnosed at second and third

endoscopy since often necrosis lacks malignant cells and thus the material is not representative for the lesion. Multiple biopsies increase the diagnostic yield in such cases, specifically at least 10 biopsies from both the center and margin of such an ulceration.

Some types of gastric vascular malformations should be biopsied to exclude or confirm the endoscopic diagnosis, although caution should be exercised in sampling a suspected Dieulafoy lesion as management may then require emergency gastrectomy! However, in gastric vascular antral vascular ectasia (GAVE, watermelon stomach) it is necessary to identify microthrombi in small subepithelial vessels. Endoscopically the antrum shows red stripes reminiscent of the outside of a watermelon pattern due to the dilated and congested subepithelial vessels. Biopsies should be taken from the red stripes.

19.2.3 Small Bowel

Duodenal biopsies could be considered to document a complete histologic evaluation in an upper gastrointestinal (GI) tract endoscopy. The clinical impact of performing duodenal biopsies is generally rather low, especially when there is no clinical suspicion for celiac disease or anemia. When celiac disease is a consideration or anemia is present, at least six biopsies (especially in celiac disease—four from the descending duodenum and two from the bulb) are recommended. Celiac disease, giardiasis, and adenoma of the papilla region or various other small bowel segments, follicular lymphoma, neuroendocrine tumors (that are very aggressive in the terminal ileum even if very small), autoimmune duodenitis, Crohn's disease, and some metabolic disorders are diagnoses that can be found in the small bowel and that have a huge clinical impact. The problem is that these diagnoses are rather rare compared to the vast majority of individuals in whom small bowel samples yield no pathologic findings. However, even if cost analysts question small bowel biopsies, the value of a correct histopathologic diagnosis can be enormous in patients in whom the endoscopic findings are negligible.

19.2.4 Colorectum

By frequency, a major symptom of colorectal injury is diarrhea. There are various etiologies for diarrhea starting from osmotic diarrhea in individuals with consumption of sugar substitutes, chronic IBD, infections, microscopic colitis, and even polyposis syndromes or stenotic tumors. As a general rule, biopsies should be taken from all colonic segments (two each) in different containers. Specifically, rectal biopsies should be submitted in separate containers to ensure that the correct etiology can be assigned. The differential diagnosis of IBD[14,15] can be difficult, especially early in its course when histologic features of chronic injury are incompletely developed. Ileal biopsies separately submitted in a different container may similarly help to differentiate Crohn's disease from ulcerative colitis. Also, in such cases, biopsies from the upper GI tract may help not to overlook Crohn's involvement of the upper GI tract and thus confirming a Crohn's diagnosis in the lower GI tract. The differential diagnosis of colitis-associated neoplasia and sporadic neoplasia often requires review by an experienced pathologist normally a second opinion outside the primary institution.

In cases for which there is a clinical suspicion for microscopic colitis, two biopsies from each colonic segment should be taken and placed in different containers according to the various

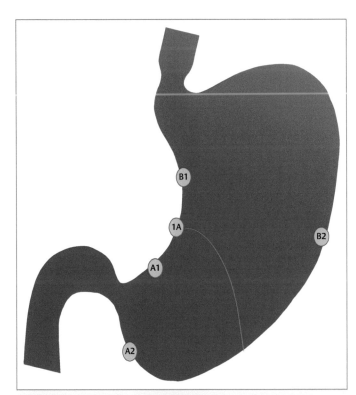

Fig. 19.5 Location of biopsies according to the updated Sydney system (Dixon MF et al) with two biopsies of antrum, lesser and greater curvature 3 cm proximal to the pylorus and two biopsies from the middle of the corpus at lesser and greater curvature (all mandatory), and one additional biopsy from the incisura angularis (optional).

colonic segments. It should be noted that patients with microscopic colitis show more prominent changes within the proximal colon than the distal colon. The leading symptom, and thus the indication for biopsies, is a rather nonsuspicious colonic endoscopic appearance in patients with watery diarrhea.

Polyps should be removed completely at first endoscopic diagnosis since the vast majority of polyps larger than 5 mm is neoplastic. As a general rule and a general convention, all of these polyps require histopathologic evaluation. Small distal hyperplastic polyps do not require removal nor histopathologic evaluation, but the endoscopist should be very sure about the endoscopic diagnosis in order to follow such a protocol. If in doubt, it would better seem to send the specimen for pathologic evaluation. Such strategies vary worldwide for both medical reasons and as a result of different reimbursement policies of national health systems. Tumors of the colorectum that cannot be removed by an endoscopic procedure should be biopsied to prove malignancy and thus arrange for the patient to have disease-specific treatment.

19.3 Endoscopic Resections

The recent development and improvement of endoscopic detection[16] and resection techniques have required a refined histopathologic evaluation. For example, the resection margin status in surgical operation specimens is measured in centimeters whereas this can be micrometers in endoscopic resections. Careful histologic evaluation[17,18] and correlation with outcome data made it possible that ever-increasing numbers of patients with early neoplastic lesions can be safely managed endoscopically rather than surgically in centers around the globe. This trend leads to lesser costs, faster recovery periods, and less invasive procedures for the price of equal survival rates compared to traditional surgery. Risk factors are continuously evaluated and refined if necessary and thus indications have widened for endoscopic procedures over the last decade.

High-quality evaluation starts in the endoscopy suite; the specimen should be orientated and pinned loosely on cork or thick paper. Appropriate fixatives should be used and a 12- to 24-hour fixation period should be ensured. In the pathology laboratory, photographic documentation is useful and help the pathologist to identify the closest margin to a tumor. Specimens should always be embedded completely. Distances to horizontal and vertical margins, as well as the largest diameter of the tumor, and in tumors that invade the submucosa, total tumor thickness, and depth of infiltration measured from the deepest portion of the muscularis mucosae into the submucosa should be given in micrometers. Risk factors such as deep submucosal invasion, lymphatic or blood vessel permeation, tumor budding, poor differentiation, or perineural invasion should be noted in the report (▶Table 19.1). If any of these factors is unfavorable, surgical therapy should be considered; preferably, this should be decided following consultation in a multidisciplinary tumor board.

19.4 Conclusion

Endoscopy and histopathology are both disciplines based on morphology. They are interdependent. Clinical patient data are extremely important for the pathologist, and as knowledge of

Table 19.1 Histologic risk factors of GI carcinomas (e.g. Esophageal Carcinoma)

- Depth of infiltration (m1–m3 in squamous mucosal carcinoma, m1–m4 in Barrett's mucosal carcinoma, sm1–sm3, T2, T3a, T3b, T4a, T4b)
- Grading (G1–G4)
- Differentiation (e.g., signet ring, intestinal, gastric, mucinous, etc.)
- Lymphatic vessel permeation
- Blood vessel permeation
- Perineural invasion
- Peritumoral inflammation
- Budding of tumor cells (including clustering)
- Resection status (complete vs. incomplete)
- Status of lymph nodes
- Distant metastasis

the endoscopic findings ensure the correct histopathologic diagnoses. The clinical impact of biopsies throughout the GI tract varies with location and indication for taking biopsies. As general rule for the endoscopist, histopathologic diagnoses should always be related to the endoscopic findings since this ensures quality of the procedure and helps the endoscopist better identify lesions correctly. This is a major contribution of histopathology to endoscopy. As a general rule for the pathologist, the etiology of changes should always be given within the final report. Cases for which there is doubt can be sent to other colleagues for second opinions.

References

[1] Virchow R. Die Cellularpathologie in ihrer Begründung auf physiologische und pathologische Gewebelehre. 1st ed. Berlin: Hirschfeld; 1858

[2] Stewart GB. Microscopes. San Diego, CA: Lucent; 1992

[3] Bichat XMF. Traité des membranes en général et de diverses membranes en particulier. Paris: Richard Caille Ravier; 1799

[4] Dohm G. Die Geschichte der Mikroskopie. Berlin: Springer; 2013:227

[5] Dohm G. Die Geschichte der Mikroskopie. Berlin: Springer; 2013:285

[6] Dejaco C, Oesterreicher C, Angelberger S, et al. Diagnosing colitis: a prospective study on essential parameters for reaching a diagnosis. Endoscopy. 2003; 35(12):1004–1008

[7] Geboes K. La collaboration entre l'endoscopiste et le pathologiste. Acta Endoscopica. 2006; 36:245

[8] Tytgat GN. The value of esophageal histology in the diagnosis of gastroesophageal reflux disease in patients with heartburn and normal endoscopy. Curr Gastroenterol Rep. 2008; 10(3):231–234

[9] Vieth M. Contribution of histology to the diagnosis of reflux disease. Best Pract Res Clin Gastroenterol. 2008; 22(4):625–638

[10] Dixon MF, Genta RM, Yardley JH, Correa P. Classification and grading of gastritis. The updated Sydney System. International Workshop on the Histopathology of Gastritis, Houston 1994. Am J Surg Pathol. 1996; 20(10):1161–1181

[11] Stolte M, Panayiotou S, Schmitz J. Can NSAID/ASA-induced erosions of the gastric mucosa be identified at histology? Pathol Res Pract. 1999; 195(3):137–142

[12] Vieth M, Müller H, Stolte M. Can the diagnosis of NSAID-induced or Hp-associated gastric ulceration be predicted from histology? Z Gastroenterol. 2002; 40(9):783–788

[13] Vieth M, Neumann H, Falkeis C. The diagnosis of gastritis. Diagn Histopathol. 2014; 20(6):213–221

[14] Vieth M, Atreja R, Neumann H. Carcinoma in inflammatory bowel disease: endoscopic advances, management, and specimen handling. A review for the pathologist. Diagn Histopathol. 2015; 21(7):290–298

[15] Vieth M, Neumann H. Current issues in inflammatory bowel disease neoplasia. Histopathology. 2015; 66(1):37–48

[16] Kiesslich R, Burg J, Vieth M, et al. Confocal laser endoscopy for diagnosing intraepithelial neoplasias and colorectal cancer in vivo. Gastroenterology. 2004; 127(3):706–713

[17] Lauwers GY, Forcione DG, Nishioka NS, et al. Novel endoscopic therapeutic modalities for superficial neoplasms arising in Barrett's esophagus: a primer for surgical pathologists. Mod Pathol. 2009; 22(4):489–498

[18] Vieth M, Langner C, Neumann H, Takubo K. Barrett's esophagus. Practical issues for daily routine diagnosis. Pathol Res Pract. 2012; 208(5):261–268

20 Endoscopic Ultrasonography

Geoffroy Vanbiervliet

20.1 Introduction

Endoscopic ultrasonography (EUS) has become indispensable and unavoidable in the diagnostic and the treatment of the digestive diseases. It is a demanding technique and learning remains long, tedious, and difficult. A prior initial experience in diagnostic and therapeutic digestive endoscopy is required in order to understand this procedure better. The high diagnostic accuracy of the technique especially in cancerous pathologies and the recent popularization of the EUS-guided sample using fine-needle aspiration (FNA) have led to the integration of this technique at the center of care in digestive oncology. This is therefore the recommended first-line investigation for the histologic diagnosis of solid and cystic pancreatic tumors and for evaluation of their locoregional extension. Nevertheless, a wide range of pathologies can be advantageously evaluated by the EUS from submucosal tumors through esophageal motility disorders or endometriosis. EUS also benefits from the latest technologies in ultrasound with exceptional resolution, elastography, and contrast EUS now possible to significantly improve the diagnostic capabilities in many fields. Recently EUS moved progressively to a unique interventional modality that offers a minimally invasive alternative to various surgical interventions with an excellent safety profile. The drainage of pancreatic pseudocysts is the historical example. However, improving the equipment now allows considering a multitude of drainage techniques sometimes see hybrid like for biliary or pancreatic duct and digestive anastomosis. A very exciting future expects this technique which is now mature. This text presents the basic principles of EUS, its validated indications, and its main outcomes.

20.2 Overview of the Procedure

EUS is a technology allowing the use of ultrasound within the upper and lower digestive lumen. The transducer is placed at the tip of the endoscope which keeps a video view of the gastrointestinal (GI) tract. The close contact with the intestinal wall allows the use of high frequency which brings the best compromise between image resolution and depth of field. This specificity makes it the technique of choice for the analysis of the bowel wall (esophagus, stomach, duodenum, rectum, and anus) and organs in contact (mediastinum, liver, biliary ducts, gallbladder, pancreas, vagina, bladder). The quality of the results of the procedure depends directly on the operator's experience.

20.3 General Diagnostic and Therapeutic Techniques

20.3.1 Conditions of Implementation

EUS allows the analysis of the upper digestive part from the esophagus to the distal duodenum and adjacent organs. The exploration of the lower part of the digestive tract is limited to anus, rectum, and sigmoid. A bowel preparation based on enema is required for the anorectal exploration. The procedure could be routinely performed under propofol sedation, but conscious sedation is still widely used in Europe and Asia.[1] The outpatient management is the rule in case of diagnostic procedure including the EUS-guided sample using FNA.[2] Room air or CO_2 insufflations are suitable for diagnostic EUS and EUS-FNA, but CO_2 is required for therapeutic process due to the risk of perforation especially in case of EUS-guided digestive anastomosis. Periprocedural antibiotic prophylaxis is suggested by international guidelines for EUS-FNA of pancreatic cysts.[3] Prophylactic antibiotics have not been studied in case of interventional EUS procedures (i.e., pseudocyst and biliary or pancreatic duct drainage, tumor destruction, vascular treatment, fiducial placement). Nevertheless, this prophylaxis is usually performed, with infectious complication infrequently reported. As recommended, no withdrawal or modification of antiplatelet agents and anticoagulation therapy are required for diagnostic EUS.[4] Aspirin alone is allowed during EUS-FNA in case of solid tumor. All antiplatelet or anticoagulation treatment should be stopped when therapeutic EUS is performed or when EUS-FNA on cystic lesion is expected.

20.3.2 Endoscopes and Probe

The radial scanning or curved linear array endoscope is used depending on local expertise, but only linear probe allows a therapeutic approach and FNA due to the large working channel (3.7–3.8 mm) and the presence of an elevator. If imaging capability of each techniques is compared, curved linear array seems to be superior in the exploration of the pancreatic head–body transition, the pancreatic tail, the hepatic hilum, and the vascular bifurcation whereas radial scanning allows a better major duodenal papilla and gallbladder delineation.[5] High frequencies (5–12 MHz) and Doppler analysis are now available in all echoendoscope. Endorectal ultrasonography could be accomplished using rigid or flexible devices: rigid linear probe presents a limited insertion but are more practical for rectal cancer staging and anal functional disorders (▶ Fig. 20.1).[6,7]

20.3.3 EUS Semiology of the Bowel Wall

The stratification of the bowel wall with EUS could be described in five, seven, or nine layers according to the type of frequency used. In low frequency (5–7.5MHz), five layers are usually visible as described in ▶ Fig. 20.2. The fourth hypoechoic layer is an essential marker since it corresponds to the muscular layer. The appearance in nine layers is possibly observed with very high-frequency probes (20 MHz) which are less used and available. These probes help to identify the muscularis mucosae (fourth hypoechoic layer with these) and its potential involvement by tumor, increases risk of cancerous lymph nodes.

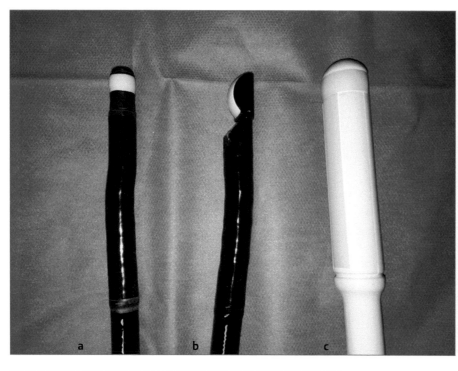

Fig. 20.1 (a) Tips of the radial scanning. (b) Curved linear array. (c) Endoscope and rectal rigid linear probe. The radial probe allows a 360-degree scanning view and the linear probe provides a large 120-degree field of view.

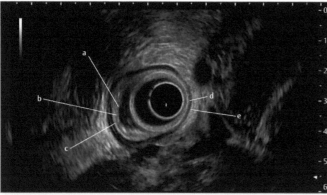

Fig. 20.2 View of the five layers of the gastrointestinal wall at the frequency of 10 MHz using a radial scanning probe: (a) the hyperechoic interface, (b) the hypoechoic layer of mucosae, (c) the hyperechoic aspect of the submucosal layer, (d) the hypoechogenicity of the muscular layer, and (e) the hyperechoic interface (serosa).

20.3.4 Techniques

The patient is placed in prone or left lateral position. Insufflation during the procedure and the introduction of the endoscope needs to be minimized in order to reduce artifact. The instillation of water should be considered to improve the resolution of the picture especially for the GI wall analysis. A close contact between probe and the target area is mandatory using the up handle of the scope.

Usually, the procedure for biliopancreatic investigation starts from the second/third duodenum to allow the inspection of the interest area with a slow withdrawal and rotation of the scope. The head of pancreas, papilla, and the distal part of common bile duct is accurately investigated by a transduodenal approach. The proximal part of the bile duct with hepatic hilum, the arterial and venous axis (portal vein, superior mesenteric artery and vein) could be explored by transduodenal and transgastric approach. The body and tail of the pancreas, the celiac trunk, and the splenic artery/vein are analyzed only by a transgastric view.

The endoscope is pushed into the sigmoid (aorta bifurcation and spine in posterior view) under video control and then the EUS exploration phase is performed after fulfilling the digestive lumen with water with a slow withdrawal of the scope.

20.4 Accessory Devices and Techniques

20.4.1 Elastography

It is a noninvasive method that can be used in combination with conventional EUS which is a measure of tissue stiffness evaluated by the application of slight pressure to the target with the ultrasonography probe (▶ Fig. 20.3). It has been demonstrated to differentiate between benign and malignant solid pancreatic masses and lymph nodes with a high accuracy, as well as normal pancreatic tissues from early chronic pancreatitis.[8]

20.4.2 Contrast-Enhanced EUS

Contrast-enhanced EUS (CE-EUS) is the intravenous use of microbubble blood pool agents to allow the real-time imaging of tumor vascularization and perfusion. The evaluation of microvascularity by CE-EUS was useful, especially for the discrimination between pancreatic adenocarcinoma (hypoenhancement) and inflammatory nodules in chronic pancreatitis.[9]

20.4.3 Needles and EUS-Guided Sample

EUS-guided needles of various diameters (19, 20, 22, and 25 gauge) are commercially available. Specific designs have been proposed to allow core tissue acquisition which provides a more representative sample and tissue architecture of the lesion with capability for immunohistochemistry or vital

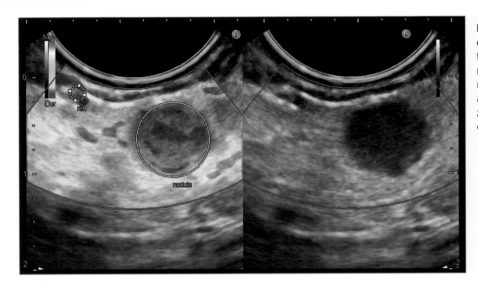

Fig. 20.3 Semiquantitative EUS elastography of a neuroendocrine tumor in the body of the pancreas. The elasticity is expressed as a relative ratio but not as an absolute value. Two nonoverlapping areas are selected, usually area A is the lesion, area B is the reference zone, and strain ratio represents the B/A quotient (5.09 here).

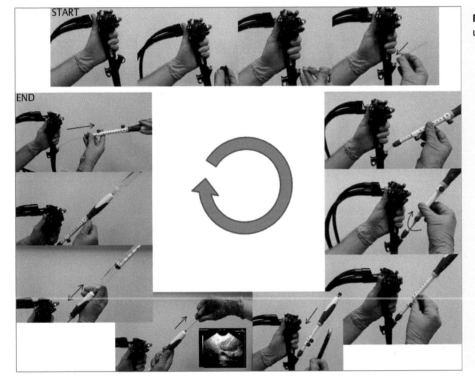

Fig. 20.4 The different steps for EUS-FNA using the classical technique.

stains: 19-gauge Trucut needle and side port (reverse cutting bevel) at the tip of the needle in different caliber (EUS–fine needle biopsy [FNB]) are available. Nevertheless, the Trucut needle did not show any improvement comparing with other needles due to a lack of flexibility and high failure rate in duodenum (40%).[10] No significant difference between the EUS-FNB and standard FNA needles is observed for sample adequacy, diagnostic accuracy, or acquisition of a core specimen.[11] However, a reduction in passes to establish the diagnosis is demonstrated with it and a higher diagnostic yield has been suggested for nonpancreatic lesion.[12]

The usual technique for EUS-FNA implicates several steps which are presented in ►Fig. 20.4. The fanning technique should be considered for each EUS sample.[13] This technique is based on the change of the axis of the needle in different areas within the mass by using the up–down dial of the echoendoscope when moving back and forth. Other variants have been

described to improve the tissue acquisition including the EUS-FNA without stylet (reduction of the procedure time and the risk of accidental needlestick injuries), the capillary or "slow-pull" technique (slow withdrawal of the stylet), and the wet-suction technique (column of air replaced by 5 mL of saline solution in the needle).

The classical suction technique improved the diagnostic yield and the adequacy of the specimen. The high negative pressure (50/60 mL) is certainly better to obtain a significant higher rate of adequate sample for histologic analysis.[10] The use of stylet does not impact the EUS-guided sampling result.[2]

Air flushing in a slow and controlled fashion is the best way to express the material from the needle. Stylet reinsertion is only required if the aspirates cannot be expelled due to clotting or drying. The collection of histopathologic specimens could be performed using smear, liquid-based cytology, and/or cell block (►Fig. 20.5). The cell block improves the diagnostic

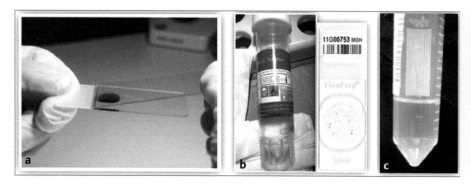

Fig. 20.5 The available techniques for the collection of histopathologic specimens: **(a)** smear for cytopathologic analysis including rapid on-site evaluation (ROSE), **(b)** liquid-based cytology for monocellular layer, **(c)** cell block using formalin 4% and allowing immunohistochemistry.

yield as it provides histologic analysis and should be considered when possible.

20.5 Accepted Indications

Diagnostic and therapeutic EUS procedures are listed in ▶Table 20.1. EUS allows the diagnosis and staging of GI tumor and mediastinal mass associated with tissue or fluid analysis by EUS-guided FNA (cytologic/histologic/chemical/molecular evaluation). Therapeutic capabilities are used for guided marking (fiducial placement), drainage (collection, obstructed duct, digestive diversion), tumoral destruction, and pharmaceutical injection (block, neurolysis, embolization).

Table 20.1 Accepted indications for EUS

Diagnostic procedures	
Staging	• Tumors of gastrointestinal tract • Tumors of biliary ducts and pancreas • Tumors of mediastinum including lung cancer
Tissular/vascular/functional abnormalities	• Abnormalities of the digestive wall • Abnormalities of the adjacent structures • Motility esophageal disorders • Portal hypertension • Evaluation of the pancreas including masses (acute/chronic pancreatitis and cysts) • Perianal and perirectal disorders (abscess, anal sphincter injuries, fistulae, endometriosis)
Pancreatic cancer screening	• Individual with two or more blood relatives and at least one first-degree relative with pancreatic cancer • Carriers of *p16*, *PALB2*, or *BRCA2* mutations with a first-degree relative with pancreatic cancer • All individuals with Peutz–Jeghers syndrome • Individuals with Lynch syndrome and a first-degree relative with pancreatic cancer
Guided sampling	• Tissue sampling of lesions within, or adjacent to, the wall of the gastrointestinal tract
Therapeutic procedures	
Guided marking	• Placement of fiducial markers
Guided drainage/access	• Treatment of symptomatic pseudocysts • Access to bile/pancreatic duct • Digestive anastomosis (gastrojejunal, excluded stomach after bypass)
Tumoral destruction	• Alcohol injection (cyst) • Radiofrequency ablation
Pharmaceutical injection	• Vascular embolization • Celiac plexus block or neurolysis • Antitumoral agents

EUS, endoscopic ultrasonography.

20.6 Quality Measures

The American Society for Gastrointestinal Endoscopy (ASGE) has recently defined the accepted quality indicators in EUS (▶Table 20.2).[14] These were selected because of their ease of establishment, monitoring, and reporting. The priority indicators are as follows:
• The frequency with which all GI cancers are staged with the AJCC/UICC TNM staging system.
• Diagnostic rates and sensitivity for malignancy in patients undergoing EUS-guided FNA of pancreatic masses.
• The incidence of adverse events after EUS-FNA (bleeding, perforation, and acute pancreatitis).

20.7 Training

The ASGE recommends a minimum of 150 supervised EUS investigations, including 75 pancreaticobiliary EUS investigations and 50 EUS-FNA procedures, to establish comprehensive competence in all aspects of EUS.[15] Specific training program including theoretical courses and hands-on courses in live pigs showed to increase competency for diagnostic and EUS-FNA.[16] Furthermore, education on various models with isolated animal organs could be the best compromise between realism, cost, and availability. Finally, European Society of Gastrointestinal Endoscopy (ESGE) guidelines recommend a combination of different simulators and if possible a live swine model to achieve training.[2] The challenging learning curve and the need to satisfy minimal thresholds justify a careful approach before practicing EUS independently.[17]

20.8 Complications and Prevention

Most of the relevant literature concluded that diagnostic EUS procedures were safe, and related complications were extremely low. ▶Table 20.3 summarizes the main adverse events, risks, and their frequency.

20.8.1 Noninterventional EUS

Duodenal perforation occurs significantly more often compared to other sites. Fatal issues due to perforation are uncommon but reported.[18] The possible risk factors for EUS-related perforation

Table 20.2 Quality indicators in EUS according to ASGE guidelines[14]

Quality indicator	Type of measure	Performance target (%)
Preprocedural		
Frequency with which EUS is performed for an indication (included in a published standard list of appropriate indications and the indication is documented)	Process	> 80
Frequency with which consent is obtained	Process	> 98
Frequency with which appropriate antibiotics are administered in the setting of FNA of cystic lesions	Process	N/A
Frequency with which EUS exams are performed by trained endosonographer	Process	> 98
Intraprocedural		
Frequency with which the appearance of relevant structures, specific to the indication for the EUS, is documented	Process	> 98
Frequency with which all gastrointestinal cancers are staged with AJCC/UICC TNM staging system	Process	> 98
Frequency with which pancreatic mass measurements are documented along with evaluation for vascular involvement, lymphadenopathy, and distant metastases	Process	> 98
Frequency with which EUS wall layers involved by subepithelial masses are documented	Process	> 98
Percentage of patients with distant metastasis, ascites, and lymphadenopathy undergoing EUS-guided FNA who have tissue sampling of both the primary tumor diagnosis and lesions outside of the primary field when this would alter patient management	Process	> 98
Diagnostic rate of adequate sample in all solid lesions undergoing EUS-FNA	Outcome	≥ 85
Diagnostic rates and sensitivity for malignancy in patients undergoing EUS-FNA of pancreatic masses	Outcome	Diagnostic rate ≥ 70 Sensitivity ≥ 85
Postprocedural		
Frequency with which the incidence of adverse events after EUS-FNA (acute pancreatitis, bleeding, perforation, and infection) is documented	Process	> 98
Incidence of adverse events after EUS-FNA (acute pancreatitis, bleeding, perforation, and infection)	Outcome	Acute pancreatitis < 2 Perforation < 0.5 Clinically significant bleeding < 1

ASGE, The American Society for Gastrointestinal Endoscopy; AJCC, American Joint Committee on Cancer; EUS, endoscopic ultrasonography; FNA, fine-needle aspiration; N/A, not applicable; TNM, tumor node metastasis; UICC, the Union for International Cancer Control.

are the operator inexperience, the presence of a stricture, a duodenal diverticulum, or a pancreatic head tumor, a dilation performed prior to EUS procedure, a difficult previous endoscopic esophageal intubation, and the use of a linear probe.[19] Bleeding and aspiration are infrequent with only few case reports. Bacteremia was prospectively evaluated and remains rare without clinical symptoms of infection developed during follow-up.

20.8.2 EUS-FNA

The risk of adverse events is higher compared with noninterventional EUS. According to a recent systematic review of 51 EUS-FNA trials, among complications the most common are postprocedural pain (34%), acute pancreatitis (34%), fever and infectious complications (16%), and bleeding (13%).[20] Perforations and bile leaks are uncommon (3%). The overall complication rate of EUS-FNA in this systematic analysis of 10,941 patients was 0.98% (1.72% in 31 prospective studies). The procedure-related mortality was estimated at 0.02%. Risk factors for EUS-FNA complications are the operator experience and presence of a liquid component (cyst) of the lesion especially in pancreas (higher risk of bleeding and infectious complications). There is no evidence to support that needle size affects complication rate.

20.8.3 Interventional EUS

Compared with diagnostic EUS and EUS-FNA, the risk of complications is considerably higher for EUS-guided interventions particularly for pancreaticobiliary drainage. The cumulative adverse event rate was 23% in a recent review including 1,192 patients who benefit from EUS-guided biliary drainage.[21] No difference between transgastric or transduodenal approach was observed in term of morbidity including rendezvous and anterograde techniques. The overall rate of complications is 16% for EUS-guided pancreatic drainage with lowest incidences of adverse events for rendezvous technique.[22]

20.9 Prevention

Several measures have been proposed to minimize the risks of EUS procedures. It includes (1) adequate training in specific and supervised programs; (2) cooperative and adequately sedated patients; (3) restrict the water filling in the upper gastrointestinal tract; (4) avoid the dilation of malignant strictures; (5) respect the recommendations for antibiotics prophylaxis and discontinuation of antiplatelet/anticoagulation agents especially for cystic lesion; (6) limit the EUS-guided sample to patients in whom cytopathology will significantly modify the management; (7) use

Table 20.3 Complications of diagnostic and therapeutic EUS

Adverse event	Frequency (%)
Diagnostic EUS	
Perforation	0.03–0.15
Bleeding	0–0.03
Aspiration	NA/5 cases reported
Bacteremia	1.9–2
EUS–fine-needle aspiration or biopsy	
Perforation	0–0.86
Bleeding	
• Extraluminal	0.15–1.4
• Intraluminal	4
Pain	0.34
Acute pancreatitis	0.44
Infection	0.55
Pancreatic leak	NA/ only case report
Therapeutic EUS	
Pseudocyst	
• Overall	8
• Infection	4
• Bleeding	2
• Perforation	1.6
Celiac plexus neurolysis	
• Overall	21
Celiac plexus block	
• Overall	7
Bile duct drainage	
• Overall	23.3
• Intrahepatic approach	25
• Extrahepatic approach	21.8
Pancreatic duct drainage	
• Overall	16
• Pancreatitis	3
• Bleeding	2
• Perforation	2
• Pain	3

EUS, endoscopic ultrasonography.

Doppler function before EUS-FNA to avoid interposition of vessels in the needle trajectory; (8) preferential use of rendezvous technique in case of duct drainage.

References

[1] van Riet PA, Cahen DL, Poley JW, Bruno MJ. Mapping international practice patterns in EUS-guided tissue sampling: outcome of a global survey. Endosc Int Open. 2016; 4(3):E360–E370

[2] Polkowski M, Larghi A, Weynand B, et al; European Society of Gastrointestinal Endoscopy (ESGE). Learning, techniques, and complications of endoscopic ultrasound (EUS)-guided sampling in gastroenterology: European Society of Gastrointestinal Endoscopy (ESGE) Technical Guideline. Endoscopy. 2012; 44(2):190–206

[3] Khashab MA, Chithadi KV, Acosta RD, et al; ASGE Standards of Practice Committee. Antibiotic prophylaxis for GI endoscopy. Gastrointest Endosc. 2015; 81(1):81–89

[4] Veitch AM, Vanbiervliet G, Gershlick AH, et al. Endoscopy in patients on antiplatelet or anticoagulant therapy, including direct oral anticoagulants: British Society of Gastroenterology (BSG) and European Society of Gastrointestinal Endoscopy (ESGE) guidelines. Endoscopy. 2016; 48(4):385–402

[5] Kaneko M, Katanuma A, Maguchi H, et al. Prospective, randomized, comparative study of delineation capability of radial scanning and curved linear array endoscopic ultrasound for the pancreaticobiliary region. Endosc Int Open. 2014; 2(3):E160–E170

[6] Colaiácovo R, Assef MS, Ganc RL, et al. Rectal cancer staging: correlation between the evaluation with radial echoendoscope and rigid linear probe. Endosc Ultrasound. 2014; 3(3):161–166

[7] Barthet M, Bellon P, Abou E, et al. Anal endosonography for assessment of anal incontinence with a linear probe: relationships with clinical and manometric features. Int J Colorectal Dis. 2002; 17(2):123–128

[8] Cui XW, Chang JM, Kan QC, et al. Endoscopic ultrasound elastography: current status and future perspectives. World J Gastroenterol. 2015; 21(47):13212–13224

[9] Alvarez-Sánchez MV, Napoléon B. Contrast-enhanced harmonic endoscopic ultrasound imaging: basic principles, present situation and future perspectives. World J Gastroenterol. 2014; 20(42):15549–15563

[10] Wani S, Muthusamy VR, Komanduri S. EUS-guided tissue acquisition: an evidence-based approach (with videos). Gastrointest Endosc. 2014; 80(6):939–59.e7

[11] Bang JY, Hawes R, Varadarajulu S. A meta-analysis comparing ProCore and standard fine-needle aspiration needles for endoscopic ultrasound-guided tissue acquisition. Endoscopy. 2016; 48(4):339–349

[12] Aadam AA, Wani S, Amick A, et al. A randomized controlled cross-over trial and cost analysis comparing endoscopic ultrasound fine needle aspiration and fine needle biopsy. Endosc Int Open. 2016; 4(5):E497–E505

[13] Bang JY, Magee SH, Ramesh J, et al. Randomized trial comparing fanning with standard technique for endoscopic ultrasound-guided fine-needle aspiration of solid pancreatic mass lesions. Endoscopy. 2013; 45(6):445–450

[14] Wani S, Wallace MB, Cohen J, et al. Quality indicators for EUS. Gastrointest Endosc. 2015; 81(1):67–80

[15] DiMaio CJ, Mishra G, McHenry L, et al; ASGE Training Committee. EUS core curriculum. Gastrointest Endosc. 2012; 76(3):476–481

[16] Barthet M, Gasmi M, Boustiere C, Giovannini M, et al. Club Francophone d'Echoendoscopie Digestive. EUS training in a live pig model: does it improve echo endoscope hands-on and trainee competence? Endoscopy. 2007; 39(6):535–539

[17] Wani S, Coté GA, Keswani R, et al. Learning curves for EUS by using cumulative sum analysis: implications for American Society for Gastrointestinal Endoscopy recommendations for training. Gastrointest Endosc. 2013; 77(4):558–565

[18] Lachter J. Fatal complications of endoscopic ultrasonography: a look at 18 cases. Endoscopy. 2007; 39(8):747–750

[19] Jenssen C, Alvarez-Sánchez MV, Napoléon B, Faiss S. Diagnostic endoscopic ultrasonography: assessment of safety and prevention of complications. World J Gastroenterol. 2012; 18(34):4659–4676

[20] Wang KX, Ben QW, Jin ZD, et al. Assessment of morbidity and mortality associated with EUS-guided FNA: a systematic review. Gastrointest Endosc. 2011; 73(2):283–290

[21] Wang K, Zhu J, Xing L, et al. Assessment of efficacy and safety of EUS-guided biliary drainage: a systematic review. Gastrointest Endosc. 2016; 83(6):1218–1227

[22] Alvarez-Sánchez MV, Jenssen C, Faiss S, Napoléon B. Interventional endoscopic ultrasonography: an overview of safety and complications. Surg Endosc. 2014; 28(3):712–734

21 Hybrid, Natural Orifice, and Laparoscopy-Assisted Endoscopy: New Paradigms in Minimally Invasive Therapy

Robert H. Hawes

21.1 Introduction

The initial concept of natural orifice transluminal endoscopic surgery (NOTES) was to pass a flexible endoscope through the gut wall and perform surgical procedures in the peritoneal cavity or mediastinum. While this concept has not yet come to full fruition, the movement should be credited with accelerating the progression of therapeutic endoscopy. Therapeutic endoscopy has a long tradition extending from polypectomy in the 60s to endoscopic retrograde cholangiopancreatography (ERCP) with sphincterotomy, stone extraction, and stent placement through hemostasis and luminal stenting. We have now entered an era of endoluminal therapy which includes treatment of gastrointestinal reflux disease (GERD), en bloc resection of early gastrointestinal cancers, obesity management, and full-thickness resection of tumors of the gut wall. The next progression is cooperative laparoscopic and endoscopic techniques (CLET). With CLET, the disciplines of minimally invasive surgery (MIS) and therapeutic endoscopy have come together to solve common problems and this has given birth to hybrid procedures; laparoscopy-assisted endoscopy and endoscopy-assisted laparoscopic surgery. This progression from standard therapeutic endoscopy through CLET will eventually culminate in a more complete realization of NOTES. It was in fact the NOTES movement that brought together therapeutic endoscopists and minimally invasive surgeons. The experience gained from this cooperation of disciplines combined with lessons learned by working through the progression of endoluminal and hybrid procedures promises to offer less invasive treatments which will hopefully lower costs and improve outcomes. The purpose of this chapter is to provide an overview of these new techniques and to provide a window into the future of therapeutic endoscopy. While attempts will be made to provide the indications, complications, and training required to perform these procedures, it must be understood that these new therapeutic domains are rapidly evolving and outcomes today will likely be different in the near future.

21.2 History of NOTES

The idea of natural orifice surgery (NOS) was conceived by Sergei Kantsevoy and Tony Kalloo in the late 1990s. While working with the Apollo Group, they introduced the concept of passing a flexible endoscope through a natural orifice and accessing the mediastinum or peritoneal cavity using the gut as a window (like the skin). The first report of their work was presented to the Society for Surgery of the Alimentary Tract (SSAT) during Digestive Disease Week (DDW) in 2000 and involved transgastric peritoneoscopy.[1] However, it was their report 2 years later at DDW describing a NOTES gastrojejunostomy in a survival swine model that really caught the attention of the MIS world.[2] The excitement (and concern) prompted the Society of American Gastrointestinal and Endoscopic Surgeons (SAGES)

and the American Society for Gastrointestinal Endoscopy (ASGE) to form a committee to oversee the responsible development of NOTES. This societal cooperation resulted in an annual meeting devoted to updating the progress of NOTES, a White Paper presenting a roadmap for the responsible development of NOTES[3] and research support to solve the obstacles to the clinical implementation of NOTES procedures. As time progressed, it became clear that flexible endoscopes and existing accessories were inadequate to implement the types of procedures that Kalloo and Kantsevoy initially conceived. Therapeutic gastroenterologists were unable to enter the operating room (OR) and were not credentialed to do surgical procedures. Surgeons, except for a chosen few, did not have the endoscopic skills to perform surgical procedures with the flexible endoscope. Minimally invasive surgeons wanted to continue to use their familiar rigid platforms and ventured into transvaginal cholecystectomy and single-port laparoscopic surgery as potentially less invasive approaches to standard laparoscopic surgery. Enthusiasm among gastroenterologists, surgeons, and industry waned and the NOTES movement lost its focus.

The idea of doing surgical procedures with the flexible endoscope through a natural orifice was resurrected by Haru Inoue when he advanced two concepts originally developed within the Apollo Group. The first concept was introduced by Chris Gostout and his group at the Mayo Clinic. Dr. Gostout's team was trying to solve the riddle of safe and easy en bloc resection. As part of this work, they developed the concept of "submucosal tunneling" to create a working area within the submucosal space.[4,5,6,7] They modified concepts developed by the Japanese for endoscopic submucosal dissection (ESD) and became proponents of using balloons to expand the submucosal space. During this time, Jay Pasricha conceived of the second concept, the idea of using Dr. Gostout's tunneling technique to perform an endoscopic myotomy as a treatment for achalasia.[8] It was the brilliance of Dr. Inoue, relying on his extensive experience in ESD and laparoscopic Heller's myotomy, that enabled him to perform the first per oral endoscopic myotomy (POEM) for the treatment of achalasia.[9,10] It was the introduction of POEM into clinical practice that initiated the concept of submucosal surgery. With the advent of POEM, it has proven the safety of making a small mucosal incision, working within the submucosal space and achieving safe and effective closure by placing clips on the mucosal incision. This has now led to a procedure called submucosal tunneling endoscopic resection (STER) which is being applied to small gastrointestinal stromal tumors (GISTs). GISTs arise from the muscularis propria and thus endoscopic resection usually results in entry into the peritoneal cavity or mediastinum. A desire to remove GISTs and early gastric cancers is what is primarily responsible for the development of laparoscopic–endoscopic and endoscopic–laparoscopic hybrid procedures. Endoscopic submucosal surgery and hybrid laparoscopic–endoscopic procedures represent the critical bridges between therapeutic endoscopy and NOTES.

21.3 Submucosal Surgery

POEM is covered more thoroughly in other areas within this textbook. Briefly, the procedure involves making a small submucosal injection in the esophageal wall followed by a vertical mucosal incision (▶Fig. 21.1; **Video 21.1**). The entry point is either anterior or posterior depending on the preference of the endoscopist and whether the patient has had prior treatment. Once the space is entered, a step-by-step dissection of the submucosal fibers is performed using various ESD instruments. This dissection is extended a few centimeters into the cardia. When the dissection is complete, the endoscope is withdrawn to a point a few centimeters distal to the mucosal incision and the myotomy is begun. There is not a uniform standard and some endoscopists perform a selective myotomy involving only the inner circular muscle layer while others purposely cut through both circular and longitudinal fibers. There are no comparative studies between these two techniques. Once the myotomy is extended into the cardia, the scope is withdrawn and the mucosal incision is closed by a series of clips. Decisions about whom to treat and the length of the myotomy are now being determined by the results of high-resolution manometry and categorizing the patient according to the Chicago Classification.[11,12] Large single-and multicenter studies have now been reported and randomized trials comparing POEM with Heller's myotomy and pneumatic dilation are nearly complete and will soon be reported. Many consider POEM to be the first natural orifice surgery. Two important concepts emerging from the POEM experience which are relevant to the advancement of therapeutic endoscopy are the safety and efficacy of working within the submucosal space and that safe and effective closure of "tunnels" can be achieved by simple closure of the mucosal incision.

Endoscopic resection of submucosal tumors came about as an extension of POEM. It is primarily applied to GISTs in the esophagus and stomach (▶Fig. 21.2). The technique is initiated in the same manner as POEM. At a certain distance from the submucosal tumor, a submucosal injection followed by a mucosal incision into the submucosal space is made. The endoscopist then tunnels down to the lesion and works within the submucosal space to dissect, isolate, and resect the tumor. The tumor is withdrawn through the tunnel and the mucosal incision is closed with clips. In the course of this procedure, entry into the mediastinum or peritoneal cavity can occur. For the mediastinum, as long as CO_2 is being used, escape of gas from the endoscope is usually not problematic. In the case of gastric GISTs, placement of a Veress needle may be required to evacuate CO_2 from the peritoneal cavity. The importance of STER is that it allows resection of submucosal tumors while preserving the stomach wall. It reinforces the safety of working within the submucosal space and has now led to exploration of endoscopic pyloromyotomy for the treatment of gastroparesis.[13] The potential for submucosal surgery is vast, and in addition to POEM and pyloromyotomy includes the smooth muscle biopsy in gut motility disorders, drug delivery, pacemaker, and neural stimulation procedures (**Video 21.2**).

21.4 Back to NOTES

The era of NOTES began in earnest when SAGES and the ASGE combined forces and formed a joint committee to oversee the responsible development of NOTES. The first and most important contribution of that committee was the publication of the first White Paper published jointly in Gastrointestinal Endoscopy and Surgical Endoscopy in 2006.[3] An important component of the White Paper was a list of obstacles that the committee felt

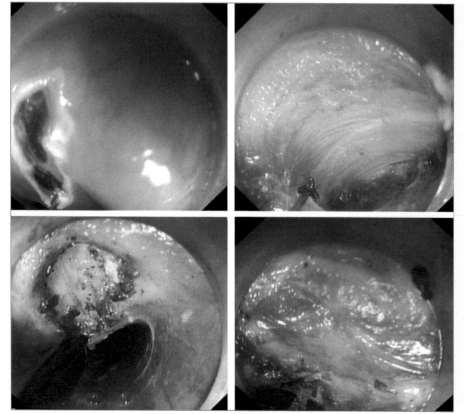

Fig. 21.1 The procedure of per oral endoscopic myotomy (POEM), including mucosal incision, development of submucosal tunnel, inner circular myotomy, and clip closure of mucosal entrance.

needed to be addressed in order for NOTES to become a clinical reality (▶Table 21.1). At the first International Summit in NOTES in 2006, working groups were formed to make recommendation on research required to overcome these obstacles.

A number of proposals were made and tested to achieve safe access to the peritoneal cavity. These included a simple incision with a needle knife–like instrument, utilizing a percutaneous endoscopic gastrostomy tube technique as well as tunneling as described under submucosal surgery section of this chapter. In the end, no single technique came to the fore.

From the beginning, there was considerable concern about safe and effective gastric closure. Some felt that the ESD experience of perforation closure with hemoclips could be translated to a NOTES closure. Most felt, however, that clips were insufficiently robust and durable to reach the very high threshold for secure closure established by surgical suturing. Investigators largely agreed that the ideal closure is the time-tested, full-thickness suturing which is well established in surgical practice. There is now an available endoscopic full-thickness suturing system (OverStitch, Apollo Endosurgery, Austin, Texas).

While there is a product for endoscopic suturing that potentially solves the issue of secure closure, there is no suturing system with the size and maneuverability to do fine suturing within the

Table 21.1 Obstacles to the clinical implementation of natural orifice transluminal endoscopic surgery

1. Access
2. Closure
3. Suturing
4. Anastomosis
5. Spatial orientation
6. Multitasking platform
7. Management of intraoperative "events"
8. Physiologic untoward events
9. Training

peritoneal cavity. Most NOTES contributors, especially minimally invasive surgeons, felt that it will be necessary to build a multitasking platform with articulating arms in order to meet the need of intraperitoneal suturing.

Surgeons were extremely concerned about spatial orientation. The "in-line" imaging provided by a flexible endoscope is completely different than the "overview" perspective provided by an umbilical camera. There is insufficient experience to determine whether this is a real issue or not but many feel that sophisticated platforms capable of doing surgical procedures in the peritoneal cavity will require separation of the optics from the end-effector functions.

One of the most intriguing obstacles to the full implementation of NOTES is the idea that it will require a multitasking platform. Minimally invasive surgeons are extremely reluctant to give up the ability to have two "arms" and have the ability to triangulate. Much of the early work in this area tested flexible direct drive systems. Olympus began testing a system they called EndoSamurai (Olympus Corporation, Tokyo). The Carl Stortz company, unveiled the Anubiscope (Karl Storz, Tuttlingen, Germany). Boston Scientific (Natick, Massachusetts) did early testing of a flexible articulating platform they called the direct drive endoscopic system (DDES) as well. All these systems, in their original form, have been abandoned. It is now felt that computer interface, motor-driven robotic systems hold the greatest promise in therapeutic endoscopy and NOTES. There are numerous companies now working on such systems but none are currently approved for use in humans and are commercially available.

A critical component of surgical practice is the management of intraoperative "issues" to avoid becoming complications. Hemostasis, closure of inadvertent perforation, and proper energy delivery to avoid excessive collateral tissue damage are all important components of surgical practice. The same "issues" could occur during NOTES procedures and techniques and instruments

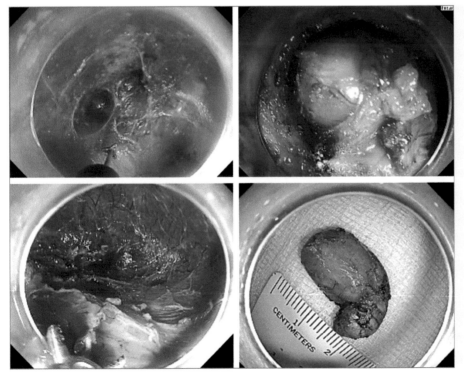

Fig. 21.2 Submucosal tunnel endoscopic resection (STER)/per oral endoscopic tunnel resection (POETR) for treatment of gastric and esophageal subepithelial tumors.

need to be available to solve these emergent issues. There is not yet a full array of laparoscopic-type instruments available on a flexible platform. Intraperitoneal suturing is not possible and a ubiquitous instrument, used in most laparoscopic surgeries, the harmonic scalpel (or a comparable technology) is not yet available in a flexible platform.

There was concern that NOTES might cause unforeseen physiologic events. It was always assumed that endoscopic systems would need to use CO_2 rather than room air when working in the peritoneal cavity and that a pneumoperitoneum would need to be maintained. However, it was not known whether intraperitoneal pressure requirements for NOTES would be higher or lower when compared to standard laparoscopic surgery. It was also not known whether transintestinal entry would lead to greater or lesser amounts of postoperative adhesions. In the course of NOTES research, no unanticipated or unique physiologic events have been encountered.

The final obstacle was training. In reality, although there has been much discussion, this issue has not been resolved or fully addressed. It is assumed that a degree of cross-training would be required; minimally invasive surgeons would require significant amount of training in flexible endoscopy and gastroenterologists would require a certain amount of general surgical training as well as some laparoscopic experience. It was hypothesized that NOTES would lead to a hybrid specialty—someone specializing in minimally invasive therapy irrespective of the specific instrument(s) required. There was general consensus that such hybrid training would not lead to board certification in both surgery and internal medicine. In the end, although not all agree, it is most likely that the majority of minimally invasive therapists of the future will come from the surgical ranks with flexible endoscopic training coming either from specialized surgical programs or specialized advanced endoscopy training centers.

Assessment depends on how physicians define the procedure. Several thousand cases of hybrid transvaginal procedures are documented in the literature including cholecystectomy, nephrectomy, and vertical sleeve gastrectomy,[14,15,16,17,18] but usually the procedure is performed with rigid instruments and often with transcutaneous laparoscopic ports. Most physicians involved with NOTES feel that POEM represents the first clinically applied NOTES procedure. It is performed through a natural orifice with a flexible instrument and mimics a surgical procedure. In this context, STER could also be considered a NOTES procedure.

Currently, the most promising pure NOTES procedure is transanal colon resection. This was introduced by Swanstom in 2007 when his group described transanal sigmoid resection in a human cadaver model.[19] Transanal access for colon resection has now been proven safe and feasible in both swine and fresh human cadaver models.[20,21] As in all NOTES procedures, limitations imposed by lack of optimal instrumentation had to be overcome. Instrument needs for transanal procedures has been solved in part by the availability of transanal endoscopic microsurgery (TEM) platforms.[22] Once the technique for transanal colon resection was established, it was necessary to determine if oncologic principles could be maintained if the resection was performed for cancer. The capability of performing an adequate oncologic resection was confirmed by Rieder in 2011 when he

randomized male cadavers to either laparoscopic or transanal sigmoid resection for simulated cancers at 25 cm.[23] Adequate proximal margins (transanal approach required laparoscopic assistance) were achieved with both techniques and lymph node yields were similar. The first hybrid NOTES transanal total mesorectal excision (TME) for rectal cancer was reported in 2010 by Sylla and Lacy.[24] The number of transanal TME cases is growing exponentially and trials are now ongoing to determine its safety and efficacy.[25]

21.5 Laparoscopy-Assisted Endoscopy

The idea of laparoscopy-assisted endoscopy probably began with laparoscopy-assisted enteroscopy before the advent of double balloon enteroscopy. However, current utilization is aimed primarily at improving the safety of ESD when performed by less experienced endoscopists or when performed in the colon. The other main application is to achieve full-thickness resection primarily for GISTs and more recently for early gastric cancer. These techniques fall under the umbrella of CLET and are listed in ▸Table 21.2. This section will concentrate on laparoscopy-assisted endoscopic resection (LAER) and combined laparoscopic–endoscopic resection (CLER).

21.6 Laparoscopy-Assisted Endoscopic Resection

LAER began in the early days of endoscopic mucosal resection (EMR) in the colon. This technique was used more frequently in the western world as EMR was applied to large colon polyps. The fear of causing perforation and inability to adequately access polyps in certain areas of the colon (hepatic and splenic flexure) prompted the use of laparoscopic guidance to control bleeding, repair perforation, or to mobilize and stretch areas of the colon to aid endoscopic resection.[26] As techniques and accessories were refined and improved, especially our ability to recognize and close perforations with clips, laparoscopic assistance to aid colonic EMR has largely been abandoned. In the western world, EMR for benign colon lesions has reached a level of safety and effectiveness that laparoscopic control should not be required.

Table 21.2 Cooperative laparoscopic and endoscopic techniques

1. Laparoscopy-assisted endoscopic resection (LAER)
   a) Endoscopic mucosal resection (EMR) and endoscopic submucosal dissection (ESD) are undertaken under laparoscopic observation/control
2. Endoscopy-assisted laparoscopic resection (EARL)
   a) Endoscopy-assisted wedge resection
   b) Endoscopy-assisted laparoscopic transluminal surgery
   c) Endoscopy-assisted laparoscopic intraluminal surgery
   d) Endoscopy-assisted laparoscopic intragastric stapling
3. Combined laparoscopic endoscopic resection (CLER)
   a) Laparoscopic–endoscopic cooperative surgery (LECS)
   b) Inverted LECS
   c) Laparoscopy-assisted endoscopic full-thickness resection (LAEFR)
   d) Clean nonexposure technique (Clean-NET)
   e) NEWS

21.7 Endoscopy-Assisted Laparoscopic Resection

There are several techniques that fall under the category of endoscopy-assisted laparoscopic resection (EARL) (▶Table 21.2) The first is *endoscopy-assisted wedge resection*. Many GISTs can be managed quite effectively by laparoscopic wedge resection. Challenges can occur when the lesion is located near the pylorus, on the posterior gastric wall and at or near the gastroesophageal junction (GEJ). The ease of the laparoscopic approach is dependent on whether the lesion is exophytic (primarily protruding into the peritoneal cavity and favors 1-degree laparoscopic resection), centered in the wall of the stomach, or endophytic (most of the lesion is protruding into the lumen of the stomach which makes the laparoscopic approach more difficult). The flexible endoscope serves to help localize the lesion, protect the integrity of the gut lumen when the lesion is near the pylorus or the GEJ, and helps assure that the entire lesion will be removed as the staple line is being positioned. The literature is relatively robust in describing the results of this technique. The R-degree resection rate (negative lateral and deep margins) is nearly 100% with a conversion rate to open surgery of about 5%. Complication rates vary between 0 and 9%.[27,28,29] Not all gastric GISTs can be removed with this technique and the median size in most series is about 4 cm. A downside of this approach is that often a significant amount of normal gastric wall is unnecessarily removed. This is the main rationale for exploring endoscopic techniques but as of 2016, endoscopically assisted laparoscopic wedge resection is considered the standard of care for small-to-medium–sized gastric GISTs.

A variant of the wedge resection technique is termed *endoscopy-assisted laparoscopic transluminal (transgastric) surgery* (▶Table 21.2). The same basic cooperation between laparoscopy and endoluminal endoscopy is applied but with this technique, a laparoscopic gastrostomy, usually along anterior wall, is made with the exact position determined by endoscopic transillumination. The mucosa surrounding the lesion is grasped and the lesion is pulled through the gastrostomy into the peritoneal cavity and then resected with an inverted wedge excision using a laparoscopic stapler. Alternatively, if this is a mucosa-based lesion, the laparoscopic team can perform a submucosal or full-thickness excision of the lesion. The gastrostomy is closed utilizing an endoscopic stapler and/or sutures. This technique is primarily applied to lesions on the posterior wall of the stomach[30,31] and duodenum.[32]

Rather than pulling the gastric wall through a gastrostomy into the peritoneal cavity, another alternative is termed *endoscopy-assisted laparoscopic intraluminal (intragastric) surgery* (▶Table 21.2). This technique was first described by Ohashi in 1995[33] and relies more on endoscopic assistance through traction and in some cases, specimen retrieval. Once the lesion is located endoscopically, an optical port and two working ports are advanced through the gastric wall into the lumen. In some cases, the gastric wall is tacked to the abdominal wall to provide added stability for the laparoscopic ports. The lesion can then be removed by laparoscopic mucosal resection, full-thickness resection, or laparoscopic stapling. This technique can be applied for removal of benign submucosal tumors and GISTs as well as early gastric cancer.[34,35,36] This approach may be particularly effective for lesions near the GEJ.[37]

A technique that can be applied to endophytic submucosal tumors is *endoscope-assisted laparoscopic intragastric stapling* (▶Table 21.2). This involves passing a 12-mm laparoscopic port into the gastric lumen. The endoscopist visualizes and exposes the tumor. A laparoscopic stapler is then employed to resect the lesion by inverted wedge resection.[38,39]

21.8 Combined Laparoscopic–Endoscopic Resection

This section comprises techniques that involve dissection and resection with both laparoscopic and endoscopic contributions. The first technique is called *laparoscopic–endoscopic cooperative surgery* (LECS) (▶Table 21.2). It was described by Hiki[40] and combines endoscopic submucosal dissection with inversion of the lesion into the peritoneal cavity followed by resection of the lesion and closure of the gastrostomy using a laparoscopic stapler. The first part of the procedure is performed by the endoscopist who makes cautery marks around the periphery of the lesion and then, after a submucosal injection, makes a 75% circumferential incision into the submucosa. The endoscopist then extends the 75% circumferential incision through the gastric wall. The tumors then grasp laparoscopically, pulled into the peritoneal cavity, and in the final 25% circumferential cut is made simultaneously with closure of the gastric defect using a laparoscopic stapler. These procedures used primarily for benign submucosal tumors of the stomach and is particularly noted for its very low reported complication rate.[40,41] There is one report of its use for duodenal tumor resection.[42]

A modification of the LECS procedure has been used for resection of early gastric cancer and avoids potential dissemination of tumor cells into the peritoneal cavity. The procedure is called *inverted LECS* and was described by Nunobe in 2012.[43] In this technique, a submucosal injection is made around the tumor. A seromuscular dissection is then performed laparoscopically down to the stained submucosal layer plane. The tumor is inverted into the gastric lumen and closure of the gastric wall is performed by laparoscopic seromuscular extramucosal suturing. With the tumor now invaginated inside the gastric lumen and the gastric wall closed, mucosal resection around the tumor can be performed in the usual ESD fashion. The tumor is extracted endoscopically.

As therapeutic endoscopy has progressed, an important goal has been made to develop a technique for full-thickness resection of the gut wall. There are many issues to resolve to make this procedure safe including management of the pneumoperitoneum and control of bleeding should it occur on the serosal surface. Until the advent of endoscopic suturing, closure was also an important issue. These obstacles can all be effectively managed with a laparoscopic–endoscopic approach. This hybrid procedure is termed *laparoscopy-assisted endoscopic full-thickness resection* (LAEFR). This was introduced by Abe in 2009.[44] With this procedure, the endoscopic team performs a full-thickness incision around the tumor. During this process, the laparoscopic team can facilitate the procedure by providing traction. Eventually, CO_2 is lost into the peritoneal cavity and endoluminal visualization and exposure become quite challenging. At this point, the laparoscopic team completes the resection and the specimen is retrieved either per oral placed in a protected plastic bag and brought through a port site. The gastric wall defect is sutured closed by the laparoscopic team. This procedure is primarily promoted for the removal of gastric GIST, but its utility has also been explored for removal of gastric cancer. When used as a cancer operation, sentinel node and lymph node dissection is performed laparoscopically.

When full-thickness resection is performed for cancer, it is important to avoid any exposure of the cancer to the peritoneal cavity. This can be accomplished by a hybrid technique called *clean nonexposure technique* (Clean-NET). This was described by Inoue in 2012.[45] The Clean-NET procedure involves tumor localization endoscopically followed by injection of the submucosal layer with a solution containing indocyanine green. Full-thickness stay sutures are then placed around the lesion to fix the mucosa to the other layers. Selective laparoscopic dissection of the serosa and muscle layer is performed down to the submucosal plane (indicated by green coloring). Using the stay sutures, the specimen

with preserved intact mucosal layer is pulled into the peritoneal cavity and produces an intact mucosal "net" within which the lesion is contained. A mechanical stapler is then used to respect the specimen which seals the gastric wall (and the lesion) within a protective "net" preventing exposure of the specimen to the peritoneal cavity. The specimen is then placed into a laparoscopic bag and withdrawn through the port hole.

The final procedure to be reviewed in this section is called *nonexposed endoscopic wall–inversion surgery* (NEWS) (▶ Fig. 21.3; **Video 21.3**). This procedure was developed with the aim to treat early gastric cancer. The two major advantages are that it preserves the integrity of the gut wall preventing leakage into the peritoneal cavity and also the specimen is kept within the gut lumen thus avoiding any potential exposure to the peritoneal cavity. The lesion as outlined endoscopically with cautery marks and a similar marking technique is used laparoscopically to mark the serosal surface. A submucosal injection of sodium hyaluronate mixed with indigo carmine is made circumferentially around the

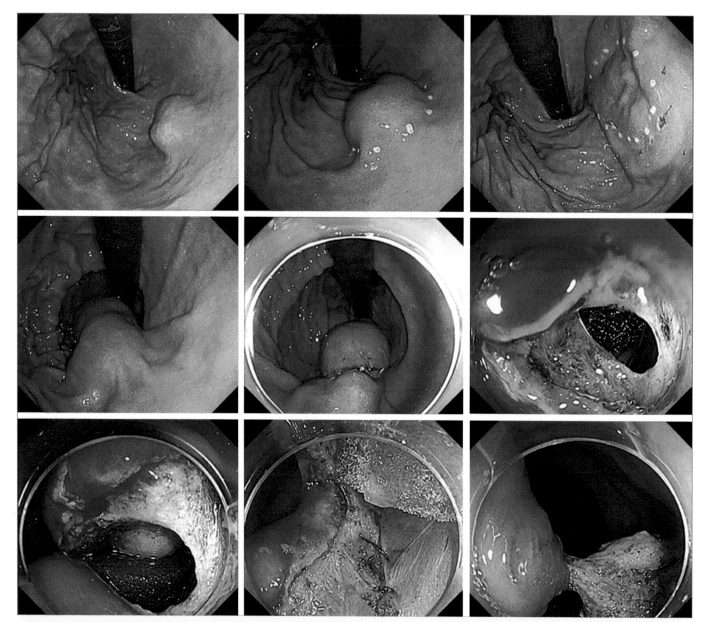

Fig. 21.3 (a) Endoscopic procedure of nonexposure wall–invasion surgery (NEWS) for treatment of gastric subepithelial tumor.

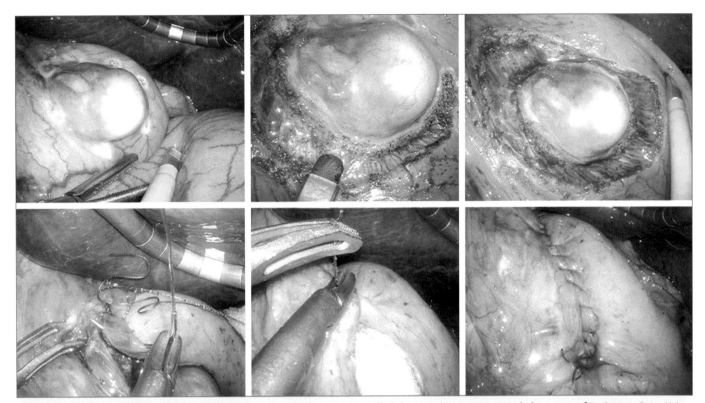

Fig. 21.3 (b) Laparoscopic procedure of NEWS for treatment of gastric subepithelial tumor. (Images are provided courtesy of Dr Osamu Goto, Keio University School of Medicine.)

tumor. Meanwhile, the whole lymph node group containing the sentinel node is dissected and sent for frozen section. Once confirmation is received that the nodes are negative, the laparoscopic team performs a circumferential seromuscular dissection down to the submucosal space. The tumor is inverted into the gastric lumen and the seromuscular layer is closed with running sutures. Prior to closure, a surgical spacer, cut to fit the resection site is placed between the tumor and the suture line. The resection is then completed by circumferential incision through the mucosa and submucosa down to the spacer. The resected specimen is retrieved to the mouth. The experimental design of this procedure was reported by Goto in 2011.[46] The procedure has been reported in a small number of gastric GISTs[47] and early gastric cancer by the same group.[48]

Hybrid laparoscopic–endoscopic procedures came about as a result of collaborative relationships between minimally invasive surgeons and therapeutic endoscopists. These procedures were developed to solve problems that could not be optimally managed by either discipline. In the process, minimally invasive surgeons have become more aware and more appreciative of the capabilities of the flexible endoscope. Alternatively, therapeutic endoscopists have come to understand the advantages that minimally invasive surgeons possess with their rigid instruments, the vast array of instruments available for dissection, resection, and hemostasis, and the perspective of approaching organs from the serosal as opposed to the mucosal surface. Hybrid procedures are currently used primarily for submucosal lesions of the upper gastrointestinal tract and early gastrointestinal cancers. Hybrid procedures, however, often require two teams and thus are inherently inefficient, difficult to coordinate, and consume excessive resources. As minimally invasive therapy progresses, we will see that some procedures will be entirely done laparoscopically while many will mature and able to be completed entirely using a flexible endoscope; these no longer require laparoscopic assistance. It is this milieu of minimally invasive surgeons and therapeutic endoscopists working together to create less invasive therapies that will further progress the concept of NOTES.

21.9 Summary

We are witnessing an unprecedented evolution in therapeutic endoscopy. Polypectomy, biliary sphincterotomy, hemostasis, and luminal stenting represented the extent of this endoscopic capability for decades. In the last 10 years, we have seen the development of endoluminal therapies for GERD, obesity, and ESD providing an en bloc curative treatment for early gastrointestinal malignancies. We are now experiencing the development of submucosal surgery which promises to further extend the capabilities of the flexible endoscope. MIS (laparoscopic) has progressed in parallel with therapeutic endoscopy. The early NOTES movement brought disciples of MIS and endoscopy together and as a result, we saw the emergence of hybrid procedures. Combining laparoscopy and flexible endoscopy has served to further accelerate both disciplines. Nevertheless, we are seeing a slow but steady conversion of surgical procedures to less invasive endoscopic procedures; ESD replacing gastrectomy, POEM replacing Heller's myotomy, and STER for the management of esophageal and gastric GISTs. Refinements in endoluminal treatments for GERD and obesity will likely erode into Nissen's fundoplication and bariatric surgery. Endoscopic manipulation of the duodenum holds promise as a treatment for type 2 diabetes and possibly other metabolic diseases such as nonalcoholic steatohepatitis (NASH). Finally, after the introduction of NOTES by Kalloo and Kantsevoy in 2002, we are now seeing the early results from basic work that has taken place since their seminal presentation at DDW in 2005. POEM issued in the true NOTES era and now transanal colon resection will accelerate the movement. Endoluminal therapies, submucosal surgery, and NOTES will ensure that the flexible endoscope will continue to play a vital role in minimally invasive therapies. The future is bright for young physicians and surgeons with imagination and energy who are willing to obtain the requisite training to become the minimally invasive therapist of the future. In this era of health care reform and lowering costs, an improving outcome is paramount, solutions can be found with minimally invasive therapies utilizing a flexible platform through a natural orifice.

References

[1] Kalloo AN, Singh VK, Jagannath SB, et al. Flexible transgastric peritoneoscopy: a novel approach to diagnostic and therapeutic interventions in the peritoneal cavity. Gastrointest Endosc. 2004; 60(1):114–117

[2] Kantsevoy SV, Jagannath SB, Niiyama H, et al. Endoscopic gastrojejunostomy with survival in a porcine model. Gastrointest Endosc. 2005; 62(2):287–292

[3] Rattner D, Kalloo A;. ASGE/SAGES Working Group. ASGE/SAGES working group on natural orifice transluminal endoscopic surgery. October 2005. Surg Endosc. 2006; 20(2):329–333

[4] Sumiyama K, Gostout CJ, Rajan E, et al. Transgastric cholecystectomy: transgastric accessibility to the gallbladder improved with the SEMF method and a novel multibending therapeutic endoscope. Gastrointest Endosc. 2007; 65(7):1028–1034

[5] Sumiyama K, Gostout CJ, Rajan E, , et al. Submucosal endoscopy with mucosal flap safety valve. Gastrointest Endosc. 2007; 65(4):688–694

[6] Sumiyama K, Tajiri H, Gostout CJ. Submucosal endoscopy with mucosal flap safety valve (SEMF) technique: a safe access method into the peritoneal cavity and mediastinum. Minim Invasive Ther Allied Technol. 2008; 17(6):365–369

[7] Gostout CJ, Knipschield MA. Submucosal endoscopy with mucosal resection: a hybrid endoscopic submucosal dissection in the porcine rectum and distal colon. Gastrointest Endosc. 2012; 76(4):829–834

[8] Pasricha PJ, Hawari R, Ahmed I, et al. Submucosal endoscopic esophageal myotomy: a novel experimental approach for the treatment of achalasia. Endoscopy. 2007; 39(9):761–764

[9] Inoue H, Kudo SE. [Per-oral endoscopic myotomy (POEM) for 43 consecutive cases of esophageal achalasia] Nihon Rinsho. 2010; 68(9):1749–1752

[10] Inoue H, Minami H, Kobayashi Y, et al. Peroral endoscopic myotomy (POEM) for esophageal achalasia. Endoscopy. 2010; 42(4):265–271

[11] Bredenoord AJ, Fox M, Kahrilas PJ, et al.; International High Resolution Manometry Working Group. Chicago classification criteria of esophageal motility disorders defined in high resolution esophageal pressure topography. Neurogastroenterol Motil. 2012; 24(suppl 1):57–65

[12] Kahrilas PJ, Bredenoord AJ, Fox M, et al; International High Resolution Manometry Working Group. The Chicago Classification of esophageal motility disorders, v3.0. Neurogastroenterol Motil. 2015; 27(2):160–174

[13] Khashab MA, Stein E, Clarke JO, et al. Gastric peroral endoscopic myotomy for refractory gastroparesis: first human endoscopic pyloromyotomy (with video). Gastrointest Endosc. 2013; 78(5):764–768

[14] Rattner DW, Hawes R, Schwaitzberg S, et al. The Second SAGES/ASGE White Paper on natural orifice transluminal endoscopic surgery: 5 years of progress. Surg Endosc. 2011; 25(8):2441–2448

[15] Zornig C, Mofid H, Emmermann A, et al. Scarless cholecystectomy with combined transvaginal and transumbilical approach in a series of 20 patients. Surg Endosc. 2008; 22(6):1427–1429

[16] Gee DW, Rattner DW. Transmediastinal endoscopic intervention. J Gastrointest Surg. 2011; 15(8):1303–1305

[17] Bazzi WM, Wagner O, Stroup SP, et al. Transrectal hybrid natural orifice transluminal endoscopic surgery (NOTES) nephrectomy in a porcine model. Urology. 2011; 77(3):518–523

[18] Fischer LJ, Jacobsen G, Wong B, et al. NOTES laparoscopic-assisted transvaginal sleeve gastrectomy in humans—description of preliminary experience in the United States. Surg Obes Relat Dis. 2009; 5(5):633–636

[19] Whiteford MH, Denk PM, Swanström LL. Feasibility of radical sigmoid colectomy performed as natural orifice transluminal endoscopic surgery (NOTES) using transanal endoscopic microsurgery. Surg Endosc. 2007; 21(10):1870–1874

[20] Sylla P, Willingham FF, Sohn DK, et al. NOTES rectosigmoid resection using transanal endoscopic microsurgery (TEM) with transgastric endoscopic assistance: a pilot study in swine. J Gastrointest Surg. 2008; 12(10):1717–1723

[21] Sylla P, Sohn DK, Cizginer S, et al. Survival study of natural orifice transluminal endoscopic surgery for rectosigmoid resection using transanal endoscopic microsurgery with or without transgastric endoscopic assistance in a swine model. Surg Endosc. 2010; 24(8):2022–2030

[22] Denk PM, Swanström LL, Whiteford MH. Transanal endoscopic microsurgical platform for natural orifice surgery. Gastrointest Endosc. 2008; 68(5):954–959

[23] Rieder E, Spaun GO, Khajanchee YS, et al. A natural orifice transrectal approach for oncologic resection of the rectosigmoid: an experimental study and comparison with conventional laparoscopy. Surg Endosc. 2011; 25(10):3357–3363

[24] Sylla P, Rattner DW, Delgado S, Lacy AM. NOTES transanal rectal cancer resection using transanal endoscopic microsurgery and laparoscopic assistance. Surg Endosc. 2010; 24(5):1205–1210

[25] https://clinicaltrials.gov/ct2/results?cond=trans+anal+TME&term=&cntry1=&state1=&Search=Search

[26] Prohm P, Weber J, Bönner C. Laparoscopic-assisted colonoscopic polypectomy. Dis Colon Rectum. 2001; 44(5):746–748

[27] Novitsky YW, Kercher KW, Sing RF, Heniford BT. Long-term outcomes of laparoscopic resection of gastric gastrointestinal stromal tumors. Ann Surg. 2006; 243(6):738–745, discussion 745–747

[28] Wilhelm D, von Delius S, Burian M, et al. Simultaneous use of laparoscopy and endoscopy for minimally invasive resection of gastric subepithelial masses—analysis of 93 interventions. World J Surg. 2008; 32(6):1021–1028

[29] Huguet KL, Rush RM, Jr, Tessier DJ, et al. Laparoscopic gastric gastrointestinal stromal tumor resection: the mayo clinic experience. Arch Surg. 2008; 143(6):587–590, discussion 591

[30] Hepworth CC, Menzies D, Motson RW. Minimally invasive surgery for posterior gastric stromal tumors. Surg Endosc. 2000; 14(4):349–353

[31] Matthews BD, Walsh RM, Kercher KW, et al. Laparoscopic vs open resection of gastric stromal tumors. Surg Endosc. 2002; 16(5):803–807

[32] Marzano E, Ntourakis D, Addeo P, et al. Robotic resection of duodenal adenoma. Int J Med Robot. 2011; 7(1):66–70

[33] Ohashi S. Laparoscopic intraluminal (intragastric) surgery for early gastric cancer. A new concept in laparoscopic surgery. Surg Endosc. 1995; 9(2):169–171

[34] Schubert D, Kuhn R, Nestler G, et al. Laparoscopic-endoscopic rendezvous resection of upper gastrointestinal tumors. Dig Dis. 2005; 23(2):106–112

[35] Privette A, McCahill L, Borrazzo E, et al. Laparoscopic approaches to resection of suspected gastric gastrointestinal stromal tumors based on tumor location. Surg Endosc. 2008; 22(2):487–494

[36] Lamm SH, Steinemann DC, Linke GR, et al. Total inverse transgastric resection with transoral specimen removal. Surg Endosc. 2015; 29(11):3363–3366

[37] Shim JH, Lee HH, Yoo HM, et al. Intragastric approach for submucosal tumors located near the Z-line: a hybrid laparoscopic and endoscopic technique. J Surg Oncol. 2011; 104(3):312–315

[38] Ridwelski K, Pross M, Schubert S, et al. Combined endoscopic intragastral resection of a posterior stromal gastric tumor using an original technique. Surg Endosc. 2002; 16(3):537

[39] Pross M, Wolff S, Nestler G, et al. A technique for endo-organ resection of gastric wall tumors using one intragastric trocar. Endoscopy. 2003; 35(7):613–615

[40] Hiki N, Yamamoto Y, Fukunaga T, et al. Laparoscopic and endoscopic cooperative surgery for gastrointestinal stromal tumor dissection. Surg Endosc. 2008; 22(7):1729–1735

[41] Kawahira H, Hayashi H, Natsume T, et al. Surgical advantages of gastric SMTs by laparoscopy and endoscopy cooperative surgery. Hepatogastroenterology. 2012; 59(114):415–417

[42] Hirokawa F, Hayashi M, Miyamoto Y, et al. Laparoscopic and endoscopic cooperative surgery for duodenal tumor resection. Endoscopy. 2014; 46(suppl 1 UCTN):E26–E27

[43] Nunobe S, Hiki N, Gotoda T, et al. Successful application of laparoscopic and endoscopic cooperative surgery (LECS) for a lateral-spreading mucosal gastric cancer. Gastric Cancer. 2012; 15(3):338–342

[44] Abe N, Takeuchi H, Yanagida O, et al. Endoscopic full-thickness resection with laparoscopic assistance as hybrid NOTES for gastric submucosal tumor. Surg Endosc. 2009; 23(8):1908–1913

[45] Inoue H, Ikeda H, Hosoya T, et al. Endoscopic mucosal resection, endoscopic submucosal dissection, and beyond: full-layer resection for gastric cancer with non-exposure technique (CLEAN-NET). Surg Oncol Clin N Am. 2012; 21(1):129–140

[46] Goto O, Mitsui T, Fujishiro M, et al. New method of endoscopic full-thickness resection: a pilot study of non-exposed endoscopic wall-inversion surgery in an ex vivo porcine model. Gastric Cancer. 2011; 14(2):183–187

[47] Mitsui T, Niimi K, Yamashita H, et al. Non-exposed endoscopic wall-inversion surgery as a novel partial gastrectomy technique. Gastric Cancer. 2014; 17(3):594–599

[48] Goto O, Takeuchi H, Kawakubo H, et al. First case of non-exposed endoscopic wall-inversion surgery with sentinel node basin dissection for early gastric cancer. Gastric Cancer. 2015; 18(2):434–439

22 Gastroesophageal Reflux Disease and Infectious Esophagitis

Hye Yeon Jhun and Prateek Sharma

Gastroesophageal reflux disease (GERD) is one of the most common reason for a patient to visit to a gastroenterologist. This is characterized as a condition when reflux of the stomach contents into the esophagus cause troublesome symptoms and complications.[1] It remains a highly prevalent disease worldwide with an estimate of 18 to 28% in North America with only East Asia showing prevalence less than 10%.[2] GERD includes a constellation of symptoms including heartburn, regurgitation, dysphagia, chest pain, and extraesophageal syndromes including chronic cough, asthma, and laryngitis that can easily affect the quality of life.[3] In addition, the spectrum of injury and long-term complications include erosive esophagitis, esophageal stricture formation, and Barrett's esophagus which can progress to esophageal adenocarcinoma.[4] Therefore, accurate diagnosis and appropriate management are imperative.

22.1 Diagnostic Approaches

A presumptive diagnosis of GERD can be made in the setting of typical symptoms including heartburn and regurgitation.[5] An empiric trial with proton pump inhibitor (PPI) can be a simple method for diagnosing GERD and assessing symptoms. GERD can be established if symptoms respond to 1 to 2 weeks of therapy and recur when medication is discontinued. Although practical, this approach has shown to have a sensitivity of 78% and a low specificity of 54% with using 24-hour pH monitoring as a reference standard, suggesting that a negative trial with PPI does not rule out GERD.[6]

Upper gastrointestinal (GI) endoscopy is the standard diagnostic method used to evaluate the esophageal mucosa in patients with GERD. This should be especially considered in patients with alarm symptoms such as dysphagia, odynophagia, involuntary weight loss, evidence of GI bleeding, anemia, abnormal imaging studies, persistent vomiting for 7 to 10 days[7] or inadequate response to appropriate medical therapy. Endoscopic findings suggestive of reflux esophagitis include the presence of definitive mucosal breaks (erosions), ulceration, peptic stricture, and Barrett's esophagus. However, more than 50% of patients with heartburn and regurgitation have normal endoscopic findings. Thus, the sensitivity of diagnosing GERD by endoscopy is low, but the specificity has been reported as high as 90 to 95%.[8]

Erosive esophagitis has been reported in up to 30 to 40% in patients with GERD symptoms.[9] However, the correlation between severity of GERD symptoms and degree of underline esophageal mucosal damage is poor. Early signs of acid reflux could potentially include subtle findings of erythema and edematous changes of the mucosa. With progressive acid injury, erosions can develop near the gastroesophageal junction (GEJ) that are characterized by a mucosal break with whitish or yellowish exudates.

There are multiple classification systems that have been developed to characterize the degree and severity of erosive esophagitis. The most commonly used classification systems are the Los Angeles (LA) classification and Savary-Miller system that have been used in multiple clinical studies and practices to document the severity of the disease. The LA classification (▶Table 22.1, ▶Fig. 22.1) has excellent intraobserver and interobserver reliability regardless of the experience of the endoscopist[10] and is commonly used in clinical practice to document disease severity.

Endoscopy also provides utility as biopsy for histology can be obtained during the procedure. It is currently recommended to take biopsies for esophagitis for immune-compromised patients, to rule out eosinophilic esophagitis in those with dysphagia, presence of irregular or deep ulcers, proximal location of esophagitis, columnar lined esophagus, presence of esophageal mass, nodularity, and irregular esophageal strictures to rule out other diagnosis including infection and malignancy.[7] Furthermore, endoscopic evaluation is recommended by several guidelines in patients with chronic GERD with multiple risk factors including male gender, age above 50 years, Caucasian race, and central obesity to screen for Barrett's esophagus.[11]

Ambulatory pH monitoring is another diagnostic test for GERD that allows correlation between symptoms and reflux episodes and determines reflux frequency and abnormal esophageal acid exposure. This can be performed by either insertion of a transnasal catheter (impedance–pH monitoring for 24 hours) or by placing a telemetry capsule (pH monitoring for 48 hours) endoscopically. Reflux monitoring is recommended while off PPI in both modalities, however, testing on PPI can be performed with impedance–pH monitoring to measure nonacid reflux.[5]

22.2 Therapeutic Approaches

Treatment for GERD should be targeted based on specific goals. For patients without erosive esophagitis, the goals are to provide complete or sufficient control of symptoms and to prevent symptomatic relapse. For patients with esophagitis, the goals are to heal the underline mucosa, maintain endoscopic remission, and to treat and prevent possible complications.[12]

Lifestyle modifications should be recommended in all patients with GERD. Several randomized control studies have

Table 22.1 Los Angeles classification of erosive esophagitis

Classification	Grade	Description
Los Angeles	A	One (or more) mucosal break not longer than 5 mm that does not extend between the tops of two mucosal folds
	B	One (or more) mucosal break longer than 5 mm that does not extend between the tops of two mucosal folds
	C	One (or more) mucosal break that is continuous between the tops of more than two mucosal folds but involves < 75% of the circumference
	D	One (or more) mucosal break that involves at least 75% of the circumference

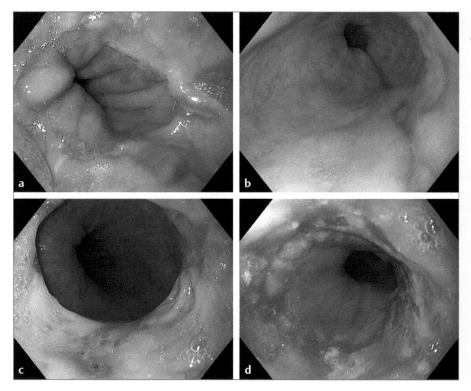

Fig. 22.1 Los Angeles classification of erosive esophagitis.

demonstrated improvement in GERD symptoms and esophageal acid exposure as measured by 24-hour pH testing when the head of the bed is elevated by wedges or blocks specially in patients that have nocturnal GERD.[13,14,15,16] Multiple case–control studies[15,16] have shown significant association between weight loss and improvement in GERD symptoms and esophageal acid exposure. Increase in body mass index (BMI), even in patients with normal BMI of more than 3.5 was associated with increased reflux symptoms. Therefore, it is recommended to encourage weight reduction in patients with BMI greater than 25 or patients with recent weight gain.[7] Smoking cessation in normal-weight individuals on antireflux therapy have also shown to reduce reflux symptoms in a large prospective cohort study.[17] Currently, there is insufficient evidence to show clinical improvement with cessation of caffeine, chocolate, or carbonated beverages, and this is not routinely recommended unless patients notice correlation of symptoms and symptom improvement with elimination.[3]

Medical options for GERD include antacids, histamine-receptor antagonists (H_2RA), or PPI therapy. PPI therapy has shown to have a significantly faster healing rate and relief of symptoms compared to H_2RA in all grades of erosive esophagitis.[18] A meta-analysis of 7,635 patients with erosive esophagitis reported overall improvement with PPI therapy in 84% of the patients compared to 52% with H_2RA therapy and 28% with placebo.[18] Currently, an 8-week course of PPI is the standard treatment for patients with erosive esophagitis. No clinically significant difference in efficacy between different PPIs have been demonstrated.[19] Maintenance therapy with PPI should be considered to those who have recurrent symptoms once PPI is discontinued and in patients with erosive esophagitis and Barrett's esophagus.[5] A double-blinded comparison study with lansoprazole and ranitidine for long-term maintenance therapy of healed erosive esophagitis after acute treatment in 1 year showed 67% treated

with lansoprazole remained healed, compared to 13% treated with ranitidine.[20]

22.3 Surgical Therapy

Surgical therapy (Nissen's fundoplication) is another long-term therapy option for patients with chronic GERD. This can be considered in patients who wish to discontinue medical therapy, who have refractory esophagitis, or persistent symptoms specifically regurgitation in those with documented GERD. The best response to surgical therapy is seen in those GERD patients with typical symptoms and those with a good response to PPI therapy. In a randomized, open study by Galmiche et al,[21] a total of 372 patients were randomized to receive either PPI or undergo laparoscopic antireflux surgery (LARS) for chronic GERD and were followed up for 5 years. Symptom remission was reported in 92% of the patients on PPI and in 85% who received surgical fundoplication at 5 years. Complication rates were similar in both groups: 24% in PPI group and 29% in LARS group. Overall, this study demonstrated that most patients remained in remission with either antireflux therapy for GERD in 5 years.

A recent advance in minimally invasive surgical approaches to GERD has been the use of the "Linx" procedure, which gives augmentation of the esophageal sphincter with a magnetic device. This can be considered in patients who have incomplete response with PPI or who are reluctant to undergo surgical fundoplication. A recent study by Ganz et al[22] prospectively assessed 100 patients with GERD before and after sphincter augmentation. This showed a decrease of acid exposure in 64% of the patients and decreased use of PPI in 93% of the patients. Most frequent adverse effects were dysphagia seen in 68% of patients postoperatively, which was 11% at 1 year and 4% at 3 years.

22.4 Endoscopic Therapy for GERD

Endoscopic therapies for GERD include radiofrequency energy, suturing, and transoral incisionless fundoplication (TIF). The "Stretta" procedure is a technique that uses radiofrequency energy to the lower esophageal sphincter. In theory, this is to induce muscle proliferation and fibrosis in the submucosa and muscle layer to create a less compliant esophagus. However, there are no human histopathologic data to indicate increase in smooth muscle density after the Stretta procedure at this time. The two main physiologic effects of the Stretta procedure are to create an increase in lower esophageal sphincter pressure and a decrease in transient lower esophageal relaxations.

An open-label trial in 118 patients observed objective improvement in esophageal acid exposure and GERD symptom scores with repeat measured analysis in 12 months.[23] Subsequent studies have demonstrated Stretta to eliminate PPI usage in 43 to 72% of the patients and achieving effective and satisfactory long-term symptom control for 5 to 10 years with infrequent adverse effects.[24,25] Corley et al[26] studied 64 patients who were randomized to receive either Stretta (n = 35) or sham (n =29) therapy. This study showed that radiofrequency energy delivery improved reflux symptoms and quality of life, but did not decrease the acid exposure time or medication use in 6 months compared to the sham group. A recent meta-analysis[27] including four randomized control trials overall demonstrated no difference with Stretta versus sham in acid exposure time, PPI withdrawal, or quality of life. Overall studies have not shown consistent efficacy with Stretta therapy and therefore, is not recommended as an alternative over medical therapy or surgery for treatment of GERD.[5]

TIF procedure has gone through a number of technical revisions since its initial approval in 2007 to closely replicate surgical fundoplication. The device is placed in the stomach to construct a full-thickness plication with polypropylene stiches 3 to 5 cm above the GEJ to create a gastroesophageal flap valve.[28] Most studies involving TIF have been based on short-term follow-up. In a recent randomized, blinded, sham-control trial with 129 patients which excluded patients with hiatal hernia greater than 2 cm in length showed TIF to eliminate troublesome regurgitation in 67% of the patients compared to 45% in patients who received sham treatment and PPI in 6 months.[29] TIF was also associated with decrease in number of reflux episodes and showed modest improvement of intraesophageal pH. However, it failed to provide improvement in heartburn symptoms suggesting this procedure may not be useful for PPI refractory heartburn patients.

Limited studies with long-term follow-up have reported that TIF may provide reduction or cessation of PPI use up to 2 to 6 years.[30,31,32] Periprocedural complication rates have been described to be low. Among 492 patients who underwent TIF procedure, both esophageal perforation and pneumothorax were reported as 0.4%.[33] Although there is no evidence to propose, TIF is more effective than surgical fundoplication. TIF can be considered most effective in a subgroup of patients with chronic GERD with hiatal hernia less than 2 cm.[31,32] Therefore, careful patient selection and experience of the endoscopist should be considered prior to receiving therapy. Further prospective studies evaluating long-term treatment efficacy and complications are needed in this field.

22.5 Infectious Esophagitis

Infectious esophagitis can be caused by fungal, bacterial, viral, or parasitic organisms. They are commonly seen in immune-compromised patients such as patients with human immunodeficiency virus infection, hematologic malignancy, or those who have received chemotherapy or organ transplantation. However, esophageal infections can still develop in immune-competent patients, especially if they have underlying esophageal disease. Diagnosis is based on endoscopic findings and confirmed by tissue sampling for histopathology.

22.5.1 Candida Esophagitis

Candida esophagitis is the most common infection of the esophagus. It has been reported to have a prevalence between 1.7 and 3.8% of patient's undergoing endoscopy for diagnostic work-ups (upper GI symptoms, abnormal test including anemia, or positive fecal occult blood testing), gastric cancer screening, and/or therapeutic endoscopy.[34,35] It mostly affects immune-compromised patients, but can also be seen in immune-competent patients with advanced age, underline history of diabetes, alcohol use, smoking, usage of glucocorticoids, acid suppression therapy, and recent exposure to antibiotics.[36,37] Underlying dysmotility of the esophagus that leads to luminal stasis has also been associated with an increased risk of infection.

Patients typically present with symptoms of odynophagia, dysphagia, epigastric pain, and heartburn and may have concomitant oral thrush. However, not all cases are symptomatic and up to 20% of healthy adults and 40% of immune-compromised patients with *Candida* esophagitis do not report any of the above-mentioned symptoms.

Diagnosis of *Candida* esophagitis is usually made based on characteristic findings seen during upper endoscopy of white plaque–like mucosal lesions that are difficult to wash away. These lesions can be sparse or may coalesce to form a white pseudomembrane carpeting the entire mucosa in severe cases (▶Fig. 22.2). Endoscopic findings can be graded using the Kodsi's classification shown in ▶Table 22.2. Multiple biopsies of the affected area and brushings for cytology should be obtained[38] for histopathology. This would typically show the presence of yeast and invasion of pseudohyphae into the mucosal cells (▶Fig. 22.3). Budding years may be seen more clearly with periodic acid–Schiff staining (▶Fig. 22.4) or methenamine silver stain (▶Fig. 22.5). Identification of a causative organ is crucial in making the diagnosis of infectious esophagitis as histopathology alone cannot sometimes differentiate between reflux esophagitis and infectious esophagitis.[39]

Empiric treatment with antifungal medication can be initiated in immune-compromised patients with classic esophageal symptoms and presence of oral thrush. However, if symptoms do not improve in 3 to 5 days, endoscopy is recommended to rule out other viral infections. Systemic antifungal therapy is always required and treatment with oral fluconazole with 200 to 400 mg (3–6 mg/kg) daily for 14 to 21 days is recommended.[40] In refractory cases, voriconazole, posaconazole, or itraconazole for 3 weeks should be administered.[40] *Candida glabrata* is a non-albicans fungal esophagitis that has up to a 20%

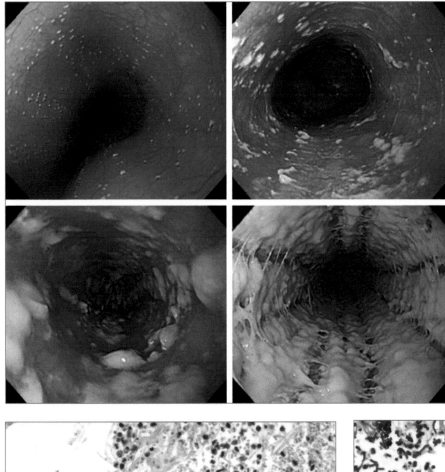

Fig. 22.2 Relationship between clinical factors and severity of esophageal candidiasis according to Kodsi's classification. Reproduced with permission from Asayama N et al. Dis Esophagus 2014;27: 214–219.

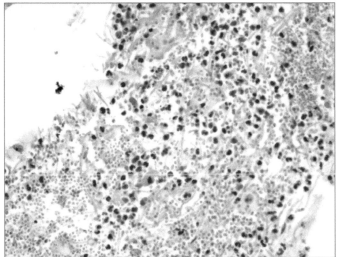

Fig. 22.3 Hematoxylin and eosin stain of *Candida* spp. (Image is provided courtesy of Sharad C. Mathur, MD; Pathology and Laboratory Medicine Service, Kansas City VA Medical Center.)

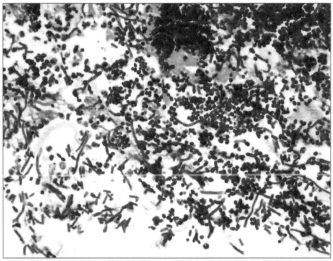

Fig. 22.4 Periodic acid–Schiff for *Candida* spp. (Image is provided courtesy of Sharad C. Mathur, MD; Pathology and Laboratory Medicine Service, Kansas City VA Medical Center.)

Table 22.2 Kodsi's classification of endoscopic grading of *Candida* esophagitis

Grade	Description
I	Raised whitish plaques < 2 mm in diameter without ulceration
II	Raised whitish plaques > 2 mm in diameter without ulceration
III	Confluent linear and nodular plaques with ulceration
IV	Grade III findings with narrowing of the esophageal ulcer

reported resistance to fluconazole.[41] Therefore, current guidelines recommend higher dosage of fluconazole 800 mg daily for fluconazole-susceptible isolates and amphotericin B (AmB) deoxycholate or oral flucytosine for fluconazole-resistant *C. glabrata*.[40]

22.5.2 Herpes Simplex Virus Esophagitis

Herpes simplex virus (HSV) infection is commonly seen throughout the world, and involvement of the esophagus has been frequently recognized. This can occur in both immune-compromised and immune-competent hosts. Typical presentation in an immune-competent patient is a young man presenting with odynophagia, chest pain, and fever. Odynophagia is the most common clinical manifestation seen in 76% of the patients. Concurrent oral lesions are less common and documented in about 21% of the patients.[42]

Early endoscopic findings of HSV esophagitis are those of small round vesicles in the mid-to-distal esophagus. As the infection

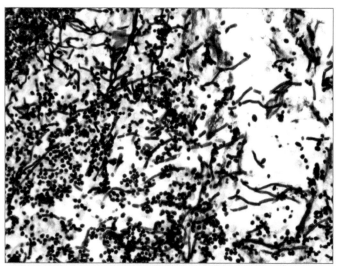

Fig. 22.5 Grocott's methenamine silver stain for *Candida* spp. (Image is provided courtesy of Sharad C. Mathur, MD; Pathology and Laboratory Medicine Service, Kansas City VA Medical Center.)

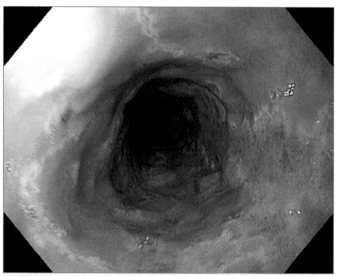

Fig. 22.6 Ulcerated lesions associated with herpes simplex virus esophagitis.

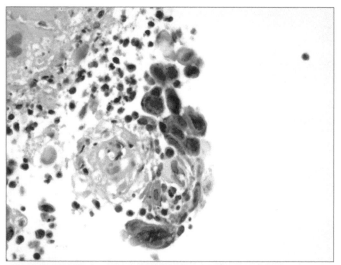

Fig. 22.7 Hematoxylin and eosin stain of herpes simplex virus. (Image is provided courtesy of Sharad C. Mathur, MD; Pathology and Laboratory Medicine Service, Kansas City VA Medical Center.)

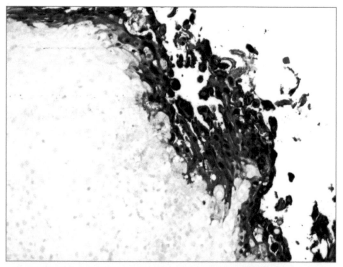

Fig. 22.8 Immunohistochemical stain for herpes simplex virus. (Image is provided courtesy of Sharad C. Mathur, MD; Pathology and Laboratory Medicine Service, Kansas City VA Medical Center.)

progresses, the vesicle centers slough to form a well-circumscribed ulcer that has a "volcano-like" appearance (▶ Fig. 22.6). These lesions can coalesce to produce friable mucosa, hemorrhage, and mucosal necrosis. HSV infects squamous epithelial cells, which is absent from ulcer craters as they tend to slough off. Therefore, biopsies should be obtained from the ulcer margins to have the highest diagnostic yield. Biopsy samples should be sent for standard histology (▶ Fig. 22.7), immunohistochemistry staining (▶ Fig. 22.8), and possibly HSV culture and HSV polymerase chain reaction (PCR). Histologically, this would show multinucleated giant cells with eosinophilic intranuclear inclusions (Cowdry A inclusion body) or ground-glass nuclei inclusions (Cowdry B inclusion body). The sensitivity of HSV PCR has been reported as more than 92%, and specificity as 100%.

Spontaneous resolution of HSV esophagitis usually occurs in immune-competent patients. Some patients may respond quickly with a short course of oral acyclovir 200 mg five times a day or 400 mg times a day administered for 7 to 10 days. In immune-compromised patients, a longer course of antiviral agents for 14 to 21 days is recommended. In cases of severe

infection, treatment can be started with intravenous (IV) acyclovir 5 mg/kg IV every 8 hours which can be changed to oral agents: acyclovir 400 mg three times a day, famciclovir 500 mg two times a day, or valacyclovir 1 g two times a day. Refractory cases are likely due to viruses that have mutations with thymidine kinase that are resistant to acyclovir. Intravenous foscarnet 80 to 120 mg/d is recommended is these cases.[43]

22.5.3 Cytomegalovirus Esophagitis

Cytomegalovirus (CMV) esophagitis is less commonly reported than *C.* esophagitis and HSV esophagitis and accounts of 0.01% of all esophageal ulcers.[44] CMV esophagitis is usually observed in patients posttransplantation, and the average time to develop CMV esophagitis after solid organ transplantation is 6 months.[44]

On endoscopy, patients with CMV infection, typically have deep ulcers in the distal esophagus and patchier and superficial ulcers in the upper and mid esophagus. In contrast to HSV infection, CMV typically involves the endothelium cells and vessels and spares epithelial cells. Therefore, biopsies should be taken from the base of the ulcers to optimize sampling and diagnostic accuracy. Taking three biopsy samples from the ulcer base has shown to have a diagnostic yield of 80%, and if up to 7 to 10 biopsies are obtained, the yield is shown to increase up to 100%.[45] Sampled tissue should be further sent for CMV PCR as this has a higher sensitivity than histopathology and also detects both latent and clinical disease. Evidence of enlarged cells with intranuclear inclusion bodies, often described as "owl's eye" appearance are diagnostic histologic findings. Serologic studies are not recommended as 80% of the world's population is seropositive for CMV infection.[46] CMV culture from tissue samples is also insufficient to establish the diagnosis as this can be positive in the absence of clinical disease.[47]

All patients diagnosed with CMV esophagitis need treatment with antiviral therapy. Intravenous ganciclovir 5 mg/kg every 12 hours is preferred as induction therapy that can be switched to oral valganciclovir 900 mg every 12 hours once patients can tolerate oral therapy. Treatment should be continued until 2 weeks after virologic clearance. In patients with relapsed disease, maintenance therapy with oral valganciclovir 900 mg twice a day should be continued.[43]

22.5.4 Other Infections

Other infections involving the esophagus include human immunodeficiency virus (HIV), *Mycobacterium tuberculosis*, *Histoplasma capsulatum*, *Treponema pallidum*, and human papilloma virus. A wide variety of esophageal ulcerations can be seen with these pathogens, and diagnosis can be made in most cases by tissue biopsies and cytologic brushings. HIV esophagitis is a diagnosis of exclusion that can be made once other infections (*Candida*, CMV, HSV) have been excluded.

References

[1] Vakil N, van Zanten SV, Kahrilas P, et al; Global Consensus Group. The Montreal definition and classification of gastroesophageal reflux disease: a global evidence-based consensus. Am J Gastroenterol. 2006; 101(8):1900–1920, quiz 1943

[2] El-Serag HB, Sweet S, Winchester CC, Dent J. Update on the epidemiology of gastro-oesophageal reflux disease: a systematic review. Gut. 2014; 63(6):871–880

[3] Becher A, El-Serag H. Systematic review: the association between symptomatic response to proton pump inhibitors and health-related quality of life in patients with gastro-oesophageal reflux disease. Aliment Pharmacol Ther. 2011; 34(6):618–627

[4] Kahrilas PJ. Clinical practice. Gastroesophageal reflux disease. N Engl J Med. 2008; 359(16):1700–1707

[5] Katz PO, Gerson LB, Vela MF. Guidelines for the diagnosis and management of gastroesophageal reflux disease. Am J Gastroenterol. 2013; 108(3):308–328, quiz 329

[6] Numans ME, Lau J, de Wit NJ, Bonis PA. Short-term treatment with proton-pump inhibitors as a test for gastroesophageal reflux disease: a meta-analysis of diagnostic test characteristics. Ann Intern Med. 2004; 140(7):518–527

[7] Muthusamy VR, Lightdale JR, Acosta RD, et al; ASGE Standards of Practice Committee. The role of endoscopy in the management of GERD. Gastrointest Endosc. 2015; 81(6):1305–1310

[8] Richter JE. Severe reflux esophagitis. Gastrointest Endosc Clin N Am. 1994; 4(4):677–698

[9] Ronkainen J, Aro P, Storskrubb T, et al. High prevalence of gastroesophageal reflux symptoms and esophagitis with or without symptoms in the general adult Swedish population: a Kalixanda study report. Scand J Gastroenterol. 2005; 40(3):275–285

[10] Lundell LR, Dent J, Bennett JR, et al. Endoscopic assessment of oesophagitis: clinical and functional correlates and further validation of the Los Angeles classification. Gut. 1999; 45(2):172–180

[11] Shaheen NJ, Falk GW, Iyer PG, Gerson LB; American College of Gastroenterology. ACG clinical guideline: diagnosis and management of Barrett's esophagus. Am J Gastroenterol. 2016; 111(1):30–50, quiz 51

[12] Labenz J, Malfertheiner P. Treatment of uncomplicated reflux disease. World J Gastroenterol. 2005; 11(28):4291–4299

[13] Hamilton JW, Boisen RJ, Yamamoto DT, et al. Sleeping on a wedge diminishes exposure of the esophagus to refluxed acid. Dig Dis Sci. 1988; 33(5):518–522

[14] Pollmann H, Zillessen E, Pohl J, et al. [Effect of elevated head position in bed in therapy of gastroesophageal reflux] Z Gastroenterol. 1996; 34(suppl 2):93–99

[15] Fraser-Moodie CA, Norton B, Gornall C, et al. Weight loss has an independent beneficial effect on symptoms of gastro-oesophageal reflux in patients who are overweight. Scand J Gastroenterol. 1999; 34(4):337–340

[16] Mathus-Vliegen LM, Tytgat GN. Twenty-four-hour pH measurements in morbid obesity: effects of massive overweight, weight loss and gastric distension. Eur J Gastroenterol Hepatol. 1996; 8(7):635–640

[17] Ness-Jensen E, Lindam A, Lagergren J, Hveem K. Tobacco smoking cessation and improved gastroesophageal reflux: a prospective population-based cohort study: the HUNT study. Am J Gastroenterol. 2014; 109(2):171–177

[18] Chiba N, De Gara CJ, Wilkinson JM, Hunt RH. Speed of healing and symptom relief in grade II to IV gastroesophageal reflux disease: a meta-analysis. Gastroenterology. 1997; 112(6):1798–1810

[19] Zheng RN. Comparative study of omeprazole, lansoprazole, pantoprazole and esomeprazole for symptom relief in patients with reflux esophagitis. World J Gastroenterol. 2009; 15(8):990–995

[20] Peura DA, Freston JW, Haber MM, et al. Lansoprazole for long-term maintenance therapy of erosive esophagitis: double-blind comparison with ranitidine. Dig Dis Sci. 2009; 54(5):955–963

[21] Galmiche JP, Hatlebakk J, Attwood S, et al; LOTUS Trial Collaborators. Laparoscopic antireflux surgery vs esomeprazole treatment for chronic GERD: the LOTUS randomized clinical trial. JAMA. 2011; 305(19):1969–1977

[22] Ganz RA, Peters JH, Horgan S, et al. Esophageal sphincter device for gastroesophageal reflux disease. N Engl J Med. 2013; 368(8):719–727

[23] Triadafilopoulos G, DiBaise JK, Nostrant TT, et al. The Stretta procedure for the treatment of GERD: 6 and 12 month follow-up of the U.S. open label trial. Gastrointest Endosc. 2002; 55(2):149–156

[24] Liang WT, Wang ZG, Wang F, et al. Long-term outcomes of patients with refractory gastroesophageal reflux disease following a minimally invasive endoscopic procedure: a prospective observational study. BMC Gastroenterol. 2014; 14:178

[25] Dughera L, Navino M, Cassolino P, et al. Long-term results of radiofrequency energy delivery for the treatment of GERD: results of a prospective 48-month study. Diagn Ther Endosc. 2011; 2011:507157

[26] Corley DA, Katz P, Wo JM, et al. Improvement of gastroesophageal reflux symptoms after radiofrequency energy: a randomized, sham-controlled trial. Gastroenterology. 2003; 125(3):668–676

[27] Lipka S, Kumar A, Richter JE. No evidence for efficacy of radiofrequency ablation for treatment of gastroesophageal reflux disease: a systematic review and meta-analysis. Clin Gastroenterol Hepatol. 2015; 13(6):1058–67.e1

[28] Auyang ED, Carter P, Rauth T, Fanelli RD; SAGES Guidelines Committee. SAGES clinical spotlight review: endoluminal treatments for gastroesophageal reflux disease (GERD). Surg Endosc. 2013; 27(8):2658–2672

[29] Hunter JG, Kahrilas PJ, Bell RC, et al. Efficacy of transoral fundoplication vs omeprazole for treatment of regurgitation in a randomized controlled trial. Gastroenterology. 2015; 148(2):324–333.e5

[30] Hopkins J, Switzer NJ, Karmali S. Update on novel endoscopic therapies to treat gastroesophageal reflux disease: a review. World J Gastrointest Endosc. 2015; 7(11):1039–1044

[31] Bell RC, Barnes WE, Carter BJ, et al. Transoral incisionless fundoplication: 2-year results from the prospective multicenter U.S. study. Am Surg. 2014; 80(11):1093–1105

[32] Testoni PA, Testoni S, Mazzoleni G, et al. Long-term efficacy of transoral incisionless fundoplication with Esophyx (Tif 2.0) and factors affecting outcomes in GERD patients followed for up to 6 years: a prospective single-center study. Surg Endosc. 2015; 29(9):2770–2780

[33] Jain D, Singhal S. Transoral incisionless fundoplication for refractory gastroesophageal reflux disease: where do we stand? Clin Endosc. 2016; 49(2):147–156

[34] Takahashi Y, Nagata N, Shimbo T, et al. Long-term trends in esophageal candidiasis prevalence and associated risk factors with or without HIV infection: lessons from an endoscopic study of 80,219 patients. PLoS One. 2015; 10(7):e0133589

[35] Asayama N, Nagata N, Shimbo T, et al. Relationship between clinical factors and severity of esophageal candidiasis according to Kodsi's classification. Dis Esophagus. 2014; 27(3):214–219

[36] Chocarro Martínez A, Galindo Tobal F, Ruiz-Irastorza G, et al. Risk factors for esophageal candidiasis. Eur J Clin Microbiol Infect Dis. 2000; 19(2):96–100

[37] Kim KY, Jang JY, Kim JW, et al. Acid suppression therapy as a risk factor for Candida esophagitis. Dig Dis Sci. 2013; 58(5):1282–1286

[38] Sharaf RN, Shergill AK, Odze RD, et al; ASGE Standards of Practice Committee. Endoscopic mucosal tissue sampling. Gastrointest Endosc. 2013; 78(2):216–224

[39] Demir D, Doğanavşargil B, et al. Is it possible to diagnose infectious oesophagitis without seeing the causative organism? A histopathological study. Turk J Gastroenterol. 2014; 25(5):481–487

[40] Pappas PG, Kauffman CA, Andes DR, et al. Clinical practice guideline for the management of candidiasis: 2016 update by the Infectious Diseases Society of America. Clin Infect Dis. 2016; 62(4):e1–e50

[41] Pfaller MA, Diekema DJ. Epidemiology of invasive candidiasis: a persistent public health problem. Clin Microbiol Rev. 2007; 20(1):133–163

[42] Ramanathan J, Rammouni M, Baran J, Jr, Khatib R. Herpes simplex virus esophagitis in the immunocompetent host: an overview. Am J Gastroenterol. 2000; 95(9):2171–2176

[43] Kaplan JE, Benson C, Holmes KK, et al; Centers for Disease Control and Prevention (CDC). National Institutes of Health. HIV Medicine Association of the Infectious Diseases Society of America. Guidelines for prevention and treatment of opportunistic infections in HIV-infected adults and adolescents: recommendations from CDC, the National Institutes of Health, and the HIV Medicine Association of the Infectious Diseases Society of America. MMWR Recomm Rep. 2009; 58(RR-4):1–207, quiz CE1–CE4

[44] Wang HW, Kuo CJ, Lin WR, et al. The clinical characteristics and manifestations of cytomegalovirus esophagitis. Dis Esophagus. 2016 May; 29(4):392–399.

[45] Wilcox CM, Straub RF, Schwartz DA. Prospective evaluation of biopsy number for the diagnosis of viral esophagitis in patients with HIV infection and esophageal ulcer. Gastrointest Endosc. 1996; 44(5):587–593

[46] Bate SL, Dollard SC, Cannon MJ. Cytomegalovirus seroprevalence in the United States: the national health and nutrition examination surveys, 1988–2004. Clin Infect Dis. 2010; 50(11):1439–1447

[47] Péter A, Telkes G, Varga M, et al. Endoscopic diagnosis of cytomegalovirus infection of upper gastrointestinal tract in solid organ transplant recipients: Hungarian single-center experience. Clin Transplant. 2004; 18(5):580–584

23 Barrett's Esophagus and Early Neoplasia

Maximilien Barret, Roos E. Pouw, Kamar Belghazi, and Jacques J. G. H. M. Bergman

23.1 Diagnostic Work-Up for Barrett's Esophagus and Early Neoplasia

23.1.1 General Approach to Barrett's Esophagus

Definitions of Barrett's Esophagus

The diagnosis of Barrett's esophagus (BE) requires the presence of endoscopically visible columnar mucosa in the tubular esophagus. There is no consensus if the presence of intestinal metaplasia (IM) in biopsies from the tubular esophagus is a prerequisite for the diagnosis of BE. Guidelines from the United States[1] require histologic confirmation of IM for the diagnosis of BE, whereas the British guidelines also accept a histologic finding of fundic- or cardia-type metaplasia.[2,3]

All guidelines agree, however, that the presence of IM is the most important risk factor for an increased risk of esophageal adenocarcinoma (EAC) (▶ Table 23.1), and only advise endoscopic surveillance for those cases where the presence of IM is confirmed.

Definition of Dysplasia and Early Cancer

Malignant progression in BE is thought to be a multistep process, with progressive grades of dysplasia and eventually invasive cancer. Grading of neoplasia is performed according to the Vienna classification of gastrointestinal epithelial neoplasia: (1) negative for neoplasia/dysplasia, (2) indefinite for neoplasia/dysplasia, (3) noninvasive low-grade neoplasia (low-grade dysplasia [LGD]), (4) noninvasive high-grade neoplasia (high-grade dysplasia [HGD], noninvasive carcinoma and suspicion of invasive carcinoma), and (5) invasive neoplasia (intramucosal carcinoma, submucosal carcinoma, or beyond).[9]

Table 23.1 Guidelines on Barrett's esophagus diagnostic and surveillance from US, British, Dutch, and European Medical Societies, and international consensus statements

	ASGE, 2012[4]	BSG, 2014,2015[2,3]	International consensus, 2012 and 2015[5,6]	ACG, 2016[1]	Dutch guidelines[7]	ESGE, 2017[8]
BE definition	IM in biopsies from the tubular esophagus.	An esophagus in which any portion of the normal distal squamous epithelial lining has been replaced by *metaplastic columnar epithelium*, which is clearly visible *endoscopically* (≥ 1 cm) above the GE junction.	Any type of columnar metaplastic epithelium.	Salmon-colored mucosa into the tubular esophagus extending ≥ 1 cm proximal to the GE junction with biopsy confirmation of IM.	Endoscopically visible columnar epithelium in the esophagus with histologic confirmation of IM in biopsies.	Distal esophagus lined with columnar epithelium with a minimum length of 1 cm (tongues or circular) containing specialized intestinal metaplasia at histopathological examination.
Management of nondysplastic BE	"Consider no surveillance; if surveillance is selected, no more frequently than every 3–5 y."	Surveillance every 3–5 y if BE < 3cm, 2–3 y if BE ≥ 3cm.	No recommendations made. No surveillance if life expectancy is < 5 y. Restricted to high-risk groups: age ≥ 50 y, white race, male sex, obesity, and symptoms.	Surveillance every 3–5 y	BE < 1 cm: no surveillance. BE 1–3 cm: surveillance at 5 y. BE 3–10 cm: surveillance at 3 y. BE > 10 cm: referral to Barrett's expert center.	An irregular Z-line/columnar-lined esophagus of < 1 cm: no routine biopsies or endoscopic surveillance. BE ≥ 1 cm and < 3 cm: surveillance every 5 y. BE ≥ 3 cm and < 10 cm: surveillance every 3 y. BE ≥ 10 cm: referral to a Barrett's expert center for surveillance endoscopies. Patients > 75 yrs and no previous evidence of dysplasia: no subsequent surveillance.

Table 23.1 (*continued*) Guidelines on Barrett's esophagus diagnostic and surveillance from US, British, Dutch, and European Medical Societies, and international consensus statements

	ASGE, 2012[4]	BSG, 2014,2015[2,3]	International consensus, 2012 and 2015[5,6]	ACG, 2016[1]	Dutch guidelines[7]	ESGE, 2017[8]
Management of BE with low-grade dysplasia (LGD)	Surveillance endoscopy at 6 mo, then every year consider endoscopic ablation therapy.	Confirmed by 2 pathologists. Second endoscopy at 6 mo. If LGD is found in one follow-up endoscopy, consider ablation or 6 monthly follow-up.	Confirmed by 2 pathologists. Surveillance endoscopy every 6–12 mo. Ablation therapy if long-segment BE, multifocal dysplasia, or persistence of dysplasia over time.	Endoscopic therapy or surveillance endoscopy every 12 mo.	Confirmed by an expert pathologist. Referral to Barrett's expert center for RFA in case of a repeated diagnosis of LGD, or endoscopic surveillance after 6 mo and yearly thereafter in experienced hands: follow up after 6 mo and yearly thereafter.	If confirmed by 2nd expert GI pathologist, referral to BE expert center. Repeat surveillance endoscopy in 6 months. If no dysplasia: surveillance endoscopy after 1 year. After 2 subsequent negative endoscopies, follow NDBE recommendation. If confirmed LGD in subsequent endoscopies: endoscopic ablation should be preferred.
Surveillance intervals for BE with high-grade dysplasia	Surveillance endoscopy in the absence of endoscopic eradication therapy.	Surveillance endoscopy in the absence of endoscopic eradication therapy.	Not recommended.	Not recommended.	Only recommended as an alternative for therapy in selected cases (severe comorbidity or short life expectance). Intervals: first year 3-monthly, second year 6-monthly, and yearly hereafter.	Not recommended.
Management of high-grade dysplasia/early cancer	Endoscopic eradication therapy.	Endoscopic eradication therapy.	Endoscopic eradication therapy.	Endoscopic eradication therapy.	Endoscopic resection of visible lesions and eradication of residual BE (preferably with RFA).	If confirmed by 2nd expert GI pathologist, referral to BE expert center for high-definition endoscopy: -Endoscopic resection of visible lesions - In absence of visible lesions, random 4-quadrant biopsies.If negative for dysplasia, endoscopy in 3 months. If HGD is confirmed, endoscopic ablation (preferably with RFA).
Surveillance after ablation therapy	Every 3 mo for the first year, every 6 mo in the second year, and annually thereafter.	Every 3 mo for the first year and yearly thereafter.	Needed (surveillance intervals not clearly stated).	Every 3 mo for the first year, every 6 mo in the second year, and annually thereafter	3, 9, and 21 mo, then annually during the first 5 y. If no more IM at that stage, follow-up can be stopped or intervals prolonged.	Surveillance intervals not stated.

ASGE, American Society of Gastrointestinal Endoscopy; BSG, British Society of Gastroenterology; ACG, American College of Gastroenterology; BE, Barrett's esophagus; ESGE, European Society of Gastrointestinal Endoscopy; IM,intestinal metaplasia; GE, gastroesophageal; RFA, radiofrequency ablation.

Importantly, the assessment of dysplasia can be troubled by the presence of inflammatory changes in the epithelium; therefore, reflux esophagitis grade C or D should be controlled prior to biopsy, and repeat endoscopic assessment after proton pump inhibitor (PPI) therapy for 8 to 12 weeks is recommended.[1]

Indefinite for dysplasia is not an intermediate step in the pathogenesis of EAC, but rather a temporary diagnosis used when the biopsies show some features of dysplasia, but when epithelial regeneration (inflammation, erosion) might account for the atypia. Close follow-up is recommended, with a repeat endoscopy after optimization of acid-suppressive medications for 3 to 6 months. If the "indefinite for dysplasia" diagnosis is confirmed on this examination, a surveillance interval of 12 months is recommended.[1]

Endoscopic Classification of Barrett's Esophagus and Early Neoplastic Lesions

Classification of Barrett's Esophagus

To describe the endoscopic extent of BE, the Prague classification was developed and validated in 2006.[10] This classification reports the circumferential extent (C) and the maximal extent of the Barrett's segment (M), measured from the upper end of the gastric folds (▶ Fig. 23.1). For example, with the top of the gastric folds measured at 38 cm of the dental arcade, circumferential Barrett's mucosa up to 36 cm, and Barrett's tongues extending up to 33 cm, the BE segment will be reported as C2M5.The Prague classification uses the proximal extent of the gastric folds as the gastroesophageal (GE) junction landmark for the distal margin of the Barrett's segment. However, the definition of the GE junction remains a matter of debate. Localizing the most proximal extent of the gastric folds can be affected by the distention of the distal esophagus and proximal stomach; for example, overinsufflation of a hiatal hernia may lead to overdiagnosis of BE. In Asia, endoscopists tend to define the GE junction at the distal extent of the palisade vessels, which are fine longitudinal veins located in superficial layers of the distal esophagus.[9,11] The working group that developed the Prague C&M criteria did consider the palisade vessels as an alternative landmark but found it not to be reliably assessable in most of the BE videos they used in the validation process.[10] In addition, studies have shown a poor interobserver agreement for determining the lower end of the palisade zone. Other studies have reported that its use is associated with a prevalence of BE greater than 15% in Japanese patients referred for standard endoscopy, a rate which virtually proves the low reliability of this landmark.[12,13]

Irrespective of the definition of the GE junction, differentiating an irregular Z-line with small triangular extensions of gastric mucosa in the tubular esophagus from an ultrashort-segment BE (< 1cm), remains a challenge for the endoscopist. Three main studies have well demonstrated the extremely low risk of neoplastic progression of IM of such findings, varying from 0 to 1.5% per year for dysplasia[14,15] and 0.01% for cancer.[16] Finally, the most recent BE guidelines advise that columnar epithelium extending above the upper end of the gastric folds less than 1 cm should not be routinely biopsied. For those cases where the presence of IM is documented in these short segments, there is no indication for surveillance.[1,2,378]

Classification of Early Barrett's Neoplasia

The macroscopic appearance of lesions in the esophagus should be described using the Paris classification.[17,18] This classification is based on a Japanese classification of the gross types of superficial neoplastic lesions, describing the following types: polypoid (pediculated: type 0–Ip and sessile: type 0–Is), flat and slightly elevated (type 0–IIa), flat and level (type 0–IIb), flat and depressed (type 0–IIc), or excavated (type 0–III). Assessment of the macroscopic type may provide important information about the possibility of endoscopic treatment. The flat-type lesions are the most prevalent lesions in BE (▶ Fig. 23.2). These lesions are associated with the most favorable infiltration depth and differentiation grade and can usually be managed endoscopically. Type 0–III lesions are always associated with deep submucosal infiltration and therefore not amenable for endoscopic treatment (**Video 23.1**).[19] Although strong data are lacking, most type 0–Is lesions are also invading into the deeper submucosal layers.

23.1.2 Endoscopic Imaging of Barrett's Esophagus

Endoscopic Imaging Techniques

White-Light Endoscopy

In recent years, several new imaging technologies have been developed with the expectation that their use would improve the detection of early neoplasia in BE.[20] However, standard white-light endoscopic (WLE) remains the most important technique to detect neoplastic lesions in BE. The development of high-definition (HD) endoscopy systems with integrated optical chromoendoscopy techniques has been the most important improvement in Barrett's endoscopy over the last decade.

Conventional Chromoendoscopy

Chromoendoscopy uses vital staining, contrast staining, or reactive staining to improve endoscopic visualization of neoplastic lesions. Vital stains (e.g., methylene blue) are actively absorbed by the epithelium. Contrast stains (e.g., indigo carmine) accumulate in mucosal pits and grooves, highlighting the superficial mucosal architecture. Reactive stains (e.g., acetic acid) react

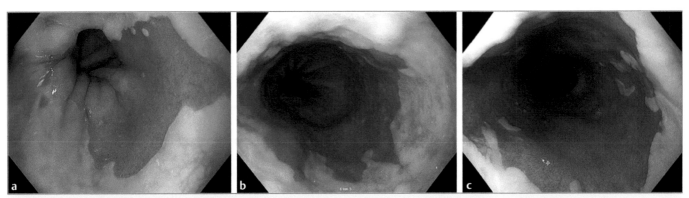

Fig. 23.1 **(a)** C2M0 Barrett's esophagus. **(b)** C3M4 Barrett's esophagus. **(c)** C14M15 Barrett's esophagus. Reproduced with permission of www.BEST-academia.eu. Copyright © 2016 BEST-Academia.

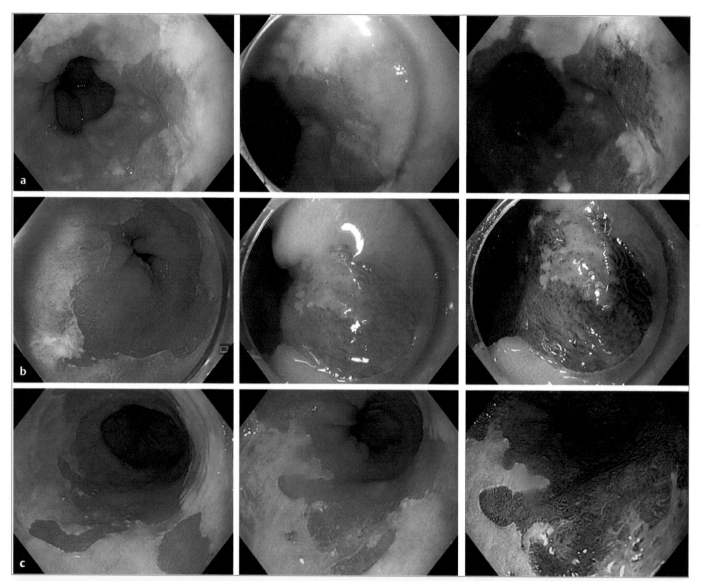

Fig. 23.2 Early neoplastic lesions imaged with high-definition white-light and narrow-band imaging. **(a)** C1M5 Barrett's esophagus with a slightly elevated lesion, type 0–IIa, between 2 and 3 o'clock (histology showed a T1m3 lesion). **(b)** C0M2 Barrett's esophagus with a flat lesion, type 0–IIb, at 3 o'clock (histology showed a T1m3 lesion). **(c)** C2M4 Barrett's esophagus with a slightly elevated and slightly depressed lesion, type 0–IIa + 0–IIc lesion between 5 and 8 o'clock (histology showed a T1m2 lesion). Reproduced with permission of www.BEST-academia.eu. Copyright © 2016 BEST-Academia.

with the epithelium to temporarily change its appearance ("acetic whitening") thus highlighting the mucosal pattern. In addition, the earlier disappearance of the whitening in early neoplasia may also improve its detection. Early studies on the use of methylene blue suggested increased detection of early neoplasia,[21] yet a recent meta-analysis of nine studies showed that there is no incremental yield for methylene blue chromoendoscopy over standard WLE.[22] In a randomized crossover study, indigo carmine did not show any benefit in terms of detection over optical chromoendoscopy and both chromoendoscopy techniques did not increase the number of patients diagnosed with neoplasia over HD-WLE.[23] Acetic acid is a cheap agent that increases the contrast of the mucosal pattern, and recent publications have suggested that it may be of aid in the identification of early neoplasia.[24,25,26] However, other studies have questioned the additional value of acetic acid over HD-WLE[27] and properly designed crossover studies, such as for methylene blue and indigo carmine, are lacking (▶ Fig. 23.3).

Optical Chromoendoscopy

Optical chromoendoscopy techniques improve the visualization of mucosal morphology without the use of dyes. Preprocessing techniques optimize mucosal and vascular imaging by adjusting the wavelength composition of the excitation light, generally by mainly using blue light. Blue light, by its shorter wavelength, only penetrates superficially into the tissue and causes less scattering. In addition, blue light is highly absorbed by hemoglobin, resulting in optimal visualization of blood vessels. Examples are narrow-band imaging (NBI; Olympus, Tokyo, Japan), or blue laser imaging (BLI; Fujifilm, Tokyo, Japan).

Postprocessing techniques use normal white-light excitation and reprocessing of the reflected images by an appropriate algorithm. Examples are Fuji intelligent chromo endoscopy (FICE, Fujifilm, Sataima, Japan), or i-Scan (Pentax, Tokyo, Japan).

Most preprocessing optical chromoendoscopy techniques also incorporate some kind of postprocessing algorithm but their

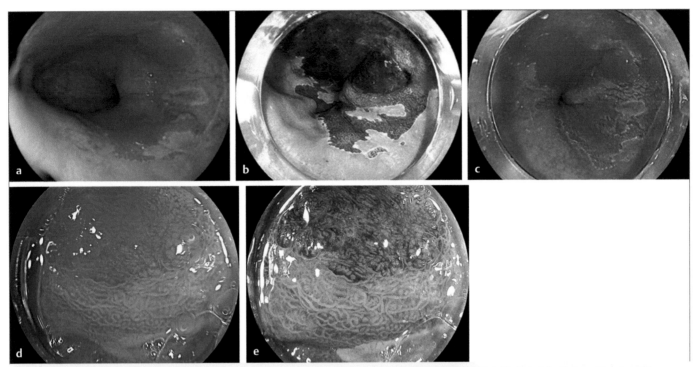

Fig. 23.3 Imaging of a well-differentiated T1m2 adenocarcinoma in a C1M5 BE. **(a)** Overview with high-resolution white-light endoscopy. **(b)** Overview with blue light imaging. **(c)** Overview after acetic acid spraying. **(d, e)** Lateral margin of the lesion in detail with white-light endoscopy and blue light imaging. Reproduced with permission of www.BEST-academia.eu. Copyright © 2016 BEST-Academia.

essential part is the adjusted excitation wavelength. Therefore, these techniques have superior resolution and brightness compared to postprocessing optical chromoendoscopy techniques.

Most studies on optical chromoendoscopy techniques in BE have used NBI, with only two small-sized studies involving i-Scan[28] or FICE.[29] BLI has only recently become available. Regular mucosal and vascular NBI patterns have been shown to correlate with nondysplastic BE, while irregular features are associated with early neoplasia.[23] Although optical chromoendoscopy may offer a more detailed inspection of the mucosal and vascular morphology than HD-WLE, clinical studies have not clearly demonstrated an additional value over HD-WLE for the detection of Barrett's neoplasia. Most experts, however, agree that the use of optical chromoendoscopy is useful in the delineation of early neoplastic lesions prior to resection.

Autofluorescence Imaging

Autofluorescence imaging (AFI) is based on the principle that certain endogenous substances, such as nicotinamide adenine dinucleotide and collagen, emit light of longer wavelengths when excited with light of shorter wavelengths. Spectroscopy studies have shown that Barrett's neoplasia has a different autofluorescence spectrum compared with nonneoplastic Barrett's mucosa.[30,31] These findings led to the development of wide-field AFI as a "red flag" technique,[32] which was later integrated with HD-WLE and NBI into an "endoscopic trimodal imaging" (ETMI) system.[33] In uncontrolled ETMI studies, AFI increased the detection of early neoplasia, while NBI reduced the false-positive rate associated with AFI.[34] However, two subsequent randomized crossover trials that compared ETMI with standard-resolution WLE with Seattle protocol biopsies, failed to show the superiority of ETMI

in detection of early neoplasia.[35,36] The use of a third-generation AFI system with a dual-band autofluorescence algorithm also showed disappointing results.[37] A critical review of the clinical impact of AFI showed that it had only limited value in identifying patients with neoplasia or detecting additional neoplastic lesions in patients already known to harbor a neoplastic lesion elsewhere in the BE.[38] AFI is barely used in clinical practice nowadays.

Confocal Laser Endomicroscopy

Confocal laser endomicroscopy (CLE) and probe-based CLE (pCLE) have the potential of providing real-time histologic data during endoscopy, using intravenous injection of fluorescein to enhance the vascular structures. This technique has the potential of providing real-time histologic data during endoscopy. CLE is currently only available with the pCLE system, since the integrated CLE (iCLE) endoscopy system by Pentax/Optiscan, which had the best resolution and frame rate, has been taken out of market. CLE allows for a reliable prediction of the presence of neoplasia on preselected still images of BE,[39,40] however, other studies have shown a lower sensitivity of only 68%.[41] The combination of pCLE with HD-WLE may increase the detection of early neoplasia compared to HD-WLE alone.[40] Theoretically, the possibility of sampling only suspicious areas on pCLE could reduce the number of random biopsies.[42,43] However, pCLE equipment is expensive and obtaining good-quality pCLE images is challenging. Given its limited scanning depth, there is no use for CLE in assessing invasion depth of neoplastic lesions. The use of CLE for follow-up after endoscopic therapy has been suggested,[44] however, controlled studies in this field are lacking. Finally, the whole concept of real-time histologic assessment during endoscopy is questionable: first, the negative predictive value of pCLE will never be high enough to withhold endoscopists from sampling an area that appears suspicious on HD-WLE; second, proceeding immediately with treatment of identified visible lesions in which pCLE confirms the diagnosis of neoplasia is restricted since generally patients need to receive information and provide consent before practicing an endoscopic resection; third, while diagnostic endoscopies can be performed in any hospital, therapeutic endoscopies should be referred to tertiary care centers, according to the guidelines.[1] Therefore, the wide-scale diffusion of pCLE in the evaluation of BE is unlikely. An optimal HD-WLE inspection allows the detection of most prevalent neoplastic lesions, to sample them for histology after which the patient is informed and referred for treatment. In the absence of morphologic abnormalities, future management of BE will probably consist of sampling the Barrett's segment, either with biopsies or brush cytology, not to detect morphologic changes (as on the biopsy samples or pCLE) but to detect molecular markers associated with an increased risk of progression, well before any morphologic abnormalities detectable on histology (or pCLE) occur.[45]

Optical Coherence Tomography

Optical coherence tomography (OCT) works analogous to ultrasound, utilizing light waves instead of sound waves to create two-dimensional images based on differences in optical scattering of tissue structures. OCT generates cross-sectional images of tissues in real-time with a resolution comparable to low-power microscopy. Volumetric laser endomicroscopy (VLE) utilizes second-generation OCT technology, which is incorporated in a novel system: Nvision VLE Imaging System (NinePoint Medical Inc., Cambridge, Massachusetts, United States). This system is capable of performing a circumferential scan of the esophagus, with a length of 6 cm and a depth of 3 mm, in just 90 seconds. Since VLE enables subsurface examination, this system has the potential to aid in early BE neoplasia detection during endoscopy. In the future, VLE might guide the endoscopist in targeting suspicious areas and avoid the need for random biopsies. In order to reach this aim, clear distinction of neoplasia in BE on VLE has to be possible. Currently, ongoing studies are developing VLE criteria and scoring systems for BE neoplasia for use in clinical practice.[46,47] Just like pCLE, VLE is currently far from guiding therapeutic interventions or withholding an endoscopist to biopsy a visible lesion. However, given its potential to scan the whole Barrett's segment and by its deeper scanning depth, it may help targeting biopsies on dysplastic areas in the future.

23.2 Endoscopic Surveillance for Barrett's Esophagus

Endoscopic Barrett's surveillance aims at identifying patients at risk for progression to EAC or at detecting Barrett's neoplasia at a curable stage. Several studies have shown that Barrett's surveillance results in the detection of earlier stages of EAC compared to patients who are diagnosed with EAC without being part of a surveillance program.[48,49] Cost-effectiveness studies have shown that surveillance strategies can be cost-effective.[50]

However, taking into account lead-time and length-time biases, retrospective studies of surveillance tests for cancer can appear more effective than they are. A case–control study from 2013 involving 351 patients with EAC did not find any difference in the risk of death by EAC between the patients who underwent surveillance endoscopy within 3 years and those who did not.[51] These data, combined with the fact that a minority of EAC arises in patients with known BE,[48,52] question the relevance of surveillance endoscopy in BE.

The estimated annual risk of neoplastic progression of non-dysplastic BE (NDBE) is about 0.3% for EAC and 0.5 to 0.8% for HGD and EAC combined.[52,53] Studies have identified some endoscopic and clinical factors that are associated with malignant progression. Examples of potential risk factors are the length of the Barrett's segment, the presence of erosive esophagitis at endoscopy, presence of a hiatal hernia, LGD, gastroesophageal reflux symptoms, smoking habits, and body mass index (BMI). The use of PPIs, statins, and nonsteroidal anti-inflammatory drugs (NSAIDs) may have a protective effect.[54,55] For the length of the BE, a number of recent studies strongly suggest that the length of the Barrett's segment is correlated with the risk of neoplastic progression. Also, the presence of confirmed LGD appears to be associated with a significant increase in risk of neoplastic progression. Therefore, current guidelines have taken BE length and presence of LGD` into account in their advised surveillance intervals. ▶Table 23.1 describes the current advice on endoscopic surveillance according to European, American, Dutch, and British guidelines.

23.3 Management of Dysplasia and Early Cancer in Barrett's Esophagus

Deciding on the best management of intraepithelial neoplasia and early cancer in BE is a two-step approach. First, one needs to assess if the neoplasia is endoscopically manageable. It is important to detect macroscopic abnormalities and remove them by endoscopic resection (ER), allowing for optimal histologic staging. Although endoscopic ultrasound (EUS) is still a widely used diagnostic modality to assess the depth of tumor invasion and detect lymph node metastases, several studies have demonstrated that EUS has virtually no clinical impact on the work-up of early esophageal neoplasia. Differentiating between T1a and T1b cancer is not reliable with EUS and the yield of finding lymph node metastasis is very low given the minimal risk of lymph node metastasis associated with early Barrett's cancer.[56,57] Thus, ER remains the crucial diagnostic step to allow for accurate T-staging and to assess other risk factors for lymph node metastasis such as differentiation grade and presence of lymphovascular invasion. If ER is performed and shows low-risk features for lymph node metastasis, that is, neoplasia confined to the mucosa, well-to-moderately differentiated cancer, radical resection, and no lymphovascular invasion, further endoscopic management is justified. Then the second step is to decide on the removal of all residual Barrett's mucosa, to avoid recurrence of dysplasia in the remainder of the Barrett's, which is described in up to 30% of patients after 5-year follow-up.[58,59]

23.3.1 Indications for Endoscopic Treatment

High-Grade Dysplasia and Mucosal Cancer

Based on a wide variety of international studies, there is now overwhelming evidence that endoscopic treatment is the treatment of choice for BE patients with HGD and mucosal cancer, with 5-year disease-free survival in over 95% of patients.[5,60,61] For flat-type HGD without visible lesions, endoscopic ablation of the Barrett's mucosa is the treatment of choice. In the case of visible lesions, no matter how subtle, ER needs to be performed for staging, and to render the mucosa flat for subsequent ablation of the residual Barrett's segment. Complete eradication of the Barrett's mucosa is indicated for most patients since focal treatment by ER is associated with recurrent lesions elsewhere in the BE in up to a third of patients during follow-up.[60,61] Stepwise radical endoscopic resection results in an effective removal of neoplasia and of the whole Barrett's segment, with a 2 to 4% recurrence rate of neoplasia after 24 to 32 months. However, circumferential ER is associated with esophageal stenosis in 37 to 88% of the patients.[62,63,64] A randomized study has shown that stepwise radical endoscopic resection of BE less than 5 cm, compared to ER of visible lesions followed by radiofrequency ablation (RFA) of residual flat mucosa, resulted in comparably high rates of eradication of neoplasia and IM. However, stepwise radical endoscopic resection was associated with a higher number of complications and therapeutic sessions.[64] Therefore, complete ER of BE is only used in selected cases, for example, in case of short-segment Barrett's with diffuse irregular mucosa or in the absence of circumferential BE. Endoscopic ablation of BE is currently the best option to handle residual BE after ER[5] and will be described in more detail below.

Low-Grade Dysplasia

The management of LGD is evolving, partly due to studies suggesting that "true-LGD" has a malignant progression rate close to that of HGD,[65,66] partly due to studies showing that RFA is a safe and effective treatment strategy for these patients.[67,68] Thus, management of LGD more and more resembles that of HGD and EAC. The first step is the confirmation of the histologic diagnosis by an expert pathologist.[2,6,65,66]

Curvers et al and Duits et al retrospectively examined the prognostic value of an expert pathology panel for reviewing the LGD diagnosis of community hospital pathologists in two separate cohorts.[65,66] They demonstrated that only 15 and 27% of the original LGD diagnoses were confirmed, while the remaining 85 and 73% were downstaged. After a median follow-up of 51 and 39 months, the risk of progression to HGD or EAC was 13.4 and 9.1% per patient-year in the confirmed LGD group. In contrast, patients with a downstaged diagnosis of NDBE had an annual neoplastic progression rate of 0.5 and 0.6%, respectively.

A confirmed diagnosis of LGD is not only a predictor for progression to HGD or cancer over time but also a marker for prevalent neoplasia that may have been overlooked at the baseline endoscopy. Therefore, patients with a confirmed diagnosis of LGD should undergo a repeat endoscopy at 6 to 12 months to rule out prevalent neoplasia, followed by either strict annual endoscopic surveillance, or ablative treatment. A recently multicenter randomized clinical trial that enrolled 136 patients with a confirmed diagnosis of LGD demonstrated that RFA reduced the risk of progression to HGD or EAC from 26.5 to 1.5% (95% confidence interval [CI], 14.1–35.9%; $p < 0.001$), and resulted in a sustained complete eradication of IM metaplasia at 3 years in 88.2% of the patients.[67] Given the durability of the results of RFA over time,[61,68] latest expert consensus and guidelines have included RFA as a treatment option for patients with confirmed LGD.[1,2,3,6,7,8]

Nondysplastic Barrett's Esophagus

Currently, an approach of endoscopic surveillance with biopsies is used to detect malignant progression in patients with NDBE. However, surveillance is limited by the difficulty to detect early neoplasia endoscopically, by biopsy sampling error, by interobserver variability between pathologists, and by questionable cost-effectiveness. The annual progression rates to HGD and EAC (0.5–0.8%) are relatively low and ablation of NDBE is not generally accepted. However, in selected high-risk patients (eg, a combination of a Barrett's segment > 5 cm, age < 50 years, or a first-degree relative with EAC), ablation may be considered in the future as an alternative to endoscopic surveillance.

23.3.2 Endoscopic Treatment Techniques

Endoscopic Resection

ER is the cornerstone of endoscopic treatment for early BE neoplasia. Since ER of visible lesions provides a large tissue specimen for accurate histologic diagnosis, ER is both the last step of the diagnostic work-up and the first step of the treatment of early neoplasia.

Multiband Mucosectomy

The most widely used ER technique nowadays is the multiband mucosectomy (MBM) technique. MBM uses a modified variceal band ligator (Duette MBM system, Cook Endoscopy, Limerick, Ireland) or more recently the Captivator System (Boston Scientific, Natick, Massachusetts, United States) with a transparent cap with six rubber bands, releasing wires, a releasing handle, and a 5 to 7 F hexagonal braided polypectomy snare. The target mucosa is sucked into a cap, and by releasing a rubber band, a pseudopolyp is created. This pseudopolyp can then be resected using the snare (▶ Fig. 23.4). Because the MBM cap holds six rubber bands, six subsequent resections can be performed without removing the endoscope and while using the same snare. It is hypothesized that the contraction force of the rubber band is not strong enough to constrain the muscularis propria, and that submucosal lifting is therefore not necessary during the use of MBM. Indeed, no perforations have been recorded in a large prospective study including 243 MBM procedures using the Duette system, with 1060 resections.[69] The MBM technique is advisable for en bloc resection of flat-type lesions (Paris type 0–IIa, 0–IIb, 0–IIc) or small elevated lesions (Paris type 0–Is) in BE with a diameter less than or equal to 15 mm, and for piecemeal resections of larger flat-type dysplastic areas (**Video 23.2**).

ER-Cap Technique

Another technique for ER of BE lesions is the ER-cap technique. The ER-cap technique involves the use of a specially designed transparent hard oblique cap (inner diameter of 12 mm) with a distal ridge, allowing for the placement of a specific asymmetrical crescent-shaped snare (ER kit, Olympus GmbH, Hamburg, Germany). After submucosal fluid injection to lift the lesion from the deeper wall layers, the snare is prelooped in the ridge of the cap. Subsequently, the lesion is sucked into the cap, and the snare is tightened, creating a pseudopolyp that can

then be resected (▶Fig. 23.5). A randomized-controlled trial comparing the MBM and ER-cap technique for piecemeal ER demonstrated that MBM was cheaper and quicker compared to ER-cap, but equally safe despite omission of the submucosal lifting step.[70] Therefore, the ER-cap technique has largely been replaced by the MBM technique in most Barrett's expert centers. For us, the only remaining indication is the en bloc resection of lesions of 15 to 20 mm, for which MBM would require piecemeal resection, whereas an ER-cap procedure with a large-caliber flexible ER-cap may remove the lesion in one piece (**Video 23.3**).

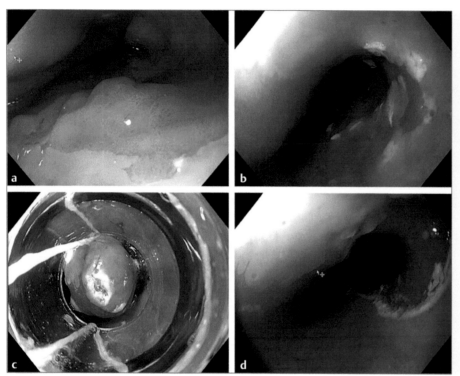

Fig. 23.4 Multiband mucosectomy (MBM) procedure. **(a)** C0M6 Barrett's esophagus with a type 0–IIa + 0–IIc lesion at 6 o'clock. **(b)** Delineation of the lesion with coagulation markings. **(c)** A pseudopolyp is created after suctioning the mucosa and releasing a rubber band around the lesion.
(d) Endoscopic resection wound after resection of the pseudopolyp with an electrocautery snare. Reproduced with permission of www.BEST-academia.eu. Copyright © 2016 BEST-Academia.

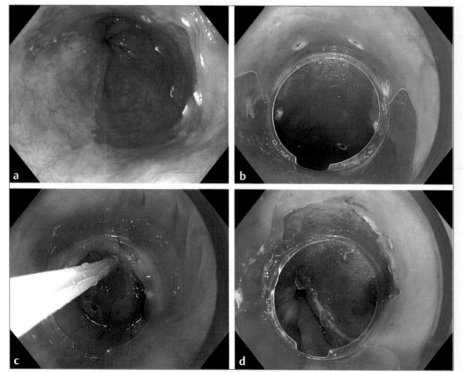

Fig. 23.5 Endoscopic resection using the ER-cap technique. **(a)** C1M5 Barrett's esophagus with a visible lesion at 2 o'clock. **(b)** Endoscopic view through the distal attachment cap on the delineated lesion. **(c)** After submucosal lifting of the lesion, the mucosa is sucked into the cap and by closing the prelooped snare, the mucosa is captured and can be resected using electrocautery. **(d)** Endoscopic resection wound. Reproduced with permission of www.BEST-academia.eu. Copyright © 2016 BEST-Academia.

Endoscopic Submucosal Dissection

Endoscopic submucosal dissection (ESD) allows for en bloc resection of superficial lesions irrespective of their size, at the cost of longer procedures, and higher complication rates (▶Fig. 23.6). ESD has proven to be superior to cap-based ER techniques in terms of recurrence rates in the management of squamous cell carcinoma of the esophagus.[71] However, ESD is technically demanding and has a flat learning curve, and is therefore currently practiced, in Western countries, only by a limited number of expert endoscopists. Prospective European studies of ESD in Barrett's early neoplasia have shown disappointing results, with 38.5 to 64% of histologically complete resection of HGD/EAC.[72,73] As a consequence, the recent European Society of Gastrointestinal Endoscopy (ESGE) guidelines recommended that piecemeal ER should be preferred over ESD in most cases of Barrett's early neoplasia.[74] We reserve ESD (i) for patients with a strong suspicion of submucosal invasion; (ii) for the resection of lesions with a large intraluminal component prohibiting a cap-based resection (i.e., the intraluminal part of the lesion would fill the cap upon suctioning and the resection of the basal mucosal layers may thus b`e irradical despite the absence of deep submucosal invasion). In our hands, less than 10% of all early Barrett's neoplasia cases require ESD (**Video 23.4**).

Endoscopic Ablation of Barrett's Esophagus

Endoscopic ablation techniques can be used to treat flat-type Barrett's mucosa, either as a secondary treatment after focal ER of visible lesions, or primarily for flat-type HGD, confirmed LGD, or in selected patients with NDBE.

Photodynamic Therapy

Photodynamic therapy was the first ablation technique to be widely studied, and gave disappointing results because of a variable depth of ablation, with a 30% stenosis rate, high rates of buried Barrett's, and 44 to 78% success rate at 5 years for eradication of HGD/EAC.[75,76] Currently, this treatment has largely been abandoned.

Argon Plasma Coagulation

Argon plasma coagulation (APC) has also been proposed for the ablation of residual BE, because of its availability and low costs. A recently published work demonstrated that APC ablation after ER reduced the recurrence rate from 37 to 3% at 2 years follow-up.[77] However, ablation using APC is operator dependent, because of a variable distance between the probe and the esophageal mucosa, time of application, and energy settings; thus, a high variability in the ablation effect is to be expected. Furthermore, ablation of circumferential BE is particularly labor intensive, likely to be incomplete, requires numerous treatment sessions, and causes esophageal stenoses in up to 9% of cases.[73] Therefore, APC ablation of residual BE is currently limited to the ablation of small residual Barrett's islands or tongues after prior ER or RFA treatment.

Recently, a modified APC probe called Hybrid APC (Erbe Elektromedizin, Tübingen, Germany) has been developed, allowing to inject 0.9% saline in the submucosal space via a waterjet channel integrated to the APC probe (▶Fig. 23.7). Achieving submucosal lifting before thermal ablation should allow to perform APC ablation at a high power, which might improve the outcomes of APC ablation, particularly in terms of safety. While the first pilot study seems to confirm this hypothesis, with a 2% stenosis rate,[78] prospective multicenter studies are currently ongoing.

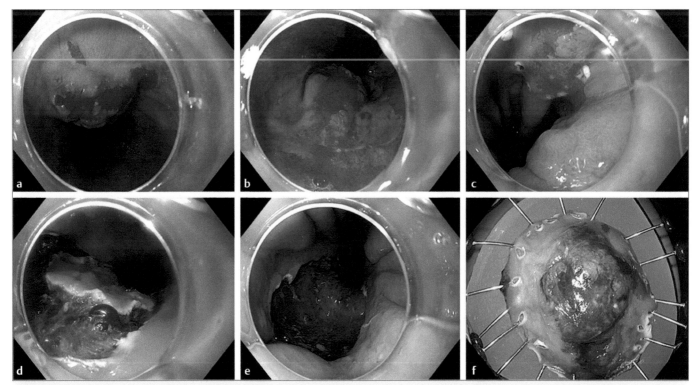

Fig. 23.6 Endoscopic submucosal dissection. (**a**) Type 0–Is lesion in a COM5 Barrett's esophagus. (**b**) Same lesion is shown in retroflexed position. (**c**) Delineation of the lesion by placing coagulation markers around the lesion. (**d**) After submucosal injection, the lesion has been incised circumferentially. (**e**) Endoscopic resection wound. (**f**) The resection specimen is pinned down on paraffin. Reproduced with permission of www.BEST-academia.eu. Copyright © 2016 BEST-Academia.

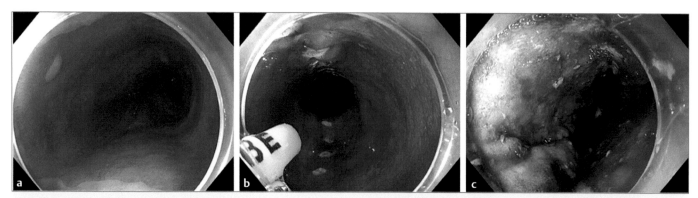

Fig. 23.7 Hybrid APC treatment. **(a)** C8M8 Barrett's esophagus with no visible lesions. **(b)** Coagulation markers are placed to delineate half of the circumference of the Barrett's segment. **(c)** Immediate effect after lifting and ablation with the hybrid-APC catheter. Reproduced with permission of www.BEST-academia.eu. Copyright © 2016 BEST-Academia.

Radiofrequency Ablation

With three randomized-controlled trials,[64,67,79] three large cohort studies,[61,68,80] and over 10 large retrospective studies,[81,82] RFA is the most widely studied ablation method for BE. A randomized multicenter trial has demonstrated equivalent results to stepwise radical endoscopic resection with better safety outcomes, particularly in terms of esophageal stenosis (14 vs. 88%, $p < 0.001$).[64] RFA is particularly interesting for long circumferential BE segment, in which a reproducible, controlled in-depth, 3-cm-long ablation can be obtained, unlike any other ablation technique. Indeed, even in BE longer than 10 cm, a complete eradication rate of IM as high as 83% can be achieved by ER followed by RFA.[83] Finally, the efficacy and durability up to 5 years of this combined management was confirmed in recent reports.[61,68,80] Complete eradication of neoplasia and IM was reached in 95 to 96% and 89 to 92% of cases at 2 years, respectively. Sustained complete remission of neoplasia and IM was found in 90% of patients at 5 years, and all recurrences could be managed endoscopically.

RFA is performed using a catheter carrying a bipolar electrode. Two main types of devices exist for RFA: a balloon-based ablation system (Barrx360, Medtronic, Minneapolis, Minnesota, United States) inserted over guidewire and followed by the endoscope in a side-to-side manner. This system allows for a quick ablation of large circumferential areas of BE, but requires a preliminary step of measurement of the esophageal diameter using a sizing balloon (▶ Fig. 23.8, ▶ Fig. 23.9). Therefore, a newly designed self-sizing RFA catheter has been developed in order to perform circumferential ablation without needing the sizing step. For circumferential ablation, the electrode is positioned 1 cm above the proximal extent of the BE, the balloon is inflated, and energy is delivered (two times 12 J/cm², 40 W/cm²), resulting in circumferential ablation of a 3-cm BE segment. For the newer self-sizing catheter ablation regimens using 10 J/cm² are advised and currently studied (**Video 23.5**).

The second type of ablation system is a focal ablation catheter, attached to the tip of the endoscope, and designed to ablate tongues or islands of BE. Various sizes of focal RFA devices exist, but the Barrx90, allowing for a 90-degree ablation is the most commonly used. In Europe, ablation is typically obtained by a double application of 15 J/cm², repeated after cleaning of the coagulated zone and the device. In the United States, the same regimen is used using a double-double 12 J/cm² energy setting. The optimal ablation regimen for focal RFA is currently being studied.

Generally, most patients require one circumferential Barrx360 ablation and two focal Barrx90 ablation treatments to achieve eradication of all IM. In all patients, the GE junction needs to be treated circumferentially with the focal (Barrx90) catheter, at least once, to ensure optimal eradication of IM at this level. More recently, a third type of device has been commercialized: a through the scope "channel" catheter, with a limited surface of ablation of 7.5 × 15.7 mm (as compared to 13 × 20 mm for the Barrx90) and a floppy electrode, and the ability to ablate in difficult areas, especially in narrowed, scarred esophagus after extensive ER.

23.3.3 Current Guidelines for Endoscopic Treatment and Subsequent Follow-Up

All recently published guidelines agree on the principle of ER of any visible lesion arising in BE followed by ablation of the residual BE with RFA.[1,2,3,4,5,6,7,8,11] Endoscopic follow-up is still recommended after BE eradication, since long-term follow-up data of this relatively new treatment modality are not yet available. As shown in ▶ Table 23.1, guidelines recommend close endoscopic surveillance 3-monthly for the first year, followed by at least yearly surveillance with targeted biopsies of any visible lesions, and systematic biopsies of the neosquamous mucosa and the GE junction.[1,2,3,4,7,8]

The fear of buried glands leading to buried dysplasia and carcinoma has probably been overrated. First, the actual occurrence of buried Barrett's after RFA is very low, and does not exceed 0.9%.[76] One study has even questioned the concept of buried Barrett's after RFA, suggesting that it would be an artifact of specimen sampling and processing.[84] Second, the neoplastic potential of buried IM is quite uncertain, and the link between buried IM and the cases of buried carcinoma has not been established.

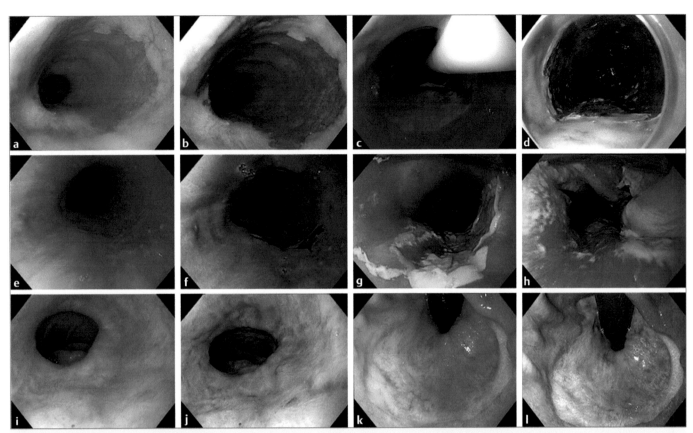

Fig. 23.8 Radiofrequency ablation (RFA) treatment. **(a, b)** C4M5 Barrett's esophagus shown with white-light endoscopy (WLE) and narrow-band imaging (NBI). **(c, d)** Coagulation effect immediately after circumferential ablation using the balloon-based electrode, shown with WLE and NBI. **(e, f)** Endoscopy 3 months later showing residual Barrett's islands (WLE and NBI). **(g, h)** Focal ablation of residual Barrett's mucosa and the neosquamocolumnar junction using the Barrx 90 catheter. **(i–l)** Control endoscopy performed 3 months later: complete eradication of endoscopically visible Barrett's mucosa (WLE and NBI). Reproduced with permission of www.BEST-academia.eu. Copyright © 2016 BEST-Academia.

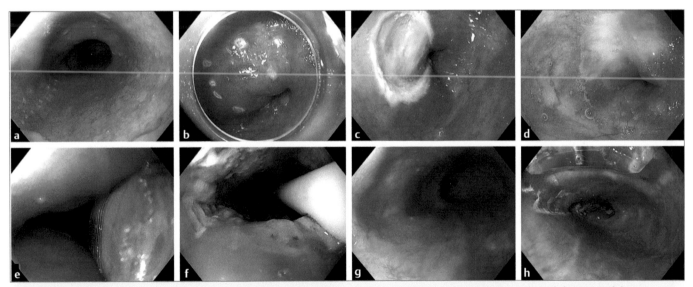

Fig. 23.9 Endoscopic resection and circumferential radiofrequency ablation (RFA). **(a)** C8M9 Barrett's esophagus with a subtle type 0–IIb lesion at 10 o'clock. **(b)** Delineation of the lesion. **(c)** Result after en bloc resection of the lesion. **(d)** After 12 weeks the endoscopic resection scar shows squamous regeneration. **(e)** Circumferential ablation with the Barrx360 system. **(f)** Coagulation effect immediately after the ablation. **(g)** Residual Barrett's mucosa (97% regression) after 3 months. **(h)** Two Barrett islands and the neosquamocolumnar junction were treated with focal RFA using the Barrx90 catheter seen at 12 o'clock in the endoscopic view. Reproduced with permission of www.BEST-academia.eu. Copyright © 2016 BEST-Academia.

23.4 Areas of Uncertainty, Experimental Techniques, and Research

23.4.1 Biological Markers in Barrett's Esophagus

Currently, the onset of morphologic changes in the BE segment or presence of LGD is the most reliable way to determine the risk of neoplastic progression in a patient. Better biomarkers are needed, fulfilling the following conditions: widely present throughout the BE segment, preceding morphologic changes, and highly associated with relevant outcomes (progression to cancer or no risk of neoplastic progression). The optimal way these markers should be sampled (endoscopic biopsies, endoscopic brushing, transoral cytology sponges, feces tests, or blood samples) as well as the composition of biomarker panels has not been established yet, but much progress has recently been made in this field.[45,85]

23.4.2 Low-Risk Submucosal Cancer

Barrett's cancer infiltrating the submucosa is still regarded as an indication for surgery, given the risk of lymph node metastasis (N+) ranging from 0 to 22% for sm1, and 36 to 54% for sm2/3 cancer.[74,86] These risk estimates are, however, based on retrospective cohorts with submucosal cancer diagnosed in surgical resection specimens. At the time these studies were performed, esophagectomy was the treatment of choice for any grade of neoplasia, ranging from a single-biopsy diagnosis of HGD to stage T3 cancer. Therefore, accurate histologic differentiation between different depths of submucosal invasion did not bear much clinical relevance. Surgical specimens were routinely cut in 5- to 10-mm slices and the area of deepest infiltration may therefore have been missed easily. This may have resulted in underestimation of invasion depth, and thus a wrong interpretation of the N+ risk corresponding with a certain depth of invasion. In contrast, when infiltration depth is assessed in ER specimens, which are routinely cut in 2-mm slices with additional cuts in case of submucosal invasion, the N+ risk for certain infiltration depths can be reported more accurately. This has already been demonstrated by the fact that the 4 to 12% risk of N+ for mucosal cancer reported in surgical series is in fact much lower (< 0.5%) when the diagnosis is based on ER specimens. As reported by Manner et al, and Alvarez Herrero et al, the risk of N+ in "low-risk" submucosal cancer diagnosed in ER specimens, may also be lower than reported thus far.[87,88] Low-risk criteria are defined as follows: well-to-moderately differentiated cancer, with submucosal invasion of less than or equal to 500 µm, without signs of lymphovascular invasion. Taking into account that the N+ risk may be lower than reported thus far, and that most patients with low-risk submucosal cancer are elderly with comorbidities, endoscopic treatment may be considered as a valid alternative to surgery in these cases.

23.4.3 Novel Developments in Endoscopic Ablation

While RFA currently appears as the simplest, most effective, and best validated ablation technique, it remains expensive, and therefore not accessible to all centers. New versions of older ablation techniques, possibly cheaper compared to RFA, have been proposed. The balloon-based cryoablation therapy has recently proved feasible and safe in a prospective multicenter study[89] (▶ Fig. 23.10). A second-generation APC,

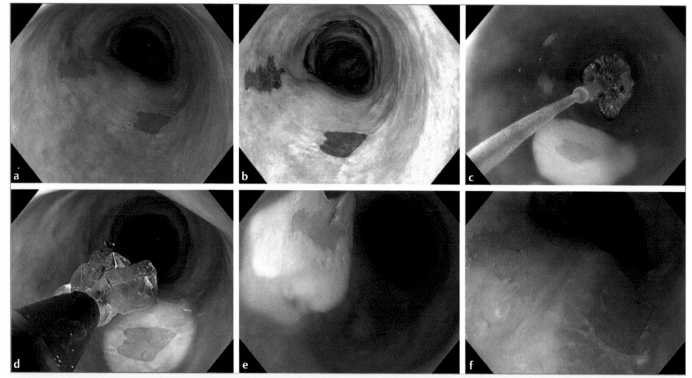

Fig. 23.10 Focal cryoablation. **(a)** After prior treatment with circumferential radiofrequency ablation, two residual Barrett's islands are seen at 6 o'clock (4 × 9 mm) and 9 o'clock (5 × 6 mm). **(b)** Islands shown with narrow-band imaging. **(c)** Cryoablation of the Barrett islands. **(d, e)** Cryoeffect immediately after ablation of the islands. **(f)** Effect after a couple of minutes. Reproduced with permission of www.BEST-academia.eu. Copyright © 2016 BEST-Academia.

termed hybrid APC—already discussed above—is also under development.[77] Currently available data are still preliminary, and the place of these alternative ablation techniques remains to be defined.

23.5 Conclusion

The diagnosis of BE relies on the presence of IM in the biopsies of a greater than or equal to 1 cm segment of salmon-colored mucosa in the tubular esophagus. Until better risk stratification of the patients using biomarkers is available, endoscopic surveillance with careful HD-WLE and systematic quadratic biopsies according to the Seattle protocol is recommended to detect early neoplasia. Any visible lesion is suspect of bearing HGD or early adenocarcinoma, and should be resected endoscopically in expert centers. ER is preferably carried out with MBM. ESD is restricted to a minority of lesions that are bulky, or judged at high risk of submucosal infiltration and should therefore be removed en bloc. In the presence of early neoplasia, the residual Barrett's mucosa should be ablated, typically by RFA, until complete eradication of IM is reached. In cases of LGD confirmed by an expert pathologist, ablation or yearly surveillance is advisable. After eradication of IM, 3-monthly endoscopic follow-up for the first year, then long-term annual follow-up is advised.

References

[1] Shaheen NJ, Falk GW, Iyer PG, Gerson LB. ACG clinical guideline: diagnosis and management of Barrett's esophagus. Am J Gastroenterol. 2016; 111(1):30–50, quiz 51

[2] Fitzgerald RC, di Pietro M, Ragunath K, et al; British Society of Gastroenterology. British Society of Gastroenterology guidelines on the diagnosis and management of Barrett's oesophagus. Gut. 2014; 63(1):7–42

[3] Tham T. Guidelines on the diagnosis and management of Barrett's oesophagus—an update. British Society of gastroenterology. http://www.bsg.org.uk/clinical-guidelines/oesophageal/guidelines-on-the-diagnosis-and-management-of-barrett-s-oesophagus.html. Accessed February 1, 2016

[4] Evans JA, Early DS, Fukami N, et al. ASGE Standards of Practice Committee. The role of endoscopy in Barrett's esophagus and other premalignant conditions of the esophagus. Gastrointest Endosc. 2012; 76(6):1087–1094

[5] Bennett C, Vakil N, Bergman J, et al. Consensus statements for management of Barrett's dysplasia and early-stage esophageal adenocarcinoma, based on a Delphi process. Gastroenterology. 2012; 143(2):336–346

[6] Bennett C, Moayyedi P, Corley DA, et al; BOB CAT Consortium. BOB CAT: a large-scale review and Delphi consensus for management of Barrett's esophagus with no dysplasia, indefinite for, or low-grade dysplasia. Am J Gastroenterol. 2015; 110(5):662–682, quiz 683

[7] Richtlijn Barrett-oesofagus (Dutch Barrett oesophagus guideline). Nederlandse Vereniging van Maag-Darm-Leverartsen. www.oncoline.nl. In press

[8] Weusten B, Bisschops R, Coron E, et al. Endoscopic management of Barrett's esophagus: European Society of Gastrointestinal Endoscopy (ESGE) Position Statement. Endoscopy 2017; 49(2):191–198

[9] Schlemper RJ, Riddell RH, Kato Y, et al. The Vienna classification of gastrointestinal epithelial neoplasia. Gut. 2000; 47(2):251–255

[10] Sharma P, Dent J, Armstrong D, et al. The development and validation of an endoscopic grading system for Barrett's esophagus: the Prague C & M criteria. Gastroenterology. 2006; 131(5):1392–1399

[11] Spechler SJ, Sharma P, Souza RF, et al; American Gastroenterological Association. American Gastroenterological Association technical review on the management of Barrett's esophagus. Gastroenterology. 2011; 140(3):e18–e52, quiz e13

[12] Amano Y, Ishimura N, Furuta K, et al. Which landmark results in a more consistent diagnosis of Barrett's esophagus, the gastric folds or the palisade vessels? Gastrointest Endosc. 2006; 64(2):206–211

[13] Azuma N, Endo T, Arimura Y, et al. Prevalence of Barrett's esophagus and expression of mucin antigens detected by a panel of monoclonal antibodies in Barrett's esophagus and esophageal adenocarcinoma in Japan. J Gastroenterol. 2000; 35(8):583–592

[14] Jung KW, Talley NJ, Romero Y, et al. Epidemiology and natural history of intestinal metaplasia of the gastroesophageal junction and Barrett's esophagus: a population-based study. Am J Gastroenterol. 2011; 106(8):1447–1455, quiz 1456

[15] Sharma P, Weston AP, Morales T. et al. Relative risk of dysplasia for patients with intestinal metaplasia in the distal oesophagus and in the gastric cardia. Gut. 2000; 46(1):9–13

[16] Pohl H, Pech O, Arash H, et al. Length of Barrett's oesophagus and cancer risk: implications from a large sample of patients with early oesophageal adenocarcinoma. Gut. 2016; 65(2):196–201

[17] The Paris endoscopic classification of superficial neoplastic lesions: esophagus, stomach, and colon: November 30 to December 1, 2002. Gastrointest Endosc. 2003; 58(s)(uppl)(6):S3–S43

[18] Endoscopic Classification Review Group. Update on the paris classification of superficial neoplastic lesions in the digestive tract. Endoscopy. 2005; 37(6):570–578

[19] Pech O, Gossner L, Manner H, et al. Prospective evaluation of the macroscopic types and location of early Barrett's neoplasia in 380 lesions. Endoscopy. 2007; 39(7):588–593

[20] Boerwinkel DF, Swager A, Curvers WL, Bergman JJ. The clinical consequences of advanced imaging techniques in Barrett's esophagus. Gastroenterology. 2014; 146(3):622–629.e4

[21] Canto MI, Setrakian S, Willis J, et al. Methylene blue-directed biopsies improve detection of intestinal metaplasia and dysplasia in Barrett's esophagus. Gastrointest Endosc. 2000; 51(5):560–568

[22] Ngamruengphong S, Sharma VK, Das A. Diagnostic yield of methylene blue chromoendoscopy for detecting specialized intestinal metaplasia and dysplasia in Barrett's esophagus: a meta-analysis. Gastrointest Endosc. 2009; 69(6):1021–1028

[23] Kara MA, Peters FP, Rosmolen WD, et al. High-resolution endoscopy plus chromoendoscopy or narrow-band imaging in Barrett's esophagus: a prospective randomized crossover study. Endoscopy. 2005; 37(10):929–936

[24] Longcroft-Wheaton G, Duku M, Mead R, et al. Acetic acid spray is an effective tool for the endoscopic detection of neoplasia in patients with Barrett's esophagus. Clin Gastroenterol Hepatol. 2010; 8(10):843–847

[25] Bhandari P, Kandaswamy P, Cowlishaw D, Longcroft-Wheaton G. Acetic acid-enhanced chromoendoscopy is more cost-effective than protocol-guided biopsies in a high-risk Barrett's population. Dis Esophagus. 2012; 25(5):386–392

[26] Pohl J, Pech O, May A. et al. Incidence of macroscopically occult neoplasias in Barrett's esophagus: are random biopsies dispensable in the era of advanced endoscopic imaging? Am J Gastroenterol. 2010; 105(11):2350–2356

[27] Curvers W, Baak L, Kiesslich R, et al. Chromoendoscopy and narrow-band imaging compared with high-resolution magnification endoscopy in Barrett's esophagus. Gastroenterology. 2008; 134(3):670–679

[28] Rey JW, Deris N, Marquardt JU, et al. High-definition endoscopy with iScan and Lugol's solution for the detection of inflammation in patients with nonerosive reflux disease: histologic evaluation in comparison with a control group. Dis Esophagus.

[29] Camus M, Coriat R, Leblanc S, et al. Helpfulness of the combination of acetic acid and FICE in the detection of Barrett's epithelium and Barrett's associated neoplasias. World J Gastroenterol. 2012; 18(16):1921–1925

[30] Georgakoudi I, Jacobson BC, Van Dam J, et al. Fluorescence, reflectance, and light-scattering spectroscopy for evaluating dysplasia in patients with Barrett's esophagus. Gastroenterology. 2001; 120(7):1620–1629

[31] Panjehpour M, Overholt BF, Vo-Dinh T. et al. Endoscopic fluorescence detection of high-grade dysplasia in Barrett's esophagus. Gastroenterology. 1996; 111(1):93–101

[32] Kara MA, Smits ME, Rosmolen WD, et al. A randomized crossover study comparing light-induced fluorescence endoscopy with standard videoendoscopy for the detection of early neoplasia in Barrett's esophagus. Gastrointest Endosc. 2005; 61(6):671–678

[33] Kara MA, Peters FP, Ten Kate FJ. et al. Endoscopic video autofluorescence imaging may improve the detection of early neoplasia in patients with Barrett's esophagus. Gastrointest Endosc. 2005; 61(6):679–685

[34] Curvers WL, Singh R, Song L-MW-K, et al. Endoscopic tri-modal imaging for detection of early neoplasia in Barrett's oesophagus: a multi-centre feasibility study using high-resolution endoscopy, autofluorescence imaging and narrow band imaging incorporated in one endoscopy system. Gut. 2008; 57(2):167–172

[35] Curvers WL, Alvarez Herrero L, Wallace MB, et al. Endoscopic tri-modal imaging is more effective than standard endoscopy in identifying early-stage neoplasia in Barrett's esophagus. Gastroenterology. 2010; 139(4):1106–1114

[36] Curvers WL, van Vilsteren FG, Baak LC, et al. Endoscopic trimodal imaging versus standard video endoscopy for detection of early Barrett's neoplasia: a multicenter, randomized, crossover study in general practice. Gastrointest Endosc. 2011; 73(2):195–203

[37] Boerwinkel DF, Holz JA, Aalders MCG, et al. Third-generation autofluorescence endoscopy for the detection of early neoplasia in Barrett's esophagus: a pilot study. Dis Esophagus. 2014; 27(3):276–284

[38] Boerwinkel DF, Shariff MK, di Pietro M, et al. Fluorescence imaging for the detection of early neoplasia in Barrett's esophagus: old looks or new vision? Eur J Gastroenterol Hepatol. 2014; 26(7):691–698

[39] Kiesslich R, Gossner L, Goetz M, et al. In vivo histology of Barrett's esophagus and associated neoplasia by confocal laser endomicroscopy. Clin Gastroenterol Hepatol. 2006; 4(8):979–987

[40] Sharma P, Meining AR, Coron E, et al. Real-time increased detection of neoplastic tissue in Barrett's esophagus with probe-based confocal laser endomicroscopy: final results of an international multicenter, prospective, randomized, controlled trial. Gastrointest Endosc. 2011; 74(3):465–472

[41] Gupta A, Attar BM, Koduru P. et al. Utility of confocal laser endomicroscopy in identifying high-grade dysplasia and adenocarcinoma in Barrett's esophagus: a systematic review and meta-analysis. Eur J Gastroenterol Hepatol. 2014; 26(4):369–377

[42] Dunbar KB, Okolo P, III, Montgomery E, Canto MI. Confocal laser endomicroscopy in Barrett's esophagus and endoscopically inapparent Barrett's neoplasia: a prospective, randomized, double-blind, controlled, crossover trial. Gastrointest Endosc. 2009; 70(4):645–654

[43] Canto MI, Anandasabapathy S, Brugge W, et al; Confocal Endomicroscopy for Barrett's Esophagus or Confocal Endomicroscopy for Barrett's Esophagus (CEBE) Trial Group. In vivo endomicroscopy improves detection of Barrett's esophagus-related neoplasia: a multicenter international randomized controlled trial (with video). Gastrointest Endosc. 2014; 79(2):211–221

[44] Wallace MB, Crook JE, Saunders M, et al. Multicenter, randomized, controlled trial of confocal laser endomicroscopy assessment of residual metaplasia after mucosal ablation or resection of GI neoplasia in Barrett's esophagus. Gastrointest Endosc. 2012; 76(3):539–47.e1

[45] Varghese S, Newton R, Ross-Innes CS, et al. Analysis of dysplasia in patients with Barrett's esophagus based on expression pattern of 90 genes. Gastroenterology. 2015; 149(6):1511–1518.e5

[46] Swager A, Boerwinkel DF, de Bruin DM, et al. Volumetric laser endomicroscopy in Barrett's esophagus: a feasibility study on histological correlation. Dis Esophagus. 2016; 29(6):505–512

[47] Leggett CL, Gorospe EC, Chan DK, et al. Comparative diagnostic performance of volumetric laser endomicroscopy and confocal laser endomicroscopy in the detection of dysplasia associated with Barrett's esophagus. Gastrointest Endosc. 2016; 83(5):880–888.e2

[48] Corley DA, Levin TR, Habel LA, et al. Surveillance and survival in Barrett's adenocarcinomas: a population-based study. Gastroenterology. 2002; 122(3):633–640

[49] van Sandick JW, van Lanschot JJ, Kuiken BW, et al. Impact of endoscopic biopsy surveillance of Barrett's oesophagus on pathological stage and clinical outcome of Barrett's carcinoma. Gut. 1998; 43(2):216–222

[50] Inadomi JM, Sampliner R, Lagergren J, et al. Screening and surveillance for Barrett esophagus in high-risk groups: a cost-utility analysis. [comment] Ann Intern Med. 2003; 138(3):176–186

[51] Corley DA, Mehtani K, Quesenberry C, et al. Impact of endoscopic surveillance on mortality from Barrett's esophagus-associated esophageal adenocarcinomas. Gastroenterology. 2013; 145(2):312–9.e1

[52] Bhat SK, McManus DT, Coleman HG, et al. Oesophageal adenocarcinoma and prior diagnosis of Barrett's oesophagus: a population-based study. Gut. 2015; 64(1):20–25

[53] Yousef F, Cardwell C, Cantwell MM, et al. The incidence of esophageal cancer and high-grade dysplasia in Barrett's esophagus: a systematic review and meta-analysis. Am J Epidemiol. 2008; 168(3):237–249

[54] Bhat S, Coleman HG, Yousef F, et al. Risk of malignant progression in Barrett's esophagus patients: results from a large population-based study. J Natl Cancer Inst. 2011; 103(13):1049–1057

[55] Bureo Gonzalez A, Bergman JJGHM, Pouw RE. Endoscopic risk factors for neoplastic progression in patients with Barrett's oesophagus. United European Gastroenterol J. 2016; 4(5):657–662

[56] Thomas T, Gilbert D, Kaye PV, et al. High-resolution endoscopy and endoscopic ultrasound for evaluation of early neoplasia in Barrett's esophagus. Surg Endosc. 2010; 24(5):1110–1116

[57] Pouw RE, Heldoorn N, Alvarez Herrero L, et al. Do we still need EUS in the workup of patients with early esophageal neoplasia? A retrospective analysis of 131 cases. Gastrointest Endosc. 2011; 73(4):662–668

[58] Peters FP, Kara MA, Rosmolen WD, et al. Endoscopic treatment of high-grade dysplasia and early stage cancer in Barrett's esophagus. Gastrointest Endosc. 2005; 61(4):506–514

[59] May A, Gossner L, Pech O, et al. Local endoscopic therapy for intraepithelial high-grade neoplasia and early adenocarcinoma in Barrett's oesophagus: acute-phase and intermediate results of a new treatment approach. Eur J Gastroenterol Hepatol. 2002; 14(10):1085–1091

[60] Pech O, May A, Manner H, et al. Long-term efficacy and safety of endoscopic resection for patients with mucosal adenocarcinoma of the esophagus. Gastroenterology. 2014; 146(3):652–660.e1

[61] Phoa KN, Pouw RE, van Vilsteren FG, et al. Remission of Barrett's esophagus with early neoplasia 5 years after radiofrequency ablation with endoscopic resection: a Netherlands cohort study. Gastroenterology. 2013; 145(1):96–104

[62] Chennat J, Konda VJ, Ross AS, et al. Complete Barrett's eradication endoscopic mucosal resection: an effective treatment modality for high-grade dysplasia and intramucosal carcinoma—an American single-center experience. Am J Gastroenterol. 2009; 104(11):2684–2692

[63] Pouw RE, Seewald S, Gondrie JJ, et al. Stepwise radical endoscopic resection for eradication of Barrett's oesophagus with early neoplasia in a cohort of 169 patients. Gut. 2010; 59(9):1169–1177

[64] van Vilsteren FG, Pouw RE, Seewald S, et al. Stepwise radical endoscopic resection versus radiofrequency ablation for Barrett's oesophagus with high-grade dysplasia or early cancer: a multicentre randomised trial. Gut. 2011; 60(6):765–773

[65] Curvers WL, ten Kate FJ, Krishnadath KK, et al. Low-grade dysplasia in Barrett's esophagus: overdiagnosed and underestimated. Am J Gastroenterol. 2010; 105(7):1523–1530

[66] Duits LC, Phoa KN, Curvers WL, et al. Barrett's oesophagus patients with low-grade dysplasia can be accurately risk-stratified after histological review by an expert pathology panel. Gut. 2015; 64(5):700–706

[67] Phoa KN, van Vilsteren FG, Weusten BL, et al. Radiofrequency ablation vs endoscopic surveillance for patients with Barrett esophagus and low-grade dysplasia: a randomized clinical trial. JAMA. 2014; 311(12):1209–1217

[68] Shaheen NJ, Overholt BF, Sampliner RE, et al. Durability of radiofrequency ablation in Barrett's esophagus with dysplasia. Gastroenterology. 2011; 141(2):460–468

[69] Alvarez Herrero L, Pouw RE, van Vilsteren FG, et al. Safety and efficacy of multiband mucosectomy in 1060 resections in Barrett's esophagus. Endoscopy. 2011; 43(3):177–183

[70] Pouw RE, van Vilsteren FG, Peters FP, et al. Randomized trial on endoscopic resection-cap versus multiband mucosectomy for piecemeal endoscopic resection of early Barrett's neoplasia. Gastrointest Endosc. 2011; 74(1):35–43

[71] Takahashi H, Arimura Y, Masao H, et al. Endoscopic submucosal dissection is superior to conventional endoscopic resection as a curative treatment for early squamous cell carcinoma of the esophagus (with video). Gastrointest Endosc. 2010; 72(2):255–264, 264.e1–264.e2

[72] Chevaux JB, Piessevaux H, Jouret-Mourin A, et al. Clinical outcome in patients treated with endoscopic submucosal dissection for superficial Barrett's neoplasia. Endoscopy. 2015; 47(2):103–112

[73] Neuhaus H, Terheggen G, Rutz EM, et al. Endoscopic submucosal dissection plus radiofrequency ablation of neoplastic Barrett's esophagus. Endoscopy. 2012; 44(12):1105–1113

[74] Pimentel-Nunes P, Dinis-Ribeiro M, Ponchon T, et al. Endoscopic submucosal dissection: European Society of Gastrointestinal Endoscopy (ESGE) Guideline. Endoscopy. 2015; 47(9):829–854

[75] Overholt BF, Wang KK, Burdick JS, et al; International Photodynamic Group for High-Grade Dysplasia in Barrett's Esophagus. Five-year efficacy and safety of photodynamic therapy with Photofrin in Barrett's high-grade dysplasia. Gastrointest Endosc. 2007; 66(3):460–468

[76] Gray NA, Odze RD, Spechler SJ. Buried metaplasia after endoscopic ablation of Barrett's esophagus: a systematic review. Am J Gastroenterol. 2011; 106(11):1899–1908, quiz 1909

[77] Manner H, Rabenstein T, Pech O, et al. Ablation of residual Barrett's epithelium after endoscopic resection: a randomized long-term follow-up study of argon plasma coagulation vs. surveillance (APE study). Endoscopy. 2014; 46(1):6–12

[78] Manner H, May A, Kouti I, et al. Efficacy and safety of hybrid-APC for the ablation of Barrett's esophagus. Surg Endosc. 2016; 30(4):1364–1370

[79] Shaheen NJ, Sharma P, Overholt BF, et al. Radiofrequency ablation in Barrett's esophagus with dysplasia. N Engl J Med. 2009; 360(22):2277–2288

[80] Phoa KN, Pouw RE, Bisschops R, et al. Multimodality endoscopic eradication for neoplastic Barrett oesophagus: results of an European multicentre study (EURO-II). Gut. 2016;65(4):555–562

[81] Bulsiewicz WJ, Kim HP, Dellon ES, et al. Safety and efficacy of endoscopic mucosal therapy with radiofrequency ablation for patients with neoplastic Barrett's esophagus. Clin Gastroenterol Hepatol. 2013; 11(6):636–642

[82] Chadwick G, Groene O, Markar SR, et al. Systematic review comparing radiofrequency ablation and complete endoscopic resection in treating dysplastic Barrett's esophagus: a critical assessment of histologic outcomes and adverse events. Gastrointest Endosc. 2014; 79(5):718–731.e3

[83] Alvarez Herrero L, van Vilsteren FG, Pouw RE, et al. Endoscopic radiofrequency ablation combined with endoscopic resection for early neoplasia in Barrett's esophagus longer than 10 cm. Gastrointest Endosc. 2011; 73(4):682–690

[84] Pouw RE, Visser M, Odze RD, et al. Pseudo-buried Barrett's post radiofrequency ablation for Barrett's esophagus, with or without prior endoscopic resection. Endoscopy. 2014; 46(2):105–109

[85] Ross-Innes CS, Becq J, Warren A, et al; Oesophageal Cancer Clinical and Molecular Stratification (OCCAMS) Study Group. Oesophageal Cancer Clinical and Molecular Stratification OCCAMS Study Group. Whole-genome sequencing provides new insights into the clonal architecture of Barrett's esophagus and esophageal adenocarcinoma. Nat Genet. 2015; 47(9):1038–1046

[86] Bollschweiler E, Baldus SE, Schröder W, et al. High rate of lymph-node metastasis in submucosal esophageal squamous-cell carcinomas and adenocarcinomas. Endoscopy. 2006; 38(2):149–156

[87] Manner H, Pech O, Heldmann Y, et al. Efficacy, safety, and long-term results of endoscopic treatment for early stage adenocarcinoma of the esophagus with low-risk sm1 invasion. Clin Gastroenterol Hepatol. 2013; 11(6):630–635, quiz e45

[88] Alvarez Herrero L, Pouw RE, van Vilsteren FG, et al. Risk of lymph node metastasis associated with deeper invasion by early adenocarcinoma of the esophagus and cardia: study based on endoscopic resection specimens. Endoscopy. 2010; 42(12):1030–1036

[89] Schölvinck DW, Künzli HT, Kestens C, et al. Treatment of Barrett's esophagus with a novel focal cryoablation device: a safety and feasibility study. Endoscopy. 2015; 47(12):1106–1112

24 Squamous Neoplasia of the Esophagus

Hassan A. Siddiki and David E. Fleischer

24.1 Introduction

24.1.1 Epidemiology and Risk Factors

Squamous cell carcinoma (SCC) of the esophagus and its precursor lesions are referred to as squamous cell neoplasia (SCN). SCC of the esophagus is one of the two main malignancies of the esophagus, the other being adenocarcinoma. Esophageal cancer makes up 3.7% of all non–skin-related cancers worldwide. Approximately 450,000 new cases are detected each year worldwide. It is the eighth most common cancer in both genders combined, and the sixth most common cancer in men. More than 80% of cases arise in less developed regions of the world and, of those, 90% are SCC.[1] Barrett's esophagus (BE), the main precursor to adenocarcinoma of the esophagus, is covered in Chapter 23. adenocarcinoma of the esophagus, is covered in Chapter 23. Advanced esophageal cancer, both SCC and adenocarcinoma, is covered in Chapter 27. This chapter focuses on squamous precursors of esophageal cancer and early SCC.

Various epidemiologic associations are known for SCC. In the United States, two major associations include smoking with a population-attributable risk (PAR) of 56% (confidence interval [CI] of 36–75) and alcohol with a PAR of 72.4% (95% CI 53–86).[2] In contrast, in the economically less developed countries in eastern and central Asia and eastern and southern Africa (the so-called esophageal cancer belt) where rates (per 100,000) of SCC are the highest in the world, alcohol and tobacco exposure have little or no role (▶Fig. 24.1).[3,4,5] Studies in high-risk areas

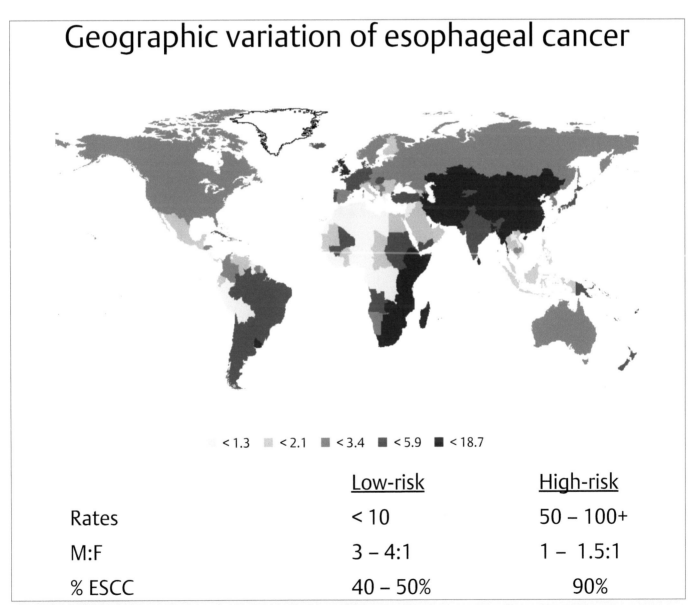

	Low-risk	High-risk
Rates	< 10	50 – 100+
M:F	3 – 4:1	1 – 1.5:1
% ESCC	40 – 50%	90%

Legend: < 1.3, < 2.1, < 3.4, < 5.9, < 18.7

Fig. 24.1 Geographic variation of esophageal cancer. The world map illustrates the areas of high and low prevalence. An esophageal cancer belt passes from China through Central Asia along the eastern and southern coasts of Africa.

suggest that the exposure to carcinogens such as polycyclic aromatic hydrocarbons, poor oral hygiene, opium, poor aromatic hydrocarbons, poor oral hygiene, opium, poor nutrition, and thermal damages are major risks, whereas tobacco exposure plays only a minor role. In certain parts of China, coal cakes are used for both cooking and heating. The inhaled smoke has a high level of polycyclic aromatic hydrocarbons which is an important risk factor for SCC in China.[6] A report from India describes poor oral hygiene as a risk for esophageal squamous cell carcinoma (ESCC) in Kashmir.[7] Drinking hot tea, a habit common in Northern Iran, has been strongly associated with a high risk of esophageal cancer.[8] A study from Tenwek Hospital in Bomet, Kenya, describes risk factors for SCC. One of the traditions is to drink mursik which is a combination of a fermented beverage with an ash-like material.[8] There is some controversy about the role of human papilloma virus (HPV). A relationship between HPV and SCN has not been shown consistently.[9] Despite these differences in etiology, both high- and low-rate SCC share dysplasia as their precursor lesion

and thus approaches to screening and treatment are common to both. ▶ Fig. 24.2 shows photograph of one of the authors DF) with colleagues and patients in China (24.2a) and Kenya (24.2b).

24.1.2 Precursor Lesions for Squamous Neoplasia

Some, but not all, of these associations exist for precursor lesions for SCC. Precursor lesions may be divided histologically into (1) mild dysplasia, (2) moderate dysplasia, and (3) severe dysplasia (▶ Fig. 24.3). Squamous dysplasia requires the presence of nuclear atypia (enlargement, pleomorphism, and hyperchromasia), loss of cell polarity, and abnormal tissue maturation without invasion of epithelial cells through the basement membrane.

Compared with normal, in mild dysplasia, the abnormalities are confined to the lower third of the epithelium; whereas in moderate dysplasia, these are present in the lower two-thirds

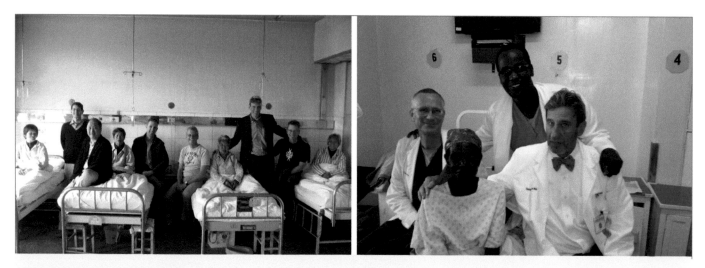

Fig. 24.2 Clinical research in high-risk populations. **(a)** The author (DF) in Feiching, China, with collaborators and patients. **(b)** With coworkers and patient in Kenya.

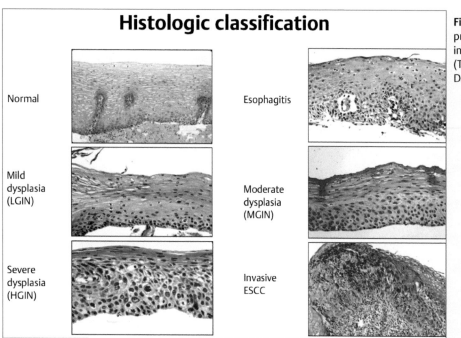

Fig. 24.3 Histologic classification of precursors of squamous cell carcinoma and invasive squamous cell carcinoma. (This image is provided courtesy of Dr. Sanford Dawsey.)

of the epithelium; and in severe dysplasia, these also involve the upper third of the epithelium. Full-thickness involvement of the epithelium is called carcinoma in situ. It is considered by some to be synonymous with severe dysplasia based on their similar histologic appearance and risk of progression to invasive SCC. Risk factors for SCC and dysplasia in high-risk populations are similar in some situations: gender (no), alcohol drinking (no), family history of cancer (yes), tooth loss (yes), water source (yes), and HPV (yes/no). These are different in that tobacco seems to be a risk for SCC and not dysplasia, and serum pepsinogen levels do not appear to be a risk for SCC but risk for dysplasia.[10]

The most definitive assessment of risk for squamous cell esophageal histology has come from the Linxian Dysplasia Nutrition Intervention Trial (NIT).[11] Over a 3.5-year period, mild dysplasia increased the risk of developing SCC by 2.2, moderate dysplasia by 15.8, and severe dysplasia by 72.6. On a follow-up study at 13.5 years, SCC developed in 8% of the participants who initially had a normal histology, but 24% with mild dysplasia, 50% with moderate dysplasia, and 74% with severe dysplasia.[12]

24.2 Diagnostic Approaches

Since most patients with squamous dysplasia of the esophagus and early esophageal cancer will be asymptomatic, the diagnoses will generally be made by screening unless the lesion is found incidentally in a patient that has unrelated symptoms. In the United States, there are no guidelines that recommend screening for SCN. In high-incidence areas (China, Iran, Japan, East Africa) screening is increasingly employed (▶Table 24.1).

24.2.1 Nonendoscopic Techniques

A common nonendoscopic screening technique for early detection of esophageal cancer is esophageal balloon cytology

Table 24.1 Diagnostic techniques to assess for squamous cell carcinoma and its precursors

Nonendoscopic techniques	Endoscopic techniques
Balloon cytology	High-resolution endoscopy with white light and magnification
Sponge cytology	Chromoendoscopy with Lugol's iodine
Molecular tumor markers	Optical chromoendoscopy
Autoantibodies	Confocal laser endoscopy
	High-resolution microendoscopy
	Endoscopic ultrasound
	Volumetric laser endomicroscopy

developed for screening in high-risk populations. To sample the esophagus blindly, an inflatable balloon covered with netting was developed in China[13,14] and later an encapsulated sponge was developed in Japan (▶Fig. 24.4).[15,16]

Balloon Cytology

This technique employs "fishing" for esophageal squamous cells. A nylon or silk mesh covering a deflated balloon is swallowed by the patient and once the balloon is in the stomach, it can be inflated and pulled proximally. The compliance of the balloon is controlled with a syringe that connects to the device via tubing. On withdrawing the balloon, the device will be pulled back. Prior to that, it will be partially deflated and then pulled through the mouth where the cells which are collected in the mesh undergo cytologic staining. The method suffers from low sensitivity, less than 50%.[17] However, the ease of use and affordability are appealing. This technique was widely used in China and accepted as a diagnostic method by the World Health Organization. A recent study of 15 years of follow-up showed

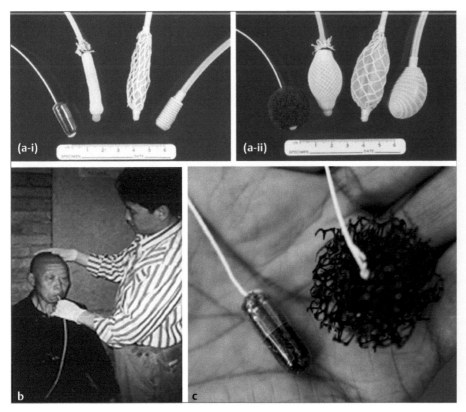

Fig. 24.4 Balloons and sponges used for nonendoscopic diagnosis. **(a–i)** Left to right: cytologic sponge; two versions of a balloon with mesh. **(a–ii)** An inflatable rubber-ribbed device. **(b)** A Chinese health care worker passing balloon into patient's esophagus for screening. **(c)** Cytologic sponge in gelatin capsule before and after release.

that balloon cytology examination remained a reliable method for early detection of esophageal cancer and has accumulated a valuable cytologic bank.[18]

Sponge Cytology

In this technique, a polyurethane mesh is compressed inside a gelatin capsule and attached to a string. The encapsulated sponge is swallowed by the patient and when the sponge enters the stomach the contents of the stomach dissolve the gelatin covering. The mesh devoid of its covering can now expand (▶ Fig. 24.4c). As the sponge is pulled up the esophagus, mucosal cells get scraped and these exfoliated cells are then collected, processed, and stained for cellular abnormalities. There are no large studies evaluating this technique for detecting dysplasia. In a smaller study using a very early version of the sponge, the sensitivity and specificity of this technique was 24 and 92%, respectively.[19] Because of blind sampling and limited morphologic evaluation of only a fraction of the cells, the accuracy of the early sponge was not precise enough for it to be recommended as a community-based screening tool. Recent studies done using the cytosponge for dysplasia related to BE have been more encouraging, demonstrating the overall sensitivity of 79% increasing to 87.2% for patients with long-segment BE, who swallowed the device and a specificity for diagnosing BE of 92.4%.[20] In a large study conducted in the United Kingdom, where the cytosponge was combined with immunohistochemical staining for trefoil factor 3 (TFF3, a biomarker for BE) the overall sensitivity was 79.9%. Compared to endoscopy, the specificity was 92.4%. Similar studies have not been conducted for SCN. In the current form, the sponge cannot replace endoscopic screening. It is being studied in parts of the world where the incidence of SCC is high. If it is shown to be sensitive and specific, it would be a "game changer" in screening for both SCC and its precursors. One aspect of this discussion relates to whether balloon and sponge techniques differ in the evaluation of patients with squamous lesions versus BE. Barrett's epithelium is thicker than squamous epithelium, is better vascularized, and has a mucus layer, all of which would seemingly make it more resistant

to ablation than squamous tissue. On the other hand, squamous epithelium (which sloughs off more easily than Barrett's tissue after ablation) may be more difficult to ablate because it may regenerate from the epithelial linings of ducts in the submucosal glands, and since neoplasia can extend down into the ducts, this may lead to recurrence.

24.2.2 Endoscopic Techniques

High-Resolution White Light with Magnification

White light high-definition endoscopy with magnification can detect advanced lesions as irregular mucosa, white patch, focal red area, erosions, or a plaque but many early cancers and precursors may be missed without the use of chromoendoscopy. This topic is covered in more detail in Chapter 18. According to the Paris Classification of superficial neoplastic lesions, an abnormal-appearing lesion is called "superficial" when its endoscopic appearance suggests that the depth of penetration in the digestive wall is not more than into the submucosa, that is, there is no infiltration of the muscularis propria.[21] All such superficial lesions come under the type "0" and can range from completely flat (0–IIB) to elevated (0–IIa) and depressed (0–IIc) (▶ Fig. 24.5).

Chromoendoscopy with Lugol's Solution

Iodine staining was first employed by Schiller in 1932 to detect abnormalities in the uterine cervix. The basic principle is that iodine stains normal squamous cells a brownish-green color, but that pathologic tissue depleted of glycogen does not pick up the stain and produces an unstained lesion. For example, dysplastic or malignant cells, which are devoid of glycogen, will not pick up the stain (▶ Fig. 24.6). Lugol's solution contains iodine and potassium iodide. The strength of the solution can vary, but commonly includes mixing 12 g of iodine with 24 g of potassium iodide in 1 L water. The formula gives the solution a strength of 1.2% by

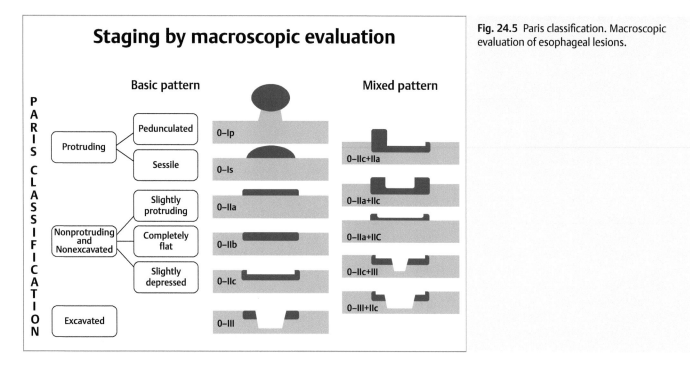

Fig. 24.5 Paris classification. Macroscopic evaluation of esophageal lesions.

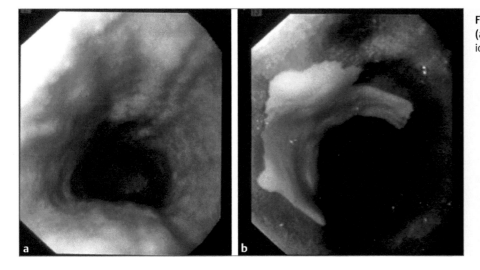

Fig. 24.6 Endoscopic view of early SCC. **(a)** White light endoscopy. **(b)** After Lugol's iodine staining.

elemental iodine content and 3% by total iodine content. Lugol's staining improves the sensitivity of detection of squamous neoplastic lesions, dysplasia and carcinoma, from 62 to 96% without any loss of specificity.[22]

Compared with cytology balloons, its sensitivity and specificity are superior, at 96 and 63%, respectively.[23] In expert centers, specificity could reach 100% after reviewing the histology. In China, a high-risk population study showed that after staining with Lugol's solution, 23% of the lesions containing high-grade dysplasia and 55% of the lesions containing low-grade dysplasia, which were missed by routine endoscopy, could be detected by Lugol's solution, suggesting a strong role in the early detection of dysplastic lesions.[22]

Twenty milliliters of dye is sprayed from the distal to proximal via biopsy channel using a spray catheter (Olympus America, Inc., Millville, New Jersey). The decision to spray from distal to proximal or proximal to distal is a matter of personal preference. Alternatively, an endoscopic retrograde cholangiopancreatography catheter could also be used. The margins of any lesion are better demarcated after staining, making it useful for therapeutic resections when feasible. The specificity of iodine for staining dysplastic lesions is compromised by inflamed mucosa, like esophagitis, which may also appear unstained. When examining the mucosa, special care must be taken not to overlook the upper third of the esophagus. Once Lugol's solution is applied, there needs to be a certain urgency in obtaining biopsies since the staining lasts for only a few minutes. Both biopsies of abnormal areas and systematic sampling of normal areas should be performed and care must be taken to keep these in separate jars.

Optical Chromoendoscopy

These techniques improve the visualization of mucosal morphology without needing the use of dyes. Narrow-band imaging (NBI) (Olympus, Tokyo, Japan) is the approach that has been best studied. Optical chromoendoscopy can be divided into two categories: (1) preprocessing and (2) postprocessing. As is described in Chapter 18, preprocessing techniques optimize mucosal and vascular imaging by adjusting the wavelength composition of the excitation light, generally by mainly using blue light. Blue light, by its shorter wavelength, only penetrates superficially in the tissue and causes less scattering. In addition, blue light is highly absorbed by hemoglobin resulting in

optimal visualization of blood vessels. This technique is utilized by both NBI and blue laser imaging (Fujifilm, Tokyo, Japan). Postprocessing techniques use normal white light excitation and reprocessing of the reflected images by an appropriate algorithm. Examples of this are Fuji intelligent chromoendoscopy (Fujifilm, Satamia, Japan) and i-Scan (Pentax, Tokyo, Japan). All of these techniques can be combined with magnifying endoscopy. The combination enables the endoscopist to visualize intrapapillary capillary loop (IPCL) patterns which are capillary loops arising perpendicularly from smooth-branching vessels in the subepithelium. In mucosal cancer, these loops dilate causing the vascular network to be less transparent than a normal mucosa (▶Fig. 24.7). In SCC, four IPCL pattern changes have been described, including dilation, weaving, change in caliber, and variety in shape. These features may be useful in estimating atypia and depth of invasion.[24] A more current classification has been described by Inoue.[25]

In a randomized-controlled trial, it was shown that NBI improved the detection rates for SCC.[26] In this study, the sensitivity of NBI for diagnosis of superficial cancer was 97.2%. The accuracy of NBI for the diagnosis of superficial esophageal cancer was 88.9%; however, no large prospective studies have shown that magnifying endoscopy with NBI is superior to Lugol's chromoendoscopy. In another more recently conducted study, changes in the morphology of IPCLs were well correlated with the depth of SCC invasion.[27]

Confocal Laser Endoscopy

This is a high-resolution imaging technique that introduced a novel endoscopic surveillance method for SCN and has the ability to detect cancer at the subcellular level (see Chapter 18). Using CLE, the mucosa can be analyzed at a magnification of 1,000 times, and with a maximum penetration depth of the scanning laser light of up to 250 microns. Changes in vessels, connective tissue, and in the cellular architecture can be evaluated during ongoing endoscopy. When confocal imaging is paired with chromoendoscopy, accuracy rates have been shown to dramatically rise, approaching more than 95%, mostly attributable to improvement of the known low specificity of chromoendoscopy alone.[28] The drawback to this technique is that existing platforms are expensive (> $150,000) and are available mainly in tertiary care centers. There is also the limitation that it is not possible to image

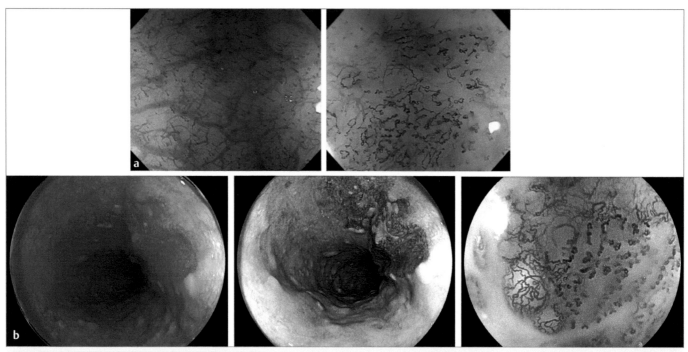

Fig. 24.7 Demonstration of normal vascular pattern and vascular pattern with early SCC. Endoscopic definition of intrapapillary capillary loops (IPCLs). (a) Olympus narrow-band imaging. (b) Fujifilm, blue light imaging. (Figure (b) is provided courtesy of Dr. Tomoyuki Kuike.

the abnormality and perform a biopsy at the same time. CLE is not a wide-view endoscopic platform like chromoendoscopy and works best for evaluating a focal lesion.

High-Resolution Microendoscopy

High-resolution microendoscopy (HRME) has the potential to provide images of the surface epithelium with similar resolution to CLE but with significantly reduced system complexity and cost. The HRME system requires fluorescent images via coherent fiber bundle placed in contact with tissue. Illumination is provided via bandpass-filtered blue light–emitting diode. The system is controlled by laptop computer which acquires and displays video at a frame rate of 15 frames per second. The cost of the system, which is not commercially available, may be less than $5,000. The feasibility of quantitative analysis of HRME images for the prediction of SCC by using the mean nuclear area to discriminate nonneoplastic and neoplastic esophageal squamous epithelium exists. Quantitative information from the high-resolution images was used to identify high-grade squamous dysplasia or invasive SCC based on the histopathologic findings. The study showed a sensitivity of 87 and specificity of 97% in a test set and a sensitivity of 84 and a specificity of 95% in a different validation. The studies published on this technique have used post hoc image analysis which limits the generalizability of the results.[29]

Endoscopic Ultrasonography

Even high-frequency ultrasound has not achieved accuracy for the staging of SCC, mainly because of its poor resolution and limited depiction with an appropriate coupler design. EUS provides suboptimal delineation of muscularis mucosa and submucosa. In 33% of SCC cases, it was difficult to draw a clear line of demarcation in the nine-layer structure with high-frequency ultrasound including the interfacial architecture.[30]

Volumetric Laser Endomicroscopy

Volumetric laser endomicroscopy (VLE) is a method of optical endomicroscopy that uses optical coherence tomography (OCT) to produce cross-sectional and subsurface images to an approximate depth of 3 mm and is being used to accurately measure, in real time, mucosal and submucosal abnormalities for the detection of focal dysplasia and neoplasia. OCT is the only technology that can depict real-time cross-sectional images of biological tissue at a near-microscopic level without contrast agents, such as required with CLE. After investigating the correlation between OCT-based staging and the histologic staging of en bloc endoscopic submucosal dissection (ESD) specimens, the criteria for OCT-based staging for early esophageal cancer was established.[31] ▶Fig. 24.8 shows VLE imaging in a case of superficial esophageal cancer. Real-time tissue marking is expected and it would greatly enhance the accuracy of tissue biopsy with VLE.

24.3 Treatment for Squamous Neoplasia of the Esophagus

The therapies for treating early SCC and its precursors are similar to the ones that are used for BE and carcinoma in Barrett's. They can be divided into two categories: (1) resective modalities and (2) ablative modalities (▶Table 24.2).

The informed decision between the patient and the endoscopist to proceed with endoscopic therapy for SCN hinges on staging (▶Fig. 24.9). When primary endoscopic therapy

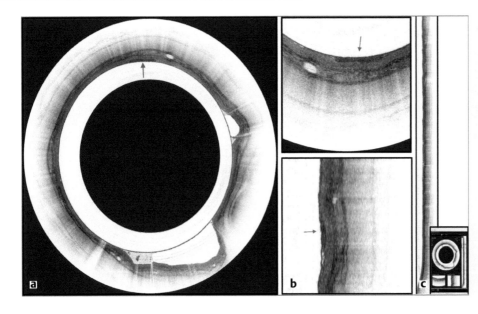

Fig. 24.8 Volumetric laser endomicroscopy demonstrating early squamous cell carcinoma. **(a)** Circumferential view, lesion at 12 o'clock/ arrow. **(b)** Close-up horizontal view, lesion at 6 o'clock/arrow. **(c)** Longitudinal view/ arrow. (This images are provided courtesy of Dr Arvind Trindade.)

Table 24.2 Endoscopic treatment modalities for squamous cell neoplasia

Resective modalities	Thermal techniques
Endoscopic mucosal resection (EMR)	Radiofrequency ablation
• Cap assisted	Cryotherapy
• Band ligation	Photodynamic therapy
Endoscopic submucosal dissection (ESD)	Argon plasma coagulation
	Bipolar coagulation

is planned for asymptomatic patients with early neoplasia, the intent is always cure. If there is a substantial risk of lymph node metastasis (LNM), then surgical resection with or without chemoradiation is appropriate. The risk of LNM is linked to the depth of tumor invasion. For T1m1 (intraepithelial neoplasia) and T1m2 lesions (limited to the lamina propria) the risk of LNM is less than 5%. Lesions invading the muscularis mucosa (T1m3) or superficial submucosa (T1sm1) carry a higher risk of distant LNM.[32] For these T1m3/T1sm1 borderline risk lesions, selecting endoscopic treatment versus surgery should be discussed in a multidisciplinary setting based on patient factors and the histologic grade of neoplasia. Poorly differentiated lesions have a higher risk of LNM as compared to well-differentiated lesions. Well-to-moderately differentiated T1m3 cancers involve lymph nodes 6 to 18%.[33,34] Regarding T1sm1 lesions, it should be understood that while endoscopic therapy may be adequate in "low-risk" sm1 adenocarcinoma, similar-depth SCN lesions are more aggressive in nature and have a higher tendency for early metastasis (as high as 53%). In a pooled outcome study of 7,645 patients with esophageal cancer involving the submucosa, the percentage of LNM was 37%. Lymph node, lymphatic, and vascular invasion in sm1 esophageal cancers was 27, 46, and 22%, respectively. Rates of LNM for sm1 and sm2 were significantly higher in SCN compared with adenocarcinoma, whereas the LNM for sm3 was comparable, with greater than 50% involvement in both histologic subtypes.[35]

When the decision is made that endoscopic therapy will be undertaken, the next decision is whether to use resective therapy or ablation. Whenever the lesion is nodular, resection is required,

at least for the component that is elevated. If it is a completely flat lesion, thermal therapies are appropriate. For larger flat lesions, thermal therapy, usually radiofrequency ablation (RFA), has the appeal that it is easier and often more efficient. It has the inherent disadvantage that no tissue is acquired. Western physicians who have seen many patients with BE are more familiar with RFA. Eastern physicians are more comfortable with resective techniques.

24.3.1 Endoscopic Resection

The goal of endoscopic resection may be either a mucosal resection or a submucosal dissection. The American Society for Gastrointestinal Endoscopy Technology Committee has recently reviewed both methods.[36,37] The first experiences of esophageal endoscopic mucosal resection (EMR) were reported 25 years ago. The technique evolved over the next 25 years from the simple lift and cut technique (strip biopsy) to more complex procedures using specifically designed resective tubes.[38] Over the past decade, it is common to perform mucosal resection with either the standard cap-assisted approach or with a band-ligation device. EMR with either a cap or band ligation is generally performed if less than 50% of the luminal circumference is involved and the total size is not more than 2 cm. With resection of circumferential lesions, stricturing almost always occurs. Lesions of 1 to 2 cm in diameter can be removed en bloc while larger lesions require a piecemeal approach. Options for both resection and thermal ablative therapies are described in ▶ Table 24.2.

Cap-Assisted Endoscopic Mucosal Resection

Cap-assisted EMR (EMRC) was described before band ligation. There are some differences. With EMRC, a submucosal injection is used to separate the mucosa from the submucosa. Slightly larger specimens are obtained with cap versus band. Many feel the cap-assisted technique is slightly more cumbersome. The

TNM Staging Of Esophageal Cancer

Primary tumor (T)*	
TX	Primary tumor cannot assessed
T0	No evidence of primary tumor
Tis	High-grade dysplasia•
T1	Tumor invades lamina propria, muscularis mucosae, or submucosa
T1a	Tumor invades lamia propria or muscularis mucosae
T1b	Tumor invades submucosa
T2	Tumor invades muscularis propria
T3	Tumor invades adventitia
T4	Tumor invades adiacent structures
T4a	Resectable tumor invading pleura, pericardium, or diaphragm
T4b	Unresectable tumor invading other adjacent structures, such as aorta, vertebral body, trachea, etc.

Regional lymph nodes (N)Δ	
NX	Regional lymph node(s) cannot be assessed
N0	No regional lymph node metastasis
N1	Metastasis in 1-2 regional lymph nodes
N2	Metastasis in 3-6 regional lymph nodes
N3	Metastasis in seven or more regional lymph nodes

Distant metastasis (M)	
M0	No distant metastasis
M1	Distant metastasis

Stage	T	N	M
0	Tis (HGD)	N0	M0
IA	T1	N0	M0
IB	T1	N0	M0
	T2-3	N0	M0
IIA	T2-3	N0	M0
	T2-3	N0	M0
IIB	T2-3	N0	M0
	T1-2	N1	M0
IIIA	T1-2	N2	M0
	T3	N1	M0
	T4a	N0	M0
IIIB	T3	N2	M0
IIIC	T4a	N1-2	M0
	T4b	Any	M0
	Any	N3	M0
IV	Any	Any	M1

Fig. 24.9 Tumor, node, and metastasis (TNM) staging for esophageal cancer.

techniques of EMR are described in more detail in Chapter 23, but the steps generally begin with Lugol's iodine to define the area of abnormality. The margin of the unstained lesion is generally marked with electrocautery because the Lugol's iodine will fade. Afterward a submucosal injection is performed for both safety and ease of resection. Afterward the cap is placed over the lesion and suction is employed. The tissue is invaginated into the cap where a snare that has been preset is used for a resection.

The largest study aimed to investigate the rates of survival and metastasis after EMR of ESCC with mucosal or submucosal invasion included 402 with a mean follow-up of 50 months.[34] The 5-year survival rate was 91% for mucosal lesions and 71% for lesions involving the submucosa. The rate of metastasis at 5 years was 0.4% for mucosal lesions and 8.7% for submucosal lesions.

Another study simultaneously evaluated long-term outcomes of EMR for early SCN and compared it to early adenocarcinoma.[39] The study included 204 patients with SCC and 26 with adenocarcinoma. Mean follow-up was 36.5 months for SCC and 26 months for adenocarcinoma. The recurrence rate of SCC was significantly higher than that of adenocarcinoma (4 local recurrence + 22 metachronous in the SCC group vs. 1 metachronous recurrence in the adenocarcinoma group). The median time to recurrence was 35 months (range, 12–85). The cumulative 5-year disease-free survival rates of SCC were significantly lower than those of adenocarcinoma (57 vs. 85.2%; $p = 0.01$). The cumulative 5-year recurrence rates of SCC were significantly higher than those of adenocarcinoma (32 vs. 4.2%; $p = 0.023$) concluding that rate of recurrence after EMR was higher in patients with SCC than in patients with adenocarcinoma. Recommendations from this paper suggested more rigorous endoscopic follow-up for patients with SCN after EMR than in those with adenocarcinoma.

Endoscopic Mucosal Resection Band Ligation

An early report of tissue band ligation followed by snare resection in patients with SCC and their precursors was described in 1996.[40] This technique has been replaced by multiband mucosectomy (MBM). This technique is especially useful in settings where resources and endoscopic expertise are less available. With this technique, there is no requirement for lifting and the snaring, once the ligation is taking place, is typical to what physicians use for polypectomies.

This technique is described in more detail in Chapter 23. Basically, the area is stained with Lugol's iodine or defined by optical chromoendoscopy. Afterward electrocautery may be used for marking. No submucosal injection is employed. The lesion with a rim of normal mucosa is sucked into the cap followed by the release of a single band. Afterward, the polyp which is created is resected with a snare (▶ Fig. 24.10).

A recent randomized trial enrolled 84 patients who underwent MBM and compared them to 42 patients who had EMRC for early SCN. An endoscopically complete resection with MBM was achieved in all patients. This study showed that at 3-month and 12-month follow-up, none of the patients had high-grade intraepithelial neoplasm (HGIN) or SCC at the resection site. Endoscopic resection with MBM led to a significant reduction both in procedure time and in the cost of disposables accessories. In both the MBM group and the EMRC group, esophageal stenosis occurred in between 19 and 22%. None of these stenoses required intervention.[41]

Endoscopic Submucosal Dissection

This technique was developed in Japan in the 1980s and is now one of the mainstay therapies for early SCC and precursor lesions. Unlike EMR, there is no maximum size limitation and due to the fact that the tumor is removed en bloc, the local recurrence after resection is lower than with EMR. The ESD requires that the endoscopist be well trained and works in a unit that deals with complex endoscopic procedures.

The indication of ESD for SCN, according to the Japanese Esophageal Society Guidelines[32] is for intramucosal cancers involving the epithelium and lamina propria occupying less than two-thirds of the circumference of the esophagus. Relative indications include cancers involving a muscularis mucosa and less than 200 μm of submucosa. A variety of dissecting knives are available. The actual procedure is described in more detail in Chapter 23, but basically it involves staining with Lugol's iodine, and then making electrocautery markings. Before making a mucosal incision, a submucosal injection is performed, generally with glycerol or hyaluronic acid. Once the fluid is injected, a hole is created in the mucosa with a knife and the tip of the knife is introduced in the submucosal space. Keeping the mucosa hooked, the direction of the knife is kept turned toward the lumen while mucosa is being cut. The knife has the ability to employ spray coagulation in order to prevent bleeding from submucosal vessels. Once the mucosal incision is performed in a circumference, submucosal deeper fibers can now be cut using the cap for countertraction. For vessels greater than 1 mm in the submucosa, coagulation can be performed using hemostatic forceps. Some authorities used a silk line with a clip to create light tension for countertraction by attaching the clip to the lesion on its submucosal side. ▶ Fig. 24.11 demonstrates the technique.

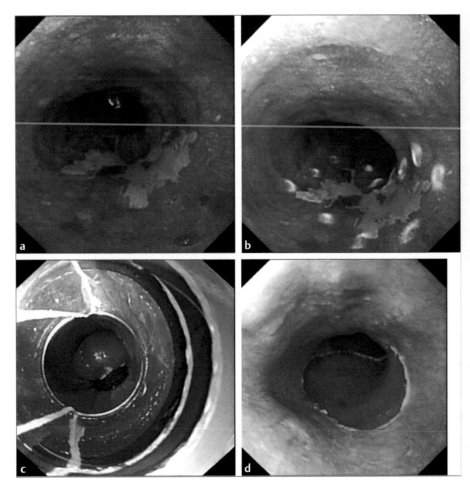

Fig. 24.10 Technique of band-ligation EMR. Band ligation for SCN. **(a)** Staining with Lugol's iodine, **(b)** close-up view, **(c)** band-ligation seen, **(d)** after endoscopic mucosal resection.

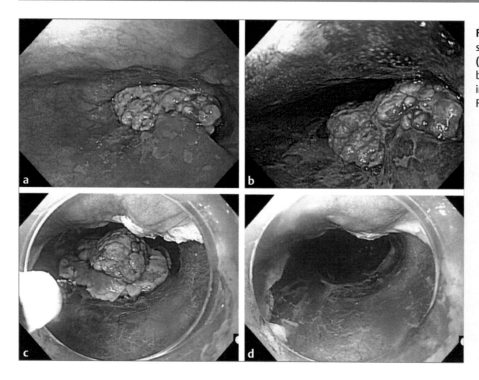

Fig. 24.11 Technique of endoscopic submucosal dissection. **(a)** White light, **(b)** Lugol's iodine stain, **(c)** needle knife beginning resection, **(d)** after ESD. (These images are provided courtesy of Dr Norio Fukami.)

A meta-analysis that included eight studies comparing ESD and EMR for endoscopic resection of superficial SCN demonstrated that ESD had a higher en bloc resection rate.[42]

The pooled analysis showed a significantly lower recurrence rate in the ESD group than in the EMR group (0.3 vs. 11.5% odds ratio [OR]−0.08; $p < 0.001$). However, subgroup analysis shows that the recurrence rate for ESD and EMR was equivalent when lesion size was smaller than 20 mm ($p = 0.25$).

Considering a higher perforation risk of ESD (0–6% vs. 0–2% for EMR), higher stricture rate of 12 to 17% for lesions greater than 75% of circumference and the need for specialized training to achieve competency, EMR is preferred over ESD for lesions less than 15 mm.[43]

The relative aggressive nature of SCN when compared to adenocarcinoma is again seen in the data generated by studies reporting the performance of ESD. T1a SCN that involves the muscularis mucosa poses a substantial risk (6–9%) for LNM that appears to be greater than esophageal adenocarcinoma of the same depth.[44,45,46] In another publication, data of a single-center cohort of 2,920 patients operated for cancers of the esophagus reported the 5-year survival rate for patients with surgically resected T1a cancer werer 78%, with notable differences between adenocarcinoma (91%) and SCC (62%).[47]

24.4 Thermal Therapy

Of the thermal therapies that are listed in ▶Table 24.2, only RFA and cryotherapy are commonly employed and the published experience with RFA is greater than that with cryotherapy for precursor lesions of SCC and also with BE for precursor lesion of adenocarcinoma.

24.4.1 Radiofrequency Ablation

For patients with early SCC and its precursors, the endoscopic pattern often shows lesions greater than 3 cm and there also

may be a mosaic pattern. If there is no nodularity and submucosal invasion, RFA can be an appealing and efficient procedure. In patients with lesions greater than 3 cm or ones that cover more than 75% of the esophagus, endoscopic resection has a high risk of causing stenosis.[48] RFA is technically less demanding than ESD and for larger lesions is more efficient than EMR.

In a large prospective cohort of 96 patients who underwent RFA for greater than or equal to 3 cm flat (0–IIb) lesions containing intraepithelial neoplasia or T1m2 invasion, complete response was achieved in 84% of patients after a mean of 1.9 RFA treatments at 12 months.[49] Multivariable analysis demonstrated that baseline grade of neoplasia, specifically SCC T1m2 (OR 0.05) and lesion length (OR 0.79) were independent negative predictors of complete response at 12 months. Two patients demonstrated neoplastic progression, of which one went from intraepithelial to T1m2 at 6 months. Stricture formation was the most common adverse event affecting 21% of patients. Since that time, different RFA doses have been utilized and the stricture rate is much less. In post hoc analysis of different circumferential RFA technique groups, application of circumferential RFA at 12 J/cm² with no cleaning had the lowest stricture rate and a similar 12-month complete response rates compared with the other groups. In a recent study it was demonstrated that RFA and ESD are equally effective in the short-term treatment of early large (> 3cm) flat large SCN[50]; however, ESD was associated with a higher rate of adverse events, especially in the lesions extending for more than 75% of the circumference. Of a total of 65 patients, 18 were treated with RFA and 47 with ESD. The complete resection rate of ESD and complete response rate at 12 months after primary RFA were 89.3 and 77.8%, respectively. However, the biggest drawback is that unlike ESD and EMR, ablation precludes an opportunity for accurate histopathologic diagnosis. In the same study, it should be noted that 14/47 (29%) post-ESD specimens had histologic upstaging compared with the pre-ESD biopsies, and 4 of them had lymphovascular invasion requiring chemoradiation or surgery, again highlighting the role of en bloc tissue retrieval. In an elegant study to quantify the rate of poor histologic features lost to pathology work-up by ablative treatment, 65 large, flat-type lesions were included that were deemed eligible for ablative treatment. The authors also recorded the pattern of neoplastic ductal extension in specimens of lesions. This was done to further understand the concept of extension of neoplastic disease along mucosal surfaces into gland orifices and ducts of esophageal submucosal glands creating a sheltered "niche" beyond the reach of ablation. Thirty-five percent (6/17) of lesions that were initially considered eligible for RFA treatment showed submucosal invasion hence confirming that histologic prognostication based on the flatness of the lesion is poor, and could place patients at risk for LNM.[51] The conclusions of this study are at variance with those by Zhang and He presented earlier. This is not uncommon when new technologies are applied. Further studies will help reconcile the differences.

Western physicians will be quite familiar with using RFA for BE. Because BE is often circumferential, for long segments a circumferential device is used (Halo 360, Covidien/Medtronic). It may also be used for SCN when there are circumferential lesions. A new 360-degree treatment device (Express catheter) allows for both sizing of the esophageal diameter and treatment with a single balloon. For noncircumferential lesions, a variety of focal treatment devices are available.

The esophagus is sprayed with Lugol's iodine and unstained lesions are marked with electrocautery. Afterward, thermal therapy with RFA is applied generally utilizing 12 J (▶ Fig. 24.12). There is some controversy as to whether it is necessary to scrape the treated area before delivering a second series of RFA. Unlike resective techniques, no tissue specimen is available and therefore follow-up is mandatory. It is typical to repeat the endoscopy 2 to 3 months after the initial procedure and reassess the situation. In many instances, a second round of treatment is necessary. Follow-up is also repeated after the complete eradication has been achieved. The exact timing of post-RFA surveillance for squamous lesions is not well established. Many of the recommendations are borrowed from the Barrett's literature,

24.4.2 Cryotherapy

Cryotherapy is an endoscopic method using a noncontact approach for tissue destruction by application of a cryogen sprayed as a gas onto the target mucosa. Both liquid nitrogen and carbon dioxide have been utilized and there is some debate about the relative advantages and disadvantages of each. Rapid freezing causes failure of cellular metabolism because of stress on lipids and proteins. Continued freezing produces extracellular ice, creating a hyperosmotic extracellular environment which draws fluid from the cells. Further freezing produces intracellular ice formation disrupting organelles and cell membrane. This leads to vascular stasis with edema, platelet aggregation, and formation of microthrombi. This results in ischemic necrosis. ▶ Fig. 24.13 shows the catheter delivering the cryogen and the ice formation after treatment.

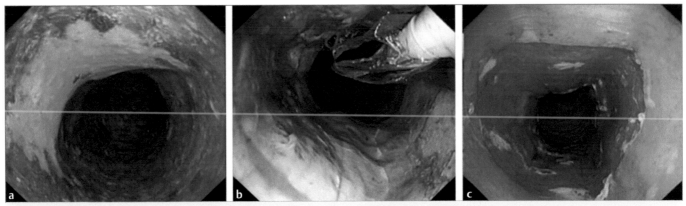

Fig. 24.12 Early SCC before and after treatment with RFA. **(a)** Lugol's iodine stain, **(b)** immediately after RFA with 360-degree circumferential balloon, **(c)** posttreatment.

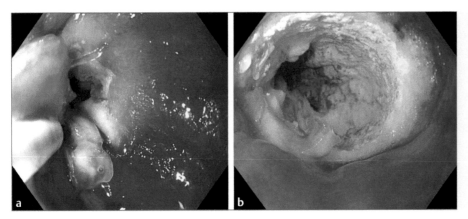

Fig. 24.13 Cryotherapy for high-grade intraepithelial neoplasia. **(a)** Spray catheter in place, **(b)** after ice formation.

Cryotherapy has been used for palliative treatment of esophageal cancer. There are no large series describing the use of cryotherapy for early esophageal cancer.

24.4.3 Other Ablative Techniques

Photodynamic therapy (PDT), multipolar electrocautery (MPEC), and argon plasma coagulation (APC) have been used for ablation for a wide variety of lesions in the gastrointestinal tract. PDT has the appeal that presumably only the pathologic lesion is affected by the light therapy, but because the procedure is much more complex than RFA and because the stricture rate is high, it is not commonly employed. For the small lesions, MPEC and APC could be utilized but the dosimetry is not as precise as with RFA and it is more time consuming to treat larger lesions.

24.5 Areas of Uncertainty, Experimental Techniques, and Research

The curse of esophageal cancer (whether SCC or adenocarcinoma) is that by the time that symptoms develop, the cancer is usually at an advanced stage. Therefore, the keys to improved survival are earlier diagnosis. In high-risk areas around the world where programs have been set up for early detection and treatment, these involve five components: (1) identification of a precursor lesion, (2) a primary screening method, (3) a method for endoscopic localization, (4) staging, and (5) utilization of the least invasive therapy (▶Table 24.3).

The counterpart to BE as a precursor for adenocarcinoma, squamous dysplasia, is the antecedent lesion. Unlike BE, which is endoscopically visible, squamous dysplasia may not be visible with routine white light endoscopy and as long as endoscopic screening is necessary, the discovery of precursor lesions will be limited by cost and the ability to screen. Therefore, the development of nonendoscopic screening is critical. The concept of balloon

cytology has been utilized for more than a half a century, but has been limited by sensitivity and specificity. The hope that sponges may improve the performance of nonendoscopic screening is encouraging but has not been established. Whereas initial nonendoscopic screening was based on cellular identification, it is hopeful that biomarkers will be even more valuable.

The hope that molecular markers will aid in the early diagnosis of esophageal cancer has not been realized. Tumor-specific genes like *p16* hypermethylation and adenomatous polyposis coli hypermethylation have been described in SCN. Hypermethylated *p16* in tumor tissue was shown to be present in 82% of SCCs; however, precursor lesions or early neoplasia are unlikely to shed altered deoxyribonucleic acid (DNA) in the serum or stool.[52,53] If a molecular signal is identified, which is truly expressed in large areas of squamous epithelium and represents a field effect, it may make this approach more feasible.

The possibility that autoantibodies could be useful as potential serum markers for SCC has been intriguing. An autoantibody blood test may be used as an aid to diagnose SCC, especially in early SCC.[54] The hope is that measurements of autoantibodies could differentiate early-stage SCC from normal controls.

Another attempt at nonendoscopic evaluation is development of a tethered capsule that captures snapshots of the esophagus with optical frequency domain imaging (OFDI) (▶Fig. 24.14). Such a capsule might reconstruct a 3D image of the esophagus and provide enough details to allow the diagnosis of abnormal

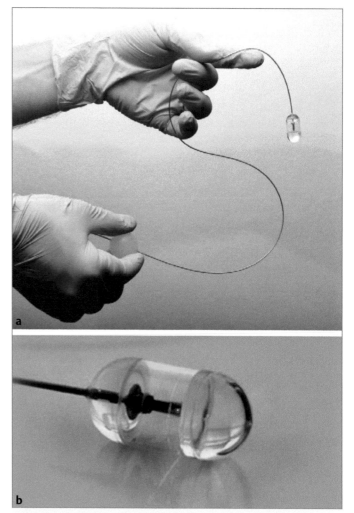

Fig. 24.14 Tethered capsule for evaluation of early changes of esophageal cancer.

Table 24.3 Components of a program for early detection and treatment of squamous cell carcinoma and its precursors

Program for early detection and treatment of SCC and its precursors	
Component	**State of the art/areas for research**
Identification of precursor lesion	Squamous dysplasia
Primary screening method	Need for nonendoscopic method • Sponge cytology • Molecular markers
Endoscopic localization	Lugol's iodine Optical chromoendoscopy
Staging	High-resolution endoscopy Optical chromoendoscopy High-resolution microendoscopy Volumetric laser endomicroscopy Imaging techniques
Utilization of the least invasive therapy	Thermal ablative therapy Endoscopic mucosal resection Endoscopic submucosal dissection Full-thickness endoscopic resection

growth patterns before something is seen microscopically.[55] After the patient is identified by some nonendoscopic screening device, endoscopy would be carried out.

Localization would need to be achieved and currently Lugol's iodine, which is low tech, low cost is the approach most commonly utilized. The hope would be that optical chromoendoscopy could give additional information. Additionally, staging would be required so the decision could be made about which therapy was best. Currently, focal resections and focal ablations are utilized with advancing depth of removal being carried out as technology advances. The advent of third-space endoscopic access (e.g., as employed with peroral endoscopic myotomy) could increase the ability for more extensive tissue removal or destruction. Ultimately, full-thickness endoscopic methods will be employed.

All of this investigation assumes that the esophageal cancer or its precursor has developed. An even more encouraging strategy would be to find a chemopreventive method. More than 10 analyses have been published from different interventions. Most of these have been carried out in China in high-risk areas. All but two of the trials evaluated nutritional intervention, including a variety of micronutrients. Evidence for a beneficial effect on premalignancy was observed in some studies with the use of a combination of retinol plus riboflavin plus zinc, multivitamins, selenomethionine, and some fruits. If such a chemo-preventive agent were developed, it would change the paradigm.

24.6 Summary

In developing countries, tobacco and alcohol are the main risk factors for esophageal cancer. In less developed countries, a number of risk factors have been identified. The divergent etiologic risk factors may be linked by the production of polycyclic aromatic hydrocarbons. Dysplasia is the precursor lesion that can progress to cancer. As with patients who have intestinal metaplasia as a risk for adenocarcinoma, it would helpful to define which patients who have dysplasia as a risk factor for SCC are likely to progress and which are not. In high-risk populations, screening programs can be implemented to intervene at a stage when a disease is potentially curable. For squamous lesions, Lugol's chromoendoscopy is helpful in both discovering premalignant lesions and demarcating them. Staging is the first step to define what the management will be. If the lesion is localized to the mucosa and flat, then both thermal therapies and resective therapies are available. RFA, which has had promising results for the management of BE, has been utilized for dysplasia and early esophageal cancer. Both EMR and ESD have shown long-term benefits and as opposed to thermal therapies offer an opportunity for the pathology to be evaluated. Attempts have been made to define a chemoprevention approach. The absence of a nonendoscopic approach to screen for SCN has been the biggest gap in finding and curtailing the disease, and the discovery of such an approach would be a game changer worldwide.

References

[1] Ferlay J, Soerjomataram I, Dikshit R, et al. Cancer incidence and mortality worldwide: sources, methods and major patterns in GLOBOCAN 2012. Int J Cancer. 2015; 136(5):E359–E386

[2] Prabhu A, Obi KO, Rubenstein JH. The synergistic effects of alcohol and tobacco consumption on the risk of esophageal squamous cell carcinoma: a meta-analysis. Am J Gastroenterol. 2014; 109(6):822–827

[3] Cook-Mozaffari PJ, Azordegan F, Day NE. et al. Oesophageal cancer studies in the Caspian Littoral of Iran: results of a case-control study. Br J Cancer. 1979; 39(3):293–309

[4] Islami F, Kamangar F, Aghcheli K, et al. Epidemiologic features of upper gastrointestinal tract cancers in Northeastern Iran. Br J Cancer. 2004; 90(7):1402–1406

[5] Tran GD, Sun XD, Abnet CC, et al. Prospective study of risk factors for esophageal and gastric cancers in the Linxian general population trial cohort in China. Int J Cancer. 2005; 113(3):456–463

[6] Deziel NC, Wei WQ, Abnet CC, et al. A multi-day environmental study of polycyclic aromatic hydrocarbon exposure in a high-risk region for esophageal cancer in China. J Expo Sci Environ Epidemiol. 2013; 23(1):52–59

[7] Dar NA, Islami F, Bhat GA, et al. Poor oral hygiene and risk of esophageal squamous cell carcinoma in Kashmir. Br J Cancer. 2013; 109(5):1367–1372

[8] Islami F, Pourshams A, Nasrollahzadeh D, et al. Tea drinking habits and oesophageal cancer in a high risk area in northern Iran: population based case-control study. BMJ. 2009; 338:b929

[9] Togawa K, Jaskiewicz K, Takahashi H, et al. Human papillomavirus DNA sequences in esophagus squamous cell carcinoma. Gastroenterology. 1994; 107(1):128–136

[10] Kamangar F, Diaw L, Wei WQ, et al. Serum pepsinogens and risk of esophageal squamous dysplasia. Int J Cancer. 2009; 124(2):456–460

[11] Wang JB, Abnet CC, Fan JH. et al. The randomized Linxian Dysplasia Nutrition Intervention Trial after 26 years of follow-up: no effect of multivitamin supplementation on mortality. JAMA Intern Med. 2013; 173(13):1259–1261

[12] Wang GQ, Abnet CC, Shen Q, et al. Histological precursors of oesophageal squamous cell carcinoma: results from a 13 year prospective follow up study in a high risk population. Gut. 2005; 54(2):187–192

[13] Shu YJ. Cytopathology of the esophagus. An overview of esophageal cytopathology in China. Acta Cytol. 1983; 27(1):7–16

[14] Shu YJ. The Cytopathology of Esophageal Carcinoma: Precancerous Lesions and Early Cancer. New York, NY: Masson; 1985

[15] Jaskiewicz K, Venter FS, Marasas WF. Cytopathology of the esophagus in Transkei. J Natl Cancer Inst. 1987; 79(5):961–967

[16] Nabeya K, Onozawa K, Ri S. Brushing cytology with capsule for esophageal cancer. Chir Gastroenterol.. 1979; 13:101–107

[17] Roth MJ, Liu SF, Dawsey SM, et al. Cytologic detection of esophageal squamous cell carcinoma and precursor lesions using balloon and sponge samplers in asymptomatic adults in Linxian, China. Cancer. 1997; 80(11):2047–2059

[18] Wang LD, Yang HH, Fan ZM, et al. Cytological screening and 15 years' follow-up (1986–2001) for early esophageal squamous cell carcinoma and precancerous lesions in a high-risk population in Anyang County, Henan Province, Northern China. Cancer Detect Prev. 2005; 29(4):317–322

[19] Wei WQ, Abnet CC, Lu N, et al. Risk factors for oesophageal squamous dysplasia in adult inhabitants of a high risk region of China. Gut. 2005; 54(6):759–763

[20] Ross-Innes CS, Debiram-Beecham I, O'Donovan M, et al; BEST2 Study Group. Evaluation of a minimally invasive cell sampling device coupled with assessment of trefoil factor 3 expression for diagnosing Barrett's esophagus: a multi-center case-control study. PLoS Med. 2015; 12(1):e1001780

[21] The Paris endoscopic classification of superficial neoplastic lesions: esophagus, stomach, and colon: November 30 to December 1, 2002. Gastrointest Endosc. 2003; 58(suppl 6):S3–S43

[22] Dawsey SM, Fleischer DE, Wang GQ, et al. Mucosal iodine staining improves endoscopic visualization of squamous dysplasia and squamous cell carcinoma of the esophagus in Linxian, China. Cancer. 1998; 83(2):220–231

[23] Davydov M, Delektorskaya VV, Kuvshinov YP, et al. Superficial and early cancers of the esophagus. Ann N Y Acad Sci. 2014; 1325:159–169

[24] Inoue H, Honda T, Nagai K, et al. Ultra-high magnification endoscopic observation of carcinoma in situ of the esophagus. Dig Endosc. 1997; 9(1):16–18

[25] Inoue H. Magnification endoscopy in the esophagus and stomach. Dig Endosc. 2001; 13:40–41

[26] Muto M, Minashi K, Yano T, et al. Early detection of superficial squamous cell carcinoma in the head and neck region and esophagus by narrow band imaging: a multicenter randomized controlled trial. J Clin Oncol. 2010; 28(9):1566–1572

[27] Sato H, Inoue H, Ikeda H, et al. Utility of intrapapillary capillary loops seen on magnifying narrow-band imaging in estimating invasive depth of esophageal squamous cell carcinoma. Endoscopy. 2015; 47(2):122–128

[28] Pech O, Rabenstein T, Manner H, et al. Confocal laser endomicroscopy for in vivo diagnosis of early squamous cell carcinoma in the esophagus. Clin Gastroenterol Hepatol. 2008; 6(1):89–94

[29] Shin D, Protano MA, Polydorides AD, et al. Quantitative analysis of high-resolution microendoscopic images for diagnosis of esophageal squamous cell carcinoma. Clin Gastroenterol Hepatol. 2015; 13(2):272–279.e2

[30] Das A, Sivak MV, Jr, Chak A, et al. High-resolution endoscopic imaging of the GI tract: a comparative study of optical coherence tomography versus high-frequency catheter probe EUS. Gastrointest Endosc. 2001; 54(2):219–224

[31] Hatta W, Uno K, Koike T, et al. Optical coherence tomography for the staging of tumor infiltration in superficial esophageal squamous cell carcinoma. Gastrointest Endosc. 2010; 71(6):899–906

[32] Kuwano H, Nishimura Y, Oyama T, et al. Guidelines for Diagnosis and Treatment of Carcinoma of the Esophagus April 2012 edited by the Japan Esophageal Society. Esophagus 2015;12:1–30

[33] Xu YW, Peng YH, Chen B, et al. Autoantibodies as potential biomarkers for the early detection of esophageal squamous cell carcinoma. Am J Gastroenterol. 2014; 109(1):36–45

[34] Yamashina T, Ishihara R, Nagai K, et al. Long-term outcome and metastatic risk after endoscopic resection of superficial esophageal squamous cell carcinoma. Am J Gastroenterol. 2013; 108(4):544–551

[35] Gockel I, Sgourakis G, Lyros O, et al. Risk of lymph node metastasis in submucosal esophageal cancer: a review of surgically resected patients. Expert Rev Gastroenterol Hepatol. 2011; 5(3):371–384

[36] Draganov PV, Gotoda T, Chavalitdhamrong D, Wallace MB. Techniques of endoscopic submucosal dissection: application for the Western endoscopist? Gastrointest Endosc. 2013; 78(5):677–688

[37] Hwang JH, Konda V, Abu Dayyeh BK, et al; ASGE Technology Committee. Endoscopic mucosal resection. Gastrointest Endosc. 2015; 82(2):215–226

[38] Makuuchi H. Esophageal endoscopic mucosal resection (EEMR) tube. Surg Laparosc Endosc. 1996; 6(2):160–161

[39] Nakagawa K, Koike T, Iijima K, et al. Comparison of the long-term outcomes of endoscopic resection for superficial squamous cell carcinoma and adenocarcinoma of the esophagus in Japan. Am J Gastroenterol. 2014; 109(3):348–356

[40] Fleischer DE, Wang GQ, Dawsey S, et al. Tissue band ligation followed by snare resection (band and snare): a new technique for tissue acquisition in the esophagus. Gastrointest Endosc. 1996; 44(1):68–72

[41] Zhang YM, Boerwinkel DF, Qin X, et al. A randomized trial comparing multiband mucosectomy and cap-assisted endoscopic resection for endoscopic piecemeal resection of early squamous neoplasia of the esophagus. Endoscopy. 2016;48(4):330 –338 8

[42] Guo HM, Zhang XQ, Chen M, et al, . Endoscopic submucosal dissection vs endoscopic mucosal resection for superficial esophageal cancer. World J Gastroenterol. 2014; 20(18):5540–5547

[43] Ishihara R, Iishi H, Uedo N, et al. Comparison of EMR and endoscopic submucosal dissection for en bloc resection of early esophageal cancers in Japan. Gastrointest Endosc. 2008; 68(6):1066–1072

[44] Akutsu Y, Uesato M, Shuto K, et al. The overall prevalence of metastasis in T1 esophageal squamous cell carcinoma: a retrospective analysis of 295 patients. Ann Surg. 2013; 257(6):1032–1038

[45] Leers JM, DeMeester SR, Oezcelik A, et al. The prevalence of lymph node metastases in patients with T1 esophageal adenocarcinoma a retrospective review of esophagectomy specimens. Ann Surg. 2011; 253(2):271–278

[46] Takahashi H, Arimura Y, Masao H, et al. Endoscopic submucosal dissection is superior to conventional endoscopic resection as a curative treatment for early squamous cell carcinoma of the esophagus (with video). Gastrointest Endosc. 2010; 72(2):255–264, 264.e1–264.e2

[47] Gertler R, Stein HJ, Langer R, et al. Long-term outcome of 2920 patients with cancers of the esophagus and esophagogastric junction: evaluation of the New Union Internationale Contre le Cancer/American Joint Cancer Committee staging system. Ann Surg. 2011; 253(4):689–698

[48] Zhang YM, Bergman JJ, Weusten B, et al. Radiofrequency ablation for early esophageal squamous cell neoplasia. Endoscopy. 2010; 42(4):327–333

[49] He S, Bergman J, Zhang Y, et al. Endoscopic radiofrequency ablation for early esophageal squamous cell neoplasia: report of safety and effectiveness from a large prospective trial. Endoscopy. 2015; 47(5):398–408

[50] Wang WL, Chang IW, Chen CC, et al. Radiofrequency ablation versus endoscopic submucosal dissection in treating large early esophageal squamous cell neoplasia. Medicine (Baltimore). 2015; 94(49):e2240

[51] Jansen M, Schölvinck DW, Kushima R, et al. Is it justified to ablate flat-type esophageal squamous cancer? An analysis of endoscopic submucosal dissection specimens of lesions meeting the selection criteria of radiofrequency studies. Gastrointest Endosc. 2014; 80(6):995–1002

[52] Hibi K, Taguchi M, Nakayama H, et al. Molecular detection of p16 promoter methylation in the serum of patients with esophageal squamous cell carcinoma. Clin Cancer Res. 2001; 7(10):3135–3138

[53] Kawakami K, Brabender J, Lord RV, et al. Hypermethylated APC DNA in plasma and prognosis of patients with esophageal adenocarcinoma. J Natl Cancer Inst. 2000; 92(22):1805–1811

[54] Xue L, Ren L, Zou S, et al. Parameters predicting lymph node metastasis in patients with superficial esophageal squamous cell carcinoma. Mod Pathol. 2012; 25(10):1364–1377

[55] Gora MJ, Sauk JS, Carruth RW, et al. Tethered capsule endomicroscopy enables less invasive imaging of gastrointestinal tract microstructure. Nat Med. 2013; 19(2):238–240

25 Benign Esophageal Strictures and Esophageal Narrowing Including Eosinophilic Esophagitis

Peter D. Siersema

25.1 Introduction

Benign esophageal strictures and narrowing are commonly seen in daily endoscopic practice. The cornerstone of the management of benign strictures is endoscopic dilation therapy. A subgroup of strictures is refractory or recurs repeatedly after initial dilation. For these so-called difficult strictures alternative treatment modalities are available, that is, steroid injections into the stricture combined with dilation, incisional therapy for refractory anastomotic strictures, stent placement, self-bougienage, or surgery as salvage treatment. The scientific background for these treatments is largely based on case series and only a few randomized studies have compared different treatment modalities.

In this chapter, the most frequently used endoscopic treatment modalities for benign strictures and narrowing are discussed and practical information for the management of some specific causes of esophageal stricturing and narrowing, that is, eosinophilic esophagitis (EoE) and post–endoscopic resection (ER) of premalignant stages and early-stage malignancies, is presented.

25.2 Diagnostic Approaches

25.2.1 General Approach Including Causes, Symptoms, and Diagnosis

Benign esophageal strictures and narrowing are caused by a variety of esophageal disorders or injuries, including gastroesophageal reflux disease (GERD), radiation therapy, or ingestion of a corrosive substance. They also occur at the anastomotic site after esophageal resection. Two relatively new kids on the block include EoE, which may lead to focal or diffuse esophageal narrowing, and stricturing due to ER or ablative therapy in the esophagus.

Dysphagia is the most common symptom in patients with a benign esophageal stricture and narrowing. Interestingly, most patients with a benign stricture do not experience severe weight loss, as is often seen in malignant esophageal strictures. Some patients have symptoms of odynophagia, mostly as a result of radiotherapy and severe reflux esophagitis. The first presentation in EoE is frequently food bolus obstruction, but patients may also have symptoms of regurgitation and sometimes aspiration (pneumonia).

Barium swallow can detect these esophageal strictures; however, most cases are nowadays detected by upper endoscopy. If the stricture diameter does not allow introduction of a normal-caliber endoscope, one should consider using a small-caliber endoscope. A combined anterograde and retrograde dilation (CARD) or rendezvous approach is useful for the treatment of a completely obstructed esophagus.[1] It should be considered to take biopsies in case malignancy is suspected and to confirm EoE.

25.3 Classification System

Benign esophageal strictures can be subdivided into simple and complex strictures. Simple strictures are short, focal, straight, and frequently allow passage of a normal-diameter endoscope. Examples include Schatzki's rings, esophageal webs, and most peptic strictures.[2] Overall, one to three dilations are sufficient to relieve dysphagia in simple strictures. Only 25 to 35% of patients require additional sessions, with a maximum of five dilations in more than 95% of patients.[3]

Complex strictures are usually longer (> 2 cm), angulated, irregular, or have a severely narrowed diameter. These strictures are more difficult to treat and have a tendency to be refractory or to recur despite dilation therapy.[2] Etiologies of complex strictures include anastomotic strictures, radiation-induced strictures, and caustic strictures. When strictures are refractory or recur frequently, dilation therapy alone is usually not sufficient to relieve dysphagia. According to the Kochman criteria, refractory or recurrent strictures are defined as an anatomical restriction because of persistent or recurrent fibrosis. This may occur as the result of either an inability to successfully remediate the anatomical problem to a diameter of at least 14 mm over five sessions at 2-week intervals (refractory); or as a result of an inability to maintain a satisfactory luminal diameter for 4 weeks once the target diameter of 14 mm has been achieved (recurrent).[2] In these cases, repeated dilations are indicated, or one of the alternative techniques described under the section *Variations of standard techniques* could be considered.

25.4 Therapeutic Approaches

25.4.1 Standard Technique

Endoscopic Dilation with an Inflatable Balloon or Bougie Dilator

Treatment aims to relieve dysphagia, with the avoidance of complications and the prevention of recurrences. In most cases this can be achieved by endoscopic dilation with an inflatable balloon or a (Savary) bougie dilator, both introduced over a guidewire (▶ Fig. 25.1). No differences have been shown between balloon and bougie dilation in safety and efficacy. For strictures in the proximal esophagus, especially for anastomotic strictures, wire-guided bougie dilators can be used as these allow sensing the degree of resistance during dilation, which may help in deciding whether further dilation with larger-diameter bougies should be considered. The most frequently reported complications associated with esophageal dilation include perforation, hemorrhage, and bacteremia. The reported rates of perforation vary between 0.1 and 0.4% and are mostly seen with complex strictures.[4]

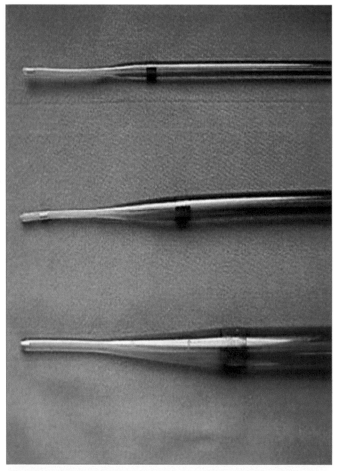

Fig. 25.1 Different-sized (Savary) bougie dilators for dilation of esophageal strictures.

It is advised to start endoscopic dilation at a balloon or bougie size that is 1 to 2 mm larger than the estimated stricture diameter and to limit initial dilation to a diameter of 8 to 12 mm. If strictures cannot be traversed with a standard endoscope, the next step is to use a small-caliber endoscope. If still not possible to traverse, it is advised to advance the guidewire under fluoroscopy. In some cases, especially when the stricture has already been dilated several times, one may consider to traverse the guidewire and the balloon or bougie "blind," that is, not using fluoroscopy.

It is generally accepted that the risk of perforation is minimal when "the rule of three" is applied, meaning that the maximum dilation diameter should not increase greater than 3 mm per session. A recent study by Grooteman et al[5] has questioned the rule of three and suggested that more than three dilation steps may be considered in benign esophageal strictures. Caution is, however, needed with the dilation of malignant strictures, as the authors found an increased risk of perforations and adverse events when the rule of three was not applied.

25.4.2 Variations of Standard Techniques

Endoscopic Dilation Combined with Steroid Injection

Endoscopic dilation combined with steroid injection has been reported to prevent stricture recurrence. Unfortunately, randomized

trials are limited and mostly not adequately powered. Camargo et al randomized 14 patients with corrosive strictures between steroid injections or placebo, both combined with dilation.[6] They found no difference in dilation frequency or recurrent dysphagia between the two groups. Ramage et al. randomized 30 patients with peptic strictures with recurrent dysphagia after at least one dilation session to dilation with or without intralesional four-quadrant injections of triamcinolone.[7] It was concluded that dilation combined with steroid injection reduced the number of repeat dilations and increased the dysphagia-free period, with redilation rates of 13% in the steroid group versus 60% in the control group ($p = 0.01$). Finally, Hirdes et al randomized 60 patients with untreated cervical anastomotic esophageal strictures after esophagostomy with gastric tube interposition and dysphagia for at least solid food to dilation with or without four-quadrant triamcinolone injections.[8] They concluded that adding intralesional steroid injections to Savary dilation in patients with benign anastomotic esophageal strictures did not result in a clinically significant benefit. The authors also noted an increased incidence of candida esophagitis in the remaining esophagus in the steroid group.

It can be concluded that steroid injection combined with dilation seems to reduce the risk of recurrent dysphagia in benign esophageal strictures of peptic origin. However, in other stricture types no significant effect was found, probably related to the underlying cause of stricturing. It is advised to repeat steroid injection up to a maximum of three sessions. Nonetheless, the optimal injection dose, technique, and frequency remain to be determined.

Needle–Knife Incision

Incisional Therapy

Incisional therapy with a needle–knife was first reported for the treatment of Schatzki rings.[9] This was followed by incisional therapy for anastomotic strictures of the esophagus. In our practice, we place a transparent hood on the tip of the endoscope to enhance control and safety when performing incisional therapy. For cutting, we use a bimodal blended electrocautery current (ERBE Electromedizin GmbH, Tübingen, Germany) with software-controlled fractionated cuts (Endocut). The effective cutting power is maximized at 120 W for 50 ms. The maximum coagulation power during the forced coagulation mode is 45 W for 750 ms. With the needle–knife catheter under direct vision, longitudinal incisions are made around the circumference of the stenotic ring. The required length of the cut is chosen according to the length of the fibrotic stricture as endoscopically determined. The depth of the incision, estimated by comparison with the length of the needle–knife, is not more than 4 mm (►Fig. 25.2).

Hordijk et al treated 24 patients with endoscopic incisional therapy using an endoscopic retrograde cholangiopancreatography (ERCP) needle–knife. After 2 years of follow-up, more than 85% of the patients were still dysphagia-free after one session.[10] This was followed by another study by the same group, in which 62 patients with a primary anastomotic stricture after esophagectomy (which were not previously treated with dilation therapy) were randomized to Savary dilation or incisional therapy using a needle–knife. No significant difference was found in the mean number of dilations (2.9; 95% confidence interval [CI], 2.7–4.1 vs. 3.3; 95% CI,

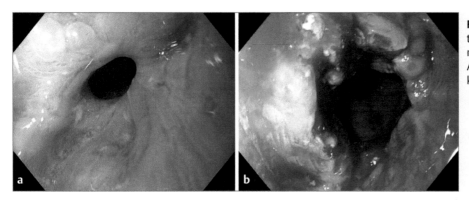

Fig. 25.2 (a) Narrow anastomotic stricture in the proximal esophagus following esophageal resection and gastric tube interposition. **(b)** As a result of incisional therapy with a needle–knife, the anastomotic site is widened.

2.3–3.6l; $p = 0.46$) or success rate (80.6 vs. 67.7%, $p = 0.26$) between the incisional and dilation therapy arms, respectively.[11] No complications were observed after incisional therapy.

From these results, it can be concluded that incisional therapy can be considered as an alternative treatment in patients with a (relatively) short stenosis. Incisional therapy should, however, only be used in esophageal strictures that consist of elevated strictures based on fibrous or scar-like tissue, such as Schatzki's rings and anastomotic strictures.

Stent Placement

Dilation of an esophageal stricture with a balloon or a bougie is usually done for a period of a few seconds or some minutes. If the dilator can be kept in place for a longer time, the benefits of dilation may be longer lasting. In the past few years, temporary stent placement has increasingly been used for refractory benign esophageal strictures (▶Fig. 25.3).

Self-Expandable Plastic Stents

Self-expandable plastic stents (SEPS) are FDA approved for this indication, and have been used for benign esophageal strictures, but the production of the only SEPS available; the Polyflex (Boston Scientific, Natick, Massachusetts) has recently been stopped. Although the Polyflex was found to be effective for the treatment of refractory esophageal strictures, it was found that the risk of migration with this stent was high.[12] Moreover, the stent had a high radial and axial force, which may result in an increased risk of stent-related complications to the esophageal wall, for example, severe bleeding.[13]

Self-Expandable Metal Stents

Partially and fully covered self-expandable metal stents (SEMS), although not FDA approved, are also frequently used for benign esophageal strictures (▶Fig. 25.3a).

One of the major drawbacks of partially covered SEMS (pcSEMS) is that these are associated with hyperplastic tissue ingrowth through the uncovered stent mesh ends resulting in embedding of the stent in the mucosa[14] (▶Fig. 25.4). The complication rate of pcSEMS has been reported to be as high as 50 to 60%. The most common complications of these stents are indeed tissue ingrowth, but include also stent migration, pain, gastroesophageal reflux if the stent is positioned across the gastroesophageal junction, and fistula formation.[15] It is important to note that minor tissue ingrowth may also reduce the risk of stent migration (12 vs. 36%)

with fully covered SEMS (fcSEMS).[16] Tissue ingrowth can successfully be treated with the stent-in-stent method described by Hirdes et al. Using this technique, a similarly sized fcSEMS is placed inside the previously placed embedded stent.[17] Over a period of 10 to 14 days, pressure necrosis of the hyperplastic tissue occurs as a result of friction. Hereafter, both stents can usually easily be removed.

To overcome the problem of stent ingrowth, fcSEMS are preferred for benign esophageal strictures (▶Fig. 25.3b). In the first study using fcSEMS, Eloubeidi et al. placed 36 stents in 31 patients. A clinical success rate of 29% was reported. A total of 47% of patients had no recurrence of dysphagia.[16] Hirdes et al. evaluated the fully covered Wallflex (Boston Scientific, Natick, Massachusetts). They included 15 patients with a refractory benign esophageal stricture. The migration rate was, however, 35%, while tissue overgrowth was seen in 20% of patients. Recurrent dysphagia occurred in all patients after a median of only 15 days after stent removal. The disappointing results in this study were most likely due to the highly refractory patient population in this study.[18]

In general, 35 to 45% of refractory benign esophageal strictures can be treated with SEMS. Particularly, stent migration is an issue with fcSEMS, while tissue ingrowth with pcSEMS makes their use less attractive for benign condition. In order to prevent stent migration when fcSEMS are placed, it has been proposed to clip the stent with the over-the-scope clip (OTSC) device (Ovesco, Tuebingen, Germany) or to use one of the recently introduced sewing devices to prevent stent migration. In our experience, standard endoclips for the prevention of stent migration are at most only effective for a (too) short period.

Biodegradable Stents

Only a small number of studies have reported on biodegradable stent placement in the esophagus. Repici et al included more than 30 patients with a refractory benign esophageal stricture and placed an Ella BD stent (Ella CS, Hradec Králové, Czech Republic) (▶Fig. 25.5a, b). Complete relief of dysphagia was seen in 43% of patients after a median follow-up of 53 weeks.[19] No major complications were seen. In a study by van Boeckel et al, complete relief of dysphagia was reported in 33% of patients treated with an Ella BD stent after a median of 166 days. In this study, major complications occurred in four (22%) patients (hemorrhage [$n = 2$] and severe retrosternal pain [$n = 2$]).[13] Recently, Hirdes et al reported the efficacy and safety of sequential Ella BD stent placement in 28 patients with highly refractory benign strictures.[20] A total of 59 biodegradable stents were placed in these patients.

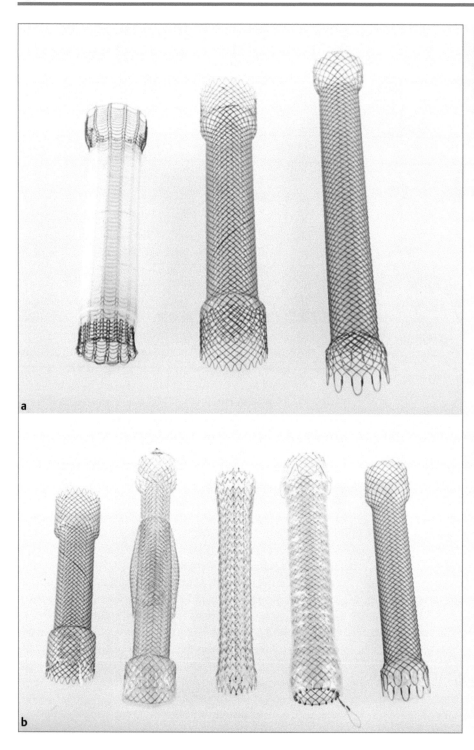

Fig. 25.3 **(a)** Selection of partially covered self-expanding metal stents for treatment of strictures in the esophagus. **(b)** Selection of fully covered self-expanding metal stents for treatment of strictures in the esophagus.

After initial stent placement, patients remained dysphagia-free for a period of 90 days, while after 6 months 25% of patients were dysphagia-free. After placement of a second biodegradable stent in patients with recurrent stricture formation, patients remained dysphagia-free for a median period of 55 days. After 6 months, only 15% of these patients were still dysphagia-free. Major complications occurred in 29 and 8%, of patients after one or two Ella BD stents, respectively.

From these studies, it can be concluded that a single biodegradable stent is only effective in approximately 30 to 40% of patients, which is not different from the results reported with SEMS. Stent placement was also found to be associated with complications, such as retrosternal pain and vomiting. Nonetheless, in selected patients with a refractory benign esophageal stricture, sequential placement of one or two biodegradable stents may be an effective alternative to avoid the burden of serial dilations or stent removal in case of SEMS placement.

Optimal Duration of Stent Placement in Refractory Benign Esophageal Strictures

The optimal duration of stent placement for treating refractory benign esophageal strictures is unknown, but probably a number of variables, such as stricture type, severity of the inflammation, stricture length, and stent type are involved.

The general principle is to leave the stent in place until the inflammation is resolved. In strictures longer than 5 cm or those due to ischemic injury, dilation with a stent for a period of at least

8 to 16 weeks is recommended. For shorter strictures and other etiologies, shorter stenting times can be recommended, but still these strictures may also be refractory. Only fcSEMS designs can safely be removed after a prolonged time of stenting. After biodegradable stent placement, follow-up can be different. Only when patients have recurrent dysphagia a repeat endoscopy is indicated. In most cases, a biodegradable stent is found to be dissolved over time and a new stent, either biodegradable stent or SEMS, can be placed.

25.5 Novel Diseases Causing Esophageal Stricturing

25.5.1 Eosinophilic Esophagitis

Stricture formation is a late complication of EoE, usually occurring in patients with an extended period of esophageal symptoms. Indications for endoscopic dilation in EoE are a tight stricture, narrow-caliber esophagus, food bolus obstruction, and failure of

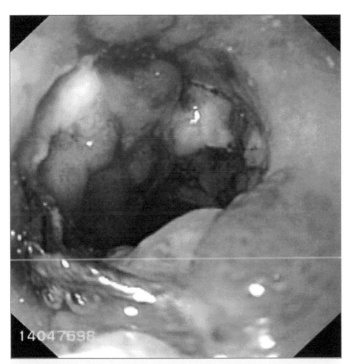

Fig. 25.4 Tissue overgrowth at the proximal end of partially covered self-expanding metal stent.

symptoms to respond to diet or drugs. If possible, treatment for EoE should already be commenced before starting dilation and should be continued afterward to prevent or delay recurrence of symptoms.

Dilation of EoE is no more dangerous than dilation for other esophageal diseases, and perforation rates are similar if experienced operators employ a safe technique and flexible endoscopy. It should be kept in mind that mucosal tears are common after dilation of EoE (8%), but these do not adversely impact outcome.[24]

It is advised to start with low bougie or balloon diameters and limit the progression of dilation per sessions when resistance is noted. After a series of dilation sessions to up to 16 to 18 mm, repeat dilations are performed based on the recurrence of dysphagia. In our experience, most patients will no longer need maintenance dilations or maximally every 1 to 2 years when this guideline is followed.[25]

Patients often experience pain during and after dilation of strictures due to EoE. It is advised to warn patients about this complication and prescribe them adequate pain-control medications prior to discharge.

25.6 Post–Endoscopic Resection

ER procedures performed in the esophagus include both endoscopic mucosal resection (EMR) and endoscopic submucosal dissection (ESD). ER in which greater than 75% of the mucosal circumference is removed are likely to result in a significant endoscopic and symptomatic stricture. Risk factors for clinically significant esophageal strictures after ER include a cervical location, a resection size greater than 75% of the esophageal circumference, and a longitudinal resection length of more than 40 mm.[26]

Repeated dilation is an effective treatment strategy for the management of post-ER symptomatic strictures. The complication rate of dilation for post-ER strictures in the esophagus is low (< 1–2%).[3] SEMS can be used in refractory strictures post-ER but may be associated with similar side effects compared to other indications.

Steroid injection into the resected area has been shown reduced to reduce the development of post-ER strictures.[27] Steroids (triamcinolone acetate) are injected in aliquots of 0.2 mL, 1 cm apart in a semicircumferential fashion up to a maximum of 20 to 60 mg depending on the size of the ER. The initial injections should be given at the margins of the ulcer. Furthermore, oral steroid therapy can also be administered prophylactically to reduce stricture formation.[28] In our experience, oral prednisolone at 30 mg/d is started on the third day post-ESD. Doses are tapered

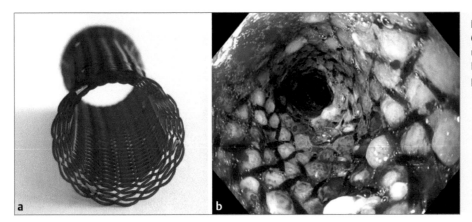

Fig. 25.5 (a) Biodegradable Ella BD stent (Ella CS, Hradec Králové, Czech Republic) to be used for benign esophageal strictures. **(b)** Endoscopic image of an Ella BD stent after placement for a benign esophageal stricture.

gradually (daily 30, 30, 25, 25, 15, and 10 mg for 7 days each), and discontinued over a period of 8 weeks.

25.7 Areas of Uncertainty, Experimental Techniques, and Research

Randomized trials are needed to determine the optimal treatment algorithm in patients with refractory and recurrent benign esophageal strictures. One such trial includes a comparison between Savary or balloon dilation therapy and stent placement, either a fully covered SEMS or biodegradable stent, to determine whether stent placement could be positioned at an earlier stage in the treatment algorithm.

Furthermore, biodegradable stents should be compared with fcSEMS. Finally, the use of a (locally applied) treatment aiming to improve oxygenation (anastomotic strictures), and/or to reduce the inflammatory process in strictures, could be an important step.

Polyglycolic acid (PGA) sheets with fibrin glue have also been evaluated in preventing post-ESD strictures. The sheets are attached with fibrin glue over the surgical wound immediately after the completion of ESD. Although the results seem favorable, more data are needed before widespread use can be advised.

References

[1] Schembre D, Dever JB, Glenn M, et al. Esophageal reconstitution by simultaneous antegrade/retrograde endoscopy: re-establishing patency of the completely obstructed esophagus. Endoscopy. 2011; 43(5):434–437

[2] Kochman ML, McClave SA, Boyce HW. The refractory and the recurrent esophageal stricture: a definition. Gastrointest Endosc. 2005; 62(3):474–475

[3] Pereira-Lima JC, Ramires RP, Zamin I, Jr, et al. Endoscopic dilation of benign esophageal strictures: report on 1043 procedures. Am J Gastroenterol. 1999; 94(6):1497–1501

[4] Saeed ZA, Winchester CB, Ferro PS, et al. Prospective randomized comparison of polyvinyl bougies and through-the-scope balloons for dilation of peptic strictures of the esophagus. Gastrointest Endosc. 1995; 41(3):189–195

[5] Grooteman KV, Wong Kee Song LM, Vleggaar FP, et al. Non-adherence to the rule of three does not increase the risk of adverse events in esophageal dilation. Gastrointest Endosc. 2017; 85:332–337

[6] Camargo MA, Lopes LR, Grangeia TdeA, et al. Use of corticosteroids after esophageal dilations on patients with corrosive stenosis: prospective, randomized and double-blind study Rev Assoc Med Bras (1992). 2003; 49(3):286–292

[7] Ramage JI, Jr, Rumalla A, Baron TH, et al. A prospective, randomized, double-blind, placebo-controlled trial of endoscopic steroid injection therapy for recalcitrant esophageal peptic strictures. Am J Gastroenterol. 2005; 100(11):2419–2425

[8] Hirdes MM, van Hooft JE, Koornstra JJ, et al. Endoscopic corticosteroid injections do not reduce dysphagia after endoscopic dilation therapy in patients with benign esophagogastric anastomotic strictures. Clin Gastroenterol Hepatol. 2013; 11(7):795–801.e1

[9] DiSario JA, Pedersen PJ, Bichiş-Canoutas C, et al. Incision of recurrent distal esophageal (Schatzki) ring after dilation. Gastrointest Endosc. 2002; 56(2):244–248

[10] Hordijk ML, Siersema PD, Tilanus HW, Kuipers EJ. Electrocautery therapy for refractory anastomotic strictures of the esophagus. Gastrointest Endosc. 2006; 63(1):157–163

[11] Hordijk ML, van Hooft JE, Hansen BE, et al. A randomized comparison of electrocautery incision with Savary bougienage for relief of anastomotic gastroesophageal strictures. Gastrointest Endosc. 2009; 70(5):849–855

[12] Repici A, Hassan C, Sharma P, et al. Systematic review: the role of self-expanding plastic stents for benign oesophageal strictures. Aliment Pharmacol Ther. 2010; 31(12):1268–1275

[13] van Boeckel PG, Vleggaar FP, Siersema PD. A comparison of temporary self-expanding plastic and biodegradable stents for refractory benign esophageal strictures. Clin Gastroenterol Hepatol. 2011; 9(8):653–659

[14] Siersema PD. Stenting for benign esophageal strictures. Endoscopy. 2009; 41(4):363–373

[15] van Boeckel PG, Siersema PD. Refractory esophageal strictures: what to do when dilation fails. Curr Treat Options Gastroenterol. 2015; 13(1):47–58

[16] Eloubeidi MA, Lopes TL. Novel removable internally fully covered self-expanding metal esophageal stent: feasibility, technique of removal, and tissue response in humans. Am J Gastroenterol. 2009; 104(6):1374–1381

[17] Hirdes MM, Siersema PD, Houben MH, et al. Stent-in-stent technique for removal of embedded esophageal self-expanding metal stents. Am J Gastroenterol. 2011; 106(2):286–293

[18] Hirdes MM, Siersema PD, Vleggaar FP. A new fully covered metal stent for the treatment of benign and malignant dysphagia: a prospective follow-up study. Gastrointest Endosc. 2012; 75(4):712–718

[19] Repici A, Vleggaar FP, Hassan C, et al. Efficacy and safety of biodegradable stents for refractory benign esophageal strictures: the BEST (Biodegradable Esophageal Stent) study. Gastrointest Endosc. 2010; 72(5):927–934

[20] Hirdes MM, Siersema PD, van Boeckel PG, Vleggaar FP. Single and sequential biodegradable stent placement for refractory benign esophageal strictures: a prospective follow-up study. Endoscopy. 2012; 44(7):649–654

[21] Runge TM, Eluri S, Cotton CC, et al. Outcomes of esophageal dilation in eosinophilic esophagitis: safety, efficacy, and persistence of the fibrostenotic phenotype. Am J Gastroenterol. 2016; 111(2):206–213

[22] Richter JE. Eosinophilic Esophagitis Dilation in the Community–Try It–You Will Like It–But Start Low and Go Slow. Am J Gastroenterol. 2016; 111(2):214–216

[23] Takahashi H, Arimura Y, Okahara S, et al. Risk of perforation during dilation for esophageal strictures after endoscopic resection in patients with early squamous cell carcinoma. Endoscopy. 2011; 43(3):184–189

[24] Hanaoka N, Ishihara R, Takeuchi Y, et al. Intralesional steroid injection to prevent stricture after endoscopic submucosal dissection for esophageal cancer: a controlled prospective study. Endoscopy. 2012; 44(11):1007–1011

[25] Yamaguchi N, Isomoto H, Nakayama T, et al. Usefulness of oral prednisolone in the treatment of esophageal stricture after endoscopic submucosal dissection for superficial esophageal squamous cell carcinoma. Gastrointest Endosc. 2011; 73(6):1115–1121

26 Achalasia

Froukje B van Hoeij, Paul Fockens, and Albert J Bredenoord

26.1 Introduction

Esophageal achalasia is a primary esophageal motor disorder characterized by aperistalsis and absent relaxation of the lower esophageal sphincter (LES). The first description of the disease is credited to Sir Thomas Willis in 1674, who resolved the symptoms by using a whale bone to dilate the LES.[1] The term achalasia, later introduced by Hurst and Rake in 1929, is derived from the ancient Greek words "*a*" and "*khalasis*" translated as "*not loosening.*" Clinically, achalasia manifests as progressive dysphagia, retrosternal pain, regurgitation, and weight loss. The diagnosis of achalasia is made using esophageal manometry. Typical endoscopic findings are stasis of food or saliva in the esophagus, a dilated lumen, and a difficult to pass LES. But achalasia can easily be missed during upper endoscopy.

In this chapter, we discuss the endoscopic findings and the endoscopic treatment modalities. All treatment modalities in achalasia are directed at lowering the pressure of the lower esophageal sphincter to improve esophageal clearance. The most used endoscopic treatment options are botulinum toxin injections, pneumatic dilations, or a myotomy of the LES. Intrasphincteric injection of botulinum toxin type A paralyzes the LES. It has a good short-term efficacy and low complication rate, but repeat injections are usually needed. Series of graded pneumatic dilations with a low-compliant polyethylene balloon have a longer efficacy, but recurrence generally occurs in half the treated patients. The most recently introduced endoscopic therapy is the peroral endoscopic myotomy (POEM). In experienced hands, it renders a very acceptable safety and efficacy at the short and medium term.

26.1.1 Epidemiology

Idiopathic or primary esophageal achalasia is a relatively rare disease with a prevalence of 10 per 100,000 individuals. The incidence has been fairly stable over the last few years, at 0.5 to 1.2 per 100,000 persons per year. The most common age of onset is around age 30 to 60 years, although an age distribution between birth and the ninth decade of life has been described. The male to female ratio is 1:1 and there is no racial predisposition.[2] General life expectancy and causes of death of achalasia patients do not differ from those of the average population.

26.1.2 Pathophysiology

The motility abnormalities of the esophageal smooth muscles occur as a result of degeneration of the myenteric (Auerbach's) plexus (▶ Fig. 26.1). Progressive decrease in number of ganglionic cells and neurons results in deranged inhibitory control.[3] This causes a varying degree of imbalance between inhibitory and excitatory function and concomitant contractility and abnormal LES relaxation. Besides this, as a result of chronic stasis of food and liquids, mucosal irritation of the distal esophagus occurs. Furthermore, some patients develop smooth muscle hypertrophy in the esophagus, secondary to the elevated LES pressure.

26.1.3 Etiology

The etiology of achalasia is still not completely elucidated, but is likely to be multifactorial. There are different hypotheses on the etiology of esophageal achalasia. The most widely accepted theory is an infectious agent causing a neurodegenerative response directly or via an autoimmune response. The autoimmune theory is based on a higher prevalence of autoimmune diseases and antineural autoantibodies in achalasia patients, and the presence of T cell infiltrates within the myenteric plexus in achalasia patients.[4,5] The infectious agent theory is based on Chagas disease with a known infectious etiology *(Trypanosoma cruzi)*, several reports on Guillain–Barré or varicella zoster preceding the onset of achalasia and increased titers of herpes viruses in achalasia patients. In some case series, achalasia is found to have a hereditary or degenerative cause. Furthermore, in some patients, an achalasia-like disorder occurs secondary to radiation damage, sarcoid infiltration, or a malignant invasion; this is called pseudoachalasia.[2]

26.1.4 Clinical Presentation

Clinically, achalasia manifests as slowly progressive dysphagia to both liquids and solids, accompanied by retrosternal pain and regurgitation of undigested food. The Eckardt score (▶ Table 26.1) is a clinical scoring system for achalasia symptoms, with a maximum score of 12. The Eckardt score is the sum of the symptom scores for dysphagia, regurgitation, chest pain, and weight loss. Patients often adapt to the slowly progressive dysphagia.[6] This

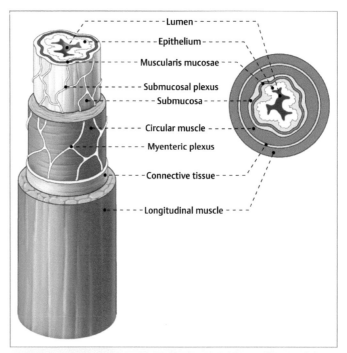

Fig. 26.1 Anatomy of the esophagogastric junction and layers of the esophageal wall. Reproduced with permission from Rogier Trompert Medical Art.

Table 26.1 The Eckardt score

Score	Dysphagia	Regurgitation	Retrosternal pain	Weight loss (kg)
0	None	None	None	None
1	Occasional	Occasional	Occasional	< 5
2	Daily	Daily	Daily	5–10
3	Each meal	Each meal	Each meal	> 10

patient delay is often exacerbated by a diagnostic delay due to unfamiliarity with the disease and frequent confusion with gastroesophageal reflux disease. In advanced disease, usually saliva regurgitation and weight loss are reported. In elderly patients with a short history of symptoms and significant weight loss, one should be aware of an underlying malignancy.

26.2 Diagnostic Approaches

26.2.1 General Approach Including Equipment and Techniques

The diagnosis is made with esophageal manometry. A barium esophagography can be very useful and provides information on esophageal emptying, luminal dilation, and shape. Sometimes endoscopic ultrasound (EUS) or computed tomography (CT) scan are used as ancillary tests.

Esophagogastroduodenoscopy

The first step in diagnostic evaluation of a patient with dysphagia will usually be an upper gastroscopy (**Video 26.1**). This is essential to rule out structural abnormalities such as a stricture or malignancy. In achalasia, typical findings on endoscopy are a dilated, atonic esophagus with retained fluid and a pinpoint LES, which

is difficult to pass (▶ Fig. 26.2). These findings are not diagnostic, however, and have a very low sensitivity and specificity. When excessive pressure is needed to pass the LES, a neoplastic process can be suspected. Sometimes smooth muscle hypertrophy occurs secondary to the elevated LES pressure. In advanced disease, a tortuous esophagus with thickened, friable, or even ulcerated mucosa can be seen secondary to chronic stasis of food and liquids. This can ultimately result in dysplasia and squamous cell carcinoma. The documented esophageal cancer risk ranges from 0-to 33-fold higher than in healthy individuals. Megaesophagus is a relatively rare complication of inadequately treated achalasia and can ultimately require esophagectomy.

Esophageal High-Resolution Manometry

Esophageal high-resolution manometry (HRM) is currently the gold standard for diagnosing achalasia. The manometry catheter is placed transnasally and measures the esophageal pressure pattern throughout the whole esophagus. In case of achalasia, the manometry will reveal aperistalsis and poor or absent LES relaxation. Depending on the type of achalasia, absent contractility (type I), panesophageal pressurization (type II), or spastic contractions (type III) will be seen during water swallows (▶ Fig. 26.3).[7]

Barium Esophagography

The barium esophagography can reveal absent or abnormal contractions, esophageal dilation, narrowing of the esophagogastric junction with a characteristic "bird-beak" appearance (▶ Fig. 26.4), and a poor esophageal emptying of the barium into the stomach. In late stages, a severely dilated, tortuous esophagus is sometimes seen, which is called a sigmoid-shaped esophagus. Another relatively rare complication of untreated achalasia is an epiphrenic

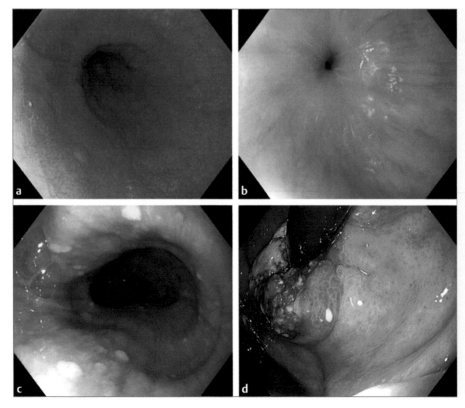

Fig. 26.2 Endoscopic findings in achalasia. (a) Red, friable, crackened mucosa due to chronic stasis of food. (b) Pinpoint lower esophageal sphincter. (c) Dilated, atonic esophagus with stasis of fluid. (d) Pseudoachalasia of an adenocarcinoma of the gastroesophageal junction.

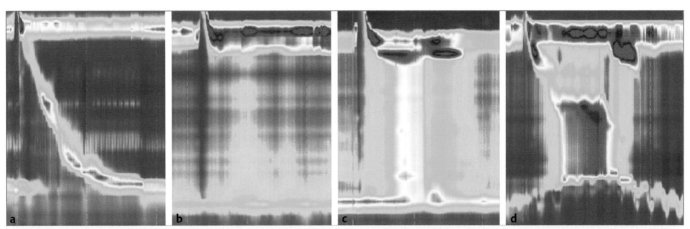

Fig. 26.3 High-resolution manometry in three different types of achalasia. (a) Normal peristalsis in a healthy subject. (b) Type I or classic achalasia with absent peristalsis. (b) Type II achalasia with panesophageal pressurization. (c) Type III or vigorous achalasia with a premature spastic contraction and esophageal shortening.

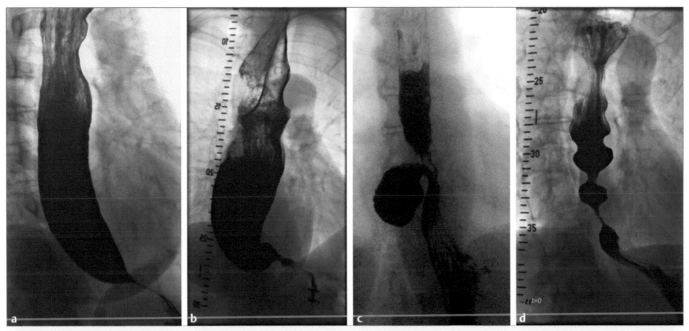

Fig. 26.4 Barium esophagography in achalasia. (a) A dilated esophagus with stasis of barium and a bird-beak appearance. (b) A tortuous, dilated esophagus with stasis of barium and a bird-beak appearance. (c) A large epiphrenic diverticulum. (d) Ladder spasm in type III achalasia.

diverticulum arising just above the LES. This is usually a herniation of the mucosa and submucosa caused by chronic elevated intraluminal pressure.

Endoscopic Ultrasound

In some cases, EUS can be used to ensure the absence of a malignancy and further examine the esophagogastric junction. Like CT scan, EUS is not recommended as a routine test in achalasia, but potentially helpful in a patient with suspected pseudoachalasia. In the presence of a neoplastic lesion, EUS can reveal asymmetric esophageal wall thickening, an extrinsic mass, and/or enlargement of adjacent lymph nodes.

26.2.2 Achalasia Subtypes

The Chicago classification represents the current state of knowledge of the primary esophageal motility disorders, including achalasia.[8] This classification is regularly updated, and comprises an algorithmic scheme for diagnosis of achalasia based on HRM criteria. Achalasia is classified in three subtypes (▶Fig. 26.3), based on characteristics of pressurization measured on HRM: type I (absent pressurization), type II (panesophageal pressurization), and type III (spastic contractions). Type II shows the best treatment response (96%), type I shows 81%, and type III shows 66%.[6] Type II achalasia likely represents early-stage achalasia with retained smooth muscle tone generating panesophageal intrabolus pressurization. Type I is generally believed to be a later phase of disease progression with complete loss of contractile activity and a dilated esophagus. Type III achalasia is considered a separate entity, characterized by premature or spastic contractions in the distal esophagus.[9]

Differential Diagnosis

In patients with typical achalasia symptoms, one should be aware of misdiagnosing another esophageal motility disorder or

Table 26.2 Differential diagnosis of achalasia

Mechanical abnormalities

Intrinsic

- Stricture, ring or web (gastroesophageal reflux disease)
- Adeno- or squamous cell carcinoma
- Eosinophilic esophagitis
- Caustic damage (sodium hydroxide ingestion or sclerotherapy)
- Radiation damage
- Diverticulum

Extrinsic

- Malignancy
- Infection (*Candida*, tuberculosis, herpes, cytomegalovirus, or histo-plasmosis)
- Cardiovascular (aneurysm, aortic dissection, or vascular anomaly)
- Mediastinal mass (lymphadenopathy or malignancy)
- Postsurgical (fundoplication)

Motility disorders

- Chagas disease
- EGJ outflow obstruction
- Absent contractility
- Distal esophageal spasm
- Ineffective esophageal motility or fragmented peristalsis
- Scleroderma

EGJ, esophagogastric junction.

a mechanical abnormality. Please see ▶Table 26.2 for the complete differential diagnosis of achalasia.

26.2.3 Guidelines and Systematic Reviews

A dominant international guideline on achalasia is lacking. In 2012, the Kagoshima consensus was established under the auspices of the International Society for Diseases of the Esophagus.[10] The most recent American College of Gastroenterology (ACG) practice guideline on diagnosis and management was updated in 2013.[11] This guideline recommends to perform an upper endoscopy in all suspected achalasia patients to rule out pseudoachalasia. Esophageal motility testing is recommended in all suspected achalasia patients without a mechanical obstruction on endoscopy. A barium esophagography is recommended in patients with ambiguous motility testing.

26.3 Therapeutic Approaches

26.3.1 Standard Techniques

Presently, there are various different treatment modalities in achalasia. All of these modalities are not curative but palliative and directed at lowering the pressure of the LES to improve esophageal clearance, while the neural degeneration cannot be corrected.

Endoscopic Botox Injections

Intrasphincteric injection of botulinum toxin type A was introduced in the 1990s.[12,13] This toxin, produced by *Clostridium botulinum*, inhibits acetylcholine release from nerve endings, preventing muscle contraction. In most centers, 100 units of botulinum toxin are dissolved in 4 mL of saline (0.9% NaCl). Using a sclerotherapy needle, 4 aliquots of 1 mL of Botox are injected intrasphincterically in each quadrant of the LES. In spastic esophageal motility disorders, 100 units of botulinum toxin are dissolved in 4 to 10 mL of 0.9% normal saline. Eight to ten separate injections, each with 10 to 12.5 units of Botox are injected distributed through the distal esophageal body or into muscular rings.[14] This leads to a short-term symptom relief in up to 90% of patients. Repeat injections are necessary in over 50% of patients, but are progressively less effective.[15] Because of the very low complication rate and short-lived effect, this treatment is reserved for elderly or otherwise high-risk patients for surgery. The most common complications are transitory chest pain and gastroesophageal reflux; both are mild complications and related to the injection procedure or decreased LES pressure.[15] Severe complications have only been reported in case reports.[16] However, one should be aware that previous Botox injections are a risk factor for development of fibrotic tissue and mucosal perforation during subsequent myotomy.

Endoscopic Pneumatic Dilation

Dilation of the LES is considered to be the eldest therapeutic approach. Several different types of dilating instruments have been used. Bougienage has been discarded due to a lower success rate and a higher incidence of perforation compared to balloon dilation. Pneumatic dilation using a low-compliant polyethylene (Rigiflex) balloon is currently the preferred method. The procedure is performed under intravenous sedation with propofol, or with midazolam and analgesia using pethidine or fentanyl. A guidewire is passed through the working channel into the stomach, over which the balloon catheter is advanced. The balloon is positioned in the esophagogastric junction and partially inflated under fluoroscopic guidance until a waist appears. The balloon is kept inflated until elimination of the waist, or for at least 1 or 2 minutes. In patients having their first balloon dilation, usually a 30-mm diameter balloon is used. In subsequent dilations, 35- or 40-mm diameter balloons are used. After the procedure, some perform an esophagogram with water-soluble barium contrast to exclude a perforation, but the authors think this should be reserved for cases with suspicion of perforation given the low perforation rate. With pneumodilation, there is frequent need for repeat dilations, although not as frequent as with Botox injections. Bleeding is the most common side effect, but it is a logical consequence of the procedure and is not associated with adverse effects. After 5 years, 70 to 90% of patients are symptom free in studies in which repeated dilations were allowed. The perforation rate after pneumodilation is 2 to 5.2%, rarely requiring surgical intervention.[17] The occurrence of gastroesophageal reflux disease is about 20 to 25%.

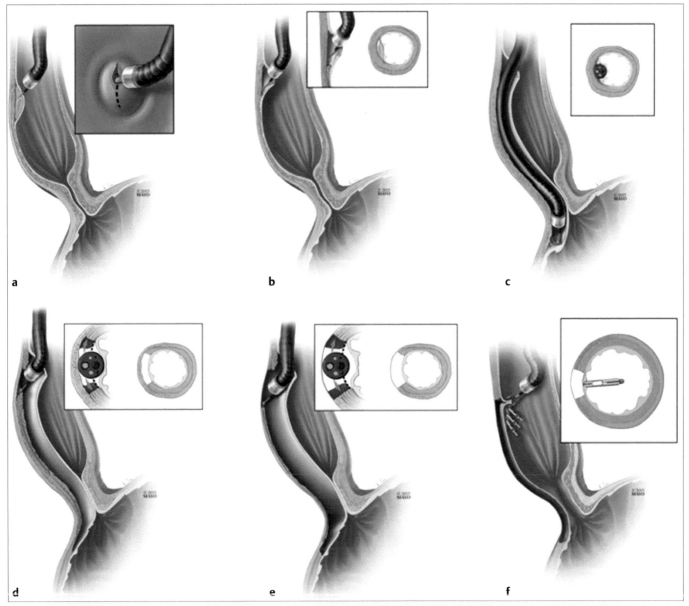

Fig. 26.5 Peroral endoscopic myotomy (POEM) in six steps. (a) Injection of methylene blue. (b) Mucosal incision. (c) Creation of submucosal tunnel. (d, e) Myotomy; (f) Closure of the incision with clips. Reproduced with permission of Mayo Foundation for Medical Education and Research.

Peroral Endoscopic Myotomy

The most recently introduced endoscopic therapeutic option has been developed by Inoue and was first published in 2010 and called POEM (**Video 26.2**).[18] After injecting the submucosa with sterile normal saline dyed with methylene blue, a 2- to 5-cm small mucosal incision in the midesophagus is made (▶ Fig. 26.5). A hybrid knife (ERBE), triangle-tip knife (Olympos), or another electrosurgical endoscopic knife, is used to create a submucosal tunnel in between the mucosa and the circular muscle layer. A conical cap on the endoscope enables optimal visualization and easier passage into the submucosal tunnel, which reaches up to and including a few centimeters of the stomach (▶ Fig. 26.6). Next, starting a few centimeters below the entrance of the submucosal tunnel, the myotomy is performed by cutting the circular muscle layer using the same knife.[18] Depending on the type of achalasia, also the longitudinal muscle layer will be removed. However, there is still debate on whether a circular myotomy, or a complete myotomy is preferable. At the end of the procedure, standard

endoscopic clips are used to close the proximal entrance of the tunnel. Prophylactic antibiotics are recommended during the POEM, as is the administration of proton pump inhibitors (PPIs). The POEM is a new treatment rapidly gaining popularity with a very good short-term safety and efficacy. The first studies report a short-term success in 82 to 100% of patients after 1 to 2 years of follow-up.[19,20,21,22] Long-term data are lacking, however. Complication rate is comparable to surgical Heller's myotomy, and POEM carries a mortality risk approaching zero.[22] The most common unwanted consequence of POEM is gastroesophageal reflux disease causing esophagitis, which can ultimately result in dysplasia and esophageal adenocarcinoma.[21] Another possible side effect is a pneumoperitoneum, sometimes requiring needle decompression. In a large meta-analysis, esophagitis was reported after 0 to 39% of procedures, adverse events requiring medical intervention in 14% of procedures, and one major adverse event requiring surgical intervention (0.2%).[22] We are currently awaiting the results of randomized comparative studies, but POEM seems a very promising treatment modality this far. POEM may be particularly

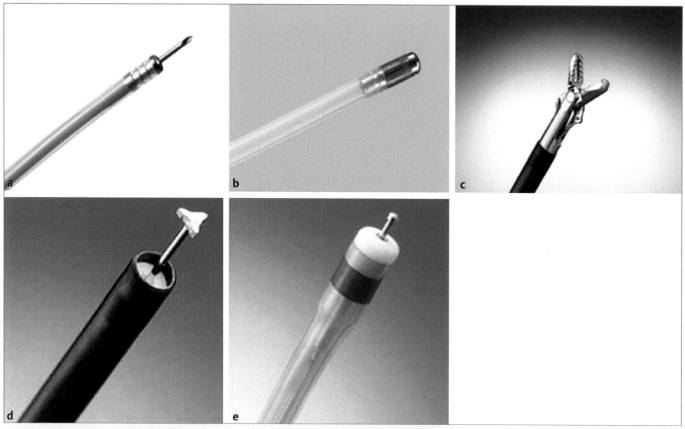

Fig. 26.6 Endoscopic material used for peroral endoscopic myotomy (POEM). **(a)** Injection needle to create a submucosal bleb. **(b)** Spray catheter to spray methylene blue to identify the submucosal tissue plane. **(c)** Coagrasper hemostatic forceps (Olympus) for monopolar coagulation in case of bleeding. **(d)** Triangle-tip knife (Olympus) for myotomy. **(e)** Dual knife (ERBE) for myotomy.

feasible in patients with type III achalasia, allowing an extended proximal myotomy.[23]

Surgical Heller's Myotomy

This surgical myotomy is named after Heller who described it first in 1913.[24] During the years, the procedure was modified from double to single myotomy and from a transthoracic approach to a minimally invasive transabdominal method with extension of the myotomy to the stomach. In this laparoscopic procedure, an anterior longitudinal myotomy of the LES is performed often combined with a Dor or Toupet fundoplication to prevent gastroesophageal reflux. After 5 years, 88 to 95% of patients are symptom free.[6] Risk for transmural perforation was estimated as 0.37% in a large systematic review.[17]

Medication

Administration of a calcium channel blocker or nitrates is generally considered to be rather ineffective, and mainly abandoned. It can be effective for persistent chest pain after endoscopic or surgical treatment in type III achalasia.

26.3.2 Guidelines and Systematic Reviews

As mentioned earlier, a dominant international guideline on achalasia is lacking. Two available guidelines are the Kagoshima

consensus from 2012[10] and the ACG practice guideline from 2013.[11] These guidelines emphasize that all treatments are palliative, since the neuronal degeneration is irreversible. Graded pneumatic dilation or a laparoscopic Heller myotomy with partial fundoplication are recommended as the initial preferred treatment of achalasia. If patients are somehow unfit or unwilling to undergo surgery, botulinum toxin is recommended. Pharmacologic treatment is only recommended after failed botulinum toxin therapy or in patients unwilling or unable to undergo surgical or endoscopic treatment. Currently, the POEM is not yet included in the guidelines.

26.4 Areas of Uncertainty, Experimental Techniques, and Research

Several new techniques are under investigation for achalasia treatment, for example, self-expandable metal stents.[25] One retrospective study comparing pneumatic dilation with stenting found a better long-term efficacy of stents,[26] while another study found no difference in long-term outcomes.[27] Thus far, no large, randomized-controlled trials have been performed evaluating the safety and efficacy of stent placement for achalasia. The possible position of stents in the therapeutic algorithm is still open for discussion.[25]

References

[1] Willis T. Pharmaceutice Rationalis Sive Diatriba de Dedicamentorum Operationibus in Humano Corpore. London, UK: Hagae Comitis; 1674:2

[2] O'Neill OM, Johnston BT, Coleman HG. Achalasia: a review of clinical diagnosis, epidemiology, treatment and outcomes. World J Gastroenterol. 2013; 19(35):5806–5812

[3] Ghoshal UC, Daschakraborty SB, Singh R. Pathogenesis of achalasia cardia. World J Gastroenterol. 2012; 18(24):3050–3057

[4] Booy JD, Takata J, Tomlinson G, Urbach DR. The prevalence of autoimmune disease in patients with esophageal achalasia. Dis Esophagus. 2012; 25(3):209–213

[5] Kraichely RE, Farrugia G, Pittock SJ, et al. Neural autoantibody profile of primary achalasia. Dig Dis Sci. 2010; 55(2):307–311

[6] Pandolfino JE, Gawron AJ. Achalasia: a systematic review. JAMA. 2015; 313(18):1841–1852

[7] Pandolfino JE, Kwiatek MA, Nealis T, et al. Achalasia: a new clinically relevant classification by high-resolution manometry. Gastroenterology. 2008; 135(5):1526–1533

[8] Kahrilas PJ, Bredenoord AJ, Fox M, et al; International High Resolution Manometry Working Group. The Chicago Classification of esophageal motility disorders, v3.0. Neurogastroenterol Motil. 2015; 27(2):160–174

[9] Gyawali CP. Achalasia: new perspectives on an old disease. Neurogastroenterol Motil. 2016; 28(1):4–11

[10] Triadafilopoulos G, Boeckxstaens GE, Gullo R, et al. The Kagoshima consensus on esophageal achalasia. Dis Esophagus. 2012; 25(4):337–348

[11] Vaezi MF, Pandolfino JE, Vela MF. ACG clinical guideline: diagnosis and management of achalasia. Am J Gastroenterol. 2013; 108(8):1238–1249, quiz 1250

[12] Pasricha PJ, Ravich WJ, Hendrix TR, et al. Intrasphincteric botulinum toxin for the treatment of achalasia. N Engl J Med. 1995; 332(12):774–778

[13] Pasricha PJ, Ravich WJ, Kalloo AN. Botulinum toxin for achalasia. Lancet. 1993; 341(8839):244–245

[14] Storr M, Allescher HD, Rösch T, et al. Treatment of symptomatic diffuse esophageal spasm by endoscopic injections of botulinum toxin: a prospective study with long-term follow-up. Gastrointest Endosc. 2001; 54(6):754–759

[15] Leyden JE, Moss AC, MacMathuna P. Endoscopic pneumatic dilation versus botulinum toxin injection in the management of primary achalasia. Cochrane Database Syst Rev. 2014; 12(12):CD005046

[16] Marjoux S, Pioche M, Benet T, et al. Fatal mediastinitis following botulinum toxin injection for esophageal spasm. Endoscopy. 2013; 45(suppl 2 UCTN):E405–E406

[17] Lynch KL, Pandolfino JE, Howden CW, Kahrilas PJ. Major complications of pneumatic dilation and Heller myotomy for achalasia: single-center experience and systematic review of the literature. Am J Gastroenterol. 2012; 107(12):1817–1825

[18] Inoue H, Minami H, Kobayashi Y, et al. Peroral endoscopic myotomy (POEM) for esophageal achalasia. Endoscopy. 2010; 42(4):265–271

[19] Von Renteln D, Fuchs KH, Fockens P, et al. Peroral endoscopic myotomy for the treatment of achalasia: an international prospective multicenter study. Gastroenterology. 2013; 145(2):309–3–11.e1, 3

[20] Kumbhari V, Khashab MA. Peroral endoscopic myotomy. World J Gastrointest Endosc. 2015; 7(5):496–509

[21] Werner YB, Costamagna G, Swanstrom LL, et al. Clinical response to peroral endoscopic myotomy in patients with idiopathic achalasia at a minimum follow-up of 2 years. Gut. 2016; 65(6):899–906

[22] Barbieri LA, Hassan C, Rosati R, et al. Systematic review and meta-analysis: Efficacy and safety of POEM for achalasia. United European Gastroenterol J. 2015; 3(4):325–334

[23] Kumbhari V, Tieu AH, Onimaru M, et al. Peroral endoscopic myotomy (POEM) vs laparoscopic Heller myotomy (LHM) for the treatment of Type III achalasia in 75 patients: a multicenter comparative study. Endosc Int Open. 2015; 3(3):E195–E201

[24] Heller E. Extra mucous cardioplasty in chronic cardiospasm with dilatation of the esophagus. Mitt Grenzgels Med Chir.. 1913; 27:141

[25] Sioulas AD, Malli C, Dimitriadis GD, Triantafyllou K. Self-expandable metal stents for achalasia: thinking out of the box! World J Gastrointest Endosc. 2015; 7(1):45–52

[26] Qian L, Wang B, Li K, et al. Long-term efficacy of pneumatic dilation and esophageal stenting for the treatment of achalasia. Digestion. 2013; 88(4):209–216

[27] Zhao H, Wan XJ, Yang CQ. Comparison of endoscopic balloon dilation with metal stent placement in the treatment of achalasia. J Dig Dis. 2015; 16(6):311–318

27 Advanced Esophageal Cancer

Sheeva K. Parbhu and Douglas G. Adler

27.1 Introduction

Esophageal cancer is the eighth most common cancer worldwide, with over 95% of cases made up of squamous cell carcinoma or adenocarcinoma.[1,2] Patients often present with complaints of rapidly progressing dysphagia, commonly associated with weight loss and fatigue.[3] Unfortunately, only a minority of patients have localized disease at the time of presentation, which limits subsequent treatment modalities.[4]

27.2 Diagnosis and Classification

While initial radiologic studies may prompt further investigation, endoscopy is necessary to establish a diagnosis. Advantages of an endoscopic examination include the ability to obtain diagnostic biopsies, as well as to more fully examine smaller lesions.[5] Single biopsies of suspicious lesions are 93% accurate, with an improvement in accuracy approaching 100% with the addition of multiple biopsies and, less commonly, brushings.[6] Endoscopic ultrasonography (EUS) is initially used for staging purposes because it is more accurate than computed tomography (CT) or positron emission tomography (PET) for evaluating tumor depth and invasion.[7] Once the diagnosis and initial staging have been made, patients often undergo CT or PET examinations to identify distant metastases.[8]

Advanced esophageal cancer, defined for our purposes as unresectable disease, corresponds with a primary tumor classification of T4b (▶Table 27.1) (▶Fig. 27.1; **Video 27.1**). This classification correlates with tumors which invade adjacent structures including the aorta, vertebral body, or trachea[9] (▶Fig. 27.2). Advanced disease includes not only patients with T4b tumor burden, but also patients who are deemed unresectable due to medical co-morbidities which preclude surgery, and patients with distant metastases. In these cases, treatment is focused on control rather than cure of disease. While prolonged progression-free survival is possible for a few patients, most therapies center around symptom palliation and quality of life improvement.

27.2.1 Malignant Dysphagia

As previously mentioned, esophageal cancer is often diagnosed at an incurable stage, with an overall 5-year survival rate as low as 20%.[10] For these patients with advanced disease, malnutrition, dysphagia, and weight loss negatively impact the quality of life. In fact, up to 80 to 90% of patients experience dysphagia during the course of their disease.[11] In these cases, relief of dysphagia

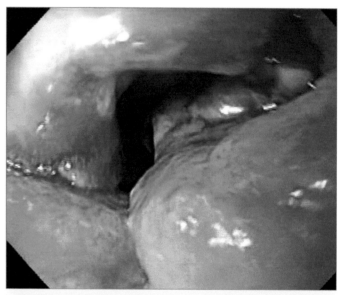

Fig. 27.1 Large esophageal cancer causing malignant dysphagia.

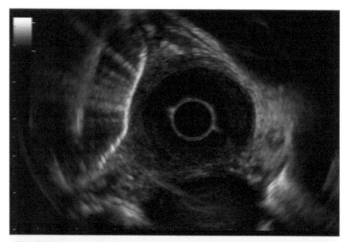

Fig. 27.2 A 7.5-MHz EUS image showing a hypoechoic esophageal cancer with local invasion into the aorta.

Table 27.1 AJCC Classification of Esophageal Cancer

Tumor staging	Description
TX	Primary tumor cannot be assessed
T0	No evidence of primary tumor
Tis	High-grade dysplasia (HGD)
T1	Invasion of lamina propria, muscularis mucosa, or submucosa
• T1a	Invasion of lamina propria or muscularis mucosa
• T1b	Invasion of submucosa
T2	Invasion of muscularis propria
T3	Invasion of adventitia
T4	Invasion of adjacent structures
• T4a	Resectable tumor with invasion of pleura, pericardium, or diaphragm
• T4b	Unresectable tumor with invasion of adjacent structures such as aorta, vertebral body, trachea, etc.

Edge SB, American Joint Committee on Cancer, American Cancer Society. AJCC Cancer Staging Handbook from the AJCC Cancer Staging Manual. New York, NY: Springer; 2010.

allowing for oral nutrition, hydration, and medication delivery becomes the primary palliative goal.

Endoscopic treatment options include dilation, placement of stents, cryotherapy ablation, and bypass of the obstruction via enteral feeding. While mechanical dilation (via balloon or bougie) can be performed, it almost never provides sustained relief of symptoms and cannot be recommended. In addition, repeated dilations of malignant stenosis can be associated with a high perforation rate.[12] Techniques such a photodynamic therapy (PDT) or laser ablation have been extensively described in the literature but are rarely used in the current era.

27.2.2 Stents

The first stents used to relieve malignant dysphagia were made of rigid plastic and were associated with poor patient tolerance and a high complication rate. These are no longer in use. In the 1990s, self-expanding metal stents (SEMS) were developed and have emerged as a cornerstone of palliative therapy for patients with malignant dysphagia (▶ Fig. 27.3).[13,14] Because these stents are constrained and have a small diameter before placement, aggressive dilation of the esophagus (and related complications) is usually avoided.[15] In the hands of experienced endoscopists, modern stents can be successfully placed in more than 90% of cases.[16] The technical aspects of placing esophageal stents and how to pick stent type and length are based on individual operator experience and can vary widely.

Partially Covered Stents

Partially covered SEMS (PCSEMS) along with uncovered SEMS were the first nonplastic stents to be used for patients with incurable esophageal malignancy. While uncovered esophageal stents are no longer available in the United States, PC stents are still widely used, usually in patients in whom no surgery is planned. They have sections of uncovered bare metal at both the proximal and distal ends of the stent, which allows the stent to embed into the esophageal wall, preventing migration.[17]

PC stents were first compared to plastic stents in a randomized-controlled fashion by Knyrim et al. Forty-two patients were studied, and both stents were found to provide similar improvement in dysphagia symptoms. The PC stents, however, were found to be associated with fewer stent migrations, fewer complications, and shorter hospitalizations, and were therefore thought to be superior.[14] These stents are susceptible to tumor ingrowth through the stent interstices (▶ Fig. 27.4).

Davies et al retrospectively studied 87 patients who had a plastic stent or a PCSEMS placed to palliate dysphagia in inoperable esophageal carcinoma. Similar to the prior study, they found that while both stents successfully relieved dysphagia, the PC stent was associated with a lower perforation rate and a reduced length of hospital stay.[18] An even larger retrospective study subsequently followed 153 patients who had had either a plastic or a PC stent. Stent placement was successful in over 90% of cases, and dysphagia was successfully treated without recurrence in more than 70% of patients in both groups. Differences were again highlighted in the rate of complications associated with the plastic stents (22%) compared to the PC stents (9%).[19] All of these studies helped usher in the era of SEMS.

PC stents have the drawbacks of not being removable due to tumor and/or tissue ingrowth of the uncovered portions. This complication can be treated with a fully covered (FC) stent placed inside the PC stent, or with ablative techniques such as argon plasma coagulation (APC) or cryotherapy.[20] Newer stent-design developments have included silicone covers attached to the inside to minimize ingrowth, "fish-scale coating" to reduce migration, and a "dog-bone" shape of the stent allowing it to better attach to the esophageal wall. One prospective trial using a newer design described improvement in patients' dysphagia scores (▶ Table 27.2) from 3 (able to tolerate liquids only) to 1 (ability to eat all liquids and some solid foods).[21] Importantly, no study has been able to describe a survival advantage with either modality, highlighting the palliative nature of this intervention.

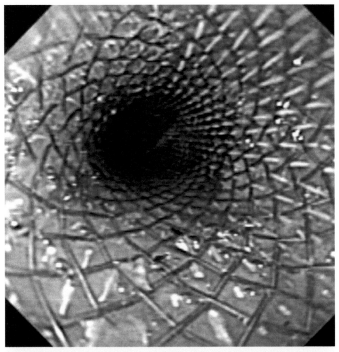

Fig. 27.3 Endoscopic image of a fully covered self-expanding metal stent (FCSEMS) in a patient with advanced esophageal cancer.

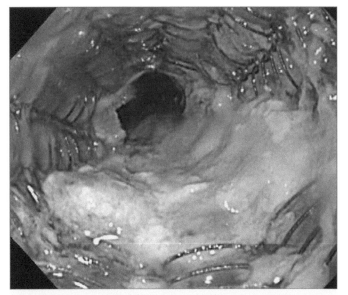

Fig. 27.4 Tumor ingrowth through a partially uncovered self-expanding metal stent (SEMS).

Table 27.2 Dysphagia Scoring System

Dysphagia score	Characteristics
Grade 0	Normal diet
Grade 1	Ability to swallow a semisolid diet (all liquids and some solid foods)
Grade 2	Ability to swallow all liquids and semisolid soft foods
Grade 3	Ability to swallow liquids only and no solid food
Grade 4	Inability to swallow saliva

Source: van Boeckel PG, Siersema PD, Sturgess R, et al. A new partially covered metal stent for palliation of malignant dysphagia: a prospective follow-up study. Gastrointest Endosc. 2010;72:1269–1273

Fully Covered Stents

Complications of PC stents include tumor ingrowth, tumor overgrowth, and food impaction related to recurrent obstruction. Food impaction is a relatively rare event, whereas tumor ingrowth is more common (▶Fig. 27.5). In addition, these stents are generally not amenable to removal after placement.[20] FC self-expanding metal stents (FCSMES) have no uncovered region that can embed into tissue, and thus are more resistant to tumor ingrowth and overgrowth. Their FC design makes these stents completely removable if needed, and have been studied in patients undergoing adjuvant chemotherapy as well as those in whom treatment of dysphagia is the only goal. As they cannot embed in the surrounding tissue, the main drawback of FCSEMS is a much higher risk of migration.

In a retrospective study of 152 patients receiving either a FC- or PCSEMS, the FC version was found to be associated with less tumor ingrowth (53–100%) as well as less incidence of recurrent dysphagia due to stenosis of the stent (8 vs. 37%). The FC stents were also found to migrate more (10 vs. 0%).[22]

Another retrospective study reported experience with 55 patients receiving FCSEMS for malignant dysphagia. These patients were also undergoing neoadjuvant therapy. In this cohort, the mean dysphagia score was improved significantly from baseline (1 vs. 2.4), and baseline body weight was able to be maintained. Thirty-one percent (17/55) patients also experienced migration of the stents, although none of these patients had adverse events related to migration or subsequent removal of the stent.[23]

A newer design with a "dog-bone" shape and internal covering is the most common FCSEMS available today. This design was prospectively studied to evaluate relief of dysphagia while avoiding stent migration. In the 33 patients who received the stent, only 3 (10%) patients experienced stent migration that was associated with recurrent dysphagia.[24]

Efficacy and Complications

While both FC- and PCSEMS are routinely used due to ease of insertion and technical success rates, various ranges of efficacy and complications have been reported in the literature.[13]

In a prospective randomized trial comparing three different types of FCSEMS, 100 patients were treated with stents for malignant dysphagia. In 4-week follow-up, all patients had an improvement in dysphagia scores by at least 1 point, with no differences found between the three stents.[25] A similar study comparing two different FCSEMS also found an improvement in dysphagia both

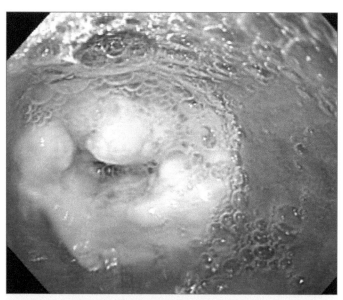

Fig. 27.5 Impacted food obstructing an esophageal stent in a patient with metastatic esophageal cancer.

immediately after stenting and in follow-up at 1 month.[26] Studies that have included PCSEMS have shown similar rates of dysphagia relief.[21,22] In general, SEMS have been shown to improve dysphagia scores (on average) between 1 to 2 points and provide immediate symptom relief in over 90% of patients.[27] In regard to palliation of symptoms, no particular FC or PC stent has been shown to be clearly superior to others. The choice of a brand, type, and size of stent for an individual is left to the endoscopist and is usually based on anatomical conditions, goals of care, and operator preference.

Complication and reintervention rates are relatively high for this group of patients, likely due to their significant disease burden, the severity of their esophageal stenosis, and the lack of a perfect or ideal esophageal stent that treats dysphagia in a manner that is free of complications. Mean survival (related to disease progression) is just over 3 months in patients with advanced esophageal cancer, with patients usually succumbing to disseminated disease—patients generally do not die from primary esophageal symptoms or difficulties.[10]

The most common early complications (occurring within 2–4 weeks of stent placement) include chest pain, nausea with or without vomiting, bleeding, gastroesophageal reflux disease (GERD), perforation, and stent migration.[10] These vary in frequency, with chest pain being relatively frequent (12–14%), and significant bleeding occurring less than 1% of the time in some studies.[28,29] GERD is very common in patients who undergo esophageal stent placement across the gastroesophageal junction (GEJ). While stents with antireflux valves are used in Europe, this technology is not yet widely available in the United States. Nausea, occasionally with vomiting, is frequently encountered in the first 24 to 72 hours and generally fades as the stent fully effaces over time.

Another common complication, stent migration, is clearly related to stent characteristics. It is commonly seen more than a week after successful stent placement, and is considered a "late" complication. Incidence of migration has been quoted as low as less than 10% (in PCSEMS) and as high as greater than 70% (in FCSEMS).[30] A more recent retrospective study of 133 patients found that stent migration occurred in 14.2% of patients with FC stents, compared to only 5.9% of patients with PC stents.[20] Strategies to help mitigate the risk of FCSEMS migration include placement of an over-the-scope clip or endoscopic sutures to anchor the stent in place.[17,31] Other risk factors associated with stent migration include placement across the GEJ (the most common site of placement), shrinkage of tumor mass with adjuvant chemotherapy or radiation, and overdilation of the esophagus before placing the stent.[13]

Other late or delayed complications of stent placement include esophagorespiratory fistula formation, bleeding, tumor overgrowth, and tumor ingrowth. While covered stents are mostly resistant to tumor ingrowth (seen rarely when the coating of the stent breaks down), this complication is seen commonly in PC stents, in as many as 10 to 18% of patients.[32] Larger-diameter stents can reduce the risk of these complications, but may increase the risk of hemorrhage, perforation, and fistula formation when compared to smaller-diameter stents.[33]

27.2.3 Cryotherapy

Cryotherapy for treatment of Barrett's esophagus was first described in 2005.[34] Cryotherapy, or cryoablation, involves the use of a cryogen (liquid nitrogen or carbon dioxide) at extremely cold temperatures to destroy tissue[35] (▶ Fig. 27.6). It has been most extensively studied in patients with Barrett's esophagus, and has been shown to be safe, well tolerated, and highly effective in eradicating high-grade dysplasia.[36] There have been a small number of studies, however, evaluating the use of cryotherapy in advanced disease.

The first report on the use of cryotherapy for palliation of malignant dysphagia reported the complete remission of recurrent squamous cell carcinoma in a patient who had been previously treated with chemotherapy and radiation.[37] In a more recent study of patients with advanced esophageal carcinoma, Greenwald et al evaluated 79 subjects to assess the safety and efficacy of cryotherapy in a randomized-controlled fashion.[38] These patients had either refused, failed, or were not candidates for standard

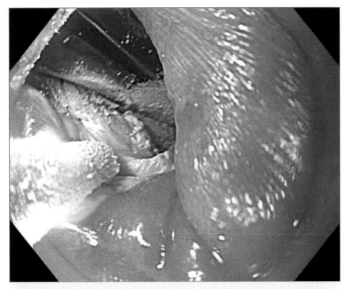

Fig. 27.6 Cryotherapy used to treat esophageal cancer in a patient with metastatic disease.

therapy (chemotherapy, radiation therapy, or esophagectomy). Although a majority of these patients had early (T1a or T1b) disease, some patients were included with more advanced malignancy, including T3 and T4 disease. Many of these patients had received or were concurrently receiving other therapies including external beam radiotherapy, APC, radiofrequency ablation, or endoscopic mucosal resection. In a median follow-up of about 11 months, confirmed tumor eradication was reported after a median of three procedures. In patients with advanced disease, tumor progression was halted for over 1 year in some cases.

The study by Greenwald et al contributes to the theory that a regimen of intermittent palliative cryotherapy ablation at intervals of 2 to 3 months may locally control disease, palliate dysphagia, and allow adequate oral intake.[38] In general, however, there are limited studies available on the use of cryotherapy to debulk advanced esophageal malignancies. In addition, this is a technically cumbersome procedure due to the need for a decompression tube in the setting of malignant luminal stenosis as the cryogens experience significant expansion with warming.[39]

27.2.4 Feeding Tubes

In patients with malignant dysphagia, the inability to take oral nutrition, hydration, and medications is a significant concern. While stents are the first-line therapy for relief, some patients have ongoing issues with oral intake and these cases may warrant consideration of some form of tube feeding. Although, in general, guidelines do not support long-term tube feeding in patients with rapidly progressive disease and extremely short life expectancy, these options are indicated for patients to prevent protein–calorie malnutrition, anorexia–cachexia syndrome, and to facilitate comfort.[40,41]

Nasoenteric tubes are useful for providing nutrition and can be placed with relative ease at the bedside.[42] These tubes, however, can give patients discomfort, promote reflux and associated esophagitis, increase risk for aspiration and sinusitis, and are most useful as a short-term solution.[43] Percutaneous endoscopic gastrostomy (PEG) tubes can also be considered for more long-term nutritional support. PEG tubes are normally well tolerated by patients for prolonged nutritional supplementation, and are most commonly placed endoscopically, although can also be placed by surgeons or interventional radiologists, especially if the tumor precludes an endoscopic approach. Some endoscopists are hesitant to endoscopically place a PEG tube with pull-through technique because of the direct contact with the tumor and concern of seeding the track and subsequent metastases. In these cases, direct-access PEG placement is preferred.[44] Complications of PEG tube placement, even in esophageal cancer patients, are relatively rare (10–15%), and include peritonitis, tube blockage or dislodgment, aspiration, and GERD.[45] Most adverse events are mild.

Since patients with advanced esophageal cancer are already at high risk for GERD, aspiration, and gastric dysmotility, some patients warrant consideration of a percutaneous jejunal tube (percutaneous endoscopic jejunostomy [PEJ]).[46] PEG-J tubes are PEG tubes that are converted to allow jejunal feeding via an internal jejunal extension. PEJ tubes can be placed by gastroenterologists, surgeons, or interventional radiologists.[47] When compared to PEG tubes, there are similar complications, although direct PEJ placement is associated with more frequent moderate-to-severe complications.[48] PEJ tubes may offer a decreased risk of aspiration, as well as increased length of patency.[49]

Few studies have examined the role of tube feeding in patients with unresectable esophageal cancer, instead studies have largely been focused on patients receiving or about to receive chemotherapy, radiation, or surgery. Siddiqui et al followed 36 patients with esophageal cancer at various stages and found that patients with stents not only had similar increases in albumin levels and body weight when compared to PEJ tube patients, but dysphagia scores, ability to tolerate oral nutrition, and overall quality of life scores were improved in patients with stents.[50]

If a patient undergoes an esophageal stent placement but still has poor oral intake, a PEG can be placed endoscopically even if the esophageal stent is still in place. One study has evaluated PEG tube placement in patients with esophageal stents. The authors showed that PEG placement was safe and effective (in all patients), with the one episode of stent migration managed without complication.[51] In patients for whom stent placement has failed, PEG/PEJ tube placement is effective in treating malnutrition in patients with unresectable disease. Unfortunately, dysphagia scores are not improved by feeding tubes, and mortality has not been shown to be significantly influenced by these interventions.[52]

27.2.5 Esophagorespiratory Fistulas

Fistulas between the gastrointestinal and respiratory tracts are sometimes encountered in patients with advanced esophageal cancer as a complication of radiation therapy, chemotherapy, or in the setting of advanced disease. Coughing, recurrent aspiration, fever, dysphagia, and pneumonia are the most common presenting symptoms, and diagnosis can be made by fluoroscopic or CT imaging, or by direct endoscopic or bronchoscopic visualization[53] (▶ Fig. 27.7). The most common fistulas, esophagotracheal (tracheoesophageal [TEF]) account for over 50% of fistulas, but esophagobronchial or esophagopulmonary fistulas (communication through lung parenchyma) can also occur.[54] TEF develop in about 5 to 15% of patients with esophageal cancer, and much less commonly (< 1%) in patients with bronchogenic carcinoma.[55] Patients with esophagorespiratory fistulae have an average survival of less than 6 weeks with supportive care alone.[54] Surgical approaches via esophageal bypass or diversion carry a very high complication and mortality rate, and for those reasons are now rarely performed. Instead, esophagorespiratory fistulas are most commonly managed by interventional modalities, such as esophageal and/or respiratory stents, clips, or suture placement.[56]

27.2.6 Stents

Esophageal Stents

The development of FC- and PCSEMS represented a significant improvement over the prior rigid and uncovered stents and allowed for successful sealing of fistulas via endoscopic stent placement[57] (▶ Fig. 27.8). Early studies describing the use of FC- or PCSEMS reported successful stent placement, fistula closure, and symptom relief in about 90% of patients.[58,59,60,61]

More recently, Ross et al retrospectively identified 97 patients with advanced esophageal cancer requiring SEMS placement, 21 of whom had malignant esophagorespiratory fistulas. In this subset of patients, 19 (90%) were found to have symptomatic improvement in dysphagia and aspiration. Median overall survival was not significantly different in patients with TEF when compared to patients with malignant dysphagia.[62] Balazs et al studied 188 patients who underwent covered stent placement for malignant esophagorespiratory fistulas, achieving successful fistula closure and symptom palliation in 144 (77%) patients.[63]

If possible, close follow-up after stent placement is integral to success, as stents can migrate, fistulas may reopen, and new fistulae can develop, all of which can lead to recurrent symptoms and infection. Some patients may be too ill to undergo repeat examinations. When compared to incompletely sealed fistulas, placement of stents which successfully seal a TEF conferred a survival benefit (15 vs. 6 weeks) in one large series.[64] Overall, in the setting of advanced terminal disease, placement of esophageal SEMS is a safe and effective palliative treatment in patients with esophagopulmonary fistulas.

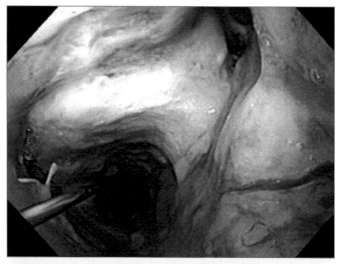

Fig. 27.7 Endoscopic image or a malignant tracheoesophageal fistula in a patient with metastatic esophageal cancer. A guidewire has been advanced through the lumen into the stomach. A surgical suture is also visible as the patient had previously undergone an esophagectomy.

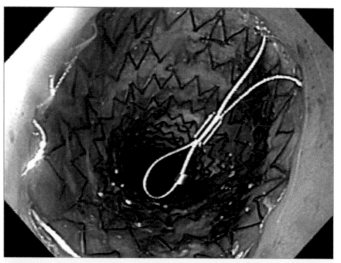

Fig. 27.8 Same patient as seen in ▶ Fig. 27.7, after placement of a fully covered self-expanding metal stent (FCSEMS) to allow oral intake and reduce the risk of aspiration.

Airway Stents

In some patients, an esophageal stent alone may be inadequate to close a TEF, or esophageal stent placement for malignant dysphagia may cause compression in the trachea, producing respiratory symptoms such as stridor or even respiratory distress. In these cases, an airway stent may be concurrently needed. In addition, although success rates greater than 90% are reported, if esophageal stenting alone does not seal a TEF, plastic stents or SEMS in the trachea or bronchus to close the fistula can also be placed (▶ Fig. 27.9, ▶ Fig. 27.10). Patients should be considered for airway stenting before or during esophageal stent placement in cases of proximal masses, or any evidence of airway compression/stridor on physical examination or imaging (▶ Fig. 27.11).

An early study by Freitag et al examined 30 patients who received just an airway stent compared to those who received both an esophageal and airway stent. Slightly greater than 50% of these patients could breathe and swallow unimpaired until shortly before their death. Mean survival time was significantly greater in the double stent group (110 days) than in the patients who received only an airway stent (24 days).[65]

Herth et al retrospectively studied 37 patients with esophageal stents, 65 patients with airway stents, and 10 patients with both esophageal and airway stents in the setting of malignant fistulas. A majority (74%) of these patients had advanced lung cancer. This study showed that survival was longer in the esophageal stent group (263 days) and the double stent group (253 days) when compared to the group of patients who received the airway stent alone (219 days).[66] Application of double stent placement was felt to be safe and effective to palliate symptoms and to successfully treat esophagorespiratory fistulas, and should be considered as first-line therapy in select patients.

27.2.7 Clips

Another therapeutic endoscopic option for TEF closure is the placement of clips. Recently, newer over-the-scope clips have been shown to have good results when compared to regular through-the-scope clips because of the ability to grip larger

amounts of tissue with a wider mouth.[67] Several case reports have reported closure of fistulas with over-the-scope clips, particularly in patients who have had nonhealing fistulas after coagulation, electrocautery, or SEMS placement.[68,69]

A large, multicenter, retrospective study of 188 patients evaluated long-term success of placement of over-the-scope clips. Of this cohort, 108 patients had clips placed for fistula, 16 of whom were esophagorespiratory fistula. Successful clip placement was shown to have immediate clinical success in 77 (90.6%) patients, with long-term clinical success at a median follow-up of 121 days achieved in 39 (42.9%) patients.[31] Although there is limited data for efficacy specifically in advanced esophageal cancer, clipping is safe and can be used effectively to close smaller esophagopulmonary fistula in certain patients.

27.2.8 Sutures

Endoscopic suturing techniques have been used in a limited but slowly expanding role over the past 10 to 15 years, with limited

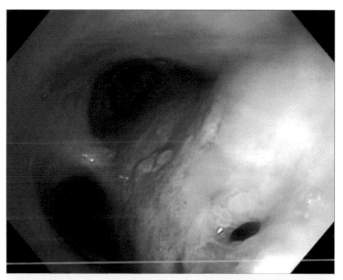

Fig. 27.9 Bronchoscopic view of a tracheoesophageal (TE) fistula in a patient with esophageal cancer.

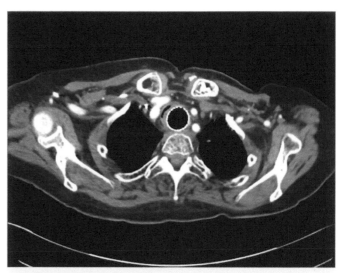

Fig. 27.11 Computed tomography (CT) scan showing tracheal compression due to an esophageal stent. The compressed trachea is deformed into a crescent shape just to the right of the esophageal stent. The stent was subsequently removed.

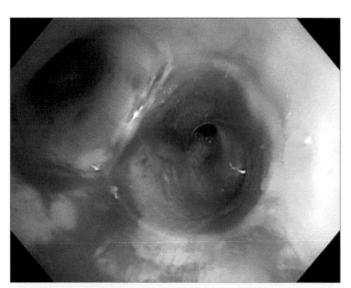

Fig. 27.10 Same patient as shown in ▶ Fig. 27.9, after placement of a plastic Y stent in the airway to attempt to close the fistula.

devices available in the United States. Suturing has been used often in the treatment of gastrointestinal perforations, fistulas, and leaks, often to treat endoscopic and surgical complications or to treat postgastrostomy gastrocutaneous fistulas or bariatric fistulas.[70,71] A few reports in the literature, including one case report, have reported closure of a persistent esophagopleural fistula via an endoscopic suturing system.[72] While an exciting new frontier, the limited available experience and evidence means endoscopic suturing has not yet arrived as a commonly used modality, but this may come as more devices appear in the market.

27.2.9 Bleeding

Although esophageal malignancy is associated with neovascularization and invasion, it has only been rarely described as a presenting symptom.[73,74] Instead, bleeding has been described more frequently after treatment with radiation or placement of plastic or metal stents, with one large case series reporting the incidence of serious bleeding after radiation or stenting at around 7%.[75] In an attempt to prevent migration of stents, newer stents have been developed with larger diameters or the addition of antimigration collars. This greater force against the esophageal wall has been reported to place patients at a higher risk of bleeding, as high as 25% in one retrospective study.[76] Most bleeding is not significant, however, and most patients with stents have no bleeding at all.[33]

Endoscopic treatment for malignant esophageal lesions that bleed has been described in only case reports or in case series involving relatively few patients. These modalities, such as APC, ethanol injection, laser therapy, cryotherapy, and clip placement have all been described as having good short-term success at stopping bleeding due to esophageal malignancy.[77,78,79,80] The use of endoscopically applied topical hemostasis agents such as Hemospray (a mineral-based powder) and EndoClot (a polysaccharide gel) has been reported in cases of nonvariceal esophageal bleeding and may serve a role in treating these lesions.[81,82] Interventional radiology techniques such as arterial embolization have also been described in managing bleeding in esophageal cancer patients.[83] Bleeding in the setting of advanced malignancy represents a severe complication of a terminal illness, and although no randomized-controlled trials exist, there are several modalities that may be successfully used depending on patient characteristics.

27.3 Conclusion

Advanced esophageal cancer is a terminal disease with a high rate of morbidity and mortality. Patients develop symptoms that compromise quality of life and severely limit essential functions. These complications, including malignant dysphagia, fistulas, and bleeding, can be effectively palliated via multiple endoscopic, surgical, and radiologic interventions. The development and placement of stents to palliate malignant dysphagia, as well as feeding tubes to provide nutrition represent pillars of treatment and, have been shown to provide symptom relief for many patients. More advanced complications such as fistulas and bleeding can also be managed endoscopically, providing some degree of palliative relief even in patients with the most devastating complications.

As technology develops and patients with advanced malignancy continue to survive longer, we will continue to learn about which interventions and devices will provide the greatest benefit and least harm for these patients.

References

[1] Kato H, Nakajima M. Treatments for esophageal cancer: a review. Gen Thorac Cardiovasc Surg. 2013; 61(6):330–335
[2] Baquet CR, Commiskey P, Mack K, et al. Esophageal cancer epidemiology in blacks and whites: racial and gender disparities in incidence, mortality, survival rates and histology. J Natl Med Assoc. 2005; 97(11):1471–1478
[3] Rubenstein JH, Shaheen NJ. Epidemiology, diagnosis, and management of esophageal adenocarcinoma. Gastroenterology. 2015; 149(2):302–3–17.e1
[4] Hur C, Miller M, Kong CY, et al. Trends in esophageal adenocarcinoma incidence and mortality. Cancer. 2013; 119(6):1149–1158
[5] Allum WH, Griffin SM, Watson A, Colin-Jones D; Association of Upper Gastrointestinal Surgeons of Great . Britain and Ireland. British Society of Gastroenterology. British Association of Surgical Oncology. Guidelines for the management of oesophageal and gastric cancer. Gut. 2002; 50(suppl 5):v1–v23
[6] Graham DY, Schwartz JT, Cain GD, Gyorkey F. Prospective evaluation of biopsy number in the diagnosis of esophageal and gastric carcinoma. Gastroenterology. 1982; 82(2):228–231
[7] Puli SR, Reddy JB, Bechtold ML, et al. Staging accuracy of esophageal cancer by endoscopic ultrasound: a meta-analysis and systematic review. World J Gastroenterol. 2008; 14(10):1479–1490
[8] van Vliet EP, Heijenbrok-Kal MH, Hunink MG, et al. Staging investigations for oesophageal cancer: a meta-analysis. Br J Cancer. 2008; 98(3):547–557
[9] Edge SB, American Joint Committee on Cancer, American Cancer Society. AJCC Cancer Staging Handbook from the AJCC Cancer Staging Manual. New York, NY: Springer; 2010
[10] Jemal A, Thomas A, Murray T, Thun M. Cancer statistics, 2002. CA Cancer J Clin. 2002; 52(1):23–47
[11] Watkinson AF, Ellul J, Entwisle K, et al. Esophageal carcinoma: initial results of palliative treatment with covered self-expanding endoprostheses. Radiology. 1995; 195(3):821–827
[12] Hernandez LV, Jacobson JW, Harris MS. Comparison among the perforation rates of Maloney, balloon, and savary dilation of esophageal strictures. Gastrointest Endosc. 2000; 51(4 pt 1):460–462
[13] Baron TH. Expandable metal stents for the treatment of cancerous obstruction of the gastrointestinal tract. N Engl J Med. 2001; 344(22):1681–1687
[14] Knyrim K, Wagner HJ, Bethge N, et al. A controlled trial of an expansile metal stent for palliation of esophageal obstruction due to inoperable cancer. N Engl J Med. 1993; 329(18):1302–1307
[15] Kozarek RA, Ball TJ, Brandabur JJ, et al. Expandable versus conventional esophageal prostheses: easier insertion may not preclude subsequent stent-related problems. Gastrointest Endosc. 1996; 43(3):204–208
[16] Siersema PD, Schrauwen SL, van Blankenstein M, et al; Rotterdam Esophageal Tumor Study Group. Self-expanding metal stents for complicated and recurrent esophagogastric cancer. Gastrointest Endosc. 2001; 54(5):579–586
[17] Irani S, Kozarek R. Esophageal stents: past, present, and future. Tech Gastrointest Endosc. 2010; 12:178–190
[18] Davies N, Thomas HG, Eyre-Brook IA. Palliation of dysphagia from inoperable oesophageal carcinoma using Atkinson tubes or self-expanding metal stents. Ann R Coll Surg Engl. 1998; 80(6):394–397
[19] Eickhoff A, Knoll M, Jakobs R, et al. Self-expanding metal stents versus plastic prostheses in the palliation of malignant dysphagia: long-term outcome of 153 consecutive patients. J Clin Gastroenterol. 2005; 39(10):877–885
[20] Homann N, Noftz MR, Klingenberg-Noftz RD, Ludwig D. Delayed complications after placement of self-expanding stents in malignant esophageal obstruction: treatment strategies and survival rate. Dig Dis Sci. 2008; 53(2):334–340
[21] van Boeckel PG, Siersema PD, Sturgess R, et al. A new partially covered metal stent for palliation of malignant dysphagia: a prospective follow-up study. Gastrointest Endosc. 2010; 72(6):1269–1273
[22] Saranovic Dj, Djuric-Stefanovic A, Ivanovic A, et al. Fluoroscopically guided insertion of self-expandable metal esophageal stents for palliative treatment of patients with malignant stenosis of esophagus and cardia: comparison of uncovered and covered stent types. Dis Esophagus. 2005; 18(4):230–238
[23] Siddiqui AA, Sarkar A, Beltz S, et al. Placement of fully covered self-expandable metal stents in patients with locally advanced esophageal cancer before neoadjuvant therapy. Gastrointest Endosc. 2012; 76(1):44–51
[24] Hirdes MM, Siersema PD, Vleggaar FP. A new fully covered metal stent for the treatment of benign and malignant dysphagia: a prospective follow-up study. Gastrointest Endosc. 2012; 75(4):712–718
[25] Siersema PD, Hop WC, van Blankenstein M, et al. A comparison of 3 types of covered metal stents for the palliation of patients with dysphagia caused by esophagogastric carcinoma: a prospective, randomized study. Gastrointest Endosc. 2001; 54(2):145–153
[26] Sabharwal T, Hamady MS, Chui S, et al. A randomised prospective comparison of the Flamingo Wallstent and Ultraflex stent for palliation of dysphagia associated with lower third oesophageal carcinoma. Gut. 2003; 52(7):922–926

[27] Martinez JC, Puc MM, Quiros RM. Esophageal stenting in the setting of malignancy. ISRN Gastroenterol. 2011; 2011:719575

[28] Conigliaro R, Battaglia G, Repici A, et al. Polyflex stents for malignant oesophageal and oesophagogastric stricture: a prospective, multicentric study. Eur J Gastroenterol Hepatol. 2007; 19(3):195–203

[29] Johnson E, Enden T, Noreng HJ, et al. Survival and complications after insertion of self-expandable metal stents for malignant oesophageal stenosis. Scand J Gastroenterol. 2006; 41(3):252–256

[30] Sharma P, Kozarek R; Practice Parameters Committee of American College of Gastroenterology. Role of esophageal stents in benign and malignant diseases. Am J Gastroenterol. 2010; 105(2):258–273, quiz 274

[31] Haito-Chavez Y, Law JK, Kratt T, et al. International multicenter experience with an over-the-scope clipping device for endoscopic management of GI defects (with video). Gastrointest Endosc. 2014; 80(4):610–622

[32] Lowe AS, Sheridan MB. Esophageal stenting. Semin Intervent Radiol. 2004; 21(3):157–166

[33] Verschuur EM, Steyerberg EW, Kuipers EJ, Siersema PD. Effect of stent size on complications and recurrent dysphagia in patients with esophageal or gastric cardia cancer. Gastrointest Endosc. 2007; 65(4):592–601

[34] Johnston MH, Eastone JA, Horwhat JD, et al. Cryoablation of Barrett's esophagus: a pilot study. Gastrointest Endosc. 2005; 62(6):842–848

[35] Erinjeri JP, Clark TW. Cryoablation: mechanism of action and devices. J Vasc Interv Radiol. 2010; 21(suppl 8):S187–S191

[36] Shaheen NJ, Greenwald BD, Peery AF, et al. Safety and efficacy of endoscopic spray cryotherapy for Barrett's esophagus with high-grade dysplasia. Gastrointest Endosc. 2010; 71(4):680–685

[37] Cash BD, Johnston LR, Johnston MH. Cryospray ablation (CSA) in the palliative treatment of squamous cell carcinoma of the esophagus. World J Surg Oncol. 2007; 5:34

[38] Greenwald BD, Dumot JA, Abrams JA, et al. Endoscopic spray cryotherapy for esophageal cancer: safety and efficacy. Gastrointest Endosc. 2010; 71(4):686–693

[39] Greenwald BD, Lightdale CJ, Abrams JA, et al. Barrett's esophagus: endoscopic treatments II. Ann N Y Acad Sci. 2011; 1232:156–174

[40] Stroud M, Duncan H, Nightingale J; British Society of Gastroenterology. Guidelines for enteral feeding in adult hospital patients. Gut. 2003; 52(suppl 7):vii1–vii12

[41] Angus F, Burakoff R. The percutaneous endoscopic gastrostomy tube. Medical and ethical issues in placement. Am J Gastroenterol. 2003; 98(2):272–277

[42] Kirby DF, Delegge MH, Fleming CR. American Gastroenterological Association technical review on tube feeding for enteral nutrition. Gastroenterology. 1995; 108(4):1282–1301

[43] Heyland DK, Drover JW, MacDonald S, et al. Effect of postpyloric feeding on gastroesophageal regurgitation and pulmonary microaspiration: results of a randomized controlled trial. Crit Care Med. 2001; 29(8):1495–1501

[44] Ellrichmann M, Sergeev P, Bethge J, et al. Prospective evaluation of malignant cell seeding after percutaneous endoscopic gastrostomy in patients with oropharyngeal/esophageal cancers. Endoscopy. 2013; 45(7):526–531

[45] Nicholson FB, Korman MG, Richardson MA. Percutaneous endoscopic gastrostomy: a review of indications, complications and outcome. J Gastroenterol Hepatol. 2000; 15(1):21–25

[46] Shike M, Latkany L. Direct percutaneous endoscopic jejunostomy. Gastrointest Endosc Clin N Am. 1998; 8(3):569–580

[47] Schattner M. Enteral nutritional support of the patient with cancer: route and role. J Clin Gastroenterol. 2003; 36(4):297–302

[48] Maple JT, Petersen BT, Baron TH, et al. Direct percutaneous endoscopic jejunostomy: outcomes in 307 consecutive attempts. Am J Gastroenterol. 2005; 100(12):2681–2688

[49] Fan AC, Baron TH, Rumalla A, Harewood GC. Comparison of direct percutaneous endoscopic jejunostomy and PEG with jejunal extension. Gastrointest Endosc. 2002; 56(6):890–894

[50] Siddiqui AA, Glynn C, Loren D, Kowalski T. Self-expanding plastic esophageal stents versus jejunostomy tubes for the maintenance of nutrition during neoadjuvant chemoradiation therapy in patients with esophageal cancer: a retrospective study. Dis Esophagus. 2009; 22(3):216–222

[51] Adler DG, Baron TH, Geels W, et al. Placement of PEG tubes through previously placed self-expanding esophageal metal stents. Gastrointest Endosc. 2001; 54(2):237–241

[52] Bower MR, Martin RC, II. Nutritional management during neoadjuvant therapy for esophageal cancer. J Surg Oncol. 2009; 100(1):82–87

[53] Burt M, Diehl W, Martini N, et al. Malignant esophagorespiratory fistula: management options and survival. Ann Thorac Surg. 1991; 52(6):1222–1228, discussion 1228–1229

[54] Kim KR, Shin JH, Song HY, et al. Palliative treatment of malignant esophagopulmonary fistulas with covered expandable metallic stents. AJR Am J Roentgenol. 2009; 193(4):W278–82

[55] Reed MF, Mathisen DJ. Tracheoesophageal fistula. Chest Surg Clin N Am. 2003; 13(2):271–289

[56] Yasuda T, Sugimura K, Yamasaki M, et al. Ten cases of gastro-tracheobronchial fistula: a serious complication after esophagectomy and reconstruction using posterior mediastinal gastric tube. Dis Esophagus. 2012; 25(8):687–693

[57] Tomaselli F, Maier A, Sankin O, et al. Successful endoscopical sealing of malignant esophageotracheal fistulae by using a covered self-expandable stenting system. Eur J Cardiothorac Surg. 2001; 20(4):734–738

[58] May A, Ell C. Palliative treatment of malignant esophagorespiratory fistulas with Gianturco-Z stents. A prospective clinical trial and review of the literature on covered metal stents. Am J Gastroenterol. 1998; 93(4):532–535

[59] Raijman I, Siddique I, Ajani J, Lynch P. Palliation of malignant dysphagia and fistulae with coated expandable metal stents: experience with 101 patients. Gastrointest Endosc. 1998; 48(2):172–179

[60] Eleftheriadis E, Kotzampassi K. Endoprosthesis implantation at the pharyngo-esophageal level: problems, limitations and challenges. World J Gastroenterol. 2006; 12(13):2103–2108

[61] Radecke K, Gerken G, Treichel U. Impact of a self-expanding, plastic esophageal stent on various esophageal stenoses, fistulas, and leakages: a single-center experience in 39 patients. Gastrointest Endosc. 2005; 61(7):812–818

[62] Ross WA, Alkassab F, Lynch PM, et al. Evolving role of self-expanding metal stents in the treatment of malignant dysphagia and fistulas. Gastrointest Endosc. 2007; 65(1):70–76

[63] Balazs A, Kupcsulik PK, Galambos Z. Esophagorespiratory fistulas of tumorous origin. Non-operative management of 264 cases in a 20-year period. Eur J Cardiothorac Surg. 2008; 34(5):1103–1107

[64] Shin JH, Song HY, Ko GY, et al. Esophagorespiratory fistula: long-term results of palliative treatment with covered expandable metallic stents in 61 patients. Radiology. 2004; 232(1):252–259

[65] Freitag L, Tekolf E, Steveling H, et al. Management of malignant esophagotracheal fistulas with airway stenting and double stenting. Chest. 1996; 110(5):1155–1160

[66] Herth FJ, Peter S, Baty F, et al. Combined airway and oesophageal stenting in malignant airway-oesophageal fistulas: a prospective study. Eur Respir J. 2010; 36(6):1370–1374

[67] Armellini E, Crinò SF, Orsello M, et al. New endoscopic over-the-scope clip system for treatment of a chronic post-surgical tracheoesophageal fistula. Endoscopy. 2015; 47(suppl 1 UCTN):E437–E438

[68] So BJ, Adler DG. Closure of a chronic, non-healing tracheoesophageal fistula with a new over-the-scope clip. ACG Case Rep J. 2014; 2(1):18–20

[69] Kirschniak A, Kratt T, Stüker D, et al. A new endoscopic over-the-scope clip system for treatment of lesions and bleeding in the GI tract: first clinical experiences. Gastrointest Endosc. 2007; 66(1):162–167

[70] Tuyama AC, Kumar N, Aihara H, et al. Endoscopic repair of gastrogastric fistula after Roux en-Y gastric bypass: a matched cohort study evaluating two methods of fistula closure. Gastroenterology. 2013; 144(5 suppl 1):S220

[71] Kantsevoy SV, Thuluvath PJ. Successful closure of a chronic refractory gastrocutaneous fistula with a new endoscopic suturing device (with video). Gastrointest Endosc. 2012; 75(3):688–690

[72] Bonin EA, Wong Kee Song LM, Gostout ZS, et al. Closure of a persistent esophagopleural fistula assisted by a novel endoscopic suturing system. Endoscopy. 2012; 44(suppl 2 UCTN):E8–E9

[73] Steffes C, Fromm D. The current diagnosis and management of upper gastrointestinal bleeding. Adv Surg. 1992; 25:331–361

[74] Sugawa C, Steffes CP, Nakamura R, et al. Upper GI bleeding in an urban hospital. Etiology, recurrence, and prognosis. Ann Surg. 1990; 212(4):521–526, discussion 526–527

[75] Nemoto K, Takai Y, Ogawa Y, et al. Fatal hemorrhage in irradiated esophageal cancer patients. Acta Oncol. 1998; 37(3):259–262

[76] Uitdehaag MJ, Siersema PD, Spaander MC, et al. A new fully covered stent with antimigration properties for the palliation of malignant dysphagia: a prospective cohort study. Gastrointest Endosc. 2010; 71(3):600–605

[77] Akhtar K, Byrne JP, Bancewicz J, Attwood SE. Argon beam plasma coagulation in the management of cancers of the esophagus and stomach. Surg Endosc. 2000; 14(12):1127–1130

[78] Tranberg KG, Stael von Holstein C, Ivancev K, et al. The YAG laser and Wallstent endoprosthesis for palliation of cancer in the esophagus or gastric cardia. Hepatogastroenterology. 1995; 42(2):139–144

[79] Loscos JM, Calvo E, Alvarez-Sala JL, Espinos D. Treatment of dysphagia and massive hemorrhage in esophageal carcinoma by ethanol injection. Endoscopy. 1993; 25(8):544

[80] Raju GS, Ahmed I, Xiao SY, et al. Graded esophageal mucosal ablation with cryotherapy, and the protective effects of submucosal saline. Endoscopy. 2005; 37(6):523–526

[81] Sung JJ, Luo D, Wu JC, et al. Early clinical experience of the safety and effectiveness of Hemospray in achieving hemostasis in patients with acute peptic ulcer bleeding. Endoscopy. 2011; 43(4):291–295

[82] Holster IL, Kuipers EJ, Tjwa ET. Hemospray in the treatment of upper gastrointestinal hemorrhage in patients on antithrombotic therapy. Endoscopy. 2013; 45(1):63–66

[83] Loffroy RF, Abualsaud BA, Lin MD, Rao PP. Recent advances in endovascular techniques for management of acute nonvariceal upper gastrointestinal bleeding. World J Gastrointest Surg. 2011; 3(7):89–100

28 Peptic Ulcer Disease and Bleeding, Including Duodenal Ulcer

Moe Kyaw, James Lau, and Joseph Jao Yiu Sung

28.1 Introduction

In peptic ulcer disease and bleeding, endoscopy has both a diagnostic and therapeutic role—diagnosis of peptic ulcer, exclusion of malignancy, identifying bleeding focus, hemostatic treatment, assessing risk of rebleeding, and prevention of further rebleeding. A variety of endoscopic therapeutic modalities for peptic ulcer bleeding have evolved which are classified into injection, thermal, mechanical, and topical. This review provides a summary of commonly used modalities and techniques to maximize their effectiveness. In addition, the role of newer therapeutic modalities such as over-the-scope clips (OTSC), and endoscopic suturing devices is discussed.

28.2 Diagnosis of Peptic Ulcer Disease and Bleeding

Signs and symptoms of peptic ulcer disease include dyspepsia, anemia, bleeding, and gastric outlet obstruction. Endoscopy is advisable for new-onset dyspepsia in patients older than age 50 or those with alarm features.[1] In uncomplicated peptic ulcer disease (absence of bleeding, obstruction, or perforation), the role of endoscopy is to provide a diagnosis and exclude malignancy. In the past, biopsies of all gastric ulcers were recommended—this was based on old data suggesting up to 11% gastric ulcers represented malignancy.[2] There are no recent data to guide recommendation to biopsy all gastric ulcers. The American Society for Gastrointestinal Endoscopy (ASGE) suggested individualized approach directed by patient symptoms and endoscopic appearance of ulcers.[3] Thus, in a young patient taking nonsteroidal anti-inflammatory drug (NSAID), with endoscopic findings of NSAID-associated ulcer appearance (shallow ulcers, with erosions), routine biopsy may not be required. Because of its very low risk of malignancy with duodenal ulcers, routine biopsy is not recommended. When endoscopic appearance of gastric ulcer does suggest malignancy, multiple biopsies should be taken from both the base and edges of ulcer. All patients confirmed with peptic ulcer disease should have endoscopic testing for *Helocobacter pylori*.

Despite unclear results on efficacy, and cost-effectiveness, plus without published recommendations, routine endoscopic surveillance of gastric ulcer continues to be a common practice due to the fact that gastric ulcers may initially appear benign on endoscopy appearance and histology. The ASGE suggested an individualized approach that might be more effective—a young patient with endoscopic appearance of benign ulcer confirmed on histology with an identifiable cause (NSAID, *H. pylori*) may not require surveillance endoscopy.[3] A second-look endoscopic surveillance for duodenal ulcer is only recommended in patients with persistent symptoms.

Endoscopy is essential for management of peptic ulcer bleeding. Endoscopy allows the identification of the bleeding focus, classification of risk of rebleeding, and treatment to halt the bleeding.

Using the Forrest classification, the endoscopic appearance of ulcer can be used to identify the risk of persistent bleeding, rebleeding, and mortality (▶Table 28.1). Those ulcers classified as FI or FIIa are at high risk for rebleeding and endoscopic therapy is advised in these patients.[4,5,6] For ulcers classified as FIIb, endoscopic treatment remains controversial.[7,8] The most recent meta-analysis did not show significant benefit of endoscopic therapy on ulcers classified as FIIb.[9] Rebleeding is rare for ulcers classified as FIIc or FIII, thus endoscopic therapy is not beneficial.[10,11]

There are also other endoscopic diagnostic findings which are not described in the Forrest classification that can be used to predict rebleeding: ulcer size greater than 2 cm, blood in the gastric lumen, location of ulcer (posterior duodenal wall; proximal lesser curvature of stomach).[12,13,14]

Not all nonbleeding visible vessels have the same risk of recurrent bleeding; pale, protuberant vessels carry a higher risk than dark, flattened vessels.[15] And at times, it can be difficult to differentiate between a nonbleeding visible vessel and an adherent clot. For ulcers with adherent clot, removal of clot should be attempted to identify underlying ulcer base and exclude any visible vessels. However, even after the removal of the clot, it can be difficult to identify those vessels that are buried in the ulcer base. In such cases, the use of magnifying endoscopy has been suggested to improve exposure and characterization of visible vessels while differentiating between slightly protuberant vessels from clots and pigmented spots.[16] Doppler ultrasound at the ulcer base has also been suggested as a method to determine whether a vessel is present—a "Doppler positive" ulcer base was noted when the Doppler identified a vessel within 1 mm from the ulcer base. Both techniques are not used in common clinical practice due to cost and technical complexity.[17,18] However, recent publication has suggested the role of Doppler endoscopic probe (Vascular Technology Inc, Nashua, New Hampshire) in risk stratification for patients to determine rebleeding risk. The tip of the Doppler endoscopic probe was placed next to the ulcer pre- and postendoscopic treatment, and blood flow in the underlying ulcer base was confirmed by auditory sound. Those patients with residual blood flow after endoscopic treatment was suggested as a potential indicator for rebleeding. The authors concluded that the Doppler endoscopic probe combined with visual endoscopic assessment (of stigmata of recent hemorrhage) was more accurate

Table 28.1 Forrest's classification and recurrent bleeding risks of bleeding peptic ulcers

Forrest class	Endoscopic appearance	Risk of recurrent bleeding (%)
I	Active bleeding	55
IIa	Nonbleeding visible vessel	43
IIb	Adherent clot	22
IIc	Flat spot	10
III	Clean base	5

Adapted from Laine et al 1994 and Forrest et al 1974.[12,13]

than visual endoscopic assessment alone for risk stratification for ulcer rebleeding and as a new potential guide for definitive endoscopic hemostasis.[19]

The role of early capsule endoscopy preformed prior to gastroscopy in patients with suspected acute upper gastrointestinal bleeding has been reported in a few case series.[20,21,22] Capsule endoscopy is usually performed within 6 hours of arrival into the emergency department. To date, risk stratification for patients presenting with upper gastrointestinal bleeding has been based on clinical judgment using validated Blatchford and Rockall scores. Capsule endoscopy may have a potential role as a triage tool for early diagnosis of upper gastrointestinal bleeding, or avoiding unnecessary admissions for a gastroscopy in those with negative findings. In addition, it can be used as alternative diagnostic tool for nonendoscopists, such as emergency care physicians, who can be trained to perform capsule endoscopy and interpret the findings to achieve an earlier diagnosis.[22]

28.3 Choice of Instrument for Peptic Ulcer Bleeding

Endoscopy in bleeding patients should always be carried out in adequately equipped settings. In high-risk patients with hemodynamic instability, endoscopy in intensive care unit (ICU) settings is recommended. The development of mobile endoscopic travel cart equipped with all the necessary accessories has resulted in avoidance of unnecessary transfer of unstable patients.

The choice of endoscope depends on the severity of the bleeding and location of the ulcer site. In patients with significant bleeding, the use of a therapeutic gastroscope can be of advantage. Olympus (Olympus Corporation, Tokyo, Japan) provides two types of therapeutic gastroscopes, a single-channel (GIF-1TH190) and a double-channel therapeutic gastroscope (GIF-2TH180). The single-channel therapeutic gastroscope has a 3.7-mm working channel allowing an improvement in lavage and use of large accessories such as 10-F heater probe. The double-channel therapeutic gastroscope with 2.8- and 3.7-mm diameter channels can accommodate two endoscopic devices simultaneously.

With peptic ulcers in unfavorable locations, a change of endoscope will provide better access to target for therapy. In patients with ulcers located in the posterior wall of duodenum or stomach, the use of a colonoscope with the working channel positioned on the right side may provide more accurate approach to the ulcer.[23] A side-viewing duodenoscope can be useful in ulcers located at the junction of the first and second parts of the duodenum or on the lesser curvature of the stomach. In certain cases, using a regular gastroscope with a smaller diameter provides more flexibility in those difficult-to-reach areas.

28.4 Therapeutic Modalities for Peptic Ulcer Bleeding

The goal of therapeutic endoscopy in patients with peptic ulcer bleeding is to prevent continued bleeding or rebleeding. Endoscopic hemostasis can be achieved with injection, thermal, mechanical, and topical modalities (▶ Table 28.2).

Table 28.2 Endoscopic hemostatic modalities

Injection	Epinephrine
	Sclerosants[a]: polidocanol, ethanolamine, ethanol
	Tissue adhesives: N-butylcyanoacrylate, thrombin/fibrin glue
Thermal	Contact: Electrocautery probes, heater probe, gold probe
	Noncontact: Argon plasma coagulation, Nd: YAG laser
Mechanical	Through-the-scope clips
	Over-the-scope clips: Ovesco
	Endoscopic suturing
Topical	Hemostatic powders: Hemospray, EndoClot, ABS

ABS, Ankaferd blood stopper; YAG, neodymium-doped yttrium aluminium garnet.

[a]Agents no longer in used for treatment of peptic ulcer bleeding.

28.4.1 Injection Therapy

Epinephrine

Injection therapy with dilute epinephrine in saline (1:10,000) is widely used as the initial method for hemostasis due to its ease of use and availability. It can be an effective initial hemostatic modality in large ulcer bleeding where the views are obscured and application of other modalities will be difficult. It is delivered through a 25-gauge retractable catheter with increments of 0.5 to 1.5 mL in all four quadrants around the ulcer base, with or without injection into ulcer base. The catheter can be positioned in tangential or en face position. Epinephrine injection achieves hemostasis through a combination of a pressure effect by local tamponade, vasospasm, and induction of thrombosis. Although epinephrine injection is effective in achieving primary hemostasis, its effect resolves after 20 minutes, thus it is recommended that a second endoscopic modality should be applied to reduce the risk of rebleeding.[24,25] Epinephrine injection should be used to slow down or stop bleeding in order to obtain a clearer view of the vessel before a second endoscopic modality is applied. Epinephrine injection can potentially cause tachycardia, hypertension, cardiac arrhythmias, and angina, but they generally do not clinically manifest if less than 12 mL of epinephrine is used.[26]

Other Injection Agents

Alternative injection agents to epinephrine include sclerosants (polidocanol, ethanolamine, ethanol), fibrin sealant, N-butylcyanoacrylate. Sclerosants are no longer used due to local side effects, and limited benefits over epinephrine.[27] Although fibrin sealant was originally shown to be more effective than sclerosants (polidocanol), it is not used in clinical practice due to requirement of multiple therapies.[28] N-butylcyanoacrylate is commonly used in treatment of variceal bleeding, and it has been used in rare cases of refractory peptic ulcer bleeding.[29]

28.4.2 Thermal

Thermal therapies can be divided into contact thermal and noncontact thermal modalities, with the former being more commonly used in peptic ulcer bleeding. Contact thermal devices include electrocautery probes, heater probes, and hemostatic

Table 28.3 Contact thermal hemostatic devices

Contact thermal device	Name of device	Manufacturer	Sheath diameter (F)	Power
Multipolar electrocautery probes	Gold Probe	Boston Scientific (Natick, Massachusetts)	7, 10	15–25 W
	Injection Gold Probe	Boston Scientific (Natick, Massachusetts)	7, 10	
	Quicksilver Bipolar Probe	Cook Medical (Winston-Salem, North Carolina)	7, 10	
	Solar Probe	Olympus America (Center Valley, Pennsylvania)	7, 10	
Heater probes	Heat Probe	Olympus America	7, 10	25–30 J
Hemostatic grasper	Coagrasper	Olympus America	7	80 W[a]

[a] Soft coagulation mode.

grasper (▶Table 28.3). Noncontact thermal modalities include argon plasma coagulation (APC) and laser phototherapy (Nd: YAG laser).

Contact Thermal Modalities

Electrocautery Probes

Electrocautery probes can be monopolar, bipolar, or multipolar. A monopolar electrocautery probe supplies only one electrode to the bleeding ulcer; an electrical grounding pad is attached to the skin to complete the circuit. As electricity flows through the body from the probe to the grounding pad, there is a risk of scatter injury, thus the use of monopolar coagulation has now become obsolete. Bipolar probes contain two electrodes on the probe tip, and electricity travels from one electrode to the other. The electric circuit terminates locally at the tip of the probe and the electrical intensity decreases as the target tissue desiccates with electrocautery, limiting the depth of penetration and reducing the risk of perforation.[30] Bipolar devices have been replaced by multipolar probes, which consist of alternating arrays of positive and negative electrodes. This allows multipolar probes to be effective in both tangential or en face positions, whereas bipolar probes have to be applied en face for maximum effectiveness.

When using either bipolar or multipolar probes, the optimal technique involves using a large-diameter probe (10 F, 3.2 mm) and applying high constant pressure of low-energy (15 W) electrocoagulation for 10 to 12 seconds. This will occlude and achieve a tamponade effect on the vessel of the bleeding ulcers. The application of mechanical pressure together with electric current or heat to coagulate the vessel is known as "coaptive coagulation" (▶Fig. 28.1). A footprint effect on the ulcer base will be seen after achievement of hemostasis with thermal therapy (▶Fig. 28.2). For optimal coaptive coagulation, long-duration (10–12 seconds) and low-energy (15 W) electrocoagulation is preferred than escalating of the watts; because of an ensuing increase in impedance, escalation of watts does not increase coagulation.[31,32]

Gold Probe (Boston scientific, Natick, Massachusetts, United States) and Injection Gold Probe (Boston scientific, Natick, Massachusetts, United States) are multipolar electrocautery probes, both available in two sizes, 7 F (2.3 mm) and 10F (3.2 mm), requiring a minimum of 2.8- or 3.7-mm working channels, respectively. Thus, a therapeutic gastroscope is required for the 10-F

probes. Injection Gold Probe offers simultaneous capability of injection, electrocoagulation, and irrigation by one device.

Heater Probe

Heater probe (7, 10 F) consists of a Teflon-coated hollow aluminum cylinder with an inner heating coil. A thermocoupling device at the tip of the probe maintains a constant temperature. Unlike the electrocautery probes, heater probe coagulation is provided in the form of direct heat energy (25–30 J) delivered in pulses (4–5 pulses). The length of activation is preset, thus once the pulse has been initiated, it cannot be stopped until the complete predetermined amount of joules has been delivered. The main advantage of heater probe (along with multipolar electrocautery probes) is that as the coagulation can be applied from both the tip and side of the probe, it can be positioned both en face and tangential to the target. A foot pedal water irrigation system is attached to the catheter. This can be used to clear the ulcer surface or to ease withdraw of the probe when there is tissue adherence of probe to the ulcer base (**Video 28.1**).

Hemostatic Grasper

Hemostatic grasper is similar to the monopolar hot biopsy forceps. It is more commonly used for hemostasis during endoscopic submucosal dissection, but may also be applied to bleeding vessels in peptic ulcers. Unlike the hot biopsy forceps, the jaws on the grasper are flat, and when closed around the target tissue, monopolar electrocautery is used to desiccate the tissue. The specialized design of the hemostatic grasper allows direct coagulation energy to the isolated area, with reduction in thermal effect to the surrounding area. The main advantage of the hemostatic grasper is that it can be opened and closed prior to application of coagulation. Halting of bleeding by initial mechanical pressure confirms correct position on the vessel, coagulation energy can then be applied more effectively.

Noncontact Thermal Modalities

APC uses electrical conductivity of argon gas, producing heat superficially. Another noncontact thermal modality is laser phototherapy (Nd: YAG laser), also creating hemostasis by generation of heat. Laser coagulation can be performed by initial injection with epinephrine near the vessel followed by application of laser

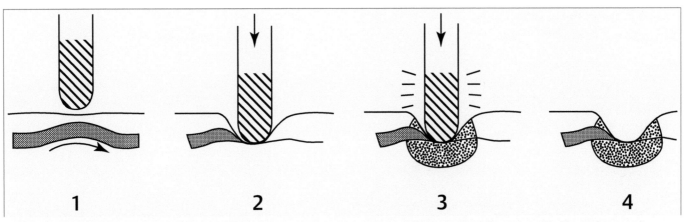

Fig. 28.1 The principle of coaptive thermocoagulation. The use of a thermal device to tamponade blood flow followed by the application of cautery to thermally seal the vessel.

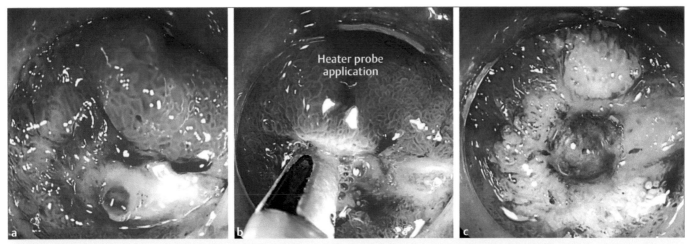

Fig. 28.2 Heater probe for peptic ulcer bleeding. **(a)** Visible vessel at ulcer base. **(b)** Application of heater probe. **(c)** Ulcer with footprint, visible vessel is ablated.

around the vessel. Care should be taken to prevent drilling of the vessel with laser as this may increase the risk of bleeding. Both modalities have limited use in hemostasis of peptic ulcer bleeding, as coaptive coagulation cannot be achieved due to lack of the compression effect. There are few data on assessing the efficacy of noncontact thermal therapy (argon plasma coagulation) in ulcer bleeding. Three small randomized-controlled studies suggested that APC has similar efficacy to injection of sclerosing agent (polidocanol) and contact thermal therapy.[9] With paucity of studies and limited evidence of their effectiveness, APC and laser phototherapy should not be considered as first-line thermal modalities.

28.4.3 Mechanical Therapy

Through-the-Scope Clips

There are several types of through-the-scope clips (▶ Table 28.4). These are all similar in design such that all of them consist of a metallic cable inside a Teflon sheath, with the clip at the distal end of cable, and a rotatable mechanism integrated into the handle.

All the devices deploy a single clip except one (Ez Clip), which is also reusable. This reusable device (Ez Clip) was the first device developed by Olympus (Olympus Corporation, Tokyo, Japan) and is available in several lengths from 4 to 9 mm. Olympus further introduced preloaded single-use devices, QuickClip and QuickClip2, QuickClip2 Long, QuickClip Pro. The QucikClip2 Long with a significantly longer prong length than its predecessors can be particularly useful when wide extra opening is required, allowing more tissue to be grabbed at one time. The latest of clips from Olympus, QuickClip Pro, has the advantage of repositioning prior to deployment with its open-and-close function and a full 360-degree rotation to ensure more precision. The Resolution Clip by Boston Scientific (Boston Scientific, Natick, Massachusetts, United States) has the advantage of being able to reopen to locate an ideal position before deployment of clip. It also has a wide jaw opening of 11 mm. The Instinct Endoscopic Hemoclip (Cook Medical Inc, Bloomington, Indiana, United States) has similarities and differences to other clips; it has 360-degree bidirectional rotation, and can be opened and closed multiple times similar to other clips, but the serrated jaw in arms can provide a more secure anchoring. In addition, the short arms and wide opening can be of advantage in difficult-to-access positions such as in the first part of the duodenum.

When using any of these clipping devices, it is most effective when there is minimum distance between the clip and the ulcer. Also, it is important for the catheter to approach perpendicular

Table 28.4 Through-the-scope clips

Manufacturer	Name of device	Clip arm length	Jaw opening angle, or width	Rotatability	Reopening capability	MRI compatibility	Additional features
Olympus	Ez Clips						
	Grey	Super short (4 mm)	135 degrees	N	N	N	Cartridge clips used in combination with reusable clip applicator
	Green	Short (6 mm)	135 degrees	N	N	N	
	Pink	Standard (7.5 mm)	135 degrees	N	N	N	
	Purple	Long (9 mm)	135 degrees	N	N	N	
	White	Short (6 mm)	90 degrees	N	N	N	
	Yellow	Standard (7.5 mm)	90 degrees	N	N	N	
	Blue	Long (9 mm)	90 degrees	N	N	N	
	White	Short (6 mm)	90 degrees	N	N	N	
	QuickClips						
	QuickClip2	7.5 mm	9 mm	Y	N	N	
	QuickClip2 Long	9 mm	11 mm	Y	N	N	Longer arm length
	QuickClip Pro	10 mm	11 mm	Y	Y	Y	360 degree rotation
Boston Scientific	Resolution Clip	NA	72 degrees,11 mm	N	Y	Y	Reopening up to five times
Cook Medical	Instinct	Short	125 degrees,16 mm	Y	Y	Y	360-degree rotation; serrated jaw; wide opening; short arms

NA, not available.

to the ulcer and minimizing tangential targeting. This will reduce scenarios where vessels are injured rather than clipped. Furthermore, it is best to open the clips just in front of the target as wavering of the opened clips can cause injury to the surrounding tissue (**Video 28.2**). In cases where visualization of the ulcer requires retroflexion, having the clips out for the scope in advance can make deployment easier. It can be difficult to deploy clips over the elevator of the duodenoscope; removing the outer sheath of the clipping catheter can facilitate easier deployment.

It is clear from several meta-analyses that epinephrine injection alone is not adequate to prevent ulcer rebleeding. Additional hemostatic modality should be used, either clip or thermal application, both with similar efficacy. Dual endoscopic therapy is not superior to thermal coagulation or clip application alone. Thus, if monotherapy is to be delivered, thermal coagulation or clips should be of choice.[33,34,35`]

Over-the-Scope Clips

Over-the-scope clip (Ovesco Endoscopy AG, Tubingen, Germany) is analogous to a bear claw (▶ Fig. 28.3). The nitinol-based OTSC is preloaded in a bent state over a clear clap and is available in three sizes (11, 12, and 14 mm in diameter) and two working depths (3 and 6 mm). The three cap sizes have been designed to accommodate various endoscope diameters: 11-mm cap for endoscope diameter 9.5 to 11 mm, 12-mm cap for endoscope diameter 10.5 to 12 mm, 14-mm cap for endoscope diameter 11.5 to 14 mm. Three types of teeth are available on the clips: atraumatic (a), traumatic (t), gastrotomy closure (gc). Both a- and t-type teeth are used in treatment of peptic ulcer bleeding. The t-type teeth are likely to provide a more secure anchoring in chronic ulcers with fibrotic

base. Its setup and deployment are similar to the endoscopic band ligation. An applicator cap is attached to the tip of the endoscope, and the release mechanism is fastened to the entrance port of the endoscope working channel. The cap is then placed over the ulcer and suction is applied before releasing the clip. The assistance of an anchor device may be useful for retracting the ulcer base into the cap (**Video 28.3**). Data from observational studies have suggested a role for OTSC in failed hemostasis with conventional endotherapies.[36,37] The challenges that users may encounter are traversing through strictures, accessing difficult locations of ulcers (posterior/inferior duodenal wall, lesser curve of gastric wall) and grasping ulcers with a fibrotic base (anchor device can be useful). Also, it may hinder accessibility by subsequent through-the-scope clips if further treatment is required.

28.4.4 Topical Hemostatic Powders

Hemospray

Hemospray (Cook Medical, Bloomington, Indiana) is an inorganic nonabsorbent powder that forms an adherent barrier at the targeted site. The delivery device consists of the Hemospray powder, delivery catheter, and an introducer handle with a built-in carbon dioxide canister, which propels the powder. The powder is delivered in short bursts by pressing a button on the introducer handle. When the powder is sprayed onto the bleeding site, it turns into a cohesive and adhesive form, becoming a barrier to cover the bleeding site (▶ Fig. 28.4). In addition, it increases the local concentration of clotting factors resulting in activation of the coagulation cascade formation of a stable fibrin plug. The coagulum usually disappears after a day. The main advantage of

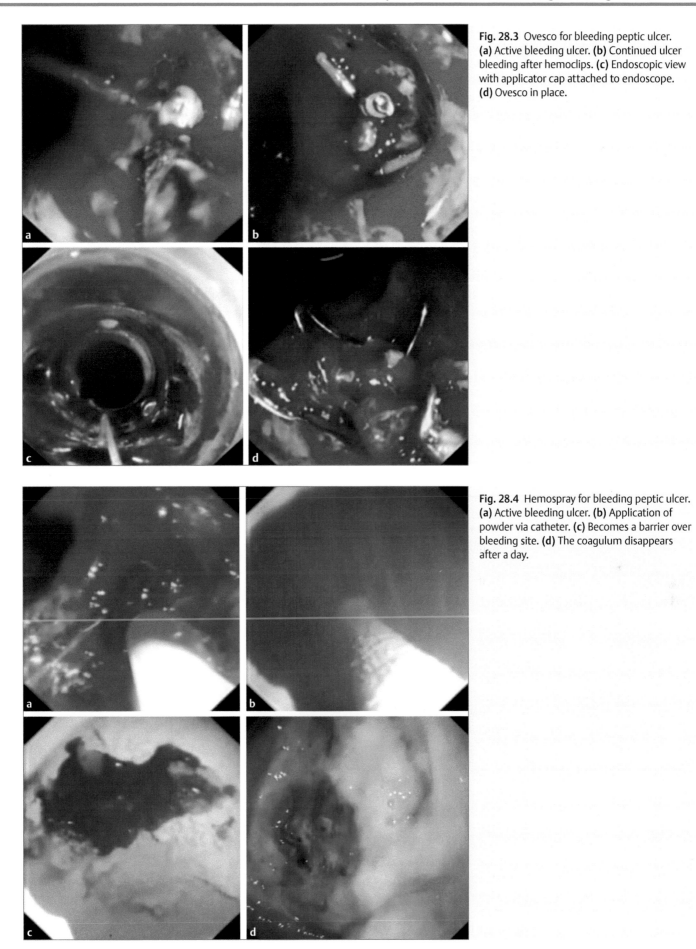

Fig. 28.3 Ovesco for bleeding peptic ulcer. **(a)** Active bleeding ulcer. **(b)** Continued ulcer bleeding after hemoclips. **(c)** Endoscopic view with applicator cap attached to endoscope. **(d)** Ovesco in place.

Fig. 28.4 Hemospray for bleeding peptic ulcer. **(a)** Active bleeding ulcer. **(b)** Application of powder via catheter. **(c)** Becomes a barrier over bleeding site. **(d)** The coagulum disappears after a day.

this modality is that it is easy to use and does not require the precision of other hemostatic modalities. Its use is only limited to actively bleeding ulcers and is considered a temporizing measure before a more definitive therapy can be applied.[38] Challenges with Hemospray include unwanted cloudy view from the dispersion of powder in the lumen, and blockage of delivery catheter by early formation of coagulum inside the catheter. The latter can be prevented by the several following steps. Before insertion of the Hemospray catheter into the accessory channel, try to keep the field dry by removing as much blood and other fluids as possible; then flush air down the accessory channel to remove any retained liquid. It is important to avoid direct catheter contact with blood or mucosa. The use of suction on the endoscope should also be avoided during delivery of the powder. Choosing an endoscope with a larger accessory channel, or a larger Hemospray delivery catheter (available in 7 and 10 F) can also minimize the risk of early formation of coagulum inside the catheter. If blockage of the catheter does occur, each Hemospray device contains an extra catheter.

The evidence for the efficacy of Hemospray for treatment of peptic ulcer bleeding has been exclusively from case series only.[39,40] Up to date, there are no comparative studies to investigate its effectiveness against existing hemostatic modalities.

Other Hemostatic Topical Agents

Other topical agents include the starch-derived polysaccharide hemostatic system (EndoClot) and the Ankaferd blood stopper (ABS; Ankaferd Health Products Ltd, Istanbul, Turkey). ABS is derived from plants' extracts.[41,42] It produces a hemostatic effect by formation of a protein network that serves as a mesh to aggravate red blood cells rather that an effect on the coagulation factors or platelets. There are still a lack of randomized-controlled trials assessing the safety and efficacy of these new topical agents in peptic ulcer bleeding.

28.5 New Hemostatic Modalities

28.5.1 Endoscopic Suturing

Several endoscopic suturing devices have been developed over the last decade, which include Bard EndoCinch (Massachusetts, United States), T-bars (Wilson Cook, North Carolina, United States), GERDIX TM (G Surg Seeon, Germany). Yet, only recently their usage is more commonly seen in clinical practice. The only device that has become widely available for clinical use and approved by the Food and Drug Administration is OverStitch (Apollo Endosurgery, Austin, Texas). It is a disposable, single-use device that is mounted onto a double-channel gastroscope (▶ Fig. 28.5, **Video 28.4**). Suturing can be interrupted or continuous and different suturing patterns can be used, each with their advantages and disadvantages.[43] It is more commonly used for closure of perforations, or full-thickness defects after resection, or fistula closure. Recently, it has been reported to have a role in peptic ulcer bleeding, by suturing the bleeding ulcer for primary hemostasis and preventing further rebleeding and excluding it from gastric lumen.[44]

Endoscopic suturing is most likely to have a role in bleeding from large ulcers where traditional modalities have failed in achieving hemostasis or unlikely to be effective in prevention of

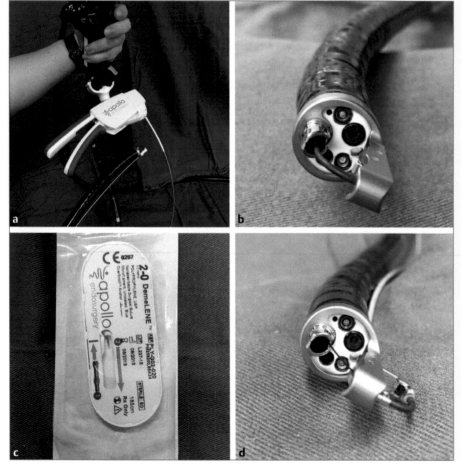

Fig. 28.5 OverStitch endoscopic suturing system (Apollo Endosurgery, Austin, Texas).

rebleeding. Closure of the ulcer may prevent the need for surgery or angiographic embolization.

28.5.2 Endoscopic Ultrasound–Guided Angiotherapy

Over the years, endoscopic ultrasound (EUS) has evolved from being a supplementary diagnostic aid to a therapeutic tool. EUS-guided angiotherapy is made possible by the close proximity of the gastrointestinal tract to the vascular structures in the abdomen. Agents used include sclerosants, N-butylcyanoacrylate, thrombin, and coils.[45] Most reports on EUS-guided angiotherapy has been in treatment of variceal bleeding.[46,47] However, there have been a few reports of EUS-guided angiotherapy in refractory peptic ulcer bleeding,[48] but feasibility and safety for its use in refractory peptic ulcer bleeding still require further studies.

28.6 Conclusion

Endoscopy allows the identification of the bleeding focus, classification of risk of rebleeding, and treatment to halt the bleeding from peptic ulcers. Using the Forrest classification, those ulcers classified as FI or FIIa are at high risk for rebleeding and endoscopic therapy is advised in these patients. There are now reports of novel techniques to provide earlier diagnosis (capsule endoscopy), or aid risk stratification (Doppler ultrasound probe) in patients presenting with upper gastrointestinal bleeding. With the current standard hemostatic modalities, epinephrine injection alone is not adequate to prevent rebleeding and additional modality; either clips or thermal devices should be used, both with similar efficacy. There are now emerging hemostatic devices such as OTSC Hemospray, OverStitch with potential benefit in selected cases. Further studies are required to compare their efficacy with existing hemostatic modalities.

Reference

[1] Shaukat A, Wang A, Acosta RD, et al; ASGE Standards of Practice Committee. The role of endoscopy in dyspepsia. Gastrointest Endosc. 2015; 82(2):227–232
[2] Stolte M, Seitter V, Müller H. Improvement in the quality of the endoscopic/bioptic diagnosis of gastric ulcers between 1990 and 1997—an analysis of 1,658 patients. Z Gastroenterol. 2001; 39(5):349–355
[3] Banerjee S, Cash BD, Dominitz JA, et al; ASGE Standards of Practice Committee. The role of endoscopy in the management of patients with peptic ulcer disease. Gastrointest Endosc. 2010; 71(4):663–668
[4] Chung IK, Kim EJ, Lee MS, et al. Endoscopic factors predisposing to rebleeding following endoscopic hemostasis in bleeding peptic ulcers. Endoscopy. 2001; 33(11):969–975
[5] Guglielmi A, Ruzzenente A, Sandri M, et al. Risk assessment and prediction of rebleeding in bleeding gastroduodenal ulcer. Endoscopy. 2002; 34(10):778–786
[6] Elmunzer BJ, Young SD, Inadomi JM, et al. Systematic review of the predictors of recurrent hemorrhage after endoscopic hemostatic therapy for bleeding peptic ulcers. Am J Gastroenterol. 2008; 103(10):2625–2632, quiz 2633
[7] Sung JJ, Chan FK, Lau JY, et al. The effect of endoscopic therapy in patients receiving omeprazole for bleeding ulcers with nonbleeding visible vessels or adherent clots: a randomized comparison. Ann Intern Med. 2003; 139(4):237–243
[8] Kahi CJ, Jensen DM, Sung JJ, et al. Endoscopic therapy versus medical therapy for bleeding peptic ulcer with adherent clot: a meta-analysis. Gastroenterology. 2005; 129(3):855–862
[9] Laine L, McQuaid KR. Endoscopic therapy for bleeding ulcers: an evidence-based approach based on meta-analyses of randomized controlled trials. Clin Gastroenterol Hepatol. 2009; 7(1):33–47, quiz 1–2
[10] Gralnek IM, Barkun AN, Bardou M. Management of acute bleeding from a peptic ulcer. N Engl J Med. 2008; 359(9):928–937
[11] Barkun AN, Bardou M, Kuipers EJ, et al; International Consensus Upper Gastrointestinal Bleeding Conference Group. International consensus recommendations on the management of patients with nonvariceal upper gastrointestinal bleeding. Ann Intern Med. 2010; 152(2):101–113
[12] Laine L, Peterson WL. Bleeding peptic ulcer. N Engl J Med. 1994; 331(11):717–727
[13] Forrest JA, Finlayson ND, Shearman DJ. Endoscopy in gastrointestinal bleeding. Lancet. 1974; 2(7877):394–397
[14] Cheng CL, Lin CH, Kuo CJ, et al. Predictors of rebleeding and mortality in patients with high-risk bleeding peptic ulcers. Dig Dis Sci. 2010; 55(9):2577–2583
[15] Freeman ML, Cass OW, Peine CJ, Onstad GR. The non-bleeding visible vessel versus the sentinel clot: natural history and risk of rebleeding. Gastrointest Endosc. 1993; 39(3):359–366
[16] Cipolletta L, Bianco MA, Salerno R, et al. Improved characterization of visible vessels in bleeding ulcers by using magnification endoscopy: results of a pilot study. Gastrointest Endosc. 2010; 72(2):413–418
[17] Kohler B, Maier M, Benz C, Riemann JF. Acute ulcer bleeding. A prospective randomized trial to compare Doppler and Forrest classifications in endoscopic diagnosis and therapy. Dig Dis Sci. 1997; 42(7):1370–1374
[18] Wong RC, Chak A, Kobayashi K, et al. Role of Doppler US in acute peptic ulcer hemorrhage: can it predict failure of endoscopic therapy? Gastrointest Endosc. 2000; 52(3):315–321
[19] Jensen DM, Ohning GV, Kovacs TO, et al. Doppler endoscopic probe as a guide to risk stratification and definitive hemostasis of peptic ulcer bleeding. Gastrointest Endosc. 2016; 83(1):129–136
[20] Gralnek IM, Ching JY, Maza I, et al. Capsule endoscopy in acute upper gastrointestinal hemorrhage: a prospective cohort study. Endoscopy. 2013; 45(1):12–19
[21] Rubin M, Hussain SA, Shalomov A, et al. Live view video capsule endoscopy enables risk stratification of patients with acute upper GI bleeding in the emergency room: a pilot study. Dig Dis Sci. 2011; 56(3):786–791
[22] Meltzer AC, Ali MA, Kresiberg RB, et al. Video capsule endoscopy in the emergency department: a prospective study of acute upper gastrointestinal hemorrhage. Ann Emerg Med. 2013; 61(4):438–443.e1
[23] Mönkemüller K, Neumann H, Bellutti M, et al. Use of a colonoscope to perform endoscopic therapy in patients with active bleeding from posterior duodenal and gastric ulcers. Endoscopy. 2009; 41(suppl 2):E93–E94
[24] Vergara M, Bennett C, Calvet X, Gisbert JP. Epinephrine injection versus epinephrine injection and a second endoscopic method in high-risk bleeding ulcers. Cochrane Database Syst Rev. 2014; 10(10):CD005584
[25] Hwang JH, Fisher DA, Ben-Menachem T, et al; Standards of Practice Committee of the American Society for Gastrointestinal Endoscopy. The role of endoscopy in the management of acute non-variceal upper GI bleeding. Gastrointest Endosc. 2012; 75(6):1132–1138
[26] Cappell MS, Iacovone FM, Jr. Safety and efficacy of esophagogastroduodenoscopy after myocardial infarction. Am J Med. 1999; 106(1):29–35
[27] Chung SC, Leong HT, Chan AC, et al. Epinephrine or epinephrine plus alcohol for injection of bleeding ulcers: a prospective randomized trial. Gastrointest Endosc. 1996; 43(6):591–595
[28] Rutgeerts P, Rauws E, Wara P, et al. Randomised trial of single and repeated fibrin glue compared with injection of polidocanol in treatment of bleeding peptic ulcer. Lancet. 1997; 350(9079):692–696
[29] Kurokohchi K, Maeta T, Ohgi T, et al. Successful treatment of a giant exposed blood vessel in a gastric ulcer by endoscopic sclerotherapy with N-butyl-2-cyanoacrylate. Endoscopy. 2007; 39(suppl 1):E250
[30] Laine L. Therapeutic endoscopy and bleeding ulcers. Bipolar/multipolar electrocoagulation. Gastrointest Endosc. 1990; 36(suppl 5):S38–S41
[31] Laine L, Long GL, Bakos GJ, et al. Optimizing bipolar electrocoagulation for endoscopic hemostasis: assessment of factors influencing energy delivery and coagulation. Gastrointest Endosc. 2008; 67(3):502–508
[32] Conway JD, Adler DG, Diehl DL, et al; ASGE Technology Committee. Endoscopic hemostatic devices. Gastrointest Endosc. 2009; 69(6):987–996
[33] Sung JJ, Tsoi KK, Lai LH, et al. Endoscopic clipping versus injection and thermo-coagulation in the treatment of non-variceal upper gastrointestinal bleeding: a meta-analysis. Gut. 2007; 56(10):1364–1373
[34] Calvet X, Vergara M, Brullet E, et al. Addition of a second endoscopic treatment following epinephrine injection improves outcome in high-risk bleeding ulcers. Gastroenterology. 2004; 126(2):441–450
[35] Marmo R, Rotondano G, Piscopo R, et al. Dual therapy versus monotherapy in the endoscopic treatment of high-risk bleeding ulcers: a meta-analysis of controlled trials. Am J Gastroenterol. 2007; 102(2):279–289, quiz 469
[36] Kirschniak A, Kratt T, Stüker D, et al. A new endoscopic over-the-scope clip system for treatment of lesions and bleeding in the GI tract: first clinical experiences. Gastrointest Endosc. 2007; 66(1):162–167
[37] Manta R, Galloro G, Mangiavillano B, et al. Over-the-scope clip (OTSC) represents an effective endoscopic treatment for acute GI bleeding after failure of conventional techniques. Surg Endosc. 2013; 27(9):3162–3164
[38] Barkun AN, Moosavi S, Martel M. Topical hemostatic agents: a systematic review with particular emphasis on endoscopic application in GI bleeding. Gastrointest Endosc. 2013; 77(5):692–700
[39] Sung JJ, Luo D, Wu JC, et al. Early clinical experience of the safety and effectiveness of Hemospray in achieving hemostasis in patients with acute peptic ulcer bleeding. Endoscopy. 2011; 43(4):291–295

[40] Chen YI, Barkun A, Nolan S. Hemostatic powder TC-325 in the management of upper and lower gastrointestinal bleeding: a two-year experience at a single institution. Endoscopy. 2015; 47(2):167–171

[41] Goker H, Haznedaroglu IC, Ercetin S, et al. Haemostatic actions of the folkloric medicinal plant extract Ankaferd Blood Stopper. J Int Med Res. 2008; 36(1):163–170

[42] Beyazit Y, Kurt M, Kekilli M, et al. Evaluation of hemostatic effects of Ankaferd as an alternative medicine. Altern Med Rev. 2010; 15(4):329–336

[43] Stavropoulos SN, Modayil R, Friedel D. Current applications of endoscopic suturing. World J Gastrointest Endosc. 2015; 7(8):777–789

[44] Chiu PW, Chan FK, Lau JY. Endoscopic suturing for ulcer exclusion in patients with massively bleeding large gastric ulcer. Gastroenterology. 2015; 149(1):29–30

[45] Saxena P, Lakhtakia S. Endoscopic ultrasound guided vascular access and therapy (with videos). Endosc Ultrasound. 2015; 4(3):168–175

[46] Binmoeller KF, Weilert F, Shah JN, Kim J. EUS-guided transesophageal treatment of gastric fundal varices with combined coiling and cyanoacrylate glue injection (with videos). Gastrointest Endosc. 2011; 74(5):1019–1025

[47] Romero-Castro R, Ellrichmann M, Ortiz-Moyano C, et al. EUS-guided coil versus cyanoacrylate therapy for the treatment of gastric varices: a multicenter study (with videos). Gastrointest Endosc. 2013; 78(5):711–721

[48] Levy MJ, Wong Kee Song LM, Farnell MB, et al. Endoscopic ultrasound (EUS)-guided angiotherapy of refractory gastrointestinal bleeding. Am J Gastroenterol. 2008; 103(2):352–359

29 Gastric Cancer Including Early Neoplasia and Preneoplastic Conditions

Takuji Gotoda

29.1 Introduction

Improvements in the recognition of premalignant lesions and the detection of early gastric cancers (EGC) will enable organ-preserving endoscopic therapy. Whereas several factors such as *Helicobacter pylori* eradication, smoking cessation, and low-salt diet might prevent gastric carcinogenesis, gastroscopy according to the proper procedure is crucial to recognize EGC. However, it is possible that even the presence of the lesion may be overlooked if the observer has no knowledge of what an EGC looks like and simply views the endoscopic images. In recent years, image-enhanced endoscopy (IEE), such as narrow-band imaging (NBI), has become more common, but high-quality white-light endoscopy should be the gold standard as a starting point for the detection of early gastric neoplasia.

With the advancement of endoscope technology in the 1980s, the number of patients diagnosed with EGC has increased. Nowadays endoscopic mucosal resection (EMR) and endoscopic submucosal dissection (ESD), which avoids the morbidity and mortality associated with gastrectomy, offer less invasive options. Endoscopic resection allows complete pathologic staging of the cancer, which is critical for risk stratification of metastatic potential, and en bloc resection with R0 (negative vertical and horizontal margins) is to protect the patient from the risk of local recurrence.

This chapter outlines the knack of steady detection of EGC without oversight by endoscopic observation under white-light and endoscopic resection strategy for EGC.

29.2 Diagnostic Approach

29.2.1 Preparation

Medical Interview Prior to Endoscopy

The most important purpose of medical interviews prior to endoscopy is to prevent morbidities associated with the examination. Obtaining a history of the use of nonsteroidal anti-inflammatory drugs (NSAIDs), anticoagulants, and antiplatelet drugs is important for deciding whether to perform a biopsy.[1] Recently, it is also necessary to interview patients about their history of examination for or eradication of *H. pylori* in countries with high rates of gastric cancer.[2,3,4]

Pretreatment

Gastroscopy is preceded by the routine administration of a mixture of mucolytic and defoaming agent to improve mucosal visualization.[5,6] Proper premedication before endoscopy is important to ensure satisfactory visualization of the gastric wall, especially before chromoendoscopy. Premedication with mucolytic agent significantly improved the visibility of the gastric mucosa during conventional endoscopy and after chromoendoscopy. Mucolytic premedication also significantly shortened the duration of endoscopy because it eliminates the need to awkwardly manipulate a wash tube during the procedure.

A standard regimen is 100 mL of water mixed with 20,000 units of mucolytic agent (Pronase MS, Kaken Pharmaceutical, Japan), 1 g of sodium bicarbonate, and 3 mL of dimethylpolysiloxane (20 mg/mL). In the West, 100 mL of water with 2 mL of acetylcysteine (200 mg/mL; Parvolex, Celltech, United Kingdom) and 0.5 mL of activated dimethicone (40 mg/mL; Infacol, Forest Laboratories, United Kingdom) can be used as an alternative.

Although it is common to use a topical pharyngeal anesthetic, its usefulness is controversial.[7,8] At least it seems clear that topical pharyngeal anesthesia does not affect patient tolerance or procedure performance in gastroscopy under sedation.[9,10]

There has been no study that demonstrated the usefulness and efficacy of antispasmodics, in particular, intramuscular or intravenous butylscopolamine bromide (hyoscine-N-butylbromide) (Buscopan 20 mg). Peppermint oil has been used as a herbal medicine since ancient times.[11] Active components of this medicine were extracted to obtain the product L-menthol (Minclea).[12,13]

Sedation

Sedation for the purpose of endoscopy is categorized as moderate sedation (conscious sedation) according to the classification of sedation and anesthesia prescribed by the American Society of Anesthesiologists.[14,15] The Ramsay sedation score is a widely used method for judging the depth of sedation and anesthesia.[16] Accidental symptoms associated with the use of sedative drugs include respiratory depression, cardiovascular depression, bradycardia, arrhythmia, anterograde amnesia, disinhibition, and hiccups.

▶ Table 29.1 shows an outline of the interview, pretreatment, and sedation procedures necessary for performing safe and effective gastroscopy.

29.2.2 Endoscopic Technique

The JAG program from United Kingdom is supported by an initial course on basic skills in upper gastrointestinal endoscopy and competence in the technique evaluated by direct observation of procedural skill (DOPS) assessments in formative and then summative appraisals.[17] DOPS descriptors basically focus on manipulative skills and disease pathology, as well as patient comfort and safety. The American Society of Gastrointestinal Endoscopy (ASGE) has a similarly outlined curriculum for gastroscopy.[18] However, in Japan, training in gastroscopy focuses on the detection of subtle mucosal changes that might indicate EGC.

In 2001, the guideline of the European Society of Gastrointestinal Endoscopy (ESGE) recommended that four images be recorded for observation of the stomach.[19] In Japan, the systematic screening

Table 29.1 Preparation for screening upper gastrointestinal endoscopy

Contents	Item	Supplement
Interview	Understanding of examination purpose	Chief complaint, screening
	Past history	Gastric cancer/ulcer, surgery, benign prostatic hyperplasia, glaucoma, serious cardio-vascular/respiratory disease
	Allergy	Drugs, soy, egg
	History of drug use	NSAIDs, anticoagulants/antiplatelet drugs
	Family history	
	Lifestyle	Tobacco, alcohol use
	H. pylori infection	History of examination/results, history of eradication
Pretreatment	Protease	Its use is desirable in countries with high rates of gastric cancer
	Antifoaming agent	Its use is desirable in countries with high rates of gastric cancer
	Pharyngeal anesthesia	Not needed under sedation
	Antispasmodics	It is not essential for screening examinations, and L-menthol can be substituted
Sedation	Midazolam	It is most frequently used. Initial dose is 2–5 mg
	Propofol	Clinical experience is increasing
	Elderly subjects	There is no reason to avoid its use
	Analgesic	May be administered in combination with sedative agents
	Patient monitor	Indispensable
	Emergency cart	Indispensable
	Ventilator	Indispensable
	Antagonists	Flumazenil, naloxone hydrochloride

NSAIDs, nonsteroidal anti-inflammatory drugs.

protocol for the stomach (SSS) has been proposed as a minimum required standard for screening procedures.[20,21] The SSS protocol should be initiated as soon as the endoscope is inserted into the gastric antrum. In the antegrade view, endoscopic images of four quadrants of the gastric antrum, incisura, lower–middle–upper body are obtained. In the retroflex view, two images of the gastric fundus and cardia by distant and closed view are taken. Overall, the SSS comprises 22 endoscopic images. However, there has been no study that actually examined the detection rate and prognosis of gastric cancer using observational procedures and the number of images recorded as key performance indicator (KPI).

29.2.3 Knowledge for Diagnosis

Mucosal Condition of *H. pylori* Infection

EGC often has only minute morphologic changes that can be difficult to detect on a background of atrophic gastritis. The detection of mild elevations or shallow depressions in the surface mucosa and subtle changes in color requires careful observation. During endoscopic examination, risk stratification should be routinely kept in mind, using specific procedures to assess the severity of a lesion and the risk of progression. This means that attention is focused on areas associated with an increased cancer risk. The presence of *H. pylori* infection, atrophy of the gastric mucosa, and intestinal metaplasia are closely related to the risk of gastric carcinogenesis.[22] Therefore, evaluation of relevant endoscopic findings is important for efficient detection of gastric cancer. A study performed in the United Kingdom also reported the detection of EGC when patients with previously diagnosed atrophic gastritis or

intestinal metaplasia were monitored in annual gastroscopy (67% of detected cancers were stage I and II in the annual follow-up group, compared with 23% in the group that was referred with symptoms; $p < 0.05$), resulting in major improvements in survival outcomes (5-year survival 50% compared with 10%; $p = 0.006$).[23]

The first step to efficient diagnosis of gastric cancer is to estimate the presence/absence of *H. pylori* infection.[24] The presence of little adhesion of mucus, regular arrangement of collecting venules (RAC), and fundic gland polyps strongly suggests, "gastric mucosa uninfected with *H. pylori*" (▶Fig. 29.1a–d). Diagnostic odds ratio as uninfected *H. pylori* status is 11.5 in patients with RAC and 34.5 in those with fundic gland polyps, respectively. In the subjects with those findings, the possibility of *H. pylori* infection is extremely low.

Conversely, atrophy of the gastric mucosa (▶Fig. 29.2a), meandering and thickening of the folds of the greater curvature of the gastric corpus (▶Fig. 29.2b, c), xanthoma (▶Fig. 29.2d), or goose flesh–like mucosa (nodular gastritis) (▶Fig. 29.2e), in the absence of the above findings, indicate a gastric mucosa currently or previously infected with *H. pylori*.[25] Attention should be paid to this finding because it is now considered to be a mucosal change associated with a higher risk of juvenile gastric cancer, particularly undifferentiated adenocarcinoma.[26,27]

Evaluation of High-Risk Mucosal Condition

The clinically most important finding in diagnosing gastric cancer is presence or absence of atrophic changes in the gastric mucosa resulting from prolonged *H. pylori* infection.[28,29,30] Atrophy of the gastric corpus and intestinal metaplasia occurs in a multifocal

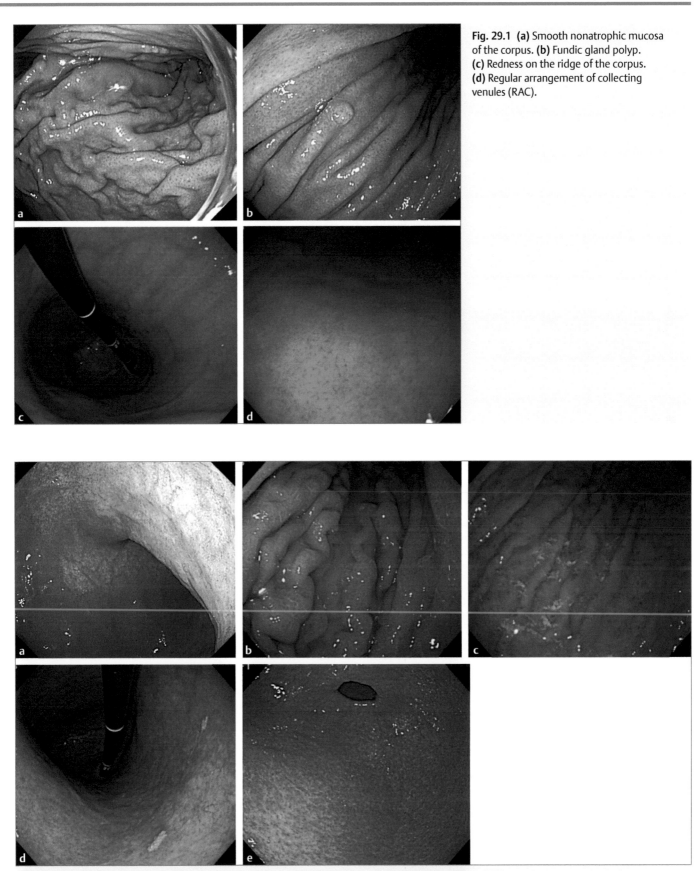

Fig. 29.1 (a) Smooth nonatrophic mucosa of the corpus. (b) Fundic gland polyp. (c) Redness on the ridge of the corpus. (d) Regular arrangement of collecting venules (RAC).

Fig. 29.2 (a) Atrophic border in the anterior wall of the lower part of the corpus. (b) Thickened folds of the greater curvature in the corpus. (c) Spotty redness and adhesion of mucus in the greater curvature of the corpus. (d) Xanthoma in the lesser curvature of the corpus. (e) Nodular gastritis in the antrum.

fashion in the fundus gland mucosa, and gradually extends to cover a greater area, eventually resulting in replacement of the entire fundus gland mucosa by atrophic and intestinal metaplastic mucosa.[31]

The borderline of the mucosa devoid of atrophy and intestinal metaplasia produced by the continuous presence of the fundus gland mucosa is almost consistent with the endoscopic atrophic border proposed by Kimura and Takemoto and Kono et al.[32,33]

The inside of the endoscopic atrophic border corresponds to the fundus gland mucosa devoid of atrophy and intestinal metaplasia. Outside the border, there is an intermediate zone consisting of a mixture of multifocal atrophic and intestinal metaplastic mucosa and normal fundus gland mucosa, in addition to areas of atrophic and intestinal metaplastic mucosa having no fundus glands (►Fig. 29.3, ►Fig. 29.4). Therefore, undifferentiated carcinoma often originates from the region inside the endoscopic atrophic border or the intermediate zone (vicinity of the atrophic border). On the other hand, well-differentiated carcinoma often arises from the external region of the endoscopic atrophic border.

Chronic infection with *H. pylori* causes molecular alterations in the gastric mucosa and transforms the mucosa into the intestinal phenotype.[34] On white-light images, some intestinal metaplasia appears slightly elevated with whitish patches (►Fig. 29.5a). NBI further reveals intestinal metaplasia by its whitish color (►Fig. 29.5b).

In magnifying NBI, a fine blue–white line of light is observed on the crests of the epithelial surface/gyri (light blue crest) of intestinal metaplasia (►Fig. 29.5c).[35] The "light blue crest" is thought to be caused by the reflection of short wavelength light at the brush border on the surface of the intestinal metaplasia.[36]

Recommended steps for diagnosing gastric cancer on the basis of *H. pylori* infection and the atrophy of gastric mucosa are shown in ►Fig. 29.6. Because the development of gastric cancer from *H. pylori* uninfected patients is extremely rare, the first step to access the risk of gastric cancer is to recognize patients with no history of *H. pylori* infection by endoscopy according to the previous description. However, we have to pay attention that one of the most typical EGC in the *H. pylori* uninfected patients is signet-ring cell carcinoma. This type of EGC, when it is discovered at very early stage, hardly shows any morphologic changes but pale faded color. Moreover, because signet-ring carcinoma sometimes exists

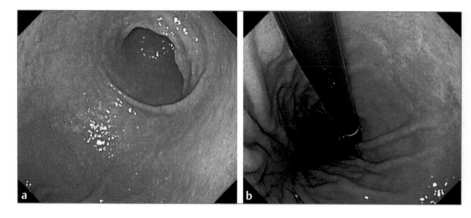

Fig. 29.3 Antral dominant atrophy (C2). **(a)** Atrophic border in the greater curvature of the antrum. **(b)** Atrophic border in the lesser curvature of the lower part of the corpus.

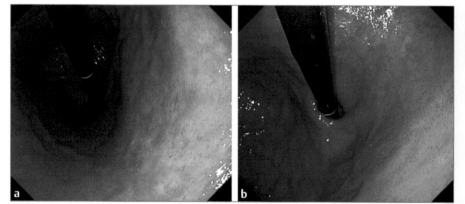

Fig. 29.4 Corpus dominant atrophy (O1). **(a)** Atrophic border in the anterior wall of the middle part of the corpus. **(b)** Atrophic border near the cardia.

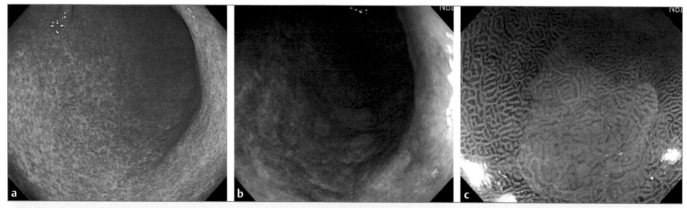

Fig. 29.5 **(a)** Atrophic mucosa of the antrum on white-light image. **(b)** Intestinal metaplasia recognized as whitish patches by narrow-band imaging (NBI). **(c)** Fine blue–white line observed on the crests of the epithelial surface/gyri (light blue crest) by magnifying NBI.

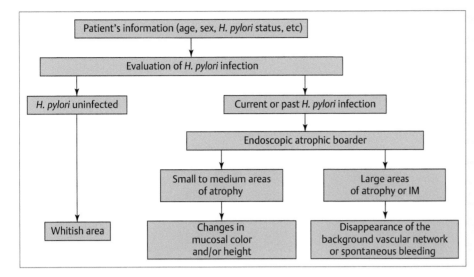

Fig. 29.6 Recommended steps for diagnosing gastric cancer on the basis of *H. pylori* infection and the atrophy of gastric mucosa.

Table 29.2 Entries in the findings record form, taking into account the diagnosis of early gastric cancer

Mucosal finding associated to *H. pylori* status	Presence/absence of regular arrangement of collecting (RAC) venules of the gastric angle		
	Presence/absence of fundus gland polyps		
	Presence/absence and severity of mucosal atrophy		
	Intestinal metaplasia		
Finding of lesion	Color tone	Redness	Pale
	Shape	Elevated	Depressed
	Site		
	Size		
Biopsy	Location/number/issue/differential diagnosis		

only in the middle layer of the lamina propria that is covered with normal foveolar epithelium, it is important to attempt obtaining enough deep biopsy specimens that contain the muscular mucosae with large forceps. Histopathologic types of EGC in *H. pylori* infected patients are associated with the morphologic type and color of EGC on white-light images. Most elevated EGC are of the differentiated type and some gastric superficial elevated type EGCs and adenomas appear whitish. Among the flat or depressed type EGCs, differentiated type cancers look reddish, whereas undifferentiated types appear whitish because of a difference in hemoglobin content (i.e., variations in vascular density).

Biopsy

There have been few reports on the clinically relevant number of biopsy specimens and suitable biopsy forceps in diagnosing early gastric cancer. Although the acquisition of six to eight biopsy specimens is recommended in Europe and the United States,[37] it has been reported in Japan and South Korea that there is no particular change in the diagnostic accuracy as long as at least two biopsy specimens are taken.[38,39] Unfortunately, biopsies have been conducted according to customary practice, and no studies have been performed to examine the number of biopsy specimens desirable as KPI for accurate diagnosis of gastric cancer.

Clinical report

At a minimum, the following information should be provided: what the endoscopic findings are, the location from which the biopsy was taken, what the endoscopic diagnosis is, and what is

being asked for in the pathologic diagnosis (▶Table 29.2). Detailed request forms enable us to review and reflect on the reasons why the biopsy was taken, and what information is needed. Following this process is very useful for improvement of diagnostic techniques.

29.3 Therapeutic Approach

29.3.1 Principle of Endoscopic Resection

EGC is defined when cancer invasion is confined to the mucosa or submucosa (T1 cancer), irrespective of the presence of lymph node metastasis (LNM).[40] Because the presence of LNM is a strong predictor on patients' prognosis, gastrectomy with lymph node dissection had been the gold standard for treatment of EGC in Japan.[42] Such an extensive surgery, however, carries a significant risk of morbidity and mortality, and is associated with long-term reduction of patients' quality of life (QOL).[42] With stratification, subgroups of patients with EGC and minimal risk of LNM could be identified.[44]

The major advantage of endoscopic resection is the ability to provide accurate pathologic staging without precluding future surgical therapy.[44,45] After endoscopic resection, pathologic assessment of depth of cancer invasion, degree of cancer differentiation, and involvement of lymphatics or vessels allow the prediction of the risk of LNM (▶Table 29.3).[46] The risk of developing LNM or distant metastasis is then weighted against the risk of surgery.[47]

Table 29.3 Independent risk factors for lymph node metastasis from submucosal invasive cancer

	Relative risk	Standard error	p
Lymphatic–vascular involvement (absence vs. presence)	6.422	0.179	< 0.001
Histologic type (differentiated vs. undifferentiated)	1.752	0.172	0.001
Tumor size (≤ 30 vs. > 30)	1.569	0.170	0.008

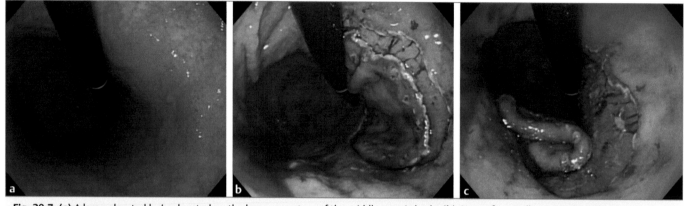

Fig. 29.7 (a) A large elevated lesion located on the lesser curvature of the middle gastric body. (b) Circumferentially mucosal cutting at the periphery of the marking dots using insulated-tip diathermic knife 2 (IT knife-2) or Dual knife with PulseCut slow (40 W). (c) Dissecting submucosal layer after additional submucosal injection.

29.3.2 Indication for Endoscopic Resection

Endoscopic resection to treat cancer is perhaps the most gratifying endoscopy to perform because of its minimally invasive curative potentials.[48,49,50] Endoscopic resection allows complete pathologic staging of the cancer, which is critical for risk stratification of metastatic potential.[51] In addition to allow pathologic staging, en bloc resection with R0 (negative vertical and horizontal margins) is to protect the patient from the risk of local recurrence.

The traditional criteria for endoscopic resection of EGC were founded on the technical limitation of traditional EMR[52] for removing gastric lesions larger than 2 cm in diameter en bloc.[53] The empirical indications for EMR were therefore[1] papillary or tubular (differentiated) adenocarcinoma,[2] less than 2 cm in diameter,[3] without ulceration within tumor,[4] and no lymphatic–vascular involvement.[54]

The subsequent advent of ESD (▶Fig. 29.7a–c)[55,56] dramatically changed the range of lesions indicated for endoscopic resection (▶Table 29.4). With an objective of expanding the indications, the risks of LNM in early gastric cancer were assessed in 5,265 cases of surgical resection performed at two major oncology centers in Tokyo.[57] In cases with undifferentiated histology, analysis of subsequently accumulated cases revealed that LNM was observed in none of the 310 cases of intramucosal cancer, 20 mm or less in size, without either lymphatic vessel invasion or ulcerated lesions (95% confidence interval [CI]: 0–0.96%).[58] Several ESD knives have since been developed and studied in detail (▶Fig. 29.8).[59,60,61,62,63]

29.3.3 Clinical Management after Endoscopic Resection

All patients with curative resection who met the traditional criteria were followed up by annual upper gastrointestinal endoscopy in order to detect local recurrence and/or metachronous gastric cancers.[65] Patients with curative resection who met the expanded criteria were additionally followed up by alternatively abdominal computed tomography (CT) and endoscopic ultrasound (EUS) every 6 months for 3 years in order to detect lymph node and distant metastases and annual gastroscopy.

Long-term outcomes after EMR for small differentiated mucosal EGC less than 2 cm in diameter have been reported to be comparable to those following gastrectomy.[65,66] Several investigators have reported that patients who underwent treatment following the expanded criteria have similar long-term survival and outcomes as patients treated according to the traditional criteria.[67,68,69,70]

Noncurative resection generally requires radical surgical resection with lymph node dissection as the standard treatment due to the possibility of LNM for a patient's prognosis.

29.4 Future Prospects

Practice guidelines and quality standards with KPIs will initiate quality assurance in gastroscopy and improve outcomes to emulate international success in the colonoscopy. However, validated KPIs for gastroscopy are not yet suited to detect EGC and this aspect is an area that should be a priority for further research.

Although IEE such as NBI is commonly employed and improves diagnostic accuracy in Japan,[71] IEE is not yet systematically applied in routine examinations worldwide. ESD has higher risk of complications such as severe bleeding or perforation, and still requires high endoscopic skills. Most Japanese experts set the level of expertise at 50 to 100 cases to become proficient in gastric ESD,[72] and require a trainee to perform at least 30 gastric ESD cases under the supervision of an expert to gain basic proficiency in this technique.[73] The low prevalence of superficial gastric epithelial neoplasms has translated into very few opportunities

Table 29.4 Early gastric cancer with no risk of lymph node metastasis (modification by ref. nos. 63 and 64)

Criteria	Incidence (No with metastasis/total number)	95% CI
Intramucosal cancer	0/1230; 0%	0–0.3
Differentiated (well and/or moderately and/or papillary adenocarcinoma) type		
No lymphatic–vascular involvement		
Irrespective of ulcer findings		
Tumor size < 3 cm		
Intramucosal cancer	0/929; 0%	0–0.4
Differentiated type		
No lymphatic–vascular involvement		
Without ulcer findings		
Irrespective of tumor size		
Intramucosal cancer	0/310; 0%	0–0.96
Undifferentiated (poorly differentiated adenocarcinoma and/or signet-ring cell carcinoma) type		
No lymphatic–vascular involvement		
Without ulcer findings		
Tumor < 2 cm		
Minute submucosal penetration (sm1)	0/145	0–2.5
Differentiated type		
No lymphatic–vascular involvement		
Tumor < 3 cm in size		

CI, confidence interval.

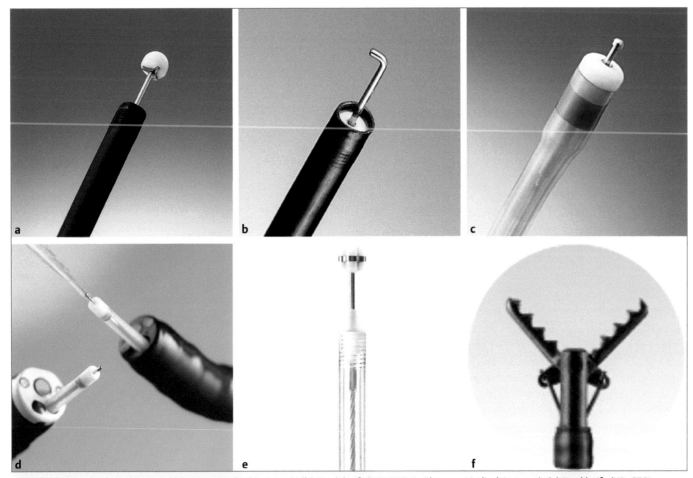

Fig. 29.8 (a) IT knife-2 (KD-611L, Olympus Medical Systems). **(b)** Hook knife (KD-620LR, Olympus Medical Systems). **(c)** Dual knife (KD-650L, Olympus Medical Systems). **(d)** Flash knife BT (Fujinon Optical Co, Ltd). **(e)** Safe knife (DK2518DV1, Fujinon Optical Co, Ltd). **(f)** Mucosectom (DP-2518, PENTAX).

for Western endoscopists to perform gastric ESD.[74] Western ESD experts to supervise ESD training are limited in number, and virtual simulators for ESD are not yet available. Proper use of ex vivo and in vivo animal models is performed in an animal facility under the direction of a veterinarian, with dedicated equipment and a standardized setup. Anyway, in order to standardize ESD procedure worldwide, more innovation and modification should be demanded.[75,76]

In cancer treatment, completely curing the illness is extremely important. However, if QOL is impaired by procedures that are superior only in terms of reducing marginal risks, patients may have difficulties in daily life and social rehabilitation after treatment.[77] The stomach not only serves as a storage compartment but also plays a role in external secretion for digestion and absorption as well as in internal secretion. Therefore, if there is no difference of curability among different treatment methods, long-term QOL should be considered seriously when we select a treatment method, especially in elderly patients.[78]

29.5 Repeat as Needed for Each Condition

In order to accurately detect initial lesions not by beginner's luck or by incidental diagnosis, but by steady techniques, it is important to implement theory-based observation (what the eyes see) and instantly relate the observation to critical analysis based on past experience and knowledge (what the brain knows) during the examination.

Medical care will always be provided with consideration of the following points: whether ESD is really minimally invasive, whether "complete" treatment attempted by physicians, such as gastrectomy, is beneficial for patients, and whether treatment that is not the best but most tolerable to the patients is an option.

References

[1] Fujimoto K, Fujishiro M, Kato M, et al; Japan Gastroenterological Endoscopy Society. Guidelines for gastroenterological endoscopy in patients undergoing antithrombotic treatment. Dig Endosc. 2014; 26(1):1–14

[2] Uemura N, Okamoto S, Yamamoto S, et al. Helicobacter pylori infection and the development of gastric cancer. N Engl J Med. 2001; 345(11):784–789

[3] Goh KL, Cheah PL, Md N, et al. Ethnicity and H. pylori as risk factors for gastric cancer in Malaysia: a prospective case control study. Am J Gastroenterol. 2007; 102(1):40–45

[4] Lee YC, Wu HM, Chen TH, et al. A community-based study of Helicobacter pylori therapy using the strategy of test, treat, retest, and re-treat initial treatment failures. Helicobacter. 2006; 11(5):418–424

[5] Fujii T, Iishi H, Tatsuta M, et al. Effectiveness of premedication with pronase for improving visibility during gastroendoscopy: a randomized controlled trial. Gastrointest Endosc. 1998; 47(5):382–387

[6] Bhandari P, Green S, Hamanaka H, et al. Use of Gascon and Pronase either as a pre-endoscopic drink or as targeted endoscopic flushes to improve visibility during gastroscopy: a prospective, randomized, controlled, blinded trial. Scand J Gastroenterol. 2010; 45(3):357–361

[7] Campo R, Brullet E, Montserrat A, et al. Topical pharyngeal anesthesia improves tolerance endoscopy: a randomized double-blind study. Endoscopy. 1995; 27(9):659–664

[8] Dhir V, Swaroop VS, Vazifdar KF, Wagle SD. Topical pharyngeal anesthesia without intravenous sedation during upper gastrointestinal endoscopy. Indian J Gastroenterol. 1997; 16(1):10–11

[9] Davis DE, Jones MP, Kubik CM. Topical pharyngeal anesthesia does not improve upper gastrointestinal endoscopy in conscious sedated patients. Am J Gastroenterol. 1999; 94(7):1853–1856

[10] Heuss LT, Hanhart A, Dell-Kuster S, et al. Propofol sedation alone or in combination with pharyngeal lidocaine anesthesia for routine upper GI endoscopy: a randomized, double-blind, placebo-controlled, non-inferiority trial. Gastrointest Endosc. 2011; 74(6):1207–1214

[11] Nair B. Final report on the safety assessment of Mentha piperita (peppermint) oil, Mentha piperita (peppermint) leaf extract, Mentha piperita (peppermint) leaf, and Mentha piperita (peppermint) leaf water. Int J Toxicol. 2001; 20(suppl 3):61–73

[12] Hiki N, Kurosaka H, Tatsutomi Y, et al. Peppermint oil reduces gastric spasm during upper endoscopy: a randomized, double-blind, double-dummy controlled trial. Gastrointest Endosc. 2003; 57(4):475–482

[13] Hiki N, Kaminishi M, Yasuda K, et al. Antiperistaltic effect and safety of L-menthol sprayed on the gastric mucosa for upper GI endoscopy: a phase III, multicenter, randomized, double-blind, placebo-controlled study. Gastrointest Endosc. 2011; 73(5):932–941

[14] American Society of Anesthesiologists Task Force on Sedation and Analgesia by Non-Anesthesiologists. Practice guidelines for sedation and analgesia by non-anesthesiologists. Anesthesiology. 2002; 96(4):1004–1017

[15] Obara K, Haruma K, Irisawa A, et al. Guidelines for sedation in gastroenterological endoscopy. Dig Endosc. 2015; 27(4):435–449

[16] Ramsay MA, Savege TM, Simpson BR, Goodwin R. Controlled sedation with alphaxalone-alphadolone. BMJ. 1974; 2(5920):656–659

[17] JAG. DOPS grade descriptors—Diagnostic upper GI endoscopy [online], https://www.thejag.org.uk/Downloads/JAG%20training%20information/DOPS%20and%20DOPyS%20form%20and%20JAG%20certification%20criteria%20update%20-%201%20February%202017.pdf. Accessed October 13, 2017.

[18] ASGE Committee on Training. Esophagogastroduodenoscopy (EGD) Core Curriculum [online], https://www.asge.org/docs/default-source/education/training/022e0f-f663bd455bb5a0476272aa871c.pdf?sfvrsn=4. Accessed October 13, 2017.

[19] Rey JF, Lambert R; ESGE Quality Assurance Committee. ESGE recommendations for quality control in gastrointestinal endoscopy: guidelines for image documentation in upper and lower GI endoscopy. Endoscopy. 2001; 33(10):901–903

[20] Yao K. The endoscopic diagnosis of early gastric cancer. Ann Gastroenterol. 2013; 26(1):11–22

[21] Uedo N, Yao K, Ishihara R. Screening and treating intermediate lesions to prevent gastric cancer. Gastroenterol Clin North Am. 2013; 42(2):317–335

[22] Dinis-Ribeiro M, Areia M, de Vries AC, et al; MAPS Participants. European Society of Gastrointestinal Endoscopy. European Helicobacter Study Group. European Society of Pathology. Sociedade Portuguesa de Endoscopia Digestiva. Management of precancerous conditions and lesions in the stomach (MAPS): guideline from the European Society of Gastrointestinal Endoscopy (ESGE), European Helicobacter Study Group (EHSG), European Society of Pathology (ESP), and the Sociedade Portuguesa de Endoscopia Digestiva (SPED). Virchows Arch. 2012; 460(1):19–46

[23] Whiting JL, Sigurdsson A, Rowlands DC, et al. The long term results of endoscopic surveillance of premalignant gastric lesions. Gut. 2002; 50(3):378–381

[24] Watanabe K, Nagata N, Nakashima R, et al. Predictive findings for Helicobacter pylori-uninfected, -infected and -eradicated gastric mucosa: validation study. World J Gastroenterol. 2013; 19(27):4374–4379

[25] Miyamoto M, Haruma K, Yoshihara M, et al. Nodular gastritis in adults is caused by Helicobacter pylori infection. Dig Dis Sci. 2003; 48(5):968–975

[26] Haruma K, Komoto K, Kamada T, et al. Helicobacter pylori infection is a major risk factor for gastric carcinoma in young patients. Scand J Gastroenterol. 2000; 35(3):255–259

[27] Miyamoto M, Haruma K, Yoshihara M, et al. Five cases of nodular gastritis and gastric cancer: a possible association between nodular gastritis and gastric cancer. Dig Liver Dis. 2002; 34(11):819–820

[28] Correa P. Human gastric carcinogenesis: a multistep and multifactorial process—First American Cancer Society Award Lecture on Cancer Epidemiology and Prevention. Cancer Res. 1992; 52(24):6735–6740

[29] Correa P. Is gastric cancer preventable? Gut. 2004; 53(9):1217–1219

[30] Naylor GM, Gotoda T, Dixon M, et al. Why does Japan have a high incidence of gastric cancer? Comparison of gastritis between UK and Japanese patients. Gut. 2006; 55(11):1545–1552

[31] Kanzaki H, Uedo N, Ishihara R, et al. Comprehensive investigation of areae gastricae pattern in gastric corpus using magnifying narrow band imaging endoscopy in patients with chronic atrophic fundic gastritis. Helicobacter. 2012; 17(3):224–231

[32] Kimura K, Takemoto T. An endoscopic recognition of the atrophic border and its significance in chronic gastritis. Endoscopy. 1969; 1(3):87–97

[33] Kono S, Gotoda T, Yoshida S, et al. Can endoscopic atrophy predict histological atrophy? Historical study in United Kingdom and Japan. World J Gastroenterol. 2015; 21(46):13113–13123

[34] Yoshimura T, Shimoyama T, Fukuda S, et al. Most gastric cancer occurs on the distal side of the endoscopic atrophic border. Scand J Gastroenterol. 1999; 34(11):1077–1081

[35] Busuttil RA, Boussioutas A. Intestinal metaplasia: a premalignant lesion involved in gastric carcinogenesis. J Gastroenterol Hepatol. 2009; 24(2):193–201

[36] Uedo N, Ishihara R, Iishi H, et al. A new method of diagnosing gastric intestinal metaplasia: narrow-band imaging with magnifying endoscopy. Endoscopy. 2006; 38(8):819–824

[37] Hale MD, Gotoda T, Hayden JD, Grabsch HI. Endoscopic biopsies from gastrointestinal carcinomas and their suitability for molecular analysis: a review of the literature and recommendations for clinical practice and research. Histopathology. 2015; 67(2):147–157

[38] Choi Y, Choi HS, Jeon WK, et al. Optimal number of endoscopic biopsies in diagnosis of advanced gastric and colorectal cancer. J Korean Med Sci. 2012; 27(1):36–39

[39] Tsuji S, Doyama H, Kaneko Y, et al. Performance of biopsy-based preoperative pathological diagnosis and optimal number of biopsy specimens for the diagnosis of early gastric cancer. Gastroenterol Endosc. 2013; 55:1796–1805

[40] Japanese Gastric Cancer Association. Japanese classification of gastric carcinoma: 3rd English edition. Gastric Cancer. 2011; 14(2):101–112

[41] Sano T, Sasako M, Kinoshita T, Maruyama K. Recurrence of early gastric cancer. Follow-up of 1475 patients and review of the Japanese literature. Cancer. 1993; 72(11):3174–3178

[42] Sasako M. Risk factors for surgical treatment in the Dutch Gastric Cancer Trial. Br J Surg. 1997; 84(11):1567–1571

[43] Tsujitani S, Oka S, Saito H, et al. Less invasive surgery for early gastric cancer based on the low probability of lymph node metastasis. Surgery. 1999; 125(2):148–154

[44] Yanai H, Matsubara Y, Kawano T, et al. Clinical impact of strip biopsy for early gastric cancer. Gastrointest Endosc. 2004; 60(5):771–777

[45] Farrell JJ, Lauwers GY, Brugge WR. Endoscopic mucosal resection using a cap-fitted endoscope improves tissue resection and pathology interpretation: an animal study. Gastric Cancer. 2006; 9(1):3–8

[46] Gotoda T, Sasako M, Ono H, et al. Evaluation of the necessity for gastrectomy with lymph node dissection for patients with submucosal invasive gastric cancer. Br J Surg. 2001; 88(3):444–449

[47] Etoh T, Katai H, Fukagawa T, et al. Treatment of early gastric cancer in the elderly patient: results of EMR and gastrectomy at a national referral center in Japan. Gastrointest Endosc. 2005; 62(6):868–871

[48] Soetikno RM, Gotoda T, Nakanishi Y, Soehendra N. Endoscopic mucosal resection. Gastrointest Endosc. 2003; 57(4):567–579

[49] Gotoda T. Endoscopic resection of early gastric cancer. Gastric Cancer. 2007; 10(1):1–11

[50] Gotoda T, Yamamoto H, Soetikno RM. Endoscopic submucosal dissection of early gastric cancer. J Gastroenterol. 2006; 41(10):929–942

[51] Hull MJ, Mino-Kenudson M, Nishioka NS, et al. Endoscopic mucosal resection: an improved diagnostic procedure for early gastroesophageal epithelial neoplasms. Am J Surg Pathol. 2006; 30(1):114–118

[52] Inoue H, Endo M, Takeshita K, et al. A new simplified technique of endoscopic esophageal mucosal resection using a cap-fitted panendoscope (EMRC) Surg Endosc. 1992; 6(5):264–265

[53] Yamao T, Shirao K, Ono H, et al. Risk factors for lymph node metastasis from intramucosal gastric carcinoma. Cancer. 1996; 77(4):602–606

[54] Japanese Gastric Cancer Association. Japanese gastric cancer treatment guidelines 2010 (ver. 3). Gastric Cancer. 2011; 14(2):113–123

[55] Ono H, Kondo H, Gotoda T, et al. Endoscopic mucosal resection for treatment of early gastric cancer. Gut. 2001; 48(2):225–229

[56] Gotoda T, Kondo H, Ono H, et al. A new endoscopic mucosal resection (EMR) procedure using an insulation-tipped electrosurgical knife knife for rectal flat lesions: report of two cases. Gastrointest Endosc. 1999; 50:560–563

[57] Gotoda T, Yanagisawa A, Sasako M, et al. Incidence of lymph node metastasis from early gastric cancer: estimation with a large number of cases at two large centers. Gastric Cancer. 2000; 3(4):219–225

[58] Hirasawa T, Gotoda T, Miyata S, et al. Incidence of lymph node metastasis and the feasibility of endoscopic resection for undifferentiated-type early gastric cancer. Gastric Cancer. 2009; 12(3):148–152

[59] Oyama T, Kikuchi Y. Aggressive endoscopic mucosal resection in the upper GI tract—Hook knife EMR method. Minim Invasive Ther Allied Technol. 2002; 11(5–6):291–295

[60] Yahagi N, Fujishiro M, Kakushima N, et al. Endoscopic submucosal dissection for early gastric cancer using the tip of an electrosurgical snare (thin type). Dig Endosc. 2004; 16:34–38

[61] Ono H, Hasuike N, Inui T, et al. Usefulness of a novel electrosurgical knife, the insulation-tipped diathermic knife-2, for endoscopic submucosal dissection of early gastric cancer. Gastric Cancer. 2008; 11(1):47–52

[62] Takeuchi Y, Uedo N, Ishihara R, et al. Efficacy of an endo-knife with a water-jet function (Flushknife) for endoscopic submucosal dissection of superficial colorectal neoplasms. Am J Gastroenterol. 2010; 105(2):314–322

[63] Toyonaga T, Man-I M, Fujita T, et al. The performance of a novel ball-tipped Flush knife for endoscopic submucosal dissection: a case-control study. Aliment Pharmacol Ther. 2010; 32(7):908–915

[64] Nakajima T, Oda I, Gotoda T, et al. Metachronous gastric cancers after endoscopic resection: how effective is annual endoscopic surveillance? Gastric Cancer. 2006; 9(2):93–98

[65] Uedo N, Iishi H, Tatsuta M, et al. Longterm outcomes after endoscopic mucosal resection for early gastric cancer. Gastric Cancer. 2006; 9(2):88–92

[66] Choi KS, Jung HY, Choi KD, et al. EMR versus gastrectomy for intramucosal gastric cancer: comparison of long-term outcomes. Gastrointest Endosc. 2011; 73(5):942–948

[67] Gotoda T, Iwasaki M, Kusano C, et al. Endoscopic resection of early gastric cancer treated by guideline and expanded National Cancer Centre criteria. Br J Surg. 2010; 97(6):868–871

[68] Chung IK, Lee JH, Lee SH, et al. Therapeutic outcomes in 1000 cases of endoscopic submucosal dissection for early gastric neoplasms: Korean ESD Study Group multicenter study. Gastrointest Endosc. 2009; 69(7):1228–1235

[69] Lee H, Yun WK, Min BH, et al. A feasibility study on the expanded indication for endoscopic submucosal dissection of early gastric cancer. Surg Endosc. 2011; 25(6):1985–1993

[70] Ahn JY, Jung HY, Choi KD, et al. Endoscopic and oncologic outcomes after endoscopic resection for early gastric cancer: 1370 cases of absolute and extended indications. Gastrointest Endosc. 2011; 74(3):485–493

[71] Ezoe Y, Muto M, Uedo N, et al. Magnifying narrowband imaging is more accurate than conventional white-light imaging in diagnosis of gastric mucosal cancer. Gastroenterology. 2011; 141(6):2017–2025.e3

[72] Kakushima N, Fujishiro M, Kodashima S. et al. A learning curve for endoscopic submucosal dissection of gastric epithelial neoplasms. Endoscopy. 2006; 38(10):991–995

[73] Gotoda T, Friedland S, Hamanaka H, Soetikno R. A learning curve for advanced endoscopic resection. Gastrointest Endosc. 2005; 62(6):866–867

[74] Draganov PV, Gotoda T, Chavalitdhamrong D, Wallace MB. Techniques of endoscopic submucosal dissection: application for the Western endoscopist? Gastrointest Endosc. 2013; 78(5):677–688

[75] Suzuki S, Gotoda T, Kobayashi Y, et al. Usefulness of a traction method using dental floss and a hemoclip for gastric endoscopic submucosal dissection: a propensity score matching analysis (with videos). Gastrointest Endosc. 2016; 83(2):337–346

[76] Yoshida M, Takizawa K, Ono H, et al. Efficacy of endoscopic submucosal dissection with dental floss clip traction for gastric epithelial neoplasia: a pilot study (with video). Surg Endosc. 2016; 30(7):3100–3106

[77] Gotoda T, Yang HK. The desired balance between treatment and curability in treatment planning for early gastric cancer. Gastrointest Endosc. 2015; 82(2):308–310

[78] Kusano C, Iwasaki M, Kaltenbach T, et al. Should elderly patients undergo additional surgery after non-curative endoscopic resection for early gastric cancer? Long-term comparative outcomes. Am J Gastroenterol. 2011; 106(6):1064–1069

30 Obesity: Endoscopic Approaches

Andrew Storm, Steven Edmundowicz, and Christopher Thompson

30.1 Introduction

Obesity is a lifelong condition that requires long-term multidisciplinary management focusing on lifestyle changes and dietary intervention and may include pharmacologic agents, endoscopic therapies, or surgery to achieve the desired outcome of weight loss and comorbidity reduction. The management of obesity is evolving and will likely be best delivered in multidisciplinary centers with expertise in all aspects of therapy. The endoscopic management of obesity is a relatively new and expanding concept in therapeutic endoscopy. Limited availability of bariatric surgeons, risk aversion for invasive surgical techniques, and rapidly increasing technology around minimally invasive endoscopic techniques are driving the field of "bariatric endoscopy." Endoscopic approaches to weight loss include gastric restriction techniques, space-occupying devices, and metabolic bypass (barrier or aspiration) devices. While long-term data for these techniques are still being pursued, endoscopists must be aware of these techniques and devices as they are likely to encounter them in clinical practice, and should be prepared to counsel patients who may inquire about them.

30.2 Obesity: Endoscopic Approaches

Just over one-third of the population of the United States is obese, and the prevalence of obesity is increasing in many countries. In the United States the cost of managing obesity and its direct complications are estimated to total US$147 billion to 210 billion, or 21% of all U.S. health expenditure, emphasizing the health and economic impact of this highly prevalent disease state.[1] While surgical approaches to morbid obesity have historically been the mainstay of procedure-induced weight loss in this population, it has become apparent that the number of patients who qualify for bariatric surgery vastly overwhelms the availability of surgeons capable of performing these procedures.[2,3] Furthermore, the morbidity of surgery may be considered unacceptably high in some obese patients, leaving something to be desired.

Over the past two decades, endoscopic weight loss techniques have been developed and are gaining popularity. Generally speaking, endoscopic procedures for bariatric patients have aimed to affect the burden of both sheer excess body weight as well as comorbid medical conditions. Population studies are clear that many medical conditions caused by or related to obesity and the metabolic syndrome are improved with modest weight loss including, but not limited to, hypertension, hyperlipidemia, obesity hypoventilation, obstructive sleep apnea, insulin resistance, hyperglycemia, and arthritis. Techniques for both endoscopic revision of previous bariatric surgery and primary antiobesity devices, platforms, and procedures are available. While the field of bariatric endoscopy is still in development, it benefits any endoscopist to understand and appreciate these technologies, as he or she will be increasingly encountered in the clinical arena. Within this chapter, we will discuss the primary and revision weight loss procedures being performed endoscopically, but do not address the complications of bariatric surgery, nor their endoscopic management, which may also be of interest to the practicing endoscopist. Finally we will report experimental techniques that are on the horizon.

30.3 Diagnostic Approach and the Multidisciplinary Obesity Center Concept

Given the relatively noninvasive techniques available to the endoscopist, most patients seeking weight loss therapy may be considered for one of several endoscopic weight loss techniques. A patient's body mass index (BMI), comorbid conditions, history of surgery, and personal weight loss goals will determine the specific technique to be used case-by-case. This is best delivered in a multidisciplinary center (either real or virtual) involving experts in obesity assessment, lifestyle management, nutritional management, pharmacologic agents, endoscopic therapies, and surgery. It should also include access to psychological support and cosmetic surgery for complete patient management. Patients must understand that obesity management is a lifelong process that requires active intervention on their part and the use of specific medications, devices, or techniques to maintain their health. Different endoscopic techniques and devices may assist in weight loss and mitigation of obesity-related complications across a wide range of BMI. Comorbid conditions, which may limit surgical techniques, should be considered when choosing candidates for bariatric endoscopic procedures. However, the minimally invasive nature of transoral flexible endoscopic therapy makes it often feasible in even the most medically complex patients.

30.3.1 General Approach, Equipment, and Techniques

Practice Setting: A Bariatric Center

An office specializing in the care of bariatric patients must incorporate larger and sturdier waiting room seating, examination tables, and stretchers, outfitted to safely and comfortably accommodate bariatric patients. A multidisciplinary approach to the bariatric patient utilizing nutritionists, behavior counselors, and multispecialty medical team is necessary to ensure 360-degree management of factors that may contribute to and complicate effective management of the patient's obesity. Having these adjunctive supports in place is critically important to the long-term success of any onetime (or repeated) surgical or endoscopic treatment.

Preprocedural Clinic Evaluation

A standardized preoperative evaluation is considered prior to bariatric surgery, and should be similarly employed prior to endoscopic bariatric procedures. Patients are evaluated for conditions that may preclude, modify, or delay their procedure.

A standard prebariatric procedure evaluation according to guideline recommendations includes the following:
1. Ruling out *Helicobacter pylori* (via endoscopic or noninvasive testing) to avoid future bleeding events, including bleeding ulceration of the excluded stomach will be more difficult to evaluate and treat postoperatively
2. Esophagogastroduodenoscopy (EGD) to evaluate for presence of esophagitis, Barrett's esophagus and varices, hiatal hernia, gastric polyps and ulcers, and tumors

When evaluating the obese patient in clinic prior to any planned surgical or endoscopic bariatric procedure, several important considerations come to the forefront. At a minimum, a onetime clinic visit to evaluate a candidate's medical history, physical examination, and commitment to lifestyle changes should occur. One should take note of comorbid conditions that may make procedural sedation more difficult for the patient. Some endoscopic techniques may be able to be safely performed with only conscious sedation. Patients should be made aware of both medical weight management techniques including pharmacotherapeutics (not discussed in this endoscopy-themed text) and surgical techniques. Dietary and lifestyle modifications are and must remain the cornerstone of obesity management. Alone, intensive lifestyle modifications have been reported to result in up to 5 to 10% total body weight loss at 1 year.[4] Bariatric surgery, including Roux-en-Y gastric bypass (RYGB), gastric banding, and sleeve gastrectomy, is superior to lifestyle interventions with

1-year percent excess weight loss of 62 to 74%, 33 to 34%, and 51 to 70%, respectively[5] (▶Fig. 30.1, ▶Fig. 30.2). While mortality rates associated with bariatric surgery are less than 0.5%, adverse event rates range from 10 to 17% and reoperation rates range from 6 to 7%. This information may help the patients in making an informed decision regarding their preferred avenue of treatment.

It is an accepted practice, if not recently completed, to check a complete blood count (CBC) and thyroid-stimulating hormone (TSH) in most patients, especially if symptoms of anemia or hypothyroidism are present. The CBC is used to screen for evidence of iron deficiency anemia, and TSH to screen for hypothyroidism, either of which may result in excess weight gain that may respond to medical supplementation.

A thorough review of the patient's diet and exercise regimen is undertaken, and the patient is counseled on appropriate dietary and exercise changes prior to any procedural intervention. We advise a strict 1,200-calorie diet (▶Table 30.1) and the United States' Centers for Disease Control and Prevention (CDC) weekly minimum exercise regimen of 2.5 hours moderate-intensity aerobic activity in addition to muscle-strengthening resistance training twice weekly. Guidelines from the American Society for Metabolic and Bariatric Surgery (ASMBS) for a patient's perioperative nutritional and medical support and evaluation exist, though these may not apply to a patient undergoing a lower-risk minimally invasive endoscopic procedure.[6]

Endoscopic Evaluation

Once a patient has been medically evaluated and has decided to pursue an endoscopic bariatric procedure, it is an accepted practice to have the patient undergo screening EGD to assess his or her anatomy and determine the procedure approach that would most benefit the patient's specific case. This screening EGD is also important if the patient previously underwent a bariatric surgical procedure in order to evaluate

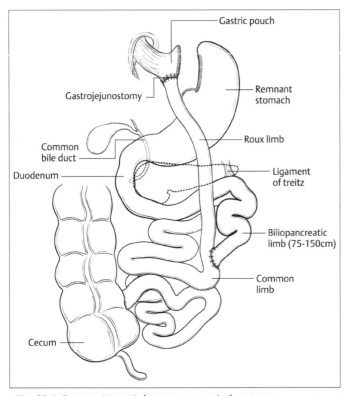

Fig. 30.1 Roux-en-Y gastric bypass postsurgical anatomy.

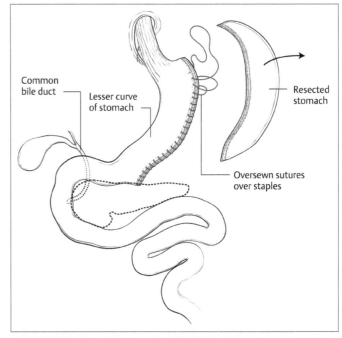

Fig. 30.2 Sleeve gastrectomy postsurgical anatomy.

Table 30.1 1,200 solid calorie diet

Diet Instructions:
- 900–1200 calories a day.
- Avoid all high-calorie and soft, mushy foods that can easily pass through a dilated gastric pouch or dilated gastrojejunal (GJ) outlet (stoma).
- Avoid any foods that dissolve in your mouth or do not require chewing (crackers or pretzels; yogurt or ice cream or soup).
- Avoid all highly refined or processed foods (protein bars, fast food, frozen meals)
- Avoid condiments (butter, gravy, cream cheese, peanut butter, oil).
- Avoid liquid calories, all beverage should have zero calories (Crystal Light, Diet Snapple, Fruit2O water are okay to drink).

Important Information:
- We encourage you to eat solid, bulky, high-fiber, low-fat foods.
- Examples of foods to avoid:
  - Beverages high in calories (fruit juice, fruit smoothie or frappes power drinks, soda, coffee with added cream or sugar)
  - Foods that do not require chewing (soups, cottage cheese, yogurt, peanut butter, mashed potato, apple sauce, pudding, ice cream)
  - Foods that dissolve in your mouth (white rice, white bread, crackers, chips, pretzel, cereal)
  - Foods that are processed (cookies, protein bar, prepackaged foods, frozen meals
  - Fast food, 100 calorie packs of any kind
  - Do not consume protein shakes unless directed to do so by your physician

for postoperative complications including gastrogastric fistula, foreign body (like suture and staples), or dilated pouch or stoma, and also serves to exclude any disorder which may limit, preclude, or delay an endoscopic bariatric procedure, for example a cancer or ulcer. Once this clinical evaluation and

EGD are completed, therapeutic planning of the endoscopic approach may ensue (▶ Fig. 30.3).

Routine Follow-Up

Given that obesity is a chronic disease, and management of obesity requires a lifelong commitment, we do also require that our patients follow up in clinic after their procedure to evaluate for any complications of therapy including malnutrition and to encourage ongoing weight loss strategies and appropriate referral to subspecialty assistance as needed (i.e., endocrinology, nutritionist, physiotherapist).

30.3.2 Therapeutic Approaches: Currently Available Techniques

Patients with Native (Nonsurgical) Anatomy

The endoscopic approach to weight loss in the obese patient depends first on their surgical history. In the patient with native gastric anatomy, several devices and primary bariatric endoscopic techniques have been developed and studied with varying rates of success. Endoscopic techniques include space-occupying devices such as an intragastric balloon, gastric aspiration devices, barrier devices including the duodenal sleeve, and gastric partitioning procedures whereby restriction of the gastric lumen is created through endoscopic suturing or tissue plication. These devices and techniques are described below.

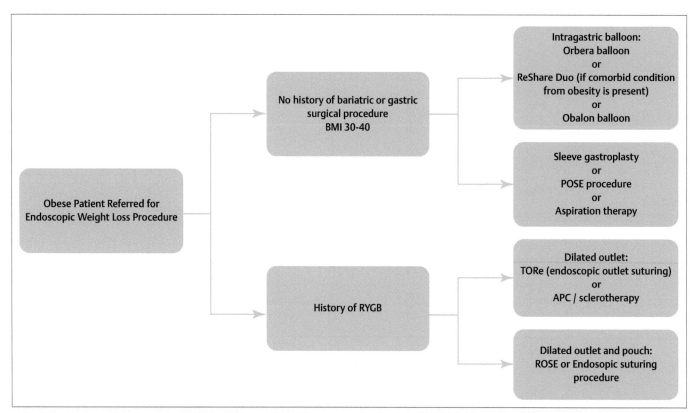

Fig. 30.3 Algorithmic approach for endoscopic bariatric therapies. APC, argon plasma coagulation; BMI, body mass index (kg/m²); POSE, Primary Obesity Surgery Endolumenal; ROSE, Revision Obesity Surgery Endolumenal; RYGB, Roux-en-Y gastric bypass; TORe, transoral outlet reduction.

30.3.3 Gastric Techniques

Intragastric Balloon

The concept of an intragastric balloon for restriction and satiety is not a new concept, and in fact one was available on the U.S. market for a short time in the 1980s, only to be withdrawn due to relatively common occurrence of serious adverse events. In the interim, device improvements aimed at reducing complications have led to two intragastric balloon devices that have been Food and Drug administration (FDA)-approved as of 2015 and are available on the market (Orbera; Apollo Endosurgery, Austin, Texas and ReShape Duo; Reshape Medical, San Clemente, California). These devices are approved for use in patients with BMI range of 30 to 40 kg/m², though the ReShape device carries the additional requirement of one or more obesity-related comorbid condition(s). These are contraindicated in patients with prior gastric surgery, bariatric surgery, inflammatory condition, mass or bleeding condition, to name a few. The intragastric balloon concept consists of a saline-filled silicone implant that is placed under endoscopic guidance into the stomach and left in place for up to 6 months, at which time the device must be removed, though it may be immediately replaced with a new balloon. Removal is accomplished with specialized retrieval tools. Intragastric balloons are considered a cosmetic implant in the United States at the time of this publication and thus require a relatively large out-of-pocket expense. This inconvenience is anticipated to change in the future, as other bariatric devices including the laparoscopic gastric band also required out-of-pocket payment at one time before gaining coverage by most insurance carriers.

The Orbera device (also known as the Bactiguard Infection Protection [BIP] balloon) is well studied and has been placed in more than 220,000 patients internationally as of 2014 (▶Fig. 30.4). A meta-analysis of 3,698 patients revealed average weight loss at 6 months of 14.7 kg or 32.1% excess weight loss and BMI reduction of 5.7 kg/m².[7] In studies to date, at least 50% of this weight loss is maintained at 12 months, but longer-term efficacy data are lacking. Orbera has also been studied as a bridge to bariatric

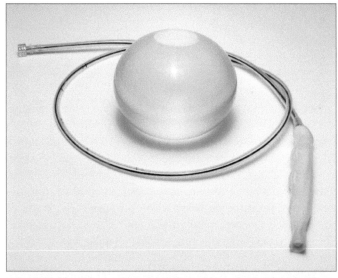

Fig. 30.4 The Orbera intragastric balloon (shown both inflated and deflated).

surgery in superobese patients (average BMI 66.5 kg/m²) resulting in average BMI loss of 5.5 kg/m², significant decrease in systolic blood pressure, decreased surgical complications, and shorter surgical procedure times.[8] Weight loss at 1 year after bariatric surgery was similar between the patients who received Orbera prior to the procedure versus those who did not. Studies have also revealed significant improvements or resolution of both diabetes and depression in patients who underwent Orbera therapy.[9,10] The ReShape balloon includes two saline-filled silicone spheres (▶Fig. 30.5a). It was FDA approved based on data from the REDUCE Pivotal trial, a prospective, sham-controlled, double-blinded randomized multicenter study in 330 obese patients. Mean BMI was 35.4, and patients who received the device experienced on average 25.1% excess weight loss at 24 weeks. Adverse events include nausea and cramping in most patients, with more serious complications including device deflation reported in 6% and gastric ulcers in 10% of patients.[11] The newest FDA-approved addition to the IGB market is the Obalon balloon system. (▶Fig. 30.5b). This device involves the sequential placement of up to 3 swallowed, gas-filled intragastric balloons, which are also approved for 6 months of therapy. Endoscopy is not required for placement of the device(s). A multicenter randomized sham controlled study of 387 patients demonstrated 24.9% total weight loss at 6 months and 24.8 percent excess weight loss at 9 months. Other competing intragastric balloon devices are likely to join the market in coming years, including models that may be swallowed like a pill and then filled with a small catheter negating the need for endoscopy or sedation.

Aspiration Therapy

The AspireAssist (Aspire Bariatrics, King of Prussia, Pennsylvania) is placed similarly to a percutaneous endoscopic gastrostomy (PEG) tube through the anterior abdominal wall leaving a low-profile port with access to the stomach. An attachable siphon-suction device is used to flush and aspirate a portion of a patient's gastric contents after a meal into the toilet. A pilot study of 18 patients with mean BMI of 43.4 were randomized to aspiration therapy (n = 11) with lifestyle therapy versus lifestyle therapy alone (n = 7). In patients who continued their assigned therapy for 1 year, aspiration patients lost 18.6 ± 2.3% body weight (49.0 ± 7.7% excess weight loss) and those receiving only lifestyle therapy lost 5.9 ± 5.0% (14.9 ± 12.2% excess weight loss).[12] This was followed with a U.S. pivotal trial that was completed and presented in 2016, with FDA approval attained in June of 2016.[13] Results in the superobese population have also been reported and are favorable.[14]

Endoscopic Sleeve Gastroplasty (Apollo OverStitch or USGI POSE)

Devices permitting transoral flexible endoscopic tissue plication and suturing have revolutionized the field of bariatric endoscopy. The endoscopic sleeve gastroplasty is a primary bariatric procedure aimed at gastric volume restriction utilizing the only widely commercially available and FDA-approved endoscopic suturing platform to date, the Apollo OverStitch (Apollo Endosurgery) (▶Fig. 30.6). A double-channel therapeutic gastroscope is fitted with the device, which is then used for deep-tissue suture placement, which may be

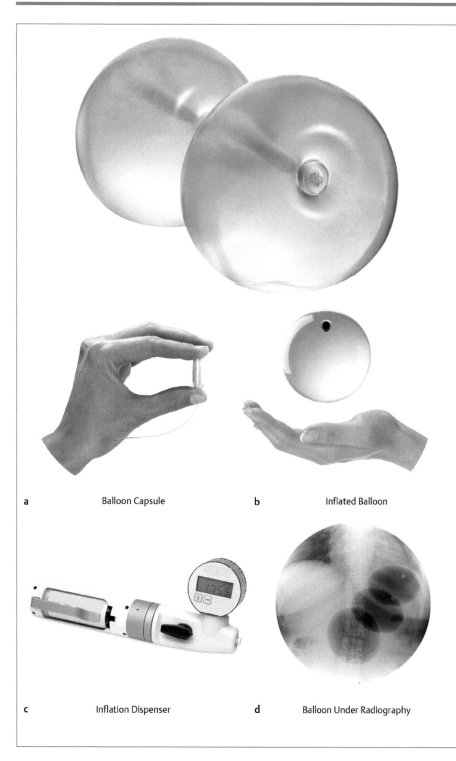

Fig. 30.5 The ReShape intragastric dual balloon system. **(a)** Obalon capsule with tether that is swallowed by patient. **(b)** Gas filled Obalon balloon. **(c)** Inflation system uses proprietary gas cartridge. **(d)** Radiograph demonstrating 3 balloons placed into the stomach

a   Balloon Capsule   b   Inflated Balloon

c   Inflation Dispenser   d   Balloon Under Radiography

assisted with the use of a supplemental tissue grasping helix device. Stitches may be placed in interrupted or running fashion and suture may be reloaded without scope or device removal. Through sequential suture placement, a fully transoral endoscopic sleeve gastroplasty may be accomplished (▶Fig. 30.7). An initial efficacy study in 23 patients reported BMI reduction from average 34.2 to 29.4 kg/m². Another single-center study of four patients with average BMI of 35.9 kg/m² established technical feasibility.[15] The Primary Obesity Multicenter Incisionless Suturing Evaluation, or "PROMISE" study of 10 patients with average BMI of 45.2 kg/m²demonstrated weight loss of 33 kg on average, with significant improvement in diabetes at 6 months.[16] Adverse events include perigastric serous fluid collection, pulmonary embolism, and pneumoperitoneum with pneumothorax.

Another pre-FDA approval device in clinical study is the Incisionless Operating Platform (IOP) (USGI Medical, San Clemente, California) (▶Fig. 30.8) that is used to accomplish Primary Obesity Surgery Endolumenal, also known as POSE (▶Fig. 30.9). The IOP platform consists of a large, green, onetime-use four-channel overtube system through which a 4.9-mm endoscope is inserted for visualization. The g-Prox tissue plication device (USGI Medical) is introduced through a separate port to place transmural tissue anchor plications. The g-Lix tissue grasping helix is used to pull tissue into the jaws of the g-Prox. Plications are placed both in the fundus (in device retroflexion) to restrict gastric accommodation, and in the distal gastric body across from the incisura to limit and slow gastric emptying, with care to avoid puncture of adjacent viscera with the g-Lix device. A study of 45 patients with average BMI of 36.7 experienced

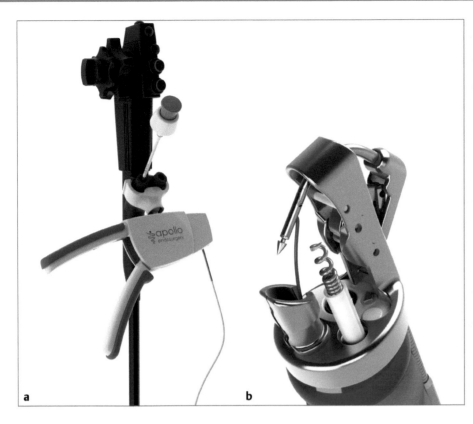

Fig. 30.6 The Apollo OverStitch device. **(a)** Handle attached to scope. **(b)** Suture driver configuration at tip of the scope.

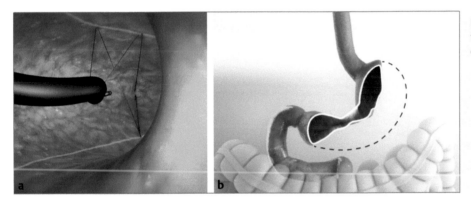

Fig. 30.7 Sleeve gastroplasty. **(a)** Intragastric full-thickness suture placement. **(b)** End result of the sleeve gastroplasty procedure.

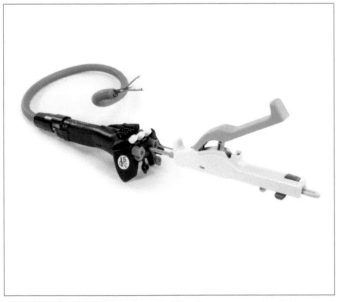

Fig. 30.8 The Incisionless Operating Platform.

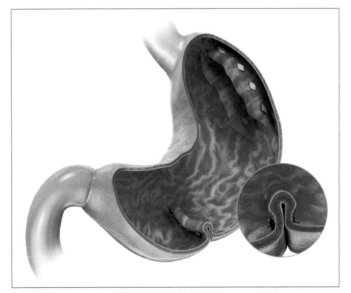

Fig. 30.9 The Primary Obesity Surgery Endolumenal (POSE) procedure intragastric view of full-thickness plication placement.

average 6-month weight loss of 16.3 kg and BMI reduction of 5.8 kg/m[2].[17] The ESSENTIAL trial, expected to lead to FDA approval of the platform, is underway at the time of this publication.

30.3.4 Small Bowel Techniques

Intraluminal Sleeve

Several iterations of small intestinal barrier devices have been studied to date. The goal of a barrier device or "sleeve" is to prevent the proximal small intestine from being exposed to caloric intake from the stomach. The best-studied device named Endo-Barrier (GI Dynamics, Lexington, Massachusetts) consists of a 60-cm polymer sleeve, anchored in the duodenal bulb and extending distally into the jejunum. The sleeve prevents absorption of caloric intake along its length, but allows pancreaticobiliary secretions to pass alongside and into the distal small bowel. Results for weight loss and comorbid conditions, especially including diabetes, were positive, however, issues with presumed anchor-associated liver abscess in the pivotal U.S. trial have delayed FDA device approval, and bleeding and sleeve migration were also reported.[18]

To our knowledge, several companies are investigating new iterations of sleeve/barrier devices that may carry a safer risk profile and could be considered for future study and clinical use, though none are available on the market as of this publication.[19] Other emerging but less studied small bowel endoscopic bariatric devices and techniques including duodenal mucosal resurfacing and magnetic anastomosis creation are discussed under "Experimental techniques."

30.3.5 Endoscopic Revision of Prior Gastric Bypass

After bariatric surgery, patients are at high risk of weight regain and other complications that may benefit from endoscopic therapy. Up to 20% of patients with RYGB fail to achieve therapeutic success (50% excess weight loss at 1 year), and another 30% will experience weight regain, defined as 15% increase from nadir.[20,21,22] Surgical revision is effective and used in up to 13% of patients but associated with complication rates of up to 50% and mortality rates more than double that of the original surgery, likely owing to the complexity of the nonnative abdominal landscape including scar, adhesions, and altered anatomy.[23,24,25,26] Endoscopic methods of revision for weight regain after surgical bypass are currently aimed at reducing dilated gastric pouch and gastrojejunal anastomosis, by means of sclerotherapy (through injection or electrocautery means) or by endoscopic suturing or plication techniques.

As a dilated (enlarged diameter) gastrojejunal anastomosis has been shown to correlate with weight regain after a bypass surgery, endoscopic revision of the anastomosis may be considered. The size of the anastomosis may be estimated using a gastroscope, and an anastomosis over 15 mm has proven to be a contributing factor to weight regain, thus indicating a role for revision of the anastomosis.[27] In the case of a dilated gastrojejunal anastomosis, endoscopic sutures may be used to reduce the aperture with the desired effect being ongoing weight loss. In the patient with a prior RYGB and a large pouch, tissue plication or endoscopic suturing to reduce the pouch diameter may be performed for further restriction in addition to revision of the dilated anastomosis. Patients with a prior sleeve gastrectomy may regain weight if the sleeve is dilated. This too may be managed with endoscopic suturing or tissue plication to reduce the sleeve diameter. Various methods of postbariatric surgery endoscopic revision are discussed in this section.

Gastrojejunal Sclerotherapy and Argon Plasma Laser Resurfacing

Given the association between dilated gastrojejunal anastomosis and weight regain after RYGB, techniques to reduce the outlet diameter through formation of scar tissue using sclerotherapy or more recently through use of argon plasma coagulation (APC) have been reported. Endoscopic sclerotherapy, similar to sclerotherapy of esophageal varices, was accomplished using submucosal needle injection of sodium morrhuate around the gastrojejunal anastomosis to create edema, scarring, and ideally reduction in aperture of the anastomosis. Because of safety concerns and decreasing availability of sodium morrhuate, as well as the availability of a new technique (APC), sclerotherapy is no longer considered advisable. A study of 28 patients demonstrated that the majority (64%) of patients lost more than 75% of their regained weight after an average 2.3 procedures spaced 3 to 6 months apart. Anastomotic diameters greater than 15 mm are less likely to benefit from this technique and may benefit more from an endoscopic suturing revision procedure. A newer technique utilizing APC has more recently gained popularity over sclerotherapy.[28] In this technique, APC resurfacing of the gastrojejunal anastomosis is accomplished through touching the tip of a straight-fire APC catheter to the gastric mucosa at the anastomosis, creating a point-coagulation injury to the mucosa and deeper submucosal layers. We use pulsed APC with settings of flow 0.8 L/s and 55 W. Circumferential resurfacing therapy is applied around the anastomosis in two to three rings (▶ Fig. 30.10).

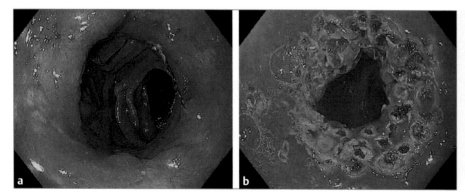

Fig. 30.10 Argon plasma coagulation (APC) resurfacing of a dilated gastrojejunal anastomosis. **(a)** Dilated gastrojejunal anastomosis. **(b)** APC is applied in concentric rings around the stoma resulting in edema, tissue contraction, and scar tissue formation ultimately resulting in reduction of the gastrojejunal aperture.

Edema, ulceration, and scar tissue formation result in aperture reduction. One international prospective nonrandomized study of 30 patients using APC at 90 W revealed that after three treatment sessions every 8 weeks, an average 15.5 kg of the 19 kg regained weight was lost.[29]

Transoral Outlet Reduction

Using the Apollo OverStitch platform, the transoral outlet reduction, or TORe procedure, is under study to reduce the aperture of the gastrojejunal anastomosis to a goal of 8-mm diameter. An overtube is placed, the gastric side of the anastomosis is treated with APC (forced coagulation, 0.8 L/min, 30 W), and then interrupted or purse string suture pattern is used to reduce the outlet diameter. With the purse string technique, the suture is tightened over an 8-mm esophageal dilation balloon to size the final outlet diameter. Studies of TORe include one with 25 patients where the gastrojejunal anastomosis, on average, was reduced from 26.4 to 6 mm with weight loss of 11.7 kg (69.5% regained weight loss) at 6 months and no adverse events.[30] Another study comparing the use of OverStitch to another endoscopic suturing device in 118 patients revealed superior weight loss in the OverStitch patients at both 6 and 12 months.[31]

Revision Obesity Surgery Endolumenal

As described earlier for the POSE procedure, the IOP platform (USGI) has been used in studies for endoscopic revision and management of weight regain after RYGB. Specifically, this procedure is considered for patients with weight regain in the setting of an enlarged pouch and dilated gastrojejunal anastomosis. Full-thickness plications are placed with the goal of reducing both pouch size and anastomosis aperture. A study of 20 patients undergoing Revision Obesity Surgery Endolumenal (ROSE) demonstrated technical success in 85%, with weight loss of 8.8 kg at 3 months.[32] A larger prospective multicenter study of 116 patients achieved technical success in 97%, with 32% of post-RYGB weight regain lost at 6 months and no significant adverse events.[33]

Sleeve Revision

In patients with weight gain after a prior sleeve gastrectomy, endoscopic repair using either a tissue plication device or endoscopic suturing device may be considered. Several small reports exist detailing the feasibility and safety of this revisional procedure, however, more data are needed before it is considered for mainstream use.[34]

30.3.6 Other Postoperative Issues That Lead to Weight Gain and May Require Endoscopic Intervention

Other complications or pathology may occur after surgical gastric bypass leading to weight regain after a bypass. These include the following:

1. Marginal ulceration

   Marginal ulcerations may occur in up to 16% of patients after gastric bypass as a result of unraveled suture material, long gastric pouch, diabetes, use of tobacco cigarettes or *H. pylori* infection.[35] Ulcerations may result in occult blood loss and iron deficiency anemia, which can cause weight regain through appetite stimulation. Healing of the ulcer(s) is of paramount importance. If the patient smokes tobacco, cessation counseling and pharmacotherapy aimed at cessation should be offered. Nonsteroidal anti-inflammatory drug (NSAID) medications should also be discontinued if possible. Additionally, we recommend using a high-dose proton pump inhibitor twice daily before meals and in addition sucralfate 1 g four times daily an hour after meals to promote healing of the ulcer. These medications should be opened or crushed, respectively, or supplied in liquid form to ensure absorption and efficacy of the medications. If foreign material (unraveled suture or staples) from the prior surgery is present at the site of ulceration, we routinely remove this endoscopically to promote healing.[36] In rare cases, nonhealing ulcers have been reported to respond to endoscopic suture overstitching.[37] Reoperation and surgical revision is reserved for the most severe and recalcitrant cases.[38]

2. Gastrogastric fistula

   Gastrogastric fistula formation was a common complication of undivided RYGB surgery, reported in up to nearly 50% of cases.[39] Over the past decade or two, routine complete transection of the stomach and gastric pouch has significantly reduced this risk to a reported incidence of 0 to 6%.[40] Gastrogastric fistulae most commonly result in weight regain due to essentially reversal of the bypass anatomy, epigastric pain, and ulceration. Endoscopic therapies for gastrogastric fistulae, including clips, glue, and endoscopic suturing are increasingly considered as the first-line approach given the increased morbidity and mortality associated with redo and revision surgery. If a fistula is discovered in the evaluation of weight regain after RYGB, correction of the fistula by endoscopic or surgical approach should be the first priority in assisting the patient with weight loss and the approach will depend on a center's expertise with these various technologies.

30.3.7 Guidelines and Systematic Reviews

The American Society for Gastrointestinal Endoscopy (ASGE) has position statements regarding bariatric endoscopy techniques and devices including the following:

- ASGE position statement: endoscopic bariatric therapies in clinical practice
- The role of endoscopy in the bariatric surgery patient

These, and other ASGE practice guidelines are available on the web at www.asge.org/publications/

The ASGE, along with the American Society for Metabolic and Bariatric Surgery (ASMBS) have also published a joint consensus statement in 2011 entitled "A Pathway to Endoscopic Bariatric Therapies." This document is also available online at https://asmbs.org/wp/uploads/2011/11/PathwayToEndoscopicBarTherapies-Nov2011.pdf

30.3.8 Experimental Techniques

With the exception of intragastric balloons, and the endoscopic plication and suturing devices described in this chapter, many of the procedures and other devices remain under investigation and their role in the management of obesity remains to be determined. As the number of patients undergoing endoscopic bariatric procedures increases, database analyses of cost benefit and efficacy will need to be undertaken to determine whether minimally invasive endoscopic techniques are overall beneficial from a systems-level standpoint.

Several additional bariatric endoscopy devices are in experimental and early FDA approval phases as of 2016 and have received attention at the international level. One of the newest and more promising technologies includes a self-assembling magnetic anastomosis system, or SAMS (GI Windows, Massachusetts, United States), which aims to allow for minimally invasive gastrojejunal anastomosis created by deploying two magnets that meet across opposing lumens to create an iatrogenic fistula. Animal and cadaveric human studies have been positive.[41,42] A human-subject pilot study is underway outside of the United States.

Another device, a percutaneous intragastric trocar (EndoTAGSS, Kansas, United States) is in animal studies and may allow for endoscopically governed bariatric procedures within the stomach.[43,44] The intragastric trocar is placed similarly to a pull-PEG tube and allows for intragastric use of laparoscopic 6- and 12-mm tools including staplers and suture drivers. The trocar is removed with external traction as with a PEG tube at the end of the procedure, and full-thickness sutures close the gastric and abdominal tract. This device is in animal studies for bariatric and other applications.

Other devices which have had varied success but have not reached the mainstream clinical arena include several stapler devices for gastric restriction (ACE stapler, Boston Scientific, Natick, Massachusetts; StomaphyX, EndoGastric Solutions, Redmond, Washington; and TransOral Gastroplasty Device, Satiety Inc, Palo Alto, California).[45,46,47] An intragastric diaphragm for restriction called TERIS (Endosense, Menlo Park, California) is not yet on the market.[48] A transpyloric shuttle (BAROnova, Goleta, California) aims to intermittently delay gastric emptying, but was complicated by gastric ulcers and is not available commercially.[49] A string of mesh spheres, anchored in the stomach but extending into the duodenum (SatiSphere; Endosphere, Columbus, Ohio) delays duodenal transit of food possibly affecting hormonally mediated satiety and glucose metabolism but is also not commercially available.[50] Another small bowel technique, known as duodenal mucosal resurfacing (Fractyl Laboratories, Cambridge, Massachusetts) uses radiofrequency ablation of the superficial small bowel mucosa with the goal of improving enteroendocrine signaling for management of diabetes.[51]

30.4 Summary

The prevalence and cost of obesity and its complications have made it a primary public health concern. Both patients and modern health care economics demand effective, accessible, less costly, and less morbid techniques and approaches for weight loss.

In the management of morbidly obese patients, endoscopic therapy is rapidly gaining traction. While we await long-term outcome studies with many of the devices mentioned above, the move to endoscopically based therapies is continuing and clear. Endoscopic approaches to weight loss and the comorbid medical conditions associated with obesity and the metabolic syndrome are now accepted and will become the preferred management option for many patients. When combined with long-term lifestyle and nutritional therapy, the safety and repeatability of endoscopic procedures make them likely candidates for long-term treatment for patients with obesity. Primary endoscopic procedures for obesity include gastroplasty with endoscopic suturing and plication devices offer intermediate-term management options that can be repeated for long-term therapy. Intragastric balloons are in use worldwide. An aspiration weight loss device and barrier devices are expected to join the market. In patients who have regained weight after surgical bypass, the associated cost and morbidity of a surgical revision procedure is high, making less-invasive endoscopic approaches more attractive. Given these exciting advances, along with high demand for weight loss treatments, the practicing endoscopist must be aware of these technologies and consider formal training to allow for implementing them in clinical practice.

References

[1] Ogden CL, Carroll MD, Kit BK, Flegal KM. Prevalence of childhood and adult obesity in the United States, 2011–2012. JAMA. 2014; 311(8):806–814

[2] Leroux EJ, Morton JM, Rivas H. Increasing access to specialty surgical care: application of a new resource allocation model to bariatric surgery. Ann Surg. 2014; 260(2):274–278

[3] Buchwald H; Consensus Conference Panel. Consensus conference statement bariatric surgery for morbid obesity: health implications for patients, health professionals, and third-party payers. Surg Obes Relat Dis. 2005; 1(3):371–381

[4] Knowler WC, Barrett-Connor E, Fowler SE, et al; Diabetes Prevention Program Research Group. Reduction in the incidence of type 2 diabetes with lifestyle intervention or metformin. N Engl J Med. 2002; 346(6):393–403

[5] Chang SH, Stoll CR, Song J, et al. The effectiveness and risks of bariatric surgery: an updated systematic review and meta-analysis, 2003–2012. JAMA Surg. 2014; 149(3):275–287

[6] Mechanick JI, Youdim A, Jones DB, et al; American Association of Clinical Endocrinologists. Obesity Society. American Society for Metabolic & Bariatric Surgery. Clinical practice guidelines for the perioperative nutritional, metabolic, and nonsurgical support of the bariatric surgery patient—2013 update: cosponsored by American Association of Clinical Endocrinologists, The Obesity Society, and American Society for Metabolic & Bariatric Surgery. Obesity (Silver Spring). 2013; 21(suppl 1):S1–S27

[7] Imaz I, Martínez-Cervell C, García-Alvarez EE, et al. Safety and effectiveness of the intragastric balloon for obesity. A meta-analysis. Obes Surg. 2008; 18(7):841–846

[8] Zerrweck C, Maunoury V, Caiazzo R, et al. Preoperative weight loss with intragastric balloon decreases the risk of significant adverse outcomes of laparoscopic gastric bypass in super-super obese patients. Obes Surg. 2012; 22(5):777–782

[9] Genco A, Bruni T, Doldi SB, et al. BioEnterics Intragastric Balloon: The Italian Experience with 2,515 Patients. Obes Surg. 2005; 15(8):1161–1164

[10] Deliopoulou K, Konsta A, Penna S, et al. The impact of weight loss on depression status in obese individuals subjected to intragastric balloon treatment. Obes Surg. 2013; 23(5):669–675

[11] Ponce J, Woodman G, Swain J, et al; REDUCE Pivotal Trial Investigators. The REDUCE pivotal trial: a prospective, randomized controlled pivotal trial of a dual intragastric balloon for the treatment of obesity. Surg Obes Relat Dis. 2015; 11(4):874–881

[12] Sullivan S, Stein R, Jonnalagadda S, et al. Aspiration therapy leads to weight loss in obese subjects: a pilot study. Gastroenterology. 2013; 145(6):1245–52.e1, 5

[13] Thompson CC, Abu Dayyeh BK, Kushner R, et al. Percutaneous Gastrostomy Device for the Treatment of Class II and Class III Obesity: Results of a Randomized Controlled Trial. *The American Journal of Gastroenterology.* 2017;112(3):447–457. doi:10.1038/ajg.2016.500.

[14] Machytka E, Buzga M, Kupka T, Bojkova M. Sa1587 aspiration therapy in super obese patients—pilot trial. Gastrointest Endosc. 2014; 79(5):AB264–AB265

[15] Abu Dayyeh BK, Rajan E, Gostout CJ. Endoscopic sleeve gastroplasty: a potential endoscopic alternative to surgical sleeve gastrectomy for treatment of obesity. Gastrointest Endosc. 2013; 78(3):530–535

[16] Abu Dayyeh BK, Acosta A, Camilleri M, et al. Endoscopic sleeve gastroplasty alters gastric physiology and induces loss of body weight in obese individuals. Clin Gastroenterol Hepatol. 2017; 15(1):37–43

[17] Espinós JC, Turró R, Mata A, et al. Early experience with the Incisionless Operating Platform™ (IOP) for the treatment of obesity: the Primary Obesity Surgery Endolumenal (POSE) procedure. Obes Surg. 2013; 23(9):1375–1383

[18] Rohde U, Hedbäck N, Gluud LL, et al. Effect of the EndoBarrier Gastrointestinal Liner on obesity and type 2 diabetes: a systematic review and meta-analysis. Diabetes Obes Metab. 2016; 18(3):300–305

[19] Sandler BJ, Rumbaut R, Swain CP, et al. One-year human experience with a novel endoluminal, endoscopic gastric bypass sleeve for morbid obesity. Surg Endosc. 2015; 29(11):3298–3303

[20] Brolin RE. Bariatric surgery and long-term control of morbid obesity. JAMA. 2002; 288(22):2793–2796

[21] McCormick JT, Papasavas PK, Caushaj PF, Gagné DJ. Laparoscopic revision of failed open bariatric procedures. Surg Endosc. 2003; 17(3):413–415

[22] Powers PS, Rosemurgy A, Boyd F, Perez A. Outcome of gastric restriction procedures: weight, psychiatric diagnoses, and satisfaction. Obes Surg. 1997; 7(6):471–477

[23] Behrns KE, Smith CD, Kelly KA, Sarr MG. Reoperative bariatric surgery. Lessons learned to improve patient selection and results. Ann Surg. 1993; 218(5):646–653

[24] Coakley BA, Deveney CW, Spight DH, et al. Revisional bariatric surgery for failed restrictive procedures. Surg Obes Relat Dis. 2008; 4(5):581–586

[25] Linner JH, Drew RL. Reoperative surgery—indications, efficacy, and long-term follow-up. Am J Clin Nutr. 1992; 55(suppl 2):606–610

[26] Buchwald H, Estok R, Fahrbach K, et al. Trends in mortality in bariatric surgery: a systematic review and meta-analysis. Surgery. 2007; 142(4):621–632, discussion 632–635

[27] Abu Dayyeh BK, Lautz DB, Thompson CC. Gastrojejunal stoma diameter predicts weight regain after Roux-en-Y gastric bypass. Clin Gastroenterol Hepatol. 2011; 9(3):228–233

[28] Aly A. Argon plasma coagulation and gastric bypass—a novel solution to stomal dilation. Obes Surg. 2009; 19(6):788–790

[29] Baretta GA, Alhinho HC, Matias JE, et al. Argon plasma coagulation of gastrojejunal anastomosis for weight regain after gastric bypass. Obes Surg. 2015; 25(1):72–79

[30] Jirapinyo P, Slattery J, Ryan MB, et al. Evaluation of an endoscopic suturing device for transoral outlet reduction in patients with weight regain following Roux-en-Y gastric bypass. Endoscopy. 2013; 45(7):532–536

[31] Kumar N, Thompson CC. Comparison of a superficial suturing device with a full-thickness suturing device for transoral outlet reduction (with videos). Gastrointest Endosc. 2014; 79(6):984–989

[32] Mullady DK, Lautz DB, Thompson CC. Treatment of weight regain after gastric bypass surgery when using a new endoscopic platform: initial experience and early outcomes (with video). Gastrointest Endosc. 2009; 70(3):440–444

[33] Horgan S, Jacobsen G, Weiss GD, et al. Incisionless revision of post-Roux-en-Y bypass stomal and pouch dilation: multicenter registry results. Surg Obes Relat Dis. 2010; 6(3):290–295

[34] Sharaiha RZ, Kedia P, Kumta N, et al. Endoscopic sleeve plication for revision of sleeve gastrectomy. Gastrointest Endosc. 2015; 81(4):1004

[35] Azagury DE, Abu Dayyeh BK, Greenwalt IT, Thompson CC. Marginal ulceration after Roux-en-Y gastric bypass surgery: characteristics, risk factors, treatment, and outcomes. Endoscopy. 2011; 43(11):950–954

[36] Lee JK, Van Dam J, Morton JM, et al. Endoscopy is accurate, safe, and effective in the assessment and management of complications following gastric bypass surgery. Am J Gastroenterol. 2009; 104(3):575–582, quiz 583

[37] Jirapinyo P, Watson RR, Thompson CC. Use of a novel endoscopic suturing device to treat recalcitrant marginal ulceration (with video). Gastrointest Endosc. 2012; 76(2):435–439

[38] Fringeli Y, Worreth M, Langer I. Gastrojejunal anastomosis complications and their management after laparoscopic Roux-en-Y gastric bypass. J Obes. 2015; 2015:698425

[39] Capella JF, Capella RF. Gastro-gastric fistulas and marginal ulcers in gastric bypass procedures for weight reduction. Obes Surg. 1999; 9(1):22–27, discussion 28

[40] Carrodeguas L, Szomstein S, Soto F, et al. Management of gastrogastric fistulas after divided Roux-en-Y gastric bypass surgery for morbid obesity: analysis of 1,292 consecutive patients and review of literature. Surg Obes Relat Dis. 2005; 1(5):467–474

[41] Ryou M, Agoston AT, Thompson CC. Endoscopic intestinal bypass creation by using self-assembling magnets in a porcine model. Gastrointest Endosc. 2016; 83(4):821–825

[42] Ryou M, Aihara H, Thompson CC. Minimally invasive entero-enteral dual-path bypass using self-assembling magnets. Surg Endosc. 2016; 30(10):4533–4538

[43] Storm AC, Aihara H, Thompson CC. A simply placed percutaneous intragastric trocar for use of laparoscopic tools in endoscopy. Gastrointest Endosc. 2016; 84(6):1051–1052

[44] Storm AC, Aihara H, Thompson CC. Novel intragastric trocar placed by PEG technique permits endolumenal use of rigid instruments to simplify complex endoscopic procedures. Gastrointest Endosc. 2016; 84(3):518–522

[45] Verlaan T, Paulus GF, Mathus-Vliegen EM, et al. Endoscopic gastric volume reduction with a novel articulating plication device is safe and effective in the treatment of obesity (with video). Gastrointest Endosc. 2015; 81(2):312–320

[46] Goyal V, Holover S, Garber S. Gastric pouch reduction using StomaphyX in post Roux-en-Y gastric bypass patients does not result in sustained weight loss: a retrospective analysis. Surg Endosc. 2013; 27(9):3417–3420

[47] Devière J, Ojeda Valdes G, Cuevas Herrera L, et al. Safety, feasibility and weight loss after transoral gastroplasty: first human multicenter study. Surg Endosc. 2008; 22(3):589–598

[48] de Jong K, Mathus-Vliegen EM, Veldhuyzen EA, et al. Short-term safety and efficacy of the trans-oral endoscopic restrictive implant system for the treatment of obesity. Gastrointest Endosc. 2010; 72(3):497–504

[49] Marinos G, Eliades C, Raman Muthusamy V, Greenway F. Weight loss and improved quality of life with a nonsurgical endoscopic treatment for obesity: clinical results from a 3- and 6-month study. Surg Obes Relat Dis. 2014; 10(5):929–934

[50] Sauer N, Rösch T, Pezold J, et al. A new endoscopically implantable device (SatiSphere) for treatment of obesity—efficacy, safety, and metabolic effects on glucose, insulin, and GLP-1 levels. Obes Surg. 2013; 23(11):1727–1733

[51] Neto MG, Coad JE, Becerra P, et al. 1141 procedure safety from first-in-human study of duodenal mucosal resurfacing as a new endoscopic treatment for type 2 diabetes. Gastroenterology. 2016; 150(4)(s)(uppl 1):S233

31 Small Intestinal Diseases Beyond the Duodenum

Jonathan A. Leighton and Lucinda A. Harris

31.1 Introduction

Endoscopically the small intestine has been a challenging part of the gastrointestinal (GI) tract to investigate. Advances in video capsule endoscopy (VCE) and the development of deep enteroscopy (single-balloon enteroscopy [SBE] and double-balloon enteroscopy [DBE]) have introduced new endoscopic modalities which can be used in the diagnosis and sometimes treatment of these diseases. ▶Table 31.1 presents an overview of categorization of small intestinal diseases used in this chapter.

The primary indications for small bowel endoscopy are evaluation of GI bleeding, identifying small bowel Crohn's disease, diagnosing small bowel tumors, and evaluation of malabsorption syndromes, particularly celiac disease. Somewhat less frequently small bowel endoscopy plays a role in identifying certain infections, congenital lesions, and miscellaneous conditions. This chapter summarizes the important diagnostic and therapeutic features of endoscopy in these areas.

31.2 Suspected Small Bowel Bleeding

Historically, bleeding in the small bowel has been difficult to diagnose and treat because of relative inaccessibility to the deep small bowel. However, with the development of newer modalities such as capsule endoscopy (CE) and deep enteroscopy, the ability to diagnose and treat bleeding lesions throughout the small bowel has improved considerably. In fact, because the ability to examine the small bowel has improved significantly, the term "obscure gastrointestinal bleeding" has evolved and the term now used is "suspected small bowel bleeding."[1] The term "obscure gastrointestinal bleeding" is reserved for truly obscure causes beyond the small bowel, such as vasculitis and hemobilia. It is important to remember that small bowel bleeding can be overt and present with melena or hematochezia or can be occult and present with iron deficiency anemia. Potential etiologies can usually be classified as vascular, inflammatory, or neoplastic (▶Table 31.1). The type of lesion correlates to some extent with age but not gender or ethnicity (▶Table 31.2). Vascular etiologies are the most common, with angioectasia being the primary lesion identified (▶Fig. 31.1). Risk factors include advancing age, aortic stenosis, chronic renal failure, and left ventricular assist devices (LVADs).[1] Inflammatory lesions of the small bowel are most often related to Crohn's disease (CD) but nonsteroidal anti-inflammatory drug (NSAID) ulcers should also be considered. The pathognomonic lesion is the diaphragm-like strictures and these can develop as multiple circumferential membranous structures after years of NSAID use. It is likely that most NSAID-induced injury is subclinical. Symptoms can include iron deficiency anemia, frank bleeding from ulcers, hypoalbuminemia, malabsorption,

Table 31.1 Diseases of the small intestine

Tumors	Congenital
Adenomas/adenocarcinoma Lymphoma Inflammatory polyps Carcinoids Lipomas Kaposi's sarcoma Stromal tumors Metastatic disease	Intestinal pseudo-obstruction Diverticula Duplication cysts Meckel's diverticulum

Malabsorption	Vascular
Celiac disease Amyloid Medication (e.g., olmesartan, valsartan) Collagenous sprue Autoimmune enteropathy Protein-losing enteropathy Scleroderma Eosinophilic gastroenteritis Graft-versus-host disease Radiation enteritis	Angioectasia Venous ectasias Telangiectasias Hemangiomas Arteriovenous malformations Aortoenteric fistula Ischemia Vasculitis

Infection	Inflammatory
Whipple's disease Tropical sprue Tuberculosis Aspergillosis Mucormycosis *Candida* *Mycobacterium-avium intracellulare* Parasites	Crohn's disease

Miscellaneous	
Lymphangiectasia Endometriosis Zollinger–Ellison syndrome Medications (NSAIDs, potassium, 6-mercaptopurine)	

NSAIDs, nonsteroidal anti-inflammatory drugs.

Table 31.2 Etiology of small bowel lesions classified by age

Younger than 40 y	Older than 40 y
Crohn's disease	Angioectasia
Dieulafoy's lesion	Dieulafoy's lesion
Neoplasia	Neoplasia
Meckel's diverticulum	NSAID enteropathy
Polyposis syndromes	

NSAID, nonsteroidal anti-inflammatory drug.
Source: Reproduced with permission from Gerson LB, Fidler JL, Cave DR, Leighton JA. ACG clinical guideline: diagnosis and management of small bowel bleeding. Am J Gastroenterol 2015;110:1265–1287

abdominal pain, and obstruction. Typical NSAID lesions on CE show circumferential symmetric ulcerating rings with usually normal intervening mucosa. They are often difficult to see with cross-sectional imaging

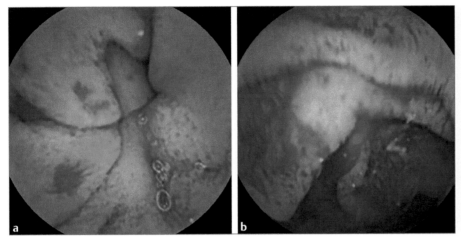

Fig. 31.1 Angioectasia image. **(a)** Small bowel angioectasia. **(b)** Associated active bleeding.

31.2.1 Diagnostic Approaches

In terms of diagnostic approach in patients with suspected small bowel bleeding, it is first important to document objective evidence of GI bleeding whenever possible, especially in those patients presenting with iron deficiency anemia. Hematologic or malabsorptive causes should always be considered in the differential diagnosis before embarking on an extensive evaluation of the small bowel. In addition, upper and lower gastrointestinal etiologies should be sufficiently ruled out, because studies have shown missed lesions in these areas. Previous studies have revealed potential bleeding sources within reach of upper endoscopy or colonoscopy in 21 to 25% of patients undergoing a small bowel evaluation.[2,3] "Second look endoscopy" is recommended whenever there is any doubt, before proceeding with a small bowel evaluation. In the case of repeat upper endoscopy, push enteroscopy should be strongly considered to evaluate the duodenal sweep and proximal jejunum.[4] Once this is completed and no source is identified, it is reasonable to evaluate the small bowel.

The two main endoscopic modalities for evaluating the small bowel include capsule endoscopy and deep enteroscopy. Capsule endoscopy is considered to be the next procedure after second look endoscopy. The diagnostic yield is highest in patients with ongoing overt bleeding as compared to occult bleeding.[5,6,7] Capsule endoscopy is an ideal screening tool prior to deep enteroscopy. Studies have shown that this approach can suggest the initial route for deep enteroscopy and also increase both the diagnostic and therapeutic yield.[8,9,10] The diagnostic yield is improved if performed within 72 hours of presentations and significantly decreases after 2 weeks of the initial bleeding.[11,12,13]

Deep enteroscopy consists of SBE and DBE and spiral enteroscopy. Deep enteroscopy methods appear to be similar in terms of diagnostic yield, safety and learning curve. While there are conflicting reports, it is believed that SBE and DBE are equally effective and performance depends on the local expertise.[14,15] Performance of deep enteroscopy within 72 hours of presentation may improve the diagnostic yield, and should be done in a timely manner.[7,16,17]

A meta-analysis comparing CE to DBE showed that there was no overall difference in diagnostic yield, however, the diagnostic yield of deep enteroscopy significantly increased after a positive capsule study.[18] Deep enteroscopy can be considered initially for those patients who present with active small bowel bleeding. Total deep enteroscopy using both the oral and anal route should be performed if there is a strong suspicion for a lesion despite previously negative studies.

It is important to remember that capsule endoscopy and deep enteroscopy are complimentary in the evaluation of suspected small bowel bleeding. Both have missed lesions found by the alternative technique. In addition, in those patients with negative studies, multidetector computed tomography (CT) scan imaging, that is, CT enterography or CT angiography, may be complimentary as well. While the overall diagnostic yield is less than capsule endoscopy, it can identify bleeding lesions when other tests are negative. Multidetector CT scanning should also be considered in those patients where capsule retention is a concern.[19, 20] An algorithm for suspected small bowel bleeding is shown in ▶ Fig. 31.2. There have been some reports on pharmacologic provocation challenges in refractory cases of small bowel bleeding. One study looking at provocative angiography when conventional angiography was normal showed good results and low complications rates.[21] Various agents have been used including anticoagulants, thrombolytics, hemodilution agents, and vasodilators. Provocative angiography can be considered in refractory cases when all other diagnostic modalities have been unsuccessful. It has also been noted that a negative capsule has a high negative predictive value.

A negative capsule study is associated with significantly lower rebleeding rates compared with those who have a positive CE.[22,23] Therefore, unless there is a high index of suspicion, further small bowel evaluation may be deferred in most patients after a negative CE, unless they present with recurrent bleeding.

31.2.2 Therapeutic Approaches

Although capsule endoscopy has been revolutionary in the evaluation and management of small bowel diseases, it is important to remember that it lacks therapeutic capabilities. The advantage to deep enteroscopy is that it allows for therapeutic intervention in those patients with small bowel bleeding. Deep enteroscopy lends itself in particular to the treatment of vascular lesions that are causing small bowel bleeding. Angioectasias are the most common lesions identified, particularly in the elderly. Rebleeding can occur in approximately one-third of patients, particularly if there are multiple lesions.[24,25]

In those patients where no definitive source for the bleeding or iron deficiency anemia is identified, and conservative observation

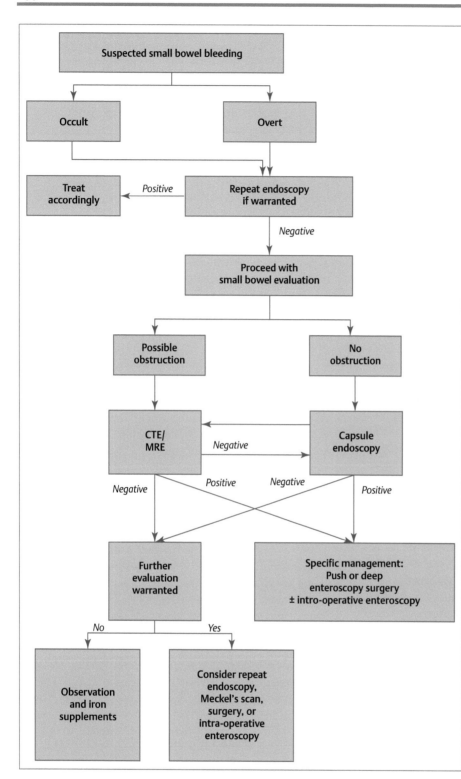

Fig. 31.2 Algorithm for suspected small bowel bleeding.

is warranted, the patient should be managed with oral or intravenous iron with blood transfusions as needed. If bleeding persists, then further diagnostic evaluations should be considered. A small bowel evaluation should be repeated as appropriate. If work-up is again nondiagnostic, and patient is on anticoagulation and/or antiplatelet therapy, then consideration to stopping one or both medications should be discussed with the appropriate physicians. With regard to angioectasias in particular, the recurrent bleeding rate is approximately 33%, but may be as high as 45%.[24,26] Recurrent bleeding from angioectasia correlates with the number of lesions, advanced age, presence of comorbid conditions, and anticoagulant therapy. It is important that if endoscopic therapy

is going to be successful, it is likely to require multiple sessions. In some patients, medical therapy will prove to be the mainstay of therapy.

In terms of medical management of angioectasias, a recent systematic review and meta-analysis again showed that up to 45% of patients may have repeat bleeding despite therapy.[26] Somatostatin analogues, such as octreotide, also showed benefit, while hormonal therapy did not.[26,27] One study suggested that thalidomide also decreases the need for blood transfusions and led to an increase in hemoglobin.[28]

In most cases, surgery is not needed in the management of patients with small bowel bleeding due to the advent of capsule endoscopy and deep enteroscopy. However, in those patients with persistent and severe suspected small bowel bleeding and negative small bowel imaging, surgery combined with intraoperative enteroscopy should be considered.

31.3 Small Bowel Crohn's Disease

Crohn's disease is an inflammatory condition that can affect the entire GI tract. Most commonly, it involves the terminal ileum and colon segmentally, but can involve only the small bowel or only the colon. As with ulcerative colitis, there is no gold standard for diagnosis and a final diagnosis is based on a comprehensive evaluation which includes history, physical examination, laboratory tests, endoscopy, pathology, and radiology. Endoscopy can play a pivotal role in the management of small bowel CD.

Isolated small bowel CD can be even more challenging to diagnose. About one-third of patients may have disease confined to the small bowel.[29] One prospective study suggested that small bowel involvement occurs more frequently than was previously recognized.[30] There are also data to suggest that localization of inflammation changes only minimally over time.[31] We also know that there is a poor correlation between symptom scores and the degree of inflammation in the bowel.[32] Because diagnosis of small bowel CD can be challenging, the average lag time between onset of symptoms and reaching a diagnosis may be as long as 35 months.[33] A comprehensive evaluation of the entire small bowel may be indicated to make a definitive diagnosis, determine disease extent and severity, and/or to evaluate for mucosal healing. The differential diagnosis of inflammation involving the small bowel can be found in ▶ Table 31.3.

31.3.1 Diagnosis

In the majority of patients with small bowel CD, the disease is localized to the terminal ileum or duodenum, and thus can be diagnosed with ileocolonoscopy and/or upper endoscopy. In the case of duodenal CD, upper endoscopy and/or push enteroscopy can be used to obtain biopsies and assess for mucosal healing. Colonoscopy with ileoscopy can assess the terminal ileum and perform similar functions. Such a traditional endoscopic evaluation allows for direct mucosal examination and biopsy and can provide valuable information on extent and severity. It can also help differentiate CD from ulcerative colitis in the appropriate setting.[34] However, it is important to realize that for isolated small bowel CD or in those with sparing of the terminal ileum, the diagnosis may be more elusive.

Table 31.3 Differential diagnosis of inflammation in the small bowel

Differential diagnosis	
Crohn's disease	Autoimmune enteropathy
NSAID enteropathy	Immune deficiency related
Celiac disease	Lymphoma/neoplasia
Radiation enteritis	Cryptogenic multifocal ulcerous stenosing enteritis
Eosinophilic enteritis	Meckel's diverticulum
Infection	
Ischemia	

The indications for a more in-depth evaluation of the small bowel in suspected CD would include the clinical or biological suspicion in the absence of lesions at ileocolonoscopy. This is particularly true in patients with negative endoscopic studies, but the presence of "alarm symptoms" such as anemia, weight loss, abdominal pain, diarrhea, and/or extraintestinal manifestations. There is evidence to suggest that a subgroup of patients will have endoscopic skipping of the terminal ileum.[35] In these situations, one must consider complimentary small bowel imaging tests such as capsule endoscopy, deep enteroscopy, and cross-sectional imaging with computed tomography enterography (CTE) or magnetic resonance enterography (MRE). The ideal test to image the small bowel in suspected CD is not known. Studies have suggested a reasonable sensitivity and specificity for CE in the evaluation of patients with suspected CD. There is evidence that CE may be more sensitive in detecting inflammatory lesions in the proximal small bowel compared with CTE or MRE.[36,37] An example of a patient with positive findings on capsule endoscopy but negative MRE and ileoscopy is shown in ▶ Fig. 31.3. In addition, the negative predictive value of CE for CD is quite high. However, the specificity of CTE for CD compared to CE appears to be better.[38] A suggested algorithm for the evaluation of a patient with suspected CD is shown in ▶ Fig. 31.4. Finally, CE and deep enteroscopy may play a role in established CD, especially in determining the extent and severity of disease, as well as providing information on mucosal healing.[39] In particular, lesions identified on capsule endoscopy can be further evaluated and biopsied if necessary. Several studies have demonstrated a significant role for deep enteroscopy in suspected CD.[40,41,42] These studies suggest that deep enteroscopy can play a role in diagnosis and management and may be complementary to capsule endoscopy and radiology. However, a complete examination may be hampered by previous surgery and active inflammation, as well as an increased risk of perforation.

In planning whether to use CE, one must consider the risk of capsule retention. Those patients with suspected small bowel bleeding or suspected CD have a low risk of retention under 2%. However, those patients with known CD have a risk of retention ranging from 5 to 13%. Risk factors for retention includes not only CD, but also use of NSAID and a history of abdominal radiation. Therefore, patients with abdominal pain, distension, suspected obstruction, or known CD should undergo cross-sectional imaging and/or a patency capsule examination of the small bowel prior to swallowing the actual capsule. If the evaluation suggests a significant risk of retention, then capsule endoscopy should not be performed.

31.3.2 Therapeutics

Up to 30% of patients with CD are prone to developing strictures in the GI tract which can lead to obstruction and abscess formation. While surgery is often indicated, endoscopy can play a role in dilating symptomatic strictures. Proximal duodenal strictures can be dilated with push enteroscopy. For CD involving the jejunum or proximal ileum, deep enteroscopy can be used for dilation of Crohn's related strictures with very good therapeutic success.[43,44] An ideal stricture for endoscopic balloon dilation is one that is 4 cm or less in length and is not complex or angulated. A recent study showed that deep enteroscopy is preferred to MRE

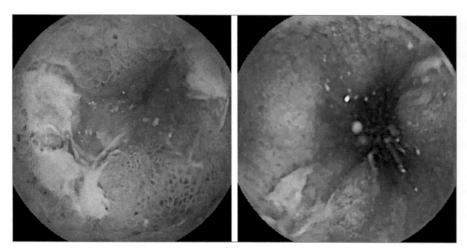

Fig. 31.3 Crohn's disease with negative magnetic resonance enterography (MRE) and ileocolonoscopy.

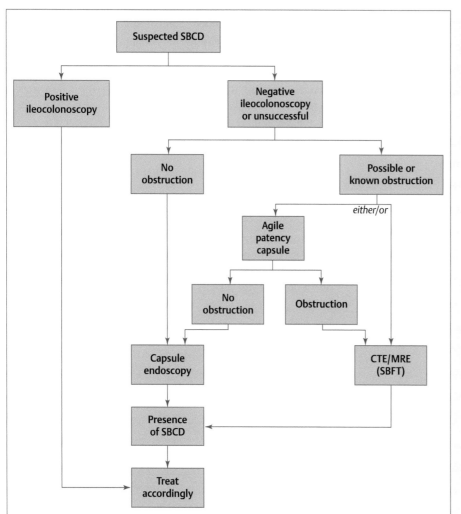

Fig. 31.4 Algorithm for the approach to suspected small bowel Crohn's disease. CTE, computed tomography enterography; MRE, magnetic resonance enterography; SBCD, small bowel Crohn's disease; SBFT, small bowel follow-through.

for identifying significant strictures.[45] Deep enteroscopy can also be used for the retrieval of retained capsule endoscopes.[46]

31.4 Dilation of Small Bowel Stricture

Deep enteroscopy allows for a more detailed examination of the small bowel stricture, to exclude malignancy and assess for possible dilation. Typically, dilation is performed using a through-the-scope balloon system. Dilations should be performed carefully in a gradual stepwise fashion 2 mm at a time up to 13 mm on the initial dilation to avoid perforation. Severe strictures should be dilated initially to 10 mm. The balloon dilator should slowly and carefully be inflated under direct vision for up to 30 to 60 seconds. Up to 50% may require repeat dilation at which time dilations can be increased up to 15 mm cautiously. Balloon dilation should be avoided when active ulcers and/or inflammation is seen at the stricture site. The injection of strictures with corticosteroids is controversial and not routinely recommended. Fully covered self-expandable metal stents in the treatment of Crohn's strictures is not currently the standard of care.

31.5 Small Bowel Tumors

Although there is approximately 20 ft of small intestine, only about 2% of GI tumors arise in the small intestine. ▶Table 31.4 outlines the most common GI tumors and their relative frequency. Adenocarcinoma, malignant carcinoids, lymphomas, and sarcomas are the most common.[47] In the western world, tumors most commonly occur in the duodenum (3 per 1, 000, 000) and less commonly in the jejunum and ileum (~ 1 per 1, 000, 000).[48] Sarcomas are fairly evenly distributed throughout the small bowel. Adenocarcinomas arising from CD, carcinoids, and lymphomas occur most commonly in the terminal ileum. Multiple tumors are suggestive of familial adenomatous polyposis (adenomas) or hamartomas (Peutz–Jeghers, Cronkhite–Canada, etc.). Tumor incidence is slightly higher in males presenting on average in people in their 60s but starting to rise in patients even in their 30s. There has been a slight rise of incidence of adenocarcinoma and malignant carcinoids, both of these have a higher incidence in African American patients more than in Caucasian patients.[48,49,50] Patients with carcinoid tumors may additionally present with diarrhea and flushing and have elevations in chromogranin A or 24-hour urinary 5-hydroxyindoleacetic acid (5-HIAA). Additionally, an octreotide scan can help identify carcinoid tumors.

31.5.1 Diagnosis

Diagnosing small bowel tumors can be challenging because clinicians can fail to consider small intestinal tumors as a source of patient's symptoms, particularly when the symptoms are rather vague. Another reason for failure to diagnose these lesions early is that diagnostic modalities, like X-rays were suboptimal in identifying tumors deep in the small bowel. In the past, endoscopy had a limited role in the diagnosis of small bowel tumors, primarily upper endoscopy (with a side-viewing endoscope) could be used to identify ampullary lesions in patients with familial adenomatous polyposis (FAP) syndromes or colonoscopy with terminal ileal intubation might identify an ileal carcinoid, adenocarcinoma, or lymphoma.

The advent of VCE and deep enteroscopy techniques has helped to expand the role of endoscopy in identifying small bowel tumors and the number of tumors and polyps that have been identified has increased.[51,52] A recent meta-analysis compared overtube-assisted enteroscopy and VCE and found that these had a high diagnostic concordance rate (80–100%—overall 93%) for small bowel polyps and tumors.[53] This is attributed to the fact that VCE is often used as the initial test to guide the direction of DBE to localize the lesion. It was also noted that overtube endoscopy was more accurate than spiral endoscopy to identify lesions. This was postulated to be the case because rotational advancement enteroscopy is not as effective as balloon-assisted enteroscopy for deep intubation.

It should be noted that both VCE and DBE can still miss lesions and there are diagnostic challenges. For instance, total small bowel enteroscopy cannot always be achieved because of technical issues or because the patient may be unwilling to undergo bidirectional endoscopy. In this meta-analysis total enteroscopy was successful in 85.7% of patients. Other endoscopic challenges include the fact that in polyposis syndromes CE can miss polyps in the periampullary area and the duodenal sweep.[54] CE has been shown though to identify more lesions and lesions that may not be reached by deep enteroscopy. CE can also have a high false-positive rate due to transient bulges that may be identified as lesions when they are not. This study demonstrated that 80% of the lesions missed by DBE were of subepithelial origin (e.g., gastrointestinal stromal tumors [GISTs] and leiomyomas). However, other lesions such as lipomas, carcinoids, and metastatic

Table 31.4 Classification of small bowel tumors[a]

Cell of origin	Type of tumor	Location	Relative frequency in small bowel
Benign epithelial lesions	Adenomas Hamartomas (Peutz–Jeghers, Cronkhite–Canada syndrome, juvenile polyposis, Cowden's disease, Bannayan–Riley–Ruvalcaba syndrome)	Most commonly duodenum Throughout the SI	Unknown Unknown
Malignant epithelial lesions	Adenocarcinoma • Primary • Secondary (metastases) Neuroendocrine (carcinoid)	Primary—(duodenum > jejunum > ileum)b Carcinoid—ileum most common site	Primary—24–52% Malignant carcinoid—17–41%
Lymphoproliferative	B-cell (mantle cell, follicular cell, diffuse large cell, marginal B cell (MALT)—type lymphoma, small bowel, immunoproliferative disorder) T cell (enteropathy-associated T-cell lymphoma)	Primary lymphoma—ileum most common site	Lymphoma—12–29%
Mesenchymal tumors	GISTs (benign and malignant) Fatty cell tumors (lipoma, liposarcoma) Neural tumors (schwannomas, intestinal autonomic tumors, ganglionomas, neurofibromas, granular cell tumors) Vascular tumors (hemangiomas, Kaposi's, angiosarcoma, lymphangioma) Smooth muscle tumors (leiomyoma, leiomyosarcoma) Paragangliomas	Sarcoma—evenly distributed in SI	Sarcoma—11–20%

GIST, gastrointestinal stromal tumor; MALT, mucosa-associated lymphoid tissue; SI, small intestine.
[a]Classification of most common small bowel tumors.
[b]In Crohn's disease, ileum is the most common site of adenocarcinoma.

disease can be submucosal as well. For FAP patients, the miss rate of polyps on CE is not known. However, a small prospective study looking at the detection of duodenal polyps with CE versus upper endoscopy suggested that CE was more accurate in detecting polyps in the third and fourth part of the duodenum.[55] The upper endoscopy was more accurate in polyp detection in the first and second portion of the duodenum, particularly at the ampulla of Vater. Another study of Peutz–Jeghers polyposis syndromes suggested that for more distal polyps (> 15 mm), MRE was a complementary procedure in detecting distal polyps because CE of larger lesions may be limited.[56] There are limited data on the miss rate of CE for single mass lesions. While CE is superior to other modalities for detection of vascular and inflammatory lesions, it does have a significant miss rate for detection of solitary lesions. One study showed a reported miss rate of 19% for neoplasms.[57]

Several tips can be useful in trying to distinguish submucosal lesions from bulges on VCE. Submucosal lesions unlike bulges due to adjacent loops of bowel may have an altered vascular pattern over the mucosa or the mucosa will be stretched, making it appear thin and translucent. A mass lesion may also have a certain white or grayish cast. "Bridging folds" are thought to be a pathognomonic feature—where the valvulae conniventes stop at the edge of the mass and form on the other side (▶ Fig. 31.5).[58] Additionally on VCE, the images must be examined over several frames. There is also the smooth protruding index on capsule endoscopy (SPICE) score that can be used to identify possible small bowel tumors (▶ Table 31.5). There are four features: (1) ill-defined boundary with the surrounding mucosa; (2) diameter larger than its height; (3) visible lumen in the frames in which it appears; and (4) image of the lesion lasting more than 10 minutes. An answer of no to features 1 and 2 is scored one point each and answer of yes to features 3 and 4 is also scored one point each with a maximum score of four. With this index, one can discriminate a mucosal bulge from a mass on VCE and a score greater than 2 has shown 83% sensitivity and 89% specificity for identifying tumors.[59] These are endoscopic criteria—for example, bleeding,

irregular surfaces—identified by a consensus group on CE in 2006 to be more likely associated with tumor and therefore likely to improve the diagnosis of tumor during CE.[60]

VCE and deep enteroscopy procedures are complimentary procedures with both false-positive and false-negative results. It is unlikely at this time that endoscopy will be the sole means of diagnosing small bowel tumors. The literature demonstrates that CT and MRE are still important modalities in identifying lesions missed by CE.[61] ▶ Fig. 31.6 demonstrates a proposed algorithm for diagnosing small bowel tumors.[62]

31.5.2 Therapeutics

Therapeutic interventions are limited to removing benign lesions such as periampullary adenomas or isolated adenomas or benign lesions such as lipomas.[63,64] Endoscopic resection of small duodenal carcinoids has been reported.[65] The data suggest poorer outcomes in periampullary lesions that have to be resected more than twice.[63] Most cancerous lesions or large deep obstructing benign lesions require surgical resection or in the case of lymphoma and advanced neuroendocrine tumors, chemotherapy may be the primary treatment. Perhaps advance in peroral endoscopic procedures will yield advances in this area.

31.6 Malabsorption Disorders of the Small Bowel

▶ Table 31.1 lists the disorders that most commonly cause malabsorption. Many of these disorders present with diarrhea and patients not uncommonly demonstrate deficiencies in iron, B_{12}, folate, vitamin D, or trace minerals. In severe cases fat malabsorption is evident as well. The prototype disorder is celiac disease, which is estimated to effect 1% of the world's population. Celiac disease can also present as a spectrum of disease with some patients presenting with mild GI symptoms of bloating or dyspepsia rather than severe diarrhea or non-GI manifestations such as recurrent aphthous ulcers, neuropathy, or associated with dermatitis herpetiformis.[66,67]

31.6.1 Diagnostics and Therapeutics

Diagnostics in the area of malabsorption will vary with the disorder. For celiac disease, serologic screening with an immunoglobulin A (IgA) level and a tissue transglutaminase (tTG) IgA is recommended as initial testing in a patient on a gluten-full diet.[68] The IgA level is performed because 2 to 3% of the population is IgA deficient. If IgA levels are low, the recommendation is to perform deamidated gliadin antibody levels raised against IgA and IgG (▶ Fig. 31.7) because tTG–IgG is less sensitive and specific for celiac disease.[69] Endoscopic biopsy is still the gold standard of diagnosis and 10% of patients with negative serology may have evidence of disease on biopsy. Endoscopic features of celiac disease can include scalloping, nodularity, or fissuring. These changes are not diagnostic of celiac disease as these can be seen in other small bowel malabsorptive disorders as well, for example, autoimmune enteropathy.[67] The disorder can have a patchy distribution in the small intestine so it is recommended that four to six single-pass biopsies of the small bowel be taken in the bulb and both proximal

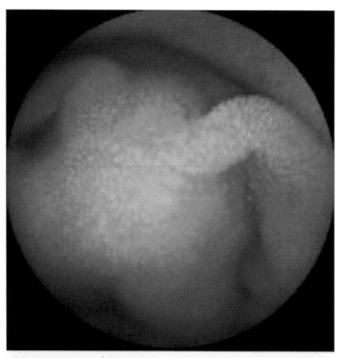

Fig. 31.5 Bridging folds image.

Table 31.5 Capsule endoscopic criteria associated with tumor likelihood[54] (major and minor)

Tumor probability	Major					Minor		
	Bleeding	Color	Disruption of mucosa	Irregular surface	Polypoid appearance	Invagination	Passage delay ≥ 30 min	White villi
High	++	++	++	++	++	++	++	++
Intermediate	+/-	+	+	+	+			
Low	-	-	-	-	+/-	-	-	-

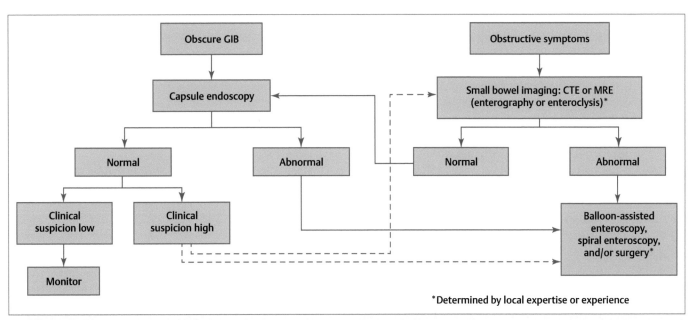

Fig. 31.6 Algorithm for diagnosis of small bowel tumors.

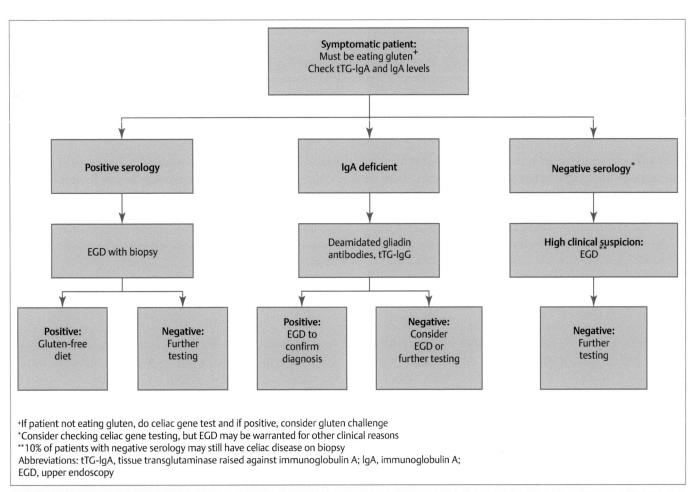

+If patient not eating gluten, do celiac gene test and if positive, consider gluten challenge
*Consider checking celiac gene testing, but EGD may be warranted for other clinical reasons
**10% of patients with negative serology may still have celiac disease on biopsy
Abbreviations: tTG-IgA, tissue transglutaminase raised against immunoglobulin A; IgA, immunoglobulin A; EGD, upper endoscopy

Fig. 31.7 Diagnosis of celiac disease.

and distal to the ampulla of Vater to help increase diagnostic yield.[70,71] A small proportion of patients may have only jejunal involvement.[72] The mainstay of therapy is a gluten-free diet.

If a patient is on a gluten-free diet prior to testing, he or she may have negative serology as antibody titers decrease with a gluten-free diet. Before offering a gluten challenge, it is reasonable to do genetic testing for HLA-DQ2 and DQ8, as almost 100% of celiac patients have one or both of the genes.[69] See ▶ Fig. 31.7 for a diagnostic algorithm.

VCE has an evolving role in the diagnosis of celiac disease when patients are resistant or unable to having upper endoscopy. Several studies have demonstrated that VCE has a very good sensitivity and specificity for diagnosing celiac disease in patients with a positive tTG.[73,74,75,76,77] In the largest study of 43 patients, VCE had sensitivity and specificity of 87.5% and 90%, respectively.[77] Not all studies have had such good results suggesting that biopsy may still be the gold standard.[78,79]

VCE can also be used to document complications of celiac disease, for example, ulcerative jejunitis or refractory celiac disease (RCD) types I and II. The endoscopic features of RCD on VCE are not clear-cut, therefore patients who are suspected of having refractory disease should also undergo small bowel imaging as well as deep enteroscopy with biopsy to diagnose RCD or enteropathy-associated T-cell lymphoma (EATL).[80] In a retrospective review of 52 patients, none of the endoscopic findings distinguished RCD type I from type 2. However two features—proximal erythema and failure of the capsule to make it to the distal intestine—were independently associated with the presence of RCD type 2 or EATL. This finding suggests that these features and others may eventually have a role in risk stratification.

Therapy for RCD I and II differs.[81] Type 1 RCD is usually treated with a continued gluten-free diet and nutritional support as well as corticosteroids. Type II disease may also be treated with corticosteroids as well as cladribine. Sometimes autologous stem cell transplant is utilized. When type II disease becomes EATL, chemotherapy for lymphoma and autologous stem cell transplant is the mainstays of therapy, but prognosis is poor.

Collagenous sprue can occur as a complication of celiac sprue without a clear trigger, but recently the angiotensin II receptor-blocking drugs, olmesartan and valsartan, have been described to cause collagenous sprue. The mechanism is not entirely understood, but a recent study suggests that olmesartan induces many of the immunopathogenic pathways of celiac disease such as increasing the number of CD8+ cells and causing an overexpression of IL15 and disrupting tight junctions.[82] Patients do not respond to a gluten-free diet nor do they all have celiac genes. The diagnosis is usually made on small bowel or colonic biopsy and regresses when the drugs are discontinued.

Autoimmune enteropathy and combined variable immunodeficiency disorder (CVID) may have serologic features of autoantibodies and low immunoglobulin levels, respectively, but small bowel biopsy can help make the diagnosis in each. Both can be associated with villous blunting and celiac atrophy but CVID has also been described to present as normal mucosal, ileal erythema, aphthous ulcer, and nodular lymphoid hyperplasia (NLH). Lesions can be patchy in this disorder as well. Treatment for autoimmune enteropathy is with steroids and for CVID, appropriate vaccinations and immunoglobulins are given. In severe cases bone marrow transplants are performed.

With the growing use of bone marrow transplants in the treatment of malignancy, gastroenterologists are encountering increasing number of patients with graft-versus-host disease (GVHD). These patients often present with diarrhea, malabsorption, and bleeding due to the invasion of donor CD8 T cells into the lining of the intestine. Grossly, GVHD can present as anything from normal-appearing tissue to ulceration to total desquamation of the mucosa, depending on the severity of the disease. It occurs in about 50% of bone marrow transplant patients and treatment is by suppression of the immune response.[83] A recent pilot study looking at 15 patients after bone marrow transplant looked at the combination of confocal endoscopy and VCE as a means of earlier detection of GVHD and found promising results.[84]

Amyloidosis often presents with bleeding but cases of malabsorption have been reported. Endoscopic features associated with amyloidosis were described as thickening of jejunal and ileal folds, but ulceration of the mucosa and mass lesions have also been reported.[85,86]

Unfortunately there are few studies that have compared enteroscopy procedures and VCE in the evaluation of malabsorption. One study has compared 25 patients with protein losing enteropathy that had DBE, VCE, and fluoroscopic enteroclysis. The diagnostic yield of DBE was 100% compared to 60% for enteroclysis for the 15 patients that had both procedures. In the 17 patients who had DBE and VCE, the diagnostic yield was not statistically significant (82% DBE vs. 76%VCE). A variety of diagnoses were found including intestinal amyloidosis, small bowel tumors, and intestinal lymphangiectasia.[87]

31.7 Small Intestinal Infections

There are many organisms that affect the small intestine and to discuss all of them is beyond the scope of this chapter. Many infections can be detected by stool–polymerase chain reaction (PCR) tests. However, the literature demonstrates that certain infections have been identified by endoscopic procedures rather than by other methods.

In patients with persistent anemia or occult bleeding, hookworm is probably the parasite most revealed by VCE (▶ Fig. 31.8).[88,89] This is likely not surprising since it is among one of the most common parasites worldwide.[90] Other parasites such as various tapeworms have also been revealed and other endoscopic techniques such as confocal laser endomicroscopy (Pentax, Tokyo) and an endocystoscopy system with a high magnification light microscopy device (Olympus Medical Systems, Tokyo) hold the potential to see organisms in vivo like *Entamoeba histolytica*.[91,92]

Other infections not only cause bleeding but also ulceration such as mycobacteria, typhoid, histoplasmosis, and syphilis. Diarrhea and fever are also commonly seen as presenting symptoms as well. *Mycobacterium tuberculosis* can present as nodularity or narrowing in the terminal ileum but has been documented in the jejunum and duodenum. Endoscopy has been used to diagnose or confirm the infection in the small bowel. *Mycobacterium avium* complex (MAC), *M. tuberculosis*, and Whipple's disease can cause tiny punctate nodules or exudate in the lining of the intestine.[93] Histologically, foamy periodic acid–Schiff (PAS)-positive macrophages can be seen in infection with these organisms in addition to Whipple's disease. Endoscopic biopsy is required to differentiate these lesions and see on histology either the gram-positive

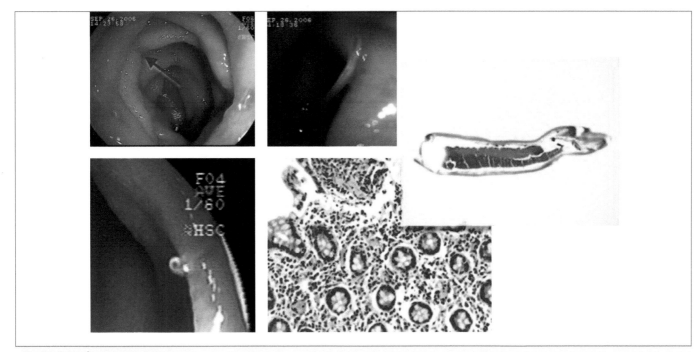

Fig. 31.8 Hookworm image.

bacillus *Tropheryma whippeli* or the acid-fast organisms that characterize MAC or *M. tuberculosis*.

Intestinal infections also present commonly in the ileum and in considering small bowel disease, it is important for the endoscopist to remember that all ileitis is not Crohn's. ▶Table 31.6 lists the organisms that have been known to cause ileitis.[94]

31.8 Congenital Lesions

Both duodenal and even jejunal diverticula are often asymptomatic. Duodenal diverticula are frequently seen on routine upper endoscopy most commonly within 2 cm of the ampulla. These are most often asymptomatic and present a challenge particularly to the therapeutic endoscopist endeavoring to cannulate the ampullary papilla during endoscopic retrograde cholangiopancreatography (ERCP) especially if these are intraluminal ("windsock") diverticula. Recently there have been case reports of endoscopic resection of these lesions.[95,96] In general, duodenal diverticular bleeding is reported more often than perforation, diverticulitis, and obstruction.[97] Endoscopic treatment of duodenal diverticular perforations via DBE is being explored but most treatment is currently either conservative or surgical.[98,99] The presence of duodenal diverticula has also been associated with increased risk of finding bacterial overgrowth when duodenal aspirates are performed.[100]

Approximately 1% of the population is estimated to have jejunal diverticula and they are most commonly found proximally on the mesenteric border of the bowel.[101] They are thought to be caused by an intestinal motility disorder and may be multiple. Nonspecific symptoms such as abdominal pain, bloating, and diarrhea can be seen and their complications are similar to duodenal diverticula. Both radiologic (CT scan and small bowel series) and endoscopy (VCE and DBE) have been used to identify diverticula.[96] Complications are similar to those of duodenal diverticula and DBE has been used to treat bleeding but with some risk of perforation.[102]

The most common congenital diverticulum is Meckel's diverticulum, a remnant of the vitelline duct. It is said to follow the "rule of 2s". Lesions (3–6 cm in length) occur in 2% of the population within 2 ft of the ileocecal valve on the antimesenteric border and contain two kinds of tissue (pancreatic or gastric). These are 3 times more likely to occur in male patients than female patients and males have more complications that often present before 2 years of age. ▶Fig. 31.9 shows a Meckel diverticulum with an ulcer. They are most often identified by 99 m-technetium pertechnetate which allows identification of the gastric mucosa if present. Endoscopic diagnosis during colonoscopy or DBE is rare. When ectopic gastric mucosa is present, bleeding can be seen. Other complications have been perforation, intussusception, diverticulitis, and occurrence of various type of cancer within the lesion have all been reported.

Duplication cysts can also be lined with ectopic gastric mucosa and therefore can be likely to have ulcers or bleed. They can occur anywhere in the GI tract.

As mentioned above jejunal diverticula may be present in intestinal dysmotility. This lesion can also be associated with intestinal pseudo-obstruction which is another congenital small bowel disorder characterized by intestinal dilation and slowing.

31.9 Miscellaneous Conditions

Some miscellaneous conditions that are not easily categorized should be mentioned. Lymphangiectasias, which represent dilated lacteals of the mucosa (sometimes extending into the submucosa) can present as incidental findings on endoscopy most commonly in the duodenum.[103] In a recent study of 1,866 consecutive endoscopies, these lesions were present in 1.9% of the procedures.[103] They may be representative of a primary process (e.g., intestinal lymphangiectasia) or a secondary process (e.g., associated with lymphoma or celiac disease).[104] Endoscopic biopsy confirms the visual impression (▶Fig. 31.10) and DBE have both been

Table 31.6 Infectious agents that can cause ileitis

Bacteria	Fungus	Parasite	Virus
Clostridium difficile	Actinomycosis	Anisakiasis	Cytomegalovirus
Salmonella spp	Histoplasma capsulatum		
Mycobacterium avium			
Mycobacterium tuberculosis			
*Typhlitis			
Yersinia spp			

*Typhilitis is a disease process caused by multiple different types of bacteria not just one type.

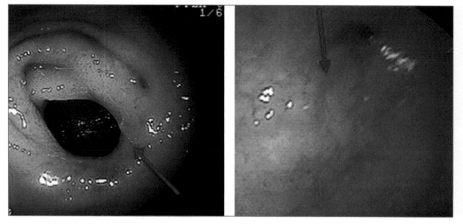

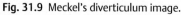
Fig. 31.9 Meckel's diverticulum image.

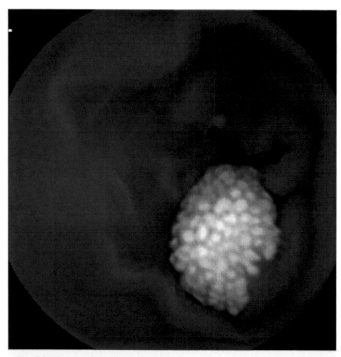

Fig. 31.10 Lymphangiectasia image.

used to demonstrate the extent of involvement of the lesions in the small bowel for diagnostic purposes.[105,106]

Endometriosis is a relatively common clinical condition whose true prevalence is not known, but its presence has been found in 12 to 32% of women undergoing laparoscopic procedures for the diagnosis of pelvic pain.[107,108] It can be found in the rectosigmoid region but another common area of occurrence is the ileum where it has presented as obstruction or fibrostenotic disease.[109,110]

Usual diagnosis has been through radiologic procedures or surgery but future diagnosis via VCE and/or DBE are conceivable and rectosigmoid resection of lesions has been performed.[111]

31.10 Conclusion

The evolution of small bowel endoscopy with the ability to perform VCE and deep enteroscopy has resulted in improved ability to diagnose and treat patients with suspected small bowel bleeding resulting in major advances in the morbidity of GI bleeding, but uncertain effects on mortality. In many cases, the ability to perform therapeutic interventions in the Small bowel has eliminated the need for invasive surgical procedures. However, larger studies are needed to determine the impact on clinical outcomes. This new technology has also improved our ability to diagnose and monitor response to new treatment modalities in CD as well. The therapeutic possibilities of deep enteroscopy have allowed treatment of strictures in CD and the potential for removal of certain tumors and obstructing growths where appropriate. Evolving technology in wireless capsule endoscopy, confocal laser endomicroscopy, and endocystoscopy as well as advances in peroral endoscopic mucosectomy promise increasing diagnostic and therapeutic capabilities. The field of small bowel enteroscopy continues to evolve rapidly, especially in the area of wireless technology. The future holds much promise for patients with suspected small bowel disease.

References

[1]   Gerson LB, Fidler JL, Cave DR, Leighton JA. ACG clinical guideline: diagnosis and management of small bowel bleeding. Am J Gastroenterol. 2015; 110(9):1265–1287, quiz 1288

[2] Kopáčová M, Bureš J, Tacheci I. Gastrointestinal lesions detected by capsule endoscopy and double-balloon enteroscopy. Video J Encyclopedia GI Endosc. 2013; 1(1):180–182

[3] Monkemuller K, Neumann H, Bellutti M, Fry LC. Missed lesion with conventional endoscopy discovered by double-balloon enteroscopy: endoscopist or instrument?—authors' reply. Aliment Pharmacol Ther. 2009; 29:919–920

[4] Robinson CA, Jackson C, Condon D, Gerson LB. Impact of inpatient status and gender on small-bowel capsule endoscopy findings. Gastrointest Endosc. 2011; 74(5):1061–1066

[5] Pennazio M, Santucci R, Rondonotti E, et al. Outcome of patients with obscure gastrointestinal bleeding after capsule endoscopy: report of 100 consecutive cases. Gastroenterology. 2004; 126(3):643–653

[6] Carey EJ, Leighton JA, Heigh RI, et al. A single-center experience of 260 consecutive patients undergoing capsule endoscopy for obscure gastrointestinal bleeding. Am J Gastroenterol. 2007; 102(1):89–95

[7] Shinozaki S, Yamamoto H, Yano T, et al. Long-term outcome of patients with obscure gastrointestinal bleeding investigated by double-balloon endoscopy. Clin Gastroenterol Hepatol. 2010; 8(2):151–158

[8] Gay G, Delvaux M, Fassler I. Outcome of capsule endoscopy in determining indication and route for push-and-pull enteroscopy. Endoscopy. 2006; 38(1):49–58

[9] Kaffes AJ, Siah C, Koo JH. Clinical outcomes after double-balloon enteroscopy in patients with obscure GI bleeding and a positive capsule endoscopy. Gastrointest Endosc. 2007; 66(2):304–309

[10] Hendel JW, Vilmann P, Jensen T. Double-balloon endoscopy: who needs it? Scand J Gastroenterol. 2008; 43(3):363–367

[11] Bresci G, Parisi G, Bertoni M, et al. The role of video capsule endoscopy for evaluating obscure gastrointestinal bleeding: usefulness of early use. J Gastroenterol. 2005; 40(3):256–259

[12] Yamada A, Watabe H, Kobayashi Y, et al Timing of capsule endoscopy influences the diagnosis and outcome in obscure-overt gastrointestinal bleeding. Hepatogastroenterology. 2012; 59(115):676–679

[13] Singh A, Marshall C, Chaudhuri B, et al. Timing of video capsule endoscopy relative to overt obscure GI bleeding: implications from a retrospective study. Gastrointest Endosc. 2013; 77(5):761–766

[14] Takano N, Yamada A, Watabe H, et al. Single-balloon versus double-balloon endoscopy for achieving total enteroscopy: a randomized, controlled trial. Gastrointest Endosc. 2011; 73(4):734–739

[15] Efthymiou M, Desmond PV, Brown G, et al. SINGLE-01: a randomized, controlled trial comparing the efficacy and depth of insertion of single- and double-balloon enteroscopy by using a novel method to determine insertion depth. Gastrointest Endosc. 2012; 76(5):972–980

[16] Aniwan S, Viriyautsahakul V, Rerknimitr R, et al. Urgent double balloon endoscopy provides higher yields than non-urgent double balloon endoscopy in overt obscure gastrointestinal bleeding. Endosc Int Open. 2014; 2(2):E90–E95

[17] Mönkemüller K, Neumann H, Meyer F, et al. A retrospective analysis of emergency double-balloon enteroscopy for small-bowel bleeding. Endoscopy. 2009; 41(8):715–717

[18] Teshima CW, Kuipers EJ, van Zanten SV, Mensink PB. Double balloon enteroscopy and capsule endoscopy for obscure gastrointestinal bleeding: an updated meta-analysis. J Gastroenterol Hepatol. 2011; 26(5):796–801

[19] Pasha SF, Hara AK, Leighton JA. Diagnostic evaluation and management of obscure gastrointestinal bleeding: a changing paradigm. Gastroenterol Hepatol (N Y). 2009; 5(12):839–850

[20] Gerson L, Kamal A. Cost-effectiveness analysis of management strategies for obscure GI bleeding. Gastrointest Endosc. 2008; 68(5):920–936

[21] Kim CY, Suhocki PV, Miller MJ, et al. Provocative mesenteric angiography for lower gastrointestinal hemorrhage: results from a single-institution study. J Vasc Interv Radiol. 2010; 21(4):477–483

[22] Kim JB, Ye BD, Song Y, et al. Frequency of rebleeding events in obscure gastrointestinal bleeding with negative capsule endoscopy. J Gastroenterol Hepatol. 2013; 28(5):834–840

[23] Riccioni ME, Urgesi R, Cianci R, et al. Negative capsule endoscopy in patients with obscure gastrointestinal bleeding reliable: recurrence of bleeding on long-term follow-up. World J Gastroenterol. 2013; 19(28):4520–4525

[24] Sakai E, Endo H, Taguri M, et al. Frequency and risk factors for rebleeding events in patients with small bowel angioectasia. BMC Gastroenterol. 2014; 14:200

[25] Rahmi G, Samaha E, Vahedi K, et al. Long-term follow-up of patients undergoing capsule and double-balloon enteroscopy for identification and treatment of small-bowel vascular lesions: a prospective, multicenter study. Endoscopy. 2014; 46(7):591–597

[26] Jackson CS, Gerson LB. Management of gastrointestinal angiodysplastic lesions (GIADs): a systematic review and meta-analysis. Am J Gastroenterol. 2014; 109(4):474–483, quiz 484

[27] Brown C, Subramanian V, Wilcox CM, Peter S. Somatostatin analogues in the treatment of recurrent bleeding from gastrointestinal vascular malformations: an overview and systematic review of prospective observational studies. Dig Dis Sci. 2010; 55(8):2129–2134

[28] Ge ZZ, Chen HM, Gao YJ, et al. Efficacy of thalidomide for refractory gastrointestinal bleeding from vascular malformation. Gastroenterology. 2011; 141(5):1629–37.e1–e4

[29] Valle J, Alcántara M, Pérez-Grueso MJ, et al. Clinical features of patients with negative results from traditional diagnostic work-up and Crohn's disease findings from capsule endoscopy. J Clin Gastroenterol. 2006; 40(8):692–696

[30] Voderholzer WA, Beinhoelzl J, Rogalla P, et al. Small bowel involvement in Crohn's disease: a prospective comparison of wireless capsule endoscopy and computed tomography enteroclysis. Gut. 2005; 54(3):369–373

[31] Vermeire S, van Assche G, Rutgeerts P. Review article: altering the natural history of Crohn's disease—evidence for and against current therapies. Aliment Pharmacol Ther. 2007; 25(1):3–12

[32] Leighton JA, Shen B, Baron TH, et al; Standards of Practice Committee, American Society for . Gastrointestinal Endoscopy. ASGE guideline: endoscopy in the diagnosis and treatment of inflammatory bowel disease. Gastrointest Endosc. 2006; 63(4):558–565

[33] Mekhjian HS, Switz DM, Melnyk CS, et al. Clinical features and natural history of Crohn's disease. Gastroenterology. 1979; 77(4 pt 2):898–906

[34] Kornbluth A, Colombel JF, Leighton JA, Loftus E; ICCE. ICCE consensus for inflammatory bowel disease. Endoscopy. 2005; 37(10):1051–1054

[35] Samuel S, Bruining DH, Loftus EV, Jr, et al. Endoscopic skipping of the distal terminal ileum in Crohn's disease can lead to negative results from ileocolonoscopy. Clin Gastroenterol Hepatol. 2012; 10(11):1253–1259

[36] Girelli CM, Porta P, Malacrida V, et al. Clinical outcome of patients examined by capsule endoscopy for suspected small bowel Crohn's disease. Dig Liver Dis. 2007; 39(2):148–154

[37] Jensen MD, Nathan T, Rafaelsen SR, Kjeldsen J. Diagnostic accuracy of capsule endoscopy for small bowel Crohn's disease is superior to that of MR enterography or CT enterography. Clin Gastroenterol Hepatol. 2011; 9(2):124–129

[38] Solem CA, Loftus EV, Jr, Fletcher JG, et al. Small-bowel imaging in Crohn's disease: a prospective, blinded, 4-way comparison trial. Gastrointest Endosc. 2008; 68(2):255–266

[39] Calabrese C, Gionchetti P, Rizzello F, et al. Short-term treatment with infliximab in chronic refractory pouchitis and ileitis. Aliment Pharmacol Ther. 2008; 27(9):759–764

[40] Mensink PB, Aktas H, Zelinkova Z, et al. Impact of double-balloon enteroscopy findings on the management of Crohn's disease. Scand J Gastroenterol. 2010; 45(4):483–489

[41] Jang HJ, Choi MH, Eun CS, et al. Clinical usefulness of double balloon enteroscopy in suspected Crohn's disease: the KASID multi-center trial. Hepatogastroenterology. 2014; 61(133):1292–1296

[42] Rahman A, Ross A, Leighton JA, et al. Double-balloon enteroscopy in Crohn's disease: findings and impact on management in a multicenter retrospective study. Gastrointest Endosc. 2015; 82(1):102–107

[43] Pohl J, May A, Nachbar L, Ell C. Diagnostic and therapeutic yield of push-and-pull enteroscopy for symptomatic small bowel Crohn's disease strictures. Eur J Gastroenterol Hepatol. 2007; 19(7):529–534

[44] Despott EJ, Gupta A, Burling D, et al. Effective dilation of small-bowel strictures by double-balloon enteroscopy in patients with symptomatic Crohn's disease (with video). Gastrointest Endosc. 2009; 70(5):1030–1036

[45] Takenaka K, Ohtsuka K, Kitazume Y, et al. Comparison of magnetic resonance and balloon enteroscopic examination of the small intestine in patients with Crohn's disease. Gastroenterology. 2014; 147(2):334–342.e3

[46] Van Weyenberg SJ, Van Turenhout ST, Bouma G, et al. Double-balloon endoscopy as the primary method for small-bowel video capsule endoscope retrieval. Gastrointest Endosc. 2010; 71(3):535–541

[47] Bresalier RS, Bechacz B. Tumors of the small intestine. In: Feldman M, Friedman LS, Brandt LJ, eds. Sleisenger and Fordtran's Gastrointestinal and Liver Diseases. 10th ed. Philadelphia, PA: Saunders; 2016:2196–2212

[48] Schottenfeld D, Beebe-Dimmer JL, Vigneau FD. The epidemiology and pathogenesis of neoplasia in the small intestine. Ann Epidemiol. 2009; 19(1):58–69

[49] Bilimoria KY, Bentrem DJ, Wayne JD, et al. Small bowel cancer in the United States: changes in epidemiology, treatment, and survival over the last 20 years. Ann Surg. 2009; 249(1):63–71

[50] Martin LF, Max MH, Richardson JD, Peterson GH. Small bowel tumors: a continuing challenge. South Med J. 1980; 73(8):981–985

[51] Moglia A, Menciassi A, Dario P, Cuschieri A. Clinical update: endoscopy for small-bowel tumours. Lancet. 2007; 370(9582):114–116

[52] Yamamoto H, Kita H, Sunada K, et al. Clinical outcomes of double-balloon endoscopy for the diagnosis and treatment of small-intestinal diseases. Clin Gastroenterol Hepatol. 2004; 2(11):1010–1016

[53] Sulbaran M, de Moura E, Bernardo W, et al. Overtube-assisted enteroscopy and capsule endoscopy for the diagnosis of small-bowel polyps and tumors: a systematic review and meta-analysis. Endosc Int Open. 2016; 4(2):E151–E163

[54] Iaquinto G, Fornasarig M, Quaia M, et al. Capsule endoscopy is useful and safe for small-bowel surveillance in familial adenomatous polyposis. Gastrointest Endosc. 2008; 67(1):61–67

[55] Yamada A, Watabe H, Iwama T. et al. The prevalence of small intestinal polyps in patients with familial adenomatous polyposis: a prospective capsule endoscopy study. Fam Cancer. 2014; 13(1):23–28

[56] Gupta A, Postgate AJ, Burling D, et al. A prospective study of MR enterography versus capsule endoscopy for the surveillance of adult patients with Peutz-Jeghers syndrome. AJR Am J Roentgenol. 2010; 195(1):108–116

[57] Lewis BS, Eisen GM, Friedman S. A pooled analysis to evaluate results of capsule endoscopy trials. Endoscopy. 2005; 37(10):960–965

[58] Lewis B, Keuchel M, Castelitz J. Malignant tumors of the small intestine. In: Keuchel M, Hagenmuller F, Fleischer DE, eds. Atlas of Video Capsule Endoscopy. Berlin: Springer; 2006:172–190

[59] Girelli CM, Porta P, Colombo E, et al. Development of a novel index to discriminate bulge from mass on small-bowel capsule endoscopy. Gastrointest Endosc. 2011; 74(5):1067–1074, quiz 1115.e1–1115.e5

[60] Mergener K, Ponchon T, Gralnek I, et al. Literature review and recommendations for clinical application of small-bowel capsule endoscopy, based on a panel discussion by international experts. Consensus statements for small-bowel capsule endoscopy, 2006/2007. Endoscopy. 2007; 39(10):895–909

[61] Postgate A, Despott E, Burling D, et al. Significant small-bowel lesions detected by alternative diagnostic modalities after negative capsule endoscopy. Gastrointest Endosc. 2008; 68(6):1209–1214

[62] Islam RS, Leighton JA, Pasha SF. Evaluation and management of small-bowel tumors in the era of deep enteroscopy. Gastrointest Endosc. 2014; 79(5):732–740

[63] Onkendi EO, Naik ND, Rosedahl JK, et al. Adenomas of the ampulla of Vater: a comparison of outcomes of operative and endoscopic resections. J Gastrointest Surg. 2014; 18(9):1588–1596

[64] Toya Y, Endo M, Orikasa S, et al, Lipoma of the small intestine treated with endoscopic resection. Clin J Gastroenterol. 2014; 7(6):502–505

[65] Scherer JR, Holinga J, Sanders M, et al. Small duodenal carcinoids: a case series comparing endoscopic resection and autoamputation with band ligation. J Clin Gastroenterol. 2015; 49(4):289–292

[66] Gujral N, Freeman HJ, Thomson AB. Celiac disease: prevalence, diagnosis, pathogenesis and treatment. World J Gastroenterol. 2012; 18(42):6036–6059

[67] Harris LA, Park JY, Voltaggio L, Lam-Himlin D. Celiac disease: clinical, endoscopic, and histopathologic review. Gastrointest Endosc. 2012; 76(3):625–640

[68] Rubio-Tapia A, Hill ID, Kelly CP, et al. American College of Gastroenterology. ACG clinical guidelines: diagnosis and management of celiac disease. Am J Gastroenterol. 2013; 108(5):656–676, quiz 677

[69] Oxentenko AS, Murray JA. Celiac disease: ten things that every gastroenterologist should know. Clin Gastroenterol Hepatol. 2015; 13(8):1396–1404, quiz e127–e129

[70] Rostom A, Murray JA, Kagnoff MF. American Gastroenterological Association (AGA) Institute technical review on the diagnosis and management of celiac disease. Gastroenterology. 2006; 131(6):1981–2002

[71] Kurien M, Evans KE, Hopper AD, et al. Duodenal bulb biopsies for diagnosing adult celiac disease: is there an optimal biopsy site? Gastrointest Endosc. 2012; 75(6):1190–1196

[72] Valitutti F, Di Nardo G, Barbato M, et al. Mapping histologic patchiness of celiac disease by push enteroscopy. Gastrointest Endosc. 2014; 79(1):95–100

[73] Petroniene R, Dubcenco E, Baker JP, et al. Given capsule endoscopy in celiac disease. Gastrointest Endosc Clin N Am. 2004; 14(1):115–127

[74] Petroniene R, Dubcenco E, Baker JP, et al. Given capsule endoscopy in celiac disease: evaluation of diagnostic accuracy and interobserver agreement. Am J Gastroenterol. 2005; 100(3):685–694

[75] Hopper AD, Sidhu R, Hurlstone DP, et al, Capsule endoscopy: an alternative to duodenal biopsy for the recognition of villous atrophy in coeliac disease? Dig Liver Dis. 2007; 39(2):140–145

[76] Rondonotti E, de Franchis R. Diagnosing coeliac disease: is the videocapsule a suitable tool? Dig Liver Dis. 2007; 39(2):145–147

[77] Rondonotti E, Spada C, Cave D, et al. Video capsule enteroscopy in the diagnosis of celiac disease: a multicenter study. Am J Gastroenterol. 2007; 102(8):1624–1631

[78] Maiden L, Elliott T, McLaughlin SD, Ciclitira P. A blinded pilot comparison of capsule endoscopy and small bowel histology in unresponsive celiac disease. Dig Dis Sci. 2009; 54(6):1280–1283

[79] El-Matary W, Huynh H, Vandermeer B. Diagnostic characteristics of given video capsule endoscopy in diagnosis of celiac disease: a meta-analysis. J Laparoendosc Adv Surg Tech A. 2009; 19(6):815–820

[80] Hadithi M, Al-toma A, Oudejans J, et al, The value of double-balloon enteroscopy in patients with refractory celiac disease. Am J Gastroenterol. 2007; 102(5):987–996

[81] Marietta EV, Nadeau AM, Cartee AK, et al. Immunopathogenesis of olmesartan-associated enteropathy. Aliment Pharmacol Ther. 2015; 42(11–12):1303–1314

[82] Rishi AR, Rubio-Tapia A, Murray JA. Refractory celiac disease. Expert Rev Gastroenterol Hepatol. 2016

[83] Ferrara JL, Levine JE, Reddy P, Holler E. Graft-versus-host disease. Lancet. 2009; 373(9674):1550–1561

[84] Coron E, Laurent V, Malard F, et al. Early detection of acute graft-versus-host disease by wireless capsule endoscopy and probe-based confocal laser endomicroscopy: results of a pilot study. United European Gastroenterol J. 2014; 2(3):206–215

[85] Harish K, Gokulan C. Selective amyloidosis of the small intestine presenting as malabsorption syndrome. Trop Gastroenterol. 2008; 29(1):37–39

[86] Bellutti M, Weigt J, Mönkemüller K, et al. Localized primary AL-type amyloidosis of the jejunum diagnosed by double-balloon enteroscopy. Endoscopy. 2007; 39(suppl 1):E134–E135

[87] Takenaka H, Ohmiya N, Hirooka Y, et al. Endoscopic and imaging findings in protein-losing enteropathy. J Clin Gastroenterol. 2012; 46(7):575–580

[88] Chen JM, Zhang XM, Wang LJ, et al. Overt gastrointestinal bleeding because of hookworm infection. Asian Pac J Trop Med. 2012; 5(4):331–332

[89] Christodoulou DK, Sigounas DE, Katsanos KH, et al. Small bowel parasitosis as cause of obscure gastrointestinal bleeding diagnosed by capsule endoscopy. World J Gastrointest Endosc. 2010; 2(11):369–371

[90] Fenwick A. The global burden of neglected tropical diseases. Public Health. 2012; 126(3):233–236

[91] Yamashita ET, Takahashi W, Kuwashima DY, et al. Diagnosis of Ascaris lumbricoides infection using capsule endoscopy. World J Gastrointest Endosc. 2013; 5(4):189–190

[92] Hosoe N, Ogata H, Hibi T. Endoscopic imaging of parasites in the human digestive tract. Parasitol Int. 2014; 63(1):216–220

[93] Makharia GK, Srivastava S, Das P, et al. Clinical, endoscopic, and histological differentiations between Crohn's disease and intestinal tuberculosis. Am J Gastroenterol. 2010; 105(3):642–651

[94] Dilauro S, Crum-Cianflone NF. Ileitis: when it is not Crohn's disease. Curr Gastroenterol Rep. 2010; 12(4):249–258

[95] Nakamura M, Nishikawa J, Hashimoto S, et al. Gastrointestinal: rare congenital abnormality of the duodenum: intraluminal duodenal diverticulum. J Gastroenterol Hepatol. 2014; 29(5):893

[96] Kumbhari V, Tieu AH, Azola A, et al. Novel endoscopic approach for a large intraluminal duodenal ("windsock") diverticulum. Gastrointest Endosc. 2015; 82(5):961

[97] Jeharajah DR, Dunbar KB. Diverticula of the pharynx, esophagus, stomach, and small intestine. Sleisenger & Fordtran's Gastrointestinal and Liver Diseases. 10th ed. Philadelphia, PA: Saunders; 2016:297–406

[98] Sasaki F, Kanmura S, Nasu Y, et al. Double-balloon enteroscopy-assisted closure of perforated duodenal diverticulum using polyglycolic acid sheets. Endoscopy. 2015; 47(suppl 1 UCTN):E204–E205

[99] Thorson CM, Paz Ruiz PS, Roeder RA, et al. The perforated duodenal diverticulum. Arch Surg. 2012; 147(1):81–88

[100] Choung RS, Ruff KC, Malhotra A, et al. Clinical predictors of small intestinal bacterial overgrowth by duodenal aspirate culture. Aliment Pharmacol Ther. 2011; 33(9):1059–1067

[101] Miller RE, McCabe RE, Salomon PF, Knox WG. Surgical complications of small bowel diverticula exclusive of Meckel's. Ann Surg. 1970; 171(2):202–210

[102] Yen HH, Chen YY, Yang CW, Soon MS. The clinical significance of jejunal diverticular disease diagnosed by double-balloon enteroscopy for obscure gastrointestinal bleeding. Dig Dis Sci. 2010; 55(12):3473–3478

[103] Kim JH, Bak YT, Kim JS, et al. Clinical significance of duodenal lymphangiectasia incidentally found during routine upper gastrointestinal endoscopy. Endoscopy. 2009; 41(6):510–515

[104] Freeman HJ, Nimmo M. Intestinal lymphangiectasia in adults. World J Gastrointest Oncol. 2011; 3(2):19–23

[105] Fang YH, Zhang BL, Wu JG, Chen CX. A primary intestinal lymphangiectasia patient diagnosed by capsule endoscopy and confirmed at surgery: a case report. World J Gastroenterol. 2007; 13(15):2263–2265

[106] Fry LC, Bellutti M, Neumann H, et al. Utility of double-balloon enteroscopy for the evaluation of malabsorption. Dig Dis. 2008; 26(2):134–139

[107] Missmer SA, Hankinson SE, Spiegelman D, et al. Incidence of laparoscopically confirmed endometriosis by demographic, anthropometric, and lifestyle factors. Am J Epidemiol. 2004; 160(8):784–796

[108] Sangi-Haghpeykar H, Poindexter AN, III. Epidemiology of endometriosis among parous women. Obstet Gynecol. 1995; 85(6):983–992

[109] Izuishi K, Sano T, Shiota A, et al. Small bowel obstruction caused by endometriosis in a postmenopausal woman. Asian J Endosc Surg. 2015; 8(2):205–208

[110] Nasr JY, Lloyd J, Yadav D. An unusual cause of fibrostenotic terminal ileal disease. Gastroenterology. 2011; 141(3):e5–e6

[111] Roman H, Abo C, Huet E, et al. Full-thickness disc excision in deep endometriotic nodules of the rectum: a prospective cohort. Dis Colon Rectum. 2015; 58(10):957–966

32 Sporadic Neoplastic Polyps of the Duodenum and Ampulla

Prashant Mudireddy and Gregory Haber

32.1 Introduction

Sporadic duodenal polyps are polyps seen in patients without a family history of genetic syndromes such as familial adenomatous polyposis (FAP). Both sporadic ampullary and nonampullary duodenal polyps are uncommon. They are usually found incidentally during upper endoscopy. With improvement in technology and devices, endoscopic resection is indicated for benign lesions. In this chapter, we discuss in detail endoscopic techniques and outcomes of endoscopic resection of both ampullary and nonampullary duodenal polyps.

32.2 Ampullary Neoplastic Polyps

The ampulla of Vater is a complex structure consisting of a papillary mound, a common pancreatobiliary channel, terminal bile duct, and terminal main pancreatic duct.[1] Ampullary neoplasms are uncommon with a reported incidence of about fewer than 1% of all gastrointestinal (GI) neoplasms and a prevalence of 0.04 to 0.12% in the general population.[2,3,4] Ampullary polyps can occur either sporadically or as a part of the genetic syndrome like FAP.[5] Endoscopic surveillance and resection remain the principal modalities for managing these patients. The surgical alternatives of a wide local excision or pancreaticoduodenal resection are reserved for those who fail or are not candidates for endotherapy.

32.2.1 Types of Ampullary Polyps

Ampullary polyps can be either benign or malignant. Adenomas are the most common benign ampullary polyps (▶Fig. 32.1).[2] Histologically, adenomas are further classified into tubular, villous, and tubulovillous. Adenomas of the ampulla follow an adenoma-to-carcinoma sequence similar to that for colon polyps.[6] The

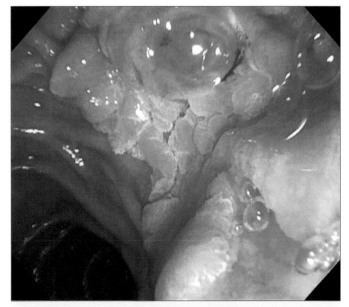

Fig. 32.1 Lateral spreading ampullary adenoma.

incidence of malignant transformation of ampullary adenomas to carcinomas ranges between 25 and 85%.[7] Adenomas and adenocarcinomas together constitute greater than 95% of ampullary tumors.[8] Less common benign ampullary tumors include gastric metaplasia, hyperplasia, lipomas, leiomyoma, lymphangioma, hamartoma, hemangioma, schwannoma, and neurogenic tumors.[2] Primary malignant lesions of the ampulla include adenocarcinoma, lymphoma, neuroendocrine, and signet-ring cell carcinoma.[2] Adenocarcinomas are the most common malignant lesions. Malignant lesions that can metastasize to the ampulla include melanoma, hypernephroma, breast carcinoma, and lymphoma.[2] See ▶Table 32.1.

32.2.2 Clinical Manifestations

Sporadic ampullary neoplasms are most commonly seen in patients in their 70s. They are usually asymptomatic and discovered incidentally on endoscopy or cross-sectional imaging. Patients may present with obstructive symptoms such as jaundice or pancreatitis, or bleeding which manifests as an obscure occult cause of anemia. Complaints of nausea, vomiting, or abdominal pain alone are uncommon manifestations of an ampullary lesion.[8,9] Jaundice is the most common symptom and seen in about 50 to 75% of patients.[8] Rarely, patients can develop cholangitis and pancreatitis.[8] In a single-center retrospective review of 157 patients with benign and malignant tumors of the ampulla, dark urine (odds ratio [OR] 14.18, 95% confidence interval [CI] 1.86–108), pruritus (OR 5.07, 95% CI 2.15–124.3), and jaundice (OR 67.24, 95% CI 15.17–297.7) were highly predictive of malignancy. Steatorrhea was moderately predictive of malignancy (OR 5.07, 95% CI 1.12–22.38). Presence of abdominal pain was more suggestive of benign tumor (OR 0.35, 95% CI 0.17–0.72).[9] See ▶Table 32.2.

In the same study, laboratory values predictive of malignancy were as follows: albumin less than 3.6 g/dL (OR 2.95, 95% CI 1.22–7.14), total bilirubin greater than 1.1 g/dL (OR 7.97, 95% CI 2.62–24.29), alkaline phosphatase greater than 126 (OR 9.73, 95% CI 3.81–24.29), alanine aminotransferase ALT greater than 47 U/L (OR 2.43, 95% CI 1.08–5.45) and aspartate aminotransferase (AST) greater than 55 U/L (OR 2.22, 95% CI 0.99–4.94). Pancreatic enzymes (amylase, lipase), white cell count, and hemoglobin were not predictive of

Table 32.1 Types of ampullary polyps

Benign	Malignant
Adenomas	Adenocarcinomas
Lipomas	Lymphomas
Fibroma	Neuroendocrine tumors
Leiomyoma	Signet-ring cell carcinoma
Lymphangioma	
Hamartoma	
Hemangioma	
Carcinoids	
Neurogenic tumors	

Table 32.2 Clinical manifestations of ampullary adenomas

Jaundice

Abdominal pain

Nausea

Vomiting

Fever, chills

Pruritus

Steatorrhea

Gastrointestinal (GI) bleed

Cholangitis

Pancreatitis

malignancy.[9] A cholestatic liver panel with elevation of liver alkaline phosphatase or gamma-glutamyl transpeptidase (GTP) is the most specific laboratory indication of an ampullary tumor. Transaminase may be mildly elevated with a spike in values associated with acute obstruction. Bilirubin elevations herald worse obstruction usually associated with malignancy. The only exception to this is cholangitis, as a manifestation of stone disease, which is a result of the stasis associated with ampullary tumors.

32.2.3 Diagnosis

Most ampullary polyps are found incidentally on endoscopy or cross-sectional imaging. With a forward-viewing endoscope it is often difficult to distinguish a duodenal polyp from an ampullary lesion. Most often duodenoscopy with a side-viewing endoscope is necessary for optimal visualization and evaluation of an ampullary lesion. Certain features of the endoscopic appearance may help predict the benign or malignant nature of the tumor. A benign ampullary lesion is characterized by a regular margins, soft consistency, and absence of ulceration or spontaneous bleeding.[8,10] On the other hand, firmness, ulceration, or friability suggest possible malignancy.[5] In a study of 56 patients with ampullary lesions failure to obtain a cleavage plane with submucosal injection was the strongest predictor of malignancy (OR 28.35, 95% CI 1.9–422.75) on multivariate analysis.[11]

Endoscopic biopsy of the ampulla is the mainstay of the histologic diagnosis. However, it is limited by high false-negative rates. In various studies the diagnostic yield of ampullary biopsies ranges from 45 to 80% with false-negative rates of 16 to 60%.[5] The difficulty in establishing a histologic diagnosis is attributable in part to a lack of an adequate specimen when the biopsy forceps are introduced across the right-angled elevator of a duodenoscope. A few strategies have been described to help improve the diagnostic yield of the endoscopic biopsy. These include obtaining at least six biopsy specimens and targeting the most suspicious areas such as depressed or ulcerated regions. Another maneuver to improve specimen acquisition is to grasp the tissue with the cup of the forceps but instead of pulling the forceps back into the channel of the scope, the tip of the scope is angled laterally away from the papilla to mechanically tear the tissue.[5] A definitive histologic evaluation may only be achieved after endoscopic ampullectomy (EA).[12] In a study by Sakorafas et al, about 50% of the ampullary tumors harbored foci of adenocarcinoma at the time of the diagnosis.[13] Endoscopic brush cytology is a helpful adjunctive technique especially when the tumor invades the wall of the bile or pancreatic duct manifests usually by the presence of a short stricture.[14,15] Diagnostic

yield of brush cytology varies from 18 to 70%.[14,15,16,17] In a study of 74 patients with pancreatobiliary strictures, brush cytology had a sensitivity of 56%, specificity of 100%, positive predictive value of 100%, negative predictive value of 51%, and accuracy of 70%.[15]

Other investigational techniques have included polymerase chain reaction (PCR) analysis of DNA for *K-Ras* gene mutations, immunohistochemical staining for p53 tumor suppressor gene, *CK7*, *CK20*, *CDX2*, *MUC1* and *MUC2*, microRNA expression, and assessment of aneuploidy by flow cytometry.[5]

Endoscopic Ultrasonography and Intraductal Ultrasound

Endoscopic ultrasonography (EUS) and intraductal ultrasound (IDUS) have been shown to be useful in the accurate T staging of the ampullary lesions. EUS operating at 7.5 to 10 MHz provides useful information as to the depth of the invasion of the duodenal wall and/or pancreatobiliary ducts, size and echogenicity of the tumor, and status of regional lymph nodes.[2,7] The reported accuracy of EUS in T staging varies between 56 and 91%, while N-stage accuracy varies between 50 and 81%.[2] EUS has been shown to be more accurate than computed tomography (CT) and magnetic resonance imaging (MRI) for T staging.

In a study of two centers comprising 50 patients, the accuracy of EUS for assessment of the T stage of ampullary neoplasms was 78% compared to 24% for CT and 46% for MRI. T-staging accuracy of EUS is decreased in the presence of a transpapillary endobiliary stent (84–72%). However, in nodal staging all three modalities were of similar efficacy (EUS 68%, CT 59%, MRI 77%, $p > 0.05$).[2,18]

IDUS utilizes frequencies between 20 and 30 MHz and is performed by advancing the ultrasound probe into the common bile duct (CBD) over a guidewire.[19] In three studies evaluating the accuracy of IDUS in T staging of ampullary neoplasms, the overall accuracy ranged between 78 and 93%.[19,20,21,22] In a prospective study of 27 patients, it was noted that IDUS was superior to EUS and CT in tumor visualization and staging (100 vs. 59.3 vs. 29.6%, respectively).[22] In another study by Ito et al, the overall accuracy of IDUS and EUS in tumor staging were similar (78 vs. 63%, respectively, $p = 0.14$).[21] Based on the limited evidence available IDUS has been shown to be slightly superior to EUS in T staging. However, IDUS is not widely utilized, is more invasive, and does not evaluate regional lymph node status.[2]

Is EUS needed in staging all the ampullary lesions? The consensus is divided among experts. In a survey of 79 expert biliary endoscopists (58% response rate), EUS was always utilized prior to ampullectomy by 67% responders, but only selectively by 31% of responders.[23] Some experts suggest foregoing EUS examination for lesions less than 1 cm in size and for those without obvious signs of malignancy as described earlier.[21] Suggested criteria for the performance of EUS/IDUS prior to therapy for ampullary lesions include size greater than 3 cm, malignant features observed on endoscopy, and biopsies showing high-grade dysplasia (HGD) or carcinoma in situ/T1 cancer.[24]

Computed Tomography, Magnetic Resonance Imaging

MRI with cholangiopancreatography provides noninvasive assessment of the distal CBD and pancreatic ducts. It provides information about intraductal extension, ductal dilation, and anatomical variants such as pancreatic divisum.[25] CT is the most suitable for evaluation of vascular invasion and distant metastasis.[7]

32.2.4 Management of Ampullary Neoplasms

Malignant ampullary lesions and benign lesions unsuitable for endoscopic therapy are treated surgically.[5] Pancreaticoduodenectomy (Whipple's) and surgical ampullectomy (SA) are the two surgical options available. Pancreaticoduodenectomy allows complete resection of the lesions and has a very low recurrence rate but is associated with considerable morbidity and a risk of mortality. The common postoperative complications include anastomotic dehiscence (up to 9%), and fistulae (up to 14%), as well as nausea, weight loss, early satiety, and altered bowel habits.[5] The mortality rates reported in literature range between 1 and 9%, although in high-volume centers performing Whipple's resection, the mortality rate is generally 2% or less.[5] Wide local excision is less invasive and involves removal of the entire ampulla of Vater with reimplantation of the CBD and pancreatic duct into the duodenal wall.[5] In a retrospective review comparing local excision to Whipple, SA was associated with statistically lower operative time (169 vs. 268 minutes), estimated blood loss (192 vs. 727 mL), mean length of stay (10 vs. 25 days), and overall morbidity (29 vs. 78%).[26] However, SA has been associated with recurrence rates ranging from 20 to as high as 50%.[27]

EA or more specifically papillectomy involves the resection of the mucosal layers and the superficial submucosal layers of the ampulla of Vater.[25,28] It is a minimally invasive technique with a high success rate and provides a safer and less invasive alternative to surgical therapy in appropriately selected cases.[5] There are no randomized trials comparing (EA to SA. However, in a retrospective study of 109 patients, EA (68 patients) was equivalent to SA (41 patients) in terms of success in the treatment for benign lesions. At the same time EA patients had a significantly reduced length of stay, lower morbidity, and readmission rates. There was no difference in the rates of mortality (0% each), margin positive excisions (20 vs. 10%, $p = 0.19$), or reinterventions (26 vs. 15%). These authors favored EA as an initial treatment strategy, reserving surgery as an option for those with unsuccessful endotherapy.[29]

32.2.5 Endoscopic Ampullectomy

EA involves resection of the ampullary lesion to the level of the submucosa. It was first described by Suzuki et al in 1983.[30] Ten years later the first case series describing the use of EA for resection of the benign ampullary adenomas was reported by Binmoeller et al. They reported a case series of 25 patients where standard snare polypectomy technique was used to resect the lesions.[31] Since then multiple case series have been reported for benign ampullary lesions.

Indications

The 2015 American Society of Gastrointestinal Endoscopy (ASGE) guidelines on the role of endoscopy in the management of ampullary adenomas do not define precise indications for EA.[5] The

general recommendations for endoscopic resection are benign histology, lack of malignant features at endoscopy, and absence of intraductal extension on EUS/IDUS. However, endoscopic techniques to manage intraductal extension have been described.

There is no consensus on the size of the ampullary adenoma that is amenable to endoscopic resection. Based on a retrospective review of 33 patients, Kim et al suggested that polyps greater than 1.5 cm or those with HGD may not be suitable for endoscopic resection due to coexistence of cancer and a high recurrence rate. In this study, polyps with low-grade dysplasia (LGD) were 1.27 +/- 0.089 cm in size, polyps with HGD were 1.81 +/- 0.99 cm in size and cancer group had a size of 1.98+/- 1.08 cm. There was a significant correlation between the size of the polyp and final pathology ($p = 0.036$).[32] In another retrospective study of 157 patients, benign ampullary lesions had a median size of 1.3 cm while adenocarcinomas had a size of 2 cm.[9] On the other hand some experts recommend that ampullary lesions up to 4 to 5 cm can be removed endoscopically as long as these are benign.[2,28,31,33,34] Although there is a correlation between size and the risk of malignancy, in the absence of evidence for invasive cancer, size alone is not a contraindication to endoscopic resection.

Another area of controversy in EA is the presence of intraductal extension. Some experts suggest that EA can be attempted when intraductal extension is limited to less than 10 mm.[2,28,35,36] In a study by Bohnacker et al, 31 patients had extension of adenomatous growth into the biliary or pancreatic ducts (two patients had extension into both the ducts) and 75 patients had no intraductal extension. The rate of curative successful endoscopic therapy in the group with intraductal extension was 43% whereas in the group without intraductal extension it was 83%. Surgery was more frequently needed in the group with intraductal extension either due to incomplete removal or recurrence (37% vs. 12%, $p < 0.001$). The authors concluded that in experienced endoscopist hands limited intraductal involvement is accessible to endoscopic removal and suitable for endoscopic therapy, because in about 50% surgery can be avoided.[37]

In summary, size alone is not a contraindication to endoscopic resection provided there is no optical or sonographic evidence for submucosal invasion, the endoscopic features of ulceration, woody hard tissue, or submucosal extension are worrisome features for invasion. Further evaluation by EUS should then be considered. As noted in the study by Kim et al, lesions with HGD may harbor foci of cancer and the pathology of the resected tumor will determine the need for subsequent surgery.[32]

EA Technique

EA is an advanced endoscopic procedure which needs considerable expertise and experience.[25] The basic technique of EA is similar to the principle used for colonoscopic polypectomy. Complete en bloc resection is preferred because it allows more accurate histologic assessment and negligible recurrence.[25] Complete en bloc resection also ensures complete removal of adenomatous tissue abutting the biliary and pancreatic orifices. For lesions with extrapapillary extension to adjacent duodenal mucosa, the papilla should be resected as a single piece and the remainder resected in as few pieces as possible (▶ Fig. 32.2).[25] Use of chromoendoscopy (using methylene blue or indigo

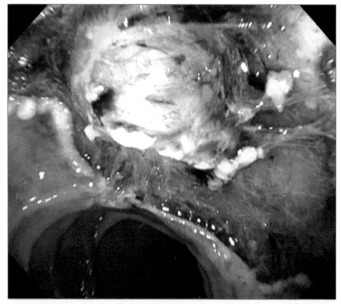

Fig. 32.2 Post endoscopic ampullectomy.

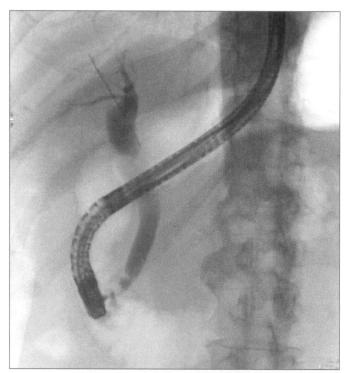

Fig. 32.3 Intraductal extension of ampullary tumor.

carmine) and narrow-band imaging (NBI) has been described to define the lateral margins of the ampullary polyps.[38,39,40,41] Itoi et al noted that NBI had a statistically significant advantage over chromoendoscopy with indigo carmine in defining the lateral margins ($p < 0.05$).[41]

Equipment

There is no evidence to suggest that one type of snare is superior to others. The snare size is chosen according to the size of the adenoma to ensure en bloc resection. A comparison of "braided" polypectomy snares and fine wire snares has been reported.[5] Use of thin wire snares is advocated by some experts because they maximize current density for swift resection of the adenoma and limit dispersion of energy.[25] We prefer soft wire oval or hexagonal snare, which facilitates positioning of the snare over the ampulla when advanced across the elevation of the duodenoscope. We also groom the snare by manually creating a gentle curve at the tip of the closed snare prior to insertion into the accessory channel to allow smooth passage of the snare across the right angle turn over the elevator of the duodenoscope.

There are no standardized electrocautery settings for EP. The goal of the thermal energy is to achieve cutting with enough coagulation to seal vessels, but avoiding thermal injury to the pancreas. We typically use an ERBE generator with a setting of Endocut Q, effect 3, duration 2, and interval 3 (ERBE USA Inc., Marietta, Georgia, United States; Olympus ESG-100, Tokyo, Japan).[25]

Technique

First step is to perform endoscopic retrograde cholangiopancreatography (ERCP) with deep cannulation and contrast injection to obtain a cholangiogram and a pancreatogram. This will identify strictures or intraductal extension of the tumor

(▶Fig. 32.3 ;**Video 32.1**, **Video 32.2**). It also helps recannulation postresection as a roadmap of the ductal anatomy is shown. In some cases cannulation is not possible prior to resection due to distortion of the anatomy and friability and bleeding in more advanced lesions may be present. In such cases postresection cannulation is often easier once the tumor bulk has been removed.[25] Some experts suggest injecting methylene blue along with contrast into the pancreatic duct to help identify the pancreatic duct orifice postpapillectomy as the flow of blue contrast marks the orifice.[42] Sphincterotomy should generally be performed postpapillectomy. Pre-EA sphincterotomy can hinder en bloc resection and complete histologic evaluation of the resected specimen due to thermal injury. It may increase the risk of bleeding, perforation, and tumor seeding.[8] Use of submucosal fluid injection prior to resection is controversial. Fluid injection may increase technical success and decrease complications.[31,43] Epinephrine helps to decrease bleeding and methylene blue or indigo carmine enhances endoscopic visualization of the margins of the adenoma. However, submucosal injection may cause difficulty in the resection of small lesions. The center of the ampullary lesion is tethered down by the biliary and pancreatic ducts and may not lift. Fluid injection results in elevation of the mucosa at the margins of the papilla with a resultant "donut" effect in which the adenoma is partially buried by the elevated surrounding mucosa. This may prevent good snare entrapment and compromise complete excision.[43]

The snare is advanced through the accessory channel of the duodenoscope. The snare is opened in a line corresponding to the long axis of the mound. The snare tip is fixed above the top of the papilla and snare is carefully opened and drawn over the papilla with the heel of the snare laid down below the inferior margin of the lesion while maintaining the position of the tip of the snare. Then snare is closed slowly entrapping the papilla and resection completed using electrocautery.[25] After the resection, the specimen should be retrieved as soon as possible before it migrates distally into the small bowel. Antiperistaltic agents such as hyoscine butylbromide 10 to 20 mg or glucagon 0.5 to 1 mg may be given intravenously prior to starting resection to decrease peristalsis.[25] Expeditious retrieval of the specimen can be achieved simply using the same snare used for resection. The specimen can be pulled up to the stomach and if it is 2 cm or greater, it is easier to drop the specimen and retrap it with a retrieval net before pulling it up through the esophagus. Alternatively, the retrieval net may be used from the outset provided the specimen is not falling down the duodenal sweep. Aspiration of the specimen through the accessory channel should be avoided to prevent fragmentation of the lesion.[5]

Pancreatic Stenting

The first priority after EP should be placement of a pancreatic duct stent.[25] EP is associated with increased risk of post-procedural pancreatitis.[5] A meta-analysis of five studies (481 patients) showed that prophylactic pancreatic duct stenting prevents post-ERCP pancreatitis. Patients in no stent group had threefold higher odds of developing pancreatitis compared to the stent group (15.5 vs. 5.8%, OR = 3.2, 95% CI 1.6–6.4).[44] In general, the PD stent is placed postampullectomy but the option of preampullectomy stent placement has been evaluated. Placing the pancreatic duct stent prior to EP might be technically easier as there is no edema or cautery-related changes. A preresection pancreatic stent may also protect the pancreatic orifice from thermal injury.[2] The problem is that a preresection stent may interfere with en bloc resection. Recently Hwang et al described use of an insulated pancreatic stent in 11 patients. They placed a 5 F polytetrafluoroethylene-insulated pancreatic stent prior to EA. Then the stent and tumor were simultaneously grasped with snare. Tumor was resected with stent in place and then specimen retrieved by perpendicular needle knife incision of the snared ampullary tumor along the edge of the stent. There was no stent migration or stent-related complications. No episodes of acute pancreatitis or perforation occurred. There were four episodes of mild bleeding and one episode of late papillary stenosis.[45] Although this approach is well crafted and a way to ensure a pancreatic stent is left in situ, it is unlikely that postampullectomy stent placement in the same patients would be a problem. The same patients in whom pancreatic stent placement is difficult postprocedure are the ones in whom preampullectomy stent placement would be difficult.

The size of the pancreatic stent is not standardized. In most reported case series 5-F stents have been used, followed by 3 F and 7 F. Placing a 5-F stent might be easier and faster.[2] The principle for pancreatic stenting is to minimize damage to the duct while maintaining adequate drainage in the immediate postampullectomy period. The stent size which best approximates the duct diameter with no internal flange is most suitable. If there is tortuosity at the genu, a shorter stent which is limited to the duct in the head of the pancreas is preferable. Duration of the pancreatic stent varies widely from 24 hours to 3 months.[2] Some experts recommend stent removal after 1 to 3 days to minimize stent-induced ductal changes, while others suggest leaving the stents for 1 to 2 months to prevent stenosis.[2] As the majority of stents will migrate out spontaneously, especially postampullectomy in which the sphincter is often removed or reduced in function, we wait 2 weeks to assess migration and if the stent is still in place, it is removed endoscopically. At the same time we will inspect the resection site and remove any residual polyp tissue.[43] In spite of the general recommendation for prophylactic pancreatic stents this is not mandatory. In patients in whom the pancreatic orifice is widely patulous postampullectomy, there is no utility in placing a pancreatic stent.

Biliary Sphincterotomy and Stenting

Routine biliary stenting is not recommended.[5] However, in certain situations biliary sphincterotomy and stenting can be performed. Biliary sphincterotomy is most useful when there is evidence of intraductal extension of the tumor. A sphincterotomy helps expose and resect the intraductal portion of the polyp using avulsion or snare excision of the tumor. A balloon-tipped catheter has been used with a dual device technique. The balloon is used to pull the polypoid tissue down out of the duct and a coaxial 5-F snare is used simultaneously to resect the intraductal portion of the polyp (**Video 32.3**).[46,47] The fully covered biliary metal stent has several benefits with respect to ampullectomy. In the event of significant bleeding, the stent effectively tamponades the vessel. If there is suspected or possible perforation, especially with intraductal resection, the fully covered self-expandable metal stent (FCSEMS) prevents extravasation and allow healing. Finally, when intraductal access is difficult, placing a FCSEMS for 6 to 8 weeks dilates the biliary orifice and permits intraductal inspection and therapy for intraductal extension of the adenoma.

Ablation of Residual Tissue

With en bloc resection, residual polyp tissue is minimal and easy to remove. The likelihood of residual tissue increases especially in the terminal ends of the ducts as the snare ampullectomy may not entrap this recessed area of polypoid tissue. Different ablative therapies have been described namely, argon plasma coagulation (APC), monopolar or bipolar electrocoagulation, laser therapy, and photocoagulation.[5] Pulsed APC at effect 2 and 20 to 25 W is the most commonly used ablative therapy as it is widely available and minimizes depth of tissue injury (▶ Fig. 32.4; **Video 32.4**, **Video 32.5**). Performing a biliary sphincterotomy exposes intraductal tumor margin. Adenoma

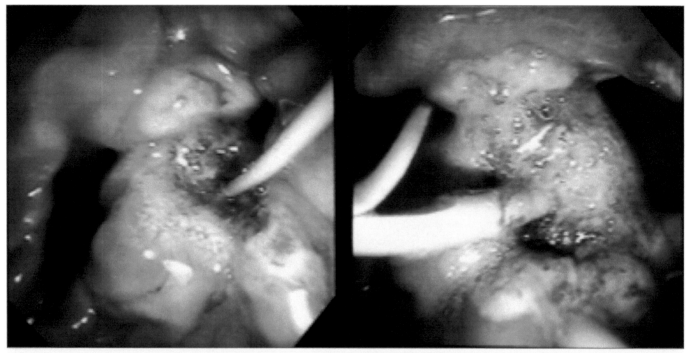

Fig. 32.4 Ablation of residual ampullary adenoma with APC.

which involves the pancreatic ductal orifice is best ablated with APC around a previously placed pancreatic duct stent.[43]

32.2.6 Endoscopic Outcomes: Clinical Success, Recurrence Rates

The reported clinical success rates of EA in literature ranges between 46 and 92% with recurrence rates between 0 and 33%, the wide divergence in results clearly related to case selection.[2,5] Moreover, the definition of clinical success and recurrence is not uniform among the published studies. In one of the large case series of 103 patients, the success rate of EA was 80%. Success in this study included patients treated with a repeat endoscopic procedure for recurrence.[48] Another large series of 106 patients included patients with intraductal growth (75) and without intraductal growth (31). The clinical success rate in patients with intraductal growth was 43% compared to 83% in the group without intraductal extension.[37]

A multicenter retrospective study evaluated the predictors of EA success. On multivariate analysis, age greater than 48 years, polyp size of 2.4 cm or less, male sex, and absence of genetic predisposition to adenoma development were predictive of success.[43] Another single-center study observed that smaller adenomas (< 2 cm) and absence of dilated ducts affected success rate.[49] See ▶ Table 32.3 for details.

Adverse Events

The overall adverse event rates reported in the literature range between 8 and 35%.[50] Underlying malignancy and lateral extension have been reported as risk factors for complications.[5] The adverse events related to EP can be divided into early and late complications. Early complications include pancreatitis, bleeding, perforation, cholangitis, and sedation-related adverse events. The major late adverse event is papillary stenosis (biliary and pancreatic).[5]

The risk of pancreatitis ranges between 5 and 15%. Most pancreatitis episodes are mild to moderate and resolve with conservative management.[50] The risk of bleeding ranges from 2 to 16%. Mild bleeding can be managed by endoscopic hemostasis, but major bleeding may need angiography and embolization. The perforation is usually retroperitoneal and risk ranges between 0 and 4%. Small perforations can be managed conservatively while large perforations or perforation in hemodynamically unstable patients may require surgery for drainage and repair.[8,25] The risk of cholangitis is 0 to 2% and repeat ERCP with sphincterotomy and/or stent resolves this problem.[8] Papillary stenosis is relatively uncommon, usually less than 2% of EA. This is managed in the usual fashion with sphincterotomy or extension of a prior cut, along with balloon dilation and FCSEMS.[50] Mortality from EA is rare but has been reported to be about 0.4% (0–7%).[5,50] See ▶ Table 32.3 for details.

32.2.7 Surveillance

Patients who have undergone EA need ongoing surveillance, the interval depending on whether the index polyp is sporadic or a manifestation of FAP. The ASGE recommends adoption of a surveillance program that is similar to patients with colon polyps with piecemeal resection taking into account degree of dysplasia, evidence of intraductal extension, and genetic predisposition.[5] In general, the first surveillance is performed 3 to 6 months after the index procedure and further surveillance endoscopies are performed from 6 to 12 months for at least 2 years and subsequently depending on the risk factors as outlined above.[5] End points of surveillance are not well established.[5] Surveillance endoscopy is best performed with a duodenoscope with biopsy of

Table 32.3 Summary of studies on endoscopic ampullectomy—outcomes, recurrence rates, complications

Study, Year (ref)	No. of patients	Success rate %	Recurrence rate %	Complica-tion %	Pancreati-tis%	Bleeding%	Perfora-tion%	Mortality%
Binmoeller et al,[a] 1993[31]	25	92	26	20	12	8	0	0
Martin et al,[b] 1997[10]	14	50	NA	13	7	7	0	7
Vogt et al,[b] 2000[51]	18	67	33	28	11	11	0	0
Desilets et al,[b] 2001[33]	13	92	0	8	8	0	0	0
Zádorová et al,[c] 2001[52]	16	81	19	25	13	13	0	0
Norton et al,[a] 2002[53]	26	46	10	35	15	8	4	0
Saurin et al,[c] 2003[54]	24	67	6	29	4	NR	NR	0
Catalano et al,[c] 2004[48]	103	80	10	10	5	2	0	0
Cheng et al,[c] 2004[34]	55	74	33	15	9	7	2	0
Bohnacker et al,[c] 2005[37]	106	73	15	33	12	25	0	0
Eswaran et al,[c] 2006[55]	51	92	NA	10	2	8	0	0
Irani et al,[c] 2009[49]	102	84	8	21	10	5	0	0
Jung et al,[b] 2009[56]	22	55	17	23	18	1	5	0
Hopper et al,[a] 2010[57]	23	91	9	20	0	16	0	0
Yamao et al,[c] 2010[58]	36	81	3	19	8	8	0	0
Jeanniard-Malet et al,[a] 2011[59]	42	88	12	24	14	7	0	0
Patel et al,[c] 2011[60]	38	81	16	16	8	5	0	0
Ito et al,[a] 2012[61]	28	86	14	53	3.5	28.5	7	0
Salmi et al,[b] 2012[62]	61	82	34	18	10	5	3	0
Napoleon et al,[c] 2014[63]	93	90	5	42	20	10	3.6	1
Ismail et al,[a] 2014[64]	61	92	20	25	10	18	0	0
Ridtitid et al,[c] 2014[65]	182	74	9	19	4	13	0	0.5

NR, not reported.

[a]Studies in which polyp was resected in single session.

[b]Studies in which number of sessions needed to complete resection not reported.

[c]Studies in which success was defined as total removal of the polyp irrespective of the number of sessions required for removal and absence of residual polyp or residual polyp during follow-up period treated completely endoscopically.

the resection scar. The need to obtain a cholangiogram and/or pancreatogram at follow-up is contingent on the presenting pathology and potential for intraductal extension.[2]

32.3 Conclusion

Sporadic ampullary neoplastic lesions are uncommon. Endoscopic and surgical options are available for management of these lesions. It is important to stage larger lesions accurately with EUS/IDUS, CT, and/or MRI. For benign lesions, EA is a safe and effective treatment option with low mortality and morbidity compared to surgical wide local excision or a Whipple operation. EA when performed by experts has a success rate of greater than 80%.

32.4 Nonampullary Sporadic Neoplastic Duodenal Polyps

Nonampullary duodenal polyps can occur as part of the genetic syndrome FAP or sporadically. The prevalence of duodenal polyps ranges between 0.3 and 1.5% based on two retrospective

studies.[66,67] However, in a prospective study of 584 patients undergoing upper endoscopy, the prevalence of duodenal polyps was 4.6%.[68] Surgery is associated with significant mortality and morbidity and recurrence rate may be high even when local excision is performed.[69] Endoscopic treatment is challenging due to the thin duodenal wall and rich vascular supply.[69] Additional challenges occur with bulky lesions, which may reduce the working space in a narrowed lumen.[70]

32.4.1 Types of Nonampullary Duodenal Polyps

Duodenal polyps can be neoplastic or nonneoplastic. In a retrospective review of 50,114 upper endoscopies, 510 patients were diagnosed to have duodenal polyps. Of these, a total of 221 lesions were biopsied. Nonneoplastic polyps were found in 196 patients and neoplastic polyps in 25 patients. On multivariate analysis, polyps greater than 10 mm and polyps in the second portion of the duodenum were independent risk factors for being neoplastic.[71] This study also noted that neoplastic polyps were larger than nonneoplastic polyps ($p < 0.01$). Neoplastic

Table 32.4 Types of nonampullary lesions

Nonneoplastic	Neoplastic
Brunner's gland hyperplasia	Adenomas
Gastric heterotopia	Carcinoids
Hyperplastic polyps	Solitary Peutz–Jeghers type polyps
Inflammatory type polyps	Metastatic cancer

duodenal polyps include adenomas, carcinoids, solitary Peutz–Jeghers type polyps, and metastatic cancer.[69,71] Nonneoplastic polyps include Brunner's gland hyperplasia, gastric heterotopia, inflammatory type polyps, and hyperplastic polyps.[69,71] See ▶ Table 32.4.

Carcinoids

These are rare and account for less than 5% of all carcinoids.[71] Most common location is the duodenal bulb. These are usually submucosal. EUS assessment helps assess the size, depth of invasion, and lymph node status. Carcinoids are challenging as a vertical R0 resection is difficult due to the submucosal location. Almost always, regardless of the resection technique, negative margins are difficult to achieve. The best method for achieving R0 resection is endoscopic submucosal dissection (ESD) with deep submucosal dissection. However, this is a high-risk procedure for perforation due to the thin muscularis propria layer. Many expert endoscopists have abandoned attempts at ESD. An alternative method is rubber band and snare, but again the risk of perforation is high. Injection, lift, and snare may be less risky, but the likelihood of R0 resection is low. Novel approaches with the over-the-scope (OTSC) clip has been introduced in an attempt to achieve complete resection with protection against perforation. The carcinoid can be suctioned into the cap and following release of the large clip, the entrapped tumor is left in situ. At follow-up endoscopy 2 weeks later, the lesion can be snared off the clip. The clip subsequently falls off or can be removed endoscopically. The new full-thickness OTSC device may prove to be useful if the size of the current colon device is reduced sufficiently to allow atraumatic passage down the upper GI tract. Lesion 1 cm or less are most suitable. Lesions 1 to 2 cm in size are somewhat more challenging. Lesions greater than 2 cm have a higher risk of nodal spread and generally require surgical excision.

Hamartomas

These are seen in patients without a history of Peutz–Jeghers syndrome. Three cases of such polyps were reported by Suzuki et al.[72] These lesions have a lobular or nodular surface. The size can vary with giant hamartomas being more challenging to excise. Endoscopic resection is indicated due to the small risk of malignant transformation.[69,72]

Adenomas

Adenomas are the most common neoplastic polyps in the duodenum. It is estimated that up to 30 to 85% of duodenal adenomas may undergo malignant transformation.[73] In a study of the natural history of sporadic nonampullary duodenal polyps, HGD and

lesion size greater than or equal to 2 cm were found to be risk factors for progression to adenocarcinoma.[74,75] Spigelman's classification is commonly used to risk stratify patients (i.e., predict the risk of developing adenocarcinoma) with duodenal polyposis. The duodenal polyposis is classified on a 5-grade scale (stages 0–4) based on number of polyps (1–4, 5–20, > 20), size of the polyps (1–4 mm, 5–10 mm, > 10 mm), histology (tubular, tubulovillous, villous), and degree of dysplasia (mild, moderate, severe). Higher the stage, greater the risk of adenocarcinoma (stage 4 has the highest risk).[76]

32.4.2 Diagnosis

As most small polyps do not cause symptoms, the diagnosis is usually made incidentally during upper endoscopy. Biopsy of enlarged folds or protuberances to confirm the nature of the polyp is obtained.[5] It is mandatory to ensure that these polyps do not involve the major papilla. Examination with a side-viewing endoscope is mandatory for those lesions located in the second portion of the duodenum, unless a clear unequivocal view is obtained with a forward-viewing scope.[5]

Endoscopic Ultrasonography

The role of EUS in the nonampullary duodenal polyps is not well defined.[5] EUS is helpful to determine the depth of invasion, lymph node status in large lesions (≥ 2 cm), and in lesions with malignant features. It may not be useful in small and benign-appearing lesions.[5]

32.4.3 Management of Nonampullary Duodenal Adenomas

Treatment options include endoscopic or surgical resection. The third option of simple observation should always be considered in patients for whom intervention is risky with endoscope resection. The ability of a patient to sustain a complication or surgical repair must be taken into account prior to embarking on resection. The method of resection is dependent on the size and histology of the polyp. Surgical options include extensive duodenal segmental resection, submucosal excision after duodenotomy, or pancreatoduodenectomy.

Indications

There are no clear guidelines suggesting which lesions should be resected endoscopically versus surgically. The 2015 ASGE guidelines suggest that in general lesions occupying greater than one-third circumference of the lumen are more challenging and the option of surgery should be considered.[5] This is due to a high rate of adverse events associated with endoscopic resection of large lesions.[5] In study by Fanning et al, lesions greater than 3 cm had significantly higher adverse events (26.3%) when compared with lesions less than 3 cm (3.2%). The most common adverse event is bleeding.[77] Surgical resection may be an alternative for massive lesions extending across several folds and with circumferential

Technique

The most commonly described technique in the literature for resection of the nonampullary duodenal polyps is endoscopic mucosal resection (EMR). Other less common techniques are ESD and APC ablation.[73]

Endoscopic Mucosal Resection

In general, EMR of duodenal polyps is similar to EMR elsewhere in the GI tract. The first step is to evaluate the location of the lesion in relation to the major papilla with a side-viewing endoscope. For lesions occupying the anterior and medial wall of the duodenum, it may be advantageous to use a side-viewing scope and for lesions occupying the lateral and posterior walls, a gastroscope or pediatric colonoscope in which the accessory channel is at 5 to 6 oclock may provide better access to the lesion.[79] The use of a 4'-mm cap is often helpful to displace folds as well as to isolate bleeding vessels when hemorrhage occurs. Injection of glucagon or hyoscine butylbromide intravenously just prior to initiating EMR is helpful if peristalsis is vigorous. The first step is to inject a solution submucosally to create a fluid cushion. We use normal saline mixed with epinephrine and methylene blue or indigo carmine (18.5-cc saline, 1.5-cc 1:10,000 epinephrine, and few a drops of dye). Methylene blue or indigo carmine helps to define the plane of resection because the injection is confined to the submucosa as the fluid disperses in this plane. In case of large lesions, it may be necessary to inject multiple times between the resections. Once an appropriate fluid cushion is achieved, the lesion can be resected using a free hand snare technique. For lesions up to 2 cm, en bloc resection can be attempted and for larger lesions piecemeal resection provides more control and a safer resection. Because of the compliance and elasticity of the duodenal submucosa, circumferential or near circumferential fluid cushions may compromise the lumen making visualization more difficult (**Video 32.6**).

For flat or carpet-like lesions, we prefer using a stiffer snare such as the Captivator II (Boston Scientific, Marlborough, Massachusetts, United States) and Histalock (US Endoscopy, Mentor, Ohio, United States) . On the other hand, when using a duodenoscope, a softer snare such as the Accusnare (Cook Medical, Bloomington, Indiana) is easier to manipulate across the elevator. EMR should be initiated at one lateral margin, usually proximal and advanced distally. In this regard, there is no absolute rule and removal of the easiest part of the polyp first allows for isolation of the difficult areas. We use an electrocautery setting of Endocut Q with effect of 3, duration 1 or 2, and interval 4 or 5 (ERBE USA Inc., Marietta, Georgia, United States). For larger lesions or if bleeding is a problem, we often "prime" the plane of resection with forced coagulation, effect 1 at 25 W. When there are small residual pieces that remain in the center and at the edges of the resection margin, we use the avulsion technique. Avulsion is a technique in which a hot biopsy forceps is used to grasp the adherent unsnareable neoplastic polyp tissue and removal is achieved with a combination of mechanical tension and application of short bursts of high energy that result in shearing of tissue. The electrocautery setting used is Endocut I with effect of 3, duration 1, and interval 2 or 3 (ERBE USA Inc., Marietta, Georgia, United States). We do not commonly use APC to ablate the residual polyp tissue as the completeness of ablation is difficult to assess. Moreover, central adherent remnants may harbor cancer and we prefer to harvest this tissue for histologic evaluation. Most lesions are resected in a single session, but for large carpet lesions multiple sessions may be needed (**Video 32.7**). Whereas in the colon multiple sessions result in scar tissue that tethers the residual polyp, in the duodenum this is less of a problem. The higher risk of bleeding in large resected areas allows for the option of partial removal and a repeat session at a later date. Given the high risk of bleeding, we often close the polypectomy defect with clips when feasible. In cases where endoscopic closure is not possible (e.g., large polypectomy defect), we use the closed end of a hot biopsy forceps to coagulate the visible vessels at the base of the polypectomy defect. We use a soft coagulation mode on the ERBE, effect 6, 60 W (ERBE USA Inc., Marietta, Georgia, United States). Gentle coaptive coagulation is achieved, but care must be taken to avoid immediate or delayed perforation as the wall is very thin.

Variations of Endoscopic Mucosal Resection

Cap-assisted EMR (EMR-C) and underwater EMR techniques have been described in the literature.[78,80] Conio et al described the use of EMR-C in 26 patients with nonampullary duodenal adenomas. An intermediate-size straight cap (MH-594, 13.9 mm; Olympus) is preloaded on the tip of a forward-viewing endoscope. Inside the distal end of the cap there is a gutter in which the opened polypectomy snare is situated. After creation of a submucosal fluid cushion, the cap is applied against the lesion and aspirated by controlled suction. To minimize the risk of perforation continuous suction was avoided. The prepositioned snare is quickly closed to secure the tissue and the polyp is resected using an Endocut polyp mode.[78]

Underwater EMR has been described by Binmoeller et al in 12 patients. The duodenal lumen is filled with sterile distilled water heated to body temperature (36°C). The lesion is marked with APC. EMR is performed using a 15-mm duckbill snare (Accusnare, Cook Medical, Winston-Salem, North Carolina, United States) with blended current (Dry Cut effect 5, 60 W on ERBE).[80] According to the authors, when the duodenal lumen is filled with water, the adenoma-bearing tissue "floats" in the water and gives an appearance similar to the submucosal lift seen after the injection. This helps in resection of the lesion without submucosal injection.[80]

32.4.4 Outcomes of Endoscopic Mucosal Resection

The success of EMR in the complete resection of the nonampullary duodenal polyps ranges between 55 and 100% among the published studies. See ▶ Table 32.5 for details. The definition of complete resection varies among these studies. Some authors suggest that the success of EMR is dependent on the experience and expertise of the endoscopist.[79] The reported recurrence rate post-EMR of the nonampullary duodenal polyps ranges between 0 and 37%. In majority of the studies the

Table 32.5 Summary of studies on nonampullary duodenal polyps—outcomes, recurrence rates, complications

Study, year (ref)	No. of patients	No. of polyps	Success rate %	Recurrence rate %	Bleeding %	Perforation %
Hirasawa et al, 1997[81]	13	14	100	0	0	0
Apel et al, 2005[82]	18	20	55	25	10	0
Lépilliez, 2008[83]	36	37	97	0	11.6	2.7
Alexander et al, 2009[79]	23	21	100	24	5	0
Honda et al, 2009[84]	14	15	100	NR	17	22
Abbass et al, 2010[85]	59	59	98	37	3	0
Conio et al, 2012[78]	26	26	96	11.5	11.5	0
Binmoeller et al, 2013[80]	12	12	92	0	25	0
Navaneethan et al, 2014[86]	54	54	73	27	4.6	2.3

recurrent adenoma was treated with either repeat endoscopic resection or ablation.[73]

Adenomas greater than 2 cm in size and those with a villous component were found to have higher recurrence rate.[85,86] Kedia et al reported the efficacy of EMR compared to the size and luminal extent of the duodenal polyps. In their study, complete endoscopic resection rate for lesions occupying less than 25% of the luminal circumference was 94.7%, while for lesions occupying greater than 25% of the circumference, the resection rate was 45.5%. Hence, they concluded that luminal extension of the lesion was the strongest predictor of the EMR success of the nonampullary duodenal polyps.[87] See ▶ Table 32.5.

32.4.5 Adverse Events

The adverse events associated with EMR of duodenal polyps include bleeding, perforation, and serositis. Bleeding can be both immediate during the index procedure or delayed. The immediate or intraprocedural bleeding rate has been reported to be about 9%.[69] Various techniques that can be employed to control bleeding include clips, coagulation with closed biopsy forceps or other thermal devices, and simple epinephrine injection.[69] The late bleeding rate reported in the literature varies between 0 and 12%. In one study of 50 nonampullary duodenal polyps, size was predictive of late bleeding. Lesions greater than 3 cm were significantly associated with bleeding compared to lesions less than 3 cm (26.3 vs. 3.2%). In this study, all the late bleeding occurred within the first 48 hours.[77] Bleeding was controlled with mono- or bipolar cautery, clips, epinephrine, or combination of these maneuvers.[77] Given the high bleeding rate, in patents with comorbidities, and large resection sites not amenable to clip closure, we admit the patient overnight for observation.

The perforation rate reported after EMR of nonampullary duodenal polyps is 0.6%.[69] This occurs more often with larger lesions. Small microperforations may be managed either conservatively by keeping the patient nil by mouth and giving intravenous antibiotics. Large perforations require surgical intervention. Serositis has been reported in 0.6% of EMRs. This is managed conservatively with antibiotics.[79] See ▶ Table 32.5.

32.4.6 Post–Endoscopic Mucosal Resection Care

An Australian group described their routine protocol after EMR of large duodenal lesions. They observe patients for 4 hours before discharge and patients are advised to follow a clear liquid diet on the day of the procedure. Patients can resume regular diet next day. Proton pump inhibitors (PPIs) are prescribed twice daily for 2 weeks postprocedure.[77] We follow a protocol similar to the above. We admit patients to hospital for overnight observation post-EMR of large polyps or if any intraprocedural complications occur. Other patients are discharged the same day especially when closure of the mucosal defect is achieved with clips. Patients are advised to maintain a liquid diet for 24 hours and advanced thereafter to a soft diet for 1 week. We prescribe PPIs twice daily for 1 month.

32.4.7 Role of Endoscopic Submucosal Dissection

ESD has been widely used in the resection of esophageal, gastric, and colon lesions; its use in duodenum is limited by a much higher risk of adverse events.[5,88] Narrow lumen, thin wall, and retroperitoneal fixation make ESD in the duodenum especially difficult.[88] In studies where ESD was used to resect duodenal adenomas, the bleeding rate was 8 to 22% and the perforation rate was 23 to 35%.[5,88] Hence, ESD is not recommended at this time for resection of duodenal lesions.[5]

32.4.8 Surveillance

There are no standardized guidelines on the surveillance protocol to be followed postresection of nonampullary duodenal polyps. ASGE recommends that surveillance intervals should be individualized based on adequacy of resection, degree of dysplasia, and underlying comorbidities. End points of surveillance are also not established.[5] Based on published literature most experts recommend surveillance endoscopy in 3 to 6 months after complete resection of the lesion, followed by surveillance endoscopies in 6 to 12 months for at least 2 years.[69,88]

32.5 Conclusion

Neoplastic nonampullary duodenal polyps are uncommon. Duodenal adenomas are the most common neoplastic lesions and are associated with risk of progression to adenocarcinoma similar to colon adenomas. Endoscopic mucosal resection is the treatment of choice for the resection of these lesions in properly selected patients.

References

[1] Blechacz B, Gores GJ. Tumors of bile ducts, gallbladder, and ampulla. In: Feldman M, Friedman LS, Brandt LJ, eds. Sleisenger and Fordtran's Gastrointestinal and Liver Disease. 9th ed. Philadelphia, PA: Saunders Elsevier; 2010:1171–1184

[2] Kim HK, Lo SK. Endoscopic approach to the patient with benign or malignant ampullary lesions. Gastrointest Endosc Clin N Am. 2013; 23(2):347–383

[3] Rosenberg J, Welch JP, Pyrtek LJ, et al, . Benign villous adenomas of the ampulla of Vater. Cancer. 1986; 58(7):1563–1568

[4] Grobmyer SR, Stasik CN, Draganov P, et al. Contemporary results with ampullectomy for 29 "benign" neoplasms of the ampulla. J Am Coll Surg. 2008; 206(3):466–471

[5] Chathadi KV, Khashab MA, Acosta RD, et al; ASGE Standards of Practice Committee. The role of endoscopy in ampullary and duodenal adenomas. Gastrointest Endosc. 2015; 82(5):773–781

[6] Fischer HP, Zhou H. Pathogenesis of carcinoma of the papilla of Vater. J Hepatobiliary Pancreat Surg. 2004; 11(5):301–309

[7] Patel R, Varadarajulu S, Wilcox CM. Endoscopic ampullectomy: techniques and outcomes. J Clin Gastroenterol. 2012; 46(1):8–15

[8] Espinel J, Pinedo E, Ojeda V, Del Rio MG. Endoscopic management of adenomatous ampullary lesions. World J Methodol. 2015; 5(3):127–135

[9] Hornick JR, Johnston FM, Simon PO, et al. A single-institution review of 157 patients presenting with benign and malignant tumors of the ampulla of Vater: management and outcomes. Surgery. 2011; 150(2):169–176

[10] Martin JA, Haber GB, Kortan PP, et al. Endoscopic snare ampullectomy for resection of benign ampullary neoplasms. Gastrointest Endosc. 1997; 45(4):AB139

[11] Kahaleh M, Shami VM, Brock A, et al. Factors predictive of malignancy and endoscopic resectability in ampullary neoplasia. Am J Gastroenterol. 2004; 99(12):2335–2339

[12] Ogawa T, Ito K, Fujita N, et al. Endoscopic papillectomy as a method of total biopsy for possible early ampullary cancer. Dig Endosc. 2012; 24(4):291

[13] Sakorafas GH, Friess H, Dervenis CG. Villous tumors of the duodenum: biologic characters and clinical implications. Scand J Gastroenterol. 2000; 35(4):337–344

[14] Tran TC, Vitale GC. Ampullary tumors: endoscopic versus operative management. Surg Innov. 2004; 11(4):255–263

[15] Ferrari Júnior AP, Lichtenstein DR, Slivka A, et al. Brush cytology during ERCP for the diagnosis of biliary and pancreatic malignancies. Gastrointest Endosc. 1994; 40(2 pt 1):140–145

[16] Macken E, Drijkoningen M, Van Aken E, Van Steenbergen W. Brush cytology of ductal strictures during ERCP. Acta Gastroenterol Belg. 2000; 63(3):254–259

[17] Stewart CJ, Mills PR, Carter R, et al. Brush cytology in the assessment of pancreatico-biliary strictures: a review of 406 cases. J Clin Pathol. 2001; 54(6):449–455

[18] Cannon ME, Carpenter SL, Elta GH, et al. EUS compared with CT, magnetic resonance imaging, and angiography and the influence of biliary stenting on staging accuracy of ampullary neoplasms. Gastrointest Endosc. 1999; 50(1):27–33

[19] Itoh A, Goto H, Naitoh Y, et al. Intraductal ultrasonography in diagnosing tumor extension of cancer of the papilla of Vater. Gastrointest Endosc. 1997; 45(3):251–260

[20] Ito K, Fujita N, Noda Y. Endoscopic diagnosis and treatment of ampullary neoplasm (with video). Dig Endosc. 2011; 23(2):113–117

[21] Ito K, Fujita N, Noda Y, et al. Preoperative evaluation of ampullary neoplasm with EUS and transpapillary intraductal US: a prospective and histopathologically controlled study. Gastrointest Endosc. 2007; 66(4):740–747

[22] Menzel J, Hoepffner N, Sulkowski U, et al. Polypoid tumors of the major duodenal papilla: preoperative staging with intraductal US, EUS, and CT—a prospective, histopathologically controlled study. Gastrointest Endosc. 1999; 49(3 pt 1):349–357

[23] Menees SB, Schoenfeld P, Kim HM, Elta GH. A survey of ampullectomy practices. World J Gastroenterol. 2009; 15(28):3486–3492

[24] Lim GJ, Devereaux BM. EUS in the assessment of ampullary lesions prior to endoscopic resection. Tech Gastrointest Endosc. 2010; 12(1):49–52

[25] Bassan M, Bourke M. Endoscopic ampullectomy: a practical guide. J Interv Gastroenterol. 2012; 2(1):23–30

[26] Clary BM, Tyler DS, Dematos P, et al. Local ampullary resection with careful intraoperative frozen section evaluation for presumed benign ampullary neoplasms. Surgery. 2000; 127(6):628–633

[27] Winter JM, Cameron JL, Olino K, et al. Clinicopathologic analysis of ampullary neoplasms in 450 patients: implications for surgical strategy and long-term prognosis. J Gastrointest Surg. 2010; 14(2):379–387

[28] Ardengh JC, Kemp R, Lima-Filho ÉR, Dos Santos JS. Endoscopic papillectomy: the limits of the indication, technique and results. World J Gastrointest Endosc. 2015; 7(10):987–994

[29] Ceppa EP, Burbridge RA, Rialon KL, et al. Endoscopic versus surgical ampullectomy: an algorithm to treat disease of the ampulla of Vater. Ann Surg. 2013; 257(2):315–322

[30] Suzuki K, Kantou U, Murakami Y. Two cases with ampullary cancer who underwent endoscopic excision. Prog Dig Endosc. 1983; 23:236–239

[31] Binmoeller KF, Boaventura S, Ramsperger K, Soehendra N. Endoscopic snare excision of benign adenomas of the papilla of Vater. Gastrointest Endosc. 1993; 39(2):127–131

[32] Kim JH, Kim JH, Han JH, et al. Is endoscopic papillectomy safe for ampullary adenomas with high-grade dysplasia? Ann Surg Oncol. 2009; 16(9):2547–2554

[33] Desilets DJ, Dy RM, Ku PM, et al. Endoscopic management of tumors of the major duodenal papilla: refined techniques to improve outcome and avoid complications. Gastrointest Endosc. 2001; 54(2):202–208

[34] Cheng CL, Sherman S, Fogel EL, et al. Endoscopic snare papillectomy for tumors of the duodenal papillae. Gastrointest Endosc. 2004; 60(5):757–764

[35] Seewald S, Omar S, Soehendra N. Endoscopic resection of tumors of the ampulla of Vater: how far up and how deep down can we go? Gastrointest Endosc. 2006; 63(6):789–791

[36] Aiura K, Imaeda H, Kitajima M, Kumai K. Balloon-catheter-assisted endoscopic snare papillectomy for benign tumors of the major duodenal papilla. Gastrointest Endosc. 2003; 57(6):743–747

[37] Bohnacker S, Seitz U, Nguyen D, et al. Endoscopic resection of benign tumors of the duodenal papilla without and with intraductal growth. Gastrointest Endosc. 2005; 62(4):551–560

[38] Yoon YS, Kim SW, Park SJ, et al. Clinicopathologic analysis of early ampullary cancers with a focus on the feasibility of ampullectomy. Ann Surg. 2005; 242(1):92–100

[39] Kim MH, Lee SK, Seo DW, et al. Tumors of the major duodenal papilla. Gastrointest Endosc. 2001; 54(5):609–620

[40] Uchiyama Y, Imazu H, Kakutani H, et al. New approach to diagnosing ampullary tumors by magnifying endoscopy combined with a narrow-band imaging system. J Gastroenterol. 2006; 41(5):483–490

[41] Itoi T, Tsuji S, Sofuni A, et al. A novel approach emphasizing preoperative margin enhancement of tumor of the major duodenal papilla with narrow-band imaging in comparison to indigo carmine chromoendoscopy (with videos). Gastrointest Endosc. 2009; 69(1):136–141

[42] Poincloux L, Scanzi J, Goutte M, et al. Pancreatic intubation facilitated by methylene blue injection decreases the risk for postpapillectomy acute pancreatitis. Eur J Gastroenterol Hepatol. 2014; 26(9):990–995

[43] Martin JA, Haber GB. Ampullary adenoma: clinical manifestations, diagnosis, and treatment. Gastrointest Endosc Clin N Am. 2003; 13(4):649–669

[44] Singh P, Das A, Isenberg G, et al. Does prophylactic pancreatic stent placement reduce the risk of post-ERCP acute pancreatitis? A meta-analysis of controlled trials. Gastrointest Endosc. 2004; 60(4):544–550

[45] Hwang JC, Kim JH, Lim SG, et al. Endoscopic resection of ampullary adenoma after a new insulated plastic pancreatic stent placement: a pilot study. J Gastroenterol Hepatol. 2010; 25(8):1381–1385

[46] Dzeletovic I, Topazian MD, Baron TH. Endoscopic balloon dilation to facilitate treatment of intraductal extension of ampullary adenomas (with video). Gastrointest Endosc. 2012; 76(6):1266–1269

[47] Kim JH, Moon JH, Choi HJ, et al. Endoscopic snare papillectomy by using a balloon catheter for an unexposed ampullary adenoma with intraductal extension (with videos). Gastrointest Endosc. 2009; 69(7):1404–1406

[48] Catalano MF, Linder JD, Chak A, et al. Endoscopic management of adenoma of the major duodenal papilla. Gastrointest Endosc. 2004; 59(2):225–232

[49] Irani S, Arai A, Ayub K, et al. Papillectomy for ampullary neoplasm: results of a single referral center over a 10-year period. Gastrointest Endosc. 2009; 70(5):923–932

[50] De Palma GD. Endoscopic papillectomy: indications, techniques, and results. World J Gastroenterol. 2014; 20(6):1537–1543

[51] Vogt M, Jakobs R, Benz C, et al. Endoscopic therapy of adenomas of the papilla of Vater. A retrospective analysis with long-term follow-up. Dig Liver Dis. 2000; 32(4):339–345

[52] Zádorová Z, Dvořák M, Hajer J. Endoscopic therapy of benign tumors of the papilla of Vater. Endoscopy. 2001; 33(4):345–347

[53] Norton ID, Gostout CJ, Baron TH, et al. Safety and outcome of endoscopic snare excision of the major duodenal papilla. Gastrointest Endosc. 2002; 56(2):239–243

[54] Saurin JC, Chavaillon A, Napoléon B, et al. Long-term follow-up of patients with endoscopic treatment of sporadic adenomas of the papilla of Vater. Endoscopy. 2003; 35(5):402–406

[55] Eswaran SL, Sanders M, Bernadino KP, et al. Success and complications of endoscopic removal of giant duodenal and ampullary polyps: a comparative series. Gastrointest Endosc. 2006; 64(6):925–932

[56] Jung MK, Cho CM, Park SY, et al. Endoscopic resection of ampullary neoplasms: a single-center experience. Surg Endosc. 2009; 23(11):2568–2574

[57] Hopper AD, Bourke MJ, Williams SJ, Swan MP. Giant laterally spreading tumors of the papilla: endoscopic features, resection technique, and outcome (with videos). Gastrointest Endosc. 2010; 71(6):967–975

[58] Yamao T, Isomoto H, Kohno S, et al. Endoscopic snare papillectomy with biliary and pancreatic stent placement for tumors of the major duodenal papilla. Surg Endosc. 2010; 24(1):119–124

[59] Jeanniard-Malet O, Caillol F, Pesenti C, et al. Short-term results of 42 endoscopic ampullectomies: a single-center experience. Scand J Gastroenterol. 2011; 46(7–8):1014–1019

[60] Patel R, Davitte J, Varadarajulu S, Wilcox CM. Endoscopic resection of ampullary adenomas: complications and outcomes. Dig Dis Sci. 2011; 56(11):3235–3240

[61] Ito K, Fujita N, Noda Y, et al. Impact of technical modification of endoscopic papillectomy for ampullary neoplasm on the occurrence of complications. Dig Endosc. 2012; 24(1):30–35

[62] Salmi S, Ezzedine S, Vitton V, et al. Can papillary carcinomas be treated by endoscopic ampullectomy? Surg Endosc. 2012; 26(4):920–925

[63] Napoleon B, Gincul R, Ponchon T, et al; Sociéte Française d'Endoscopie Digestive (SFED, French Society of Digestive Endoscopy). Endoscopic papillectomy for early ampullary tumors: long-term results from a large multicenter prospective study. Endoscopy. 2014; 46(2):127–134

[64] Ismail S, Marianne U, Heikki J, et al. Endoscopic papillectomy, single-centre experience. Surg Endosc. 2014; 28(11):3234–3239

[65] Ridtitid W, Tan D, Schmidt SE, et al. Endoscopic papillectomy: risk factors for incomplete resection and recurrence during long-term follow-up. Gastrointest Endosc. 2014; 79(2):289–296

[66] Höchter W, Weingart J, Seib HJ, Ottenjann R. [Duodenal polyps. Incidence, histologic substrate and significance] Dtsch Med Wochenschr. 1984; 109(31–32):1183–1186

[67] Reddy RR, Schuman BM, Priest RJ. Duodenal polyps: diagnosis and management. J Clin Gastroenterol. 1981; 3(2):139–147

[68] Jepsen JM, Persson M, Jakobsen NO, et al. Prospective study of prevalence and endoscopic and histopathologic characteristics of duodenal polyps in patients submitted to upper endoscopy. Scand J Gastroenterol. 1994; 29(6):483–487

[69] Basford PJ, Bhandari P. Endoscopic management of nonampullary duodenal polyps. Therap Adv Gastroenterol. 2012; 5(2):127–138

[70] Hoteya S, Yahagi N, Iizuka T, et al. Endoscopic submucosal dissection for nonampullary large superficial adenocarcinoma/adenoma of the duodenum: feasibility and long-term outcomes. Endosc Int Open. 2013; 1(1):2–7

[71] Jung SH, Chung WC, Kim EJ, et al. Evaluation of non-ampullary duodenal polyps: comparison of non-neoplastic and neoplastic lesions. World J Gastroenterol. 2010; 16(43):5474–5480

[72] Suzuki S, Hirasaki S, Ikeda F. Three cases of solitary Peutz-Jeghers-type hamartomatous polyp in the duodenum. World J Gastroenterol. 2008; 14(6):944–947

[73] Lim CH, Cho YS. Nonampullary duodenal adenoma: current understanding of its diagnosis, pathogenesis, and clinical management. World J Gastroenterol. 2016; 22(2):853–861

[74] Sellner F. Investigations on the significance of the adenoma-carcinoma sequence in the small bowel. Cancer. 1990; 66(4):702–715

[75] Okada K, Fujisaki J, Kasuga A, et al. Sporadic nonampullary duodenal adenoma in the natural history of duodenal cancer: a study of follow-up surveillance. Am J Gastroenterol. 2011; 106(2):357–364

[76] Spigelman AD, Williams CB, Talbot IC, et al. Upper gastrointestinal cancer in patients with familial adenomatous polyposis. Lancet. 1989; 2(8666):783–785

[77] Fanning SB, Bourke MJ, Williams SJ, et al. Giant laterally spreading tumors of the duodenum: endoscopic resection outcomes, limitations, and caveats. Gastrointest Endosc. 2012; 75(4):805–812

[78] Conio M, De Ceglie A, Filiberti R. Cap-assisted EMR of large, sporadic, nonampullary duodenal polyps. Gastrointest Endosc. 2012; 76(6):1160–1169

[79] Alexander S, Bourke MJ, Williams SJ, et al. EMR of large, sessile, sporadic nonampullary duodenal adenomas: technical aspects and long-term outcome (with videos). Gastrointest Endosc. 2009; 69(1):66–73

[80] Binmoeller KF, Shah JN, Bhat YM, Kane SD. "Underwater" EMR of sporadic laterally spreading nonampullary duodenal adenomas (with video). Gastrointest Endosc. 2013; 78(3):496–502

[81] Hirasawa R, Iishi H, Tatsuta M, Ishiguro S. Clinicopathologic features and endoscopic resection of duodenal adenocarcinomas and adenomas with the submucosal saline injection technique. Gastrointest Endosc. 1997; 46(6):507–513

[82] Apel D, Jakobs R, Spiethoff A, Riemann JF. Follow-up after endoscopic snare resection of duodenal adenomas. Endoscopy. 2005; 37(5):444–448

[83] Lépilliez V, Chemaly M, Ponchon T, et al. Endoscopic resection of sporadic duodenal adenomas: an efficient technique with a substantial risk of delayed bleeding. Endoscopy. 2008; 40(10):806–810

[84] Honda T, Yamamoto H, Osawa H, et al. Endoscopic submucosal dissection for superficial duodenal neoplasms. Dig Endosc. 2009; 21(4):270–274

[85] Abbass R, Rigaux J, Al-Kawas FH. Nonampullary duodenal polyps: characteristics and endoscopic management. Gastrointest Endosc. 2010; 71(4):754–759

[86] Navaneethan U, Lourdusamy D, Mehta D. Endoscopic resection of large sporadic non-ampullary duodenal polyps: efficacy and long-term recurrence. Surg Endosc. 2014; 28(9):2616–2622

[87] Kedia P, Brensinger C, Ginsberg G. Endoscopic predictors of successful endoluminal eradication in sporadic duodenal adenomas and its acute complications. Gastrointest Endosc. 2010; 72(6):1297–1301

[88] Marques J, Baldaque-Silva F, Pereira P. Endoscopic mucosal resection and endoscopic submucosal dissection in the treatment of sporadic nonampullary duodenal adenomatous polyps. World J Gastrointest Endosc. 2015; 7(7):720–727

33 Malabsorption and Food Allergy/Intolerance

Alberto Rubio-Tapia and Joseph A Murray

33.1 Introduction

Small bowel disorders causing malabsorption represent a clinical challenge. Celiac disease (CD) is the most common small bowel disorder causing malabsorption. Standard endoscopy is the method of choice to take samples of the duodenum for histologic analysis in the diagnosis of small bowel disorders. Standard endoscopy without routine biopsy has a limited capability to detect subtle alterations of the small bowel mucosa because of the low-magnification view, patchy nature of intestinal lesions, and dependency of macroscopic features on degree/severity of mucosal lesion. Currently, routine intestinal biopsies are recommended for evaluation of small bowel disorders and malabsorption including CD. Over the past decade, technology development has greatly improved our capability to examine the small bowel broadening the diagnostic role of endoscopy.

The aim of this chapter is to review the new endoscopic tools available in the diagnosis of small bowel disorders with emphasis on celiac disease (as a prototype) including water-immersion technique, capsule endoscopy (CE), enteroscopy, narrow-band imaging, confocal laser endomicroscopy, and chromoendoscopy.

33.2 Standard Endoscopy

Villous atrophy is the usual hallmark histologic abnormality for most small bowel mucosal disorders causing malabsorption (▶Table 33.1). Characteristic endoscopic findings of villous atrophy include reduced duodenal folds, scalloping of folds, fissures, mosaic pattern, and nodularity (▶Fig. 33.1).[1,2] Sensitivity for diagnosis of CD is low (50–94%), but when the endoscopic signs are present, these have a high specificity (95–100%) for villous atrophy and hence CD.[3] Low sensitivity for CD diagnosis may be explained because endoscopic markers are absent with lesser degrees of intestinal damage.[4] Thus, a normal macroscopic appearance of the small bowel mucosa does not necessarily imply normality. Low sensitivity implicates that duodenal biopsies should always be taken when the diagnosis of a malabsorption disorder is suspected. These endoscopic features have been reported in other small bowel disorders other than CD but their

sensitivity and/or specificity have not been estimated. Detection of visible villous atrophy does not determine the etiology.

Several endoscopic technologies and techniques have been developed to improve the visualization of the intestinal mucosa compared to standard endoscopy (▶Table 33.2).[3,5,6,7,8,9,10,11,12,13,14]

33.2.1 Water-Immersion Technique

Water-immersion technique is based on magnification of intestinal villi when the duodenum is filled with water. This is an easy and safe procedure that adds very little time to a standard upper endoscopy.[5,15] The simple technique consists of removal of air from the duodenum lumen by suction followed by rapid instillation of 90 to150 cc of water. This procedure has been useful to increase diagnostic yield during initial investigation of CD by standard upper endoscopy, targeting duodenal biopsy sites, and CD follow-up[5] (▶Fig. 33.2).

33.3 Chromoendoscopy and Magnification Endoscopy

Dye-staining chromoendoscopy with indigo carmine or methylene blue enhances the visualization of the mucosal surface.

Table 33.1 Conditions other than celiac disease with endoscopic features of villous atrophy

- Tropical sprue
- Small bowel bacterial overgrowth
- Sprue-like enteropathy associated with medications (e.g., olmesartan)
- Giardiasis
- Eosinophilic enteritis
- Crohn's disease
- Collagenous sprue
- Whipple's disease
- Autoimmune enteropathy
- Common variable immunodeficiency
- Malnutrition
- Graft-versus-host disease
- Lymphoma
- Intestinal tuberculosis

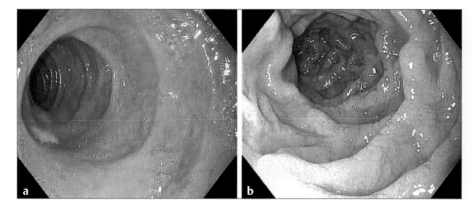

Fig. 33.1 Standard endoscopy shows reduced duodenal folds **(a)** and fissuring/scalloping **(b)** characteristic of villous atrophy in a patient with tropical sprue.

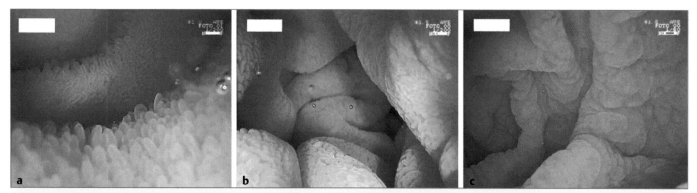

Fig. 33.2 Water-immersion technique with optical magnification shows normal villi **(a)**, partial villous atrophy **(b)**, and total villous atrophy **(c)** in a patient with celiac disease. (Images are provided courtesy of Dr Giovanni Cammarota, Rome, Italy.)

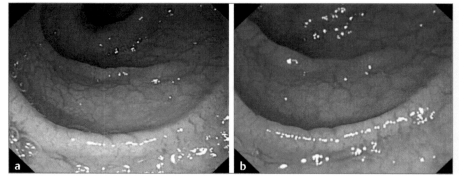

Fig. 33.3 Device-assisted enteroscopy (double-balloon) view of proximal jejunum shows classic signs of villous atrophy such as scalloping of circular folds **(a)** and a mosaic pattern **(b)** in a patient with refractory celiac disease.

Table 33.2 Sensitivity and specificity among diverse endoscopic tools for the detection of villous atrophy

Endoscopic tool	Sensitivity	Specificity
Standard endoscopy[3]	59	92
Water-immersion endoscopy[5]	91	99
Enhanced-magnification endoscopy[6]	96	-
Magnification endoscopy with dye[7]	94	88
Zoom endoscopy[8]	90	62
Capsule endoscopy[9,10,11]	70–89	95–100
Narrow-band imaging[12]	83	100
Confocal laser endomicroscopy[13]	100	80
Optical coherence tomography[14]	82	100

However, dye-staining chromoendoscopy alone was not useful to increase the detection of CD.[16] Enhanced magnification endoscopy (e.g., acetic acid + magnification) has superior accuracy compared to standard endoscopy for CD diagnosis.[6]

33.4 Narrow-Band Imaging

Narrow-band imaging uses a narrowing of the bandwidths of the blue and green filters enhancing visualization with a deeper superficial penetration than white light. Narrow-band imaging can help detect villous atrophy (sensitivity > 93%) and grade (sensitivity 83%).[12]

33.5 Confocal Laser Endomicroscopy

This novel technology allows in vivo imaging of the mucosa at 1000× magnification. It has been explored in CD with good

correlation between endoscopic findings and histology. A small study in children showed good interobserver agreement among endoscopists (Kappa 0.76).[13] Confocal laser microscopy offers the promise of diagnosis of CD during ongoing endoscopy or at the very least a more precise targeting of the abnormal small bowel mucosa.

33.6 Optical Coherence Tomography

Optical coherence tomography relies on the in vivo evaluation of duodenal mucosa using light waves echo. Among 18 patients with positive serologies for CD and 22 dyspeptic patients, there was excellent concordance between optical coherence tomography and histology for villi morphology in both CD and controls.[17] In a larger study from the same group that included 134 children (67 with positive serologies for CD), sensitivity and specificity were 82 and 100%, respectively.[14]

33.7 Device-Assisted Enteroscopy

Device-assisted enteroscopy is an invasive endoscopic method with the potential for examination of the whole intestine, which has the advantage of direct biopsy sampling and therapeutic intervention.[18,19] Mastering device-assisted enteroscopy requires considerable training and experience. Highly experience endoscopists can examine the entire intestine in about 50 to 86% of cases.[19] Device-assisted enteroscopy can be used to target areas beyond the reach of other endoscopic methods (▶ Fig. 33.3).[20,21] The indications for device-assisted enteroscopy in small bowel disorders are not standardized. However, it may be helpful to exclude/confirm complications of CD such as malignancies or ulcerative jejunitis in patients with refractory celiac disease.[22,23,24]

33.7.1 Capsule Endoscopy

CE has potential for evaluation of the whole small bowel.[25] Integrated optical magnification allows for excellent evaluation of the villous pattern. CE has good sensitivity and specificity (> 85%) for detection of villous atrophy as compared to histology (▶ Fig. 33.4)[11,26] CE could be useful for evaluation of refractory CD or when a severe complication is suspected such as lymphoma or cancer.[27,28] CE may replace diagnostic biopsy when upper endoscopy is either declined or contraindicated.[29]

33.8 Selected Small Bowel Diseases

33.8.1 Celiac Disease

CD is an immune-mediated disorder of the small bowel induced by the ingestion of a group of proteins collectively called gluten (the storage protein component of wheat, barley, and rye) in genetically susceptible individuals.[30] The small intestinal damage is characterized by villous atrophy, crypt hyperplasia, and chronic inflammation, which usually reverts to normal after gluten exclusion. The endoscopic appearance is similar to other small bowel disorders causing malabsorption associated with villous atrophy.

CD affects almost 1% of the North American general population with increasing incidence over time.[31]

The clinical presentation varies from a malabsorption syndrome with diarrhea and involuntary loss of weight to "silent" without significant symptoms even though villous atrophy is found in the intestine in both scenarios.[32] The diagnosis of CD is supported by the presence of disease-specific autoantibodies (tissue transglutaminase antibodies [tTGA] or/and endomysial antibodies [EMA]), confirmed by an abnormal intestinal biopsy and the clinical response to gluten exclusion.[33] Lifelong medically supervised gluten-free diet is very effective to control symptoms and prevent complications.

Diagnostic Approaches

CD is characterized by the development of diverse antibodies that are made against the components of the environmental factor (gliadin) (antigliadin antibodies) or connective tissue (tTGA and EMA) Diagnostic performance of serology is affected by reduced gluten ingestion. It is recommended that serology testing is done when the patient is on a regular gluten-containing diet. Total immunoglobulin A (IgA) testing is usually performed to exclude IgA deficiency that make IgA-based serology useless from a diagnostic perspective (▶ Table 33.3).

Antigliadin Antibodies

The low sensitivity/specificity of antibodies against unaltered gliadin along with the existence of alternative serologic tests with better diagnostic performance has rendered the standard antigliadin antibodies obsolete and therefore are not recommended.[33] However, a new generation of antigliadin antibody assays has been developed to detect antibodies to synthetic deamidated gliadin peptides with a high sensitivity and specificity (similar to tTGA).[34]

Endomysial Antibodies

EMA could be measured using an immunofluorescence technique with human jejunum, human umbilical cord, but most often monkey esophagus as the tissue substrate. The overall sensitivity and specificity for IgA EMA using monkey esophagus as substrate was 97 and 99.6%, respectively.[35] The tests using human umbilical cord as substrate have a lower sensitivity (90%). While the very high specificity makes EMA a very powerful serologic test, there

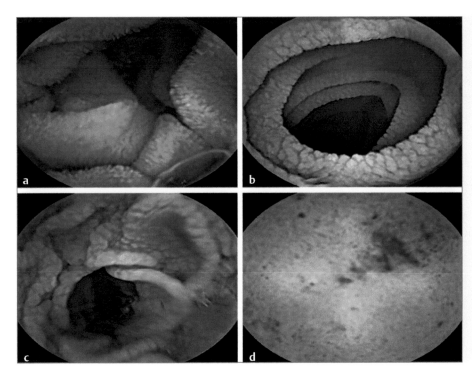

Fig. 33.4 Wireless capsule endoscopy shows normal villi (a), scalloping of folds (b) in a patient with common variable immunodeficiency and sprue, nodularity and mosaic pattern (c), and steatorrhea (d) in a patient with collagenous sprue.

Table 33.3 Serologic test and their diagnostic accuracy in celiac disease

Test	Sensitivity	Specificity
Antigliadin	< 80%	~ 80%
DGP antibodies α	84%	> 90%
EMA[a]	90–97%	99–100%
tTGA[b]	95–98%	90–98%

DGP, deamidated gliadin peptide antibodies; EMA, endomysial antibodies; tTGA, tissue transglutaminase antibodies.

[a]Sensitivity and specificity varies between studies, and according to the immunoglobulin isotype of the antibody or antigenic substrate used.

[b]Sensitivity of the IgG isotype is very low (~ 40%) in the absence of selective IgA deficiency.

are some important clinical disadvantages: results obtained in research settings are better than ones in clinical practice, EMA titers correlate with the degree of mucosal damage; the test is time-consuming, semiquantitative, and operator dependent.[36]

Tissue Transglutaminase Antibodies

The enzyme tTGA is the autoantigen for EMA, thus, a wide variety of kits with different characteristics measure tTGA by enzyme-linked immunosorbent assay with guinea pig, human red cell–derived and human recombinant substrate. The diagnostic performance is slightly better using human or human recombinant substrate (new-generation kits) than when guinea pig is used. Overall, the tTGA sensitivity is in the range of 90 to 96% and the specificity is greater than 95%.[36] tTGA has the advantage of technical simplicity.

Genetic Testing

The risk of developing CD is strongly associated with two human leukocyte antigen (HLA) haplotypes: DQ2 (encoded by the gene pair *DQA1*05* and *DQB1*02*) and/or DQ8 (encoded by a different

gene pair *DQA1*03* and *DQB1*0302*). Indeed, CD patients carry at least one of those two gene pairs (90–95% of patients have DQ2).[37] Typing of DNA from patients with CD can be easily performed from whole blood using sequence-specific primers or allele-specific oligonucleotide probes. Although approximately 35 to 40% of the general population in Caucasian countries carries either the HLA-DQ2 or HLA-DQ8 haplotypes, only a small subset of these subjects have CD. Thus, HLA genotyping in a clinical setting is useful to practically exclude the diagnosis of CD when the at-risk gene pairs are absent, especially when the diagnosis is uncertain.[32,33] Cases of CD in the absence of at-risk gene pairs have been described, but this clinical scenario is very unusual.

Endoscopy and Histopathology

The confirmation of CD requires a characteristic appearance on histologic examination of mucosal biopsy specimens obtained from the small intestine. These findings include the combination of the following: increased number of intraepithelial lymphocytes, villous atrophy, and crypt hyperplasia. Several histologic classification systems have been proposed but the most frequently used in the literature are the Marsh/Oberhuber (modified Marsh classification) and more recently Corazza's classification (▶ Fig. 33.5).[38,39] Multiple biopsies of the duodenum are recommended (one or two from bulb and four from distal duodenum) as the disease lesion can be patchy and to maximize the chances of getting well-oriented samples by endoscopy.[33] A single-biopsy technique (one biopsy specimen per pass of the forceps) may increase the yield of well-oriented duodenal samples (66% as compared to 42% with double-biopsy technique).[40] A targeted duodenal bulb biopsy from either the 9- or 12-o'clock position in addition to distal duodenal biopsies may improve diagnostic yield for CD.[41] Unfortunately, poor adherence to quality sampling recommendations is common place in the United States contributing to the observed underdiagnosis of CD.[42,43] Although various emerging endoscopy modalities (e.g., magnification endoscopy, narrow-band imaging, confocal laser endomicroscopy)

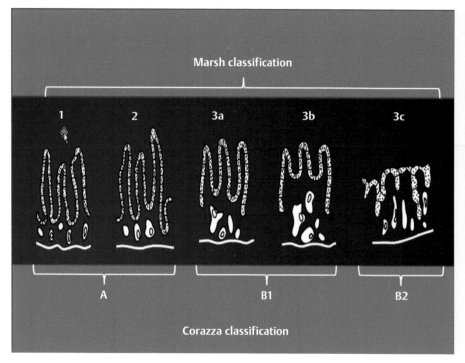

Fig. 33.5 Modified Marsh's and Corazza's classifications. Modified Marsh type 1 (infiltrative) is characterized by increased number of intraepithelial lymphocytes, type 2 (hyperplastic) is characterized by increase in crypt depth without villous atrophy, type 3 (destructive) is characterized by mild-partial (3a), marked-subtotal (3b), and complete (3c) villous atrophy. Corazza's classification may have better agreement between pathologists than modified Marsh. Grade A includes Marsh I and II, grade B1 includes Marsh 3a and 3b, and grade B2 includes Marsh 3c. Copyright Mayo Clinic Foundation.

have good test characteristics, these have yet to be adopted as part of a standard diagnostic work-up for CD.

Therapeutic Approaches

Gluten-free diet is the only available treatment for CD. Lifelong medical follow-up is necessary.[33] Early consultation with a dietitian with expertise in gluten-free diet is highly recommended. Initial treatment includes correction of nutritional deficiencies if present. Goals of therapy include control of symptoms (days to weeks), seroconversion (months to a year), and small bowel mucosal healing (years). Yearly medical follow-up is the standard of care. A small group of CD patients have recurrent and/or persistent symptoms despite good adherence to the gluten-free diet, so called refractory CD.[44] There are two types of refractory CD: type 1 immune-mediated refractory CD and type 2 characterized by the presence of aberrant intraepithelial lymphocytes (T-cell clonal disorder). Clonal type 2 refractory CD has high risk of progression to overt lymphoma. Steroids, such as budesonide, are usually effective for type 1 refractory CD.[45] Treatment options for type 2 refractory CD include steroids, azathioprine, cladribine, and for selected cases stem cell transplantation.[46,47]

Areas of Uncertainty

Nonbiopsy diagnosis has been proposed for selected symptomatic children with high titer of tTGA (> 10 times upper limit of normal) with a subsequent positive antiendomysial antibody in a separate blood sample and genetic risk consistent with CD.[48]

Summary

CD is the most common cause of villous atrophy. Diagnosis relies on serology and duodenal biopsy confirmation. A lifelong gluten-free diet is the treatment of choice. Where the diagnosis is first made by biopsy, it is important to do serology (tTGA and/or EMA) to confirm the diagnosis and to provide a baseline to follow up the gluten-free diet.

33.8.2 Tropical Sprue

Tropical sprue is a cause of malabsorption syndrome in certain tropical countries characterized by villous atrophy and clinical response to a combination of antibiotics and folic acid.[49] The etiology of tropical sprue is unknown but gut dysbiosis has been proposed. Tropical sprue presents with chronic diarrhea and symptoms related to a severe malabsorption syndrome in people living in or returning from travel to the tropical sprue locations such as Latin America, Caribbean, India, and some countries of Africa and Asia.

Diagnostic Approaches

There is not a pathognomonic test for tropical sprue. The most important factor in diagnosis is seeking the travel history. Documentation of malabsorption by nonspecific test such as fecal fat, low serum folate, serum carotene, and D-xylose is reasonable.

Exclusion of other causes of malabsorption syndrome such as CD is necessary. Small bowel biopsy findings are similar to fully developed CD though celiac-specific serology should discriminate. Clinical response to a combination of antibiotics and folic acid may help to confirm the diagnosis.

Therapeutic Approaches

Treatment of tropical sprue requires aggressive correction of malnutrition. Prolonged course of antibiotics (3–6 months) such as tetracycline and sulfonamides with folic acid have been shown to be effective.[50] High cost and lack of availability of tetracycline have been a problem in the United States.

Areas of Uncertainty

Epidemiology of tropical sprue in the developed world is poorly described. Etiology of tropical sprue remains to be elucidated. The exact duration of therapy is unknown due to lack of randomized-control studies and reports of recurrence.

Summary

Tropical sprue should be considered in patients with malabsorption syndrome living in an endemic area or with a travel history to tropical countries.

33.8.3 Small Bowel Bacterial Overgrowth

Small bowel bacterial overgrowth (SBBO) is characterized by an abnormal number of bacteria in the small bowel. SBBO can present with diarrhea, bloating, weight loss, flatulence, and malabsorption. Anemia and vitamin deficiencies are common. Folate is usually normal or elevated. Risk factors for SBBO include older age, surgically altered anatomy of the gastrointestinal (GI) tract (e.g., Billroth's surgery), alkaline gastric fluid (achlorhydria), diverticulosis of the small bowel, and delayed bowel transit as observed in motility disorders.

Diagnostic Approaches

Culture of intestinal fluid aspirate is considered as the gold standard for SBBO. Microbiological diagnosis requires greater than or equal to 10^5 colony-forming units per µL. Intestinal fluid aspirate for bacteriologic culture is obtained by endoscopy. A disinfected endoscope is advanced without suction to the level of the distal duodenum, then a long sterile catheter is introduced through the working channel of the endoscope, intestinal fluid (up to 2 mL) is obtained using gentle suction applied with a sterile syringe. Duodenal biopsy plays a limited role on SBBO diagnosis although a decreased villous to crypt ratio (consistent with villous atrophy) can be seen in up to 24% of patients with culture-confirmed SBBO.[51] Hydrogen/methane breath tests can be a noninvasive alternative. Overall, breath tests have wide variability on diagnostic accuracy due to variations on technique and/or SBBO criteria but it is accepted that breath tests have a low sensitivity (16–62%)

compared to culture of intestinal aspirate.[52] Glucose-based testing may have slightly better sensitivity than lactose-based testing.[52]

Therapeutic Approaches

The cornerstone of SBBO treatment is antibiotic therapy. There is no antibiotic of choice. Reasonable options are tetracycline, quinolones (e.g., norfloxacin), metronidazole, rifaximin, neomycin, and amoxicillin–clavulanic acid. Duration of treatment is not well defined. Short course (e.g., 10 days), cyclic (e.g., 10-day course every month of rotating antibiotics), and continuous regimens have been reported.[53] It is the authors' preference to use a short course first and to reserve cyclic and continuous regimens for patients with frequent relapse or those with severe clinical presentations and/or untreatable underlying condition. Treatments of the underlying condition (if possible) and nutritional support are key management interventions.

Areas of Uncertainty

There is no agreement as to which test should be preferred for the diagnosis of SBBO.

Summary

SBBO is defined by an altered small bowel microbiome. Endoscopy plays a limited role in diagnosis of SBBO. Treatment of SBBO includes correction of predisposing risk factors, nutritional support, and antibiotics.

33.8.4 Sprue-Like Enteropathy Associated with Olmesartan

Sprue-like enteropathy associated with olmesartan is a newly described entity characterized by severe diarrhea, weight loss, dehydration, electrolyte imbalance, and acute kidney injury in patients taking olmesartan.[54] Sprue-like enteropathy associated with olmesartan was first described by Rubio-Tapia et al,[54,55] multiple case reports and/or case-series from all around the world have since been reported.[56] Laboratory reveals nonspecific anemia and vitamin deficiencies. Celiac serologies are negative and patients have no clinical response to a gluten-free diet. Histopathologic findings include villous atrophy with or without increased intraepithelial lymphocytes; a thickened subepithelial collagen layer can be seen (collagenous sprue). Emerging evidence supports an immune-based pathophysiology with increased CD8+cells, FoxP3+ cells, and IL15R in intestinal biopsies of patients taking olmesartan.[57] Olmesartan induced increased expression of IL15 and causes disruption of tight junction proteins (e.g., Zo-1) in Caco-2 cells.

Diagnostic Approaches

Diagnosis of sprue-like enteropathy associated with olmesartan should be considered in symptomatic patients taking olmesartan with villous atrophy and negative celiac serology (seronegative villous atrophy). Upper endoscopy with duodenal biopsies is needed to document villous atrophy. Optimal method to take biopsies in sprue-like enteropathy associated with olmesartan is unknown, but we used the same protocol as recommended for CD. Capsule endoscopy shows nonspecific endoscopic findings of villous atrophy (▶ Fig. 33.6).

Confirmation of diagnosis requires resolution of symptoms after olmesartan withdrawal. Full mucosal recovery is expected and a follow-up endoscopy with duodenal biopsies is reasonable 6 to 12 months after olmesartan withdrawal.

Therapeutic Approaches

Olmesartan withdrawal is the treatment of choice for sprue-like enteropathy associated with olmesartan. Patients with severe clinical presentation, recurrent hospitalization, and partial/slow clinical response may benefit of oral (budesonide) or short course of intravenous (IV) steroid. After suspension of olmesartan, it is mandatory to fully understand the clinical indication for olmesartan and to make a careful reassessment of the need for alternative medication with the help of primary care physician. If an alternative medication is needed, a different drug class should be preferred in all cases.

Areas of Uncertainty

Although fully developed sprue-like enteropathy associated with olmesartan appears to be rare, a spectrum of disease severity is

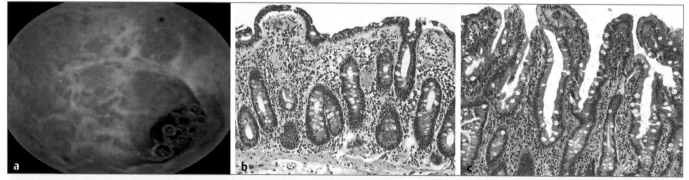

Fig. 33.6 Wireless capsule endoscopy shows total villous atrophy of proximal jejunum in a patient with sprue-like enteropathy associated with olmesartan **(a)**, duodenal biopsy specimen while the patient was taking olmesartan shows total villous atrophy and subepithelial collagen deposition (collagenous sprue) **(b)**, and biopsy specimen obtained 10 months after withdrawal of olmesartan shows mucosal recovery with near normal villi to crypt ratio **(c)**.

possible. The underlying mechanisms of the disease remain to be fully elucidated.

Summary

Sprue-like enteropathy associated with olmesartan is an emerging entity that needs to be considered early in the differential of seronegative villous atrophy. Olmesartan should be added to the list of other well-established drugs capable to produce small bowel injury such as nonsteroidal anti-inflammatory drugs and mycophenolate mofetil.

33.9 Conclusion

Endoscopy plays a central role in the diagnosis of malabsorption. Standard endoscopy with biopsy of the duodenum for microscopy/pathology examination remains the method of choice for investigation of small bowel mucosal disorders. Advanced endoscopy techniques may improve visualization of the proximal small bowel mucosa and/or target areas beyond the reach of standard endoscopy. Recent endoscopy advances made possible the direct evaluation of the whole intestine for the first time in medical history.

References

[1] Jabbari M, Wild G, Goresky CA, et al. Scalloped valvulae conniventes: an endoscopic marker of celiac sprue. Gastroenterology. 1988; 95(6):1518–1522

[2] Brocchi E, Corazza GR, Caletti G, et al. Endoscopic demonstration of loss of duodenal folds in the diagnosis of celiac disease. N Engl J Med. 1988; 319(12):741–744

[3] Oxentenko AS, Grisolano SW, Murray JA, et al. The insensitivity of endoscopic markers in celiac disease. Am J Gastroenterol. 2002; 97(4):933–938

[4] Dickey W, Hughes D. Disappointing sensitivity of endoscopic markers for villous atrophy in a high-risk population: implications for celiac disease diagnosis during routine endoscopy. Am J Gastroenterol. 2001; 96(7):2126–2128

[5] Cammarota G, Pirozzi GA, Martino A, et al. Reliability of the "immersion technique" during routine upper endoscopy for detection of abnormalities of duodenal villi in patients with dyspepsia. Gastrointest Endosc. 2004; 60(2):223–228

[6] Lo A, Guelrud M, Essenfeld H, Bonis P. Classification of villous atrophy with enhanced magnification endoscopy in patients with celiac disease and tropical sprue. Gastrointest Endosc. 2007; 66(2):377–382

[7] Siegel LM, Stevens PD, Lightdale CJ, et al. Combined magnification endoscopy with chromoendoscopy in the evaluation of patients with suspected malabsorption. Gastrointest Endosc. 1997; 46(3):226–230

[8] Badreldin R, Barrett P, Wooff DA, et al. How good is zoom endoscopy for assessment of villous atrophy in coeliac disease? Endoscopy. 2005; 37(10):994–998

[9] Petroniene R, Dubcenco E, Baker JP, et al. Given capsule endoscopy in celiac disease: evaluation of diagnostic accuracy and interobserver agreement. Am J Gastroenterol. 2005; 100(3):685–694

[10] Hopper AD, Sidhu R, Hurlstone DP, et al. Capsule endoscopy: an alternative to duodenal biopsy for the recognition of villous atrophy in coeliac disease? Dig Liver Dis. 2007; 39(2):140–145

[11] Rokkas T, Niv Y. The role of video capsule endoscopy in the diagnosis of celiac disease: a meta-analysis. Eur J Gastroenterol Hepatol. 2012; 24(3):303–308

[12] Singh R, Nind G, Tucker G, et al. Narrow-band imaging in the evaluation of villous morphology: a feasibility study assessing a simplified classification and observer agreement. Endoscopy. 2010; 42(11):889–894

[13] Venkatesh K, Abou-Taleb A, Cohen M, et al. Role of confocal endomicroscopy in the diagnosis of celiac disease. J Pediatr Gastroenterol Nutr. 2010; 51(3):274–279

[14] Masci E, Mangiavillano B, Barera G, et al. Optical coherence tomography in pediatric patients: a feasible technique for diagnosing celiac disease in children with villous atrophy. Dig Liver Dis. 2009; 41(9):639–643

[15] Cammarota G, Cuoco L, Cesaro P, et al. A highly accurate method for monitoring histological recovery in patients with celiac disease on a gluten-free diet using an endoscopic approach that avoids the need for biopsy: a double-center study. Endoscopy. 2007; 39(1):46–51

[16] Kiesslich R, Mergener K, Naumann C, et al. Value of chromoendoscopy and magnification endoscopy in the evaluation of duodenal abnormalities: a prospective, randomized comparison. Endoscopy. 2003; 35(7):559–563

[17] Masci E, Mangiavillano B, Albarello L, et al. Pilot study on the correlation of optical coherence tomography with histology in celiac disease and normal subjects. J Gastroenterol Hepatol. 2007; 22(12):2256–2260

[18] Yamamoto H, Sekine Y, Sato Y, et al. Total enteroscopy with a nonsurgical steerable double-balloon method. Gastrointest Endosc. 2001; 53(2):216–220

[19] Yamamoto H, Kita H, Sunada K, et al. Clinical outcomes of double-balloon endoscopy for the diagnosis and treatment of small-intestinal diseases. Clin Gastroenterol Hepatol. 2004; 2(11):1010–1016

[20] May A, Nachbar L, Pohl J, Ell C. Endoscopic interventions in the small bowel using double balloon enteroscopy: feasibility and limitations. Am J Gastroenterol. 2007; 102(3):527–535

[21] Leighton JA. The role of endoscopic imaging of the small bowel in clinical practice. Am J Gastroenterol. 2011; 106(1):27–36, quiz 37

[22] Heine GD, Hadithi M, Groenen MJ, et al. Double-balloon enteroscopy: indications, diagnostic yield, and complications in a series of 275 patients with suspected small-bowel disease. Endoscopy. 2006; 38(1):42–48

[23] Tomba C, Sidhu R, Sanders DS, et al. Celiac disease and double-balloon enteroscopy: what can we achieve?: The experience of 2 European Tertiary Referral Centers. J Clin Gastroenterol. 2016; 50(4):313–317

[24] Hadithi M, Al-toma A, Oudejans J, et al. The value of double-balloon enteroscopy in patients with refractory celiac disease. Am J Gastroenterol. 2007; 102(5):987–996

[25] Iddan G, Meron G, Glukhovsky A, Swain P. Wireless capsule endoscopy. Nature. 2000; 405(6785):417

[26] Murray JA, Rubio-Tapia A, Van Dyke CT, et al. Mucosal atrophy in celiac disease: extent of involvement, correlation with clinical presentation, and response to treatment. Clin Gastroenterol Hepatol. 2008; 6(2):186–193, quiz 125

[27] Barret M, Malamut G, Rahmi G, et al. Diagnostic yield of capsule endoscopy in refractory celiac disease. Am J Gastroenterol. 2012; 107(10):1546–1553

[28] Atlas DS, Rubio-Tapia A, Van Dyke CT, et al. Capsule endoscopy in nonresponsive celiac disease. Gastrointest Endosc. 2011; 74(6):1315–1322

[29] Chang MS, Rubin M, Lewis SK, Green PH. Diagnosing celiac disease by video capsule endoscopy (VCE) when esophagogastroduodenoscopy (EGD) and biopsy is unable to provide a diagnosis: a case series. BMC Gastroenterol. 2012; 12:90

[30] Green PH, Cellier C. Celiac disease. N Engl J Med. 2007; 357(17):1731–1743

[31] Ludvigsson JF, Rubio-Tapia A, van Dyke CT, et al. Increasing incidence of celiac disease in a North American population. Am J Gastroenterol. 2013; 108(5):818–824

[32] Rostom A, Murray JA, Kagnoff MF. American Gastroenterological Association (AGA) Institute technical review on the diagnosis and management of celiac disease. Gastroenterology. 2006; 131(6):1981–2002

[33] Rubio-Tapia A, Hill ID, Kelly CP, et al; American College of Gastroenterology. ACG clinical guidelines: diagnosis and management of celiac disease. Am J Gastroenterol. 2013; 108(5):656–676, quiz 677

[34] Rashtak S, Ettore MW, Homburger HA, Murray JA. Comparative usefulness of deamidated gliadin antibodies in the diagnosis of celiac disease. Clin Gastroenterol Hepatol. 2008; 6(4):426–432, quiz 370

[35] Lewis NR, Scott BB. Systematic review: the use of serology to exclude or diagnose coeliac disease (a comparison of the endomysial and tissue transglutaminase antibody tests). Aliment Pharmacol Ther. 2006; 24(1):47–54

[36] Leffler DA, Schuppan D. Update on serologic testing in celiac disease. Am J Gastroenterol. 2010; 105(12):2520–2524

[37] Jabri B, Sollid LM. Mechanisms of disease: immunopathogenesis of celiac disease. Nat Clin Pract Gastroenterol Hepatol. 2006; 3(9):516–525

[38] Marsh MN. Gluten, major histocompatibility complex, and the small intestine. A molecular and immunobiologic approach to the spectrum of gluten sensitivity ('celiac sprue'). Gastroenterology. 1992; 102(1):330–354

[39] Corazza GR, Villanacci V, Zambelli C, et al. Comparison of the interobserver reproducibility with different histologic criteria used in celiac disease. Clin Gastroenterol Hepatol. 2007; 5(7):838–843

[40] Latorre M, Lagana SM, Freedberg DE, et al. Endoscopic biopsy technique in the diagnosis of celiac disease: one bite or two? Gastrointest Endosc. 2015; 81(5):1228–1233

[41] Kurien M, Evans KE, Hopper AD, et al. Duodenal bulb biopsies for diagnosing adult celiac disease: is there an optimal biopsy site? Gastrointest Endosc. 2012; 75(6):1190–1196

[42] Lebwohl B, Tennyson CA, Holub JL, et al. Sex and racial disparities in duodenal biopsy to evaluate for celiac disease. Gastrointest Endosc. 2012; 76(4):779–785

[43] Lebwohl B, Kapel RC, Neugut AI, et al Adherence to biopsy guidelines increases celiac disease diagnosis. Gastrointest Endosc. 2011; 74(1):103–109

[44] Rubio-Tapia A, Murray JA. Classification and management of refractory celiac disease. Gut. 2010; 59(4):547–557

[45] Malamut G, Afchain P, Verkarre V, et al. Presentation and long-term follow-up of refractory celiac disease: comparison of type I with type II. Gastroenterology. 2009; 136(1):81–90

[46] Rubio-Tapia A, Kelly DG, Lahr BD, et al. Clinical staging and survival in refractory celiac disease: a single center experience. Gastroenterology. 2009; 136(1):99–107, quiz 352–353

[47] Al-Toma A, Verbeek WH, Hadithi M, et al. Survival in refractory coeliac disease and enteropathy-associated T-cell lymphoma: retrospective evaluation of single-centre experience. Gut. 2007; 56(10):1373–1378

[48] Husby S, Koletzko S, Korponay-Szabó IR, et al; ESPGHAN Working Group on Coeliac Disease Diagnosis. ESPGHAN Gastroenterology Committee. European Society for Pediatric Gastroenterology, Hepatology, and Nutrition. European Society for Pediatric Gastroenterology, Hepatology, and Nutrition guidelines for the diagnosis of coeliac disease. J Pediatr Gastroenterol Nutr. 2012; 54(1):136–160

[49] Ghoshal UC, Srivastava D, Verma A, Ghoshal U. Tropical sprue in 2014: the new face of an old disease. Curr Gastroenterol Rep. 2014; 16(6):391

[50] Rickles FR, Klipstein FA, Tomasini J, et al. Long-term follow-up of antibiotic-treated tropical sprue. Ann Intern Med. 1972; 76(2):203–210

[51] Lappinga PJ, Abraham SC, Murray JA, et al. Small intestinal bacterial overgrowth: histopathologic features and clinical correlates in an underrecognized entity. Arch Pathol Lab Med. 2010; 134(2):264–270

[52] Gasbarrini A, Corazza GR, Gasbarrini G, et al; 1st Rome H2-Breath Testing Consensus Conference Working Group. Methodology and indications of H2-breath testing in gastrointestinal diseases: the Rome Consensus Conference. Aliment Pharmacol Ther. 2009; 29(suppl 1):1–49

[53] Bures J, Cyrany J, Kohoutova D, et al. Small intestinal bacterial overgrowth syndrome. World J Gastroenterol. 2010; 16(24):2978–2990

[54] Rubio-Tapia A, Herman ML, Ludvigsson JF, et al. Severe spruelike enteropathy associated with olmesartan. Mayo Clin Proc. 2012; 87(8):732–738

[55] Rubio-Tapia A, Talley NJ, Gurudu SR, et al. Gluten-free diet and steroid treatment are effective therapy for most patients with collagenous sprue. Clin Gastroenterol Hepatol. 2010; 8(4):344–349.e3

[56] Burbure N, Lebwohl B, Arguelles-Grande C, et al. Olmesartan-associated spruelike enteropathy: a systematic review with emphasis on histopathology. Hum Pathol. 2016; 50:127–134

[57] Marietta EV, Nadeau AM, Cartee AK, et al. Immunopathogenesis of olmesartan-associated enteropathy. Aliment Pharmacol Ther. 2015; 42(11–12):1303–1314

34 Portal Hypertension, Varices, Gastropathy, and Gastric Antral Vascular Ectasia

Ibrahim Mostafa Ibrahim, Mostafa Ibrahim, and Nancy N. Fanous

34.1 Introduction

The term "portal hypertension" was first introduced by Gilbert and Carnot in 1902. Substantial progress has been achieved in understanding the pathophysiology of portal hypertension over the past decades. This progress has led to the development of new therapeutic approaches such as pharmacological and endoscopic therapies, as well as surgical and radiological shunting procedures. Portal hypertension remains one of the most serious sequelae of chronic liver disease. Complications of portal hypertension such as gastrointestinal hemorrhage, hepatic encephalopathy, hepatorenal syndrome, and ascites continue to be the cause of significant morbidity and mortality in many countries.

34.2 Portal Hypertension: What Do We Need to Know?

34.2.1 Pathophysiology of Portal Hypertension

Portal hypertension (PHT) is a clinical syndrome defined by pathologic increase of portal venous pressure gradient (PVPG) between the portal vein (PV) and the inferior vena cava (IVC) to greater than 5 mm Hg. The hepatic venous pressure gradient (HVPG) accurately reflects the portal pressure gradient in the most common causes of cirrhosis,[1] and summarizes in a single measurement the interplay between two factors: hepatic resistance to portal flow and increased portal venous blood flow.[2]

34.2.2 Noncirrhotic Portal Hypertension

The diseases leading to noncirrhotic portal hypertension (NCPH) are primarily vascular in nature and classified anatomically on the basis of site of resistance to blood flow as prehepatic, hepatic, and posthepatic; hepatic causes are further subdivided into presinusoidal, sinusoidal, and postsinusoidal (▶Table 34.1).[2,3,4]

In NCPH, HVPG is normal or only mildly elevated and is significantly lower than PV pressure.[1,2] Schistosomiasis is one of the most common causes of NCPH worldwide. Two disease entities in NCPH, noncirrhotic portal fibrosis/idiopathic PHT (NCPF/IPH) and extrahepatic PV obstruction (EHPVO) are distinct diseases presenting with features of PHT but without evidence of significant parenchymal dysfunction.[3,4,5] Doppler ultrasound (US) is the first-line radiologic investigation in both disorders. Management in both NCPF/IPH and EHPVO is focused on management of acute variceal bleeding (AVB).[3,6]

34.2.3 Cirrhotic Portal Hypertension: Natural History, Risk Stratification, and Individualizing Care

PHT is the main driving factor in the natural history of cirrhosis. HVPG measurement is the gold-standard method to assess the presence of clinically significant portal hypertension (CSPH), which is defined as HVPG greater than or equal to 10 mm Hg. Patients without CSPH have no gastroesophageal varices, and have a low 5-year risk of developing them. Ascites and gastroesophageal varices are the most frequent manifestations of CSPH.[6,7]

For patients with compensated cirrhosis, the alternative term "compensated advanced chronic liver disease (cACLD)" has been proposed by Baveno VI to better reflect the ongoing progression of severe fibrosis to cirrhosis. In asymptomatic patients with known causes of chronic liver disease (CLD), liver stiffness by transient elastography (TE) is sufficient to *suspect* cACLD. Values less than 10 kPa in the absence of other clinical signs can exclude cACLD; values 10 to 15 kPa are suggestive of cACLD; values greater than 15 kPa are highly suggestive of cACLD. In patients with virus-related cACLD, noninvasive tests as TE greater than or equal to 20 to 25 kPa, alone or combined to platelets and spleen size are sufficient to diagnose CSPH. Confirmation of cACLD can be done by liver biopsy, upper gastrointestinal (GI) endoscopy, and HVPG.[7]

Three different risk stages have been proposed based on 1-year mortality data: low-, intermediate-, and high-risk cirrhosis. Each category of risk is presented with the clinical features, HVPG value, the main outcome to prevent, the main pathophysiologic factor related with that category of risk. The 1-year mortality in these stages is less than or equal to 1%, 1 to 20%, and greater than or equal to 20%, respectively (▶Table 34.2).[8]

34.3 Diagnosis of Portal Hypertension

34.3.1 Hepatic Venous Pressure Gradient

PHT is present if the HVPG is greater than or equal to 6 mm Hg; it typically becomes clinically significant with HVPG greater than or equal to 10 mm Hg, at which point varices may develop. Once the HVPG is greater than or equal to 12 mm Hg, patients are at risk for variceal bleeding and the development of ascites.[9]

34.3.2 Noninvasive Tests

Transabdominal Ultrasound with Doppler Imaging

It may support a diagnosis of portal hypertension, but lack sensitivity.[10]

Table 34.1 Causes of noncirrhotic portal hypertension

Pre-hepatic

FHVP normal, RAP normal, WHVP normal, HVPG normal, PVP high, ISP high
Extrahepatic portal vein obstruction (EHPVO)
Portal vein thrombosis
Splenic vein thrombosis
Splanchnic arteriovenous fistula
Massive splenomegaly
- Infiltrative diseases-Lymphoma, myeloproliferative disorders
- Storage diseases-Gaucher's disease

Hepatic

*FHVP normal, RAP normal, WHVP high, HVPG normal or high, PVP high, ISP high

Pre-sinusoidal	Sinusoidal	Post-sinusoidal
Developmental abnormalities	Sinusoidal fibrosis	Venoocclusive disease
• Adult polycystic disease	• Alcoholic hepatitis	• Hepatic irradiation
• Hereditary hemorrhagic disease	• Drugs (methotrexate, amiodarone)	• Toxins-Pyrrolizidine alkaloids
• Arteriovenous fistulas	• Toxins (vinyl chloride, copper)	• Drugs-Gemtuzumab. ozogamicin.
• Congenital hepatic fibrosis	• Metabolic (NASH. Gaucher's disease)	actinomycin D. dacarbazine. cytosine
Biliary diseases	• Inflammatory (viral hepatitis. Q fever, healed	arabinoside. mithramycin, 6-thioguanine.
• Primary biliary cirrhosis	cytomegalovirus, secondary typhfc)	azathioprine. busulfan plus cyclophosphamide
• Sclerosing cholangitis	Sinusoidal collapse	Phlebosclerosis of hepatic veins
• Autoimmune cholangiopathy	• Acute necro-inflammatory diseases	• Alcoholic liver disease
• Toxic-Vinyl chloride	Sinusoidal defenestration	• Chronic radiation injury
Neoplastc occlusion of portal vein	• Alcoholic liver disease (early phase)	• Hypervitaminosis A
• Lymphoma	Sinusoidal infiltration	• E-ferol injury
• Epithelioid hemangioendothelioma	• Mastocytosis	Primary vascular malignancies
• Epithelial malignancies	• Agnogenic myeloid metaplasia	• Epithelioid hemangioendothelioma
• Chronic lymphocytic leukemia	• Gaucher's disease	• Angiosarcoma
Granulomatous lesions	• Amyloidosis	Granulomatous phlebitis
• Schistosomiasis	Sinusoidal compression	• Sarcoidosis
• Mineral oil granuloma	• By enlarged Kupffer cells (Gaucher's disease,	• Mycobacterium species
• Sarcoidosis	visceral Leishmaniasis)	• Lipogranulomas
Hepatoportal sclerosis	• By enlarged fat-laden hepatocytes (Alcoholic	• Mineral oil granuloma
Peliosis hepatitis	hepatitis. AFLP)	Hepatic vein outflow tract obstruction
Partial nodular transformation		(HVOTO, Budd-Chiari syndrome)-Idiopathic.
Noncirrhotic portal fibrosis (NCPF)/ Idiopathic		prothnombotic states
portal hypertension (IPH)		

Post-hepatic

**FHVP high, RAP normal or high, WHVP high, HVPG normal or high, PVP high, ISP high
Inferior vena cava obstruction-web, thrombosis, tumour, enlarged caudate lobe
Constrictive pericarditis
Tricuspid regurgitation
Severe right-sided heart failure
Restrictive cardiomyopathy

*HVPG not feasible in HVOTO with ocdusion of all 3 hepatic veins, or supra- and intrahepatic inferior vena cava obstruction.

**Inferior vena cava pressure should also be taken both above and below the opening of hepatic veins.

AFLP, acute fatty liver of pregnancy; FHVP, free hepatic venous pressure; HVPG, hepatic venous pressure gradient (difference between FHVP and WHVP); ISP, intrasplenic pressure; KAP, right atrial pressure; NASH, non-akoholic steatohepatitis; PVP, portal vein pressure; WHVP, wedged hepatic venous pressure.

Adapted from Khanna R and Sarin SK.[2]

Transient Elastography

A noninvasive technique to assess the stage of hepatic fibrosis and degree of PHT. Results are expressed in kilopascal and can range from 2.5 to 75 kPa.[11,12]

TE values higher than 15 kPa could be used to diagnose cA-CLD. Values greater than or equal to 20 to 25 kPa are sufficient to rule in CSPH; and less than 20 kPa associated with platelet count greater than 150,000 could safely avoid screening of esophageal varices by endoscopy.[7]

The cutoff values for patients with hepatitis C virus (HCV) infection and cirrhosis range from 11 to 17 kPa. The sensitivity and specificity are approximately 70 to 80% for F2 to F4 fibrosis.[13,14] Diagnostic accuracy is similar in patients with advanced-stage nonalcoholic fatty liver disease (NAFLD), with an area under the receiver operating characteristic (AUROC) curve of 0.94, sensitivity of 94%, and specificity of 95%.[15] In patients with autoimmune liver diseases, TE is very sensitive and specific for predicting advanced fibrosis in patients with primary biliary cholangitis and primary sclerosing cholangitis[16] however, it is less reliable than in autoimmune hepatitis due to significant hepatic inflammation that can overestimate stiffness.[17] There have been several meta-analyses of transient elastography testing, with a summary AUROC curve for diagnosing cirrhosis ranging from 0.90 to 0.95.[13,14,18] A meta-analysis of 40 studies of patients with CLD found a sensitivity of 83% and specificity of 89% for cirrhosis; however, for stage 2 fibrosis, the sensitivity was only 79% and specificity was 78%.[19]

Table 34.2 Natural history of cirrhosis and the prognostic contribution of HVPG measurement

	Stages of cirrhosis Mortality risk at 1 yr		
Clinical features	Low ≤ 1% Asymptomatic no varices	Intermediate 1%-20% Varices/ ascites or both	High > 20% Bleeding/re-bleeding SBP Refractory ascites HRS/AKI
HVPG of risk	10 mmHg		Infection other than SBP 12/16/20 mmHg
Main outcome to prevent Main pathophysiologic factor	Decompensation and/or HCC and/ or varices Intrahepatic structural and hemo- dynamic changes Portal pressure	Decompensation and/ or HCC mortality Extrahepatic hemodynamic changes Portal pressure	HCC and/ or mortality Hepatocellualr dysfunction Portal pressure Cytokine release Peripheral perfusion Coagulopathy? Other?

Each category of risk is presented with the clinical features, the hepatic venous pressure gradient value, the main outcome to prevent, the main pathophysiologic factor related with that categoiy of risk. ACLF, Acute on chronic liver failure; AKI, Acute kidney injury; HCC, Hepatocellular carcinoma; HRS, Hepato-renal syndrome; HVPG, Hepatic venous pressure gradient; SEP, Spontaneous bacterial peritonitis.

Adapted from La Mura et al.[8]

- **Evaluation for the underlying cause**: For causes of cirrhotic and noncirrhotic PHT.

34.4 Treatment of Portal Hypertension

Therapies are aimed at achieving one of the following results:

a) *Treatment of the Underlying Cause*

In the era of new antiviral drugs, cirrhosis should be regarded as a disease whose mortality risk can be significantly reduced by a specific tailored approach.[7]

b) *Prevention and Management of the Other Complications of Portal Hypertension*

Other complications of portal hypertension include spontaneous bacterial peritonitis (SBP), portal hypertensive gastropathy, hepatic hydrothorax, hepatopulmonary syndrome, portopulmonary hypertension.

c) *Decreasing Portal Hypertension and Direct Treatment of Varices*

Natural History of Varices

Varices are present in 50% of patients with cirrhosis and these form at a rate of 5 to 15% per year. Variceal bleeding occurs in one-third of patients with varices, and causes 70% of all upper gastrointestinal bleeding (UGIB) episodes in cirrhotic patients. Standardization of supportive care and new therapeutic options reduced bleeding-related mortality from about 50 to 15%—20% in the last three decades.[20,21,22]

Screening and Surveillance

In patients with cirrhosis, the risk of varices is very low in patients with platelet count greater than or equal to 150,000 and the liver stiffness less than 20 kPa on TE, those patients may be followed up with annual platelet count and TE.[7] Endoscopic screening for varices should be performed if platelet count is less than 150,000 and TE is greater than 20 kPa: every 2 to 3 years in patients with compensated cirrhosis and no varices; 1 to 2 years in small Upper

Table 34.3 Classification of esophageal varice

	Two-size classification	Three-size classification
Small	< 5 mm	Minimally elevated straight veins above the esophageal mucosal surface
Medium	-	Tortuous veins occupying less than one-third of the lumen
Large	> 5 mm	Occupying more than one-third of the lumen

Adapted from LaBrecqu D et al.[24]

Gastrointestinal Tract Disease varices; and yearly or at the time of first decompensation in decompensated cirrhosis.[20]

Esophageal varices (EV) are long columns of dilated veins, usually occurring within the lower third of the esophagus, immediately above the gastroesophageal junction (GEJ). EV are endoscopically graded according to the size (▶Table 34.3;▶Fig. 34.1)[23]; however, the American Association of Study of Liver Disease (AASLD) recommends the classification into small and large esophageal varices based on a cutoff of 5 mm. In practice, the recommendations for medium-sized varices in the three-size classification are the same as for large varices in the two-size classification.[24]

Gastric varices are supplied by the short gastric veins and drain into the deep intrinsic veins of the lower esophagus. These are classified according to site by the Sarin classification (▶Fig. 34.2, ▶Table 34.4).[25] Gastric varices account for 10 to 30% of variceal haemorrhage and can occur in up to 20% of patients with portal hypertension.[26] In our experience, the location of gastric varices according to the Sarin classification has no impact on management of acute gastric variceal bleeding (**Video 34.1**).

The predictors of variceal bleeding include presence of decompensated cirrhosis (Child–Turcotte–Pugh [CTP] class B or C), size of varices, and presence of high-risk stigmata upon endoscopy (red wale marks/cherry red spots).[27] The 1-year rate of recurrent variceal hemorrhage is approximately 60%.[28] The 6-week mortality with each episode of variceal hemorrhage is approximately 15 to 20%.[29]

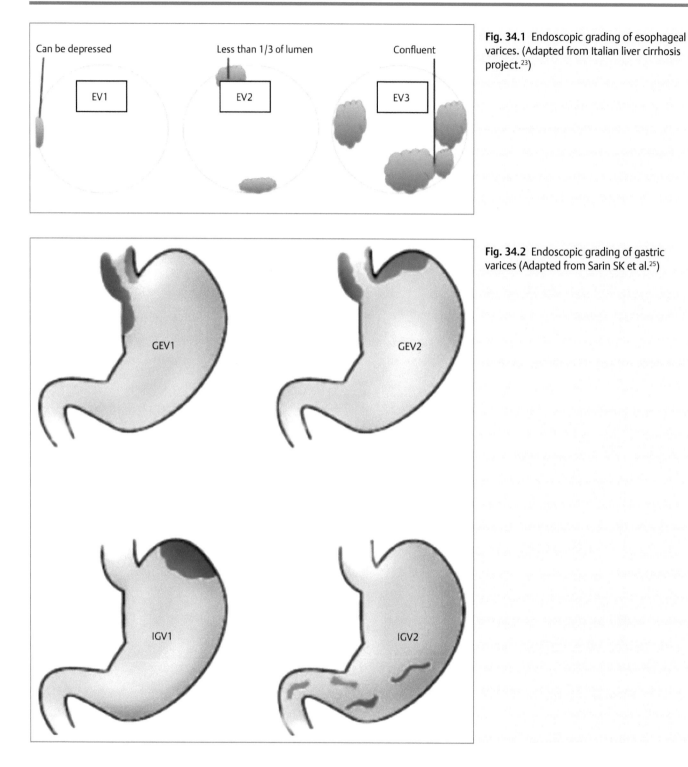

Fig. 34.1 Endoscopic grading of esophageal varices. (Adapted from Italian liver cirrhosis project.[23])

Fig. 34.2 Endoscopic grading of gastric varices (Adapted from Sarin SK et al.[25])

Table 34.4 Sarin's classification of gastric varices

Sarin's type of gastric varix	Description/location
Gastroesophageal varices-1 (GEV-1)	Continue from esophageal varices and extend on lesser curve 2–5 cm below the GE junction (75% of all gastric varices)
Gastroesophageal varices-2 (GEV-2)	Extend beyond the GE junction into the fundus of the stomach and are continuous with esophageal varices (21% of all gastric varices), and more tortuous than GEV-1
Isolated gastric varices-1 (IGV-1)	Occur in absence of esophageal varices, and occur in the fundus, and are tortuous and complex
Isolated gastric varices-2 (IGV-2)	Occur in absence of esophageal varices, in the body, antrum, or pylorus

Adapted from Sarin SK et al.[25]

Preprimary Prophylaxis

Treatment of the etiologic agent is expected to improve both liver structure and function, and this could reflect on reduction of PHT and development of varices. Treatment with nonselective β-blockers (NSBB) is *not* recommended in those patients.[20]

34.4.1 Primary Prophylaxis

Primary prophylaxis refers to the prevention of a first variceal hemorrhage in a patient with varices. Guidelines recommend usage of one of two approaches: ***pharmacologic prophylaxis using NSBB, or endoscopic prophylaxis using endoscopic variceal ligation (EVL).*** Both NSBB and EVL are superior to no treatment for the prevention of a first variceal hemorrhage in patients with medium- and large-sized varices and patients with small varices who have red signs or are Child's score B or C (**Video 34.2**).[7]

Pharmacologic Treatment

According to Baveno VI, traditional NSBB (propranolol, nadolol) and carvedilol are valid first-line treatments for primary prophylaxis of variceal hemorrhage. Carvedilol proved to be more effective than traditional NSBB in reducing HVPG, but has not been adequately compared head-to-head to traditional NSBB in clinical trials.[7]

Nadolol and propranolol at a starting dose of 20 to 40 mg/d, respectively are used in patients with good tolerability and no contraindication to β-blockers. A meta-analysis that included seven trials with 797 patients found that patients treated with β-blockers had improved outcomes compared with controls.[30] **Carvedilol** has been recommended in a dose of 12.5 mg twice daily for patients with Child A cirrhosis, and 6.25 mg twice daily for patients with Child B or C cirrhosis.[31] **Other drugs** such as simvastatin, clonidine, molsidomine, metoclopramide, pentoxifylline, verapamil, and losartan are being evaluated.[32] The effect of NSBB can be monitored through either starting at a low dose then increasing to a maximum tolerated dose as needed to achieve a resting heart rate of about 55 to 60 beats/min[33]; or a decrease in HVPG of at least 10% from baseline or to less than or equal to 12 mm Hg after chronic treatment with

NSBB is clinically relevant and is associated with a significant reduction in risk of variceal bleeding and decompensation. Similarly, acute HVPG response to intravenous propranolol may be used to identify responders to β-blockers.[7] HVPG measurements may be useful in clinical trials; however, it is not feasible for routine practice.

Endoscopic Management

EVL is recommended for patients with medium or large varices who are intolerant of or have contraindications to β-blockers, or if a goal reduction in HVPG cannot be achieved. Effectiveness of EVL versus NSBB for primary prophylaxis has been studied and several meta-analyses have been published. The overall data suggest that EVL is as effective as NSBB with somewhat less hemorrhage but no changes in overall mortality.[34,35,36,37,38]

NSBB do not prevent development or progression from small to large varices and have significant side effects. On the other hand, EVL should be performed by expert endoscopists to avoid complications including banding-induced ulcerations and bleeding (**Video 34.3**). Also, patients require routine endoscopic surveillance post-EVL due to the probability of variceal recurrence.[39] The frequency of endoscopic evaluation depends on multiple factors such as whether the patient has varices, size of varices and risk signs, and if the patient had compensated or decompensated liver disease (▶ Fig. 34.3). In general, patients require three

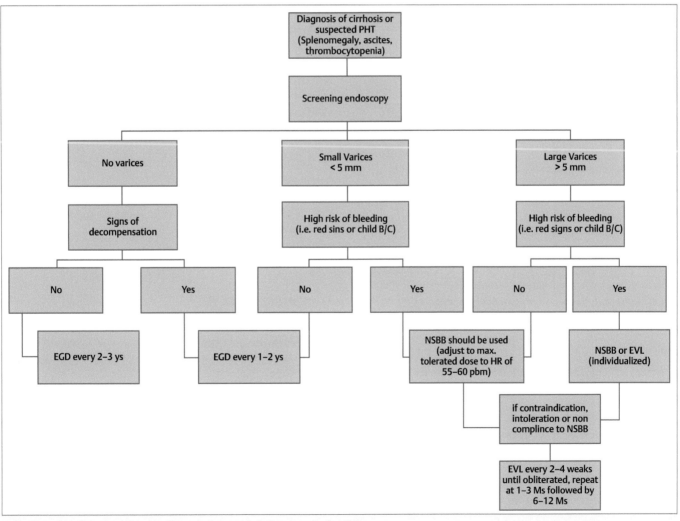

Fig. 34.3 Flow diagram demonstrating primary prophylaxis strategies for AVB.

to four sessions for eradication of varices. Combination therapy was not more effective than EVL alone in preventing hemorrhage or death.[40] Therefore, decision to choose either option should be individualized based on local resources and level of experience.

Prophylactic endoscopic sclerotherapy (ES) for esophageal varices is not recommended as it carries higher rates of complications without substantial benefit.[41,42] Though it has been studied for this use in patients with large gastric varices,[7] the Baveno consensus guidelines did not recommend cyanoacrylate injection for primary prophylaxis of gastric varices. For the time being, patients with gastric varices should continue to receive NSBB for primary prophylaxis. Surgical shunts and transjugular intrahepatic portosystemic shunt (TIPS) have been proposed for primary prophylaxis; however, the available data do not support their use.

In our experience, we do prophylactic ES for gastric varices by glue only in two situations: (1) management of acute esophageal variceal bleeding if associated with gastric varices of any type; (2) during prophylactic EVL for esophageal varices in a patient with associated gastric varices. Theoretically, obliteration of esophageal varices may lead to increased pressure in gastric varices thus increasing the possibility of gastric hemorrhage.

34.4.2 Management of Acute Variceal Bleeding

Management of AVB necessitates the work of a multidisciplinary team, and works simultaneous on four axes: initial resuscitation, treatment of acute bleeding, secondary prophylaxis, and management of treatment failure.

Risk Stratification and Resuscitation

Evaluation of hemodynamic status and intravascular volume monitoring is crucial through careful history taking, vital signs with measuring orthostatic hemodynamic changes, and laboratory testing (complete blood count [CBC], coagulation parameters, blood grouping and cross-matching of 2–4 blood units, liver and kidney function) is initially performed.

Risk stratification into low- and high-risk patients on admission according to validated prognostic scales should be done. High-risk patients can be identified for early intervention, thus reducing morbidity and mortality. Low-risk patients can be discharged safely. The *Glasgow–Blatchford score (GBS)* should be used in every patient on initial presentation.[43] The *Rockall score* can also be used, but requires knowledge of endoscopic findings to be fully completed.[44]

Airway protection up to endotracheal intubation may be considered in patients with massive bleeding and/or hepatic encephalopathy.[45] Routine use of nasogastric tube (NGT) in patients with AVB is controversial. It is unclear whether NGT placement aggravates hemorrhage from varices or Mallory–Weiss tears. Although studies have failed to demonstrate a benefit with regard to clinical outcomes[46]; however, in our experience a NGT placement and washing with cold saline together with the start of pharmacologic therapy can help decompress the stomach, help prevent aspiration, and assist in clearing the field before endoscopy.

Circulatory support is done through two large-bore peripheral intravenous lines or a central line. Replacement is done by packed red blood cells (RBCs) following the restrictive transfusion strategy aiming for a hemoglobin level of 7 to 8 g/L.[6] A study by Villanueva et al compared the efficacy and safety of a restrictive transfusion strategy (transfusion when the hemoglobin level fell below 7 g/L) with those of a liberal transfusion strategy (transfusion when the hemoglobin level fell below 9 g/L) in a total of 921 patients with severe acute upper GI bleeding. The probability of survival at 6 weeks was higher in the restrictive-strategy group than in the liberal-strategy group (95 vs. 91%). Further bleeding occurred in 10% of the patients in the restrictive-strategy group as compared with 16% of the patients in the liberal-strategy group ($p = 0.01$), and adverse events occurred in 40% as compared with 48% ($p = 0.02$). The probability of survival was significantly higher in the subgroup of patients with cirrhosis and Child–Pugh class A or B disease, but not in those with cirrhosis and Child–Pugh class C disease. Within the first 5 days, the portal-pressure gradient increased significantly in patients assigned to the liberal strategy, but not in those assigned to the restrictive strategy.[47]

Coagulopathy should be corrected as needed with fresh frozen plasma and platelet transfusion. The role of recombinant factor VIIa cannot yet be recommended for routine clinical use in patients with variceal hemorrhage.[48]

Antibiotic prophylaxis is recommended in AVB (▶ Table 34.5). A systematic review including eight placebo-controlled trials in 864 patients found the antibiotics were associated with a significant reduction in mortality and bacterial infections as bacteremia, pneumonia, SBP, and urinary tract infections.[49] Intravenous ceftriaxone (1 g/d for 7 days) proved superior to norfloxacin in a randomized-controlled trial (alternatives include trimethoprim-sulfamethoxazole [one double-strength tablet twice daily]or ciprofloxacin [500 mg orally every 12 hours]).[50] Antibiotics may also reduce the risk of recurrent bleeding in hospitalized patients who bled from esophageal varices.[51] Guidelines recommend that short-term (maximum 7 days) antibiotic prophylaxis should be instituted in any patient with cirrhosis and GI hemorrhage. In patients with advanced cirrhosis, intravenous ceftriaxone may be preferable, particularly in centers with a high prevalence of quinolone-resistant organisms.[52]

Hepatic encephalopathy (HE) prevention in patients with cirrhosis and upper GI bleeding may be achieved by either lactulose or rifaximin.[7]

Thiamine should be given in alcoholic subjects monitored for withdrawal symptoms.[53]

Treatment of AVB

Pharmacologic therapy should be started in all patients with advanced cirrhosis and UGIB who have varices or who are at risk for having varices. Upper endoscopy should be performed within 12

Table 34.5 Antibiotic prophylaxis in AVB

Antibiotic	Dose	Duration
Norfloxacin (not available in the U.S. anymore)	400 mg PO q12h	Maximum of 7 d
Ciprofloxacin	500 mg PO or IV q12h	Maximum of 7 d
Trimethoprim–sulfamethoxazole	160/800 mg PO q12h	Maximum of 7 d
Ceftriaxone	1 g IV q24h	Maximum of 7 d

AVB, acute variceal bleeding.

hours of presentation. Early rebleeding may occur 120 hours–6 weeks from time of presentation after initial hemostasis. Child–Pugh class C, the updated model for end-stage liver disease (MELD) score, and failure to achieve initial hemostasis are the variables most consistently found to predict 6-week mortality (**Video 34.4**).[7]

Acid Suppressive Therapy: Clot dissolution and platelet aggregation are pH-dependent processes. Proton pump inhibitor (PPI) treatment (an intravenous bolus followed by continuous infusion) reduces rebleeding and surgery compared with placebo or H2 receptor antagonist (H2RA) in nonvariceal UGIB.[54,55] However, PPIs' role in AVB is controversial. A systematic review aimed to assess the efficacy and safety of PPIs in gastroesophageal varices demonstrated that level I evidence suggested that PPIs reduce esophageal ulcer size postelective esophageal ligation. The clinical importance of such findings is not known given the self-limiting nature of esophageal ulcer. Available evidence does not support a role of PPIs for long-term prophylaxis of PHT-related bleeding, and high-dose infusion for acute management of gastroesophageal variceal (GEV) hemorrhage. The best available evidence supports the use of short-course (10 days) PPI postendoscopic variceal ligation to reduce ulcer size if ulcer healing is a concern. Practices such as high-dose infusion and prolonged use should be discouraged until evidence of benefit becomes available.[56]

Vasoconstrictors: Vasoactive medications selectively constrict mesenteric arterioles thus decreasing portal blood flow and are used as initial treatment of AVB before endoscopy. Randomized-controlled trials demonstrated that the early use of vasoactive drugs reduces the rate of active bleeding, making endoscopy easier to perform for diagnostic and therapeutic purposes.[57] These include vasopressin, somatostatin, and their analogs (terlipressin and octreotide, respectively). In a meta-analysis of 30 randomized trials in 3,111 patients with AVB, the use of vasoactive medications was associated with improved hemostasis and decreased 7-day mortality, transfusion requirement, and duration of hospitalization as compared with placebo.[58] Terlipressin is initially given as 2 mg intravenous (IV) bolus every 4 hours. Octreotide is given as a 50 µg IV bolus, followed by a continuous infusion at a rate of 50 µg/h. Intravenous vasopressin (0.4-unit bolus followed by an infusion of 0.4–1 units/min) can also be used. Somatostatin is given IV bolus 250 mg followed by infusion of 250 to 500 mg/h. Vapreotide as IV bolus of 50 mg followed by infusion of 50 mg/h. Vasoconstrictors should be started at the time of presentation in patients with suspected variceal bleeding and should be continued for 3 to 5 days.[7]

A systematic review found that combining somatostatin or octreotide with EVL improved the 5-day success rate compared with EVL alone.[59,60] Terlipressin is the preferred agent in many countries outside of the United States, and is the only agent individually shown to reduce mortality.[61] A meta-analysis found a statistically significant reduction in all-cause mortality with terlipressin compared with placebo. Hyponatremia has been described in patients under terlipressin, especially in patients with preserved liver function. Therefore, sodium levels must be monitored (**Video 34.5**).[7]

Endoscopy: Sedation usage before diagnostic endoscopy is routine in North America and Australia, but varies considerably among countries in Europe, Asia, and Africa.[62] Both midazolam and propofol are used for therapeutic endoscopy. As compared to midazolam, propofol was proved superior in facilitating

endoscopy, better patient satisfaction, and more rapid recovery.[63] A prospective randomized-controlled trial on 210 patients to compared sedation with a combination of propofol plus fentanyl versus midazolam plus fentanyl in cirrhotic outpatients undergoing UGIE showed that both sedation schemes were safe in this setting. Sedation with propofol plus fentanyl was more effective with a shorter recovery time compared with midazolam plus fentanyl.[64] A comparative meta-analysis of pooled data aimed to evaluate the safety of nonanesthesia provider (NAAP)-administered propofol sedation for advanced endoscopic procedures with those of anesthesia provider (AAP). Data were analyzed for hypoxia rate, airway intervention rates, endoscopist and patient satisfaction scores, and total propofol administered. The safety of NAAP sedation compared favorably with AAP sedation in patients undergoing advanced endoscopic procedures. However, it came at the cost of decreased patient and endoscopist satisfaction.[65,66]

The two endoscopic methods available for AVB are ES and EVL. ES complies the injection of a sclerosing agent intravariceal or paravariceal. A variety of sclerosant solutions are used, the most common of them are ethanolamine oleate (5%), polidocanol (1–2%), and cyanoacrylate, which proved equally effective for bleeding esophageal varices.[67] Emergency ES for bleeding esophageal varices was proved an effective and safe procedure.[68] A study compared intravariceal ethanolamine oleate and peri- and intravariceal polidocanol alone or in combination concluded that ethanolamine with or without polidocanol was safe and effective, but needs more injection sessions as compared with polidocanol. The use of polidocanol, however, is limited for its ulcerogenic effect.[69] ES is easy to use leading to rapid formation of thrombus and subsequently hemostasis. Disadvantages include variety of local and systemic complications as substernal chest pain, fever, dysphagia, and pleural effusion. Esophageal ulcers are common, and may bleed in 20% of patients.[70] Bacteremia is reported in up to 35% and may lead to SBP or distal abscesses.[71,72]

EVL works by banding all or part of a varix resulting in thrombosis and occlusion, leading to tissue necroses and sloughs in a few days to weeks, leaving a superficial mucosal ulceration which rapidly heals.[73] Actively bleeding varices or those with stigmata indicating recent bleeding (such as a fibrin plug or a "red wale" sign) should be primary targets even if they are not located at the gastroesophageal junction.

The original banding device (Stiegmann–Goff ligator) required the use of an overtube.[74] The multiple-band ligating systems produced by Conmed (Stiegmann–Goff endoscopic ligator), Boston-Scientific (SpeedBand), and Cook Medical (Saeed multiband ligators) provide 4 to 10 bands that can be deployed in one session without having to remove the endoscope.[75] The use of ligating devices may be limited in patients with severe bleeding due to limited visibility by blood accumulating in the tip of the device. We recommend using narrow-band imaging (NBI), i-Scan, and flexible spectral imaging color enhancement (FICE) to detect the gastroesophageal junction in patients with acute bleeding. This helps precise application of bands at the Z-line and improves the procedure outcomes (**Video 34.6**).

Banding is started in the most distal portion of the esophagus near the gastroesophageal junction. Bands are applied in a spiral pattern up the esophagus until 28 cm from incisors, banding all major columns of varices. In our experience, banding above 28 cm causes more pain and dysphagia; moreover, it is above the site of perforating feeding vessels. A randomized, prospective study showed that placement of more than six bands per session did not improve patient outcomes but prolonged procedure time and increase in the number of misfired bands.[76] In our experience, up to 12 bands may be placed in one session, and this decreases the total number of sessions. One-week ligation intervals led to more rapid eradication than 2-week intervals without an increase in complications, number of endoscopies, and without a reduction in rebleeding or other clinical outcomes as dysphagia/odynophagia/chest pain, strictures, and mortality. The decision regarding ligation intervals may be individualized based on physician and patient preferences and local logistics and resources.[77] In our experience, ligation after 1 week before band sloughing decreases the incidence of rebleeding due to postband ulcer. Common complications of EVL include chest pain and transient dysphagia, which respond well to analgesics.

The comparison between ES and EVL has been thoroughly evaluated. A meta-analysis and prospective randomized study showed that EVL was superior than ES for all major outcomes including initial control of bleeding, recurrent bleeding, side effects, time to variceal obliteration, and survival.[78,79] The incidence of bacteremia is less common after EVL than ES, which makes it a safer procedure specially in patients with high risk of infections.[80,81] Both EVL and ES induce inconsistent degrees of portal hypertensive gastropathy (PHG); however ES induced more fibrosis which might reduce bleeding recurrence.[82]

Combination Therapy: Is There a Role?

Combining EVL and ES has been proposed to speed variceal eradication and reduce the likelihood of rebleeding.[83] There is no advantage to combining EVL and ES for management of variceal bleeding at each and every session, a conclusion also reached in a meta-analysis.[84] Argon plasma coagulation (APC) or microwave cautery may improve the treatment of esophageal varices when combined with EVL.[85] Endoscopic clipping was proved ineffective and carries high risk of rebleeding, and therefore not recommended.[86]

EVL combined with a vasoactive drug is considered the standard of care for AVB and it is currently recommended by guidelines.[7]

34.5 Secondary Prophylaxis

Multiple sessions are required to eradicate varices. In our experience, we recommend repeating EVL within 7 to 10 days, with addition to PPIs and semisolid diet. However, there is limited published data to support this timing interval. In the second session, bands should be applied to any persistent varices. There is no concern about banding close to an ulcer from a fallen off band. After achieving variceal eradication, we suggest a follow-up endoscopy in 1 month, followed by an examination in every 3 months for 6 to 9 months; and the interval can be increased to 6 to 12 months as needed. The average eradication time is approximately 3.7 sessions with EVL and 4.9 sessions with ES.[87] Rebleeding after elective EVL appears to be considerably lower than after emergent EVL (0.5 vs. 7.1%).[88]

34.6 Management of Treatment Failure

Treatment failure occurs in 15 to 20% of patients with AVB, and is defined by the occurrence of any of the following during the acute bleeding episode (first 5 days): fresh hematemesis or greater than 100 mL of blood in the nasogastric aspirate more than 2 hours after the start of pharmacologic or endoscopic treatment; development of hypovolemic shock; or drop in hemoglobin of greater than or equal to 3 g within 24 hours.[59]

Balloon Tamponade

Three balloons have been used: the Sengstaken–Blakemore tube (which has a gastric and an esophageal balloon, and a single gastric suction port), the Minnesota tube (a modified Sengstaken–Blakemore tube with an esophageal suction port above the esophageal balloon), and the Linton–Nachlas tube (with a single 600-cc gastric balloon). The tube can be left in place for 24 to 48 hours to stabilize the patient. Major complications, such as esophageal rupture, have been observed in 6 to 20% of patients.[89]

A fully covered self-expandable metallic stent (SEMS) (Ella-Danis, Hradec Kralove, Czech Republic) may also be useful in those cases where balloon tamponade is considered.[90] In a meta-analysis that included patients with refractory esophageal variceal bleeding, a SEMS was successfully placed in 95% of patients, but with failure to control bleeding in 18%.[91] Retrieval of the stent is recommended within 7 days to avoid development of pressure-induced ulceration of the esophageal wall.[92,93] Using Histoacryl injection in esophageal variceal bleeding (as per our experience), and the availability of Hemospray will, in our opinion, reduce the use of SEMS significantly.

These methods are temporary and used to stabilize patients, before definitive therapy (surgery or TIPS).

TIPS

Positioning of TIPS as a rescue treatment has been challenged in recent studies, which recommend TIPS as the initial treatment of choice in high-risk patients that improve their prognosis.[94] TIPS with polytetrafluoroethylene PTFE-covered stents is the rescue therapy of choice if combined pharmacologic and endoscopic treatment has failed. Rebleeding during the first 5 days may be managed by a second attempt at endoscopic therapy, and if severe, PTFE-covered TIPS is likely the best option.[7] In nine randomized controlled trials in cirrhotic patients, TIPS placement within 5 days after AVB proved superior to endoscopic treatment in reducing the incidence of rebleeding, showing a significant risk reduction in 1-year mortality without significant increased incidence of hepatic encephalopathy.[95]

The success rate of hemostasis is greater than 90%,[21] but mortality is high owing to the underlying severity of cirrhosis and the added complications of uncontrolled bleeding, especially renal failure.[96] Absolute contraindications to TIPS placement include severe pulmonary hypertension (mean pulmonary pressure > 45 mm Hg), severe tricuspid regurgitation, congestive heart failure, severe liver failure, polycystic liver disease, and patients with active sepsis. Relative contraindications include severe obstructive arteriopathy, hepatic artery and celiac trunk stenosis (which may prevent adequate sinusoidal perfusion by the hepatic artery), HE, hepatocellular carcinoma, and other liver tumors and bile duct dilation.[97]

Surgery

Surgery is indicated in patients with well-preserved liver function who fail emergent endoscopic treatment. There are two basic types of surgery: shunt operation (nonselective and selective) and nonshunt operation (esophageal transection or devascularization of the gastroesophageal junction). Both are highly effective in achieving hemostasis.[98] Shunt surgery significantly increases the incidence of chronic or recurrent portal systemic encephalopathy and complicates future liver transplant surgery.[89]

In Egypt, we rarely use TIPS and surgery, and depend mostly on EVL and ES. This may be attributed to the large number of patients with variceal bleeding and our growing experience in using the different endoscopic techniques with high success rates.

34.7 New Modality in Management of AVB: Hemospray

Hemospray (Cook Medical) is a novel hemostatic nanopowder licensed for endoscopic hemostasis of nonvariceal UGIB and has been shown to be effective in preliminary studies for the management of patients with peptic ulcer bleeding.[99] A pilot study reported that hemostatic powder may be useful in emergency management of variceal rebleeding until a more definitive therapy can be provided.[100]

A recent prospective trial, conducted at two hospitals in Belgium and Egypt, included 30 cirrhotic patients with confirmed AVB. Hemospray application was safe and effective at short-term follow-up for emergency treatment of AVB in cirrhotic patients.[101]

Hemospray offers a new therapeutic option that, in our experience, could bridge the gap that exists in our daily practice between admission of a patient with AVB and more definitive management.

34.8 Management of Gastric Varices

Bleeding intragastric varices should be treated with octreotide (or somatostatin or terlipressin) and balloon tamponade followed by cyanoacrylate injection, with TIPS placement or surgery in refractory cases. Cyanoacrylate injection is highly satisfactory in controlling gastric variceal bleeding and is the preferred approach.[102] It appeared to be more effective and safer than band ligation in this subset of patients.[103] Injection can be done with patients on the right side in acute gastric variceal bleeding to provide clearer field and easier procedure.[104] Combining cyanoacrylate injection with endoscopic ultrasound–guided coil placement is sometimes done to prevent embolization.[105]

Other therapeutic options include variceal band ligation, intravariceal injection of other sclerosants, absolute alcohol, thrombin, fibrin glue, Hemospray, and balloon-occluded retrograde

transvenous obliteration (BRTO).[106,107,108,109,110,111,112] BRTO is an interventional radiologic technique that involves occluding blood flow by inflation of a balloon catheter within a draining vessel, followed by instillation of a sclerosant proximal to the site of balloon occlusion. BRTO requires the presence of a spontaneous shunt into which a balloon catheter is introduced retrograde. Observational studies suggest that patients with gastric varices treated with BRTO have good long-term bleeding control (90%).[112] Technical failure occurs in approximately 10% of cases.[112,113] Complications of BRTO include increased portal pressure with worsening of esophageal varices and ascites and systemic vein thrombosis.[114]

34.9 Management of Ectopic Varices

A guideline issued by the AASLD recommends TIPS as the preferred approach for prevention of rebleeding in patients with ectopic varices (duodenal, rectal, small intestinal, and peristomal).[115] We use cyanoacrylate injection for duodenal and rectal varices with good results.

34.10 Portal Hypertensive Gastropathy and Gastric Antral Vascular Ectasia

PHG and gastric antral vascular ectasia (GAVE) are two distinct entities and are important causes of gastrointestinal bleeding.[116] PHG, by definition, requires the presence of PHT either cirrhotic or noncirrhotic. GAVE requires neither cirrhosis nor PHT, but can occur in both. About 30% of patients with GAVE are cirrhotic and it is more frequent in patients with advanced liver disease.[117,118]

These can be differentiated by their location, endoscopic appearance, and histopathology (▶ Table 34.6).[119]

Management of PHG: During acute bleeding somatostatin, octreotide, terlipressin,[120] APC,[121] and Hemospray may be useful.[122] Current guidelines suggest using NSBB for secondary prophylaxis in patients with PHG and chronic gastrointestinal bleeding.[7] Refractory cases may require TIPS or surgical shunts as salvage therapy.[123,124]

Table 34.6 Characteristics of PHG and GAVE

	PHG	GAVE
Location	Fundus and body	Antrum
Endoscopy	Mosaic/snakeskin mucosa (mild) with red or brown spots (severe)	"Watermelon" or diffuse pattern of ectatic vessels; erythematous (mild) or hemorrhagic (severe)
Biopsy	Nonspecific Dilated mucosal and submucosal veins and ectatic capillaries	Characteristic • Dilated mucosal capillaries with fibrin thrombi • Fibromuscular hyperplasia and spindle cell proliferation of the lamina propria

GAVE, gastric antral vascular ectasia; PHG, portal hypertensive gastropathy.

Adapted from Patwardhan VR and Cardenas A.[119]

Management of GAVE: APC is effective in 90 to 100% of cases.[125] APC requires multiple sessions every 2 to 6 weeks. Recurrence mostly occurs because GAVE involves deeper submucosal structures that may not be adequately reached with coagulation. Band ligation obliterates vascular structures in the deep mucosa and submucosa, thus reducing the need for further treatments, hospital admission, and recurrent bleeding. It also required less treatment sessions than APC.[126]

In our experience, EVL proved superior to APC in treatment of GAVE.[127] We band vascular ectasias in the most distal antrum closest to the pylorus and then moved proximally until the entire affected areas were treated (up to 16 bands placed in a single session). Patients required between two and four sessions of band ligations for resolution of GAVE.

Additional therapies for refractory GAVE include radiofrequency ablation, cryotherapy, cyanoacrylate spray, endoscopic mucosectomy, and surgical antrectomy.[128,129,130,131,132]

34.11 Areas of Uncertainty, Experimental Techniques, and Research

1. The role of treatment of the etiologic agents on the long-term outcome of PHT.
2. The clinical effectiveness of intravenous PPI initiated before endoscopy in patients with AVB.
3. Evaluation of cost-effectiveness of video capsule endoscopy in screening of esophageal varices.
4. Role of endoscopic ultrasound in variceal injection therapy.
5. Effectiveness of novel endoscopic hemostasis techniques in acute esophageal and gastric and variceal bleeding by Hemospray as a bridge before more definitive therapy.
6. Effectiveness of Hemospray in management of postbanding ulceration and PHG.
7. Optimal use of glue injection in esophageal variceal bleeding.

34.12 Conclusion

- PHT is defined by increase of PVPG greater than 5 mm Hg and maybe due to cirrhotic or noncirrhotic causes. Diagnosis of PHT is done by HVPG, transabdominal ultrasound with Doppler imaging, and recently by TE where values greater than or equal to 20 to 25 kPa are sufficient to rule in CSPH. Treatment of PHT aims at decreasing PHT and direct treatment of varices, treatment of the underlying cause, and other complications of PHT.
- Varices are present in 50% of patients with cirrhosis and form at a rate of 5 to 15% per year, where one-third of patients with varices develop AVB. Endoscopic screening for varices should be performed if platelet count less than 150,000 and TE greater than 20 kPa. EVL is as effective as NSBB for primary prophylaxis of AVB; however, prophylactic ES is not recommended due to higher complication rates without substantial benefit.
- Management of AVB necessitates the work of a multidisciplinary team and works simultaneously on four axes: initial resuscitation, treatment of acute bleeding, secondary prophylaxis, and management of treatment failure. Evaluation of hemodynamic status and intravascular volume monitoring are crucial, and risk stratification by using scoring systems is important for early intervention to reduce morbidity and mortality. Airway protection, correction of coagulopathy, and blood volume replacement by packed RBCs following the restrictive

transfusion strategy are mandatory. Antibiotic prophylaxis is recommended using IV ceftriaxone, or oral norfloxacin, ciprofloxacin, or trimethoprin–sulfamethoxazole. Lactulose or rifaximin can be used to prevent HE. Pharmacologic therapy with PPIs and vasoconstrictors should be started in all patients with advanced cirrhosis and AVB who have varices or who are at risk for having varices where vasoconstrictors are associated with improved hemostasis and decreased 7-day mortality, transfusion requirement, and duration of hospitalization. Upper endoscopy should be performed within 12 hours of presentation.
- The two endoscopic methods available for AVB are ES and EVL, and are done after sedation with propofol. Injection of a sclerosing agent intravariceal or paravariceal was proved safe and effective in AVB formerly; however, EVL proved superior to ES for all major outcomes including initial hemostasis, rebleeding, side effects, time to variceal obliteration, and survival. Also, the incidence of bacteremia is less common after EVL than ES. The multiple band-ligating devices provide 4 to 10 bands for deployment in one session. NBI, i-Scan, and FICE facilitate detection of gastroesophageal junction in patients with AVB may improve the procedure outcomes. Combining somatostatin or octreotide with EVL improved the 5-day success rate compared with EVL alone. There is no advantage in combining EVL and ES for management of AVB.
- For secondary prophylaxis, multiple sessions are required to eradicate varices. Management of treatment failure may be done temporarily by balloon tamponade and fully covered SEMS before more definitive therapy (surgery or TIPS). TIPS may be the initial treatment of choice in high-risk patients, and surgery as salvage therapy in patients with preserved liver functions.
- Gastric varices are managed by cyanoacrylate injection, TIPS, or surgery. Cyanoacrylate injection is highly satisfactory in controlling gastric variceal bleeding, and can be done with patient on the right side in acute gastric variceal bleeding to provide clearer field and easier procedure. Management of ectopic varices is done by TIPS and cyanoacrylate injection. PHG and GAVE are two distinct entities and are important causes of gastrointestinal bleeding. Management of PHG is mainly medical, whereas GAVE is treated by APC or band ligation.
- Hemospray offers a new therapeutic option that, in our experience, could bridge the gap that exists in our daily practice between admission of a patient with gastroesophageal bleeding and more definitive management.

References

[1] Perelló A, Escorsell A, Bru C, et al. Wedged hepatic venous pressure adequately reflects portal pressure in hepatitis C virus-related cirrhosis. Hepatology. 1999; 30(6):1393–1397

[2] Khanna R, Sarin SK. Non-cirrhotic portal hypertension—diagnosis and management. J Hepatol. 2014; 60(2):421–441

[3] Sarin SK, Kumar A. Noncirrhotic portal hypertension. Clin Liver Dis. 2006; 10(3):627–651, x

[4] Schouten JNL, Garcia-Pagan JC, Valla DC, Janssen HLA. Idiopathic noncirrhotic portal hypertension. Hepatology. 2011; 54(3):1071–1081

[5] Garcia-Pagán JC, Hernández-Guerra M, Bosch J. Extrahepatic portal vein thrombosis. Semin Liver Dis. 2008; 28(3):282–292

[6] de Franchis R; Baveno V Faculty. Revising consensus in portal hypertension: report of the Baveno V consensus workshop on methodology of diagnosis and therapy in portal hypertension. J Hepatol. 2010; 53(4):762–768

[7] de Franchis R; Baveno VI Faculty. Expanding consensus in portal hypertension: report of the Baveno VI Consensus Workshop: stratifying risk and individualizing care for portal hypertension. J Hepatol. 2015; 63(3):743–752

[8] La Mura V, Nicolini A, Tosetti G, Primignani M. Cirrhosis and portal hypertension: the importance of risk stratification, the role of hepatic venous pressure gradient measurement. World J Hepatol. 2015; 7(4):688–695

[9] Berzigotti A, Seijo S, Reverter E, Bosch J. Assessing portal hypertension in liver diseases. Expert Rev Gastroenterol Hepatol. 2013; 7(2):141–155

[10] Berzigotti A, Piscaglia F; EFSUMB Education and Professional Standards Committee. Ultrasound in portal hypertension—part 2—and EFSUMB recommendations

for the performance and reporting of ultrasound examinations in portal hypertension. Ultraschall Med. 2012; 33(1):8–32, quiz 30–31

[11] Castera L, Forns X, Alberti A. Non-invasive evaluation of liver fibrosis using transient elastography. J Hepatol. 2008; 48(5):835–847

[12] Zarski JP, Sturm N, Guechot J, et al; ANRS HCEP 23 Fibrostar Group. Comparison of nine blood tests and transient elastography for liver fibrosis in chronic hepatitis C: the ANRS HCEP-23 study. J Hepatol. 2012; 56(1):55–62

[13] Talwalkar JA, Kurtz DM, Schoenleber SJ, et al. Ultrasound-based transient elastography for the detection of hepatic fibrosis: systematic review and meta-analysis. Clin Gastroenterol Hepatol. 2007; 5(10):1214–1220

[14] Friedrich-Rust M, Ong M-F, Martens S, et al. Performance of transient elastography for the staging of liver fibrosis: a meta-analysis. Gastroenterology. 2008; 134(4):960–974

[15] Musso G, Gambino R, Cassader M, Pagano G. Meta-analysis: natural history of non-alcoholic fatty liver disease (NAFLD) and diagnostic accuracy of non-invasive tests for liver disease severity. Ann Med. 2011; 43(8):617–649

[16] Corpechot C, El Naggar A, Poujol-Robert A, et al. Assessment of biliary fibrosis by transient elastography in patients with PBC and PSC. Hepatology. 2006; 43(5):1118–1124

[17] Grunwald D, Kothari D, Malik R. Noninvasive markers in the assessment and management of autoimmune liver diseases. Eur J Gastroenterol Hepatol. 2014; 26(10):1065–1072

[18] Shaheen AAM, Wan AF, Myers RP. FibroTest and FibroScan for the prediction of hepatitis C-related fibrosis: a systematic review of diagnostic test accuracy. Am J Gastroenterol. 2007; 102(11):2589–2600

[19] Tsochatzis EA, Gurusamy KS, Ntaoula S, et al. Elastography for the diagnosis of severity of fibrosis in chronic liver disease: a meta-analysis of diagnostic accuracy. J Hepatol. 2011; 54(4):650–659

[20] Garcia-Tsao G, Sanyal AJ, Grace ND, Carey W; Practice Guidelines Committee of the American Association for the Study of Liver Diseases. Practice Parameters Committee of the American College of Gastroenterology. Prevention and management of gastroesophageal varices and variceal hemorrhage in cirrhosis. Hepatology. 2007; 46(3):922–938

[21] Habib A, Sanyal AJ. Acute variceal hemorrhage. Gastrointest Endosc Clin N Am. 2007; 17(2):223–252, v

[22] D'Amico G, De Franchis R; Cooperative Study Group. Upper digestive bleeding in cirrhosis. Post-therapeutic outcome and prognostic indicators. Hepatology. 2003; 38(3):599–612

[23] Reliability of endoscopy in the assessment of variceal features. Italian Liver Cirrhosis Project. J Hepatol. 1987; 4:93–98

[24] LaBrecqu D, Khan AG, Sarin SK, Le Mair AW. Esophageal Varices. WGO Practice Guideline. 2013:5

[25] Sarin SK, Lahoti D, Saxena SP, et al. Prevalence, classification and natural history of gastric varices: a long-term follow-up study in 568 portal hypertension patients. Hepatology. 1992; 16(6):1343–1349

[26] Feu F, García-Pagán JC, Bosch J, et al. Relation between portal pressure response to pharmacotherapy and risk of recurrent variceal haemorrhage in patients with cirrhosis. Lancet. 1995; 346(8982):1056–1059

[27] North Italian Endoscopic Club for the Study and Treatment of Esophageal Varices. Prediction of the first variceal hemorrhage in patients with cirrhosis of the liver and esophageal varices. A prospective multicenter study. N Engl J Med. 1988; 319(15):983–989

[28] Bosch J, García-Pagán JC. Prevention of variceal rebleeding. Lancet. 2003; 361(9361):952–954

[29] Abraldes JG, Villanueva C, Bañares R, et al; Spanish Cooperative Group for Portal Hypertension and Variceal Bleeding. Hepatic venous pressure gradient and prognosis in patients with acute variceal bleeding treated with pharmacologic and endoscopic therapy. J Hepatol. 2008; 48(2):229–236

[30] Hayes PC, Davis JM, Lewis JA, Bouchier IA. Meta-analysis of value of propranolol in prevention of variceal haemorrhage. Lancet. 1990; 336(8708):153–156

[31] Bañares R, Moitinho E, Matilla A, et al. Randomized comparison of long-term carvedilol and propranolol administration in the treatment of portal hypertension in cirrhosis. Hepatology. 2002; 36(6):1367–1373

[32] Schneider AW, Kalk JF, Klein CP. Effect of losartan, an angiotensin II receptor antagonist, on portal pressure in cirrhosis. Hepatology. 1999; 29(2):334–339

[33] D'Amico G, Garcia-Pagan JC, Luca A, Bosch J. Hepatic vein pressure gradient reduction and prevention of variceal bleeding in cirrhosis: a systematic review. Gastroenterology. 2006; 131(5):1611–1624

[34] Gluud LL, Krag A. Banding ligation versus beta-blockers for primary prevention in oesophageal varices in adults. Cochrane Database Syst Rev. 2012; 8(8):CD004544

[35] Li J, Yu C, Li Y. Endoscopic band ligation versus pharmacological therapy for variceal bleeding in cirrhosis: a meta-analysis. Can J Gastroenterol. 2011; 25(3):147–155

[36] Imperiale TF, Chalasani N. A meta-analysis of endoscopic variceal ligation for primary prophylaxis of esophageal variceal bleeding. Hepatology. 2001; 33(4):802–807

[37] Khuroo MS, Khuroo NS, Farahat KL, et al. Meta-analysis: endoscopic variceal ligation for primary prophylaxis of oesophageal variceal bleeding. Aliment Pharmacol Ther. 2005; 21(4):347–361

[38] Gluud LL, Klingenberg S, Nikolova D, Gluud C. Banding ligation versus beta-blockers as primary prophylaxis in esophageal varices: systematic review of randomized trials. Am J Gastroenterol. 2007; 102(12):2842–2848, quiz 2841, 2849

[39] Sarin SK, Lamba GS, Kumar M, et al. Comparison of endoscopic ligation and propranolol for the primary prevention of variceal bleeding. N Engl J Med. 1999; 340(13):988–993

[40] Sarin SK, Wadhawan M, Agarwal SR, et al. Endoscopic variceal ligation plus propranolol versus endoscopic variceal ligation alone in primary prophylaxis of variceal bleeding. Am J Gastroenterol. 2005; 100(4):797–804

[41] Hunter MS, Omar MM, Mostafa I, et al. Prophylactic sclerotherapy: a prospective controlled trial in non alcoholic liver cirrhosis and/or schistosomal hepatic fibrosis. J Trop Med (Cairo). 1992; 2(1)

[42] Stiegmann GV, Goff JS, Michaletz-Onody PA, et al. Endoscopic sclerotherapy as compared with endoscopic ligation for bleeding esophageal varices. N Engl J Med. 1992; 326(23):1527–1532

[43] Blatchford O, Murray WR, Blatchford M. A risk score to predict need for treatment for upper-gastrointestinal haemorrhage. Lancet. 2000; 356(9238):1318–1321

[44] Rockall TA, Logan RF, Devlin HB, Northfield TC. Risk assessment after acute upper gastrointestinal haemorrhage. Gut. 1996; 38(3):316–321

[45] Rudolph SJ, Landsverk BK, Freeman ML. Endotracheal intubation for airway protection during endoscopy for severe upper GI hemorrhage. Gastrointest Endosc. 2003; 57(1):58–61

[46] Pallin DJ, Saltzman JR. Is nasogastric tube lavage in patients with acute upper GI bleeding indicated or antiquated? Gastrointest Endosc. 2011; 74(5):981–984

[47] Villanueva C, Colomo A, Bosch A, et al. Transfusion strategies for acute upper gastrointestinal bleeding. N Engl J Med. 2013; 368(1):11–21

[48] Martí-Carvajal AJ, Karakitsiou DE, Salanti G. Human recombinant activated factor VII for upper gastrointestinal bleeding in patients with liver diseases. Cochrane Database Syst Rev. 2012; 3(3):CD004887

[49] Soares-Weiser K, Brezis M, Tur-Kaspa R, Leibovici L. Antibiotic prophylaxis for cirrhotic patients with gastrointestinal bleeding. Cochrane Database Syst Rev. 2002(2):CD002907

[50] Fernández J, Ruiz del Arbol L, Gómez C, et al. Norfloxacin vs ceftriaxone in the prophylaxis of infections in patients with advanced cirrhosis and hemorrhage. Gastroenterology. 2006; 131(4):1049–1056, quiz 1285

[51] Hou MC, Lin HC, Liu TT, et al. Antibiotic prophylaxis after endoscopic therapy prevents rebleeding in acute variceal hemorrhage: a randomized trial. Hepatology. 2004; 39(3):746–753

[52] Hwang JH, Shergill AK, Acosta RD, et al; American Society for Gastrointestinal Endoscopy. The role of endoscopy in the management of variceal hemorrhage. Gastrointest Endosc. 2014; 80(2):221–227

[53] Knochel JP. Hypophosphatemia in the alcoholic. Arch Intern Med. 1980; 140(5):613–615

[54] Leontiadis GI, Sharma VK, Howden CW. Proton pump inhibitor treatment for acute peptic ulcer bleeding. Cochrane Database Syst Rev. 2006(1):CD002094

[55] Leontiadis GI, Sharma VK, Howden CW. Proton pump inhibitor therapy for peptic ulcer bleeding: Cochrane collaboration meta-analysis of randomized controlled trials. Mayo Clin Proc. 2007; 82(3):286–296

[56] Lo EA, Wilby KJ, Ensom MH. Use of proton pump inhibitors in the management of gastroesophageal varices: a systematic review. Ann Pharmacother. 2015; 49(2):207–219

[57] Escorsell A, Ruiz del Arbol L, Planas R, et al. Multicenter randomized controlled trial of terlipressin versus sclerotherapy in the treatment of acute variceal bleeding: the TEST study. Hepatology. 2000; 32(3):471–476

[58] Wells M, Chande N, Adams P, et al. Meta-analysis: vasoactive medications for the management of acute variceal bleeds. Aliment Pharmacol Ther. 2012; 35(11):1267–1278

[59] Bañares R, Albillos A, Rincón D, et al. Endoscopic treatment versus endoscopic plus pharmacologic treatment for acute variceal bleeding: a meta-analysis. Hepatology. 2002; 35(3):609–615

[60] D'amico G, Criscuoli V, Fili D, et al. Meta-analysis of trials for variceal bleeding. Hepatology. 2002; 36(4 pt 1):1023–1024, author reply 1024–1025

[61] Ioannou G, Doust J, Rockey DC. Terlipressin for acute esophageal variceal hemorrhage. Cochrane Database Syst Rev. 2003(1):CD002147

[62] Ladas SD, Satake Y, Mostafa I, Morse J. Sedation practices for gastrointestinal endoscopy in Europe, North America, Asia, Africa and Australia. Digestion. 2010; 82(2):74–76

[63] Kamel H, Kamal N, Helmy H, Mostafa I. Midazolam versus propofol sedation for therapeutic upper gastrointestinal endoscopy. Egyptian Journal of Anaesthesia. 1995; 11(2)

[64] Correia LM, Bonilha DQ, Gomes GF, et al. Sedation during upper GI endoscopy in cirrhotic outpatients: a randomized, controlled trial comparing propofol and fentanyl with midazolam and fentanyl. Gastrointest Endosc. 2011; 73(1):45–51, 51.e1

[65] Goudra BG, Singh PM, Gouda G, et al. Safety of non-anesthesia provider-administered propofol (NAAP) sedation in advanced gastrointestinal endoscopic procedures: comparative meta-analysis of pooled results. Dig Dis Sci. 2015; 60(9):2612–2627

[66] Lera dos Santos ME, Maluf-Filho F, Chaves DM, et al. Deep sedation during gastrointestinal endoscopy: propofol-fentanyl and midazolam-fentanyl regimens. World J Gastroenterol. 2013; 19(22):3439–3446

[67] Omar MM, Fakhry SM, Mostafa I. Immediate endoscopic injection therapy of bleeding oesophageal varices: a prospective comparative evaluation of injecting materials in Egyptian patients with portal hypertension. J Egypt Soc Parasitol. 1998; 28(1):159–168

[68] Hunter MS, Omar MM, Mostafa I, et al. Emergency sclerotherapy for bleeding oeophageal varices in patients with hepatic schistosomiasis and/or non-alcoholic cirrhosis. J Trop Med (Cairo). 1992; 2(2)

[69] Omar MM, Hunter MS, Mostafa I, et al. Endoscopic variceal sclerotherapy: ethanolamine (ETH), polidocanole (POL) alone or in combination? Journal of Hepatology, Gastroenterology &Infectious Diseases (JHGID). 1996; 4(2)

[70] Lee JG, Lieberman DA. Complications related to endoscopic hemostasis techniques. Gastrointest Endosc Clin N Am. 1996; 6(2):305–321

[71] Rolando N, Gimson A, Philpott-Howard J, et al. Infectious sequelae after endoscopic sclerotherapy of oesophageal varices: role of antibiotic prophylaxis. J Hepatol. 1993; 18(3):290–294

[72] Selby WS, Norton ID, Pokorny CS, Benn RA. Bacteremia and bacterascites after endoscopic sclerotherapy for bleeding esophageal varices and prevention by intravenous cefotaxime: a randomized trial. Gastrointest Endosc. 1994; 40(6):680–684

[73] Wiechowska-Kozłowska A, Białek A, Raszeja-Wyszomirska J, et al. Ligation of oesophageal varices may increase formation of "deep" gastric collaterals. Hepatogastroenterology. 2010; 57(98):262–267

[74] Stiegmann GV, Goff JS, Sun JH, et al. Technique and early clinical results of endoscopic variceal ligation (EVL). Surg Endosc. 1989; 3(2):73–78

[75] Saeed ZA. The Saeed Six-Shooter: a prospective study of a new endoscopic multiple rubber-band ligator for the treatment of varices. Endoscopy. 1996; 28(7):559–564

[76] Ramirez FC, Colon VJ, Landan D, et al. The effects of the number of rubber bands placed at each endoscopic session upon variceal outcomes: a prospective, randomized study. Am J Gastroenterol. 2007; 102(7):1372–1376

[77] Sheibani S, Khemichian S, Kim JJ, et al. Randomized trial of 1-week vs. 2-week intervals for endoscopic ligation in the treatment of patients with esophageal variceal bleeding. Hepatology. 2016; 64(2):549–555

[78] Laine L, el-Newihi HM, Migikovsky B, et al. Endoscopic ligation compared with sclerotherapy for the treatment of bleeding esophageal varices. Ann Intern Med. 1993; 119(1):1–7

[79] Fakhry S, Omar M, Al Ghannam M, et al. Endoscopic sclerotherapy versus endoscopic variceal ligation in the management of bleeding esophageal varices: a prospective randomized study in schistosomal hepatic fibrosis. Endoscopy. 2000; 1:39–44– (Arab edition)

[80] Mostafa I, Omar MM, Hassan M, et al. Bacteremia after injection sclerotherapy and band ligation for esophageal varices: a comparative study. Egypt J Med Microbiol. 1996; 5(2)

[81] Mostafa I, Omar M. Incidence of spontaneous bacterial peritonitis (SBP) after injection sclerotherapy and band ligation for esophageal varices. Egypt J Schistosomiasis Infect Endem Dis. 2000; •••:22

[82] Mostafa I, Omar MM, Akl M, et al. Changes in gastric and oesophageal mucosa after endoscopic variceal injection sclerotherapy or band ligation: a comparative study. Journal of Hepatology, Gastroenterology & Infectious diseases (JHGID). 1996; 4(2)

[83] Cotton P. Combination therapies may speed healing, reduce rebleeding of esophageal varices. JAMA. 1991; 266(2):187–188

[84] Karsan HA, Morton SC, Shekelle PG, et al. Combination endoscopic band ligation and sclerotherapy compared with endoscopic band ligation alone for the secondary prophylaxis of esophageal variceal hemorrhage: a meta-analysis. Dig Dis Sci. 2005; 50(2):399–406

[85] Meirelles-Santos JO, Montes CG, Guerrazzi F, et al. Treatment of esophageal varices using band ligation followed by microwave coagulation (abstract). Gastrointest Endosc. 2001; 53:AB120

[86] Mostafa I. Endoscopic clipping in management of acute gastroesophageal variceal bleeding—a preliminary report. Gastroenterology. 1994; 106(4):A946–A946

[87] Gimson AE, Ramage JK, Panos MZ, et al. Randomised trial of variceal banding ligation versus injection sclerotherapy for bleeding oesophageal varices. Lancet. 1993; 342(8868):391–394

[88] Petrasch F, Grothaus J, Mössner J, et al. Differences in bleeding behavior after endoscopic band ligation: a retrospective analysis. BMC Gastroenterol. 2010; 10:5

[89] D'Amico G, Pagliaro L, Bosch J. The treatment of portal hypertension: a meta-analytic review. Hepatology. 1995; 22(1):332–354

[90] Hubmann R, Bodlaj G, Czompo M, et al. The use of self-expanding metal stents to treat acute esophageal variceal bleeding. Endoscopy. 2006; 38(9):896–901

[91] Marot A, Trépo E, Doerig C, et al. Systematic review with meta-analysis: self-expanding metal stents in patients with cirrhosis and severe or refractory oesophageal variceal bleeding. Aliment Pharmacol Ther. 2015; 42(11–12):1250–1260

[92] Hubmann R, Bodlaj G, Czompo M, et al. The use of self-expanding metal stents to treat acute esophageal variceal bleeding. Endoscopy. 2006; 38(9):896–901

[93] McCarty TR, Njei B. Self-expanding metal stents for acute refractory esophageal variceal bleeding: a systematic review and meta-analysis. Dig Endosc. 2016; 28(5):539–547

[94] Monescillo A, Martínez-Lagares F, Ruiz-del-Arbol L, et al. Influence of portal hypertension and its early decompression by TIPS placement on the outcome of variceal bleeding. Hepatology. 2004; 40(4):793–801

[95] Halabi SA, Sawas T, Sadat B, et al. Early TIPS versus endoscopic therapy for secondary prophylaxis after management of acute esophageal variceal bleeding in cirrhotic patients: a meta-analysis of randomized controlled trials. J Gastroenterol Hepatol. 2016; 31(9):1519–1526

[96] Chau TN, Patch D, Chan YW, et al. "Salvage" transjugular intrahepatic portosystemic shunts: gastric fundal compared with esophageal variceal bleeding. Gastroenterology. 1998; 114(5):981–987

[97] Copelan A, Kapoor B, Sands M. Transjugular intrahepatic portosystemic shunt: indications, contraindications, and patient work-up. Semin Intervent Radiol. 2014; 31(3):235–242

[98] Henderson JM. Salvage therapies for refractory variceal hemorrhage. Clin Liver Dis. 2001; 5(3):709–725

[99] Sung JJ, Luo D, Wu JC, et al. Early clinical experience of the safety and effectiveness of Hemospray in achieving hemostasis in patients with acute peptic ulcer bleeding. Endoscopy. 2011; 43(4):291–295

[100] Ibrahim M, El-Mikkawy A, Mostafa I, Devière J. Endoscopic treatment of acute variceal hemorrhage by using hemostatic powder TC-325: a prospective pilot study. Gastrointest Endosc. 2013; 78(5):769–773

[101] Ibrahim M, El-Mikkawy A, Abdalla H, et al. Management of acute variceal bleeding using hemostatic powder. United European Gastroenterol J. 2015; 3(3):277–283

[102] Mostafa I, Omar MM, Nouh A. Endoscopic control of gastric variceal bleeding with butyl cyanoacrylate in patients with schistosomiasis. J Egypt Soc Parasitol. 1997; 27(2):405–410

[103] Sarin SK, Jain AK, Jain M, Gupta R. A randomized controlled trial of cyanoacrylate versus alcohol injection in patients with isolated fundic varices. Am J Gastroenterol. 2002; 97(4):1010–1015

[104] Mostafa I. How I do it. Glue treatment of gastric varices. World organization of digestive endoscopy OMED, 2008. http://www.worldendo.org/resource-libraries.html

[105] Binmoeller KF, Weilert F, Shah JN, Kim J. EUS-guided transesophageal treatment of gastric fundal varices with combined coiling and cyanoacrylate glue injection (with videos). Gastrointest Endosc. 2011; 74(5):1019–1025

[106] Lo GH, Lai KH, Cheng JS, et al. A prospective, randomized trial of butyl cyanoacrylate injection versus band ligation in the management of bleeding gastric varices. Hepatology. 2001; 33(5):1060–1064

[107] Kind R, Guglielmi A, Rodella L, et al. Bucrylate treatment of bleeding gastric varices: 12 years' experience. Endoscopy. 2000; 32(7):512–519

[108] Seewald S, Ang TL, Imazu H, et al. A standardized injection technique and regimen ensures success and safety of N-butyl-2-cyanoacrylate injection for the treatment of gastric fundal varices (with videos). Gastrointest Endosc. 2008; 68(3):447–454

[109] Datta D, Vlavianos P, Alisa A, Westaby D. Use of fibrin glue (beriplast) in the management of bleeding gastric varices. Endoscopy. 2003; 35(8):675–678

[110] Holster IL, Poley JW, Kuipers EJ, Tjwa ET. Controlling gastric variceal bleeding with endoscopically applied hemostatic powder (Hemospray™). J Hepatol. 2012; 57(6):1397–1398

[111] Przemioslo RT, McNair A, Williams R. Thrombin is effective in arresting bleeding from gastric variceal hemorrhage. Dig Dis Sci. 1999; 44(4):778–781

[112] Akahoshi T, Hashizume M, Tomikawa M, et al. Long-term results of balloon-occluded retrograde transvenous obliteration for gastric variceal bleeding and risky gastric varices: a 10-year experience. J Gastroenterol Hepatol. 2008; 23(11):1702–1709

[113] Cho SK, Shin SW, Lee IH, et al. Balloon-occluded retrograde transvenous obliteration of gastric varices: outcomes and complications in 49 patients. AJR Am J Roentgenol. 2007; 189(6):W365–W372

[114] Yoshimatsu R, Yamagami T, Tanaka O, et al. Development of thrombus in a systemic vein after balloon-occluded retrograde transvenous obliteration of gastric varices. Korean J Radiol. 2012; 13(3):324–331

[115] Boyer TD, Haskal ZJ; American Association for the Study of Liver Diseases. The role of transjugular intrahepatic portosystemic shunt (TIPS) in the management of portal hypertension: update 2009. Hepatology. 2010; 51(1):306

[116] Merli M, Nicolini G, Angeloni S, et al. The natural history of portal hypertensive gastropathy in patients with liver cirrhosis and mild portal hypertension. Am J Gastroenterol. 2004; 99(10):1959–1965

[117] Sarin SK, Misra SP, Singal A, et al. Evaluation of the incidence and significance of the "mosaic pattern" in patients with cirrhosis, noncirrhotic portal fibrosis, and extrahepatic obstruction. Am J Gastroenterol. 1988; 83(11):1235–1239

[118] Spahr L, Villeneuve JP, Dufresne MP, et al. Gastric antral vascular ectasia in cirrhotic patients: absence of relation with portal hypertension. Gut. 1999; 44(5):739–742

[119] Patwardhan VR, Cardenas A. Review article: the management of portal hypertensive gastropathy and gastric antral vascular ectasia in cirrhosis. Aliment Pharmacol Ther. 2014; 40(4):354–362

[120] Bruha R, Marecek Z, Spicak J, et al. Double-blind randomized, comparative multicenter study of the effect of terlipressin in the treatment of acute esophageal variceal and/or hypertensive gastropathy bleeding. Hepatogastroenterology. 2002; 49(46):1161–1166

[121] Herrera S, Bordas JM, Llach J, et al. The beneficial effects of argon plasma coagulation in the management of different types of gastric vascular ectasia lesions in patients admitted for GI hemorrhage. Gastrointest Endosc. 2008; 68(3):440–446

[122] Smith LA, Morris AJ, Stanley AJ. The use of Hemospray in portal hypertensive bleeding; a case series. J Hepatol. 2014; 60:457–460 Pubmed

[123] Kamath PS, Lacerda M, Ahlquist DA, et al. Gastric mucosal responses to intrahepatic portosystemic shunting in patients with cirrhosis. Gastroenterology. 2000; 118(5):905–911

[124] Helton WS, Maves R, Wicks K, Johansen K. Transjugular intrahepatic portasystemic shunt vs surgical shunt in good-risk cirrhotic patients: a case-control comparison. Arch Surg. 2001; 136(1):17–20

[125] Sebastian S, McLoughlin R, Qasim A, et al. Endoscopic argon plasma coagulation for the treatment of gastric antral vascular ectasia (watermelon stomach): long-term results. Dig Liver Dis. 2004; 36(3):212–217

[126] Sato T, Yamazaki K, Akaike J. Endoscopic band ligation versus argon plasma coagulation for gastric antral vascular ectasia associated with liver diseases. Dig Endosc. 2012; 24(4):237–242

[127] Abdelhalim H, Mostafa I, Abdelbary MS, et al. Endoscopic band ligation versus argon plasma coagulation for the treatment of gastric antral vascular ectasia in egyptian patients with liver cirrhosis. World J Med Sci. 2014; 10(3):357–361

[128] McGorisk T, Krishnan K, Keefer L, Komanduri S. Radiofrequency ablation for refractory gastric antral vascular ectasia (with video). Gastrointest Endosc. 2013; 78(4):584–588

[129] Cho S, Zanati S, Yong E, et al. Endoscopic cryotherapy for the management of gastric antral vascular ectasia. Gastrointest Endosc. 2008; 68(5):895–902

[130] Walia SS, Sachdeva A, Kim JJ, et al, Cyanoacrylate spray for treatment of difficult-to-control GI bleeding. Gastrointest Endosc. 2013; 78(3):536–539

[131] Katsinelos P, Chatzimavroudis G, Katsinelos T, et al. Endoscopic mucosal resection for recurrent gastric antral vascular ectasia. Vasa. 2008; 37(3):289–292

[132] Mann NS, Rachut E. Gastric antral vascular ectasia causing severe hypoalbuminemia and anemia cured by antrectomy. J Clin Gastroenterol. 2002; 34(3):284–286

Section V

Lower Gastrointestinal Tract Disease

35 Colorectal Polyps and Cancer Screening/Prevention

Douglas K. Rex

35.1 Introduction

The two major classes of precancerous colorectal lesions are the conventional adenomas and the serrated lesions. Effective colonoscopy requires detailed understanding of the spectrum of appearances of these precancerous colorectal lesions. Precancerous lesions must be effectively recognized and completely resected during colonoscopy. This chapter reviews basic knowledge needed to perform effective colonoscopy, and also reviews the fundamentals of colorectal cancer screening and surveillance.[1]

35.2 Polyp Classification and Polyp Cancer Sequences

Nearly all colorectal cancers are believed to arise from an endoscopically detectable benign precursor. The Paris classification (▶Fig. 35.1) divides the precursors into Paris type I lesions (polyps), which protrude into the colon lumen more than the diameter of a standard biopsy forceps, and the flat and depressed lesions (Paris type II), which project into the lumen less than the diameter of a standard 2.5-mm biopsy forceps.[1] Detailed

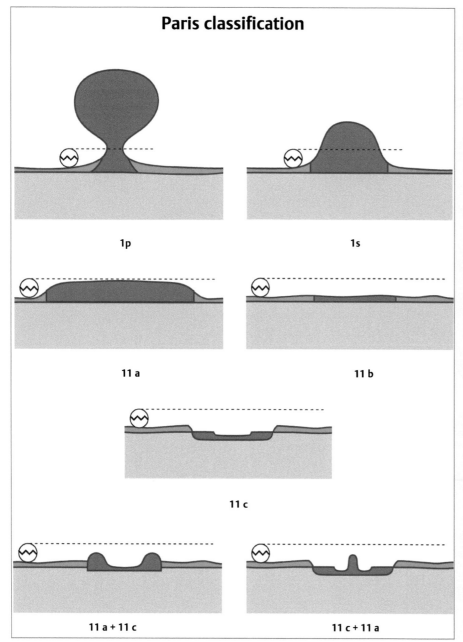

Paris classification

1p

1s

11 a

11 b

11 c

11 a + 11 c

11 c + 11 a

Fig. 35.1 The Paris classification.[1] Type I lesions are polyps. Type IIa and IIb are flat lesions. Type IIc and its variants are depressed.

knowledge of the Paris classification is useful to heighten awareness of the need to search for subtle precancerous and malignant lesions (▶Table 35.1).

The progression of polyps and flat lesions to cancer is generally referred to as the "polyp-cancer sequence." The two main histologic classes of precursor lesions are the conventional adenomas and the serrated lesions. These two classes of lesions also account for more than 90% of all colorectal polyps and flat lesions (▶Table 35.2).

Conventional adenomas are the precursor lesion of 70 to 85% of sporadically occurring colorectal cancers, as well as cancers arising in the major inherited syndromes with a defined genetic basis including Familial Adenomatous Polyposis and Lynch Syndrome (discussed in Chapter 37). Tumors arising from conventional adenomas are said to pass through the "adenoma–carcinoma sequence," which is a subtype of the polyp cancer sequence. ▶Table 35.2 shows a classification of the two major groups of precancerous colorectal polyps and flat lesions.

Colorectal cancers arising through serrated class lesions account for 15 to 30% of all cancers. Serrated class lesions are distinct from conventional adenomas endoscopically, histologically, and in their molecular features. Serrated class lesions are missed more frequently during colonoscopy than conventional adenomas,[2,3] and account for a disproportionate percentage of cancers that occur after colonoscopy.[4,5] Because recognition and understanding of the serrated pathway is more recent than the adenoma–carcinoma sequence, the effective modern colonoscopist is characterized to a substantial degree by his or her ability to detect and effectively resect serrated class lesions.

Other types of colorectal polyps are infrequently encountered, including carcinoid tumors (largely submucosal and usually located in the rectum), inflammatory polyps, hamartomas, normal structures that mimic polyps such as "mucosal polyps" (an excrescence of normal mucosa) and lymphoid follicles, and rare growths such as leiomyoma, ganglioneuroma, cystic structures (e.g., pneumatosis cystoides intestinalis), and metastatic tumors to the colon. Although the expert colonoscopist should understand these uncommon and rare lesions, the expert is also often surprised by the pathology report of some of these lesions. These lesions are not discussed in detail here, because the greatest benefit to patients accrues when the endoscopist masters understanding of the conventional adenomas and serrated class lesions.

35.3 Conventional Adenomas

35.3.1 Low-Risk versus Advanced Conventional Adenomas

By definition all conventional adenomas are dysplastic and the degree of dysplasia should be characterized as low grade or high grade. The degree of dysplasia is subject to marked interobserver variation between pathologists.[6] Classification schemes such as mild, moderate, or severe dysplasia are unacceptable since these are subject to even greater interobserver variation than the two-category scheme of low versus high grade. The separation of low versus high grade is best made based on the low-power magnification morphologic characteristics. The use of cytologic criteria to designate high-grade dysplasia leads to a much higher percentage of adenomas having high-grade dysplasia compared to when only morphologic criteria are used.[6]

Conventional adenomas can also be categorized as tubular versus tubulovillous (synonymous with villoglandular) versus villous. The great majority of conventional adenomas are tubular, which refers to an organized pattern of glands, and only a tiny fraction is villous (which refers to a frond-like growth pattern of glands). Polyps containing more than 25% villous elements should be designated tubulovillous, and more than 75% villous elements should be called villous. Villous histology is associated with a greater risk of high-grade dysplasia compared to tubular histology. As with dysplasia grade, there is marked interobserver variation between pathologists in designation of tubular versus tubulovillous, even when using identical definitions.[6]

The magnitude of the problem with interobserver variation in pathologist interpretation of dysplasia grade and tubular versus villous is such that some postpolypectomy surveillance guidelines, particularly the British guideline,[7] do not acknowledge dysplasia grade and villous elements. Nevertheless, across a population of patients there is some association of both villous elements and high-grade dysplasia with the subsequent occurrence of advanced lesions at follow-up colonoscopy.[8]

Tubular adenomas with low-grade dysplasia less than 1 cm in size are considered "low-risk" adenomas. Adenomas greater than or equal to 10 mm in size, or which have high-grade dysplasia, or have villous elements (either tubulovillous or villous histology)

Table 35.1 The four key elements of effective and cost-effective colonoscopy

- The endoscopist understands the full spectrum of endoscopic appearances of precancerous lesions in the colon and can recognize and characterize precancerous lesions when these are exposed by the colonoscope.
- The endoscopist is trained in detailed exposure of colonic mucosa, including prescription of effective bowel preparation, seeing behind folds, flexures, and valves, thorough intraprocedural cleansing of mucosal surfaces during examination, and adequate colonic distention.
- The colonoscopist effectively resects precancerous lesions.
- Postcolonoscopy the endoscopist assigns an appropriate screening or surveillance interval based on examination findings.

Table 35.2 Histologic classification of the two main classes of precancerous colorectal lesions

Conventional adenomas (all are dysplastic)
- Dysplasia grade
  - High
  - Low
- Villous elements
  - Tubular (< 25% villous)
  - Tubulovillous (25–75% villous)
  - Villous (> 75% villous
Serrated class lesions
- Hyperplastic polyps
- Sessile serrated polyp
  - Without cytological dysplasia
  - With cytological dysplasia
- Traditional serrated adenoma

are considered "advanced adenomas." In observational studies of colonoscopy findings after a baseline clearing examination, advanced adenomas are commonly used as a surrogate for cancer, because the incidence of colorectal cancer in observational postpolypectomy studies is typically low.[8] In postpolypectomy studies, three or more baseline adenomas, even if all were low-risk adenomas, are associated with the subsequent occurrence of advanced adenomas,[8] although a recent study found that at least five low-risk adenomas were needed before an increased risk of advanced adenomas at follow-up was present.[9] The occurrence of three or more adenomas is often referred to as "multiple" adenomas and is considered a "high-risk finding" even when constituted entirely from low-risk adenomas.

35.3.2 Shape and Colonic Distribution of Conventional Adenomas

As noted above, precursor lesions, including conventional adenomas can be classified as polyps versus flat lesions versus depressed lesions. Polyps are also categorized as pedunculated or sessile. Pedunculated adenomas can occur in any section of the colon, but predominate in the sigmoid. Pedunculated lesions comprise 5 to 10% of all conventional adenomas. Sessile (Paris Is shape) comprises 40 to 50% of conventional adenomas, and approximately 40 to 50% have flat (Paris IIa) shape. Although flat shape has been associated with worse histology, the bulk of evidence suggests that the risk of high-grade dysplasia and invasive cancer is no higher or even less in flat (Paris IIa) lesions compared with sessile (Is) conventional adenomas.[10] Flat lesions are skewed in distribution toward the right colon compared to sessile lesions, which may contribute to the observation that proximal cancer location is more common in interval cancers compared to cancers diagnosed during a first colonoscopy. By far the most dangerous shape for conventional adenomas is the depressed lesion, which occurs in probably 1 in every 800 to 1,000 screening

colonoscopies in persons age 50 and older.[11] Depressed lesions are at least 1 to 1.5 cm in diameter, and have a substantial surface area that is depressed compared to the rim or perimeter of the lesion. Further, the transition from the perimeter to the depressed portion is typically sharp rather than sloping. The risk of high-grade dysplasia or invasive cancer in depressed lesions is as great as 50%, which is at least 50 times higher than that of flat or sessile lesions of comparable size.

The modern expert colonoscopist is highly attuned to the shape classification of colorectal cancer precursors, and constantly attuned to subtle variations in mucosal color, surface texture, and disruption of normal mucosal vasculature that could signal the presence of a flat or depressed precursor.

35.3.3 Surface Features of Conventional Adenomas

Approximately 80 to 85% of conventional adenomas have a characteristic surface pattern that includes thick blood vessels that surround white structures that are variable in shape, but most characteristically are tubular (▶Fig. 35.2, **Video 35.1**). The Narrow-band imaging International Colorectal Endoscopic (NICE) classification scheme permits differentiation of conventional adenomas from serrated class lesions based on these features[12] (▶Table 35.3). A lesion that demonstrates a disrupted or amorphous vascular pattern, often in an area of relative depression, has a high risk of deeply invasive submucosal cancer, and should be biopsied and referred directly for surgical resection. This disrupted pattern is the NICE type III[13] (▶Table 35.3, **Video 35.2**).

35.3.4 Resection of Conventional Adenomas

Resection of large conventional adenomas that are flat or sessile can be technically challenging, and is the subject of Chapter 36.

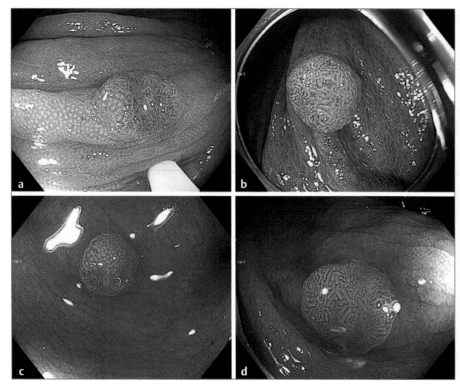

Fig. 35.2 (a–d) Typical conventional adenomas in narrow-band imaging.

Table 35.3 The NICE classification for differentiation of serrated class lesions (type I) from conventional adenomas (type II) from cancer with deep submucosal invasion (type III)

**Narrow-band imaging International Colorectal Endoscopic classification			
	Type I	**Type II**	**Type III**
Color	Same or lighter than background	Browner relative to background (verify color arises from vessels)	Brown to dark brown relative to background; sometimes patchy whiter areas
Vessels	None, or isolated lacy vessels may be present coursing across the lesion	Thick brown vessels surrounding white structures	Has area(s) with markedly distorted or missing vessels
Surface pattern	Dark or white spots of uniform or relatively uniform size	Oval, tubular, or branched white structure surrounded by brown vessels	Distortion or absence of pattern
Most likely pathology	Hyperplastic or sessile serrated polyp (adenoma)	Conventional adenoma	Deep submucosal invasive cancer

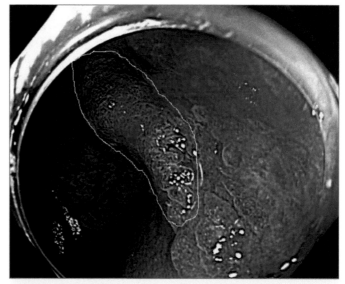

Fig. 35.3 A sessile serrated polyp with cytological dysplasia in narrow-band imaging. The dysplastic portion (outlined by the *yellow line*) has NICE type II features. The rest of the lesion to the right is NICE type I and is the sessile serrated polyp region of the lesion.

Approximately 80% of conventional adenomas are less than 1 cm in size, and many of these lesions are candidates for resection using cold techniques, which effectively remove lesions and nearly eliminate the risk of delayed hemorrhage and the rare perforation associated with thermal injury. Diminutive snares, or specialized snares made specifically for cold snaring can provide an advantage in resection. Cold snaring is the most efficient method for resection for most lesions in the 4- to 10-mm range, as the lesion can be resected in a single bite including a rim of normal tissue, which assures effective resection.[14] With larger lesions, mechanical resection without electrocautery is more difficult, and may leave a cord of submucosal tissue that has been trapped and elongated by the snare (**Video 35.3**). However, after mechanically pulling the snare through entrapped submucosa, the residual submucosa does not demonstrate polyp tissue on biopsy (▶ Fig. 35.3). Polyps less than or equal to 3 mm are commonly identified with high-definition scopes, and if determined to be conventional adenomas, these are resected in most western countries. Cold snaring is still a very efficient method, but for very flat lesions, particularly if located in the upper left endoscopic field and rotation of the colonoscope to achieve 5 o'clock positioning is difficult, such tiny polyps can be engulfed and removed with cold forceps. Use of a jumbo or large-capacity forceps helps to ensure resection in a single bite.[15] Piecemeal resection of polyps using cold forceps is never advisable, since the risk of residual polyp is substantially greater compared to cold snaring.[14] For polyps that are pedunculated or bulky, the use of electrocautery is often preferred for polyps of 5- to 10-mm size, and electrocautery is used for most such polyps greater than 10 mm in size regardless of shape.

35.4 Serrated Class Lesions

35.4.1 Terminology and Histology

The World Health Organization (WHO) classifies the serrated lesions as hyperplastic, sessile serrated polyp (SSP) (sessile serrated adenoma), and traditional serrated adenoma.[15] The term SSP and sessile serrated adenoma are synonymous, but the term SSP will be used in this chapter, because the author considers it less confusing to clinicians. More than 95% of SSPs contained no dysplasia, and the term "adenoma" is typically associated by clinicians with dysplasia because all of the conventional adenomas are dysplastic. The WHO recommends that SSP be characterized by the pathologist as without cytological dysplasia or with cytological dysplasia.

Hyperplastic polyps can be characterized as goblet cell rich, microvesicular, and mucin poor. In clinical practice, these distinctions are rarely used by pathologists. The microvesicular hyperplastic polyp can be similar to the SSP in its histologic appearance, creating substantial interobserver variation between pathologists in the interpretation of these two lesions.[16] The chief differentiating factors are that the crypts of the microvesicular hyperplastic polyp are straight, whereas in the SSP, there is crypt distortion, consisting either of dilation or lateral growth (▶ Fig. 35.4). When a substantial portion of the polyp is occupied with distorted crypts, the interpretation of SSP is straightforward. When the changes of crypt distortion are mild and confined to only one or two crypts, significant interobserver variation develops. Further, the precise definition of the number of crypts needed to establish an SSP varies between the WHO, European pathologists, and Japanese pathologists. Hyperplastic polyps and SSPs have some common molecular features, including a propensity to hypermethylation and mutation in the *BRAF* oncogene. Whether the microvesicular hyperplastic polyp is a precursor of SSP remains uncertain.

In the absence of a region of dysplasia, the pathologist should designate the SSP as "SSP without cytological dysplasia." If a region of SSP contains dysplasia, the lesion is designated "SSP with cytological dysplasia." The region of dysplasia typically has the histologic appearance of a conventional adenoma (▶ Fig. 35.3, **Video 35.4**). In the past, such lesions were often termed by pathologists as "mixed hyperplastic–adenomatous polyp." Microdissection studies show that the dysplastic area commonly has

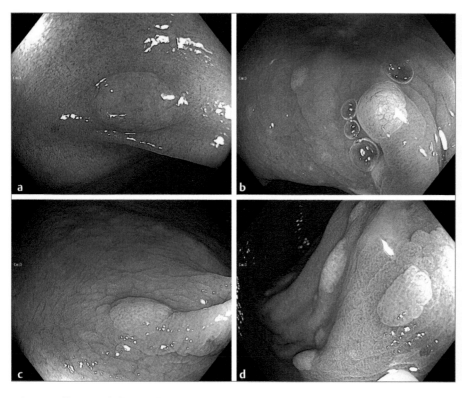

Fig. 35.4 (a–d) Hyperplastic polyps. Part **(d)** shows a small cluster of hyperplastic polyps. In part **(b)** tiny vessels are visible around the pits, but the pits are uniform in size (indicating NICE type I).

microsatellite instability.[17] It is not clear that the degree of dysplasia (low grade vs. high grade) in an SSP with cytological dysplasia has the same clinical importance that it has in conventional adenomas. Therefore, any SSP with cytological dysplasia, regardless of the dysplasia grade, should be considered an advanced lesion relative to SSP without cytological dysplasia.

Traditional serrated adenoma (TSA) is a rare left-sided lesion that is often bulky. TSAs are considered to be dysplastic in all cases though the dysplasia has unique features compared to that in conventional adenomas. Because TSA is dysplastic and has a frond-like growth pattern in many cases, it is commonly interpreted as a conventional tubulovillous adenoma by pathologists.

From a quantitative standpoint, the SSP is the major cancer precursor of the serrated class and a lesion that must be identified with high sensitivity and effectively resected.

35.4.2 Endoscopic Presentation

Hyperplastic polyps can be identified throughout the colon but predominate in the rectosigmoid. The great majority are less than or equal to 5 mm in size, and they typically have a smooth surface (▶Fig. 35.4) and may disappear with sufficient gas insufflation. Detection is enhanced by narrow-band imaging as well as postprocessing image alterations.

Compared to hyperplastic polyps, SSPs are distributed more toward the right colon and tend to be larger. SSPs are almost invariably flat or sessile in shape, and pedunculated SSPs are rare. As noted above, TSAs are most commonly left sided and tend to be bulkier than other serrated class lesions.

The NICE classification (▶Table 35.3) allows differentiation of conventional adenomas from serrated class lesions (here meaning hyperplastic polyps [HPs] and SSPs). Compared to conventional adenomas, serrated class lesions have either no blood vessels visible on their surface or have a few lacy vessels visible on the surface that seem to course past multiple pits (▶Fig. 35.5). Visualized in NBI, the pits of serrated class lesions are typically dark but in some

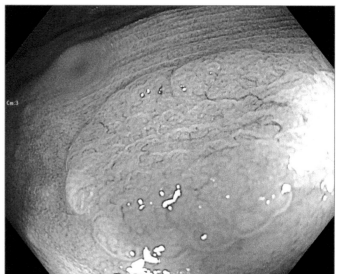

Fig. 35.5 Long lacy vessels are visible coursing past multiple pits in a hyperplastic polyp.

Table 35.4 The WASP criteria for endoscopic prediction of sessile serrated polyp (from hyperplastic polyp)[17]

- Large open pits
- Indiscrete edges
- Irregular shape
- "Cloud-like" appearance

cases are white and are uniform or relatively uniform in size. Visualized with magnification, a very thin vessel can often be seen surrounding the pits of serrated class lesions (▶Fig. 35.4b). The NICE classification does not provide for or attempt to differentiate HPs from SSPs. The WASP classification (▶Table 35.4) has been recently introduced to assist endoscopists in predicting HP versus SSP.[17] Endoscopic features that favor SSP over HP include indiscrete edges, large open pits, irregular surface, and a "cloud-like" appearance (▶Fig. 35.6, **Video 35.5**). Polyps that have all of these features,

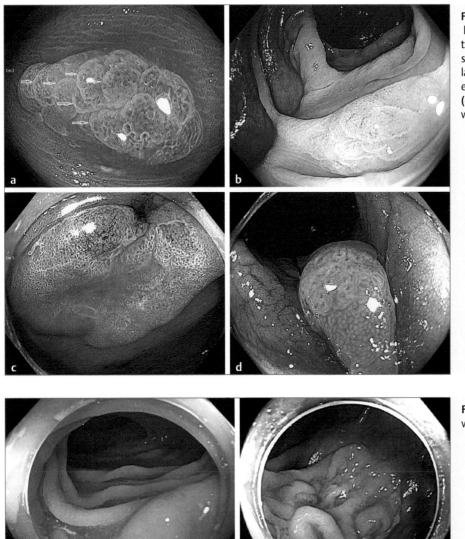

Fig. 35.6 (a) Yellow arrows indicate the bumpy surface and white lines that comprise the "cloud-like" appearance of a sessile serrated polyp (SSP). The red arrow indicates a large open pit. **(b)** Shows "cloud-like" features especially on the left side and indiscrete edges. **(c)** An SSP with irregular shape. **(d)** A small SSP with large open pits (*red arrows*).

Fig. 35.7 (a, b) Large sessile serrated polyps with adherent yellow mucus.

and particularly if they are large and located in the right colon, are almost invariably SSPs. Admittedly, any study of endoscopic features seeking to differentiate HP from SSP is hampered by high pathologist interobserver variation in differentiating the two lesions.

Additional endoscopic features common to HP and SSP include pale color, flat or sessile shape, and an adherent cap of mucus (▶ Fig. 35.7), though the mucous cap is generally more common with SSP.[18]

35.4.3 Resection of Serrated Lesions

The CARE study evaluated rates of incomplete polyp resection for lesions 5 to 20 mm in size.[19] Larger polyp size, endoscopist, and serrated histology were all associated with incomplete resection. The rate of incomplete resection overall for serrated class lesions was 31% compared to 7% for conventional adenomas. The exact methods of polypectomy employed in the trial were not stated. The reason for incomplete resection of serrated lesions almost certainly relates to the indistinct edges, which causes the endoscopist to leave residual glands particularly during piecemeal resection.

Recent studies have shown that serrated lesions greater than or equal to 10 and 20 mm in size[20,21,22] can be resected as effectively as conventional adenomas when a high-definition

colonoscope is used and the lesion is injected submucosally with a contrast agent. The combination of the contrast agent and the high-definition image allows the endoscopist to effectively track the lesion margin throughout resection. Therefore, compared to conventional adenomas, endoscopists should have a lower-size threshold for performing endoscopic mucosal resection (probably 10 mm), using a contrast agent in the submucosal injection fluid.

35.5 Colorectal Cancer Screening

Colorectal cancer screening is the search for early curable colorectal cancer and precursor lesions of cancer in asymptomatic patients. Screening prevents incident cancer, and mortality from cancer. The mechanism of prevention of incident cancer is polypectomy.

Programs for colorectal cancer screening can be established at the national level or by a health care insurance provider. When the decision to perform colorectal cancer screening is left to individual physicians and patients, screening is termed "opportunistic." In general, programmatic screening is considered superior to opportunistic screening in terms of adherence. Despite this, the United States has the highest rates of cancer screening adherence, has achieved the greatest impact on colorectal cancer incidence and mortality via screening, and screening in the United States is almost entirely opportunistic.

35.5.1 Approaches to Offering Screening

Programmatic screening usually employs an offer of a single best test, usually fecal occult blood test (FOBT), and particularly the fecal immunochemical test (FIT). For opportunistic screening guidelines often present a "menu of options," in which several tests are presented to patients. Patients and physicians then choose the test deemed most appropriate for the patient based on the pros and cons of sensitivity, cost, and risk. Although there are numerous adherents of presenting multiple options, randomized-controlled trials have generally not established that multiple options increase overall adherence rates. Another approach to testing is "sequential testing," in which patients are first offered one test (usually the most effective test) and then another test if they decline the more effective test. In some randomized-controlled trials sequential testing has maximized overall rates of adherence, and maximized adherence to the most effective test.[23] Sequential testing is the strategy used most commonly in the United States, where the test offered first is colonoscopy, and if patients decline that they are most commonly offered FIT. A seldom used approach to screening employs risk stratification, in which features such as age, sex, body mass index (BMI), and smoking history are used to construct a risk score.[24] Patients at higher risk undergo colonoscopy, and lower-risk patients are diverted to sigmoidoscopy or noninvasive strategies.

35.5.2 Factors That Affect Colorectal Cancer Risk

The clearest factors associated with colorectal cancer risk are age and male gender (▶ Table 35.5). The median age to develop colorectal cancer in the United States is 70 years. Age-adjusted risk is consistently higher for men than women, but the lifetime incidence of colorectal cancer in men and women is equal because women live longer. Age is accounted for in screening guidelines by the recommendation to begin colorectal cancer screening at 50. About 7% of all colorectal cancers occur in persons under the age of 50, and the incidence of colorectal cancer in the United States is rising in persons under age 50,[25] where it has been declining in persons over age 50, the latter largely because of screening. Persons under age 50 should be aggressively evaluated for bleeding symptoms, particularly hematochezia with blood in the toilet, iron deficiency anemia, and melena with negative upper endoscopy. Nonbleeding symptoms such as constipation, diarrhea, abdominal pain, and weight loss are also commonly subjected to colon evaluation in persons of any age but are not associated with an increased risk of colorectal cancer in the absence of bleeding symptoms, including anemia and positive occult blood tests.[26,27] Cigarette smoking, obesity, and diabetes mellitus are associated with colorectal cancer and may justify initiation of screening persons under age 50 in individual circumstances, though this is not recommended in current guidelines. African Americans have a higher incidence of colorectal cancer, develop colorectal cancer at an earlier age than whites, and are less likely to undergo screening. The American College of Gastroenterology, the American Society for Gastrointestinal Endoscopy, and the American College of Obstetrics and Gynecology all recommend that African Americans beginning screening at age 45 rather than age 50[26](▶ Table 35.6). The cost-effectiveness of this recommendation is widely debated, but the potential for its educational value is considerable since it highlights to physicians and screenees the need for strong screening policies in African Americans.

The risk of colorectal cancer is increased in the first-degree relatives of patients with colorectal cancer. Current guidelines recommend that persons with two or more first-degree relatives with colorectal cancer or any first-degree relative diagnosed with colorectal cancer at age less than 60 years should undergo colonoscopy beginning at age 40 and at a frequency of every 5 years. Persons with a single first-degree relative with colorectal cancer diagnosed after age 60 can generally undergo average risk screening, and guidelines consistently recommend a 10-year screening interval, though these differ as to whether to begin screening at age 40[28] versus 50[29] years.

Recent information suggests that an increased yield of screening in first-degree relatives of patients with colorectal adenomas occurs only in subjects with advanced adenomas (▶ Table 35.6). The American College of Gastroenterology guideline recommends that when patients have clear documentation that a first-degree relative has had an advanced adenoma (a pathology report or report of surgical resection for a benign polyp), then that individual warrants more intense screening.

Table 35.5 Factors increasing the risk for colorectal cancer (other than inherited syndromes and chronic inflammatory bowel disease of the colon)

- Older age
- Male gender
- Cigarette smoking
- Obesity
- Diabetes mellitus
- African American race
- Family history of colorectal cancer in first-degree relative

Table 35.6 Composite of general screening guidelines for U.S. population

Risk group	Age to begin	Screening options
Average risk African Americans	45[a]	1. Colonoscopy every 10 y *or* 2. Annual fecal immunochemical test *or* 3. Flexible sigmoidoscopy every 5–10 y *or* 4. Option 2 + 3 *or* 5. CT colonography every 5 y *or* 6. Fecal DNA every 3 y
Average risk all other races	50	Options same as above
First-degree relative (FDR) with colorectal cancer or advanced adenoma at age < 60 or 2 FDRs with same	40 or 10 y before age when first relative was diagnosed	Colonoscopy every 5 y Consider Lynch testing

[a]Recommended by American College of Gastroenterology and The Multi-Society Task force on Colorectal Cancer.

35.5.3 Choices of Individual Screening Tests

No single colorectal cancer screening test is dominant in all relevant features, including sensitivity, patient acceptance, cost, cost-effectiveness, and risk. ▶ Table 35.7 lists some of the advantages and disadvantages of individual screening tests.

In the United States, colonoscopy dominates colorectal cancer screening, and national colonoscopy programs have been established in Germany and Poland. Average-risk colorectal cancer screening by colonoscopy is commonly utilized by privately insured patients in Australia and some European countries.

Most nationally based programs have utilized primarily FOBT for screening, in the United Kingdom with guaiac-based testing (gFOBT) and in other countries usually FIT. Several randomized-controlled trials are under way to directly compare colonoscopy and FIT for end points of adherence and efficacy, but none of the currently established trials evaluate colonoscopy as first sequential screening.

Flexible sigmoidoscopy has been demonstrated to be effective in randomized-controlled trials in reducing left-sided cancer incidence and mortality, and has some impact on right-sided cancer if a low threshold of findings is used to stimulate colonoscopy.[30] Flexible sigmoidoscopy has fallen out of favor in many countries, because the concept of screening only a portion of the colon endoscopically is inherently weak, because the procedure is performed without sedation and produces reluctance to repeat, and because physician reimbursement is often poor.

Double-contrast barium enema is no longer included in most screening guidelines, because computed tomography (CT) colonography is more effective and better tolerated.[31,32] However, CT colonography has had minimal impact on screening worldwide. When performed with thorough bowel cleansing, CT colonography seems both costly and burdensome for a diagnosis-only test. The radiation exposure is a significant concern,[33] and the detection of extracolonic findings can produce cost and psychological burdens, though in some cases there is early detection of extracolonic cancers (particularly renal and ovarian) and large abdominal aortic aneurysms.[33]

A new combined test for fecal blood and abnormal fecal DNA has high sensitivity for cancer, improved sensitivity for large precancerous polyps, and much better sensitivity than FIT for serrated class lesions.[34] However, the FIT component accounts for most of the cancer sensitivity, and the incorporation of DNA test triples the false-positive rate, while increasing the cost by as much as 20-fold compared to FIT. Given these trade-offs, most programmatic testing will continue to rely on FIT rather than the combined FIT-fecal DNA test.

35.5.4 Surveillance after Cancer Resection

The final step in the cost-effective prevention of colorectal cancer by colonoscopy is the selection of safe and appropriate intervals until the next examination. For average-risk screening, colonoscopy should be performed at 10-year intervals. As noted above, a subset of patients with a positive family history that does not meet criteria for inherited cancer syndromes should be examined at 5-year intervals (▶ Table 35.6). Postresection of stage II or III colorectal cancer, colonoscopy should be performed to identify synchronous and metachronous cancers. In the nonobstructed patient, colonoscopy is performed to the cecum and the colon cleared prior to surgery. In the obstructed patient, CT colonography with intravenous (IV) contrast should be obtained. Three to 6 months after resection, colonoscopy is completed to detect any flat lesions that might have been missed by CT colonography. The preoperative colonoscopy or the postoperative colonoscopy in the obstructed patient conclude the initial phase of searching for synchronous lesions. As an additional check on missed synchronous lesions, colonoscopy should be performed 1 year later, and if negative, in 3 years and then at 5-year intervals, unless earlier examinations are dictated by polyp findings or evidence of an inherited syndrome.

Patients with rectal cancer should undergo the same surveillance for metachronous lesions, but in some cases examinations of the rectum by flexible sigmoidoscopy or endoscopic ultrasound are warranted every 3 to 6 months in the first 2 years after surgery.[35] Appropriate neoadjuvant chemoradiation for advanced-stage cancers, followed by surgery using the total mesorectal excision technique, can reduce the need for these measures. In this author's opinion, endoscopic ultrasound is the better choice, because recurrences can be detected outside the rectum before these are detectable by flexible sigmoidoscopy.

Table 35.7 Strengths and weaknesses of the current major colorectal cancer screening tests

	Strengths	Weaknesses
Colonoscopy	Highest sensitivity for polyps and flat lesions Only test that can remove polyps Only test recommended at 10-y intervals	Highly operator dependent Highest risk (perforation, splenic injury, aspiration) High cost Requires bowel preparation
Flexible sigmoidoscopy	Proven effective in randomized trials Inexpensive	Poor acceptance Poor sensitivity for proximal cancer and advanced lesions
CT colonoscopy	Good sensitivity for cancer and large polyps Does not require sedation Detects extracolonic cancers Detects large abdominal aortic aneurysms Low procedure risk	High cost Requires bowel preparation for high sensitivity Detects incidental extracolonic findings Recommended at 5-y intervals
Fecal immunochemical test	Noninvasive Inexpensive	Low sensitivity for advanced adenomas Does not detect serrated class lesions Recommended at 1–2-y intervals
Fecal DNA/FIT	Noninvasive Very high sensitivity for cancer Much better than FIT for detection of serrated lesions	High cost Program sensitivity unknown High false-positive rate (12%) relative to FIT (4%) Recommended at 3-y intervals

CT, computed tomography; FIT, fecal immunochemical test.

Table 35.8 Composite recommendations for surveillance colonoscopy after resection of precancerous lesions

Colonoscopy findings	Recommended intervals
1 or 2 tubular adenomas < 10 mm with only low-grade dysplasia	5–10 y
1 or 2 sessile serrated polyps without cytological dysplasia and < 10 mm in size	5 y
Any conventional adenoma ≥ 10 mm in size, or with high-grade dysplasia or with villous elements, or 3–10 conventional adenomas of any size, or SSP ≥ 10 mm, or SSP with cytological dysplasia	3 y
> 10 adenomas	< 3 y
Any conventional adenoma or SSP ≥ 20 mm removed piecemeal	3–6 mo

SSP, sessile serrated polyp.

▶ Table 35.8 summarizes current US, European, and Australian recommendations for polyp surveillance, at least generally. More significant variations from these recommendations can be found in the UK guidelines.

35.6 Conclusion

Critical steps in the prevention of colon cancer are to encourage colorectal cancer screening, and to evaluate positive tests by colonoscopy. Colonoscopy must be performed in the screening, surveillance, and diagnostic setting by an examiner who understands the entire range of endoscopic appearances of precancerous lesions (including conventional adenomas and serrated class lesions), performs a meticulous examination after achieving adequate bowel preparation, resects precancerous lesions fully and as safely as possible, and directs follow-up screening or surveillance colonoscopy at intervals that are cost-effective and reflect current guidelines.

References

[1] The Paris endoscopic classification of superficial neoplastic lesions: esophagus, stomach, and colon: November 30 to December 1, 2002. Gastrointest Endosc. 2003; 58(suppl 6):S3–S43

[2] Hetzel JT, Huang CS, Coukos JA, et al. Variation in the detection of serrated polyps in an average risk colorectal cancer screening cohort. Am J Gastroenterol. 2010; 105(12):2656–2664

[3] Kahi CJ, Hewett DG, Norton DL, et al, Prevalence and variable detection of proximal colon serrated polyps during screening colonoscopy. Clin Gastroenterol Hepatol. 2011; 9(1):42–46

[4] Sawhney MS, Farrar WD, Gudiseva S, et al. Microsatellite instability in interval colon cancers. Gastroenterology. 2006; 131(6):1700–1705

[5] Arain MA, Sawhney M, Sheikh S, et al. CIMP status of interval colon cancers: another piece to the puzzle. Am J Gastroenterol. 2010; 105(5):1189–1195

[6] Lasisi F, Mouchli A, Riddell R, et al. Agreement in interpreting villous elements and dysplasia in adenomas less than one centimetre in size. Dig Liver Dis. 2013; 45(12):1049–1055

[7] Cairns SR, Scholefield JH, Steele RJ, et al; British Society of Gastroenterology. Association of Coloproctology for Great Britain and Ireland. Guidelines for colorectal cancer screening and surveillance in moderate and high risk groups (update from 2002). Gut. 2010; 59(5):666–689

[8] Lieberman DA, Rex DK, Winawer SJ, et al. Guidelines for colonoscopy surveillance after screening and polypectomy: a consensus update by the US Multi-Society Task Force on Colorectal Cancer. Gastroenterology. 2012; 143(3):844–857

[9] Vemulapalli KC, Rex DK. Risk of advanced lesions at first follow-up colonoscopy in high-risk groups as defined by the United Kingdom post-polypectomy surveillance guideline: data from a single U.S. center. Gastrointest Endosc. 2014; 80(2):299–306

[10] Rex DK. Preventing colorectal cancer and cancer mortality with colonoscopy: what we know and what we don't know. Endoscopy. 2010; 42(4):320–323

[11] Soetikno RM, Kaltenbach T, Rouse RV, et al. Prevalence of nonpolypoid (flat and depressed) colorectal neoplasms in asymptomatic and symptomatic adults. JAMA. 2008; 299(9):1027–1035

[12] Hewett DG, Kaltenbach T, Sano Y, et al. Validation of a simple classification system for endoscopic diagnosis of small colorectal polyps using narrow-band imaging. Gastroenterology. 2012; 143(3):599–607.e1

[13] Hayashi N, Tanaka S, Hewett DG, et al. Endoscopic prediction of deep submucosal invasive carcinoma: validation of the narrow-band imaging international colorectal endoscopic (NICE) classification. Gastrointest Endosc. 2013; 78(4):625–632

[14] Kim JS, Lee BI, Choi H, et al. Cold snare polypectomy versus cold forceps polypectomy for diminutive and small colorectal polyps: a randomized controlled trial. Gastrointest Endosc. 2015; 81(3):741–747

[15] Rex DK, Ahnen DJ, Baron JA, et al. Serrated lesions of the colorectum: review and recommendations from an expert panel. Am J Gastroenterol. 2012; 107(9):1315–1329, quiz 1314, 1330

[16] Khalid O, Radaideh S, Cummings OW, et al. Reinterpretation of histology of proximal colon polyps called hyperplastic in 2001. World J Gastroenterol. 2009; 15(30):3767–3770

[17] Jspeert JE, Bastiaansen BA, van Leerdam ME, et al. Development and validation of the WASP classification system for optical diagnosis of adenomas, hyperplastic polyps and sessile serrated adenomas/polyps. Gut. 2016

[18] Tadepalli US, Feihel D, Miller KM, et al. A morphologic analysis of sessile serrated polyps observed during routine colonoscopy (with video). Gastrointest Endosc. 2011; 74(6):1360–1368

[19] Pohl H, Srivastava A, Bensen SP, et al. Incomplete polyp resection during colonoscopy-results of the complete adenoma resection (CARE) study. Gastroenterology. 2013; 144(1):74–80.e1

[20] Rex KD, Vemulapalli KC, Rex DK. Recurrence rates after EMR of large sessile serrated polyps. Gastrointest Endosc. 2015; 82(3):538–541

[21] Pellise M, Burgess NG, Tutticci N, et al. Endoscopic mucosal resection for large serrated lesions in comparison with adenomas: a prospective multicentre study of 2000 lesions. Gut. 2017; 66(4):644–653

[22] Rao AK, Soetikno R, Raju GS, et al. Large sessile serrated polyps can be safely and effectively removed by endoscopic mucosal resection. Clin Gastroenterol Hepatol. 2016; 14(4):568–574

[23] Senore C, Ederle A, Benazzato L, et al. Offering people a choice for colorectal cancer screening. Gut. 2013; 62(5):735–740

[24] Imperiale TF, Monahan PO, Stump TE, et al. Derivation and validation of a scoring system to stratify risk for advanced colorectal neoplasia in asymptomatic adults: a cross-sectional study. Ann Intern Med. 2015; 163(5):339–346

[25] Siegel R, Desantis C, Jemal A. Colorectal cancer statistics, 2014. CA Cancer J Clin. 2014; 64(2):104–117

[26] Rex DK, Mark D, Clarke B, Lappas JC, Lehman GA. Flexible sigmoidoscopy plus air-contrast barium enema versus colonoscopy for evaluation of symptomatic patients without evidence of bleeding. Gastrointest Endosc. 1995; 42(2):132–138.

[27] Lieberman DA, de Garmo PL, Fleischer DE, et al, Colonic neoplasia in patients with nonspecific GI symptoms. Gastrointest Endosc. 2000; 51(6):647–651

[28] Rex DK, Boland CR, Dominitz JA, et al; Colorectal cancer screening: Recommendations for physicians and patients from the US Multi-Society Task Force on Colorectal Cancer Gastrointest Endosc 2017; 86:18–33

[29] Rex DK, Johnson DA, Anderson JC, et al, American College of Gastroenterology. American College of Gastroenterology guidelines for colorectal cancer screening 2009 [corrected]. Am J Gastroenterol. 2009; 104(3):739–750

[30] Schoen RE, Pinsky PF, Weissfeld JL, et al; PLCO Project Team. Colorectal-cancer incidence and mortality with screening flexible sigmoidoscopy. N Engl J Med. 2012; 366(25):2345–2357

[31] Halligan S, Wooldrage K, Dadswell E, et al; SIGGAR investigators. Computed tomographic colonography versus barium enema for diagnosis of colorectal cancer or large polyps in symptomatic patients (SIGGAR): a multicentre randomised trial. Lancet. 2013; 381(9873):1185–1193

[32] von Wagner C, Smith S, Halligan S, et al; SIGGAR Investigators. Patient acceptability of CT colonography compared with double contrast barium enema: results from a multicentre randomised controlled trial of symptomatic patients. Eur Radiol. 2011; 21(10):2046–2055

[33] U.S. Preventive Services Task Force. Screening for colorectal cancer: U.S. Preventive Services Task Force recommendation statement. Ann Intern Med. 2008; 149(9):627–637

[34] Imperiale TF, Ransohoff DF, Itzkowitz SH, et al. Multitarget stool DNA testing for colorectal-cancer screening. N Engl J Med. 2014; 370(14):1287–1297

[35] Rex DK, Kahi CJ, Levin B, et al; American Cancer Society. US Multi-Society Task Force on Colorectal Cancer. Guidelines for colonoscopy surveillance after cancer resection: a consensus update by the American Cancer Society and the US Multi-Society Task Force on Colorectal Cancer. Gastroenterology. 2006; 130(6):1865–1871

36 Advanced Colorectal Polyps and Early Cancer Resection

David James Tate and Michael John Bourke

36.1 Introduction

The incidence and mortality[1] of colorectal cancer can be significantly decreased by colonoscopy and polypectomy.[2] Most colorectal polyps are small (< 10 mm) and can be easily treated by endoscopists with the relevant degree of training using cold snare polypectomy[3,4] or conventional electrosurgical polypectomy where necessary. ACPs are generally considered as those greater than or equal to 20 mm and these larger lesions have a much greater frequency of advanced histology and invasive cancer, are more challenging and hazardous to completely remove endoscopically, and require special techniques to safely achieve this. Some smaller lesions also fall into this group due to morphologic features suggesting advanced histology (e.g. depressed component). Approximately 2% of colorectal lesions are flat, 20 mm or larger, and termed laterally spreading lesions (LSLs).[5] Even very large LSLs limited to the mucosa are resectable endoscopically due to the lack of lymphatic drainage from this area. LSLs were traditionally managed surgically, but a growing body of evidence supports the similar efficacy[6] and durability[7] of ER versus surgery and more recently the superior cost-effectiveness[8] and safety profiles of ER, particularly in dedicated tertiary centers. Once SMIC has developed, there is still a possibility for ER if certain criteria are met, although this is more controversial. ▶Box 36.1 lists the indications for endoscopic therapy of advanced colorectal polyps. Over the last decade, high-quality prospective studies have emerged that provide an evidence base for the technique and safety of ER for ACPs. Two techniques exist: endoscopic mucosal resection (EMR) and endoscopic submucosal dissection (ESD). The main benefit of ESD is en bloc resection providing accurate histopathologic assessment of submucosal invasive cancer (SMIC), but this is at the expense of significantly greater complications. EMR is the main technique used in Western centers to resect large LSLs in the colon. Complications of EMR are infrequent and, in the vast majority of cases are controlled endoscopically; these include intraprocedural bleeding (11.3%), clinically significant postendoscopic bleeding (CSPEB, 6%), and perforation (1.3%). Adenoma recurrence rates of 10 to 20% are reported in high-volume centers, but this is easily resected endoscopically at surveillance procedures. Novel techniques promise to reduce the rate of recurrent adenoma and further predict those lesions that will recur. Novel procedural techniques in ER are promising, but require validation in prospective, multicenter randomized trials.

36.2 Technical Aspects and Preparation

ER of colonic ACPs requires training, adequate case volume to maintain skills, tertiary-level radiology and surgical support and a histopathologist with a dedicated interest in colorectal neoplasia.

36.2.1 Patient Preparations

Outcomes are optimized when patients are managed within an advanced tissue resection network. Research infrastructure is also highly desirable as many important clinical questions remain unanswered. Prospective monitoring of procedural and clinical outcomes with benchmarking against accepted standards is a minimum requirement.[9] Regular clinical meetings between stakeholders with discussion of interesting and challenging cases facilitate best patient care.

Seamless referral pathways that facilitate rapid and accurate transfer of data are preferable. This should include detailed imaging, a description of the lesion and comorbidities of the patient including anticoagulant medications and the indication for their use.[10] Biopsy prior to the referral of a colonic LSL is not necessary unless invasive cancer is strongly suspected; extensive photodocumentation provides more useful information. Biopsy commonly results in submucosal fibrosis, increasing the complexity of ER. Endoscopic tattoo placed on the opposite wall to the lesion for ER is encouraged to mark lesions that may be difficult to locate later.

Informed consent is vital. Complications of endoscopic mucosal resection (EMR) include deep injury to the colonic wall (deep mural injury [DMI]), bleeding, postprocedural pain, serositis, and recurrent or residual adenoma (RRA). For EMR of large colonic LSLs, rates of 1.3%[6] for colonic perforation, and up to 7% for post-EMR bleeding are quoted. Pain after EMR is uncommon and usually self-limiting, but must be reported. Patients are given contact details such that timely advice may be given should complications occur once they have left the endoscopy unit.

36.2.2 Techniques of Endoscopic Resection

Two established techniques exist for the ER of large LSLs: EMR and ESD. EMR has been refined extensively since its inception in 1977.[11] The technique involves expansion of the submucosal layer with a chromoinjectate, and placement of a snare over the target lesion. Closure of the snare with the addition of microprocessor-controlled fractionated current transects the tissue and the submucosal cushion provides a heat sink and safety barrier against ensnaring and damaging deeper structures. Lesions up to 20 mm in size can be removed en bloc, with larger lesions usually requiring piecemeal resection.

ESD was initially developed in Japan for the en bloc excision of early gastric cancer, avoiding the morbidity associated with surgery. The technique involves expansion of the submucosal plane with chromoinjectate, use of an endoscopic knife to incise the margin of the lesion (incision phase), and then separation of the lesion from the deeper structures in the submucosal plane (dissection phase) using various types of electrosurgical current and the endoscopic knife.

The main advantages afforded by ESD over EMR are derived from en bloc resection of the target lesion. This results in reduced recurrence in short- and medium-term follow-up, possible cure in low-risk submucosal invasive cancer, and a superior specimen for histologic assessment. Long-term follow-up studies of EMR for LSL greater than 20 mm, however, show that if the initial EMR was technically successful, then after two follow-up procedures at intervals of 4 and 12 months more than 98% of patients are free of recurrence and considered cured.

ESD can be used to treat LSLs with potential superficial SMIC to achieve cure. However, in large Japanese series, the number of such patients is approximately 10% and thus a universal ESD strategy does not offer a true benefit to the majority.[12] Moreover, this benefit only applies if both patient and physician decide and agree that surgery is not necessary despite submucosal invasive cancer.

These benefits come at a cost. ESD is technically challenging, significantly more time consuming, and is associated with a significantly higher rate of complications in comparison to EMR; even in expert Japanese centers, perforation rates are higher (5.7 vs. 1.4%) and mean procedure durations significantly longer (65.9–108 minutes vs. 29–30 minutes).[13] In addition, multinight hospital stay is mandated for all lesions removed by ESD whereas it is required for fewer than 5%[6] of those removed by EMR. However, the strongest argument against a universal ESD approach for all LSLs is that it does not decrease the rate of additional surgery after ER. In Japanese centers, an ESD-only approach was associated with a significantly higher rate of surgery (9.9 vs. 5.8%) than EMR.[13]

36.2.3 Equipment Required

Submucosal Injectate

Historically, the submucosal injectate for EMR was normal saline (NS), however, it results in a nonsustained mucosal lift and does not delineate the lesion margin. The optimal submucosal injectate contains three constituents:

1. **A colloid solution**, for example, succinylated gelatin (e.g., Gelofusine; B. Braun, Sempach, Switzerland) has been shown to be superior to NS in a double-blind randomized trial,[14] resulting in significantly fewer injections and resections, and a halving of the procedure time. Other solutions have also been described including hyaluronic acid, dextrose solution, and hydroxyethyl starch.
2. The addition of **an inert dye** to the injectate (chromoinjectate) allows for accurate delineation of the lesion margin; this is particularly useful for lesions with serrated or nongranular morphology to ensure complete resection. It also shows the extent of the submucosal cushion, the safe zone for EMR. Methylene blue and indigo carmine (e.g., 80 mg of indigo carmine or 20 mg of methylene blue in a 500-mL solution) are in commonplace use. They are avid for the submucosal areolar tissue and create a relatively homogeneous "blue mat" appearance when resection is within the submucosal plane (▶ Fig. 36.1).
3. Dilute **adrenaline** (1: 100,000 solution) added to the injectate reduces intraprocedural bleeding maintaining a clean EMR field and delays the dispersion of the submucosal injectate. It may also reduce the rate of CSPEB.[15]

Electrosurgical Generators

The use of a microprocessor-controlled electrosurgical generator capable of delivering fractionated current in short cutting bursts interspersed with longer coagulation pulses is essential for safe ER. These are now commonplace in tertiary endoscopy units and include, for example, ERBE VIO 300 (ERBE, Tübingen, Germany) or Olympus ESG 100 (Olympus, Tokyo, Japan). The return electrode senses tissue impedance and modifies current delivery to achieve the desired result.

Insufflation of Carbon Dioxide

The superiority of carbon dioxide insufflation over air during gastrointestinal (GI) endoscopy is firmly established, particularly with regard to decreased postprocedural pain, flatus, and bowel distension.[16] During EMR for large LSLs, carbon dioxide insufflation resulted in significantly less postprocedural admissions for pain in a large prospective series.[17]

Snares for Endoscopic Resection

A complete suite of snares of various sizes, shapes, stiffness, and wire diameters is necessary. Snares with a thinner wire diameter provide greater current density and owing to this and their narrower caliber, more swiftly transect the target tissue. The workhorse for EMR of LSLs is the 20-mm "spiral" snare (0.48-mm wire diameter). This snare has a series of serrations covering the wire and facilitates the capture of normal tissue at the lesion margin.

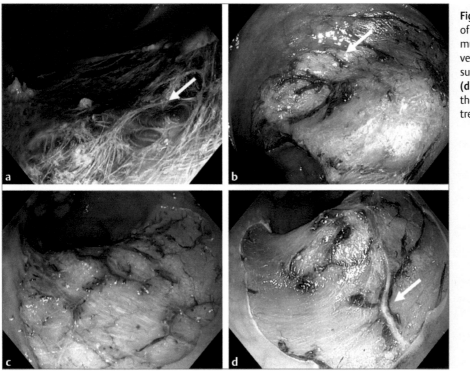

Fig. 36.1 Uncomplicated appearances of the mucosal defect after endoscopic mucosal resection. **(a)** Large herniating veins (*arrow*). **(b)** Large veins and nonstained submucosa (*arrow*). **(c)** Large branching veins. **(d)** Artery (*arrow*). Herniating vessels within the post-EMR defect do not require endoscopic treatment.

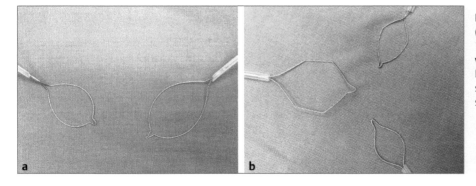

Fig. 36.2 Types of snare available for EMR. **(a)** Serrated 20-mm snare (right) and braided 15-mm snares (left), both thick (0.48-mm) wire, are the commonest snares used for EMR. **(b)** Thin (0.30-mm) wire monofilament snares of different shapes are used in specific situations, see text for details.

Increasingly, there are a range of alternatives available and there is renewed interest in the performance characteristics of various snares for particular indications. Commonly, in the right colon we use a 15-mm braided snare; the smaller size is possibly safer. Different wire stiffness, snare shape (oval, hexagonal), and performance characteristics can facilitate removal of a variety of potentially refractory lesions. Stiff thin-wire snares (0.3 mm) can allow tissue capture of residual adenoma at resection margins or previously attempted adenoma associated with significant submucosal fibrosis (▶ Fig. 36.2). Larger snares may be required for pedunculated or bulky exophytic lesions.

36.3 Lesion Assessment

Techniques to interrogate LSLs in real time prior to ER and determine the presence and degree of SMIC have been developed in recent years.

Overview assessment of the lesion is performed using high-definition white light (HD-WL). Lesion morphology should be described using the Paris classification.[18] This describes a flat lesion with less than or equal to 2.5-mm elevation above the surrounding mucosa as 0–IIa, with a central depression as 0–IIc, and a completely flat lesion as 0–IIb. 0–Is lesions are broad based but

elevated greater than 2.5 mm above the surrounding mucosa. Combinations of these terms exist (▶ Fig. 36.3). 0–Ip and 0–Isp lesions are polypoid and semipolypoid, respectively, and classified separately. Sessile lesions are also labelled based on their surface morphology as granular (G) or nongranular (NG) (▶ Fig. 36.4).

Focal interrogation of the lesion is then performed with HD-WL and image enhancement techniques such as narrow-band imaging (NBI)[19] (Olympus) or FICE (Fujifilm Medical, Saitama, Japan). The intention is to assess the pit pattern and vascular pattern of the lesion. Areas suspicious for SMIC, which are commonly demarcated, are identified and interrogated in turn, possibly with the addition of magnification (▶ Fig. 36.5).

Three systems exist for such assessment (▶ Table 36.1). **Kudo**[20] described five types of pit pattern; types III and IV indicate noninvasive disease and are suitable for ER. Experts suggest that the combination of chromic dye and magnification is required to assess the Kudo pit pattern. The **Sano classification**[21] is based on the capillary pattern as observed under NBI. Three types are recognized. Sano type II indicates noninvasive disease suitable for ER. Recently, the NBI International Colorectal Endoscopic (**NICE**)[19] criteria have been described. These are based on a combination of color, vessel, and surface pattern. The score has been reported to have a sensitivity of 94.9% and negative predictive value of

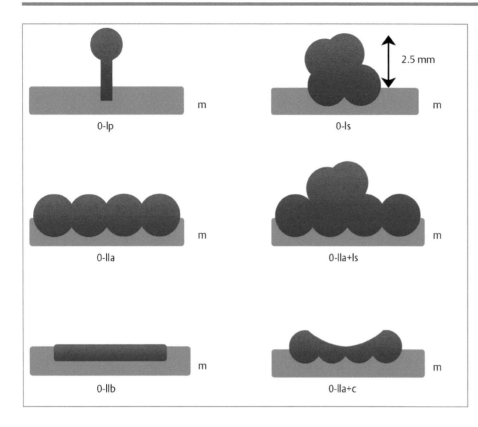

Fig. 36.3 Common Paris morphologies of laterally spreading colonic lesions referred for endoscopic resection. m, mucosa. After Paris consortium.[19]

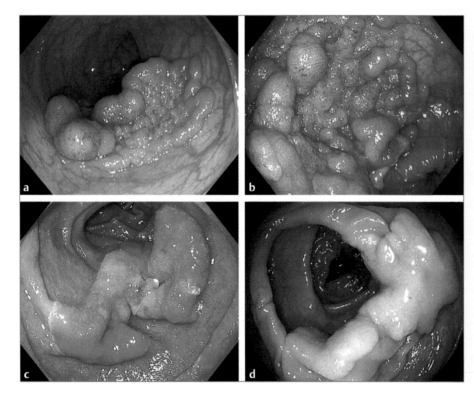

Fig. 36.4 Lesion morphology. Granular laterally spreading lesions (LSLs) in the rectum. **(a)** Paris 0–IIa/Is lesion with a dominant nodule. **(b)** Paris 0–IIa lesion. **(c, d)** Nongranular LSLs in the transverse colon. None of these lesions have suspicious features for submucosal invasive cancer, and can be stratified for such risk by the scheme in ►Fig. 36.6.

95.9% when any one of the three criteria demonstrate evidence of submucosal invasion, with substantial interobserver agreement (Kappa value 0.70).

Combining Paris classification, surface morphology, and lesion location is very useful for stratifying the risk of SMIC. Distal colonic lesions in general have a higher risk of SMIC. In large Japanese and Western[6,22] studies, 90% of lesions greater than or equal to 20 mm presenting for endoscopic resection are granular and greater than 75% are Paris 0–IIa class. In the absence of Kudo V pit pattern

or a depressed "c" component, both strong predictors of invasive disease, the risk of SMIC varies with LSL morphology[23] (►Fig. 36.6). In granular lesions, the risk is 0.9% for 0–IIa, 2.9% for 0–Is, and 7.1% for 0–IIa/Is lesions, with a greater risk in the distal colon. Nongranular lesions are at higher risk for SMIC with a 4% risk for 0–IIa NG lesions, 12.8% for 0–IIa + Is NG, and 16.7% for 0–Is NG. Again, there is generally a greater risk in the distal colon. This information can inform a targeted approach to ER, employing en bloc excision in the case of those lesions with a predicted high risk for SMIC.

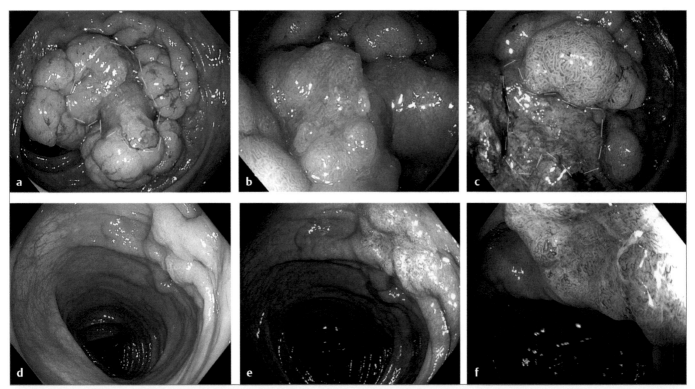

Fig. 36.5 High-definition imaging and prediction of submucosal invasive cancer (SMIC). **(a)** 50-mm granular laterally spreading lesion (LSL) in the sigmoid colon with a central demarcated area (*white dash line*) suggestive of focal submucosal invasive cancer. **(b)** White light magnification of the central area. **(c)** Narrow-band imaging (NBI) demonstrating NICE III and Sano IIIb vascular pattern within the demarcated area. **(d)** Nongranular LSL in the midtransverse colon with central depression. **(e)** NBI imaging suggesting a demarcated area concerning for submucosal invasive cancer. **(f)** Magnification demonstrating Sano IIIb vascular, NICE III, and Kudo Vn pit pattern. Histopathology confirmed SMIC in both cases.

Table 36.1 Significant features of Kudo, Sano, and NICE classifications of colorectal lesions and their relationship to endoscopic resectability

Image enhancement	HD-WL/NBI/chromoendoscopy	NBI	NBI	
Management	Kudo	Sano	NICE	Examples
Normal	I			
Endoscopic resection not required (hyperplastic) N.B. SSA/P fits this classification but requires endoscopic resection, see Section 5.7	II—stellar or open pits	I—invisible capillary pattern	**Type I**—Lighter than background, no visible vessels	
Endoscopic resection advised	IIIs/IIIL—tubular short or long pits IV—gyriform pits	II—structured capillary pattern	**Type II**—Brown relative to background, color arising from vessels. Vessels surround white, regular structures	
Likely SMIC; **consider surgery or en bloc endoscopic resection for staging**	Vi—disordered pit pattern with some maintained structure Vn—completely disordered pit pattern	III—disordered or absent capillary pattern	**Type III**—Dark brown relative to background. Areas of absent vessels and amorphous surface pattern	

NBI, narrow-band imaging; NICE, NBI International Colorectal Endoscopic Criteria; SMIC, submucosal invasive cancer; SSA/P, sessile serrated adenoma/polyp.

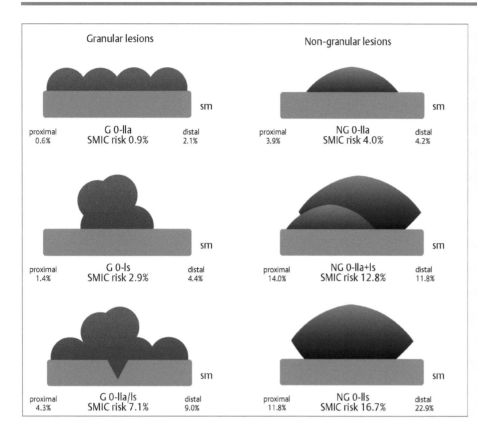

Fig. 36.6 Combining lesion morphology and granularity can predict risk of submucosal invasive cancer (SMIC). Granular (G, red color) lesions are lower risk for SMIC than nongranular (NG, green color) lesions (data from the ACE cohort).* Triangular penetration into the submucosa (sm) is the likeliest site of SMIC in lesions with a dominant nodule.[24] *(Data presented is in the absence of a depressed component or a Kudo type V pit pattern within the target lesion).

36.4 Resection Technique

36.4.1 Endoscopic Mucosal Resection

Injection Technique

An adequate submucosal cushion is required for safe EMR, and is used to improve access to the lesion. A deficient cushion risks deep injury to the colonic wall; an excessive cushion creates tension and can impede snare capture and visibility during the resection (▶ Fig. 36.7).

The **technique for injection** is as follows:

- Position the lesion at 6 o'clock in the colonoscopic view.
- Place the tip of the catheter at 30 to 45 degrees tangential to the lesion.
- Ask the assistant to extend the needle.
- Ask the assistant to commence injection while simultaneously stabbing the mucosa with the needle tip. Confirmation that the submucosal plane has been entered is with immediate and swift elevation of the lesion.
- Dynamic movement of the catheter during injection can be used to elevate the lesion to the required orientation with the needle tip anchored in the submucosal cushion. The most inaccessible portion of the lesion can often be exposed in this manner.

If the lesion does not lift, consider the following:

- **Extramural needle placement:** Gentle pulling back on the injection catheter will usually locate the submucosal plane.
- **Needle tip remaining within the colonic lumen:** Recognized by visualization of chromoinjectate spilling into the lumen.
- **Nonlifting lesion:** This can be caused by submucosal fibrosis from a previous resection attempt, previous biopsy, or lesion biology (SMIC). The appearances of **canyoning** (lifting of the surrounding normal mucosa without lifting of the lesion) and the **"jet sign"** (rapid ejection of the chromoinjectate from the lesion) are confirmatory signs associated with nonlifting.

Intramucosal injection is another type of failed injection. This can be recognized by immediate bleb-like elevation of the mucosa with no simultaneous lifting of the lesion. The bleb can be punctured with the needle tip and the injection repeated.

Resection Technique

One injection is suggested per one to three resections. The principles of snare placement and resection are detailed below (▶ Fig. 36.7):

- The lesion is sited at 6 o'clock. The snare is opened fully above the lesion and then aligned with the margin of the lesion, taking care to capture a 2- to 3-mm margin of normal mucosa, the remainder being adenoma.
- Firm pressure is applied with the snare onto the lesion with the up–down control and suction of luminal gas is performed to tent the lesion into the snare.
- The assistant closes the snare slightly until the target tissue is seen to seat within the snare. Once visually confirmed, the snare is then closed until resistance is felt.
- The assistant passes the snare to the endoscopist who uses tactile feedback to sense the amount of tissue captured. The snare can be opened slightly under direct vision to release a portion of the captured tissue if required.
- The snare is closed tight to within 1 cm to ensure swift tissue transection at the time of snare excision which preserves the endoscopic delineation within and between the tissue planes and resection margins. With this approach the layered anatomical structures of the colonic wall are easily identified.
- The mobility of the captured tissue with relation to the colonic wall is checked by rapidly moving the snare catheter back and forth within the working channel.
- The endoscopist applies one to three pulses of fractionated current with alternating cutting and coagulating cycles (e.g., EndoCut mode Q, effect 3, cut duration 1, cut interval 6; ERBE, Tübingen, Germany), to transect the tissue. This phase should be quick and there should be immediate evidence that the

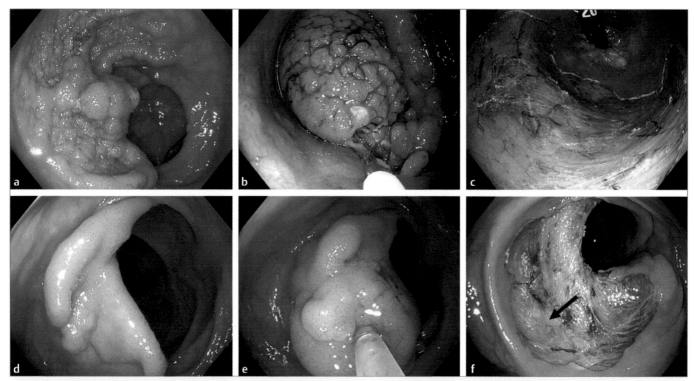

Fig. 36.7 Stages of EMR. **(a)** 50-mm Paris 0–IIa/Is granular laterally spreading lesion (LSL) in the proximal rectum with a dominant nodule. **(b)** Snare placement (20 mm, serrated) after chromogelofusine injection. **(c)** Uncomplicated bland blue mat defect after completed EMR. **(d)** 40-mm Paris-IIa nongranular LSL in the midtransverse colon. **(e)** Injection of chromogelofusine. **(f)** Hemicircumferential uncomplicated mucosal defect with golden adipose tissue (*arrow*).

snare has bedded in with each pulse. There are occasions when longer application of fractionated current may be required including lesions with significant submucosal fibrosis and resections involving adipose tissue, for example, around the ileocecal valve (ICV).

- The resected specimen is pushed aside with the snare catheter.
- Water-jet irrigation expands the mucosal defect, tamponades bleeding, and allows assessment of the plane of resection.
- For subsequent resections the free edge of the snare is aligned precisely with the edge of the mucosal/lesion incision to minimize the possibility of residual adenoma islands.

36.4.2 Endoscopic Submucosal Dissection

The technique of ESD involves the creation of a submucosal cushion, incision of the lesion margin with an endoscopic knife, and dissection beneath the lesion in the submucosal plane leading to an en bloc resection. The injectate is similar to that used for EMR with a colloid solution plus an inert dye. Most Japanese centers use 0.4% hyaluronic acid (MucoUp, Johnson and Johnson, Tokyo, Japan) as the basis of the injectate,[24] due to its superior retention in the submucosal space, particularly in the colon. Use in Western centers is limited by availability and cost.

Different knives are available for ESD and have different properties. The dual knife (Olympus, Tokyo, Japan) allows for precise dissection, but requires exchange of knife and injection catheters, whereas the hybrid knife (ERBE, Tübingen, Germany) requires no such exchange, speeding up the ESD procedure,[25,26] greatly improving the ease of further submucosal

injections and potentially increasing safety,[27] perhaps at the expense of precise dissection due to the larger size of the cutting tip. Other knives are available.[28] In the future even more tapered and precise knives with the ability to inject without device exchange have the potential to greatly speed up the technique of ESD.

The technique for ESD is as follows:

- A transparent cap is applied to the endoscope to aid separation of the mucosal and submucosal layers and to exert traction on the lesion.
- The lesion is marked with the knife tip. This is often unnecessary in the colon but of paramount importance in the stomach and esophagus as lesions can be subtly demarcated.
- Chromic solution is injected to lift the lesion.
- The lesion is isolated from the surrounding mucosa with the knife using cutting current, for example, ERBE Dry Cut (30 W, effect 2). Ultimately a circumferential mucosal incision is required, although the timing to fully complete this depends on anatomical and lesion factors.
- The lesion is dissected in the submucosal plane using cutting current, for example, ERBE Dry Cut (30 W, effect 2). Diathermy power settings can be adjusted to achieve the desired result. The division of tissue in the submucosal plane must be precisely controlled to avoid inadvertent muscle layer injury.
- Bleeding within the defect is controlled using either Swift Coagulation (e.g., ERBE effect 3, 30 W) or soft coagulation (e.g., ERBE effect 4, maximum 80 W) with the knife tip. More substantial bleeding can be controlled with hemostatic forceps using soft coagulation.
- Prophylactic coagulation of large blood vessels in the ESD defect is a common practice.[29]
- Consideration is made to the direction of gravity as the dissection progresses such that the lesion falls in a direction that aids the procedure, and patient position is changed as necessary to achieve this (▶Fig. 36.8).

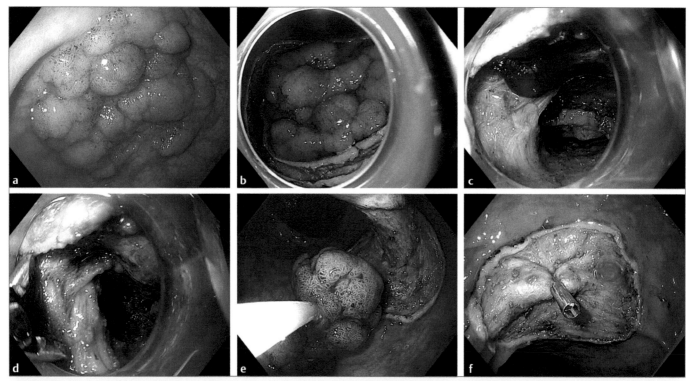

Fig. 36.8 ESD of a 35-mm rectal 0–IIa + Is LSL **(a)** with amorphous surface pattern and areas of disrupted vessels suggesting en bloc endoscopic excision would be preferable. **(b)** The lesion is isolated from the surrounding normal mucosa. **(c)** During the dissection, significant bleeding is encountered and controlled with the hemostatic forceps **(d)**. **(e)** The specimen is retrieved en bloc for histopathologic analysis. **(f)** A clip is placed over an area of muscularis propria (MP) injury within the defect.

36.5 Unique Situations

36.5.1 EMR of LSLs at the Anorectal Junction

LSLs that extend to or involve the anorectal junction (ARJ) are challenging to remove endoscopically and have traditionally been managed surgically. The ARJ has unique anatomical and physiologic characteristics which necessitate modifications to the standard EMR technique[30]:

- **Endoscopic access may be difficult and visualization impaired**. This can be improved by the use of a gastroscope or pediatric colonoscope and a short 4-mm transparent cap.
- **The area has rich somatic nervous innervation and therefore ER is often painful**. A long-acting local anesthetic is added to the submucosal injectate. We use ropivacaine final concentration 0.5% to a maximum dose of 40 mg with electrocardiographic monitoring. This provides local anesthesia for 4 hours and analgesia for up to 12 hours.
- In contrast to the more proximal colorectum **the lymphatic and venous drainage of the ARJ and distal 5 cm of rectum enters directly into the systemic circulation** bypassing the filtering function of the reticuloendothelial system/portal venous circulation and thus there is a risk of significant systemic bacteremia with repeated submucosal injection and extensive resection. Broad-spectrum antibiotics are given to all patients undergoing ER at the ARJ.
- **EMR over the hemorrhoidal plexus is considered potentially hazardous**. In practice, these thick-walled vascular columns are resistant to entrapment via the snare. Tangential injection of dye solution in the forward view into the submucosal plane elevates the mucosa away from the hemorrhoidal columns and creates a cushion over which snare resection can commence.

Postprocedure, the patient should be advised to maintain soft stools for 1 to 2 weeks and use simple analgesia, for example, paracetamol 1 g every 6 hours.

36.5.2 EMR of LSLs at the Ileocecal Valve

Involvement of the ICV has been identified as an independent risk factor for failure of EMR.[6,31] This is often due to challenging endoscopic access and complete visualization of the extent of the lesion. A transparent endoscope cap can be invaluable in this context, enabling fold deflection and visualization of LSLs extending into the ileum. Small stiff, thin-wire snares may optimize tissue capture in tight spaces and angles. ICV LSLs are at greater risk of recurrence than lesions elsewhere in the colon (17.5 vs. 11.5%),[32] but in a prospective series, surgery was ultimately avoided in 43/53 (81.1%) of cases attempted. Risk factors for failure were identified as ileal infiltration and involvement of both lips of the ICV.

36.5.3 EMR of Circumferential LSLs

LSLs involving the full circumference of the colonic wall can be removed by EMR (▶ Fig. 36.9). These lesions are uncommon and have previously been a relative contraindication to ER. A recent case series indicates that resection of such lesions is safe and, particularly in the rectum, prevents exposure of the patient to the significant morbidity risk and the potential poor long-term functional outcome of surgery.[33]

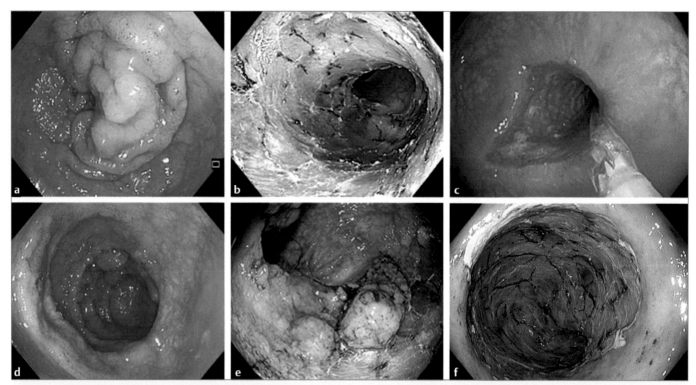

Fig. 36.9 **(a)** EMR of a fully circumferential granular 100-mm Paris 0–IIa/Is granular laterally spreading lesion (LSL) in the proximal rectum. **(b)** Completed uncomplicated mucosal defect. **(c)** Surveillance procedure at 2 months; uncomplicated EMR scar which was passable by the pediatric colonoscope after balloon dilatation. **(d)** 90-mm Paris 0–IIa/Is granular fully circumferential LSL in the proximal rectum. **(e)** Progressive EMR procedure. **(f)** Completed uncomplicated mucosal defect.

Normal bowel function is demonstrated after resection of such extensive lesions. Transient luminal stenosis may arise and steroid enemas with preemptive balloon dilation at intervals of 1 to 2 weeks for the first 6 weeks may be necessary.

36.5.4 EMR of Lumen Filling Lesions

LSLs with very large Is components occur and can fill the entire colonic lumen extending over multiple folds. These lesions are highly vascular and are often difficult to approach endoscopically due to their bulk and the potential invagination of the colonic wall into the lumen that risks deep mural injury with snare resection.

- Commence the resection at the anal end of the lesion involving a 2- to 3-mm rim of normal mucosa to enter the submucosal plane.
- Continue to inject and resect EMR, expanding the submucosal plane, carefully following the resected edge of the lesion and the plane of the colonic wall for each subsequent snare placement, "up and over" the Is component. This approach aims to avoid cutting across folds and deep mural injury.
- Tactile feedback prior to each snare resection is essential to avoid capture of excessive tissue or deeper structures within the snare.

36.5.5 EMR of Periappendiceal LSLs

LSLs involving the appendiceal orifice (or within 5 mm thereof) pose unique challenges. A single series of lesions removed by underwater EMR has been described.[34] These lesions can be safely resected by conventional EMR provided that they do not extend

deeply (beyond endoscopic vision) into the appendiceal orifice and in general do not involve more than 50% of the circumference of the appendiceal orifice. These often have substantial submucosal fibrosis and are best approached with small stiff, thin-wire snares (▶Fig. 36.10). By contrast, patients who have undergone prior appendectomy can often safely have fully circumferential lesions involving the prior appendiceal orifice carefully resected endoscopically.

36.5.6 EMR of Multiple Recurrent LSLs

LSLs with a previous resection attempt present particular challenges since there is often significant submucosal fibrosis beneath the lesion. Some modifications to the standard EMR technique are often required:

- It is often difficult to obtain adequate lifting of the target lesion due to submucosal fibrosis. Start the injection/resection in the nonfibrotic area, even outside the lesion if necessary. Areas that lift should be resected first with the goal of isolating the fibrotic area. This frees up the lateral attachments of the fibrotic area and creates a "step" adjacent to it to allow seating of the snare for tissue capture. Again small stiff, thin-wire snares are preferred.
- Areas that cannot be resected by snare can be treated by hot or cold avulsion.[35] We use the cold avulsion and adjuvant snare tip soft coagulation (CAST) technique. A cold serrated cup biopsy forceps is used to systematically avulse the residual tissue which now only has its deep attachment. Such tissue often peels off easily. This is repeated until no further adenomatous tissue remains.
- The area that was resected by cold avulsion is then treated with snare tip soft coagulation (STSC) (e.g., ERBE effect 4, maximum 80 W) to residual microadenoma.

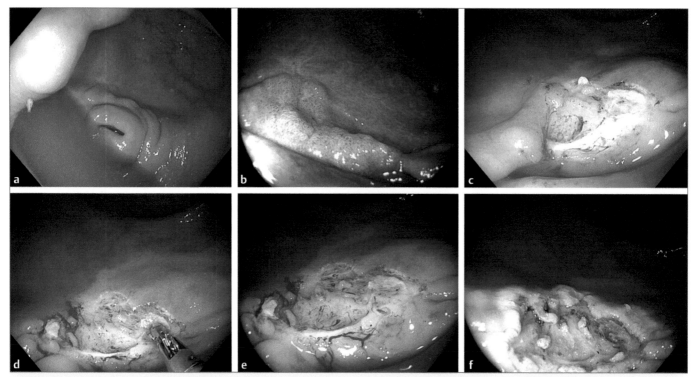

Fig. 36.10 **(a)** EMR of a previously attempted periappendiceal laterally spreading lesion (LSL). **(b)** A small (10-mm) thin wire snare is used for optimal resection. **(c)** Significant fibrosis associated with the previous resection preventing complete snare excision. **(d)** Cold avulsion of remaining adenoma that is subsequently treated with adjuvant snare tip soft coagulation (CAST). **(f)** Completed resection defect.

36.5.7 Sessile Serrated Lesions

The serrated neoplasia pathway accounts for 20 to 30% of sporadic colon cancers. Sessile serrated adenomas/polyps (SSAs/Ps) are difficult to detect endoscopically[36] and often incompletely resected (▶ Fig. 36.11).[37] Approximately 30% of SSAs/Ps greater than or equal to 20 mm contain a dysplastic focus (which endoscopically and histologically resembles adenoma). If this dysplastic focus is large or conspicuous, it can distract the endoscopist from a larger underlying serrated lesion.[38] Failure to recognize the full extent of the lesion may predispose to incomplete resection.[39] Chromoinjection can be used to better delineate the lesion margin. Care should be taken to recognize the patients who fulfil criteria for serrated polyposis syndrome.[40] They require regular colonoscopic surveillance and familial screening.[41] Recent large studies suggest that in tertiary centers SSA/P can be treated by EMR with equivalent outcomes and rates of recurrence to conventional adenomas.[42,43]

36.5.8 Endoscopic Resection of Large Pedunculated Lesions

Pedunculated lesions represent less than one-third of all polyps in the colon and those less than 20 mm in diameter with stalks less than 5 mm in diameter are safe to resect with hot snare polypectomy. Larger pedunculated adenomas with broad stalks (≥ 5 mm) can be safely resected, but often have large feeding blood vessels in their stalk which, if not prophylactically treated, may lead to postprocedural bleeding and thus mechanical hemostasis of the stalk with either clip or detachable loop is recommended.[44] Prophylactic placement of a detachable nylon loop (Endoloop [Ethicon], Polyloop [Olympus]) has been shown to reduce postpolypectomy bleeding in pedunculated lesions greater than or equal to 20 mm with stalks greater than or equal to 5 mm from 15.1% (control group) to 2.7%.[45] Adrenaline injection into the stalk reduced bleeding to 2.9% in the same study.

Lipomas and other submucosal lesions can also herniate into the lumen resembling a pedunculated polyp or adenoma; the clue to the nature of the lesion is the normal overlying mucosa. While such lesions can be safely resected if symptomatic, extreme care should be taken due to the possibility of invaginating muscularis propria (MP) and the large amount of current required to transect the fatty tissue due to the poor conduction of electrosurgical energy. Detachable nylon loop ligation of the stalk mitigates against the risk of perforation in cases where the MP may be invaginated.[46]

Resection of these lesions should employ the "snare traction" technique, particularly where there is a loop at the base of the stalk, whereby the snare is placed over the lesion and the snare catheter pulled back into the endoscope to exert traction on the stalk. This allows direct visualization of the exact point of snare closure on the proximal side of the lesion, which generally should be midstalk, to ensure that neither the loop or surrounding tissue is captured.

36.6 Endoscopy versus Surgery

The emergence of ER as a safe alternative to surgery for colonic LSLs over the last decade has stimulated comparative modeling of mortality, morbidity, and cost. For lesions limited to the mucosa there is no doubt that ER is safe, effective, and durable with a low rate of complications in large prospective series.[6,7] A large prospective multicenter study of 1,050 patients with LSL greater than or equal to 20 mm comparing actual EMR outcomes against

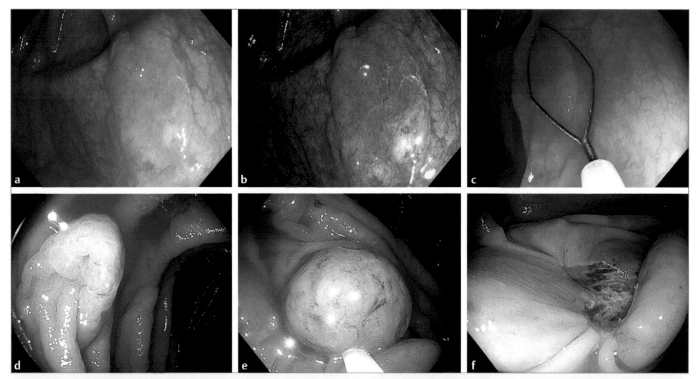

Fig. 36.11 Typical appearances of a sessile serrated adenoma (SSA/P). **(a)** The lesion is barely visible under high-definition white light. Under close inspection there is often adherent mucus and stool debris, lacy capillary structure, and a cloud-like appearance. Colonic vessels cannot be followed into the lesion. **(b)** The same lesion seen under narrow-band imaging (NBI) demonstrating superior delineation. **(c)** Lesions up to 15 mm in size can be safely removed by cold snare polypectomy, in a piecemeal fashion, avoiding the risks of EMR. **(e, f)** Larger lesions should be removed by EMR; the chromic dye sharply delineates the lesion margins.

predicted surgical outcomes using two independent and well-validated surgical scoring systems[47] showed that there was 0% mortality for EMR,[8] versus a predicted surgical mortality of 3.3% ($p < 0.0001$). The number needed to treat (NNT) to prevent one death was 30. Furthermore endoscopic management has recently been shown to be significantly more cost-effective than surgery with a mean cost saving per patient treated of U.S. $7,602 ($p < 0.001$) and a saving of 2.81 nights of hospital inpatient stay per patient.[48] A U.S. center has recently reported similar cost saving.[49] Given the ease of treatment of recurrent or residual adenoma (RRA) (94.5% in one recent study)[7] at surveillance endoscopy, there would appear to be little benefit of surgery over EMR for colonic LSLs limited to the mucosa.

Lesions which have invaded the submucosa (SMIC, the hallmark of colorectal cancer) are at risk for lymph node metastasis (LNM) at a rate of approximately 6 to 12%.[50,51] Such lesions are T1 cancers and are divided into low and high risk for LNM: **Low-risk lesions** invade less than 1 mm into the submucosa, do not demonstrate lymphovascular invasion (LVI), are well differentiated in grade, and do not demonstrate tumor budding at histologic assessment. Such lesions can be considered for curative endoscopic therapy by en bloc excision. Therefore, particularly when in vivo real-time imaging suggests the presence of **high risk for SMIC** (see Section 3 and ▶ Box 36.1), consideration of either en bloc endoscopic resection for accurate histologic assessment or surgery should be made. With LSLs larger than 20 to 25 mm, en bloc ER is often only achievable endoscopically with ESD. There are no cost or mortality studies comparing ESD with surgery; however, at least in Western centers, the technique is not readily available. Even in Japanese centers, where ESD is performed routinely, the majority of patients do not have SMIC. Of the minority that

do (10%), only 50% with superficial SMIC (SM1) are theoretically cured by ESD.[12] When **high-risk histologic features for LNM** are present in the resection specimen, then surgically fit patients should be referred for consideration of surgical resection.

36.7 Complications

Bleeding occurs in 7 to 9% of ER for colonic LSLs removed by EMR and ESD, respectively,[12,52] and can be divided into intraprocedural bleeding (IPB) or CSPEB. CSPEB is defined as bleeding after completion of endoscopic resection which necessitates presentation to the emergency department or reintervention.

36.7.1 Intraprocedural Bleeding

IPB is to be expected during ER as submucosal vessels are exposed that may be injured and bleed. In a large prospective study, the rate of IPB during EMR was 11.3%.[15] Independent predictors of bleeding included increasing lesion size, Paris 0–IIa + Is morphology and tubulovillous or villous histology. In addition, IPB was associated with an increased risk of RRA at surveillance colonoscopy. All episodes of IPB in this cohort were controlled endoscopically.

Control of IPB is easily achieved with STSC using the tip (1–2 mm extended) of the snare with short pulses of soft coagulation (e.g., ERBE effect 4, maximum 80 W). It is a light touch technique. This is convenient, inexpensive, and efficient as device exchange is not required. In a prospective study of EMR for LSL greater than or equal to 20 mm, hemostasis was achieved in 91% of IPB cases.[53] As the tissue is dessicated, the resistance to current flow rises exponentially limiting deep injury and ensuring safety. With brisk bleeding, vessels greater than 2 mm in caliber or if STSC fails to control bleeding after three to four applications, hemostatic forceps should be used, generally with the same settings. The causative vessel is grasped and cessation of bleeding confirms correct placement; the tissue is then tented slightly and soft coagulation applied. Endoscopic clips can also be used to treat IPB but are often ineffective and impair further tissue resection.

36.7.2 Clinically Significant Postendoscopic Bleeding

CSPEB occurs in 6% of patients after EMR, and two-thirds of cases occur within 48 hours.[52] ▶Fig. 36.12 demonstrates techniques for the treatment of CSPEB. Risk factors for CSPEB are right colon EMR, IPB, and use of a non microprocessor-controlled current for resection.[15] Use of anticoagulant medication according to guidelines was not significant at multivariable analysis. A study from the same group showed that 55% of cases of CSPEB settled spontaneously.[52] Factors associated with the need for intervention were hourly or more frequent hematochezia, higher ASA grade, features of shock at presentation, and transfusion requirement.

Prophylactic coagulation of visible vessels within the EMR defect did not reduce the rate of CSPEB in a large multicenter randomized-control trial.[54] Clip closure of the EMR defect showed a trend toward significance in a retrospective study,[55] however, lesions in difficult-to-access locations were not clipped; it is also difficult to close defects greater than 40 mm in our experience, thus potentially confounding these results. Techniques to improve clip closure require further study. In any event the ideal solution to CSPEB is not defined and patients should be aware of who to contact should it occur.

36.7.3 Deep Injury

The safety of endoscopic resection in the colon in part rests on the ability to detect resection that is deeper than the submucosal layer and apply endoscopic closure techniques. Inspection of the post-EMR defect is a critical component of the procedure. Generally, one should see a relatively homogeneous blue mat of intersecting submucosal connective tissue fibers. Resection deeper than the submucosa is termed deep mural injury and has recently been graded in the Sydney classification (▶Fig. 36.13).

- **Type 1:** Visible muscularis propria (MP) injury but no visible mechanical injury
- **Type 2:** Focal or generalized loss of the submucosal plane raising concern for MP injury or rendering the MP defect uninterpretable.
- **Type 3:** MP injured, specimen target sign[56] (STS) or defect target sign (DTS) identified
- **Type 4:** Actual hole within a white cautery ring, no observed contamination
- **Type 5:** Actual hole within a white cautery ring, observed contamination

Type 1 injuries do not require closure, types 3 to 5 mandate closure of the injury to the MP. It is generally not necessary to close the whole mucosal defect. Closure of the focal area of concern, that is, the area of submucosal fibrosis may be wise in type 2 injuries (▶Fig. 36.14). In a large multicenter prospective series of EMR for LSL greater than 20 mm, the rate of frank perforation was 1.3%.[6] After endoscopic closure and if the patient is stable, the resection can often be continued. A repeat procedure at a later date for two-stage resection is also possible. If there is uncertainty regarding deep injury, irrigation of chromic dye into the submucosa with the injection catheter without using the needle (topical submucosal chromoendoscopy [TSC])[57] can identify areas of

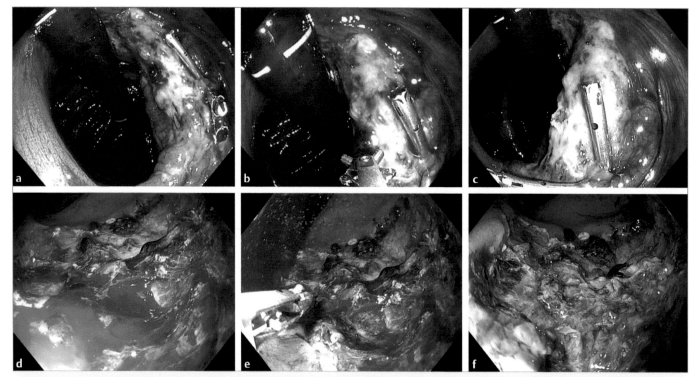

Fig. 36.12 Control of clinically significant postendoscopic bleeding (CSPEB). **(a)** A partially clipped EMR defect is seen with a clot overlying the responsible vessel. Hemostatic forceps are applied to the vessel **(b)** with obliteration of the target vessel **(c)**. **(d)** Significant bleeding from a vessel within an EMR defect; the apex of the bleeding indicates the site of the vessel. **(e)** The vessel has been grasped with hemostatic forceps; confirmation of the correct target is by cessation of bleeding **(f)** completed defect with no further bleeding.

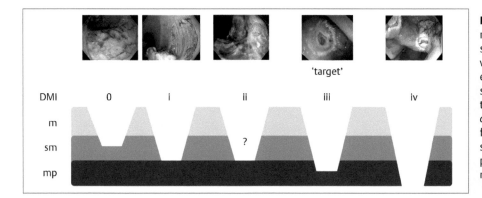

'target'

DMI   0   i   ii   iii   iv

m

sm   ?

mp

Fig. 36.13 The Sydney classification of deep mural injury (DMI) after EMR.[1] Schematic showing the depth of injury to the colonic wall with each type of DMI. Representative endoscopic images are presented above the schematic. See text for descriptions of the types of DMI (Section 6.3). Types 3 to 5 *require definitive endoscopic closure*. Closure is suggested for type 2 injury, which represents loss of the submucosal plane, often due to fibrosis from previous resection or lesion biology. m, mucosa; mp, muscularis propria; sm, submucosa.

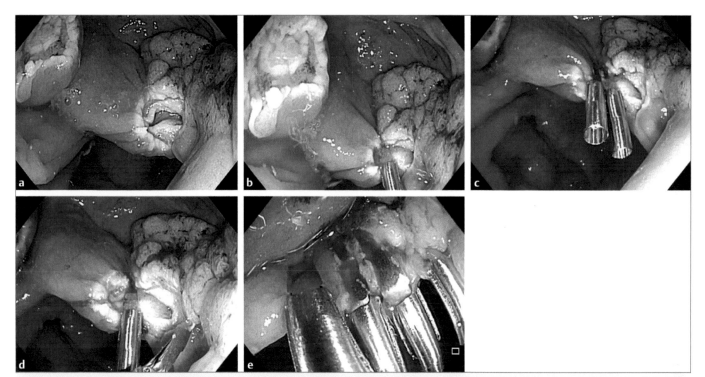

Fig. 36.14 Endoscopic closure of deep mural injury (DMI) type 4 at EMR. **(a)** Full-thickness perforation is identified at the site of EMR. This is mirrored by a specimen showing a target sign. **(b)** Initial clip placement to close the defect. **(c–e)** Further clips are placed to fully close the defect. The lesion was successfully resected endoscopically by EMR at a subsequent procedure.

nonstaining. The loose areolar tissue of the submucosa is avid for the dye unlike the MP and so unstained areas within the defect may be injured MP.

36.7.4 Postprocedural Pain

Pain is uncommon after EMR. When it does occur it does not necessarily represent deep mural injury to the colonic wall. Other causes include deep thermal injury, excessive transmural chromoinjection, and serositis. We suggest the following algorithm for managing patients post-EMR (▶ Fig. 36.15).

A two-stage recovery process is in place at our center with patients remaining in first stage recovery for 1 to 2 hours until they are ambulant. Once in the second stage recovery, the endoscopist should discuss the outcome of the case with the patient and reinforce the guidance to maintain a clear fluid diet until the next morning, symptoms to watch for requiring medical assistance, and the follow-up plan.

36.8 Residual and Recurrent Disease

36.8.1 Recurrence and EMR

A recent meta-analysis including 6,442 patients from 50 studies demonstrated a rate of endoscopic recurrence of 13.8% at first surveillance endoscopy after piecemeal ER of colonic LSLs, 95% confidence interval (CI) 12.9 to 14.7%.[58] If the EMR scar is clear at 3 to 6 months, the likelihood of late recurrence is low (4%).[7] Such high rates of early recurrence have led to international guidance recommending surveillance procedures 4 to 6 months, then 18 months post-ER for colonic LSLs.[59] This is a significant burden on patients and health care systems alike and there is thus a drive to define techniques that may reduce this rate, improve the endoscopic detection and treatment of adenoma recurrence, and triage patients who are unlikely to experience adenoma recurrence to later follow-up.

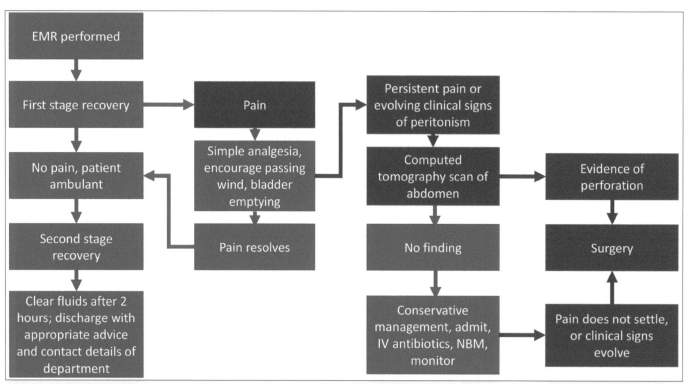

Fig. 36.15 Management of pain post-EMR and the suggested recovery procedure. EMR, endoscopic mucosal resection; IV, intravenous; NBM, nil by mouth.

36.8.2 Techniques at the Initial EMR to Prevent Recurrence

Care to resect a border of normal mucosa (2–3 mm) at the edge of an LSL undergoing EMR and inspection of the post-EMR defect for residual adenoma is paramount to prevent adenoma recurrence. Argon plasma coagulation (APC) ablation systematically applied to the edge or base of a polypectomy site in lesions greater than 15 mm was shown to reduce adenoma recurrence (1/10 recurrences APC group, 7/11 non-APC group, $p = 0.02$) in an older small study.[60] STSC applied systematically to the margin of EMR defects of lesions greater than or equal to 20 mm is the subject of a current Australian randomized-controlled trial (SCAR) which is due to report shortly; interim results are promising.

36.8.3 Triaging Patients to Follow Up Based on Risk of Recurrence

Size of LSL greater than or equal to 40 mm, intraprocedural bleeding requiring endoscopic control, and use of APC to complete initial ER were identified as predictors of recurrence at first surveillance colonoscopy.[7] The future of EMR will likely involve evidence-based staged surveillance procedures depending on individual risk factors identified at the time of the initial EMR.

36.8.4 Accurate Assessment of the Post-EMR Scar

EMR scars are identified by a pale area of colonic mucosa with disruption of the normal vascular pattern, sometimes with puckering of the mucosa at the edges of the scar (▶Fig. 36.16). We suggest a standard scar assessment protocol to maximize the sensitivity and specificity of endoscopic analysis of the post-EMR scar:[1]

- Interrogate the edges of the scar using HD-WL, followed by the center of the scar.
- The same routine is performed using NBI.
- Careful inspection of the scar includes the search for a transition point, where a nonneoplastic pit or vascular pattern (Kudo I or II) becomes a neoplastic pit pattern (Kudo III or IV). Examples of RRA within post-EMR scars are shown in ▶Fig. 36.17.

Areas of concern are always treated endoscopically as follows, even if not particularly suspicious to avoid the need to repeat the examination based on histology.

36.8.5 Endoscopic Treatment of Post-EMR Recurrence

Post-EMR RRA is easily and successfully treated endoscopically in the vast majority of cases, 90.3% in a recent meta-analysis[58] and 94.5% in a large prospective multicenter Australian series.[7]

Chromoinjection of RRA is not performed since injection often leads to a canyon effect with marked elevation of the normal nonfibrotic mucosa around the target area making it harder to resect.[61] Instead a small, stiff, thin-wire snare is used to resect RRA with a coagulating current (e.g., forced coagulation ERBE effect 2, 30 W). Difficult to ensnare areas of RRA can be removed with biopsy forceps and cold avulsion. The area of RRA is then treated liberally with STSC (CAST, described in Section 4.6). ▶Fig. 36.18 shows the endoscopic treatment of RRA within a post-EMR scar. RRA is retrieved and sent for histopathologic assessment.

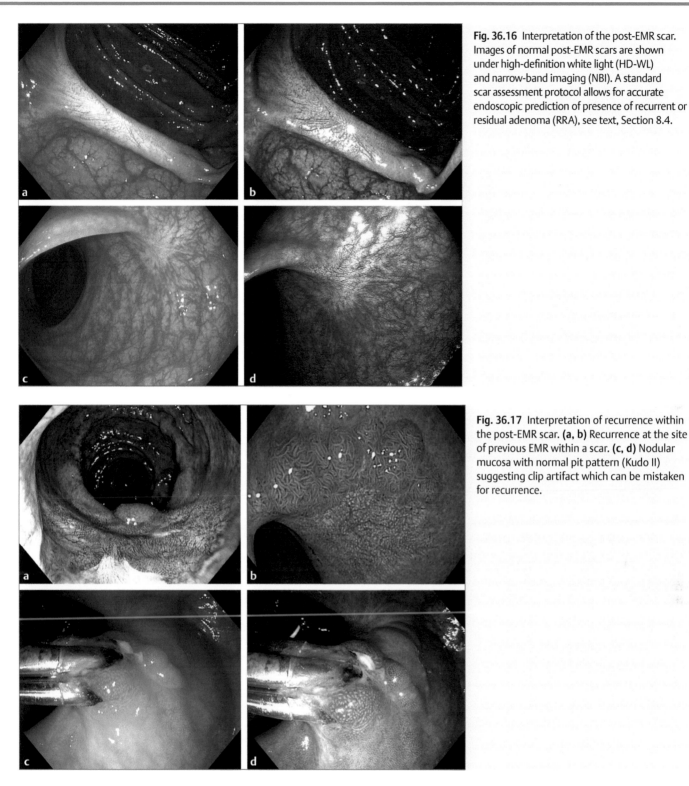

Fig. 36.16 Interpretation of the post-EMR scar. Images of normal post-EMR scars are shown under high-definition white light (HD-WL) and narrow-band imaging (NBI). A standard scar assessment protocol allows for accurate endoscopic prediction of presence of recurrent or residual adenoma (RRA), see text, Section 8.4.

Fig. 36.17 Interpretation of recurrence within the post-EMR scar. **(a, b)** Recurrence at the site of previous EMR within a scar. **(c, d)** Nodular mucosa with normal pit pattern (Kudo II) suggesting clip artifact which can be mistaken for recurrence.

Recently the phenomenon of clip artifact has been described[62, 63]; this describes nodular mucosa around endoscopic clips that were used in the initial ER (▶ Fig. 36.18); this mucosa can be differentiated reliably with endoscopic imaging from recurrence by its normal vascular pattern, but if there is doubt, the scar should be treated.

36.9 Future Direction of ER

Endoscope imaging and postprocessing techniques are evolving rapidly and now enable high-quality assessment of lesions preresection and EMR scars for RRA. These techniques will likely make biopsies of lesions preresection obsolete. Standardizing the interpretation of such imaging will allow more accurate prediction of SMIC with less interobserver variability.

Multiple modifications to the technique of EMR have been proposed. Underwater EMR[64] involves full immersion of the colonic lumen with water and dispenses with the need for submucosal chromoinjection. This is based on the endoscopic ultrasound (EUS) observation that water distension allows the mucosa to float on the submucosa during EMR. One problem with the technique is the lack of a chromic dye to interpret the submucosal defect. Good success rates have been reported, but the technique needs standardization and validation in prospective multicenter studies.

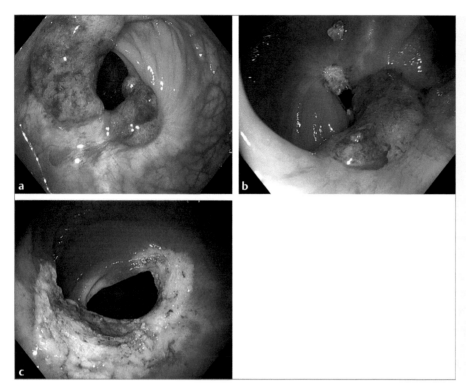

Fig. 36.18 Treatment of large multifocal recurrent adenoma after EMR of a 100-mm 90% circumferential proximal rectal lesion. This patient presented late for surveillance at 12 months post-EMR. **(a)** Multifocal recurrent adenoma in the EMR scar under high-definition white light. **(b)** First snare excision of recurrent adenoma with a thin wire snare. **(c)** Result of snare tip soft coagulation applied to the scar.

Full-thickness resection techniques for removal of invasive disease and submucosal lesions exist but are in their infancy, and are mainly limited by unreliable defect closure techniques.[65] Further prospective randomized studies comparing these techniques with surgery and ESD for the treatment of T1 cancers are required.

Much is now known about the molecular basis of colorectal cancer. Association studies between patients with AMN and normal controls may allow screening of at-risk patients, and knowledge of the molecular profile of resected lesions may lead to personalized surveillance intervals.

References

[1] Zauber AG, Winawer SJ, O'Brien MJ, et al. Colonoscopic polypectomy and long-term prevention of colorectal-cancer deaths. N Engl J Med. 2012; 366(8):687–696

[2] Winawer SJ, Zauber AG, Ho MN, et al; The National Polyp Study Workgroup. Prevention of colorectal cancer by colonoscopic polypectomy. N Engl J Med. 1993; 329(27):1977–1981

[3] Gupta N, Bansal A, Rao D, et al. Prevalence of advanced histological features in diminutive and small colon polyps. Gastrointest Endosc. 2012; 75(5):1022–1030

[4] Repici A, Hassan C, Vitetta E, et al. Safety of cold polypectomy for <10mm polyps at colonoscopy: a prospective multicenter study. Endoscopy. 2012; 44(1):27–31

[5] Rotondano G, Bianco MA, Buffoli F, et al. The Cooperative Italian FLIN Study Group: prevalence and clinico-pathological features of colorectal laterally spreading tumors. Endoscopy. 2011; 43(10):856–861

[6] Moss A, Bourke MJ, Williams SJ, et al. Endoscopic mucosal resection outcomes and prediction of submucosal cancer from advanced colonic mucosal neoplasia. Gastroenterology. 2011; 140(7):1909–1918

[7] Moss A, Williams SJ, Hourigan LF, et al. Long-term adenoma recurrence following wide-field endoscopic mucosal resection (WF-EMR) for advanced colonic mucosal neoplasia is infrequent: results and risk factors in 1000 cases from the Australian Colonic EMR (ACE) study. Gut. 2015; 64(1):57–65

[8] Ahlenstiel G, Hourigan LF, Brown G, et al; Australian Colonic Endoscopic Mucosal Resection (ACE) Study Group. Actual endoscopic versus predicted surgical mortality for treatment of advanced mucosal neoplasia of the colon. Gastrointest Endosc. 2014; 80(4):668–676

[9] Holt BA, Bourke MJ. Wide field endoscopic resection for advanced colonic mucosal neoplasia: current status and future directions. Clin Gastroenterol Hepatol. 2012; 10(9):969–979

[10] Baron TH, Kamath PS, McBane RD. New anticoagulant and antiplatelet agents: a primer for the gastroenterologist. Clin Gastroenterol Hepatol. 2014; 12(2):187–195

[11] Christie JP. Colonoscopic excision of large sessile polyps. Am J Gastroenterol. 1977; 67(5):430–438

[12] Saito Y, Uraoka T, Yamaguchi Y, et al. A prospective, multicenter study of 1111 colorectal endoscopic submucosal dissections (with video). Gastrointest Endosc. 2010; 72(6):1217–1225

[13] Fujiya M, Tanaka K, Dokoshi T, et al. Efficacy and adverse events of EMR and endoscopic submucosal dissection for the treatment of colon neoplasms: a meta-analysis of studies comparing EMR and endoscopic submucosal dissection. Gastrointest Endosc. 2015; 81(3):583–595

[14] Moss A, Bourke MJ, Metz AJ. A randomized, double-blind trial of succinylated gelatin submucosal injection for endoscopic resection of large sessile polyps of the colon. Am J Gastroenterol. 2010; 105(11):2375–2382

[15] Burgess NG, Metz AJ, Williams SJ, et al. Risk factors for intraprocedural and clinically significant delayed bleeding after wide-field endoscopic mucosal resection of large colonic lesions. Clin Gastroenterol Hepatol. 2014; 12(4):651–61.e1–e3

[16] Dellon ES, Hawk JS, Grimm IS, Shaheen NJ. The use of carbon dioxide for insufflation during GI endoscopy: a systematic review. Gastrointest Endosc. 2009; 69(4):843–849

[17] Bassan MS, Holt B, Moss A, et al. Carbon dioxide insufflation reduces number of postprocedure admissions after endoscopic resection of large colonic lesions: a prospective cohort study. Gastrointest Endosc. 2013; 77(1):90–95

[18] The Paris endoscopic classification of superficial neoplastic lesions: esophagus, stomach, and colon: November 30 to December 1, 2002. Gastrointest Endosc. 2003; 58(suppl 6):S3–S43

[19] Hayashi N, Tanaka S, Hewett DG, et al. Endoscopic prediction of deep submucosal invasive carcinoma: validation of the narrow-band imaging international colorectal endoscopic (NICE) classification. Gastrointest Endosc. 2013; 78(4):625–632

[20] Kudo S, Hirota S, Nakajima T, et al. Colorectal tumours and pit pattern. J Clin Pathol. 1994; 47(10):880–885

[21] Katagiri A, Fu KI, Sano Y, et al. Narrow band imaging with magnifying colonoscopy as diagnostic tool for predicting histology of early colorectal neoplasia. Aliment Pharmacol Ther. 2008; 27(12):1269–1274

[22] Uraoka T, Saito Y, Matsuda T, et al. Endoscopic indications for endoscopic mucosal resection of laterally spreading tumours in the colorectum. Gut. 2006; 55(11):1592–1597

[23] Burgess NG, Hourigan LF, Zanati SA, et al. Gross morphology and lesion location stratify the risk of invasive disease in advanced mucosal neoplasia of the colon: results from a large multicenter cohort. Gastrointest Endosc. 2014; 79(5):AB556

[24] Lingenfelder T, Fischer K, Sold MG, et al. Combination of water-jet dissection and needle-knife as a hybrid knife simplifies endoscopic submucosal dissection. Surg Endosc. 2009; 23(7):1531–1535

[25] Yamamoto H, Yahagi N, Oyama T, et al. Usefulness and safety of 0.4% sodium hyaluronate solution as a submucosal fluid "cushion" in endoscopic resection for gastric neoplasms: a prospective multicenter trial. Gastrointest Endosc. 2008; 67(6):830–839

[26] Ciocîrlan M, Pioche M, Lepilliez V, et al. The ENKI-2 water-jet system versus dual knife for endoscopic submucosal dissection of colorectal lesions: a randomized comparative animal study. Endoscopy. 2014; 46(2):139–143

[27] Fukami N, Ryu CB, Said S, et al. Prospective, randomized study of conventional versus HybridKnife endoscopic submucosal dissection methods for the esophagus: an animal study. Gastrointest Endosc. 2011; 73(6):1246–1253

[28] Maple JT, Abu Dayyeh BK, Chauhan SS, et al; ASGE Technology Committee. Endoscopic submucosal dissection. Gastrointest Endosc. 2015; 81(6):1311–1325

[29] Saito Y, Matsuda T, Fujii T. Endoscopic submucosal dissection of non-polypoid colorectal neoplasms. Gastrointest Endosc Clin N Am. 2010; 20(3):515–524

[30] Holt BA, Bassan MS, Sexton A, et al. Advanced mucosal neoplasia of the anorectal junction: endoscopic resection technique and outcomes (with videos). Gastrointest Endosc. 2014; 79(1):119–126

[31] Buchner AM, Guarner-Argente C, Ginsberg GG. Outcomes of EMR of defiant colorectal lesions directed to an endoscopy referral center. Gastrointest Endosc. 2012; 76(2):255–263

[32] Nanda KS, Tutticci N, Burgess NG, et al. Endoscopic mucosal resection of laterally spreading lesions involving the ileocecal valve: technique, risk factors for failure, and outcomes. Endoscopy. 2015; 47(8):710–718

[33] Tutticci N, Klein A, Sonson R, Bourke MJ. Endoscopic resection of subtotal or completely circumferential laterally spreading colonic adenomas: technique, caveats, and outcomes. Endoscopy. 2016; 48(5):465–471

[34] Binmoeller KF, Hamerski CM, Shah JN, et al. Underwater EMR of adenomas of the appendiceal orifice (with video). Gastrointest Endosc. 2016; 83(3):638–242

[35] Andrawes S, Haber G. Avulsion: a novel technique to achieve complete resection of difficult colon polyps. Gastrointest Endosc. 2014; 80(1):167–168

[36] Hetzel JT, Huang CS, Coukos JA, et al. Variation in the detection of serrated polyps in an average risk colorectal cancer screening cohort. Am J Gastroenterol. 2010; 105(12):2656–2664

[37] Pohl H, Srivastava A, Bensen SP, et al. Incomplete polyp resection during colonoscopy-results of the complete adenoma resection (CARE) study. Gastroenterology. 2013; 144(1):74–80.e1

[38] Burgess NG, Pellise M, Nanda KS, et al. Clinical and endoscopic predictors of cytological dysplasia or cancer in a prospective multicentre study of large sessile serrated adenomas/polyps. Gut.

[39] Burgess NG, Tutticci NJ, Pellise M, Bourke MJ. Sessile serrated adenomas/polyps with cytologic dysplasia: a triple threat for interval cancer. Gastrointest Endosc. 2014; 80(2):307–310

[40] Snover DC, Ahnen DJ, Burt RW. Serrated polyps of the colon and rectum and serrated polyposis. In: Bosman T, Carneiro F, Hruban R, eds. WHO Classification of Tumours of the Digestive System. Lyon, France: IARC Press. 2010:160–165

[41] Vemulapalli KC, Rex DK. Failure to recognize serrated polyposis syndrome in a cohort with large sessile colorectal polyps. Gastrointest Endosc. 2012; 75(6):1206–1210

[42] Pellise M, Burgess NG, Tutticci N, et al. Endoscopic mucosal resection for large serrated lesions in comparison with adenomas: a prospective multicentre study of 2000 lesions. Gut. 2017; 66(4):644–653

[43] Rex KD, Vemulapalli KC, Rex DK. Recurrence rates after EMR of large sessile serrated polyps. Gastrointest Endosc. 2015; 82(3):538–541

[44] Dobrowolski S, Dobosz M, Babicki A, et al. Blood supply of colorectal polyps correlates with risk of bleeding after colonoscopic polypectomy. Gastrointest Endosc. 2006; 63(7):1004–1009

[45] Kouklakis G, Mpoumponaris A, Gatopoulou A, et al; Lirantzopoulos N. Endoscopic resection of large pedunculated colonic polyps and risk of postpolypectomy bleeding with adrenaline injection versus endoloop and hemoclip: a prospective, randomized study. Surg Endosc. 2009; 23(12):2732–2737

[46] Murray MA, Kwan V, Williams SJ, Bourke MJ. Detachable nylon loop assisted removal of large clinically significant colonic lipomas. Gastrointest Endosc. 2005; 61(6):756–759

[47] Tekkis PP, Poloniecki JD, Thompson MR, Stamatakis JD. Operative mortality in colorectal cancer: prospective national study. BMJ. 2003; 327(7425):1196–1201

[48] Jayanna M, Burgess NG, Singh R, et al. Cost analysis of Endoscopic Mucosal Resection vs Surgery for Large Laterally Spreading Colorectal Lesions. Clin Gastroenterol Hepatol. 2016; 14(2):271–27–8.e1, 2

[49] Law R, Das A, Gregory D, et al. Endoscopic resection is cost-effective compared with laparoscopic resection in the management of complex colon polyps: an economic analysis. Gastrointest Endosc. 2016; 83(6):1248–1257

[50] Bosch SL, Teerenstra S, de Wilt JH, et al. Predicting lymph node metastasis in pT1 colorectal cancer: a systematic review of risk factors providing rationale for therapy decisions. Endoscopy. 2013; 45(10):827–834

[51] Kitajima K, Fujimori T, Fujii S, et al. Correlations between lymph node metastasis and depth of submucosal invasion in submucosal invasive colorectal carcinoma: a Japanese collaborative study. J Gastroenterol. 2004; 39(6):534–543

[52] Burgess NG, Williams SJ, Hourigan LF, et al. A management algorithm based on delayed bleeding after wide-field endoscopic mucosal resection of large colonic lesions. Clin Gastroenterol Hepatol. 2014; 12(9):1525–1533

[53] Fahrtash-Bahin F, Holt BA, et al. Snare tip soft coagulation achieves effective and safe endoscopic hemostasis during wide-field endoscopic resection of large colonic lesions (with videos). Gastrointest Endosc. 2013; 78(1):158–163.e1

[54] Bahin FF, Naidoo M, Williams SJ, et al. Prophylactic endoscopic coagulation to prevent bleeding after wide-field endoscopic mucosal resection of large sessile colon polyps. Clin Gastroenterol Hepatol. 2015; 13(4):724–7–30.e1, 2

[55] Liaquat H, Rohn E, Rex DK. Prophylactic clip closure reduced the risk of delayed postpolypectomy hemorrhage: experience in 277 clipped large sessile or flat colorectal lesions and 247 control lesions. Gastrointest Endosc. 2013; 77(3):401–407

[56] Swan MP, Bourke MJ, Moss A, et al. The target sign: an endoscopic marker for the resection of the muscularis propria and potential perforation during colonic endoscopic mucosal resection. Gastrointest Endosc. 2011; 73(1):79–85

[57] Holt BA, Jayasekeran V, Sonson R, Bourke MJ. Topical submucosal chromoendoscopy defines the level of resection in colonic EMR and may improve procedural safety (with video). Gastrointest Endosc. 2013; 77(6):949–953

[58] Hassan C, Repici A, Sharma P, et al. Efficacy and safety of endoscopic resection of large colorectal polyps: a systematic review and meta-analysis. Gut. 2016; 65(5):806–820

[59] Hassan C, Quintero E, Dumonceau J-M, et al; European Society of Gastrointestinal Endoscopy. Post-polypectomy colonoscopy surveillance: European Society of Gastrointestinal Endoscopy (ESGE) Guideline. Endoscopy. 2013; 45(10):842–851

[60] Brooker JC, Saunders BP, Shah SG, et al. Treatment with argon plasma coagulation reduces recurrence after piecemeal resection of large sessile colonic polyps: a randomized trial and recommendations. Gastrointest Endosc. 2002; 55(3):371–375

[61] Klein A, Bourke MJ. Advanced polypectomy and resection techniques. Gastrointest Endosc Clin N Am. 2015; 25(2):303–333

[62] Pellise M, Desomer L, Burgess NG, et al. The influence of clips on scars after EMR: clip artifact. Gastrointest Endosc. 2016; 83(3):608–616

[63] Sreepati G, Vemulapalli KC, Rex DK. Clip artifact after closure of large colorectal EMR sites: incidence and recognition. Gastrointest Endosc. 2015; 82(2):344–349

[64] Curcio G, Granata A, Ligresti D, et al. Underwater colorectal EMR: remodeling endoscopic mucosal resection. Gastrointest Endosc. 2015; 81(5):1238–1242

[65] Fujihara S, Mori H, Kobara H, et al. Current innovations in endoscopic therapy for the management of colorectal cancer: from endoscopic submucosal dissection to endoscopic full-thickness resection. BioMed Res Int. 2014; 2014(3):925058

37 Inheritable Cancer Syndromes

Evelien Dekker, Frank G.J. Kallenberg, Joep E.G. IJspeert, and Barbara A.J. Bastiaansen

37.1 Introduction

Colorectal cancer (CRC) results from genetic factors as well as environmental influences and their interaction. Most CRC cases are so called "sporadic" and seem mainly caused by interplay of environmental influences such as diet, smoking, and lifestyle factors. In a small proportion of patients, the CRC is caused by a genetic predisposition.

A family history of CRC is common among the general population. In the Western world, approximately 5 to 10% of adults have a first-degree relative with colorectal cancer, resulting in an increased risk for CRC depending on the number and age of affected relatives.[1] Up to one-third of patients with CRC appear to have increased familial risk, likely related to inheritance ("familial CRC"), but only approximately 5% of all colorectal cancers have a clear, well-defined, inherited genetic predisposition.

Inheritable cancer syndromes can be subdivided in nonpolyposis and polyposis syndromes (▶ Fig. 37.1). Lynch syndrome is a nonpolyposis syndrome caused by a dysfunction of the DNA mismatch repair system as a result of a germline mutation. Multiple adenomatous polyps may be caused by familial adenomatous polyposis (FAP), with a classical type (classical FAP) and a les profound type (attenuated FAP [AFAP]), and MUTYH-associated polyposis (MAP). Serrated polyposis syndrome (SPS) is a clinical diagnosis in patients with many serrated polyps, but the genetics are not yet known. Other, rare types of inheritable hamartomatous polyposis syndromes are Peutz–Jeghers syndrome (PJS), juvenile polyposis syndrome (JPS), and Cowden's syndrome (CS).

Diagnosing an inheritable cancer syndrome is important for several reasons: to provide an optimal surveillance strategy to prevent CRC, to provide optimal surveillance for extracolonic cancers if applicable, to provide optimal treatment in case of incident CRC, and to provide appropriate advice for relatives at risk to prevent CRC.

In general, polyposis syndromes are easily diagnosed as the number of polyps alerts the physician to think of a genetic

syndrome, and the type of polyps might lead directly to the diagnosis. Lynch's syndrome, however, is easily missed as those patients have few adenomas and those adenomas morphologically resemble sporadic lesions. Therefore, besides a family history for CRC and Lynch-associated cancers as well as the age of the patient having cancer as hallmarks for Lynch's syndrome, systematic molecular analysis of tumor tissue is nowadays used to improve the diagnosis of this genetic syndrome.

Once diagnosed, each syndrome has its specific risks and appropriate surveillance strategy in an effort to prevent CRC and extracolonic cancers, also discussed in this chapter (▶ Table 37.1).

37.2 Nonpolyposis Syndromes

37.2.1 Lynch's syndrome

Genetics

Lynch's syndrome is the most common inherited CRC syndrome and accounts for approximately 3% of newly diagnosed cases of CRC and 2% of endometrial cancer. It is an autosomal dominant disorder that is caused by a germline mutation in one of several DNA mismatch repair (MMR) genes (*MLH1, MSH2, MSH6, PMS2*) or loss of expression of *MSH2* due to a deletion in the *EPCAM* gene. The term hereditary nonpolyposis colorectal cancer (HNPCC) refers to patients and/or families who fulfill the Amsterdam criteria for Lynch's syndrome, and stems from the era when the genetic cause for this condition was unknown.

The role of the DNA MMR system is to maintain genomic integrity by correcting errors in base pairing during DNA replication. Inactivation of both alleles of one of the MMR genes leads to defective MMR and microsatellite instability (MSI). Patients with Lynch's syndrome and CRC have a germline mutation in one allele of a MMR gene; the second allele is inactivated by mutation, loss of heterozygosity, or epigenetic silencing by promoter hypermethylation. Biallelic inactivation of MMR genes in a cell results in

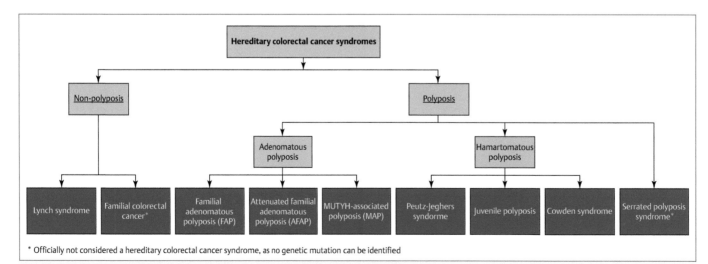

Fig. 37.1 Flowchart showing inheritable cancer syndromes subdivided into polyposis and nonpolyposis syndromes.

Table 37.1 Mutation, risks, and surveillance recommendations for each syndrome

Syndrome	Genetic mutation	Lifetime cancer risk	%	Surveillance strategies
Lynch	MLH1, MSH2, MSH6, PMS2, EPCAM	Colon Endometrium Stomach Ovary Hepatobiliary tract Upper urinary tract Pancreas Small bowel CNS (glioblastoma)	25–70 15–55 11–19 9–12 2–7 4–5 3–4 1–4 1–3	– Colonoscopy every 1–2 y, beginning at age 20–25 y – Consider annual gynecologic surveillance (CA-125 testing, transvaginal ultrasound, and endometrial biopsy), beginning between age 25 and 40 y – Consider prophylactic TAH/BSO[a] after childbearing age No data to support routine screening for other related cancers, but may be considered after counseling about the risks and benefits of available methods
Familial adenomatous polyposis (FAP)	APC	Colon Duodenum/ampullary Stomach Miscellaneous (pancreas, thyroid, CNS, liver)	100 4–36 < 1 < 2	– Colonoscopy yearly, beginning at age 10–12 y; prophylactic colectomy when indicated; if remaining rectum or pouch, surveil every 0.5–1 y – EGD with side-viewing examination every 0.5–5 y (based on Spigelman's classification), beginning at age 25–30 y No data to support routine screening for other related cancers, but may be considered after counseling about the risks and benefits of available methods
Attenuated familial adenomatous polyposis (AFAP)	APC	Colon duodenum/ampullary	70 4–12	– Colonoscopy every 1–2 y, beginning at age 18 y; prophylactic colectomy when indicated; if remaining rectum or pouch, surveil every 0.5–1 y – EGD with side-viewing examination every 0.5–5 y, beginning at age 25–30 y No data to support routine screening for other related cancers, but may be considered after counseling about the risks and benefits of available methods
MUTYH-associated polyposis (MAP)	MUTYH	Colon Duodenum	80 4	– Colonoscopy every 1–2 y, beginning at age 18 y; prophylactic colectomy when indicated; if remaining rectum or pouch, surveil every 0.5–1 y – EGD with side-viewing examination every 0.5–5 y, beginning at age 25–30 y
Serrated polyposis syndrome (SPS)	?	Colon	15–30[b]	– Colonoscopy every 1–2 y from diagnosis
Peutz–Jeghers syndrome (PJS)	STK11	Colon Pancreas Stomach Small bowel Breast	39 11–36 29 13 50	– Colonoscopy every 2–3 y, beginning in childhood/teenage years – EGD every 2–3 y, beginning in childhood/teenage years – MR/CT enterography or double-balloon enteroscopy, every 2–3 y, beginning in childhood/teenage years – Annual mammography and breast MRI, beginning at age 25 y – Annual pelvic examination, Pap smear and transvaginal ultrasound beginning at age 18 y – Consider annual MRCP and/or endoscopic ultrasound of the pancreas beginning at age 30 (although exact benefit is largely unknown)
Juvenile polyposis syndrome (JPS)	SMAD4, BMPR1A	Colon Stomach	≤ 68 ≤ 21	– Colonoscopy every 1–3 y, beginning at age 12 y – EGD every 1–3 y, beginning at age 12 y Small bowel examinations are not routinely recommended SMAD4 germline mutation carriers should be screened for hereditary hemorrhagic telangiectasia
Cowden's syndrome (CS)	PTEN	Colon Thyroid Breast Endometrium Renal cell	9 δ35 67–85 28 34	– Colonoscopy every 5 y, beginning at age 40 y Intensive cancer surveillance programs are generally coordinated by the medical oncologist

CT, computed tomography; CNS, central nervous system; EGD, esophagogastroduodenoscopy; MRI, magnetic resonance imaging; MRCP, magnetic resonance cholangiopancreatography.

Data based on Jasperson KW, Tuohy TM, Neklason DW, Burt RW. Hereditary and familial colon cancer. Gastroenterology. 2010;138:2044–2058.

[a]Total abdominal hysterectomy and bilateral salpingo-oophorectomy.

[b]Risk unknown, but 15 to 30% of SPS patients present with CRC.

defective repair of DNA mismatches occurring during replication, causing genomic instability. DNA mismatches most commonly occur in regions of repetitive nucleotide sequences, which are called microsatellites. Thus, a characteristic of loss of mismatch repair in cancers is the expansion or contraction of these microsatellite regions in the tumor compared with normal tissue. This is called MSI, and characteristic of Lynch-associated cancers.

However, MSI is not specific for Lynch's syndrome, and approximately 15% of sporadic CRCs also demonstrate MSI. Sporadic MSI-high cancers develop through somatic promoter methylation of

MLH1, leading to loss of MLH-1 function and frequently carry mutations in the *BRAF* gene.

Characteristics

Individuals with Lynch's syndrome are at an increased risk of CRC, endometrial cancer, and several other malignancies.

The lifetime risk of CRC in Lynch's syndrome is between 25 and 70%, varies by genotype, and may be influenced by ascertainment bias.[2,3] It is diagnosed at a considerably younger age than sporadic cancer, with an average 44 to 61 years versus 69 years.[4] Besides, individuals with Lynch's syndrome are at increased risk for synchronous and metachronous CRCs.

Most CRCs in Lynch's syndrome are located in the right colon. It develops from adenomas, which have no specific endoscopic hallmarks to be discriminated from sporadic adenomas. The most important feature to be considered for adequate preventive measures is their behavior: in Lynch's syndrome, the adenoma–carcinoma sequence is accelerated and estimated at 3 years, as opposed to 10 to 15 years for sporadic lesions.[5] CRCs in patients with Lynch's syndrome show a diminished response of 5-fluorouracil–based chemotherapy, but interestingly, the overall 5-year survival from CRC in Lynch's syndrome is higher when compared with sporadic CRC.

The most common extracolonic tumor in Lynch's syndrome is endometrial cancer. The risk of endometrial cancer varies depending on the MMR mutation, and is highest for MSH-2 mutation carriers.[3] Individuals with Lynch's syndrome are also at increased risk of cancer of the small bowel, stomach, ovaries, transitional cell cancer of the renal pelvis and ureter, hepatobiliary system, brain (glioma), and sebaceous neoplasms.

Diagnosis

Lynch's syndrome should be suspected in patients with synchronous or metachronous CRC, CRC before the age of 50, multiple Lynch's syndrome–associated cancers and in families showing clustering of Lynch's syndrome–associated cancers. A pathogenic germline mutation in the MMR or *EPCAM* gene makes a definitive diagnosis of Lynch's syndrome.

However, Lynch's syndrome is largely underdiagnosed. Traditionally, a family history of colorectal and other Lynch-associated cancers was the primary tool to identify Lynch's syndrome (Amsterdam criteria and Bethesda criteria, ▶ Table 37.2). Nowadays, tumor testing for MSI and immunohistochemistry for loss of MMR proteins can be used as an additional tool for identification of Lynch's syndrome. To optimize detection of Lynch's syndrome,

prediction models (e.g., PREMM) or systematic tumor testing for all newly diagnosed CRCs or all CRCs under age 70 are advocated.[6]

Screening, Surveillance, and Treatment

Individuals with Lynch's syndrome are advised to undergo CRC surveillance colonoscopies every 1 to 2 years beginning at age 20 to 25, or 5 years prior to the earliest age of CRC diagnosis in the family, whichever comes first. The main reason for frequent endoscopies is the accelerated adenoma–carcinoma pathway, and frequent colonoscopy screening, one or two yearly, was associated with a lower risk of CRC than colonoscopy screening every 2 to 3 years.[7] Quality of the colonoscopy is of utmost importance, ensuring optimal detection and complete resection of all precursor lesions. Upon detection of a CRC in a Lynch patient, a more radical surgical resection (e.g., subtotal colectomy in case of a right-sided carcinoma) should be discussed to prevent a metachronous CRC.

Women with Lynch's syndrome are also advised regular surveillance for endometrial and ovarian cancer by a gynecologist. Optimal surveillance strategies are debated and evidence is very limited, but generally include pelvic examinations, cancer antigen 125 (CA-125) testing, transvaginal ultrasound, and endometrial biopsy. The advised frequency is yearly, starting between the age of 25 and 40 years. As surveillance strategies for endometrial carcinoma are unreliable, prophylactic hysterectomy with or without ovariectomy should be discussed with female Lynch's patients after childbearing age.

Data on the effectiveness of surveillance programs for other Lynch-associated cancers are lacking. Surveillance schemes may include upper endoscopy and treatment of *Helicobacter pylori* infection when detected (once or regularly), urinalysis for tumor cells, and careful skin examination.

37.2.2 Familial CRC

Whereas one in four patients with CRC have a family history for this type of cancer, only approximately 4% are diagnosed with an inheritable cancer syndrome (▶ Fig. 37.2). Individuals from families not diagnosed with an inheritable syndrome are at increased risk of developing CRC, but not as high as with the inheritable syndromes. Having a single affected first-degree relative (i.e., parent, child, sibling) increases the risk of developing CRC approximately twofold over that of the general population.[8,9,10] The risk is further increased if two first-degree relatives have CRC or if the index case is diagnosed before the age of 50, and those families have a clinical diagnosis of "familial CRC."

Table 37.2 Amsterdam II and revised Bethesda criteria

Amsterdam II criteria (all criteria must be met)
- Three or more relatives with histologically verified colorectal cancer, one of whom is a first-degree relative of the other two; familial adenomatous polyposis should be excluded
- Colorectal cancer involving at least two successive generations
- One or more colorectal cancer cases diagnosed before the age of 50

Revised Bethesda criteria for microsatellite instability testing in colorectal tumors (one of the criteria must be met)
- Colorectal cancer diagnosed in a patient under 50 years of age
- Presence of synchronous or metachronous colorectal, or other Lynch's syndrome–related tumors, regardless of age
- Colorectal cancer diagnosed in one or more first-degree relatives with a Lynch syndrome–related tumor, with one of the cancer being diagnosed under the age of 50
- Colorectal cancer diagnosed in two or more first-degree or second-degree relatives with Lynch's syndrome–related tumors, regardless of age

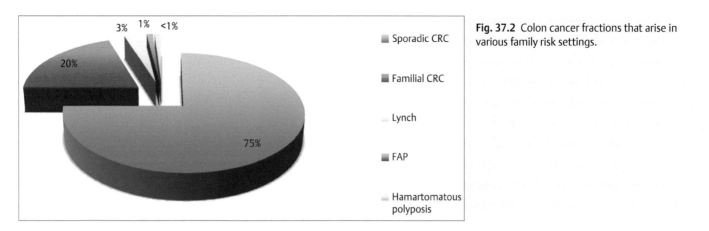

Fig. 37.2 Colon cancer fractions that arise in various family risk settings.

As the adenoma–carcinoma sequence is not accelerated in these patients, surveillance colonoscopies are advised with 5-yearly intervals. Starting age is debated in literature, but generally 45 years with 5-yearly intervals.

37.3 Polyposis Syndromes

37.3.1 Familial Adenomatous Polyposis

Genetics

Familial adenomatous polyposis (FAP) has an incidence of 1:6,850 to 1:23,700 live births.[11,12,13] It is an autosomal dominantly inherited disease, caused by a germline mutation in the *adenomatous polyposis coli* (*APC*) gene, located on chromosome 5q21–q22.[14] In most cases, FAP is inherited from one of both parents, but in 25% cases it is caused by a "de novo" mutation.[11] In 20% of these "de novo" patients the *APC* mutation is found in only a part of all body cells, which is called mosaicism.[15,16] Furthermore, in approximately 20% of patients with a clinical diagnosis of FAP, no APC mutation can be identified.[17,18]

Characteristics

FAP is characterized by the development of hundreds to thousands colorectal adenomas starting from puberty, which, without preventive measures, in nearly 100% will progress to CRC at the average age of 39 years (▶ Fig. 37.3a, b).[19] This high cancer risk is not caused by an accelerated adenoma–carcinoma sequence (such as in Lynch's syndrome), but is due to the high number of colorectal adenomas.

In many of these patients, extracolonic manifestations are also present. Of these, duodenal adenomas are most frequently encountered with a lifetime prevalence up to 90%.[20] These adenomas can be found throughout the duodenum and even in the proximal jejunum, but these usually appear at the ampulla of Vater or the periampullary region (▶ Fig. 37.3c).[21] Likewise, this results in an increased lifetime risk of both duodenal and ampullary cancer of 3 to 10% at an average age of 44 years.[22,23,24] Another frequent finding in the upper gastrointestinal (GI) tract is fundic gland polyps, located in the fundus or body of the stomach (▶ Fig. 37.3d).[25] These are small and sessile dilated glands, which rarely progress to cancer. Gastric adenomas are less common than fundic gland polyps, are typically located in the antrum, and have a low risk

of progression to cancer. The most severe extraintestinal manifestations are desmoid tumors, occurring in approximately 15% of patients with FAP. These lesions are found in the skin or abdomen, where they can obstruct or perforate organs. Today, this is the leading cause of death in FAP patients together with duodenal cancer.[26] Other, but less frequent, extracolonic manifestations associated with FAP are, among others, sebaceous or epidermoid cysts, lipomas, osteomas, fibromas, supernumerary teeth, juvenile nasopharyngeal angiofibromas, adrenal adenomas, and congenital hypertrophy of the retinal pigment epithelium.

Diagnosis

FAP should be suspected in patients with multiple colorectal adenomas or in first-degree relatives of patients diagnosed with FAP. For classical FAP, the number is usually more than 100. In these cases genetic testing needs to be performed. In case no germline *APC* mutation is identified, a search for less prevalent mutations causing polyposis (such as *POLE*, *POLD1*, *MUTYH*) can be performed, before the diagnosis of FAP is made on a clinical basis.[27,28,29,30] In case of extracolonic manifestations that raise the suspicion of FAP, a colonoscopy can be performed and if adenomas are identified, genetic testing should be done.

Screening, Surveillance, and Treatment

Patients with FAP should have annual sigmoidoscopies or colonoscopies from the age of 10 to 12 years, preferably performed in a specialized center. A preventive colectomy is performed when the number and size of adenomas impede proper and safe surveillance, which is usually by the age of 20 years. A subtotal colectomy with an ileorectal anastomosis or a proctocolectomy with an ileoanal pouch anastomosis are the preferred operations and the type of surgery depends on the age of the patient, the wish to have children, the severity of rectal polyposis, the presence or risk of developing desmoids, and the exact location of the mutation on the *APC* gene. After surgery, surveillance of the pouch or rectum remains necessary, as adenomas will reappear eventually (▶ Fig. 37.3e). Surveillance intervals of every 6 months to 1 year are advised. Polypectomies of large or suspicious polyps can be done at the discretion of the endoscopist.[27,28,29,30]

Duodenal surveillance should start at age of 25 to 30 years, and should be continued for life.[27,28,29,30] It is usually performed with a standard gastroscope combined with a side-viewing instrument to visualize the ampulla of Vater. The frequency of surveillance is

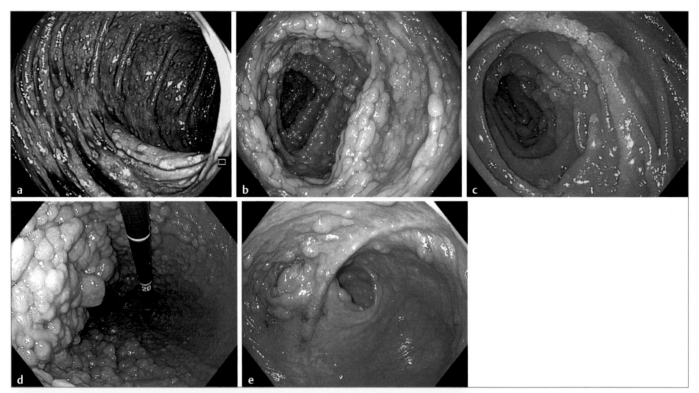

Fig. 37.3 Endoscopic images in patients with familial adenomatous polyposis. **(a)** Colonic adenomas, visualized using chromoendoscopy. **(b)** Colonic adenomas. **(c)** Duodenal adenomas. **(d)** Fundic gland polyps. (e) Adenomas in ileoanal pouch.

determined by the severity of the duodenal polyposis assessed by the Spigelman classification, based on size, number, histology, and degree of dysplasia of duodenal polyps (▶ Table 37.3).[21,31] The Spigelman stage indicates the risk of developing duodenal cancer within 10 years, ranging from 0% at stage 0 to 36% at stage IV. Therefore, the surveillance interval depends on the patient's Spigelman stage, ranging from 6 months to 5 years. Of note, the risk of developing stage IV duodenal disease is high; by the age of 60 years the risk is 43% and it increases to 50% by the age of 70 years.[31] To avoid the risk of malignant progression, endoscopic resection of large or high-grade dysplastic adenomas can be performed, which might also result in a lower Spigelman stage. In case of extensive and severe polyposis, endoscopic surveillance might no longer be reliable and duodenectomy should be considered. Several studies have evaluated effect of drugs (such as sulindac or celecoxib) on polyp burden, showing an effect on the prevention and regression of adenomas. However, the effect on cancer prevention remains unknown and, unfortunately,

celecoxib has a significant cardiovascular risk. Studies evaluating chemoprevention continue to hopefully delay surgery and prevent cancer.

No consensus exists for screening for extraintestinal manifestations, such as desmoid tumors and thyroidal disease, but screening can be considered.[27,28,29,30]

37.3.2 Attenuated Familial Adenomatous Polyposis

AFAP differs from FAP by having fewer colonic adenomas, a smaller risk of developing CRC and a later age of onset of colorectal adenomas (~ 44 years). If CRC occurs, it is usually diagnosed at the age of around 55 years. The cumulative risk of CRC at the age of 80 years is estimated at 70%.[32,33,34] Colonic adenomas are usually located in the right colon and the rectum is often relatively spared. In one-third of patients with clinical signs of AFAP, a mutation close to the proximal end of the *APC* gene can be identified, in one-third a *MUTYH* mutation is found and in the remaining patients no genetic cause can be identified.[35] Moreover, AFAP can occur in families where other family members have FAP. Duodenal adenomas and carcinomas and extraintestinal manifestations also occur, although less frequent and at a higher age compared to FAP.[33]

Screening, Surveillance, and Treatment

As the emergence of adenomas and cancer is delayed by 10 to 20 years compared with FAP, onset of colonoscopy screening can be delayed until the age of 18 years and should be performed annually or biannually. There is an indication for prophylactic surgery if the number and size of adenomas impair adequate surveillance. In contrast to colorectal adenomas and cancer, the expression of

Table 37.3 Modified Spigelman's score, classification, and advised surveillance intervals[11,21]

Factor	Score		
	1 Point	2 Points	3 Points
No. of polyps	1–4	5–20	> 20
Polyp size, mm	1–4	5–10	> 10
Histology	Tubular	Tubulovillous	Villous
Dysplasia	Low grade	-	High grade

Classification and Surveillance
- No polyps, stage 0: surveillance every 5 y
- 1–4 points, stage I: surveillance every 5 y
- 5–6 points, stage II: surveillance every 3 y
- 7–8 points, stage III: annual surveillance
- 9–12 points, stage IV: surveillance every 6–12 mo

duodenal polyposis does not appear to be attenuated in number, age at emerge or cancer risk in patients with AFAP compared with FAP. Therefore, upper gastrointestinal tract surveillance recommendations are the same as for patients with FAP. Screening for extraintestinal manifestations, such as desmoid tumors and thyroidal disease, can be considered.[27,28,29,30]

37.3.3 *MUTYH*-Associated polyposis

MAP is an autosomal recessive disorder, caused by biallelic mutations in the *MUTYH* gene.[36] As a result, this disorder is usually found in one generation among siblings. It causes fewer than 1% of all CRC cases and 5 to 10% of patients with up to 100 adenomas have a homozygote or compound heterozygote *MUTYH* mutation.[18,37] MAP is clinically comparable to AFAP, with patients usually having 10 to several hundreds of colonic adenomas by the fifth or sixth decade.[18,36] However, the clinical presentation can vary and those patients with biallelic *MUTYH* mutations can also have less than 10 or even no polyps, but still develop CRC.[38,39,40] Frequently these patients are also found to have multiple hyperplastic and/or sessile serrated polyps.[41] MAP is usually diagnosed around the age of 48 years and 60% of patients have a simultaneous CRC.[36,42,43] This could be explained by the lack of a suspicious family history in most cases resulting in a late onset of screening. In addition, the adenoma–carcinoma sequence could be increased, comparable to Lynch's syndrome.[44]

Extracolonic cancers occur, although in a smaller number, and at a higher age compared to FAP. The prevalence of duodenal adenomas is approximately 17% and the cumulative risk of duodenal carcinoma is 4%. These patients also seem to be at increased risk of cancers of the ovaries, bladder, and skin, among others.[45]

Screening, surveillance, and treatment recommendations for patients with MAP are identical to those for AFAP.[27,28,29,30,46]

37.3.4 Serrated Polyposis Syndrome

Diagnostic Approaches

SPS is a clinical diagnosis, as defined by the World Health Organization criteria (▶Table 37.4, ▶Fig. 37.4a, b).[47] Individuals with cumulatively at least five serrated polyps proximal to the sigmoid colon, of which two greater than or equal to10 mm in diameter (criterion 1), at least one serrated polyp proximal to the sigmoid, and a first-degree relative with SPS (criterion 2), and/or at least 20 serrated polyps, irrespective of size, but located throughout the colon (criterion 3) meet the criteria for SPS.[47] No germline mutations for SPS have been detected.[48] In a recent systematic review the prevalence of SPS was estimated below 0.09% in an average-risk screening population.[49] However, several studies showed that only a minority of patients with SPS are diagnosed at initial screening colonoscopy and true prevalence of disease might be higher.[50,51,52] Within the two largest cohorts described, mean age at diagnosis of SPS varied between 57 and 61 years and no gender preferences were found.[53,54] Patients with SPS have an increased risk of CRC, although the lifetime risk is largely unknown.[53,54] Approximately 15 to 30% of patients diagnosed with SPS are also diagnosed with CRC.[53,54] Patients with SPS do not seem to possess an increased extracolonic cancer risk.[55]

Up to date, no studies have showed an incremental value of advanced imaging techniques for the diagnosis of SPS. Narrow-band imaging did not show any effect on the detection rate of polyps in SPS patients.[56] Chromoendoscopy showed to increase the detection of serrated polyps in a general population and might help less experienced endoscopists to identify patients with SPS.[57] However, an increase in general awareness seems to be the most important factor to enhance SPS diagnosis.[51,52] Endoscopists should especially be keen on diagnosing SPS in case one large or several small serrated polyps are detected in the proximal colon.[52]

Therapeutic Approaches

Treatment of patients with SPS can be separated in an initial clearing phase and a surveillance phase.[58,59] During clearing all polyps greater than or equal to 5 mm, and all polyps less than 5 mm with the optical aspect of an adenoma or sessile serrated adenoma/polyp should be removed.[58,59] Among others, endoscopists might especially be keen on the real-time detection and complete resection of sessile serrated adenomas/polyps with dysplasia.[53,54] These high-risk lesions seem difficult to find due to their innocuous morphology and size and are suggested to be frequently incompletely resected.[60,61] This might be due to the fact that only the dysplastic component of the lesion was

Table 37.4 WHO criteria for the diagnosis of serrated polyposis syndrome

WHO 1	At least five serrated polyps proximal to rectosigmoid, of which at least two of which are ≥ 10 mm in size
WHO 2	Any serrated polyps proximal to rectosigmoid and a first-degree relative with serrated polyposis syndrome
WHO 3	At least 20 serrated polyps of any size distributed throughout the colon

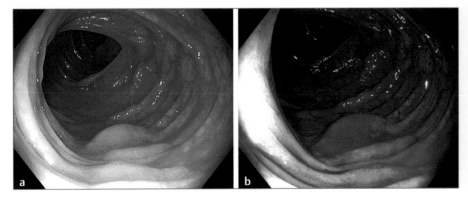

Fig. 37.4 Endoscopic images in patients with serrated polyposis syndrome. **(a)** High-resolution white-light image of a patient with serrated polyposis syndrome. **(b)** Narrow-band image of a patient with serrated polyposis syndrome.

recognized (mimicking adenomatous dysplasia) and delineated by the endoscopist, although evidence for this hypothesis is lacking.[60] A sufficient withdrawal time, proper bowel preparation, and complete colonoscopy are mandatory to detect all relevant lesions.[62,63,64] In case endoscopic clearing is not feasible and/or if CRC is diagnosed, subtotal colectomy with an ileosigmoidal or ileorectal anastomosis seems indicated.[58,59,62]

During surveillance, all polyps greater than or equal to 5 mm and all polyps less than 5 mm with the optical aspect of an adenoma or sessile serrated adenoma/polyp should be removed.[58,59] If this is not possible during one procedure, additional colonoscopies should be performed.[58,59] Again, a subtotal colectomy is indicated if endoscopic clearing is not feasible and/or if CRC is diagnosed.[58,59] Yearly surveillance, following above-mentioned approach showed to be safe and feasible in the only prospectively performed surveillance study up to date.[58,59]

37.3.5 Hamartomatous Polyposis Syndromes

Peutz–Jeghers Syndrome

PJS is a rare, autosomal dominantly inherited disorder, which is characterized by typical mucocutaneous pigmentations, childhood onset of multiple hamartomatous polyps in the GI tract (most commonly in the small bowel), and an increased risk of gastrointestinal and extraintestinal cancers (▶ Fig. 37.5a–c). The incidence of this condition is estimated to be between 1 in 50,000 and 1 in 200,000 live births.[65,66] It is caused by germline mutations in the serine threonine kinase 11 (STK11, also known as LKB1) tumor suppressor gene, which are found in 70% of PJS

patients.[66,67] The classical presentation in adolescence is with small bowel obstruction, intussusception, and GI bleeding leading to anemia. Later in life PJS patients have an increased risk of developing cancer (81–93% lifetime risk), including a 70% risk of GI cancer, a 50% risk of breast cancer, and a 11 to 36% risk of pancreatic cancer.[67,68]

Surveillance strategies usually recommend starting small bowel visualization (e.g., magnetic resonance/computed tomography [MR/CT] enterography or double-balloon enteroscopy) in order to remove larger small bowel polyps (> 1.5 cm) to prevent intestinal invagination. Upper and lower endoscopies with polypectomies are advised, but starting ages vary widely from 8 years to adulthood. Women are advised regular breast and gynecologic screening starting at age 25 years. The effectiveness of pancreas surveillance programs is not yet known.[67,68,69,70]

Juvenile Polyposis Syndrome

JPS is an autosomal dominant condition characterized by multiple juvenile polyps, most prominently in the colon, but also in the stomach, duodenum, and small bowel (▶ Fig. 37.6a, b). JPS is caused by mutations in the SMAD4 or BMPR1A gene, identified in approximately 50 to 60% of JPS patients. Approximately 25% of patients have de novo mutations. The incidence of JPS is between 1 in 100,000 and 1 in 160,000 individuals.[69,70,71,72,73,74] The generally accepted clinical criteria for JPS include (1) more than or equal to 5 juvenile polyps in the colorectum, (2) juvenile polyps in the entire GI tract, (3) or any number of polyps in a patient with a positive family history for polyposis syndrome are present.[29,71,72]

Polyps are mainly located in the colon and stomach and the syndrome is associated with an enhanced risk for GI malignancies

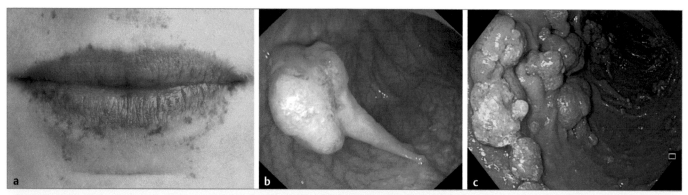

Fig. 37.5 Endoscopic images in patients with Peutz–Jeghers syndrome. (a) Mucocutaneous pigmentations. (b) Colonic hamartoma. (c) Gastric hamartomas.

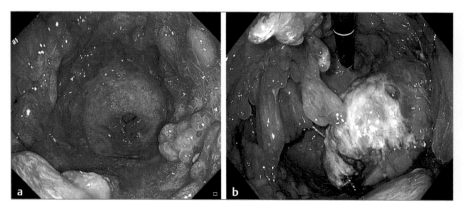

Fig. 37.6 Endoscopic images in a patient with juvenile polyposis syndrome. (a) Juvenile polyps in the stomach. (b) Juvenile polyps in the stomach, with a carcinoma in situ.

with a lifetime risk up to 68% for colorectal cancer and 21% for stomach cancer in case of severe polyposis.[71,72,73,74] Patients with *SMAD4* germline mutations may have massive polyposis limited to the stomach. Moreover, recent data demonstrated that almost all *SMAD4* germline mutation carriers fulfill the criteria for hereditary hemorrhagic telangiectasia (HHT), which is described as the JPS-HHT overlap syndrome. Such patients often have mucocutaneous telangiectasias leading to nose bleeds, as well as GI and pulmonary arteriovenous malformations.[75,76]

Endoscopic surveillance with polypectomy by gastroscopy and colonoscopy is generally recommended every 1 to 3 years (depending on the severity of polyposis) beginning at age 12 years, or earlier in case of symptoms. Small bowel investigations are not routinely recommended in JPS. Complete or partial colectomy/gastrectomy may be indicated in patients with massive polyposis that cannot effectively be controlled or surveilled endoscopically or in patients with advanced dysplasia. Finally, all *SMAD4* germline mutation carriers should be screened for HHT.[29,77]

Cowden's Syndrome

CS and its variants like Bannayan–Riley–Ruvalcaba syndrome and PTEN hamartoma tumor syndrome (PHTS) are rare highly genetically penetrant hamartomatous polyposis syndromes with a phenotypically heterogenous presentation. The estimated incidence is 1 in 200,000 live births.[78] The diagnosis of CS is made either genetically by testing germline mutations in the *PTEN* gene or clinically based on a set of clinical criteria like macrocephaly (75–97%), multiple colonic polyps including juvenile polyps and ganglioneuromas, dysplastic ganglyocytomas of the cerebellum, breast cancer (lifetime risk 85%), nonmedullary (follicular) thyroid carcinoma (lifetime risk 35%), endometrial cancer (lifetime risk 28%), macular pigmentation of the glans penis, and mental retardation (IQ ≤ 75).

Patients are at an increased risk of breast, endometrial, thyroid, kidney, and colorectal cancer. Intensive cancer surveillance programs are advised and generally coordinated by the medical oncologist. Gastrointestinal surveillance includes 5-yearly colonoscopy starting at age 40 years.[29,77,79]

References

[1] Wilschut JA, Steyerberg EW, van Leerdam ME, et al. How much colonoscopy screening should be recommended to individuals with various degrees of family history of colorectal cancer? Cancer. 2011; 117(18):4166–4174

[2] Quehenberger F, Vasen HF, van Houwelingen HC. Risk of colorectal and endometrial cancer for carriers of mutations of the hMLH1 and hMSH2 gene: correction for ascertainment. J Med Genet. 2005; 42(6):491–496

[3] Bonadona V, Bonaïti B, Olschwang S, et al; French Cancer Genetics Network. Cancer risks associated with germline mutations in MLH1, MSH2, and MSH6 genes in Lynch syndrome. JAMA. 2011; 305(22):2304–2310

[4] Hampel H, Stephens JA, Pukkala E, et al. Cancer risk in hereditary nonpolyposis colorectal cancer syndrome: later age of onset. Gastroenterology. 2005; 129(2):415–421

[5] Edelstein DL, Axilbund J, Baxter M, et al. Rapid development of colorectal neoplasia in patients with Lynch syndrome. Clin Gastroenterol Hepatol. 2011; 9(4):340–343

[6] Giardiello FM, Allen JI, Axilbund JE, et al; US Multi-Society Task Force on Colorectal Cancer. Guidelines on genetic evaluation and management of Lynch syndrome: a consensus statement by the US Multi-Society Task Force on colorectal cancer. Gastroenterology. 2014; 147(2):502–526

[7] Vasen HF, Abdirahman M, Brohet R, et al. One to 2-year surveillance intervals reduce risk of colorectal cancer in families with Lynch syndrome. Gastroenterology. 2010; 138(7):2300–2306

[8] Johns LE, Houlston RS. A systematic review and meta-analysis of familial colorectal cancer risk. Am J Gastroenterol. 2001; 96(10):2992–3003

[9] Baglietto L, Jenkins MA, Severi G, et al. Measures of familial aggregation depend on definition of family history: meta-analysis for colorectal cancer. J Clin Epidemiol. 2006; 59(2):114–124

[10] Butterworth AS, Higgins JP, Pharoah P. Relative and absolute risk of colorectal cancer for individuals with a family history: a meta-analysis. Eur J Cancer. 2006; 42(2):216–227

[11] Bisgaard ML, Fenger K, Bülow S, et al. Familial adenomatous polyposis (FAP): frequency, penetrance, and mutation rate. Hum Mutat. 1994; 3(2):121–125

[12] Björk J, Akerbrant H, Iselius L, et al. Epidemiology of familial adenomatous polyposis in Sweden: changes over time and differences in phenotype between males and females. Scand J Gastroenterol. 1999; 34(12):1230–1235

[13] Bülow S, Faurschou Nielsen T, Bülow C, et al. The incidence rate of familial adenomatous polyposis. Results from the Danish Polyposis Register. Int J Colorectal Dis. 1996; 11(2):88–91

[14] Burt RW, DiSario JA, Cannon-Albright L. Genetics of colon cancer: impact of inheritance on colon cancer risk. Annu Rev Med. 1995; 46:371–379

[15] Hes FJ, Nielsen M, Bik EC, et al. Somatic APC mosaicism: an underestimated cause of polyposis coli. Gut. 2008; 57(1):71–76

[16] Aretz S, Stienen D, Friedrichs N, et al. Somatic APC mosaicism: a frequent cause of familial adenomatous polyposis (FAP). Hum Mutat. 2007; 28(10):985–992

[17] Galiatsatos P, Foulkes WD. Familial adenomatous polyposis. Am J Gastroenterol. 2006; 101(2):385–398

[18] Grover S, Kastrinos F, Steyerberg EW, et al. Prevalence and phenotypes of APC and MUTYH mutations in patients with multiple colorectal adenomas. JAMA. 2012; 308(5):485–492

[19] Jang YS, Steinhagen RM, Heimann TM. Colorectal cancer in familial adenomatous polyposis. Dis Colon Rectum. 1997; 40(3):312–316

[20] Bülow S, Björk J, Christensen IJ, et al; DAF Study Group. Duodenal adenomatosis in familial adenomatous polyposis. Gut. 2004; 53(3):381–386

[21] Spigelman AD, Williams CB, Talbot IC, et al. Upper gastrointestinal cancer in patients with familial adenomatous polyposis. Lancet. 1989; 2(8666):783–785

[22] Brosens LA, Keller JJ, Offerhaus GJ, et al. Prevention and management of duodenal polyps in familial adenomatous polyposis. Gut. 2005; 54(7):1034–1043

[23] Bülow S, Christensen IJ, Højen H, et al. Duodenal surveillance improves the prognosis after duodenal cancer in familial adenomatous polyposis. Colorectal Dis. 2012; 14(8):947–952

[24] Groves CJ, Saunders BP, Spigelman AD, Phillips RK. Duodenal cancer in patients with familial adenomatous polyposis (FAP): results of a 10 year prospective study. Gut. 2002; 50(5):636–641

[25] Cruz-Correa M, Giardiello FM. Familial adenomatous polyposis. Gastrointest Endosc. 2003; 58(6):885–894

[26] Arvanitis ML, Jagelman DG, Fazio VW, et al. Mortality in patients with familial adenomatous polyposis. Dis Colon Rectum. 1990; 33(8):639–642

[27] Balmaña J, Balaguer F, Cervantes A, Arnold D; ESMO Guidelines Working Group. Familial risk-colorectal cancer: ESMO Clinical Practice Guidelines. Ann Oncol. 2013; 24(suppl 6):vi73–vi80

[28] Stoffel EM, Mangu PB, Gruber SB, et al; American Society of Clinical Oncology. European . Society of Clinical Oncology. Hereditary colorectal cancer syndromes: American Society of Clinical Oncology Clinical Practice Guideline endorsement of the familial risk-colorectal cancer: European Society for Medical Oncology Clinical Practice Guidelines. J Clin Oncol. 2015; 33(2):209–217

[29] Syngal S, Brand RE, Church JM, et al; American College of Gastroenterology. ACG clinical guideline: genetic testing and management of hereditary gastrointestinal cancer syndromes. Am J Gastroenterol. 2015; 110(2):223–262, quiz 263

[30] Dutch Society For Clinical Genetics. CBO Guideline Hereditary Colorectal Cancer. 2015. http://oncoline.nl/erfelijke-darmkanker. Accessed August 23, 2017

[31] Saurin JC, Gutknecht C, Napoleon B, et al. Surveillance of duodenal adenomas in familial adenomatous polyposis reveals high cumulative risk of advanced disease. J Clin Oncol. 2004; 22(3):493–498

[32] Sieber OM, Segditsas S, Knudsen AL, et al. Disease severity and genetic pathways in attenuated familial adenomatous polyposis vary greatly but depend on the site of the germline mutation. Gut. 2006; 55(10):1440–1448

[33] Burt RW, Leppert MF, Slattery ML, et al. Genetic testing and phenotype in a large kindred with attenuated familial adenomatous polyposis. Gastroenterology. 2004; 127(2):444–451

[34] Hernegger GS, Moore HG, Guillem JG. Attenuated familial adenomatous polyposis: an evolving and poorly understood entity. Dis Colon Rectum. 2002; 45(1):127–134, discussion 134–136

[35] Nielsen M, Hes FJ, Nagengast FM, et al. Germline mutations in APC and MUTYH are responsible for the majority of families with attenuated familial adenomatous polyposis. Clin Genet. 2007; 71(5):427–433

[36] Sieber OM, Lipton L, Crabtree M, et al. Multiple colorectal adenomas, classic adenomatous polyposis, and germ-line mutations in MYH. N Engl J Med. 2003; 348(9):791–799

[37] Cleary SP, Cotterchio M, Jenkins MA, et al. Germline MutY human homologue mutations and colorectal cancer: a multisite case-control study. Gastroenterology. 2009; 136(4):1251–1260

[38] Wang L, Baudhuin LM, Boardman LA, et al. MYH mutations in patients with attenuated and classic polyposis and with young-onset colorectal cancer without polyps. Gastroenterology. 2004; 127(1):9–16

[39] Balaguer F, Castellví-Bel S, Castells A, et al; Gastrointestinal Oncology Group of the Spanish Gastroenterological Association. Identification of MYH mutation carriers in colorectal cancer: a multicenter, case-control, population-based study. Clin Gastroenterol Hepatol. 2007; 5(3):379–387

[40] Terdiman JP. MYH-associated disease: attenuated adenomatous polyposis of the colon is only part of the story. Gastroenterology. 2009; 137(6):1883–1886

[41] Boparai KS, Dekker E, Van Eeden S, et al. Hyperplastic polyps and sessile serrated adenomas as a phenotypic expression of MYH-associated polyposis. Gastroenterology. 2008; 135(6):2014–2018

[42] Nielsen M, Weiss MM, Vasen HF, Hes FJ. [From gene to disease; MutYH-associated polyposis coli (MAP)] Ned Tijdschr Geneeskd. 2005; 149(53):2970–2972

[43] Sampson JR, Dolwani S, Jones S, et al. Autosomal recessive colorectal adenomatous polyposis due to inherited mutations of MYH. Lancet. 2003; 362(9377):39–41

[44] Nieuwenhuis MH, Vogt S, Jones N, et al. Evidence for accelerated colorectal adenoma–carcinoma progression in MUTYH-associated polyposis? Gut. 2012; 61(5):734–738

[45] Vogt S, Jones N, Christian D, et al. Expanded extracolonic tumor spectrum in MUT-YH-associated polyposis. Gastroenterology. 2009; 137(6):1976:1985–.e1–e10

[46] Vasen HF, Möslein G, Alonso A, et al. Guidelines for the clinical management of familial adenomatous polyposis (FAP). Gut. 2008; 57(5):704–713

[47] Snover DC, Ahnen DJ, Burt RW, Odze RD; Serrated polyps of the colon and rectum and serrated polyposis. In: Bosman T, Carneiro F, Hruban R, et al. WHO Classification of Tumours of the Digestive System 2010. World Health Organization, Lyon, 2010; 160 -5.

[48] Clendenning M, Young JP, Walsh MD, et al. Germline mutations in the polyposis-associated genes, and are not common in individuals with serrated polyposis syndrome. PLoS One. 2013; 8(6):e66705

[49] van Herwaarden YJ, Verstegen MH, Dura P, et al. Low prevalence of serrated polyposis syndrome in screening populations: a systematic review. Endoscopy. 2015; 47(11):1043–1049

[50] IJspeert JE, Bevan R, Senore C, et al. Detection rate of serrated polyps and serrated polyposis syndrome in colorectal cancer screening cohorts: a European overview. Gut. 2017; 66(7):1225 – 1232

[51] Edelstein DL, Axilbund JE, Hylind LM, et al. Serrated polyposis: rapid and relentless development of colorectal neoplasia. Gut. 2013; 62(3):404–408

[52] Vemulapalli KC, Rex DK. Failure to recognize serrated polyposis syndrome in a cohort with large sessile colorectal polyps. Gastrointest Endosc. 2012; 75(6):1206–1210

[53] IJspeert JE, Rana SA, Atkinson NS, et al. Clinical risk factors of colorectal cancer in patients with serrated polyposis syndrome: a multicentre cohort analysis. Gut. 2017; 66(2):278–284

[54] Carballal S, Rodriguez-Alcalde D, Moreira L, et al. Colorectal cancer risk factors in patients with serrated polyposis syndrome: a large multicentre study. Gut. 2016; 65(11):1829–1837

[55] Hazewinkel Y, Reitsma JB, Nagengast FM, et al. Extracolonic cancer risk in patients with serrated polyposis syndrome and their first-degree relatives. Fam Cancer. 2013; 12(4):669–673

[56] Hazewinkel Y, Tytgat KM, van Leerdam ME, et al. Narrow-band imaging for the detection of polyps in patients with serrated polyposis syndrome: a multicenter, randomized, back-to-back trial. Gastrointest Endosc. 2015; 81(3):531–538

[57] East JE, Saunders BP, Jass JR. Sporadic and syndromic hyperplastic polyps and serrated adenomas of the colon: classification, molecular genetics, natural history, and clinical management. Gastroenterol Clin North Am. 2008; 37(1):25–46, v

[58] La Nauze R, Suzuki N, Saunders B, et al. The endoscopist's guide to serrated polyposis. Colorectal Dis. 2014; 16(6):417–425

[59] Hazewinkel Y, Tytgat KM, van Eeden S, et al. Incidence of colonic neoplasia in patients with serrated polyposis syndrome who undergo annual endoscopic surveillance. Gastroenterology. 2014; 147(1):88–95

[60] Burgess NG, Tutticci NJ, Pellise M, Bourke MJ. Sessile serrated adenomas/polyps with cytologic dysplasia: a triple threat for interval cancer. Gastrointest Endosc. 2014; 80(2):307–310

[61] Bouwens MW, van Herwaarden YJ, Winkens B, et al. Endoscopic characterization of sessile serrated adenomas/polyps with and without dysplasia. Endoscopy. 2014; 46(3):225–235

[62] East JE, Vieth M, Rex DK. Serrated lesions in colorectal cancer screening: detection, resection, pathology and surveillance. Gut. 2015; 64(6):991–1000

[63] Butterly L, Robinson CM, Anderson JC, et al. Serrated and adenomatous polyp detection increases with longer withdrawal time: results from the New Hampshire Colonoscopy Registry. Am J Gastroenterol. 2014; 109(3):417–426

[64] de Wijkerslooth TR, Stoop EM, Bossuyt PM, et al. Differences in proximal serrated polyp detection among endoscopists are associated with variability in withdrawal time. Gastrointest Endosc. 2013; 77(4):617–623

[65] Utsunomiya J, Gocho H, Miyanaga T, et al. Peutz-Jeghers syndrome: its natural course and management. Johns Hopkins Med J. 1975; 136(2):71–82

[66] Giardiello FM, Trimbath JD. Peutz-Jeghers syndrome and management recommendations. Clin Gastroenterol Hepatol. 2006; 4(4):408–415

[67] Latchford AR, Phillips RKS. Gastrointestinal polyps and cancer in Peutz-Jeghers syndrome: clinical aspects. Fam Cancer. 2011; 10(3):455–461

[68] Jasperson KW, Tuohy TM, Neklason DW, Burt RW. Hereditary and familial colon cancer. Gastroenterology. 2010; 138(6):2044–2058

[69] Beggs AD, Latchford AR, Vasen HFA, et al. Peutz-Jeghers syndrome: a systematic review and recommendations for management. Gut. 2010; 59(7):975–986

[70] van Lier MG, Wagner A, Mathus-Vliegen EM, et al. High cancer risk in Peutz-Jeghers syndrome: a systematic review and surveillance recommendations. Am J Gastroenterol. 2010; 105(6):1258–1264, author reply 1265

[71] Brosens LA, Langeveld D, van Hattem WA, et al. Juvenile polyposis syndrome. World J Gastroenterol. 2011; 17(44):4839–4844

[72] Dahdaleh FS, Carr JC, Calva D, Howe JR. Juvenile polyposis and other intestinal polyposis syndromes with microdeletions of chromosome 10q22–23. Clin Genet. 2012; 81(2):110–116

[73] Samadder NJ, Jasperson K, Burt RW. Hereditary and common familial colorectal cancer: evidence for colorectal screening. Dig Dis Sci. 2015; 60(3):734–747

[74] Latchford AR, Neale K, Phillips RK, Clark SK. Juvenile polyposis syndrome: a study of genotype, phenotype, and long-term outcome. Dis Colon Rectum. 2012; 55(10):1038–1043

[75] Gallione CJ, Repetto GM, Legius E, et al. A combined syndrome of juvenile polyposis and hereditary haemorrhagic telangiectasia associated with mutations in MADH4 (SMAD4). Lancet. 2004; 363(9412):852–859

[76] O'Malley M, LaGuardia L, Kalady MF, et al. The prevalence of hereditary hemorrhagic telangiectasia in juvenile polyposis syndrome. Dis Colon Rectum. 2012; 55(8):886–892

[77] National Comprehensive Cancer Network (NCCN). Clinical practice guidelines in oncology: colorectal cancer screening. http://www.nccn.org. Accessed March 23, 2016

[78] Ngeow J, Eng C. PTEN hamartoma tumor syndrome: clinical risk assessment and management protocol. Methods. 2015; 77–78:11–19

[79] Eng C. Will the real Cowden syndrome please stand up: revised diagnostic criteria. J Med Genet. 2000; 37(11):828–830

38 Inflammatory Bowel Disease and Microscopic Colitis

Marjolijn Duijvestein and Geert R. D'Haens

38.1 Introduction

Inflammatory bowel diseases (IBDs) are chronic inflammatory disorders of the gastrointestinal (GI) tract that comprise Crohn's disease (CD) and ulcerative colitis (UC). Endoscopy not only plays an essential role in the diagnosis and characterization, enabling biopsy sampling of the affected digestive tract, but also contributes to the evaluation, monitoring, and management of the disease. Furthermore, endoscopy is used to detect dysplasia contributing to the surveillance of long-standig disease.

The direct visual appreciation of lesions, so much more accurate than radiologic studies, and the ability to collect biopsy samples have made endoscopic examinations the first-line procedures in the initial evaluation of patients with unexplained chronic diarrhea and suspected IBD. The need for an unpleasant bowel preparation, the high cost, and the discomfort sometimes caused by endoscopic procedures should nevertheless force the clinician to limit the indications as strictly and correctly as possible.

This chapter describes the endoscopic characteristics of CD and UC lesions, the role for endoscopy in the evaluation of disease severity using endoscopic indices, the use of endoscopic surveillance, indications for pre- and postoperative endoscopy in IBD, endoscopy in ileoanal pouches and pouchitis, and therapeutic endoscopic interventions. Furthermore, the clinical features and role of endoscopy in the diagnosis of microscopic colitis will be reviewed.

38.2 Endoscopic Characteristics of IBD

38.2.1 Lower Endoscopy

Crohn's Disease

Endoscopically, CD is often characterized by areas of inflammation separated by normal-appearing mucosa, which are called skip lesions. Any part of the GI tract from mouth to anus can be affected, although most commonly the ileum is involved (▶ Fig. 38.1). Early mild lesions include small (< 5 mm) aphthous ulcers (▶ Fig. 38.2). In more severe disease deep irregular and longitudinal ulcerations (▶ Fig. 38.3, ▶ Fig. 38.4) can be seen as well as a cobblestone appearance of the mucosa (▶ Fig. 38.5). As the inflammation is transmural, it can result in strictures and fistulae. Often rectal sparing is seen. Biopsy specimens to confirm the diagnosis should be taken from the edges of ulcers and aphthous erosions (▶ Table 38.1). Specific guidelines on how many biopsies should ideally be taken are lacking.

Ulcerative Colitis

Inflammation in UC tends to be continuous, confluent, and concentric. Characteristically, inflammation commences proximal to the anus. The demarcation between inflamed and normal

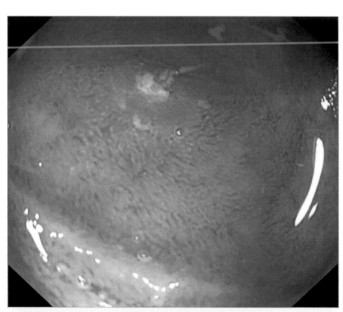

Fig. 38.1 Crohn's aphthous ulcers in the terminal ileum.

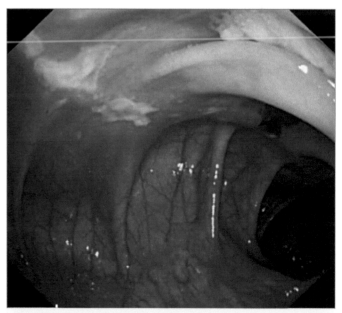

Fig. 38.2 Crohn's ulcers with normal surrounding mucosa in the colon.

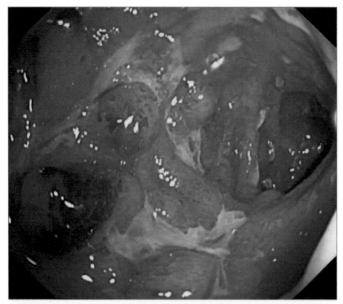

Fig. 38.3 Deep ulcerations and spontaneous hemorrhage in a patient with severe Crohn's disease (CD).

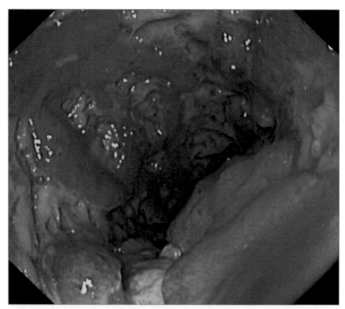

Fig. 38.4 Deep ulcerations with granular friable mucosa in a patient with severe Crohn's disease (CD).

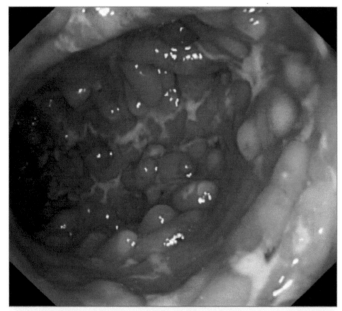

Fig. 38.5 Mucosal pattern with nodular appearance referred to as a "cobblestone-like" mucosa in a patient with severe Crohn's disease (CD).

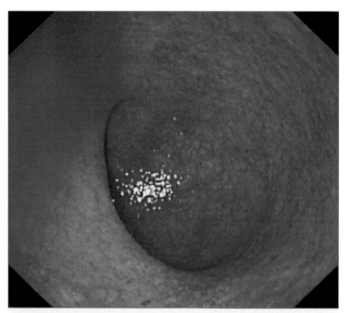

Fig. 38.6 Granular colonic mucosa in a patient with ulcerative colitis (UC), with a faded vascular pattern, mild friability, and erythema (Mayo 1).

areas is usually clear and in general there are no skip lesions. Initial lesions include loss of vasculature and hyperemia of the colonic mucosa (▶Fig. 38.6, ▶Fig. 38.7). In moderate disease, discrete ulcers surrounded by inflamed mucosa develop progressing to large, continuous ulcers with increasing severity of the disease (▶Fig. 38.8). "Backwash ileitis," extension of macroscopic or histologic inflammation from the cecum into the most distal ileum, has been reported in up to 20% of patients with pancolitis[2,3] and is associated with a more refractory course of disease.[4]

38.2.2 Upper Endoscopy

Crohn's Disease

At least half of pediatric-onset CD patients have an upper GI localization, which is associated with a more severe disease course, therefore requiring more aggressive therapy.[5] In the pediatric and adolescent population, upper GI endoscopy is therefore routinely performed in the assessment of IBD.[6] In the adult population, the prevalence of upper GI involvement is suggested to be around

Table 38.1 Terminology of endoscopic lesions in Inflammatory Bowel Disease, from the ECCO guideline.[1]

Mucosal damage	Description	Grading
Loss of vascular pattern	Loss of normal mucosal appearance without well-demacated, arborizing capillaries	From patchy or blurred to complete loss
Erythema	Unnaturally reddened mucosa	From discrete or punctiform to diffuse erythema
Granularity	Mucosal pattern produced by a reticular network of radiolucent foci of 0.5–1 mm of diameter with a sharp light reflex	From fine to coarse or nodular, due to abnormal light reflection
Friability/bleeding	Bleeding or intramucosal hemorrhage before or after the passage of the endoscope	From contact bleeding (bleeding with light touch) to spontaneous bleeding
Erosion	A definite discontinuation of mucosa < 3 mm in size. Also described as pinpoint ulceration	Isolated, diffuse
Aphthous ulcer	White depressed center surrounded by a halo of erythema; (some consider this synonymous with "erosion")	Isolated, multiple
Ulcer	Any lesion of the mucosa of unequivocal depth, with or without reddish halo	Isolated or multiple based on morphology: circular, linear, stellar, serpiginous, irregular shape. Superficial or deep
Ulcer size (no underscore)	Defined in millimeter or classified as ≤ 5 mm; 5–20 mm; > 20 mm	Diffuse, mucosal abrasion with residual mucosa producing a polypoid appearance
Ulcer depth (no underscore)	Shallow (localized to submucosa)—no border. Deep (beyond muscularis propria)—e.g., edges elevated > 1 mm	
Stenosis	Narrowing of the lumen	Single, multiple, passable (by standard adult endoscope), unpassable, passable after dilation. Ulcerated, nonulcerated
Postinflammatory polyps (previously "pseudopolyp")	Polypoid lesion, usually small, glistering, isolated or multiple, scattered throughout the colon. Sometimes cylindrical or giant (> 2 cm) in size	Isolated, diffuse, occluding ("giant")
Cobblestone	Mucosal pattern with raised nodules, resembling the paving of a "Roman" road	With or without ulceration

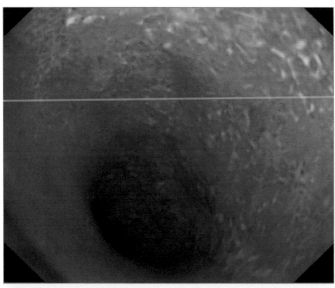

Fig. 38.7 Moderate inflammation with an absence of vascular pattern, marked friability, and erosions seen in an ulcerative colitis (UC) patient (Mayo 2).

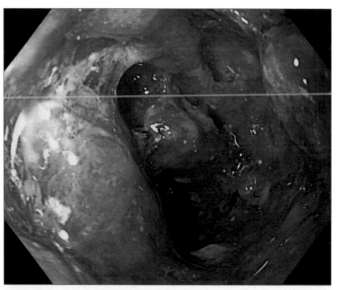

Fig. 38.8 Severe inflammation with large ulcerations and spontaneous bleeding in a patient with ulcerative colitis (UC) (Mayo 3).

16%, of which only one-third of the patients are symptomatic.[7] It is to be debated if upper endoscopy should be in the diagnostic work-up of CD patients, but it should at least be performed in CD patients with dyspepsia, abdominal pain, and vomiting in order to rule out other causes for the symptoms and to correctly classify the distribution and extent of the disease.

In the esophagus, Crohn's lesions can present as aphthous ulcerations, "punched-out" ulcers or larger perforating lesions. In the stomach inflammation is present as focal erythema with or without ulcerations and in the duodenum frank ulcerations are often seen, quite commonly complicated by stenosis at the level of the gastric outlet or in the midduodenum.

Ulcerative Colitis

Upper endoscopy is not routinely performed in patients with UC. Occasionally, diffuse duodenitis can develop in patients with severe UC, even after proctocolectomy.

38.2.3 Small Bowel Imaging

CD can affect segments of the small bowel out of reach of the colonoscope. Small bowel video capsule endoscopy should be considered in patients with suspected CD and negative ileocolonoscopy.[8] The Lewis score (LS)[9] has been developed to assess mucosal inflammatory disease in the small bowel. This scoring index is based on three capsule endoscopic variables: villous appearance, ulceration, and stenosis. In addition, each variable is assessed by other parameters including size and extent of the change. Using these parameters, a score range of 8 to 4,800 points was established: LS less than 135 reflects normal mucosal appearances, LS 135 to 790 mild mucosal inflammatory change, and an LS value greater than or equal to 790 moderate-to-severe mucosal inflammatory changes.

In patients with obstructive features or known stenosis, a cross-sectional imaging modality such as magnetic resonance enterography (MRE) or computed tomography enterography (CTE) should be the method of choice.[10] Furthermore, MRE can objectify the transmural nature of the disease, its anatomical distribution as well as the presence of extraluminal disease.

38.2.4 Endoscopic Ultrasonography

The cumulative incidence of perianal fistulas in CD range from 23 to 38%.[4,11] Perianal fistula are often diagnosed and classified by using a combination of both clinical and imaging findings. Endoscopic ultrasound (EUS), magnetic resonance imaging (MRI), and examination under anesthesia (EUA) are accurate tests for determining fistula anatomy in patients with perianal CD.[12] Combining two of the three modalities gives an accuracy of 100%. Examination under anesthesia in the hands of an experienced surgeon has been considered the gold standard in the assessment of perianal CD, with the advantage that surgical drainage of any abscesses and placement of noncutting setons can be performed as required.[13] Currently, it is advised to first perform a noninvasive procedure such as MRI to visualize perianal fistula unless there is a need for immediate drainage of sepsis.[14] For endoscopic ultrasonography endoanal probes are used transrectally. Fistulas are visible as hyperechoic tracks or beads within a larger hypoechoic tract consistent with surrounding inflammation.[15] Data from three small clinical trials suggest that fistula imaging by EUS can guide in medical decision making with better clinical outcomes.[16,17,18]

38.2.5 Endoscopic Retrograde Cholangiopancreatography

Primary sclerosing cholangitis (PSC) is a chronic, cholestatic liver disease characterized by chronic inflammation and fibrosis of the biliary tract affecting both intrahepatic and extrahepatic bile ducts leading to the formation of bile duct strictures. The vast majority of patients with PSC have accompanying IBD. The presence of PSC increases the risk of colorectal cancer (CRC) development almost by a 10-fold,[19] furthermore PSC patients are at increased risk of developing cholangiocarcinoma with a 20% lifetime risk.[20] Endoscopic retrograde cholangiopancreatography (ERCP) is the gold standard for diagnosing PSC. ERCP is used for diagnostic (brush cytology) and therapeutic purposes, that is, balloon dilation or stent placement.

38.3 Endoscopy in Established IBD

38.3.1 Acute Colitis

In patients with chronic bloody diarrhea, endoscopy with mucosal biopsies is an important tool to evaluate the severity of disease[21] and to exclude other (infectious) causes of acute colitis,[22] such as cytomegalovirus (CMV) colitis, rectal mucosal prolapse, malignancy, and hemorrhoidal bleeding.[23] In most cases unprepped sigmoidoscopy with minimal inflation is sufficient. Biopsies are particularly useful to exclude CMV colitis in patients with prolonged exposure to steroids and/or azathioprine.[24] Furthermore, the endoscopic appearance predicts the course of the disease and may guide treatment intensification. For example, in UC it is known that the presence of extensive and deep ulcerations at endoscopy is associated with an increased risk of colectomy.[25,26]

38.3.2 Routine Endoscopy

Routine endoscopy in IBD patients in clinical remission, besides surveillance for dysplasia and after surgery, has been considered to be unnecessary. In these cases, noninvasive tests and surrogate markers of disease activity,[27] such as fecal levels of calprotectin[28] or lactoferrin,[29,30] can be used to assess disease activity. Whether treatment intensification to attain "mucosal healing" despite the absence of symptoms is to be recommended remains to be studied. In the cases of a suspected relapse, refractory disease, new/unexplained symptoms, change of medical therapy, or when surgery is considered, endoscopy should be seriously performed.

38.4 Endoscopic Evaluation of IBD Disease Activity

Mucosal healing is generally defined as the absence of all ulcerative lesions and is an important indicator of efficacy of treatment. Achieving mucosal healing is becoming an important objective in the management of inflammatory bowel diseases as it is associated with improved disease outcome.[31]

Endoscopic activity may be reliably scored using endoscopic scoring indexes. In CD, the CD endoscopic index of severity (CDEIS)[32] or simple endoscopic score for CD (SES-CD)[33] are often used. Both tools have been prospectively validated and shown to be reproducible and have good interobserver agreement.[1,33,34] After ileocecal resection, the Rutgeerts' score[35] is used to determine postsurgical recurrence severity of disease.

Endoscopic activity in UC is commonly scored using the Mayo endoscopic subscore,[36] endoscopic healing is generally accepted as Mayo grade 0 or 1 (although any friability should be considered as nonhealed mucosa).[37] Recently, the new UCEIS has been validated as an alternative instrument to measure UC disease severity.[38,39]

38.4.1 Crohn's Disease

For luminal CD, two endoscopic activity scores (CDEIS[32] and SES-CD)[33] have been developed. These scores have been prospectively validated, have shown to be reproducible and have good interobserver agreement.[1,33,34] Both scores divides the colon in five segments: rectum, sigmoid and left colon, transverse colon, right colon, and ileum. The CDEIS requires scoring of the following endoscopic parameters per segment: (1) presence or absence of ulcers, distinguished as superficial or deep, (2) percentage of surface ulcerated and/or affected, and (3) presence of stenosis, classified as ulcerated or nonulcerated stenosis. All of these scores together provide the CDEIS score, with a range between 0 and 44. The other endoscopic score, known as the SES-CD scores on a scale from 0 to 3 selected endoscopic parameters (ulcer size, ulcerated and affected surfaces, strictures) in each of the five bowel segments to give a total score of 0 to 60. Nevertheless, both scores are somewhat complicated, and therefore their use has been restricted to clinical trials at most sites. In routine clinical care reporting of endoscopic activity should include accurate descriptions of any abnormalities in each segment.

38.4.2 Ulcerative Colitis

Several endoscopic indices have been developed to assess disease activity in UC. In 1955, Truelove and Witts[40] were the first to measure UC endoscopic activity in a clinical trial. The Baron index,[41] introduced in 1964, evaluates the mucosa of the rectosigmoid area using a 4-point scale (▶Table 38.2). The UC endoscopic index of severity (UCEIS)[39] and UC colonoscopic index of severity (UCCIS)[42] underwent formal (preliminary) validation. Several other endoscopic scoring systems for disease severity are available,[43] but lack formal validation. The Mayo endoscopic subscore[36] has been extensively used in clinical trials to evaluate treatment efficacy in terms of endoscopic remission. Higher scores indicate more severe disease, with a maximum total score of 3 (▶Fig. 38.8). Although not formally validated, endoscopic remission has been defined as a Mayo subscore less than or equal to 1, however, complete endoscopic remission should be restricted only to score 0.

38.5 Endoscopy after Surgery
38.5.1 Lower Endoscopy
Postoperative Crohn's Disease

In CD patients, ileocolonoscopy is the gold standard to diagnose postoperative recurrence after ileocecal resection. Routine ileocolonoscopy should be performed 6 to 12 months after surgery.[1] It has been shown that selective immune suppression started after early endoscopic assessment of recurrence, leads to better disease control.[44]

Postsurgical measurement of disease activity at the ileocolonic anastomosis can be recorded using the Rutgeerts score for postsurgical recurrence.[45] The score was developed and validated in order to predict the postoperative disease course.[35] Patients with recurrence graded i2 or more were shown to present with a more severe course of disease in terms of clinical and surgical recurrence, while patients with no (i0) or minimal (i1, e.g., < 5 aphthoid ulcers with normal mucosa) endoscopic activity are at minimal risk of recurrence (▶Table 38.3).

Table 38.2 Endoscopic scoring systems commonly used in current clinical trials of Ulcerative Colitis

Score [ref.]	Description
Mayo endoscopic subscore[36] Range: 0–3	0. Normal: normal or healed mucosa 1. Mild: erythema, decreased vascular pattern 2. Moderate: marked erythema, absent vascular pattern, friability, erosions 3. Severe: spontaneous bleeding, large ulcers
Modified Baron Score[41] Range: 0–4	0. Normal mucosa 1. Granular mucosa with an abnormal vascular pattern 2. Friable mucosa 3. Microulceration of the mucosa with spontaneous bleeding 4. Denuded mucosa (gross ulceration)
Ulcerative colitis endoscopic index of severity (UCEIS)[39] Range: 0–8	Vascular pattern 0. Normal: clear vascular pattern 1. Patchy obliteration: partially visible vascular pattern 2. Obliterated: complete loss of vascular pattern Bleeding 0. None: no visible blood 1. Mucosal: some spots or streaks of coagulated blood on the surface of the mucosa ahead of the scope, which can be washed away 2. Luminal mild: some free liquid blood in the lumen 3. Luminal moderate or severe: frank blood in the lumen ahead of endoscope or visible oozing from mucosa after washing intraluminal blood, or visible oozing from a hemorrhagic mucosa Erosions and Ulcers 0. Normal mucosa: no visible erosions or ulcers 1. Erosions: tiny (< 5 mm) defects in the mucosa, of a white or yellow color with a flat edge 2. Superficial ulcer: larger (> 5 mm) defects in the mucosa, which are discrete fibrin-covered ulcers when compared to erosions, but remain superficial 3. Deep ulcer: deeper excavated defects in the mucosa, with a slightly raised edge

Postoperative Ulcerative Colitis

In the case of UC, surgical treatment is considered curative when the entire colon and rectum are removed. For this, conservative proctocolectomy with ileal pouch–anal anastomosis (IPAA) is the method of choice leaving no stoma and a preserved anal route of defecation. Although IPAA preserves quality of life,[46] pouch failure is seen in up to 8.5% of the cases.[47] Endoscopy plays a role in diagnosing underlying pathology in these patients. Furthermore, endoscopy can play a role in surveillance of dysplasia.

Pouchitis

The term pouchitis refers to nonspecific inflammation of the pouch (▶ Fig. 38.9) and is a common complication in patients with IPAA. In patients with UC without associated PSC, the cumulative prevalence of pouchitis at 1, 5, and 10 years has been reported to be 15.5, 36, and 45.5%, respectively.[48] The diagnosis of pouchitis is based on the presence of symptoms (typically increased stool frequency, abdominal cramping, urgency, tenesmus, and pelvic discomfort), together with endoscopic (erythema, granularity, friability, bleeding, erosions, ulcerations) and histologic alterations (nonspecific acute inflammation with polymorphonuclear leukocyte infiltration, crypt abscesses, ulcerations, in association with a chronic inflammatory

Table 38.3 Rutgeerts score to classify neoterminal ileum disease activity following ileocolonic resection

	Description
i0	No lesions
i1	≤ 5 aphthoid ulcers
i2	> 5 aphthoid ulcers with normal mucosa in between, or skip areas with larger lesions, or lesions/ulcers (< 1 cm) confined to ileocolonic anastomosis
i3	Diffuse aphthous ileitis with extensively inflamed mucosa
i4	Diffuse inflammation with large ulcers, nodules, and/or stenosis

infiltrate). A digital examination is recommended prior to the insertion of the scope into the anus to evaluate the condition of the anastomosis, and to rule out the presence of a stricture.

Dysplasia

In general, the risk for neoplasia in patients with UC and IPAA is low.[49] Dysplasia can develop in either the ileal pouch mucosa or any retained anorectal mucosa. Currently, no clear consistent recommendations for pouch surveillance are available in the current IBD guidelines.[50] In general, yearly pouch endoscopy has been advised in high-risk patients, that is, patients with previous rectal dysplasia or dysplasia/cancer at the time of pouch surgery, PSC, type C pouch mucosa (permanent persistent atrophy and severe inflammation), or refractory pouchitis.[1,51,52,53]

38.6 Endoscopic Surveillance in IBD

Patients with IBD are at increased risk of developing CRC compared with the general population and therefore undergo surveillance endoscopy. Meta-analysis of population-based cohort studies determined that UC increases the risk of CRC 2.4-fold[54] and CD up to 2.2-fold.[55] Especially patients with long-standing and extensive colitis,[56] colitis-associated patients,[57] the presence of postinflammatory polyps (reflecting previous severe inflammation) (▶ Table 38.1) (▶ Fig. 38.10)[58] and patients with a family history of CRC[59] have an increased risk of CRC development.

Surveillance endoscopy should be performed under optimal conditions with high-resolution endoscopic equipment[60] and during disease remission to be able to discriminate between inflammatory and neoplastic changes. Chromoendoscopy increases the diagnostic yield for detection of dysplasia in patients with colonic inflammatory bowel disease.[61] Either methylene blue or indigo carmine is sprayed on the mucosa, thereby highlighting the borders and surface architecture of neoplastic lesions, hereby

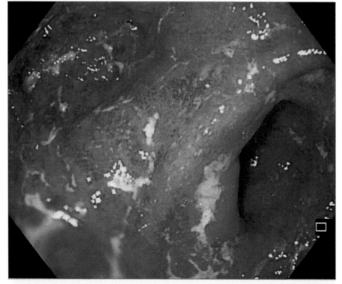

Fig. 38.9 An ileal pouch–anal anastomosis (IPAA) with evidence of chronic pouchitis. The mucosa is friable and erythematous.

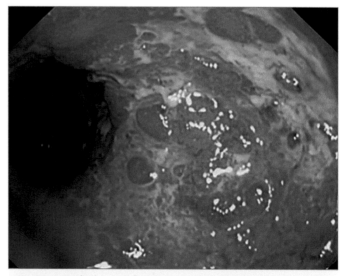

Fig. 38.10 Multiple postinflammatory polyps (previously "pseudopolyps"), large ulcerations, and markedly friable erythematous mucosa in a patient with ulcerative colitis (UC) (Mayo 3).

aiding in the differentiation of neoplastic versus nonneoplastic tissue. Any visible lesion is biopsied, leading to higher detection rates of intraepithelial neoplasia.[62,63] In general, surveillance starts 8 to 10 years from the onset of disease, and the interval is based on patient's risk factors and current guidelines.[64] Other image enhancement techniques such as narrow-band imaging, autofluorescence, and endomicroscopy for IBD surveillance are currently under investigation but have so far not been superior to classic methods.

38.7 Therapeutic Endoscopic Approaches in IBD

Strictures in IBD can occur because of long-standing inflammation and at sites of bowel anastomosis. Intestinal strictures, more commonly seen in CD compared with UC, are a major cause for morbidity and need for surgery in CD. These are often classified into either inflammatory or fibrotic.[65] Traditionally, inflammatory strictures have been treated with medical therapy of which the majority required surgery over time,[66] whereas fibrotic strictures are mostly treated surgically, which is associated with an overall recurrence rate of approximately 23%.[67] Successful (repetitive) balloon dilation of obstructive gastroduodenal strictures in patients with CD has been reported in case reports and small series.[68,69,70]

Most available data about endoscopic dilation in CD is of ileocecal and anastomotic strictures (▶ Fig. 38.11), although balloon dilation of small intestinal strictures with double-balloon enteroscopy (DBE) has also been described. In general, studies are small and include a heterogeneous group of patients and dilation techniques. The technical success of endoscopic balloon dilation (defined as being able to pass with the endoscope directly

after dilation) is reported to vary between 86 and 95%, and the clinical success (defined as resolution of obstructive symptoms) is 64 to 70%, increasing to 78% when patients with failed procedures due to technical reasons are excluded.[71,72] Best results are obtained when stricture length is less than 4 cm and when there is no ulcer present in the stricture. Strictures often recur requiring redilation. Because of the high recurrence rate after balloon dilation of CD strictures, intralesional injection of medication (being steroids or anti–tumor necrosis factor [anti-TNF] agents) has been studied but with no clear clinical effect. A literature review in 2010 comparing strictureplasty to endoscopic balloon showed a surgical recurrence rate of 24% after a median follow-up of 46 months in the strictureplasty group and a median surgical recurrence rate, that is, the need for surgery after dilation, of 27.6% in the endoscopic balloon dilation group.[73] However, a more recent meta-analysis with 25 studies including 1,089 patients and 2,664 dilations of both de novo and anastomotic strictures showed a cumulative surgery rate of 75% at 5-year follow-up (341 of 455 patients).[74] This same meta-analysis showed an overall complication rate of 6.4% (95% confidence interval [CI]: 5–8.2), which is higher than complication rates of 2 to 3% reported in earlier studies. More complications seem to occur with use of the larger balloons (diameter of 25 mm) compared to the use of smaller balloons (diameter of < 20 mm).[75]

38.8 Microscopic Colitis

Microscopic colitis causes chronic, watery, diarrhea and occurs more frequently in middle-aged females. The etiology is believed to be multifactorial, and is associated with autoimmune disorders such as celiac disease, polyarthritis, and thyroid disorders,

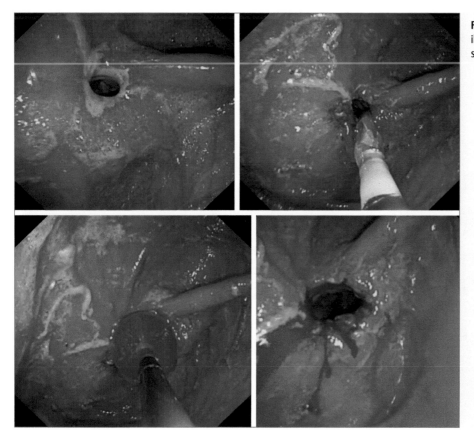

Fig. 38.11 Balloon dilation of a stenotic ileocolonic anastomosis in a patient with severe CD.

smoking, and medications, such as nonsteroidal anti-inflammatory drugs, proton pump inhibitors, and selective serotonin reuptake inhibitors.[76] The term microscopic colitis is used as a common denominator of both collagenous colitis and lymphocytic colitis, differentiated by specific histologic features. A colonoscopy with mucosal biopsies is necessary to establish the diagnosis of microscopic colitis. On endoscopy, patients with microscopic colitis usually have normal-appearing colonic mucosa, although nonspecific findings including slight edema, erythema, and friability may be seen. Biopsies should be obtained from the right side of the colon as the highest yield was in transverse colon (83%), right colon (70%), and lowest in rectosigmoid colon (66%).[77] Lymphocytic colitis is characterized by an intraepithelial lymphocytic infiltrate (> 20 per high-power field), whereas collagenous colitis is characterized by colonic subepithelial collagen band (>10 μm in thickness).

References

[1] Annese V, Daperno M, Rutter MD, et al; European Crohn's and Colitis Organisation. European evidence based consensus for endoscopy in inflammatory bowel disease. J Crohns Colitis. 2013; 7(12):982–1018

[2] Haskell H, Andrews CW, Jr, Reddy SI, et al. Pathologic features and clinical significance of "backwash" ileitis in ulcerative colitis. Am J Surg Pathol. 2005; 29(11):1472–1481

[3] Goldstein N, Dulai M. Contemporary morphologic definition of backwash ileitis in ulcerative colitis and features that distinguish it from Crohn disease. Am J Clin Pathol. 2006; 126(3):365–376

[4] Abdelrazeq AS, Wilson TR, Leitch DL, et al. Ileitis in ulcerative colitis: is it a backwash? Dis Colon Rectum. 2005; 48(11):2038–2046

[5] Crocco S, Martelossi S, Giurici N, et al. Upper gastrointestinal involvement in paediatric onset Crohn's disease: prevalence and clinical implications. J Crohns Colitis. 2012; 6(1):51–55

[6] Hummel TZ, ten Kate FJ, Reitsma JB, et al. Additional value of upper GI tract endoscopy in the diagnostic assessment of childhood IBD. J Pediatr Gastroenterol Nutr. 2012; 54(6):753–757

[7] Annunziata ML, Caviglia R, Papparella LG, Cicala M. Upper gastrointestinal involvement of Crohn's disease: a prospective study on the role of upper endoscopy in the diagnostic work-up. Dig Dis Sci. 2012; 57(6):1618–1623

[8] Dionisio PM, Gurudu SR, Leighton JA, et al. Capsule endoscopy has a significantly higher diagnostic yield in patients with suspected and established small-bowel Crohn's disease: a meta-analysis. Am J Gastroenterol. 2010; 105(6):1240–1248, quiz 1249

[9] Gralnek IM, Defranchis R, Seidman E, et al. Development of a capsule endoscopy scoring index for small bowel mucosal inflammatory change. Aliment Pharmacol Ther. 2008; 27(2):146–154

[10] Bourreille A, Ignjatovic A, Aabakken L, et al; World Organisation of Digestive Endoscopy (OMED) and the European Crohn's and Colitis Organisation (ECCO). Role of small-bowel endoscopy in the management of patients with inflammatory bowel disease: an international OMED-ECCO consensus. Endoscopy. 2009; 41(7):618–637

[11] Schwartz DA, Loftus EV, Jr, Tremaine WJ, et al. The natural history of fistulizing Crohn's disease in Olmsted County, Minnesota. Gastroenterology. 2002; 122(4):875–880

[12] Schwartz DA, Wiersema MJ, Dudiak KM, et al. A comparison of endoscopic ultrasound, magnetic resonance imaging, and exam under anesthesia for evaluation of Crohn's perianal fistulas. Gastroenterology. 2001; 121(5):1064–1072

[13] Tozer PJ, Burling D, Gupta A, et al. Review article: medical, surgical and radiological management of perianal Crohn's fistulas. Aliment Pharmacol Ther. 2011; 33(1):5–22

[14] Panes J, Bouhnik Y, Reinisch W, et al. Imaging techniques for assessment of inflammatory bowel disease: joint ECCO and ESGAR evidence-based consensus guidelines. J Crohns Colitis. 2013; 7(7):556–585

[15] Schwartz DA, Harewood GC, Wiersema MJ. EUS for rectal disease. Gastrointest Endosc. 2002; 56(1):100–109

[16] Schwartz DA, White CM, Wise PE, Herline AJ. Use of endoscopic ultrasound to guide combination medical and surgical therapy for patients with Crohn's perianal fistulas. Inflamm Bowel Dis. 2005; 11(8):727–732

[17] Spradlin NM, Wise PE, Herline AJ, et al. A randomized prospective trial of endoscopic ultrasound to guide combination medical and surgical treatment for Crohn's perianal fistulas. Am J Gastroenterol. 2008; 103(10):2527–2535

[18] Lahat A, Assulin Y, Beer-Gabel M, Chowers Y. Endoscopic ultrasound for perianal Crohn's disease: disease and fistula characteristics, and impact on therapy. J Crohn's Colitis. 2012; 6(3):311–316

[19] Singh S, Talwalkar JA. Primary sclerosing cholangitis: diagnosis, prognosis, and management. Clin Gastroenterol Hepatol. 2013; 11(8):898–907

[20] Claessen MM, Vleggaar FP, Tytgat KM, et al. High lifetime risk of cancer in primary sclerosing cholangitis. J Hepatol. 2009; 50(1):158–164

[21] Nahon S, Bouhnik Y, Lavergne-Slove A, et al. Colonoscopy accurately predicts the anatomical severity of colonic Crohn's disease attacks: correlation with findings from colectomy specimens. Am J Gastroenterol. 2002; 97(12):3102–3107

[22] Surawicz CM. What's the best way to differentiate infectious colitis (acute self-limited colitis) from IBD? Inflamm Bowel Dis. 2008; 14(suppl 2):S157–S158

[23] Dignass A, Lindsay JO, Sturm A, et al. Second European evidence-based consensus on the diagnosis and management of ulcerative colitis part 2: current management. J Crohns Colitis. 2012; 6(10):991–1030

[24] Van Assche G, Vermeire S, Rutgeerts P. Management of acute severe ulcerative colitis. Gut. 2011; 60(1):130–133

[25] Buckell NA, Williams GT, Bartram CI, Lennard-Jones JE. Depth of ulceration in acute colitis: correlation with outcome and clinical and radiologic features. Gastroenterology. 1980; 79(1):19–25

[26] Carbonnel F, Gargouri D, Lémann M, et al. Predictive factors of outcome of intensive intravenous treatment for attacks of ulcerative colitis. Aliment Pharmacol Ther. 2000; 14(3):273–279

[27] Sands BE. Biomarkers of inflammation in inflammatory bowel disease. Gastroenterology. 2015; 149(5):1275–1285.e2

[28] Kristensen V, Klepp P, Cvancarova M, et al. Prediction of endoscopic disease activity in ulcerative colitis by two different assays for fecal calprotectin. J Crohns Colitis. 2015; 9(2):164–169

[29] Sipponen T, Savilahti E, Kolho KL, et al. Crohn's disease activity assessed by fecal calprotectin and lactoferrin: correlation with Crohn's disease activity index and endoscopic findings. Inflamm Bowel Dis. 2008; 14(1):40–46

[30] Wang Y, Pei F, Wang X, et al. Diagnostic accuracy of fecal lactoferrin for inflammatory bowel disease: a meta-analysis. Int J Clin Exp Pathol. 2015; 8(10):12319–12332

[31] Frøslie KF, Jahnsen J, Moum BA, Vatn MH; IBSEN Group. Mucosal healing in inflammatory bowel disease: results from a Norwegian population-based cohort. Gastroenterology. 2007; 133(2):412–422

[32] Mary JY, Modigliani R. Development and validation of an endoscopic index of the severity for Crohn's disease: a prospective multicentre study. Groupe d'Etudes Thérapeutiques des Affections Inflammatoires du Tube Digestif (GETAID). Gut. 1989; 30(7):983–989

[33] Daperno M, D'Haens G, Van Assche G, et al. Development and validation of a new, simplified endoscopic activity score for Crohn's disease: the SES-CD. Gastrointest Endosc. 2004; 60(4):505–512

[34] Tontini GE, Bisschops R, Neumann H. Endoscopic scoring systems for inflammatory bowel disease: pros and cons. Expert Rev Gastroenterol Hepatol. 2014; 8(5):543–554

[35] Rutgeerts P, Geboes K, Vantrappen G, et al. Predictability of the postoperative course of Crohn's disease. Gastroenterology. 1990; 99(4):956–963

[36] Schroeder KW, Tremaine WJ, Ilstrup DM. Coated oral 5-aminosalicylic acid therapy for mildly to moderately active ulcerative colitis. A randomized study. N Engl J Med. 1987; 317(26):1625–1629

[37] Daperno M, Castiglione F, de Ridder L, et al; Scientific Committee of the European Crohn's and Colitis Organization. Results of the 2nd part Scientific Workshop of the ECCO. II: Measures and markers of prediction to achieve, detect, and monitor intestinal healing in inflammatory bowel disease. J Crohn's Colitis. 2011; 5(5):484–498

[38] Travis SP, Schnell D, Krzeski P, et al. Reliability and initial validation of the ulcerative colitis endoscopic index of severity. Gastroenterology. 2013; 145(5):987–995

[39] Travis SP, Schnell D, Krzeski P, et al. Developing an instrument to assess the endoscopic severity of ulcerative colitis: the Ulcerative Colitis Endoscopic Index of Severity (UCEIS). Gut. 2012; 61(4):535–542

[40] Truelove SC, Witts LJ. Cortisone in ulcerative colitis; final report on a therapeutic trial. BMJ. 1955; 2(4947):1041–1048

[41] Baron JH, Connell AM, Lennard-Jones JE. Variation between observers in describing mucosal appearances in proctocolitis. BMJ. 1964; 1(5375):89–92

[42] Samuel S, Bruining DH, Loftus EV, Jr, et al. Validation of the ulcerative colitis colonoscopic index of severity and its correlation with disease activity measures. Clin Gastroenterol Hepatol. 2013; 11(1):49–54.e1

[43] Walsh A, Palmer R, Travis S. Mucosal healing as a target of therapy for colonic inflammatory bowel disease and methods to score disease activity. Gastrointest Endosc Clin N Am. 2014; 24(3):367–378

[44] De Cruz P, Kamm MA. Reply: To PMID 25542620. Gastroenterology. 2015; 148(7):1475–1476

[45] Rutgeerts P, Geboes K, Vantrappen G, et al. Natural history of recurrent Crohn's disease at the ileocolonic anastomosis after curative surgery. Gut. 1984; 25(6):665–672

[46] Berndtsson I, Oresland T. Quality of life before and after proctocolectomy and IPAA in patients with ulcerative proctocolitis—a prospective study. Colorectal Dis. 2003; 5(2):173–179

[47] Hueting WE, Buskens E, van der Tweel I, et al. Results and complications after ileal pouch anal anastomosis: a meta-analysis of 43 observational studies comprising 9,317 patients. Dig Surg. 2005; 22(1–2):69–79

[48] Penna C, Dozois R, Tremaine W, et al. Pouchitis after ileal pouch-anal anastomosis for ulcerative colitis occurs with increased frequency in patients with associated primary sclerosing cholangitis. Gut. 1996; 38(2):234–239

[49] Derikx LA, Kievit W, Drenth JP, et al; Dutch Initiative on Crohn and Colitis. Prior colorectal neoplasia is associated with increased risk of ileoanal pouch neoplasia in patients with inflammatory bowel disease. Gastroenterology. 2014; 146(1):119–1–28.e1

[50] Derikx LA, Nissen LH, Oldenburg B, Hoentjen F. Controversies in pouch surveillance for patients with inflammatory bowel disease. J Crohns Colitis. 2016; 10(6):747–751

[51] Shergill AK, Lightdale JR, Bruining DH, et al; American Society for Gastrointestinal Endoscopy Standards of Practice Committee. The role of endoscopy in inflammatory bowel disease. Gastrointest Endosc. 2015; 81(5):1101–1121.e1–13

[52] Cairns SR, Scholefield JH, Steele RJ, et al; British Society of Gastroenterology. Association of Coloproctology for Great Britain and Ireland. Guidelines for colorectal cancer screening and surveillance in moderate and high risk groups (update from 2002). Gut. 2010; 59(5):666–689

[53] Farraye FA, Odze RD, Eaden J, Itzkowitz SH. AGA technical review on the diagnosis and management of colorectal neoplasia in inflammatory bowel disease. Gastroenterology. 2010; 138(2):746–774, 774.e1–774.e4, quiz e12–e13

[54] Jess T, Gamborg M, Matzen P, et al. Increased risk of intestinal cancer in Crohn's disease: a meta-analysis of population-based cohort studies. Am J Gastroenterol. 2005; 100(12):2724–2729

[55] Jess T, Rungoe C, Peyrin-Biroulet L. Risk of colorectal cancer in patients with ulcerative colitis: a meta-analysis of population-based cohort studies. Clin Gastroenterol Hepatol. 2012; 10(6):639–645

[56] Rutter M, Saunders B, Wilkinson K, et al. Severity of inflammation is a risk factor for colorectal neoplasia in ulcerative colitis. Gastroenterology. 2004; 126(2):451–459

[57] Jayaram H, Satsangi J, Chapman RW. Increased colorectal neoplasia in chronic ulcerative colitis complicated by primary sclerosing cholangitis: fact or fiction? Gut. 2001; 48(3):430–434

[58] Velayos FS, Loftus EV, Jr, Jess T, et al. Predictive and protective factors associated with colorectal cancer in ulcerative colitis: a case-control study. Gastroenterology. 2006; 130(7):1941–1949

[59] Askling J, Dickman PW, Karlén P, et al. Family history as a risk factor for colorectal cancer in inflammatory bowel disease. Gastroenterology. 2001; 120(6):1356–1362

[60] Subramanian V, Ramappa V, Telakis E, et al. Comparison of high definition with standard white light endoscopy for detection of dysplastic lesions during surveillance colonoscopy in patients with colonic inflammatory bowel disease. Inflamm Bowel Dis. 2013; 19(2):350–355

[61] Subramanian V, Mannath J, Ragunath K, Hawkey CJ. Meta-analysis: the diagnostic yield of chromoendoscopy for detecting dysplasia in patients with colonic inflammatory bowel disease. Aliment Pharmacol Ther. 2011; 33(3):304–312

[62] Günther U, Kusch D, Heller F, et al. Surveillance colonoscopy in patients with inflammatory bowel disease: comparison of random biopsy vs. targeted biopsy protocols. Int J Colorectal Dis. 2011; 26(5):667–672

[63] van den Broek FJ, Stokkers PC, Reitsma JB, et al. Random biopsies taken during colonoscopic surveillance of patients with longstanding ulcerative colitis: low yield and absence of clinical consequences. Am J Gastroenterol. 2014; 109(5):715–722

[64] Mowat C, Cole A, Windsor A, et al; IBD Section of the British Society of Gastroenterology. Guidelines for the management of inflammatory bowel disease in adults. Gut. 2011; 60(5):571–607

[65] Lichtenstein GR, Olson A, Travers S, et al. Factors associated with the development of intestinal strictures or obstructions in patients with Crohn's disease. Am J Gastroenterol. 2006; 101(5):1030–1038

[66] Samimi R, Flasar MH, Kavic S, et al. Outcome of medical treatment of stricturing and penetrating Crohn's disease: a retrospective study. Inflamm Bowel Dis. 2010; 16(7):1187–1194

[67] Yamamoto T, Fazio VW, Tekkis PP. Safety and efficacy of strictureplasty for Crohn's disease: a systematic review and meta-analysis. Dis Colon Rectum. 2007; 50(11):1968–1986

[68] Kelly SM, Hunter JO. Endoscopic balloon dilatation of duodenal strictures in Crohn's disease. Postgrad Med J. 1995; 71(840):623–624

[69] Matsui T, Hatakeyama S, Ikeda K, et al. Long-term outcome of endoscopic balloon dilation in obstructive gastroduodenal Crohn's disease. Endoscopy. 1997; 29(7):640–645

[70] Rana SS, Bhasin DK, Chandail VS, et al. Endoscopic balloon dilatation without fluoroscopy for treating gastric outlet obstruction because of benign etiologies. Surg Endosc. 2011; 25(5):1579–1584

[71] Hassan C, Zullo A, De Francesco V, et al. Systematic review: endoscopic dilatation in Crohn's disease. Aliment Pharmacol Ther. 2007; 26(11–12):1457–1464

[72] Mueller T, Rieder B, Bechtner G, Pfeiffer A. The response of Crohn's strictures to endoscopic balloon dilation. Aliment Pharmacol Ther. 2010; 31(6):634–639

[73] Wibmer AG, Kroesen AJ, Gröne J, et al. Comparison of strictureplasty and endoscopic balloon dilatation for stricturing Crohn's disease—review of the literature. Int J Colorectal Dis. 2010; 25(10):1149–1157

[74] Morar PS, Faiz O, Warusavitarne J, et al; Crohn's Stricture Study (CroSS) Group. Systematic review with meta-analysis: endoscopic balloon dilatation for Crohn's disease strictures. Aliment Pharmacol Ther. 2015; 42(10):1137–1148

[75] Gustavsson A, Magnuson A, Blomberg B, et al. Endoscopic dilation is an efficacious and safe treatment of intestinal strictures in Crohn's disease. Aliment Pharmacol Ther. 2012; 36(2):151–158

[76] Masclee GM, Coloma PM, Kuipers EJ, Sturkenboom MC. Increased risk of microscopic colitis with use of proton pump inhibitors and non-steroidal anti- inflammatory drugs. Am J Gastroenterol. 2015; 110(5):749–759

[77] Surawicz CM. Collating collagenous colitis cases. Am J Gastroenterol. 2000; 95(1):307–308

39 Lower Intestinal Bleeding Disorders

Alexander Meier and Helmut Messmann

39.1 Introduction

Gastrointestinal bleeding from the colon is a common reason for hospitalization, and endoscopic hemostasis is the daily challenge that must be mastered by gastroenterologists. For this, many different endoscopic techniques are available (injection therapy, hemoclips, thermal coagulation, topical hemostatic substances). Depending on the source of bleeding, the suitable and most effective method must be chosen. In this chapter, we discuss the diagnostic approach and definitive treatment of colonic hemorrhage.

The following definitions will guide you while you go through the rest of the chapter.

- *Lower gastrointestinal (GI) bleeding* is defined as acute or chronic abnormal blood loss originating from the colon.
- *Acute lower intestinal bleeding* is arbitrarily defined as bleeding of less than 78 hours duration resulting in instability of vital signs, anemia, and/or a need for blood transfusion.
- *Chronic lower intestinal bleeding* is defined as slow blood loss over a period of several days or longer presenting with symptoms of occult fecal blood, intermittent melena, or scant hematochezia.
- *Occult gastrointestinal bleeding* means that the amounts of blood in the feces are too small to be seen but are detectable by chemical tests.
- *Obscure gastrointestinal bleeding* often presents as lower intestinal bleeding and means bleeding from an unclear site that persists or recurs after a negative initial or primary endoscopy.

39.2 General Aspects

39.2.1 Epidemiology

The incidence of lower gastrointestinal bleeding is only one-fifth of that in the upper gastrointestinal tract and is estimated at 21 to 27 cases per 100,000 adults/year. Lower intestinal bleeding is usually chronic and self-limiting. Twenty-one of 100,000 adults/year require hospitalization due to severe bleeding. Among these, men and older patients suffer from more severe lower intestinal bleeding. There is a 200-fold increase in the incidence from the third to the ninth decade, due to diverticulosis and angiodysplasia.[1] In a cross-sectional survey, it was found that 15.5% of the population in the United States suffered from rectal bleeding, but only 13.9% of those affected sought medical care.[2]

Some 20% of all gastrointestinal bleeding disorders occur from colonic and anorectal sources. A small bowel source is less common. Studies of lower gastrointestinal bleeding have noted 0.5 to 12% of recurrent bleeding after an initial nondiagnostic colonoscopy result. However, some have estimated that a source in the small bowel is the cause of gastrointestinal bleeding in up to 5% of cases.[3]

39.2.2 Clinical Course and Prognosis

There is evidence that upper gastrointestinal bleeding differs in acuteness and severity from lower intestinal bleeding. Patients with lower intestinal bleeding are in shock significantly less often (19 vs. 35%, respectively), require fewer blood transfusions (36 vs. 64%), and have a significantly higher hemoglobin level (84 vs. 61%).[4] Patients with colonic bleeding require fewer blood transfusions in comparison with those who have bleeding from the small intestine. As in upper gastrointestinal bleeding, the majority (80–85%) of cases of bleeding in the lower intestinal tract stop spontaneously. The mortality and morbidity rates increase with age. The overall mortality rate varies between 2 and 3.6%. Patients with bleeding episodes after hospital admission have significantly higher mortality rates (23.1%) in comparison with those who bleed before hospital admission.[5]

Several studies have identified clinical features that predict the risk of complications in patients with presumed acute lower GI bleeding. These features can be used to help categorize patients either as low or high risk.[6,7,8] High-risk features include the following:

- Hemodynamic instability (hypotension, tachycardia, orthostasis, syncope)
- Persistent bleeding
- Significant comorbid illnesses
- Advanced age
- Bleeding that occurs in a patient who is hospitalized for another reason
- A prior history of bleeding from diverticulosis or angiodysplasia
- Current anticoagulant or antiplatelet use
- Prolonged prothrombin time
- A nontender abdomen
- Anemia
- An elevated blood urea nitrogen level
- An abnormal white blood cell count

The likelihood of a poor outcome correlates with the number of high-risk features present.[6] Velayos et al[8] identified the following risk factors indicating severe lower intestinal bleeding:

- Hemodynamic instability (blood pressure < 100 mm Hg, heart rate > 100 beats/min) 1 hour after initial medical evaluation
- Active gross bleeding per rectum
- Initial hematocrit less than or equal to 35%

39.3 Diagnostic Approach

39.3.1 History

A focused history helps differentiate the causes of lower intestinal bleeding. Important points include the duration of bleeding, stool color (melena; massive, intermittent, or scant hematochezia; small quantities of blood in the stool), and frequency. Lower intestinal bleeding is usually suspected when hematochezia is present. This means the passage of maroon or bright red blood or blood clots per rectum. This is different from upper gastrointestinal bleeding, which often presents with hematemesis (vomiting blood) and melena. However, massive upper gastrointestinal bleeding can also present with bright red stool; up to 11% of patients with hematochezia may have upper gastrointestinal bleeding. Zuckerman et al reported that melena as a sign of upper gastrointestinal bleeding is correctly described and diagnosed in the acute setting by most physicians, as well as hematochezia for the incidence of a lower gastrointestinal bleeding.[9]

Clinical symptoms such as pain, weight loss, changes in bowel habits, or fever are helpful in planning the next diagnostic steps. When the patient's medical history is being investigated, note should be made of previous bleeding episodes, abdominal and vascular operations, radiotherapy of the pelvic organs, a history of peptic ulcer disease or inflammatory bowel disease (IBD), medication (especially acetylsalicylic acid, nonsteroidal anti-inflammatory drugs [NSAIDs], and anticoagulation treatment), a family history of malignant disease, and comorbidity.

39.3.2 Physical Examination

The physical examination helps differentiate acute from chronic bleeding and includes assessment of circulatory stability. Blood loss of less than 250 mL has no influence either on heart rate or blood pressure. Blood loss of more than 800 mL induces a fall in blood pressure of about 10 mm Hg and a heart rate increase of 10 beats/min. Paleness, weakness, and dizziness are frequent symptoms. Extensive` blood loss of more than 1,500 mL usually presents with shock symptoms, tachypnea, and depressed mental status. Digital rectal examination in combination with a test for occult blood helps confirm the patient's description of stool color. A digital rectal examination can also detect 40% of rectal carcinomas; in 2% of patients with massive rectal bleeding, the digital rectal examination detected a rectal cancer.[10]

39.3.3 Laboratory Studies

The initial laboratory work-up should include the following:
- Complete blood count (including hemoglobin, hematocrit, and thrombocytes)
- Coagulation profile
- Serum chemistry (electrolytes and creatinine)
- Sample for type and cross-match

39.3.4 Endoscopy

Flexible Endoscopy

Flexible endoscopy is considered the mainstay for evaluation of lower intestinal bleeding. The incidence of serious complications is approximately one in 1,000 procedures. Elderly patients and those with cardiovascular or pulmonary diseases are at special risk for cardiopulmonary complications. Aspiration (in upper endoscopy), oversedation, hypoventilation, and vasovagal events are the major problems. Perforation rarely occurs, even in urgent colonoscopy. Patients should be continuously monitored during urgent endoscopy using electrocardiography and noninvasive measurement of oxygen saturation. If there are unstable vital signs, patients must receive resuscitation before endoscopy. Recently guidelines for sedation in endoscopy were published.[11]

Esophagogastroduodenoscopy. In patients with hematochezia and hemodynamic instability, esophagogastroduodenoscopy should be undertaken first to exclude an upper gastrointestinal source (▶ Fig. 39.1). Particularly in patients with a history of peptic ulcer and portal hypertension, this should be considered in any case.

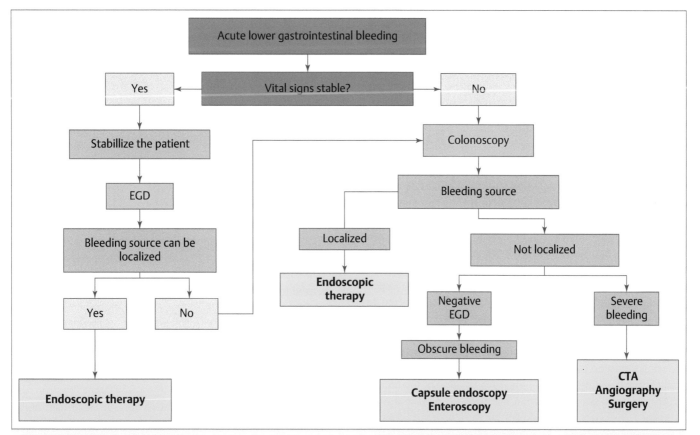

Fig. 39.1 Algorithm for diagnosis and therapy in patients with acute lower gastrointestinal bleeding with hematochezia (adapted from Gölder S. Untere gastrointestinale Blutung. In: Messmann H, ed. Lehratlas der Koloskopie. Stuttgart: Thieme; 2015:194–218[19]). CTA, computed tomographic angiography; EGD, esophagogastroduodenoscopy.

Colonoscopy. It has been demonstrated that in experienced hands, colonoscopy plays the same role in acute lower intestinal bleeding as esophagogastroduodenoscopy does in acute upper gastrointestinal bleeding. Advantages of colonoscopy compared with other tests for lower GI bleeding include its potential to precisely localize the site of the bleeding regardless of the etiology or rate of bleeding, the ability to collect pathologic specimens, and the potential for therapeutic intervention. As in upper gastrointestinal bleeding, there are three main principles underlying early or urgent colonoscopy:

• Determination of the location and type of the bleeding source
• Identification of patients with ongoing hemorrhage and those who are at high risk for rebleeding
• Assessment of the potential for endoscopic intervention

All patients with acute lower intestinal bleeding must be stabilized. Contraindications for colonoscopy are severe active inflammation and also inadequate visibility conditions. The colonoscopy should be aborted if the patient becomes unstable, the bleeding is so severe that identification of a bleeding source is impossible, or the risk of perforation is too high. The diagnostic yield for urgent (within 12 hours after admission) colonoscopy in acute lower intestinal bleeding is in the range of 48 to 90%.[10] Other publications have reported diagnostic yields of 89 to 97%,[12] which is perhaps a reflection of more consistent use of urgent colonoscopy.

Studies demonstrated that early colonoscopy (examination conducted within 24 hours of admission) is significantly associated with a shorter hospital stay.[5,13] Navaneethan et al reported that there was no difference in mortality in patients with lower GI bleeding who had early versus delayed colonoscopy (0.3 vs. 0.4%, $p = 0.24$), however, patients who underwent early colonoscopy had a shorter length of hospital stay (2.9 vs. 4.6 days, $p < 0.001$), a decreased need for blood transfusion (44.6 vs. 53.8%, $p < 0.001$), and lower hospitalization costs (U.S. $22,142 vs. U.S.$28,749, $p < 0.001$).[5] Some studies suggested that the risk of rebleeding and surgery in patients with severe diverticular hemorrhage can be reduced by early colonoscopy with endoscopic treatment compared with patients treated conservatively.[14] Endoscopic therapy was also more likely to be performed during early examinations.[5,15]

Urgent colonoscopy is defined as within 12 hours after hospitalization. A randomized trial of patients found that a strategy of urgent colonoscopy improved detection of the source of bleeding compared with expectant/elective colonoscopy alone or with radiographic interventions. But mortality, hospital stay, transfusion requirements, or the need for surgery were not significantly reduced.[16] A concern in urgent colonoscopy is bowel preparation. Chaudhry et al[17] showed that in patients with acute lower intestinal bleeding, a high diagnostic yield (97%) and effective hemostasis was possible even without bowel preparation. They were able to control active bleeding in 17 of 27 patients (63%) by endoscopic intervention. However, other recommendations instead advise cleansing the colon as thoroughly as possible in acute lower gastrointestinal bleeding, which improves evaluation of the mucosa and in turn enhances recognition of smaller lesions and minimizes the risk of complications resulting from poor visualization. However, the role of urgent colonoscopy in lower gastrointestinal bleeding remains controversial.[18] In our institution, bowel cleansing is performed with a polyethylene glycol electrolyte solution.

For optimal colon preparation, the patient must consume 4 to 6 L of the solution.[19] In some cases it may be helpful to administer a prokinetic antiemetic drug such as metoclopramide or to administer the solution via a nasogastric tube if the patient has problems with swallowing the fluid.

The segmental location of fresh blood, or the level above which no blood is present, should be carefully documented by the endoscopist. An attempt should be made to reach the cecum whenever possible. This is important as a substantial proportion of bleeding sites are located in the right hemicolon. In addition, the endoscopist should try to intubate the terminal ileum. Blood flowing from above is a clear sign of a more proximal bleeding site. Ohyama et al[12] reported that even in conditions of urgent colonoscopy, it was possible to inspect the cecum in 56% of patients and that advancement as far as the terminal ileum was achieved in 27%.

A case series of colonoscopy with unprepared conditions located the bleeding lesion in 39% of patients and the cecum was reached in 69%.[20] Immediate colonoscopy was performed after tap water enema without oral bowel preparation, aided by waterjet pumps and mechanical suction devices.

Repeated Endoscopy

In patients with nondiagnostic upper endoscopy and colonoscopy, a repeated endoscopy is helpful in identifying lesions missed at the time of the initial endoscopic evaluation. Studies have reported that lesions within the range of a conventional endoscope were detected by small bowel endoscopy or by a second-look endoscopy in 6 to 20% of cases.[21,22,23] Repeated capsule endoscopy is acceptable in patients with obscure gastrointestinal bleeding and negative capsule endoscopy findings. Jones et al[24] reported a high yield (75%) with repeated capsule endoscopy in patients with obscure gastrointestinal bleeding when the first examination was negative. In addition, these findings led to a change in management in 62.5% of repeated studies. Limited visualization due to blood and debris during the initial capsule endoscopy appears to be a common reason for repeated studies. Recurrent bleeding is another reason.

39.3.5 Nonendoscopic Methods

Computed Tomographic Angiography

Several reports have described computed tomographic angiography (CTA) for the localization of active hemorrhage.[25,26] As CTA is widely available, fast, and minimally invasive, it is an appealing diagnostic modality. In addition, anatomical details that may be helpful for subsequent interventions such as angiography are delivered.

Bleeding at a rate of 0.3 to 0.5 mL/min can be detected with CTA, typically using multidetector-row helical computed tomography (CT). Compared with single-detector–row helical CT, multidetector-row helical CT permits markedly increased resolution and shortens scanning time.

Several studies have examined CTA for the detection of GI bleeding:

• A meta-analysis of 22 studies with 672 patients found that CTA had a sensitivity of 85% and a specificity of 92% for detecting active GI bleeding.[27]

- In a study of 161 patients, CTA was similar to radionuclide imaging for detecting bleeding on subsequent angiography (sensitivity of 90%, specificity of 20%), but with more precision when it came to localizing the site of the bleeding.[28]

Potential drawbacks of CTA include the high-contrast volume that is administered to the patient if angiography is performed after CT.

Visceral Angiography

It is estimated that visceral angiography can only detect active bleeding of at least 0.5 to 1 mL/min. The specificity of this procedure is 100%, but the sensitivity varies with the pattern of bleeding, ranging in one study from 47% with acute to 30% with recurrent bleeding.[29] Data on the clinical utility of angiography in obscure gastrointestinal bleeding are very limited. Advantages of angiography include the lack of a need for bowel preparation, the ability to localize the bleeding source exactly (if identified), and the potential for therapy. Angiography should be reserved for patients who have massive bleeding that precludes colonoscopy or in whom endoscopy has failed to identify the bleeding source. A study group from Hong Kong compared immediate capsule endoscopy (CE) and mesenteric angiography in patients with acute, overt, obscure gastrointestinal bleeding. The diagnostic yield of immediate CE was significantly higher than angiography (53.3 vs. 20.0%, p = 0.016). The cumulative risk of rebleeding in the angiography and CE group was 33.3 and 16.7%, respectively (p = 0.10, log-rank test), and there was no significant difference in the long-term outcomes between the two groups including further transfusion, hospitalization for rebleeding, and mortality.[30]

Transcatheter embolization is a more definitive means of controlling hemorrhage and has largely replaced vasopressin infusion. The risk of bowel infarction was decreased with the use of superselective embolization of distal vessels using coaxial catheters. In patients found to have active bleeding, superselective embolization is feasible in 80%, and bleeding is successfully controlled in 97%.[31] However, the embolization procedure is associated with a risk of intestinal infarction of up to 20%, as well as other serious complications including arterial injury, thrombus formation, and renal failure.

A retrospective study analyzed 53 cases of lower intestinal bleeding (20 patients with colonoscopy and 20 patients with visceral angiography and nuclear scintigraphy). Performance of colonoscopy showed a broad diagnostic yield in the urgent setting, with consecutive shorter hospital stays and a less transfusion rate. There was no difference relating to necessity of surgical intervention.[32]

Nuclear Scintigraphy

Nuclear scintigraphy is a sensitive method of detecting gastrointestinal bleeding at a rate of 0.1 mL/min, but has largely been replaced by CT scan that is more practical and the diagnostic method of choice. The role of nuclear scans, and in particular of technetium-99m (99mTc)-labeled red blood cells, is limited in patients with obscure gastrointestinal bleeding and has substantially declined with the advent of complete endoscopic imaging of the small bowel. A major disadvantage of nuclear imaging is that it localizes bleeding only to an area of the abdomen. For example, bleeding from a redundant sigmoid may appear in the right lower quadrant, suggesting bleeding in the right colon. Another problem is colonic motility, which can move blood in either a peristaltic or antiperistaltic direction. When scans are positive within 2 hours, localization is correct in 95 to 100% of cases, but with positive scans after 2 hours, the accuracy decreases to 57 to 67%.[10] Scintigraphy may be a useful tool for intermittent gastrointestinal bleeding, when endoscopic methods have failed. It is strongly recommended that every positive radionuclide imaging examination should be confirmed by endoscopy or angiography before definitive therapy is considered—such as surgery, for example. Two types of nuclear scans have been used: 99mTc sulfur colloid and 99mTc pertechnetate-labeled autologous red blood cells. Both techniques are noninvasive and sensitive for GI bleeding.

Exploratory Laparotomy

Currently, exploratory laparotomy is seldom performed without intraoperative enteroscopy. Lesions have to be identified by simple palpation and transillumination. In two reports, diagnosis was possible at surgery in 64 and 65% of cases, respectively.[33]

39.4 Differential Diagnosis

The colon accounts for one-third of cases of gastrointestinal bleeding. The frequency of colonic bleeding sources reported varies among publications. One reason for this could be that studies often fail to differentiate between probable and definite sources of bleeding. In addition, the definitions of acute lower intestinal bleeding used are far from uniform. A source of lower intestinal bleeding cannot be definitively identified in up to 25% of patients.[34] Age can provide a clue to the cause of acute lower gastrointestinal bleeding as younger patients tend to bleed from hemorrhoids, vascular malformations, and rectal ulcers, while older patients tend to bleed from diverticula, vascular malformations, and neoplasms.

An analysis of 1,159 patients with lower gastrointestinal bleeding identified the following sources of bleeding[32]:
- Diverticula (5–42%)
- Colonic ischemia (6–18%)
- Anorectal diseases (6–16%)
- Neoplasia (3–11%)
- Angiodysplasia (0–3%)
- Following polypectomy (0–13%)
- Inflammation (2–4%)

▶ Table 39.1 provides an overview of the frequencies of bleeding sources in patients presenting with hematochezia.

Table 39.1 Distribution of sources of hematochezia reported in the literature

Source of bleeding	Frequency (%)
Diverticula	5–42%
Colonic ischemia	6–18%
Anorectal diseases	6–16%
Neoplasia	3–11%
Angiodysplasia	0–3%
Following polypectomy	0–13%
Inflammation	2–4%

Based on Strate LL, Saltzman JR, Ookubo R, Mutinga ML, Syngal S. Validation of a clinical prediction rule for severe acute lower intestinal bleeding. Am J Gastroenterol 2005;100(8):1821–1827.

39.4.1 Diverticula

Diverticula (▶Fig. 39.2) are the reported source of gastrointestinal bleeding in 5 to 42% of patients with lower gastrointestinal bleeding. Although most diverticula are located in the left hemicolon, especially in the sigmoid colon, diverticula in the right hemicolon appear to have a greater bleeding tendency. However, the correlation may not always be causal, as diverticula are often cited as the bleeding source in the colon due to lack of evidence of another source.

Among patients with diverticulosis, the risk of bleeding is approximately 0.5 per 1,000 person-years.[35] In a study of 1,514 asymptomatic patients with diverticulosis, the cumulative incidence of bleeding was 0.2% at 12 months, 2.2% at 60 months, and 9.5% at 120 months. Risk factors for bleeding included age greater than or equal to 70 years (adjusted hazard ratio [aHR] 3.7) and bilateral diverticulosis (aHR 2.4). Interestingly, obesity also appears to increase the risk of diverticulitis and colonic diverticular bleeding.[36]

39.4.2 Vascular Diseases

Angiodysplasias are cited as the source of lower intestinal bleeding in up to 3 to 12% of patients. The majority of angiodysplasias are located in the right hemicolon, and often occur several at a time. The frequency increases with age. In colonoscopic studies, these are found in 0.83 to 1.4% of the patients examined.[1] Angiodysplasias appear endoscopically as red, circumscribed mucosal lesions (▶Fig. 39.3) with a diameter of 1 mm to a few centimeters. The vast majority of affected individuals do not bleed,[37] and therapy is not always indicated for every angiodysplasia detected on colonoscopy. In consequence, angiodysplasias detected during emergency colonoscopy are not automatically the source of bleeding unless these are bleeding or show stigmata (visible vessel, adherent clot, or submucosal bleeding). It is important to avoid the use of opiates[38] and cold water lavage[39] during colonoscopy as these reduce blood flow in the mucosa, decreasing the diagnostic yield.

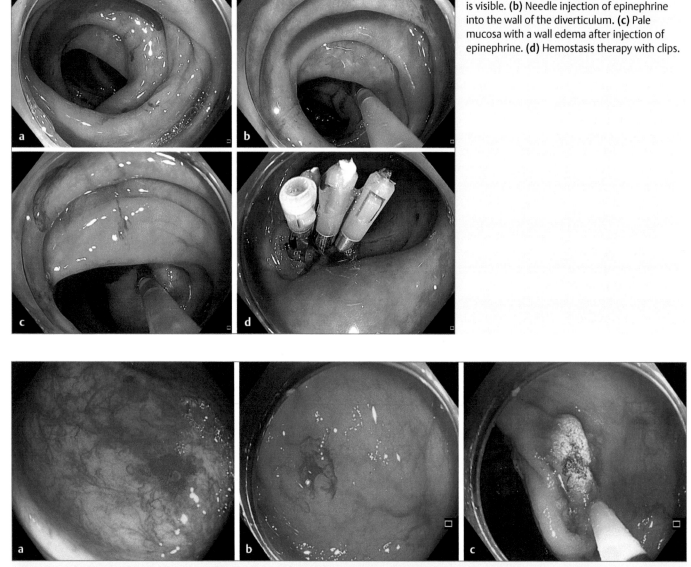

Fig. 39.2 A bleeding sigmoid diverticulum. **(a)** A streak of blood from the diverticulum is visible. **(b)** Needle injection of epinephrine into the wall of the diverticulum. **(c)** Pale mucosa with a wall edema after injection of epinephrine. **(d)** Hemostasis therapy with clips.

Fig. 39.3 **(a)** Angiodysplasia in the cecum. **(b)** Bleeding angiodysplasia in the ascending colon. **(c)** Hemostasis therapy with argon plasma coagulation (APC).

Angiodysplasias manifest in the colon in association with numerous syndromes, the most well-known of which is hereditary hemorrhagic telangiectasia (HHT), also known as Osler–Weber–Rendu syndrome. HHT is an autosomal dominant disease characterized by the formation of abnormal blood vessels. The clinical picture shows attacks involving various organs, primarily the brain, lungs, skin, nose, liver, and gastrointestinal tract. Two clear genetic defects related to hereditary hemorrhagic telangiectasia have been identified. Unlike usual angioectasias, HHT affects younger people as well, with involvement of the entire gastrointestinal tract. The diagnosis should be made on the basis of the Curaçao criteria (▶Table 39.2). Gastrointestinal bleeding occurs in one-third of patients with HHT[40] and patients over the age of 60 are particularly at risk. The most common localization of HHT is the stomach and proximal small bowel; the colon is less often affected.[41]

Rectal varices. Bleeding, especially from rectal varices is not uncommon in patients with portal hypertension. Rectal varices have a gray–blue color and may be confused with mucosal folds.

Radiation injury. Radiation proctitis due to radiotherapy for pelvic tumors can lead to blood loss, but bleeding generally does not present a problem. A more serious problem is neovascularization resulting from tissue ischemia in radiation-induced endarteritis obliterans. This can lead to considerable morbidity due to recurrent blood loss. Following radiotherapy for prostate carcinoma, 13% of patients report more or less pronounced rectal blood loss over a period of 4 to 41 months.[42] Patients with chronic radiation proctitis have similar symptoms as patients with acute radiation proctitis. If bleeding occurs, it is usually more severe. In addition, patients may have symptoms of obstructed defecation due to strictures with symptoms of constipation, rectal pain, urgency, and, rarely, fecal incontinence due to overflow. Chronic radiation injury usually presents endoscopically with multiple telangiectasias, often extending into the anal canal. The mucosa is pale, lacking vessels, and vulnerable. In severe cases, there can also be ulcerations and massive hemorrhage.

Dieulafoy lesion. Bleeding from a Dieulafoy lesion in the stomach is not an unusual finding, but it is an unexpected cause of colonic bleeding. Small mucosal lesions with subsequent erosion of an underlying vessel can lead to spurting hemorrhage.

Colonic ischemia. Hematochezia is not infrequently caused by colonic ischemia. Older patients are most likely to experience ischemia-related colitis because of underlying risk factors

such as arrhythmias, relative hypotension, and heart failure. Often there is no clear precipitating event, and young patients can present with ischemic colitis, particularly those with a hypercoagulable state.[43] In most cases patients have associated abdominal pain, although its absence does not preclude the diagnosis. Ischemic colitis tends to be continuous and left-sided. Distinguishing features may include a clear demarcation between involved and normal mucosa, rectal sparing, and a single longitudinal ulcer.[44] In most cases the bleeding is self-limited (85–90%) and do resolve with correction of the underlying cause and volume repletion.[45]

39.4.3 Inflammation

Massive hemorrhage leads to hospitalization in 0.1% of patients with ulcerative colitis and 1.2% of patients with Crohn's disease.[46] Among Crohn's patients, bleeding locations have been described in one report as being evenly distributed between the small bowel and colon. In half of all patients with bleeding related to chronic IBD, bleeding stops spontaneously. However, the rebleeding rate is 35%[46] (▶Fig. 39.4).

Although infectious colitis and pseudomembranous colitis can present with bloody diarrhea, life-threatening hemorrhage is rare. NSAIDs can promote bleeding from any number of possible lesions in the gastrointestinal tract. NSAIDs also induce colitis, which may not be visibly discernible from infectious colitis or chronic IBD. The endoscopic appearance can also include flat and usually irregularly bordered erosions and ulcerations, which are surrounded by an otherwise normal-appearing mucosa.

39.4.4 Neoplasia

Carcinomas range from 3 to 11% as the source of hematochezia. Bleeding is the result of erosions on the surface of the tumor. Colon polyps are reported to be the source of lower intestinal bleeding in 5 to 11% of patients. Larger polyps with a diameter

Table 39.2 Criteria for clinical diagnosis of hereditary hemorrhagic telangiectasia

Findings
Epistaxis (spontaneous or recurrent)
Telangiectasias on skin and mucosa: multiple, characteristic localizations (face, lips, oral cavity, and fingers)
Visceral arteriovenous malformations (lung, brain, liver, spine) or gastrointestinal telangiectasias (with or without bleeding)
Family history: immediate family member with HHT (according to the above criteria)
Probability of diagnosis
Definitive diagnosis: three or more criteria
Probable diagnosis: two criteria
Improbable: less than two criteria
HHT, hereditary hemorrhagic telangiectasia

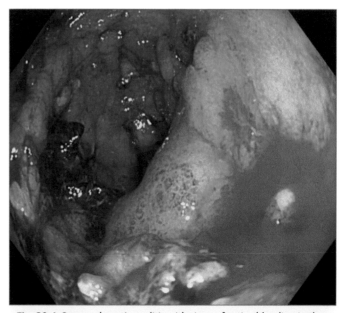

Fig. 39.4 Severe ulcerative colitis with signs of active bleeding in the right hemicolon.

of more than 1 cm bleed more often. By far the most common cause of lower gastrointestinal bleeding from benign polyps is polypectomy (see Section Bleeding after Colonic Polypectomy).

39.4.5 Anorectal Diseases

Hemorrhoids are the source in 2 to 9% of patients with acute lower gastrointestinal bleeding.[47] Although anal fissures often cause bloodstained stools, acute bleeding is rare. Fissures are relatively easily diagnosed by inspecting the anus. The patient typically has severe pain upon spreading the anus, but the lesion can be carefully and painlessly inspected after injecting a few milliliters of a local anesthetic. Bleeding from fissures usually ceases spontaneously.

Local ischemia appears to play a role in the pathogenesis of solitary rectal ulcers. Internal rectal prolapse or lack of inhibition of the puborectalis muscle during straining are thought to be responsible. Heavy bleeding is rare.

39.5 Therapy

39.5.1 Initial Resuscitation

There are no clear recommendations regarding which patients should be admitted to an intensive care unit. However, it appears reasonable to monitor patients closely if there is ongoing bleeding and they are at high risk on the basis of the factors mentioned earlier. In addition, patients with a transfusion requirement greater than 2 units of packed red blood cells and those with significant comorbidity should be considered for admission to an intensive care unit. Patients with congestive heart failure or valvular disease may benefit from close monitoring (central venous pressure, pulse contour continuous cardiac output) to minimize the risk of fluid overload. Two large-diameter peripheral catheters or a central venous catheter should be placed for intravenous access. Any coagulopathy (prothrombin time international normalized ratio [INR] > 1.5) should be corrected using fresh frozen plasma or prothrombin complex concentrate and vitamin K. In patients with significant thrombocytopenia (< 50,000/μL), platelet transfusions can be considered. Rapid fluid replacement is indicated in patients with severe hypovolemia or shock. The ideal hemoglobin concentration/hematocrit depends on the patient's age, the rate of bleeding, and the presence of comorbid conditions. The ACG clinical guideline recommends that packed red blood cells should be transfused to maintain the hemoglobin greater than 7 g/dL. For patients with massive bleeding, significant comorbid illness (especially cardiovascular ischemia) or a possible delay in receiving therapeutic interventions a threshold of 9 g/dL should be considered.[37] Villanueva et al reported that as compared with a liberal transfusion strategy, a restrictive strategy significantly improved the outcomes in patients with upper gastrointestinal bleeding.[48]

39.5.2 Endoscopy

The efficacy of endoscopic intervention in patients with upper gastrointestinal bleeding is beyond doubt. These benefits have also been demonstrated in lower intestinal bleeding.[14]

39.6 Injection Therapy

Injection therapy is an inexpensive and easy-to-learn method to achieve hemostasis (▶ Fig. 39.2). The injection needles consist of a Teflon sheath with an extendable needle at the tip. For treatment in the colon, a needle extension length of 4 mm should be used in order to limit the depth of penetration. Usually, epinephrine (Suprarenin, Adrenaline) is used. This causes vasoconstriction and physical compression of the vessel. The individual injection dose should be as low as possible (e.g., 1–2 mL, 1:10,000–1:100,000 dilution). Alternative agents (absolute alcohol, sodium tetradecyl sulfate, ethanolamine, and polidocanol) are not superior to epinephrine and can also cause mucosal injury. The simple method can also be applied without optimal vision or if the position of the endoscope and instrument are tangential to the bleeding lesion. Hemostasis is achieved by compression and vasoconstriction. Injection often is used for primary hemostasis therapy to attain an interruption of the blood flow and thus to achieve a better accessibility. If consecutive, a circumscribed bleeding source (e.g., a visible vessel) is identified, additive mechanical methods are used for definitive hemostasis (see mechanical hemostasis). If that is not the case or the lesion is not accessible to clip therapy, injection of fibrin can be performed.

39.7 Thermocoagulation

Heat application causes edema, coagulation of tissue protein, and contraction of vessels in the tissue, resulting in hemostasis. In bipolar circumactive probe (BICAP) and monopolar electrocoagulation, electrical current is passed through the tissue and heats it up. In the bipolar modality, the current flows between the two electrodes in the probe tip, and in the monopolar method, it is necessary to place a neutral electrode on the patient's body. The coagulation depth is greater with monopolar coagulation than with bipolar. Some monopolar probes have holes in the probe tip for irrigation for example, electrohydrothermal (EHT) probes. A major problem with contact electrocoagulation is the fact that the probe may stick to the tissue; removing the probe entails a risk of tearing off tissue and subsequently inducing bleeding. Perforation occurs in up to 2.5% of patients in whom bipolar coagulation is used in the thin-walled right hemicolon.

Argon plasma coagulation (APC) transmits energy from ionized argon gas to the tissue without contact between the probe and tissue (▶ Fig. 39.3). The flexible application probe is inserted into the working channel of the endoscope. The penetration depth is 0.8 to 3 mm and it is automatically limited by the desiccation of the tissue. Although valid figures for perforation rates are lacking, these are probably well below 1%.

There are few studies that directly compare APC to other methods for achieving hemostasis. A systematic review published in 2005 identified only two randomized-controlled trials (with only 121 individuals) in nonvariceal upper GI bleeding.[49] However, APC is used widely due to its ease of use and perceived safety advantages.[50]

39.8 Topical Agents

39.8.1 Hemospray (Cook Medical) TG 325

Hemospray is a nonorganic substance that is sprayed via a non-contact method on the bleeding lesion with a 7- to 10-F catheter. The application system contains a CO_2 cartridge that generates the pressure for the substance application (▶ Fig. 39.5). Hemospray presents the following features: The powder forms a mechanical barrier over the bleeding lesion; it absorbs the liquid and causes a serum separation with concentration of clotting factors and activates the intrinsic coagulation cascade.[51]

39.8.2 EndoClot (EndoClot Plus Inc.)

EndoClot is a polysaccharide that accelerates the coagulation cascade by binding in the wound area. There is no sufficient data for use in the lower GI tract and handling with adequate dosage is difficult because of the type of application (compressor with manual dosing). Huang et al report an effective application to prevent bleeding after endoscopic mucosal resection (EMR) in the gastrointestinal tract.[52]

39.8.3 Ankaferd Blood Stopper (Ankaferd Health Products)

Ankaferd Blood Stopper is a mix of traditional Turkish herbal components and is so far only available in Turkey.[53] The powder initiates the coagulation cascade and leads to the activation of plasma coagulation.

39.9 Mechanical Methods

Metal clips allow definitive and secure closure of bleeding vessels. The endoscopist can immediately recognize whether a vessel has been occluded. Various clips are available, with various jaw angles (9–12 mm) and lengths. The sheath with the clip is advanced through the working channel of the endoscope. If a distinct bleeding source is visible, clips are placed directly to the vessel to stop the bleeding. In case of elongated vessel opening, each of the inflow and outflow of the vessel must be treated with a clip for definitive hemostasis. Ligation using rubber bands is used for bleeding hemorrhoids. This is a simple and inexpensive treatment method, but it may be complicated by pain and the risk of rebleeding after the band has fallen off.

39.9.1 Over-the-scope Clip System (OTSC) (Ovesco, Tübingen, Germany)

The OTSC was developed primarily for the closure of perforations and fistulae. The Nitinol clip is placed on a transparent cap at the distal end of the endoscope. After suction or gapping, the lesion is pulled into the cap and the OTSC is released. In a case series, Kirschniak et al successfully treated 27 patients with bleeding episodes in the upper and lower GI tract.[54] These results were confirmed by the work of Manta et al who successfully treated 30 patients with OTSC.[55] Nevertheless the method is not the first-choice procedure because of the available alternative therapies, the challenging procedure technique and the need of changing to a special endoscope.

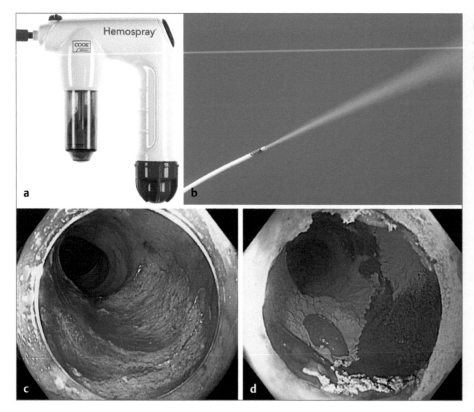

Fig. 39.5 (a) Hemospray (Cook Medical) TG 325 Application Device. **(b)** The powder is sprayed toward the bleeding lesion. **(c)** Bleeding after endoscopic mucosa resection. **(d)** After therapy with Hemospray.

39.10 Differential Endoscopic Therapy

39.10.1 Diverticula

Jensen et al[14] showed that in acute lower gastrointestinal bleeding emanating from colonic diverticula in which active bleeding (▶Fig. 39.2) or stigmata such as a visible vessel or an adherent clot were identified, patients with endoscopic therapy (epinephrine injection and bipolar coagulation) had less rebleeding, in comparison with 53% of those who did not undergo endoscopic intervention. However, these excellent results are contradicted by another study,[56] in which a retrospective analysis of diverticular bleeding was conducted. Using the same endoscopic interventional techniques, this study observed early rebleeding in 38% of cases and late rebleeding in 23%. At first glance, the results of these two studies appear contradictory. A closer look, however, reveals that Jensen et al[14] consistently advised their patients to discontinue the use of NSAIDs or acetylsalicylic acid and to follow a high-fiber diet. It is therefore possible that these additional factors help explain the divergent results and that nonendoscopic factors also play an important role in the treatment outcome. The colonic diverticular bleeding stops spontaneously in over 80% of the patients, but a rebleeding is not rare. Nowadays, interventional endoscopy and angiographic treatment have gained a leading role and surgery is only performed in case of failure of the former therapy[57] or can be for patients who are good surgical candidates and have recurrent episodes of bleeding. Shibata et al reported their experience performing a cap-assisted colonoscopy. In case of diverticular bleeding, the authors could identify a relevant diverticulum in 49% of the investigations.[58] There is no consensus regarding which endoscopic treatment is optimal. In addition to epinephrine injection and coagulation methods, mechanical hemostasis with metal clips is widely used.[14] Again, Japanese studies show effectiveness of endoscopic band ligation for colonic diverticular hemorrhage.[59] Over 3 years, the group performed endoscopy with a transparent cap at the top of the endoscope to diagnose diverticular hemorrhage in 53 patients and applied endoscopic band ligation for hemostasis in 27 patients with an identified bleeding diverticulum. A hemostasis rate of 96.3% was achieved and in 9 of 12 patients treated with endoscopic band ligation and follow-up colonoscopy revealed resolution of the responsible diverticula. Caution with use in the right-sided colon as injuries of the muscularis propria are described.[60]

Nagata et al reported the use of endoscopic detachable snare ligation (EDSL) to treat diverticular hemorrhage. The definitive bleeding diverticulum was ligated with a detachable snare, instead of a rubber band. Because of the procedure technic removal of the scope to attach the ligation device and reinsertion for treatment are not needed. Sustained hemostasis was achieved in 7 patients (88%), and early rebleeding occurred in 1 patient, in whom the applied suction seemed inadequate. No complications occurred in any patient.[61]

Recently a case report with the use of OTSC (Ovesco, Tübingen, Germany) to archive stable hemostasis for recurrent diverticular bleeding was published.[62]

39.10.2 Vascular Diseases

Endoscopic thermocoagulation has proved effective in the treatment of angiodysplasias in the colon and rectum. Successful use of heater probes, monopolar and bipolar electrocautery, Nd:YAG laser, and APC has been reported (▶Fig. 39.3). May et al[63] treated angiodysplasias in the small bowel most frequently using APC, with or without injection of a diluted epinephrine–saline solution (1:100,000) during double-balloon enteroscopy. Other groups[64,65,66] have also used APC (with a maximum energy output of 20 W)[65] to treat angiodysplasias in the small bowel. Successful injection of fibrin glue has also been reported for bleeding angiodysplasias.[64]

Three items should be noted with regard to practical application of thermocoagulation:

- Low power and short application times should be used, especially in the cecum, ascending colon, and small bowel, in order to limit the depth of coagulation. Laser coagulation is not without risk in the right hemicolon and small bowel.
- Larger vascular malformations should first be coagulated around their periphery and then in the center.
- Contact thermocoagulation procedures involve a risk of bleeding, as adherent tissue may be torn off when the probe is withdrawn. Noncontact procedures such as APC have a distinct advantage.

The treatment of vascular angioectasias in patients with chronic rectal radiation injury is a special problem. Among contact procedures, bipolar probes and heater probes were equally successful.[67] A small case series reported the efficacy of radiofrequency ablation (RFA) with the BarRx Halo (90) system in three patients with bleeding from chronic radiation proctitis. In all cases, the procedure was well tolerated and hemostasis was achieved after 1 or 2 RFA sessions. Reepithelialization of squamous mucosa was observed over areas of prior hemorrhage and no stricturing or ulceration was seen on follow-up up to 19 months after RFA treatment.[68]

39.10.3 Inflammation

In patients with IBD, circumscribed colonic bleeding sources can be treated endoscopically. Epinephrine injection, bipolar coagulation, and application of clips[46] have been successfully used in achieving hemostasis.

Schäfer et al[64] reported successful endoscopic treatment of larger erosions and ulcers in patients with CD in the proximal ileum. There are no recommendations for endoscopic therapy of colonic bleeding emanating from NSAID-induced erosions or ulcers. In practice, injection (epinephrine) therapy or clipping devices have been effective in colonic lesions. However, in the majority, bleeding in IBD patients is most often diffuse making endoscopic treatment sometimes very difficult. Application of powder could be an alternative, however, no data exist so far regarding the same.

39.10.4 Neoplasia

Both laser and APC allow endoscopic hemostasis in bleeding carcinomas. Contact methods are less suitable, as tearing off tissue after coagulation is completed can cause hemorrhagic oozing. Injection of absolute alcohol into the tumor has also been successful

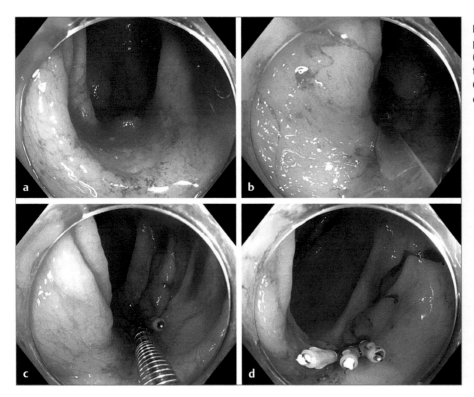

Fig. 39.6 (a) Active bleeding after polypectomy with a visible central vessel. **(b)** Needle injection of epinephrine into the wall. **(c)** Placement of clips (Olympus QuickClip2). **(d)** Successful hemostasis with clips.

in achieving hemostasis.[69] Metal clips can be tried in circumscribed bleeding sources. Endoscopically applied TC-325 (Hemospray) is a promising agent for bleeding from diffuse, vulnerable sources such as colon cancer.[70] In our department we use topical agents (Hemospray, Endoclot) to control diffuse tumor-related bleeding (▶ Fig. 39.5).

39.10.5 Bleeding after Colonic Polypectomy

Postpolypectomy bleeding is the most common complication of colonic polypectomy, occurring in 0.3 to 6.1% of polypectomies in various reports.[71,72]

Bleeding after polypectomy in the colon may occur immediately, although the time between polypectomy and bleeding can vary and may occasionally be up to 2 weeks. In the event of postpolypectomy bleeding, a variety of endoscopic techniques have proved to be safe and effective. These include loop or rubber band ligation of the remaining polyp stalk, thermocoagulation with or without preceding epinephrine injection, and application of metal clips. Bleeding can be controlled endoscopically in the majority of patients. Thus, those who perform polypectomy should also have the ability to perform hemostasis and should have the necessary tools available (▶ Fig. 39.6).

Independent risk factors for immediate bleeding after polypectomy included age greater than or equal to ≥ 65 years, cardiovascular or chronic renal disease, the use of anticoagulants, polyp size greater than 1 cm, polyp morphology, poor bowel preparation, cutting mode of electrosurgical current, and inadvertent cutting of a polyp before current application.[73] The ASGE recommends the continuation of low doses of ASA. In case of high-risk endoscopic procedures as polypectomy thienopyridine should be switched at least 5 to 7 days before to ASA monotherapy.[74]

References

[1] Qayed E, Dagar G, Nanchal RS. Lower gastrointestinal hemorrhage. Crit Care Clin. 2016; 32(2):241–254

[2] Talley NJ, Jones M. Self-reported rectal bleeding in a United States community: prevalence, risk factors, and health care seeking. Am J Gastroenterol. 1998; 93(11):2179–2183

[3] Lewis BS. Small intestinal bleeding. Gastroenterol Clin North Am. 1994; 23(1):67–91

[4] Pasha SF, Shergill A, Acosta RD, et al; ASGE Standards of Practice Committee. The role of endoscopy in the patient with lower GI bleeding. Gastrointest Endosc. 2014; 79(6):875–885

[5] Navaneethan U, Njei B, Venkatesh PG, Sanaka MR. Timing of colonoscopy and outcomes in patients with lower GI bleeding: a nationwide population-based study. Gastrointest Endosc. 2014; 79(2):297–306.e12

[6] Strate LL, Orav EJ, Syngal S. Early predictors of severity in acute lower intestinal tract bleeding. Arch Intern Med. 2003; 163(7):838–843

[7] Das A, Ben-Menachem T, Cooper GS, et al. Prediction of outcome in acute lower-gastrointestinal haemorrhage based on an artificial neural network: internal and external validation of a predictive model. Lancet. 2003; 362(9392):1261–1266

[8] Velayos FS, Williamson A, Sousa KH, et al. Early predictors of severe lower gastrointestinal bleeding and adverse outcomes: a prospective study. Clin Gastroenterol Hepatol. 2004; 2(6):485–490

[9] Zuckerman GR, Trellis DR, Sherman TM, Clouse RE. An objective measure of stool color for differentiating upper from lower gastrointestinal bleeding. Dig Dis Sci. 1995; 40(8):1614–1621

[10] Zuckerman GR, Prakash C. Acute lower intestinal bleeding: part I: clinical presentation and diagnosis. Gastrointest Endosc. 1998; 48(6):606–617

[11] Obara K, Haruma K, Irisawa A, et al. Guidelines for sedation in gastroenterological endoscopy. Dig Endosc. 2015; 27(4):435–449

[12] Ohyama T, Sakurai Y, Ito M, et al. Analysis of urgent colonoscopy for lower gastrointestinal tract bleeding. Digestion. 2000; 61(3):189–192

[13] Nagata N, Niikura R, Sakurai T, et al. Safety and effectiveness of early colonoscopy in management of acute lower gastrointestinal bleeding on the basis of propensity score matching analysis. Clin Gastroenterol Hepatol. 2016; 14(4):558–564

[14] Jensen DM, Machicado GA, Jutabha R, Kovacs TO. Urgent colonoscopy for the diagnosis and treatment of severe diverticular hemorrhage. N Engl J Med. 2000; 342(2):78–82

[15] Strate LL, Syngal S. Timing of colonoscopy: impact on length of hospital stay in patients with acute lower intestinal bleeding. Am J Gastroenterol. 2003; 98(2):317–322

[16] Green BT, Rockey DC, Portwood G, et al. Urgent colonoscopy for evaluation and management of acute lower gastrointestinal hemorrhage: a randomized controlled trial. Am J Gastroenterol. 2005; 100(11):2395–2402

[17] Chaudhry V, Hyser MJ, Gracias VH, Gau FC. Colonoscopy: the initial test for acute lower gastrointestinal bleeding. Am Surg. 1998; 64(8):723–728

[18] Strate LL. Editorial: urgent colonoscopy in lower GI bleeding: not so fast. Am J Gastroenterol. 2010; 105(12):2643–2645

[19] Gölder S. Untere gastrointestinale Blutung. In: Messmann H, ed. Lehratlas der Koloskopie. Stuttgart: Thieme; 2015:194–218

[20] Repaka A, Atkinson MR, Faulx AL, et al. Immediate unprepared hydroflush colonoscopy for severe lower GI bleeding: a feasibility study. Gastrointest Endosc. 2012; 76(2):367–373

[21] Delvaux M, Fassler I, Gay G. Clinical usefulness of the endoscopic video capsule as the initial intestinal investigation in patients with obscure digestive bleeding: validation of a diagnostic strategy based on the patient outcome after 12 months. Endoscopy. 2004; 36(12):1067–1073

[22] Kitiyakara T, Selby W. Non-small-bowel lesions detected by capsule endoscopy in patients with obscure GI bleeding. Gastrointest Endosc. 2005; 62(2):234–238

[23] Tang SJ, Christodoulou D, Zanati S, et al. Wireless capsule endoscopy for obscure gastrointestinal bleeding: a single-centre, one-year experience. Can J Gastroenterol. 2004; 18(9):559–565

[24] Jones BH, Fleischer DE, Sharma VK, et al. Yield of repeat wireless video capsule endoscopy in patients with obscure gastrointestinal bleeding. Am J Gastroenterol. 2005; 100(5):1058–1064

[25] Scheffel H, Pfammatter T, Wildi S, et al. Acute gastrointestinal bleeding: detection of source and etiology with multi-detector-row CT. Eur Radiol. 2007; 17(6):1555–1565

[26] Yoon W, Jeong YY, Shin SS, et al. Acute massive gastrointestinal bleeding: detection and localization with arterial phase multi-detector row helical CT. Radiology. 2006; 239(1):160–167

[27] García-Blázquez V, Vicente-Bártulos A, Olavarria-Delgado A, et al; EBM-Connect Collaboration. Accuracy of CT angiography in the diagnosis of acute gastrointestinal bleeding: systematic review and meta-analysis. Eur Radiol. 2013; 23(5):1181–1190

[28] Jacovides CL, Nadolski G, Allen SR, et al. Arteriography for lower gastrointestinal hemorrhage: role of preceding abdominal computed tomographic angiogram in diagnosis and localization. JAMA Surg. 2015; 150(7):650–656

[29] Walker TG, Salazar GM, Waltman AC. Angiographic evaluation and management of acute gastrointestinal hemorrhage. World J Gastroenterol. 2012; 18(11):1191–1201

[30] Leung WK, Ho SS, Suen BY, et al. Capsule endoscopy or angiography in patients with acute overt obscure gastrointestinal bleeding: a prospective randomized study with long-term follow-up. Am J Gastroenterol. 2012; 107(9):1370–1376

[31] Strate LL, Naumann CR. The role of colonoscopy and radiological procedures in the management of acute lower intestinal bleeding. Clin Gastroenterol Hepatol. 2010; 8(4):333–343, quiz e44

[32] Strate LL, Saltzman JR, Ookubo R, et al. Validation of a clinical prediction rule for severe acute lower intestinal bleeding. Am J Gastroenterol. 2005; 100(8):1821–1827

[33] Lau WY, Fan ST, Wong SH, et al. Preoperative and intraoperative localisation of gastrointestinal bleeding of obscure origin. Gut. 1987; 28(7):869–877

[34] Rockey DC. Lower gastrointestinal bleeding. Gastroenterology. 2006; 130(1):165–171

[35] Niikura R, Nagata N, Shimbo T, et al. Natural history of bleeding risk in colonic diverticulosis patients: a long-term colonoscopy-based cohort study. Aliment Pharmacol Ther. 2015; 41(9):888–894

[36] Strate LL, Liu YL, Aldoori WH, et al. Obesity increases the risks of diverticulitis and diverticular bleeding. Gastroenterology. 2009; 136(1):115–122.e1

[37] Strate LL, Gralnek IM. ACG Clinical Guideline: Management of Patients With Acute Lower Gastrointestinal Bleeding. Am J Gastroenterol. 2016; 111(4):459 –474

[38] Brandt LJ, Spinnell MK. Ability of naloxone to enhance the colonoscopic appearance of normal colon vasculature and colon vascular ectasias. Gastrointest Endosc. 1999; 49(1):79–83

[39] Brandt LJ, Mukhopadhyay D. Masking of colon vascular ectasias by cold water lavage. Gastrointest Endosc. 1999; 49(1):141–142

[40] Kjeldsen AD, Kjeldsen J. Gastrointestinal bleeding in patients with hereditary hemorrhagic telangiectasia. Am J Gastroenterol. 2000; 95(2):415–418

[41] Longacre AV, Gross CP, Gallitelli M, et al. Diagnosis and management of gastrointestinal bleeding in patients with hereditary hemorrhagic telangiectasia. Am J Gastroenterol. 2003; 98(1):59–65

[42] Teshima T, Hanks GE, Hanlon AL, et al. Rectal bleeding after conformal 3D treatment of prostate cancer: time to occurrence, response to treatment and duration of morbidity. Int J Radiat Oncol Biol Phys. 1997; 39(1):77–83

[43] Theodoropoulou A, Sfiridaki A, Oustamanolakis P, et al. Genetic risk factors in young patients with ischemic colitis. Clin Gastroenterol Hepatol. 2008; 6(8):907–911

[44] Zuckerman GR, Prakash C, Merriman RB, et al. The colon single-stripe sign and its relationship to ischemic colitis. Am J Gastroenterol. 2003; 98(9):2018–2022

[45] Chavalitdhamrong D, Jensen DM, Kovacs TO, et al. Ischemic colitis as a cause of severe hematochezia: risk factors and outcomes compared with other colon diagnoses. Gastrointest Endosc. 2011; 74(4):852–857

[46] Pardi DS, Loftus EV, Jr, Tremaine WJ, et al. Acute major gastrointestinal hemorrhage in inflammatory bowel disease. Gastrointest Endosc. 1999; 49(2):153–157

[47] Zuckerman GR, Prakash C. Acute lower intestinal bleeding. Part II: etiology, therapy, and outcomes. Gastrointest Endosc. 1999; 49(2):228–238

[48] Villanueva C, Colomo A, Bosch A, et al. Transfusion strategies for acute upper gastrointestinal bleeding. N Engl J Med. 2013; 368(1):11–21

[49] Havanond C, Havanond P. Argon plasma coagulation therapy for acute non-variceal upper gastrointestinal bleeding. Cochrane Database Syst Rev. 2005(2):CD003791

[50] Rey JF, Beilenhoff U, Neumann CS, Dumonceau JM; European Society of Gastrointestinal Endoscopy (ESGE). European Society of Gastrointestinal Endoscopy (ESGE) guideline: the use of electrosurgical units. Endoscopy. 2010; 42(9):764–772

[51] Wong Kee Song LM, Banerjee S, Barth BA, et al; ASGE Technology Committee. Emerging technologies for endoscopic hemostasis. Gastrointest Endosc. 2012; 75(5):933–937

[52] Huang R, Pan Y, Hui N, et al. Polysaccharide hemostatic system for hemostasis management in colorectal endoscopic mucosal resection. Dig Endosc. 2014; 26(1):63–68

[53] Holster IL, Brullet E, Kuipers EJ, et al. Hemospray treatment is effective for lower gastrointestinal bleeding. Endoscopy. 2014; 46(1):75–78

[54] Kirschniak A, Subotova N, Zieker D, et al. The Over-the-scope clip (OTSC) for the treatment of gastrointestinal bleeding, perforations, and fistulas. Surg Endosc. 2011; 25(9):2901–2905

[55] Manta R, Galloro G, Mangiavillano B, et al. Over-the-scope clip (OTSC) represents an effective endoscopic treatment for acute GI bleeding after failure of conventional techniques. Surg Endosc. 2013; 27(9):3162–3164

[56] Bloomfeld RS, Rockey DC, Shetzline MA. Endoscopic therapy of acute diverticular hemorrhage. Am J Gastroenterol. 2001; 96(8):2367–2372

[57] Cirocchi R, Grassi V, Cavaliere D, et al. New Trends in Acute Management of Colonic Diverticular Bleeding: A Systematic Review. Medicine (Baltimore). 2015; 94(44):e1710

[58] Shibata S, Shigeno T, Fujimori K, et al. Colonic diverticular hemorrhage: the hood method for detecting responsible diverticula and endoscopic band ligation for hemostasis. Endoscopy. 2014; 46(1):66–69

[59] Ishii N, Setoyama T, Deshpande GA, et al. Endoscopic band ligation for colonic diverticular hemorrhage. Gastrointest Endosc. 2012; 75(2):382–387

[60] Barker KB, Arnold HL, Fillman EP, et al. Safety of band ligator use in the small bowel and the colon. Gastrointest Endosc. 2005; 62(2):224–227

[61] Akutsu D, Narasaka T, Wakayama M, et al. Endoscopic detachable snare ligation: a new treatment method for colonic diverticular hemorrhage. Endoscopy. 2015; 47(11):1039–1042

[62] Kassab I, Dressner R, Gorcey S. Over-the-scope clip for control of a recurrent diverticular bleed. ACG Case Rep J. 2015; 3(1):5–6

[63] May A, Nachbar L, Pohl J, Ell C. Endoscopic interventions in the small bowel using double balloon enteroscopy: feasibility and limitations. Am J Gastroenterol. 2007; 102(3):527–535

[64] Schäfer C, Rothfuss K, Kreichgauer HP, Stange EF. Efficacy of double-balloon enteroscopy in the evaluation and treatment of bleeding and non-bleeding small bowel disease. Z Gastroenterol. 2007; 45(3):237–243

[65] Heine GD, Hadithi M, Groenen MJ, et al. Double-balloon enteroscopy: indications, diagnostic yield, and complications in a series of 275 patients with suspected small-bowel disease. Endoscopy. 2006; 38(1):42–48

[66] Suzuki T, Matsushima M, Okita I, et al. Clinical utility of double-balloon enteroscopy for small intestinal bleeding. Dig Dis Sci. 2007; 52(8):1914–1918

[67] Kwan V, Bourke MJ, Williams SJ, et al. Argon plasma coagulation in the management of symptomatic gastrointestinal vascular lesions: experience in 100 consecutive patients with long-term follow-up. Am J Gastroenterol. 2006; 101(1):58–63

[68] Zhou C, Adler DC, Becker L, et al. Effective treatment of chronic radiation proctitis using radiofrequency ablation. Therap Adv Gastroenterol. 2009; 2(3):149–156

[69] Beejay U, Marcon NE. Endoscopic treatment of lower gastrointestinal bleeding. Curr Opin Gastroenterol. 2002; 18(1):87–93

[70] Soulellis CA, Carpentier S, Chen YI, et al. Lower GI hemorrhage controlled with endoscopically applied TC-325 (with videos). Gastrointest Endosc. 2013; 77(3):504–507

[71] Levin TR, Zhao W, Conell C, et al. Complications of colonoscopy in an integrated health care delivery system. Ann Intern Med. 2006; 145(12):880–886

[72] Sorbi D, Norton I, Conio M, et al. Postpolypectomy lower GI bleeding: descriptive analysis. Gastrointest Endosc. 2000; 51(6):690–696

[73] Kim HS, Kim TI, Kim WH, et al. Risk factors for immediate postpolypectomy bleeding of the colon: a multicenter study. Am J Gastroenterol. 2006; 101(6):1333–1341

[74] Acosta RD, Abraham NS, Chandrasekhara V, et al; ASGE Standards of Practice Committee. The management of antithrombotic agents for patients undergoing GI endoscopy. Gastrointest Endosc. 2016; 83(1):3–16

40 Anorectal Diseases

Disaya Chavalitdhamrong and Rome Jutabha

40.1 Introduction

Anorectal disease refers to diseases of the anus and rectum such as hemorrhoids, anal fissures, anorectal abscesses, anal fistulas, and anal cancer. Inspection, perianal palpation, digital examination, abdominal examination, and rectovaginal palpation provide initial assessment. In cases of painful anal lesions, topical, regional, or even general anesthesia may be required. Anoscopy and sigmoidoscopy are often required for further evaluation. Rectal endoscopic ultrasound is particularly important in certain conditions. Patients may delay seeking medical advice because of embarrassment. Understanding of the pathophysiology and anatomy is critical to success in management of anorectal disease. We herein review anorectal diseases including its pathophysiology; inflammation, infection, vascular cause, neoplasm, and mechanical cause.

40.2 Inflammation

40.2.1 Crohn's Disease

Symptoms and signs related to perianal disease occur in 35 to 45% of patients with Crohn's disease (CD). The major perianal complications include anal fissures, anorectal fistulae, and abscesses. Conservative treatment of anorectal diseases in CD patients has been advocated given the high risk of complications and the evidence that spontaneous healing may also occur.[1]

Anal Fissure

Diagnosis

Fissures are present in up to 19% of patients with CD.[2] Anal fissure in CD may be asymptomatic or present with bleeding, deep ulceration, or anal pain, which may be worsened during evacuation. Nonhealing fissures or deeper ulcers may lead to fistula or perianal abscess formation. Chronic fissure can lead to stricture formation.

Treatment

Treatments consist of keeping the area clean and dry. The first line of treatment should be medical management including nitroglycerin paste, topical calcium channel blockers, and botulinum toxin.[3] These treatments are successful in up to 80% of cases.[3] In the case of nonhealing symptomatic fissure, proctitis should be ruled out.[3] Topical nitroglycerin 0.2% has not been evaluated in anal fissure in CD. Surgery such as lateral internal sphincterotomy may require in fissures that are resistant to conservative treatment, but it should be reserved to carefully selected patients.[4] It was reported that 40% of patients suffered from postoperative complications even without active rectal disease.[4]

Perianal Fistula

Anorectal fistula develops in 20 to 30% of patients with CD.[2] Fistulae are usually the consequence of penetration of an abscess. The fistulous openings most commonly involve the perianal skin but can also be in the groin, vulva, and scrotum. Fistulae can be classified as simple (superficial, inter-, or transsphincteric fistula below the dentate line, with a single opening and no anorectal stricture or abscess), or complex (trans-, supra-, or extrasphincteric fistula above the dentate line, or a fistula with multiple external openings, associated abscess, or stricture, or rectovaginal fistula).[5]

Diagnosis

Fistula can present with anal pain, painful defecation, and perianal opening with purulent discharge. Physical examination may reveal perianal openings, pneumaturia, and passage of stool through the vagina if urinary bladder or vagina is involved, respectively. Evaluation of the anatomy includes probing under general anesthesia, fistulography, barium studies, ultrasound, computed tomography (CT), and magnetic resonance imaging (MRI).[6] The combination of different imaging modalities appears to be more accurate than any one modality alone.[6]

Treatment

Treatment of the underlying CD is needed. A combined medical and surgical approach offers the best chance for success. Medication options include antibiotics (such as metronidazole and ciprofloxacin), immunosuppressives (6-mercaptopurine and azathioprine, cyclosporine, and tacrolimus), and immunomodulators (infliximab and adalimumab).[3] In the presence of proctitis, medical therapy should be continued until there is adequate resolution of proctitis. Surgery should be considered in patients with simple low intersphincteric fistulae or fistulae refractory to medical therapy or with severe symptoms.

Anorectal Abscesses

Diagnosis

Anorectal abscesses develop in 50% of patients with perianal CD especially in patients with anal fistulae. The abscesses can be seen at perianal area or can be felt via digital rectal examination or seen on CT scan.

Treatment

Prompt surgical incision and drainage and treatment with broad-spectrum antibiotics are mandatory. In the presence of a fistula, a noncutting seton can be placed to prevent recurrence and facilitate drainage.[3]

40.2.2 Perianal Abscesses

A perianal abscess is a collection of purulent material that arises from glandular crypts in the anus or rectum.

Diagnosis

Patients with a perianal abscess often present with severe pain in the anal or rectal area. Purulent rectal drainage may be noted. Physical examination may reveal palpable perirectal mass. It is important to distinguish anorectal abscess from other perianal suppurative processes.[7]

Treatment

Anal abscesses should be drained early. The placement of a seton should be considered when the internal opening is identifiable. Antibiotic therapy is unnecessary in uncomplicated anorectal abscess.[7] The key to successful treatment is the eradication of the primary tract. As surgery may lead to a disturbance of continence, several sphincter-preserving techniques have been developed.[7]

40.2.3 Anorectal Fistula

The most common etiology of an anorectal fistula is an anorectal abscess. Other causes of anorectal fistulae include CD, lymphogranuloma venereum, radiation proctitis, rectal foreign bodies, and actinomycosis.

Diagnosis

A fistula can be explored with a fistula probe. The internal opening in the anus can be viewed by an anoscopic examination, while a sigmoidoscope may be required to view the internal opening in the rectum.

Treatment

Surgical treatment is the mainstay of therapy and is required in patients with symptomatic anorectal fistulae. The goal of surgical therapy is to eradicate the fistula while preserving fecal continence. Fistulotomy is the main surgical therapy. Fistulectomy and primary sphincteroplasty could be the therapeutic options for complex anal fistula. Reported success rates were very high and the risk of postoperative fecal incontinence was lower than after simple fistulotomy.[8] Permacol collagen paste and fibrin glue are new options for the treatment of anorectal fistula.[9,10] Permacol paste functions by filling the fistula tract with an acellular cross-linked porcine dermal collagen matrix suspension. It is shown to be effective in treating primary and recurrent anorectal fistula.[9] Fibrin glue is a novel treatment for anal fistulae.[10] Fibrin glue has shown to heal more complex fistulae than fistulotomy.[10]

40.3 Infection

Infectious proctitis is the rectal inflammation caused by the infectious pathogens typically being sexually acquired. Among men who have sex with men (MSM) with clinical proctitis, chlamydia and gonorrhea are the most frequently identified pathogens in the rectum.[11] Approximately 85% of rectal gonorrhea and chlamydia infections are asymptomatic, and many patients who are infected rectally are not simultaneously infected at other anatomical sites.[12] The Centers for Disease Control and Prevention (CDC) recommends at least annual screening for chlamydia and gonorrhea in MSM at the urethral, pharyngeal, or rectal site based on recent exposure.[13]

40.3.1 Chlamydial Infection

Diagnosis

Chlamydia is the most frequently reported bacterial sexually transmitted infection. Chlamydial proctitis occurs primarily in MSM who engage in receptive anal intercourse, with a positivity in a screening population of 3 to 10.5%.[14] Chlamydia can also infect the rectum in women, either through receptive anal sex or spreading from the cervix and vagina. It can cause symptoms of proctitis including rectal pain, discharge, or bleeding. The incubation period for Chlamydia is 5 to 14 days. Infection can be caused by D–K and L serovars. Obtaining a diagnosis for rectal chlamydia can be challenging. Culture is limited to research and reference laboratories. Serology can support the diagnosis, but is not standardized and requires a high level of expertise to interpret. Antigen detection by swab has generally shown good sensitivity and specificity for urogenital chlamydia; however, for rectal swab, the limited data suggest a sensitivity of less than 50%.[15] Several studies have shown that nucleic acid amplification tests (NAATs) on rectal specimens are more sensitive than culture in detecting rectal chlamydia and still have high specificity. In particular, the use of a transcription-mediated amplification method seems to show consistently strong results.[16]

Treatment

Empiric therapy for both chlamydia and gonorrhea is indicated for acute proctitis. A regimen of doxycycline (100 mg twice daily for 7 days) or azithromycin (1 g orally once) plus a single intramuscular dose of ceftriaxone (250 mg) is active against both. Abstaining from sex for 1 week after initiation of treatment decreases transmission, and treatment of partners decreases reinfection.[17]

40.3.2 Gonococcal Proctitis

Diagnosis

Neisseria gonorrhoeae can be transmitted by oral–anal, anoreceptive intercourse, or spreading from cervical or urethral gonorrhea. Most women and approximately half of men with anorectal gonorrhea are asymptomatic.[18] The classic anoscopic examination of gonorrhea includes thick purulent discharge. NAATs are preferred tests. The transcription-mediated amplification shows greater sensitivity compared with culture and similar specificity.[19] NAATs do not require the careful handling required for culture and can detect both gonorrhea and chlamydia.[17] These are more expensive than culture and cannot provide information on antibiotic susceptibility.[17]

Treatment

Therapy for both gonorrhea and chlamydia with ceftriaxone and doxycycline is indicated for the treatment of patients with acute proctitis.

40.3.3 Herpes Simplex Virus

Diagnosis

Both herpes simplex viruses 1 and 2 (HSV-1 and HSV-2) can cause genital herpes (▶ Fig. 40.1).[17] Transmission is via anal, vaginal, or oral sex.[17] Most people with HSV are asymptomatic. Clinical manifestations include vesicles, ulcers on or near the anus, genitals, or mouth. It can also manifest as proctitis. The first outbreak may be associated with fever, lymphadenopathy, or body aches. Recurrences are typical, shorter in duration and less severe. The standard diagnostic test is viral culture.[17] Polymerase chain reaction (PCR) test is more accurate and rapid.[17] Serologic tests are for recurrent disease.[17]

Treatment

There is no cure for herpes. Antiviral medications prevent or shorten outbreaks, reduce transmission rates, and decrease the duration of viral shedding.[17] Acyclovir 400 mg five times a day for 10 days is for herpes proctitis. Acyclovir 400 mg three times a day for 7 to 10 days is for perianal lesions (5 days for recurrent disease). Acyclovir 400 mg two times a day is for suppression. Antiviral alternatives include famciclovir and valacyclovir.[20]

40.3.4 Syphilis

Diagnosis

Anal chancres are painful and resolve after 3 to 6 weeks whether treated or not. Secondary syphilis may also include mucous membrane lesions of the anus and rectum. Condyloma lata may also develop in areas including the groin. The screening tests are venereal disease research laboratory (VDRL) and rapid plasma reagin (RPR).[17] The confirmation test is a treponemal test such as fluorescent treponemal antibody absorption (FTA-ABS) test.[17]

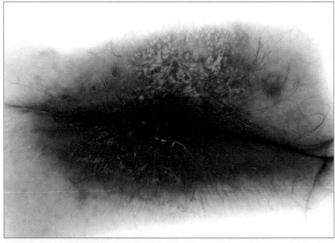

Fig. 40.1 Anal herpes.

Treatment

A single intramuscular (IM) dose of 2.4 million units of benzathine penicillin G cures a person with syphilis for less than a year.[17] Additional doses are needed for those with syphilis for longer than a year.[17] All patients should undergo testing for human immunodeficiency virus (HIV). Follow-up should occur at 6 and 12 months after treatment.[17]

40.3.5 Lymphogranuloma Venereum

Diagnosis

It is caused by the species *Chlamydia trachomatis*. The serovars are most commonly L1, L2, or L3. Lymphogranuloma venereum (LGV) can result in proctocolitis with anal pain via anal receptive sex. It can progress to colorectal fistulae and strictures if not treated early. Diagnosis is generally based on clinical suspicion and can be verified by NAATS.[17]

Treatment

Doxycycline 100 mg orally twice daily for 21 days.[17] An alternative regimen is erythromycin base 500 mg orally four times a day for 21 days.[17]

40.4 Vascular Cause

40.4.1 Ischemic Proctitis

Diagnosis

Ischemic proctitis commonly occurs at the splenic, descending, and sigmoid colon (▶ Fig. 40.2).[21] The rectum is involved in only 2 to 5% of cases because of its abundant collateral blood supply.[21] Risk factors include major vascular occlusive disease, disruption of collateral circulation, and low-flow state.[21] Although CT scan can suggest the diagnosis and identify other causes of clinical deterioration, colonoscopy remains the key test in diagnosing and determining the extent of ischemic change.[21]

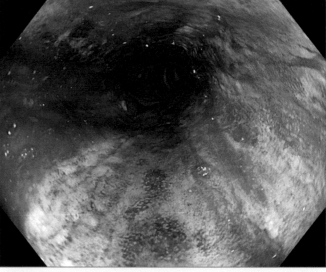

Fig. 40.2 Ischemic proctitis.

Treatment

Treatment is nonoperative for nongangrenous ischemic proctocolitis, whereas surgery is necessary for gangrenous, transmural rectal ischemia. The extent of resection will be determined intraoperatively by the appearance of the bowel.[21]

40.4.2 Radiation Proctitis

Diagnosis

Acute radiation proctitis occurs during or within 6 months of radiation therapy.[22] Chronic radiation proctitis often occurs 9 to 14 months following radiation exposure, but can occur any time postirradiation up to 30 years after exposure.[23] Endoscopic findings are nonspecific such as pallor, friability, and telangiectasias. Findings may include strictures, ulcerations, fistulae, and areas of mucosal hemorrhage in chronic radiation proctitis. In the acute phase of radiation proctitis, extensive mucosal inflammation, eosinophilic infiltration of the submucosa, crypt atrophy, and crypt abscesses are observed on histology.[22] Chronic damage is characterized by obliterative enteritis with ulceration and fibrous induration of the gut.[24] The cardinal sign of chronic radiation proctitis that distinguishes it from acute radiation proctitis is the presence of small-vessel vasculopathy.[25]

Treatment

Acute radiation proctitis needs supportive treatment consisting of hydration and antidiarrheals as needed and butyrate enemas, as these may accelerate healing in acute radiation proctitis. Chronic radiation proctitis may need sucralfate or glucocorticoid enemas (e.g., hydrocortisone enema 100 mg twice daily). Most instances of proctitis are self-limited and respond to medical management. Endoscopic therapy may be required in patients who fail to medical treatments. Currently available endoscopic modalities are formalin instillation, potassium titanyl phosphate (KTP) laser, neodymium:yttrium-aluminum-garnet (Nd:YAG) laser, argon laser, bipolar electrocoagulation, heater probe, argon plasma coagulation (APC), and newer methods including cryotherapy, and radiofrequency ablation.[26] The paucity of well-controlled, blinded, randomized studies makes it impossible to fully assess the comparative efficacy of the different endoscopic and medical therapies for chronic radiation proctitis.[25] APC seems to be the most effective and the main endoscopic therapy in managing bleeding from radiation proctitis.[25,26]

Complications of endoscopic therapy have been reported. Balloon dilation for radiation-related strictures is associated with increased risk of perforation in patients with long or angulated strictures. It is therefore suitable for short strictured segment.[22] Transmural necrosis, fibrosis, stricture formation, and rectovaginal fistula have been reported with use of lasers.[27] The risk of necrosis or stricture is less with KTP laser compared to Nd:YAG laser.[22] Bipolar electrocoagulation and the heater probe cause less tissue injury compared to laser therapy.[22] The APC causes limited depth of coagulation (0.5–3 mm) that minimizes the risks of perforation, stenosis, and fistulization. Radiofrequency ablation and cryotherapy are newer methods that cover larger area per application. Radiofrequency ablation is limited to the superficial mucosa (0.5–1 mm), thereby avoiding deep tissue injury.[28] Cecal perforation caused by gas overdistention has been reported with cryotherapy.[29] Surgery should be reserved for patients who have intractable symptoms such as a stricture, pain, bleeding, perforation, or a fistula.

40.5 Neoplasm

40.5.1 Anal Cancer

Diagnosis

Rectal bleeding, anorectal pain, or sensation of a rectal mass are among the most common initial symptoms of anal cancer (▶ Fig. 40.3). Major contributing factors for the increase in anal cancer incidence include increasing receptive anal intercourse, increasing human papillomavirus (HPV) infections, and longer life expectancy of treated people who are seropositive for HIV.[30] High-risk populations include HIV-positive MSM, HIV-negative MSM, HIV-positive individuals, and women with a history of cervical cancer.[31] HPV has been detected in over 90% of anal cancers.[31] A tumor node metastasis (TNM) staging system for anal canal cancers is based on tumor size/invasion of adjacent structures and the presence or absence of nodal or distant metastases.

Treatment

Combined chemoradiotherapy has emerged as the preferred method of treatment for anal canal cancer because it can cure many patients while preserving the anal sphincter. Surgical therapy is reserved for recurrent or persistent disease after chemoradiotherapy. HPV vaccine may be useful as prevention of anal cancer and adjuvant therapy for anal cancer.[30,31]

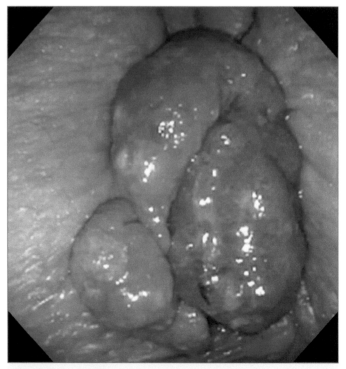

Fig. 40.3 Anal cancer.

40.5.2 Anal Intraepithelial Neoplasia

Diagnosis

The prevalence of anal intraepithelial neoplasia has been increasing, especially in high-risk patients, including MSM, HIV-positive patients, and those who are immunosuppressed.[32] The histopathologic manifestations of HPV in anal intraepithelial neoplasia are most apparent at the anal transition zone. The progression from low-grade to high-grade anal intraepithelial neoplasia includes HIV-related immunosuppression with a lower CD4 cell count, anal HPV infection, and the presence of multiple HPV types including the high-risk types. The rate of progression from high-grade anal intraepithelial neoplasia to invasive anal cancer is about 5%.[32] Anal intraepithelial neoplasia is usually asymptomatic although it may be associated with local symptoms. The diagnosis requires anal cytology and biopsy specimens.

Treatment

Trichloroacetic acid, infrared coagulation, or electrocautery can be used for intra-anal lesions. Topical imiquimod or 5-fluorouracil may be used intra-anally or prior to surgical intervention for perianal lesions.[32] Wide local excision and targeted ablation with electrocautery, infrared coagulation, or cryotherapy are treatments for perianal lesions.[32] Recurrence rates remain high regardless of treatment delivered and surveillance is paramount.[32] The HPV vaccine is approved for prevention of the HPV infection and development of HPV-related anal cancer.[30]

40.6 Mechanical Cause

40.6.1 Hemorrhoids

Internal Hemorrhoids

The cardinal signs of internal hemorrhoids are painless bleeding with bowel movements and intermittent, reducible protrusion.

Diagnosis

Hemorrhoids should be diagnosed by history and physical examination. The source of bleeding requires confirmation by endoscopic studies. Physical examination should include visual inspection of the anus, both at rest and while straining, and digital examination for other anal pathology.[33] Internal hemorrhoids can be graded based on their history: first-degree hemorrhoids

Table 40.1 Medical therapy for hemorrhoids

Stop aspirin and NSAIDs

Avoid straining with bowel movements, prolong standing, or heavy lifting

Use fiber supplementation and drink extra, nonalcoholic fluids

Take daily stool softeners during severe episodes

Use hydrocortisone suppositories or creams

Use frequent sitz baths (warm water without soap or irritants)

Reduce prolapsing hemorrhoids after bowel movements or exercise

Avoid dietary irritants such as pepper, spices, coffee, or caffeine

NSAIDs, nonsteroidal anti-inflammatory drugs.

do not prolapse, second-degree hemorrhoids prolapse but self-reduce, third-degree hemorrhoids protrude and require manual reduction, and fourth-degree hemorrhoids protrude and cannot be reduced.[33]

Treatment

Patient should be instructed to avoid prolonged straining or sitting during bowel movements, minimize heavy weight lifting or prolonged standing, decrease constipation by taking supplement fiber, stool softeners, and extra water, cleanse the anorectal area with sitz baths, use topical agents to reduce hemorrhoid size (suppositories or creams), and avoid dietary irritants or condiments (such as caffeine, spicy food, and pepper) that may contribute to pruritus. Summaries of the medical treatment of hemorrhoids are shown in ▶ Table 40.1.

Endoscopic treatments usually reserved for patients with grades 1 to 3 internal hemorrhoids, who do not respond to medical management. Hemorrhoid grade is the most important factor in selecting the optimal treatment modality. A total of three segments are usually treated during each session. Treatment of contiguous segments should be avoided because it can result in large confluent ulcers, severe rectal bleeding, pain, or spasm. Symptoms are usually improved in 85 to 90% of patients. Treatment is usually three to five sessions. Recurrences can be reduced by strict adherence to medical therapies. Complications include rectal pain or spasm, bleeding, ulceration (▶ Fig. 40.4), urinary retention, and stricture formation. Surgical referral should be considered for those who are refractory to or cannot tolerate office procedures or who have fourth-degree hemorrhoids.[33,34]

Procedures including bipolar electrocoagulation (electrical energy), direct current electrocoagulation (electrical energy), infrared coagulation (light energy), heat probe coagulation (thermal energy), injection sclerotherapy, and band ligation should be considered in grades 1 to 3 hemorrhoids that remain symptomatic after medical therapy.[35,36,37,38,39,40,41,42]

Bipolar electrocoagulation is quickly and easily performed with minimal pain.[35,38] The probes are inexpensive. Treatments are performed through a slotted anoscope at a generator setting

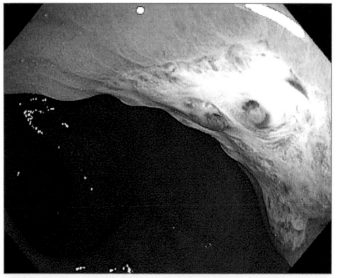

Fig. 40.4 Rectal ulcer following hemorrhoid band ligation.

of between 12 and 16 W with 1-second pulse duration. The base of the internal hemorrhoid segment above the dentate line is coagulated with 4 to 7 pulses per hemorrhoid segment. Treatments are separated at 4- to 6-week interval for a treatment end point of hemorrhoid grade 1 and resolution of bleeding. The response rate is more than 90%. The recurrence rate is 10 to 20% per year and be treated with repeated bipolar electrocoagulation.

Infrared coagulation using Infrared Coagulator IRC2100 probe is another widely used method.[39,40] The tip of the IRC probe is gently placed in contact with the tissue and then three to five applications of 1.5-second pulses are applied to each hemorrhoid above the dentate line. Repeat treatments are recommended at 4 to 6 weeks. The main advantages of infrared coagulation are its ease of use, low cost, minimal complication rate.

Injection sclerotherapy uses for grades 1 to 3 internal hemorrhoids.[43,44] Submucosal injections of various sclerosing agents such as phenol in almond oil, aluminum potassium sulfate and tannic acid, quinine, ethanolamine, or diluted alcohol have the advantage of being an easy, fast, and inexpensive procedure. However, serious complications have been reported including severe rectal pain, hematoma, perirectal abscesses, and sepsis.

Band ligation is a safe, effective, and widely available treatment for grades 2 and 3 internal hemorrhoids.[35,36,37,40] Because of its low cost, ease of use, low rate of adverse events, and relative effectiveness, band ligation is currently the most widely used technique.[41] Treatment can be performed in an antegrade or retroflexed position by using single or multishot devices. Banding in retroflexion with a diagnostic endoscope might be preferred. Bands are released around the hemorrhoid base above the dentate line. An average of three to four bands are placed during each session. Treatments are repeated at 4- to 6-week intervals until symptoms are controlled and hemorrhoids are reduced to grade 0 to 1. There may be self-limited bleeding for 3 to 5 days after banding. Patients may also experience a dull ache or fullness.

A comparative study of bipolar versus direct current electrocoagulation for treatment of bleeding internal hemorrhoids showed that both were effective for control of chronic bleeding from grades 1 to 3 internal hemorrhoids.[45] Bipolar probe was significantly faster than direct current probe.[45] A comparative study of heater and bipolar coagulation revealed that the techniques and complications of heater and bipolar probes were similar.[38] Failures and crossovers were less frequent, and the time to symptom relief was shorter with the heater probe than with the bipolar probe.[38] New bipolar tissue ligator combines constant tissue compression and temperature guidance accomplished the desired histologic changes with less muscular damage at much lower temperatures than the infrared coagulator.[46] Band ligation is more effective but associated with more pain and discomfort to the patient compared to infrared coagulation.[40] Infrared coagulation could be considered to be a suitable alternative office procedure for the treatment of early-stage hemorrhoids.[40]

Recommendations

Bipolar probe electrocoagulation and infrared coagulation are the endoscopic treatments of choice for symptomatic grades 1 and 2 bleeding internal hemorrhoids because of their well-established safety, efficacy, and ease of application. Grade 3 internal hemorrhoids are best treated by endoscopic band ligation.[35] Grade 4 internal hemorrhoids require surgical intervention. Surgical intervention should be considered for patients who fail endoscopic treatments or for those who cannot return for serial treatments or if endoscopic treatments are contraindicated.

External Hemorrhoids

Diagnosis

External hemorrhoid is recognized on physical examination. Symptomatic external hemorrhoids typically cause thrombosis and pain.[42] Thrombosed external hemorrhoids reveal tender blue lump at the anal verge.

Treatment

External hemorrhoids are not amenable to anoscopic or endoscopic treatment and require surgical intervention for severe or persistent symptoms. Surgery may be superior to conservative treatment, but there is no evidence regarding the optimal period of conservative management.[47] It depends on the time of identification for a thrombosed external hemorrhoid. Most patients who present urgently within 3 days of onset of pain benefit from excision.[33]

40.6.2 Rectal Prolapse

Diagnosis

Rectal prolapse is a pelvic floor disorder that typically occurs in elderly women, but can occur in men and women of all ages (▶ Fig. 40.5). Rectal prolapse results in local symptoms and bowel dysfunction. A complete rectal prolapse is the protrusion of all layers of the rectum through the anus. Partial prolapse involves prolapse of the mucosa only. The diagnosis is typically made by the clinical evaluation. The protrusion may be intermittent.

Treatment

Surgical repair procedure either by an intra-abdominal or perineal approach is the main therapy.[48] The range of surgical methods available to correct the underlying pelvic floor defects in full-thickness rectal prolapse reflects the lack of consensus regarding the best operation.[49] Perineal stapled prolapse resection is a relatively newly reported technique that appears to be an easy, fast, and safe procedure.[50] Indications for surgery include the presence of rectal prolapse, the sensation of a mass from the prolapsed bowel, fecal incontinence, and/or constipation associated with rectal prolapse.

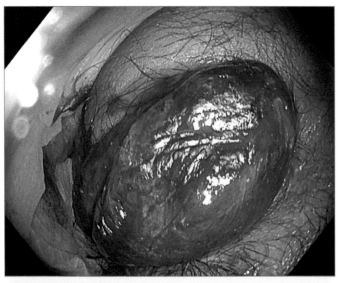

Fig. 40.5 Rectal prolapse.

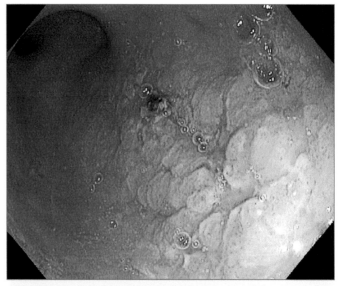

Fig. 40.6 An endoscopic appearance of solitary rectal ulcer syndrome (SRUS) as a polypoidal growth.

40.6.3 Solitary Rectal Ulcer Syndrome

Diagnosis

Solitary rectal ulcer syndrome (SRUS) is associated with reduced blood perfusion of the rectal mucosa, leading to local ischemia and ulceration.[51] It is frequently associated with pelvic floor disorders.[52] It can present with rectal bleeding, mucous discharge, prolonged excessive straining during defecation, perineal and abdominal pain, pelvic fullness and a sense of incomplete evacuation, and constipation.[52] The endoscopic appearance is not specific and may manifest as a solitary ulcer (20%), multiple ulcers (40%), polypoidal growth, and erythematous patches[52,53] (▶ Fig. 40.6). The diagnosis is made on the basis of histopathologic findings of fibromuscular obliteration of the lamina propria with splaying of the muscularis mucosae upward between the crypts, thickened mucosa, and glandular distortion.[51] Diffuse collage deposition in the lamina propria and abnormal smooth muscle fiber extensions are sensitive markers for differentiating SRUS from other conditions.[52] Rectal endoscopic ultrasonography can be useful in the evaluation of SRUS and ruling out an associated malignancy.[54] The characteristic findings are thick hyperechoic submucosa and thick hypoechoic muscularis propria with an intermediate hyperechoic layer.[54]

Treatment

Conservative management includes bulk laxatives, retraining of bowel habits using biofeedback in patients with dyssynergic defecation.[55] Treatment with topical glucocorticoids, salicylates, sucralfate enemas, botulinum toxin, and APC has been described.[56] Surgical options are for nonhealing SRUS and include local excision, rectopexy, fecal diversion, or combined laparoscopic resection rectopexy and transanal endoscopic microsurgery.[57]

40.6.4 Anal Fissure

Diagnosis

Anal fissure, acute or chronic, may result from high anal pressure, local trauma, or secondary to an underlying medical/surgical condition. The diagnosis is based on the history of painful defecation and the physical examination finding of a superficial tear in the anoderm. The pathognomonic feature of an acute fissure is a superficial tear, while a chronic fissure appears hypertrophied with skin tags and/or papillae.

Treatment

Most acute anal fissures respond to conservative treatment including high-fiber diet, sitz baths, topical analgesic, and one of the topical vasodilators (nifedipine or nitroglycerin) for I to 2 months. Colonoscopy to rule out Crohn's disease is required for patients with persistent symptoms for more than 2 months. Relief of constipation should also be addressed. Conservative treatments result in healing in up to 70% of fissures.[58] Either botulinum toxin injection or a lateral internal sphincterotomy, or both therapies are the options for the patients who fail medical treatment.[58,59] In patients with Crohn's disease or HIV, maximizing medical therapy is the mainstay of treatment.[58] Surgery such as fissurectomy is a primary treatment option for the chronic anal fissure.[60]

40.6.5 Stercoral Ulcer

Diagnosis

Stercoral ulceration originates in severe chronic constipation.[61] The clinical presentation is nonspecific with lower abdominal pain and rectal bleeding. The large bowel, usually the sigmoid colon, is subjected to ischemia, ulceration, necrosis, and

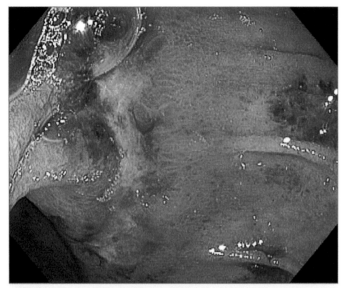

Fig. 40.7 Stercoral ulcer in sigmoid colon.

perforation (▶Fig. 40.7).[51] Stercoral ulcer perforation most frequently occurs at the antimesenteric border of the sigmoid colon and rectosigmoid junction. These areas have relatively decreased blood flow, are subject to increased pressure as a result of the narrower lumen, and the location of the most dehydrated stool.[62] The rectum and descending colon are the next most common locations of perforation.[62]

Treatment

Treatment of constipation helps prevent the stercoral ulcer. Treatment of stercoral ulcer perforation is a surgical emergency and generally consists of broad-spectrum parenteral antibiotics and urgent resection of the affected colorectal segment with Hartmann's procedure.[62]

References

[1] D'Ugo S, Franceschilli L, Cadeddu F, et al. Medical and surgical treatment of haemorrhoids and anal fissure in Crohn's disease: a critical appraisal. BMC Gastroenterol. 2013; 13:47

[2] Keighley MR, Allan RN. Current status and influence of operation on perianal Crohn's disease. Int J Colorectal Dis. 1986; 1(2):104–107

[3] Lewis RT, Maron DJ. Anorectal Crohn's disease. Surg Clin North Am. 2010; 90(1):83–97 Table of Contents

[4] Cracco N, Zinicola R. Sphincterotomy for anal fissure in Crohn's disease: is it dangerous? Int J Colorectal Dis. 2016; 31(3):761

[5] Sandborn WJ, Fazio VW, Feagan BG, Hanauer SB; American Gastroenterological Association Clinical Practice Committee. AGA technical review on perianal Crohn's disease. Gastroenterology. 2003; 125(5):1508–1530

[6] Schwartz DA, Wiersema MJ, Dudiak KM, et al. A comparison of endoscopic ultrasound, magnetic resonance imaging, and exam under anesthesia for evaluation of Crohn's perianal fistulas. Gastroenterology. 2001; 121(5):1064–1072

[7] Amato A, Bottini C, De Nardi P, et al; Italian society of colorectal surgery. Evaluation and management of perianal abscess and anal fistula: a consensus statement developed by the Italian Society of Colorectal Surgery (SICCR). Tech Coloproctol. 2015; 19(10):595–606

[8] Ratto C, Litta F, Donisi L, Parello A. Fistulotomy or fistulectomy and primary sphincteroplasty for anal fistula (FIPS): a systematic review. Tech Coloproctol. 2015; 19(7):391–400

[9] Giordano P, Sileri P, Buntzen S, et al. A prospective multicentre observational study of Permacol collagen paste for anorectal fistula: preliminary results. Colorectal Dis. 2016; 18(3):286–294

[10] Lindsey I, Smilgin-Humphreys MM, Cunningham C, et al. A randomized, controlled trial of fibrin glue vs. conventional treatment for anal fistula. Dis Colon Rectum. 2002; 45(12):1608–1615

[11] Klausner JD, Kohn R, Kent C. Etiology of clinical proctitis among men who have sex with men. Clin Infect Dis. 2004; 38(2):300–302

[12] Kent CK, Chaw JK, Wong W, et al. Prevalence of rectal, urethral, and pharyngeal chlamydia and gonorrhea detected in 2 clinical settings among men who have sex with men: San Francisco, California, 2003. Clin Infect Dis. 2005; 41(1):67–74

[13] Workowski KA, Berman SM; Centers for Disease Control and Prevention. Sexually transmitted diseases treatment guidelines, 2006. MMWR Recomm Rep. 2006; 55(RR-11):1–94

[14] Marcus JL, Bernstein KT, Stephens SC, et al. Sentinel surveillance of rectal chlamydia and gonorrhea among males—San Francisco, 2005–2008. Sex Transm Dis. 2010; 37(1):59–61

[15] Tay YK, Goh CL, Chan R, et al. Evaluation of enzyme immunoassay for the detection of anogenital infections caused by Chlamydia trachomatis. Singapore Med J. 1995; 36(2):173–175

[16] Cosentino LA, Campbell T, Jett A, et al. Use of nucleic acid amplification testing for diagnosis of anorectal sexually transmitted infections. J Clin Microbiol. 2012; 50(6):2005–2008

[17] Cone MM, Whitlow CB. Sexually transmitted and anorectal infectious diseases. Gastroenterol Clin North Am. 2013; 42(4):877–892

[18] Klein EJ, Fisher LS, Chow AW, Guze LB. Anorectal gonococcal infection. Ann Intern Med. 1977; 86(3):340–346

[19] Bachmann LH, Johnson RE, Cheng H, et al. Nucleic acid amplification tests for diagnosis of Neisseria gonorrhoeae and Chlamydia trachomatis rectal infections. J Clin Microbiol. 2010; 48(5):1827–1832

[20] Workowski KA, Berman S; Centers for Disease Control and Prevention (CDC). Sexually transmitted diseases treatment guidelines, 2010. MMWR Recomm Rep. 2010; 59(RR-12):1–110

[21] Sharif S, Hyser M. Ischemic proctitis: case series and literature review. Am Surg. 2006; 72(12):1241–1247

[22] Sarin A, Safar B. Management of radiation proctitis. Gastroenterol Clin North Am. 2013; 42(4):913–925

[23] Gilinsky NH, Burns DG, Barbezat GO, et al. The natural history of radiation-induced proctosigmoiditis: an analysis of 88 patients. Q J Med. 1983; 52(205):40–53

[24] Haboubi NY, Schofield PF, Rowland PL. The light and electron microscopic features of early and late phase radiation-induced proctitis. Am J Gastroenterol. 1988; 83(10):1140–1144

[25] Hasleton PS, Carr N, Schofield PF. Vascular changes in radiation bowel disease. Histopathology. 1985; 9(5):517–534

[26] Lenz L, Rohr R, Nakao F, et al. Chronic radiation proctopathy: a practical review of endoscopic treatment. World J Gastrointest Surg. 2016; 8(2):151–160

[27] Rustagi T, Mashimo H. Endoscopic management of chronic radiation proctitis. World J Gastroenterol. 2011; 17(41):4554–4562

[28] Patel A, Pathak R, Deshpande V, et al. Radiofrequency ablation using BarRx for the endoscopic treatment of radiation proctopathy: a series of three cases. Clin Exp Gastroenterol. 2014; 7:453–460

[29] Hou JK, Abudayyeh S, Shaib Y. Treatment of chronic radiation proctitis with cryoablation. Gastrointest Endosc. 2011; 73(2):383–389

[30] Mensah FA, Mehta MR, Lewis JS, Jr, Lockhart AC. The human papillomavirus vaccine: current perspective and future role in prevention and treatment of anal intraepithelial neoplasia and anal cancer. Oncologist. 2016; 21(4):453–460

[31] Stier EA, Chigurupati NL, Fung L. Prophylactic HPV vaccination and anal cancer. Hum Vaccin Immunother. 2016; 12(6):1348–1351

[32] Long KC, Menon R, Bastawrous A, Billingham R. Screening, surveillance, and treatment of anal intraepithelial neoplasia. Clin Colon Rectal Surg. 2016; 29(1):57–64

[33] Wald A, Bharucha AE, Cosman BC, Whitehead WE. ACG clinical guideline: management of benign anorectal disorders. Am J Gastroenterol. 2014; 109(8):1141–1157, (Quiz) 1058

[34] Lohsiriwat V. Treatment of hemorrhoids: a coloproctologist's view. World J Gastroenterol. 2015; 21(31):9245–9252

[35] Jutabha R, Jensen DM, Chavalitdhamrong D. Randomized prospective study of endoscopic rubber band ligation compared with bipolar coagulation for chronically bleeding internal hemorrhoids. Am J Gastroenterol. 2009; 104(8):2057–2064

[36] Paikos D, Gatopoulou A, Moschos J, et al. Banding hemorrhoids using the O'Regan Disposable Bander. Single center experience. J Gastrointestin Liver Dis. 2007; 16(2):163–165

[37] Iyer VS, Shrier I, Gordon PH. Long-term outcome of rubber band ligation for symptomatic primary and recurrent internal hemorrhoids. Dis Colon Rectum. 2004; 47(8):1364–1370

[38] Jensen DM, Jutabha R, Machicado GA, et al. Prospective randomized comparative study of bipolar electrocoagulation versus heater probe for treatment of chronically bleeding internal hemorrhoids. Gastrointest Endosc. 1997; 46(5):435–443

[39] Gupta PJ. Infra red photocoagulation of early grades of hemorrhoids--5-year follow-up study. Bratisl Lek Listy. 2007; 108(4–5):223–226

[40] Gupta PJ. Infrared coagulation versus rubber band ligation in early stage hemorrhoids. Braz J Med Biol Res. 2003; 36(10):1433–1439

[41] Siddiqui UD, Barth BA, Banerjee S, et al; ASGE Technology Committee. Devices for the endoscopic treatment of hemorrhoids. Gastrointest Endosc. 2014; 79(1):8–14

[42] Hall JF. Modern management of hemorrhoidal disease. Gastroenterol Clin North Am. 2013; 42(4):759–772

[43] Yano T, Yano K. Comparison of injection sclerotherapy between 5% phenol in almond oil and aluminum potassium sulfate and tannic acid for grade 3 hemorrhoids. Ann Coloproctol. 2015; 31(3):103–105

[44] Tomiki Y, Ono S, Aoki J, et al. Treatment of internal hemorrhoids by endoscopic sclerotherapy with aluminum potassium sulfate and tannic acid. Diagn Ther Endosc. 2015; 2015:517690

[45] Randall GM, Jensen DM, Machicado GA, et al. Prospective randomized comparative study of bipolar versus direct current electrocoagulation for treatment of bleeding internal hemorrhoids. Gastrointest Endosc. 1994; 40(4):403–410

[46] Piskun G, Tucker R. New bipolar tissue ligator combines constant tissue compression and temperature guidance: histologic study and implications for treatment of hemorrhoids. Med Devices (Auckl). 2012; 5:89–96

[47] Chan KK, Arthur JD. External haemorrhoidal thrombosis: evidence for current management. Tech Coloproctol. 2013; 17(1):21–25

[48] Murphy PB, Schlachta CM, Alkhamesi NA. Surgical management for rectal prolapse: an update. Minerva Chir. 2015; 70(4):273–282

[49] Tou S, Brown SR, Nelson RL. Surgery for complete (full-thickness) rectal prolapse in adults. Cochrane Database Syst Rev. 2015; 11(11):CD001758

[50] Mistrangelo M, Tonello P, Brachet Contul R, et al. Perineal stapled prolapse resection for full-thickness external rectal prolapse: a multicentre prospective study. Colorectal Dis. 2016; 18(11):1094–1100

[51] Edden Y, Shih SS, Wexner SD. Solitary rectal ulcer syndrome and stercoral ulcers. Gastroenterol Clin North Am. 2009; 38(3):541–545

[52] Zhu QC, Shen RR, Qin HL, Wang Y. Solitary rectal ulcer syndrome: clinical features, pathophysiology, diagnosis and treatment strategies. World J Gastroenterol. 2014; 20(3):738–744

[53] Abid S, Khawaja A, Bhimani SA, et al. The clinical, endoscopic and histological spectrum of the solitary rectal ulcer syndrome: a single-center experience of 116 cases. BMC Gastroenterol. 2012; 12:72

[54] Sharma M, Somani P, Patil A, et al. Endoscopic ultrasonography of solitary rectal ulcer syndrome. Endoscopy. 2016; 48(suppl 1 UCTN):E76–E77

[55] Rao SS, Benninga MA, Bharucha AE, et al. ANMS-ESNM position paper and consensus guidelines on biofeedback therapy for anorectal disorders. Neurogastroenterol Motil. 2015; 27(5):594–609

[56] Waniczek D, Rdes J, Rudzki MK, et al. Effective treatment of solitary rectal ulcer syndrome using argon plasma coagulation. Prz Gastroenterol. 2014; 9(4):249–253

[57] Ihnat P, Martinek L, Vavra P, Zonca P. Novel combined approach in the management of non-healing solitary rectal ulcer syndrome—laparoscopic resection rectopexy and transanal endoscopic microsurgery. Wideochir Inne Tech Malo Inwazyjne. 2015; 10(2):295–298

[58] Beaty JS, Shashidharan M. Anal fissure. Clin Colon Rectal Surg. 2016; 29(1):30–37

[59] Whatley JZ, Tang SJ, Glover PH, et al. Management of complicated chronic anal fissures with high-dose circumferential chemodenervation (HDCC) of the internal anal sphincter. Int J Surg. 2015; 24(pt A):24–26

[60] Vershenya S, Klotz J, Joos A, et al. Combined approach in the treatment of chronic anal fissures. Updates Surg. 2015; 67(1):83–89

[61] Hussain ZH, Whitehead DA, Lacy BE. Fecal impaction. Curr Gastroenterol Rep. 2014; 16(9):404

[62] Baltazar G, Sahinoglu S, Betler M, et al. Rectal stercoral ulcer perforation. Am Surg. 2012; 78(12):E515–E516

Section VI

Biliopancreatic, Hepatic, and Peritoneal Diseases

41 Benign Biliary Disorders

Guido Costamagna, Pietro Familiari and Cristiano Spada

41.1 Introduction

Benign biliary disorders may occur in various traumatic and nontraumatic conditions. In daily practice, the most common situation of benign biliary disorders is benign biliary strictures. Benign biliary strictures account for significant morbidity and mortality and are difficult to treat. These originate from a variety of etiologies, most commonly postoperative injury (e.g., postcholecystectomy), orthotopic liver transplantation (OLT), chronic pancreatitis, and chronic cholangiopathies (e.g., primary sclerosing cholangitis [PSC]).

Accurate diagnosis and management of benign biliary disorders are based on correlating imaging findings with epidemiologic, clinical, and laboratory data.

41.2 Postoperative Biliary Stricture

Benign biliary strictures are rarely encountered in the general population and require coordinated care between medical, surgical, pathologic, and radiologic specialties for appropriate evaluation and management. Benign biliary stricture can be the result of a wide array of nonneoplastic causes. In Western countries, iatrogenic stricture is the most common benign biliary stricture

and accounts for up to 80% of all benign strictures. The incidence of iatrogenic injuries of the bile ducts has increased two- to threefold (0.3–0.7%) after the advent of laparoscopic cholecystectomy.[1,2] This is mostly due to misidentification of anatomical structures during laparoscopic surgery, acute inflammation, or fibrous adhesions in the gallbladder fossa, excessive use of electrocautery, inaccurate placement of clips, sutures, and ligations.[1,3] Postcholecystectomy strictures often involves the common hepatic duct or the common bile duct (CBD). The clinical and biochemical manifestations may be evident early in the postoperative period, and may be associated with jaundice and cholangitis, or with peritonitis caused by a bile leak. Delayed presentation is commonly related to ischemic injury or reanastomosis of the CBD, with the time to presentation dependent on the individual rate of fibrosis.[3]

The main classification used to evaluate biliary duct strictures is the Bismuth classification (▶ Fig. 41.1) that is based on stricture location.[4]

Several biliary complications may develop following OLT, including the formation of strictures, bile leaks, and biliary filling defects. Benign biliary strictures are the most common complication of OLT. Patients who undergo liver transplantation are at highest risk of developing biliary strictures with a rate of about 20 to 30%. Biliary strictures can occur during` the early (< 30 days) or late (> 30 days) posttransplantation time and may be anastomotic or nonanastomotic. (▶ Fig. 41.2). Early strictures may

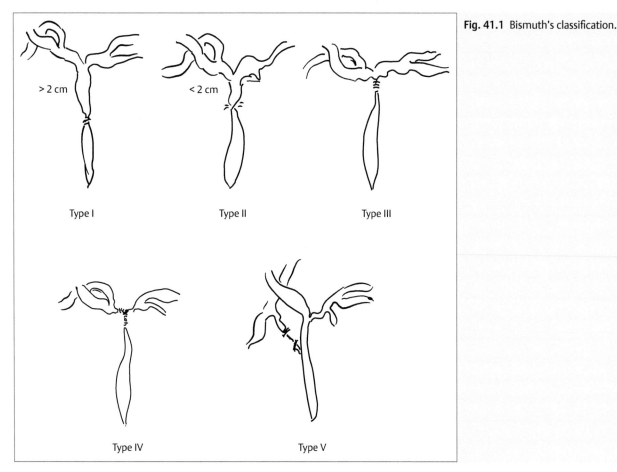

Fig. 41.1 Bismuth's classification.

Type I   Type II   Type III

Type IV   Type V

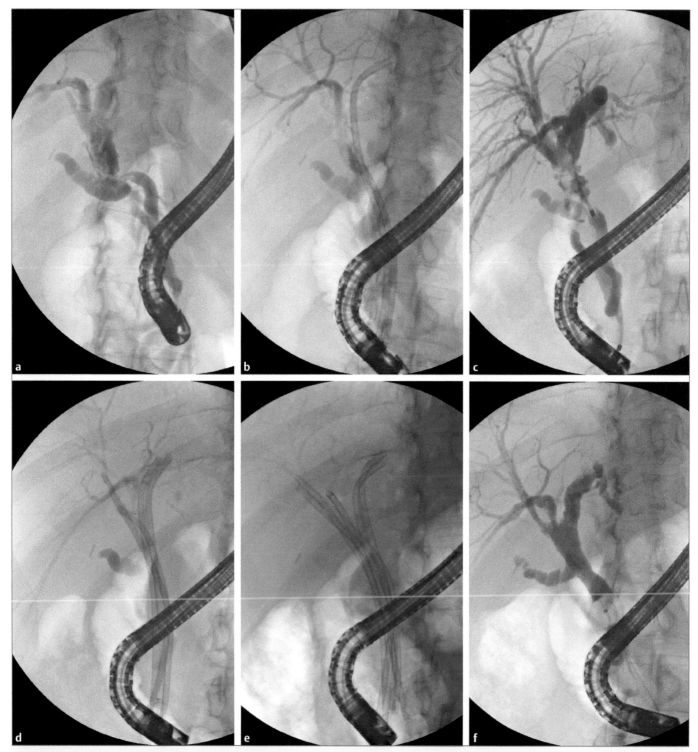

Fig. 41.2 Anastomotic biliary stricture after liver transplantation. The patient underwent progressive dilation of the stricture with the placement of multiple plastic stents. **(a)** ERCP shows an anastomotic stricture. The donor common bile duct is dilated above the stricture. In the cholangiogram, please note the two cystic duct stumps, the donor one and the recipient one. **(b)** Two plastic stents are inserted side-by-side to dilate the stricture. **(c)** After 3 months the anastomotic stricture still persists. **(d)** Four plastic stents are placed side-by-side. **(e)** After 3 months, a total of six stents are placed to additionally dilate the stricture. **(f)** After additional 3 months, 9 months after the first ERCP, the anastomotic stricture is completely resolved, and the stents are removed.

be the result of CBD size mismatch between the donor and the recipient. These may also be caused by surgical technique and are often anastomotic. Hepaticojejunostomy is more likely to result in early stricture development than duct-to-duct anastomosis. Late strictures are usually associated with ischemic damage and result in a higher rate of retransplantation or surgical revision.[3] Anastomotic strictures develop secondary to fibrosis and are caused by

focal stenosis at the junction of the recipient's CBD with donor's common hepatic duct. About 80% of post-OLT bile duct strictures are anastomotic. Nonanastomotic strictures result from biliary ischemia induced by hepatic artery thrombosis or stenosis and prolonged donor organ ischemic time. Typically, they start at the hilum and may progress to the intrahepatic ducts. Nonanastomotic strictures after OLT respond less favorably to endoscopic therapy than anastomotic strictures, with up to 25 to 50% of patients expiring or undergoing retransplantation.

Clinically, benign biliary strictures may present with pain, jaundice, cholangitis, pruritus, or only with alteration of liver function tests (bilirubin, alkaline phosphatase, and gamma-glutamyl transferase). In patients with OLT, the clinical presentation of biliary strictures may occur during the early posttransplantation time or even several years after surgery.

Ultrasound is the initial imaging modality of choice for the detection of biliary dilation. Ultrasound is also useful and accurate to detect the level of obstruction. Computed tomography (CT) scan is indicated to show bile duct dilation and the underlying cause of biliary obstruction, and potential complications (i.e., cholangitic abscess).[5] In addition, CT scan may help in differentiating benign from malignant biliary strictures. Magnetic resonance cholangiopancreatography (MRCP) can accurately delineate the biliary anatomy, site and length of the stenosis, being therefore very useful before endoscopic retrograde cholangiopancreatography (ERCP) for planning therapy. Unlike ERCP, MRCP offers the advantage of noninvasive imaging without the risk of any procedure-related complications, allows evaluation of the biliary system beyond a tight stricture. In patients with a nonanastomotic stricture following OLT, the evaluation for hepatic artery thrombosis or stenosis by Doppler ultrasound and/or angiography by CT scan or magnetic resonance imaging (MRI) should be considered. Flow-limiting hepatic artery disease is a known cause of nonanastomotic stricture and may require endovascular stenting, thrombolysis, or surgery.[3] Endoscopic ultrasound (EUS) has been shown to improve the accuracy of ERCP in differentiating benign from malignant strictures, including also the feasibility of EUS-guided fine-needle aspiration (FNA). The combination of endoscopic ultrasound with ERCP results in higher accuracy for diagnosis (up to 85%) compared with EUS-guided FNA or ERCP-guided biopsy alone (70 and 67%, respectively).[6,7] Several diagnostic tools for assessment of biliary strictures and for intraluminal tissue characterization have been developed in the last few years. These are mainly indicated in case of uncertainty and when a differential diagnosis between malignant and benign stricture is required. These include intraductal ultrasound, peroral videocholangioscopy, confocal laser endomicroscopy, and optical coherence tomography. The majority of these techniques are still under evaluation in clinical trials.[1,3]

Minimally invasive procedures such as endoscopic or percutaneous transhepatic biliary dilation and stenting are considered treatments of choice for iatrogenic strictures.[8] Nevertheless, considering the access route, endoscopy is preferred to the percutaneous approach due to a reduced morbidity, better efficacy, and increased comfort for the patient. ERCP has emerged as the therapeutic intervention of choice for managing biliary strictures. Postoperative biliary strictures benefit from an "aggressive" endoscopic approach, with the insertion of an increasing number of plastic stents at 3-monthly stent exchange intervals until there is complete morphologic disappearance of the stricture, independent of the duration of treatment.[1,9,10] Placing multiple side-by-side, large-bore plastic stents has been shown to improve long-term outcomes of benign biliary strictures compared with placing one or two stents alone (with a 3-monthly exchanges for a period of 1 year). Anastomotic strictures following liver transplantation can also benefit from this aggressive

approach. This strategy results in very high efficacy (80–90%) for postoperative strictures.[3,11,12] Patients who are candidates to the endoscopic treatment, a complete sphincterotomy is necessary stent placement, to allow stent insertion. Despite the high success rate of multiple plastic stent therapy, multiple treatment sessions are required. Because placement of a single, fully covered, self-expandable metallic stent (cSEMS) results in radial dilation of a stricture equivalent to that of at least three side- by-side plastic stents, preliminary studies including small clinical trials were designed to support the hypothesis that deployment of cSEMS would be beneficial in patients with benign strictures. Results of these studies have generally been contradictory, with high long-term morbidity rates. Moreover, these have been limited by retrospective and nonrandomized design, small sample sizes, and inclusion of patients with partially treated strictures.[13,14,15] Recently in a well-designed trial,[16] patients were randomized to receive multiple plastic stents or a single cSEMS, stratified by stricture etiology and with endoscopic reassessment for resolution every 3 months (plastic stents) or every 6 months (cSEMS). Patients were followed up for 12 months after stricture resolution to assess for recurrence. Among patients with benign biliary strictures and a bile duct diameter 6 mm or more in whom the covered metallic stent would not overlap the cystic duct, cSEMS were not inferior to multiple plastic stents after 12 months in achieving stricture resolution. In specific settings, therefore, metallic stents should be considered an appropriate option in patients with benign biliary stricture. In case of endoscopic/percutaneous treatment failure, surgery represents a valid treatment alternative.

41.3 Chronic Pancreatitis and Biliary Strictures

Chronic pancreatitis (CP) may result in obstruction of the intrapancreatic part of the CBD and accounts for up to 10% of benign biliary strictures. A stricture of the intrapancreatic bile duct develops in approximately 3 to 46% of patients with CP[17,18,19,20,21] and can seriously compromise the clinical course of disease. Biliary strictures usually complicate a long-lasting disease, as a result of severe fibrosis of the pancreatic head parenchyma, which compresses and narrows the distal CBD. Parenchymal fibrosis in CP is a slow, irreversible process, and these strictures usually occur late in the natural history of the disease. However, CP-related bile duct strictures may also be seen in patients with a recently diagnosed disease and can be the result of an acute pancreatic inflammation, being the final consequence of the edema of the pancreatic head that compresses the intrapancreatic bile duct. These strictures may resolve spontaneously or, in more severe cases, be persistent and require biliary drainage. Biliary strictures in patients with CP can also be the result of an extrinsic compression from a pancreatic pseudocyst, retention cyst, or a walled-off pancreatic necrosis. These strictures usually disappear after the drainage of the pancreatic fluid collection. It is of paramount importance to reasonably rule out malignancy before embarking on the endoscopic treatment of presumed CP-related biliary strictures, as such a treatment usually lasts for 1 year and the course of pancreatic cancer is rapid. Patients with CP have a higher risk of pancreatic cancer compared to reference population. CT scan and/or EUS should be periodically performed in patients with CP, to early identify suspected nodules and masses.

Biliary strictures have a broad spectrum of presentation, varying from mildly elevated levels in liver function tests to severe jaundice in case of complete biliary obstruction. The incidental finding of a CP-related biliary stricture accounts for up to 17% of cases.[17] Abdominal pain is usually considered the predominant symptom in most patients, but is mainly caused by a bout of acute pancreatitis rather than by a biliary stricture per se. Jaundice may be present in 30 to 50% of patients at diagnosis.[5,17] Alteration of liver function test results and biochemical markers of cholestasis, including alkaline phosphatase and gamma-glutamyl transferase, may be persistent for some weeks after the normalization of bilirubin levels. A small proportion of patients with a biliary stricture secondary to CP may develop secondary biliary cirrhosis. The combination of a dilated CBD at abdominal ultrasound and elevation of levels of biochemical markers of cholestasis usually allows to make a diagnosis of a biliary stricture. CT-scan is usually required to exclude neoplasms, evaluate the severity of chronic pancreatitis, to identify stones and calcifications, and to plan the necessary treatment. MRCP may be helpful to differentiate a benign from a malignant biliary stricture. However, cholangiographic features are unreliable because of a wide variability of the radiologic appearance of the stricture. Cytologic and histologic confirmation is often indicated to rule out the presence of malignancy. Brush cytology and endobiliary biopsies can be obtained during ERCP, but the sensitivity of the sampling is low. EUS-guided FNA is the option of choice to obtain cytologic and histologic sampling from biliary duct thickening and/or pancreatic masses because of its safety profile and diagnostic accuracy.[17,22]

Patients with CP-related bile duct strictures are recommended to receive treatment in cases of symptoms (i.e., cholangitis, jaundice), secondary biliary cirrhosis, bile duct stones, progression of biliary stricture, or when anicteric cholestasis (a serum alkaline phosphatase level greater than twice the upper limit) persists for more than 1 month. The management of CP-related biliary strictures should be carefully evaluated and tailored on the patient conditions and needs. CP-related biliary strictures are more difficult to be dilated than other benign biliary strictures. The presence of parenchymal calcifications and stones increases the fibrosis and tightness of the strictures, which are often permanent with only partial and not sustained benefits after simple dilation. Furthermore the risk of incidental pancreatic cancer should be taken into the account. The possibility of surgical management of CP-related biliary strictures should be conscientiously considered, especially in young patients in good health conditions and with a long life expectancy. In such patients surgical drainage is still considered the gold standard. However, comorbidities and local consequences of repeated attacks of pancreatitis, or patient's preferences may contraindicate surgery. ERCP and stent placement may be the therapeutic intervention of choice for managing biliary strictures secondary to CP only in selected patients. If the stricture does not disappear after a 1-year treatment, the patients should undergo surgical hepaticojejunostomy. When a CBD stricture caused by chronic pancreatitis has been treated endoscopically using a single biliary plastic stent, the long-term success has been disappointing.[23] Stenting with multiple plastic stents has led to success in

60 to 92% of cases.[24,25] Every biliary stricture that persists and is associated with alteration of biochemical markers of cholestasis is indicated for drainage by either surgery or endoscopy.[17] Biliary drainage is also indicated when frequent relapses of biliary obstruction occur in order to reduce the risk of secondary biliary cirrhosis and cholangitis. In asymptomatic patients or in patients with a slight increase of biochemical markers of cholestasis, a conservative management is indicated with close monitoring of liver functions tests. Endoscopic bile duct stricture dilation with stent placement is one of the therapeutic option. Usually, biliary strictures disappear in about one-third of patients who undergo single plastic stenting for 3 to 6 months. An aggressive approach with multiple simultaneous side-by-side stents to obtain calibration of the biliary tract appears to be superior to single stent placement, providing the long-term benefit. Self-expandable metal stents in patients with CP-related biliary strictures show good outcomes at midterm follow-up, and might be proposed for patients unfit for surgery as a more effective treatment to plastic stenting.[14,26,27,28] The role of fully covered, removable, self-expandable metal stent in patients with CP-related strictures, who are unfit for surgery, is particularly interesting. These patients may need a prolonged stenting period: differently from patients with malignancies these patients have a longlife expectancy, and plastic stents do not usually offer sustained benefits in case of tight and fibrotic strictures. Fully covered SEMS, with their large diameter, can improve dilation of the stricture, facilitate bile drainage for a long time, and reduce the number of hospitalization due to stent exchange and cholangitis. Fully covered SEMS can be very easily removed and exchanged, and their placement do not require very special skills[26] (▶ Fig. 41.3). Unfortunately, some complications caused by long-term stenting with SEMS have been observed and include SEMS migration, embedding into the CBD and consequent difficulties at SEMS removal, and hyperplastic overgrowth above the proximal end of the SEMS that may result in creation of de novo strictures.

41.4 Primary Sclerosing Cholangitis

PSC is a chronic cholestatic hepatic disease characterized by progressive fibrosing inflammatory involvement of intrahepatic and extrahepatic bile ducts, leading to cholestasis and cirrhosis. The fibrosing inflammatory process is responsible for the development of fibrotic strictures and saccular dilations of the intrahepatic and extrahepatic bile ducts resembling beads on a string that are diagnosed radiographically.[3,29,30,31] The majority of patients suffering from PSC are also affected by inflammatory bowel disease (i.e., ulcerative colitis). No medical treatments have been demonstrated to be effective in PSC that may lead to end-stage liver disease and need for transplantation. Approximately 40% of patients with PSC develop so-called dominant strictures, which can cause biliary obstruction that require endoscopic treatment.[3,32,33,34] Despite the variability in clinical presentation, endoscopy plays a role in the management of patients with PSC when they present with clinical and biochemical deterioration and severe cholestasis caused by a dominant biliary stricture involving either the CBD or the right or left main intrahepatic ducts. These strictures are well diagnosed

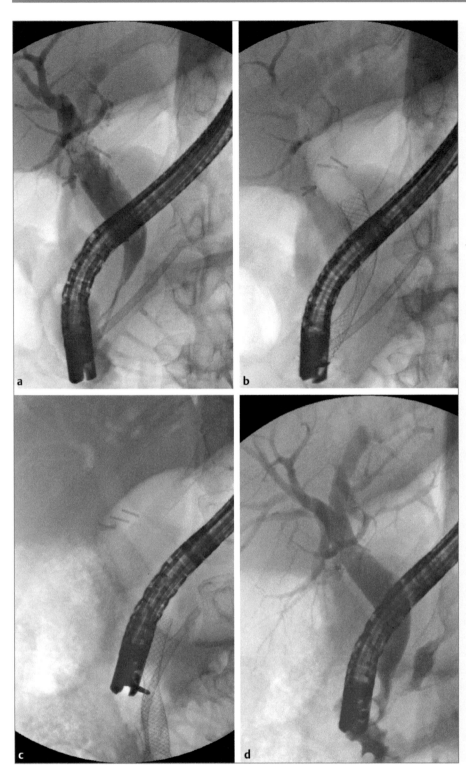

Fig. 41.3 Chronic pancreatitis-related biliary stricture.
(a) ERCP shows a regular distal common bile duct stricture. A plastic stent has been already placed into the pancreatic duct to treat a stricture.
(b) A fully covered self-expanding metal sent is deployed into the common bile duct.
(c) After 1 year the self-expanding metal stent is easily removed with a foreign body forceps.
(d) Final cholangiography demonstrates the resolution of the bile duct stricture.

by MRI and can be treated endoscopically using pneumatic dilation or stenting. None of the treatments currently available is definitively effective in the long term. The true impact of endoscopic stent placement is uncertain because the evidence is mainly based on small, retrospective studies and there are no prospective randomized-controlled trial comparing balloon dilation with endoscopic stent placement. Stent placement may be detrimental in some patients because complications including stent occlusion and cholangitis may occur more frequently than in patients who receive balloon dilation alone.[3,35,36,37] The goal of endoscopic dilation is to dilate the strictures and to reduce the serum alkaline phosphatase level to 1.5 times the upper limit of normal.[3,38,39,40] Short-term stenting (2 weeks) with a single plastic stent is suggested for patients with PSC if hydrostatic dilation alone is unsuccessful; longer periods of stenting increase the risk of cholangitis. During ERCP, strictures should be routinely brushed for cytology because patients with PSC have a 20 to 30% risk of developing cholangiocarcinoma.[41,42] ERCP should be performed carefully and only when strictly indicated in patients with PSC. Severe deterioration of health status has been observed after ERCP, balloon dilation, or stent placement (more likely because of introduction of contamination above strictures) in patients with end-stage liver disease.[12,35,43]

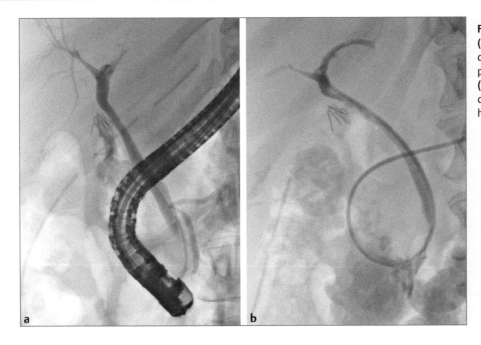

Fig. 41.4 Bile leak after cholecystectomy. **(a)** ERCP shows a bile leak from the cystic duct stump. An endoscopic sphincterotomy is performed, and a nasobiliary drain placed. **(b)** Cholangiography through the nasobiliary drain after 5 days demonstrates the complete healing of the bile leak.

41.5 Bile Duct Leaks

Bile leaks are most often a consequence of surgery or trauma. Healing of biliary leaks is achieved by reducing the pressure gradient between the biliary tree and the duodenum. Nearly all postoperative biliary leaks, with the exception of complete transection of the CBD, are amenable to endoscopic treatment. Different techniques can be used: biliary sphincterotomy, nasobiliary drainage, biliary stenting, or a combination of these techniques. These treatments are equally effective for the closure of a biliary leak within a few days.[12,44,45,46] Endoscopic sphincterotomy is associated with immediate, short-term, and long-term complications, but is necessary when residual CBD stones are present.[46] Sphincterotomy without stent insertion is inferior to stent placement alone.[47] Temporary placement of a nasobiliary drainage is also an option. Its main advantage is maintenance of access for repeat cholangiography to confirm leak closure[12] (▶Fig. 41.4). Disadvantages of nursing nasobiliary drainage include prolonged hospitalization while awaiting leak closure, patient discomfort, and tube migration or inadvertent dislodgment.[12] Biliary stenting with or without sphincterotomy is the most widely accepted technique. Although, stent placement requires at least one repeated procedure for stent removal, it is associated with less discomfort for the patient than a nasobiliary catheter. Stents are necessary when a biliary stricture is associated with the leak. Different stent strategies to manage biliary leaks (i.e., stenting with or without sphincterotomy, different stent sizes and stent duration) have been described and compared, all showing similar results.[12,48,49,50] The use of large-bore stents (> 10 F) is preferred to avoid early clogging and to improve bile flow. Stents are usually removed 4 to 8 weeks after insertion.[12,51]

References

[1] Costamagna G, Boškoski I. Current treatment of benign biliary strictures. Ann Gastroenterol. 2013; 26(1):37–40

[2] Tee HP, James MW, Kaffes AJ. Placement of removable metal biliary stent in post-orthotopic liver transplantation anastomotic stricture. World J Gastroenterol. 2010; 16(28):3597–3600

[3] Baron TH, Sr, Davee T. Endoscopic management of benign bile duct strictures. Gastrointest Endosc Clin N Am. 2013; 23(2):295–311

[4] Bismuth H, Majno PE. Biliary strictures: classification based on the principles of surgical treatment. World J Surg. 2001; 25(10):1241–1244

[5] Shanbhogue AK, Tirumani SH, Prasad SR, et al. Benign biliary strictures: a current comprehensive clinical and imaging review. AJR Am J Roentgenol. 2011; 197(2):W295–W306

[6] Domagk D, Wessling J, Reimer P, et al. Endoscopic retrograde cholangiopancreatography, intraductal ultrasonography, and magnetic resonance cholangiopancreatography in bile duct strictures: a prospective comparison of imaging diagnostics with histopathological correlation. Am J Gastroenterol. 2004; 99(9):1684–1689

[7] Eloubeidi MA, Chen VK, Jhala NC, et al. Endoscopic ultrasound-guided fine needle aspiration biopsy of suspected cholangiocarcinoma. Clin Gastroenterol Hepatol. 2004; 2(3):209–213

[8] Memeo R, Piardi T, Sangiuolo F, et al. Management of biliary complications after liver transplantation. World J Hepatol. 2015; 7(29):2890–2895

[9] Costamagna G, Pandolfi M, Mutignani M, et al. Long-term results of endoscopic management of postoperative bile duct strictures with increasing numbers of stents. Gastrointest Endosc. 2001; 54(2):162–168

[10] Costamagna G, Tringali A, Mutignani M, et al. Endotherapy of postoperative biliary strictures with multiple stents: results after more than 10 years of follow-up. Gastrointest Endosc. 2010; 72(3):551–557

[11] Tringali A, Barbaro F, Pizzicannella M, et al. Endoscopic management with multiple plastic stents of anastomotic biliary stricture following liver transplantation: long-term results. Endoscopy. 2016; 48(6):546–551

[12] Perri V, Familiari P, Tringali A, et al, Plastic biliary stents for benign biliary diseases. Gastrointest Endosc Clin N Am. 2011; 21(3):405–433, viii

[13] Park JS, Lee SS, Song TJ, et al. Long-term outcomes of covered self-expandable metal stents for treating benign biliary strictures. Endoscopy. 2016; 48(5):440–447

[14] Oh D, Park DH, Cho MK, et al. Feasibility and safety of a fully covered self-expandable metal stent with antimigration properties for EUS-guided pancreatic duct drainage: early and midterm outcomes (with video). Gastrointest Endosc. 2016; 83(2):366–73.e2

[15] Devière J, Nageshwar Reddy D, Püspök A, et al; Benign Biliary Stenoses Working Group. Successful management of benign biliary strictures with fully covered self-expanding metal stents. Gastroenterology. 2014; 147(2):385–395, quiz e15

[16] Coté GA, Slivka A, Tarnasky P, et al. Effect of covered metallic stents compared with plastic stents on benign biliary stricture resolution: a randomized clinical trial. JAMA. 2016; 315(12):1250–1257

[17] Familiari P, Boškoski I, Bove V, Costamagna G. ERCP for biliary strictures associated with chronic pancreatitis. Gastrointest Endosc Clin N Am. 2013; 23(4):833–845

[18] Afroudakis A, Kaplowitz N. Liver histopathology in chronic common bile duct stenosis due to chronic alcoholic pancreatitis. Hepatology. 1981; 1(1):65–72

[19] Huizinga WK, Thomson SR, Spitaels JM, Simjee AE. Chronic pancreatitis with biliary obstruction. Ann R Coll Surg Engl. 1992; 74(2):119–123, discussion 123–125

[20] Petrozza JA, Dutta SK. The variable appearance of distal common bile duct stenosis in chronic pancreatitis. J Clin Gastroenterol. 1985; 7(5):447–450

[21] Sand JA, Nordback IH. Management of cholestasis in patients with chronic pancreatitis: evaluation of a treatment protocol. Eur J Surg. 1995; 161(8):587–592

[22] Lewis JJ, Kowalski TE. Endoscopic ultrasound and fine needle aspiration in pancreatic cancer. Cancer J. 2012; 18(6):523–529

[23] Haapamäki C, Kylänpää L, Udd M, et al. Randomized multicenter study of multiple plastic stents vs. covered self-expandable metallic stent in the treatment of biliary stricture in chronic pancreatitis. Endoscopy. 2015; 47(7):605–610

[24] Pozsár J, Sahin P, László F, et al. Medium-term results of endoscopic treatment of common bile duct strictures in chronic calcifying pancreatitis with increasing numbers of stents. J Clin Gastroenterol. 2004; 38(2):118–123

[25] Catalano MF, Linder JD, George S, et al. Treatment of symptomatic distal common bile duct stenosis secondary to chronic pancreatitis: comparison of single vs. multiple simultaneous stents. Gastrointest Endosc. 2004; 60(6):945–952

[26] Perri V, Boškoski I, Tringali A, et al. Fully covered self-expandable metal stents in biliary strictures caused by chronic pancreatitis not responding to plastic stenting: a prospective study with 2 years of follow-up. Gastrointest Endosc. 2012; 75(6):1271–1277

[27] Behm B, Brock A, Clarke BW, et al. Partially covered self-expandable metallic stents for benign biliary strictures due to chronic pancreatitis. Endoscopy. 2009; 41(6):547–551

[28] Cahen DL, Rauws EA, Gouma DJ, et al. Removable fully covered self-expandable metal stents in the treatment of common bile duct strictures due to chronic pancreatitis: a case series. Endoscopy. 2008; 40(8):697–700

[29] Pitt HA, Thompson HH, Tompkins RK, Longmire WP, Jr. Primary sclerosing cholangitis: results of an aggressive surgical approach. Ann Surg. 1982; 196(3):259–268

[30] Wiesner RH, LaRusso NF. Clinicopathologic features of the syndrome of primary sclerosing cholangitis. Gastroenterology. 1980; 79(2):200–206

[31] Chandok N, Hirschfield GM. Management of primary sclerosing cholangitis: conventions and controversies. Can J Gastroenterol. 2012; 26(5):261–268

[32] Stiehl A, Rudolph G, Klöters-Plachky P, et al. Development of dominant bile duct stenoses in patients with primary sclerosing cholangitis treated with ursodeoxycholic acid: outcome after endoscopic treatment. J Hepatol. 2002; 36(2):151–156

[33] Björnsson E, Lindqvist-Ottosson J, Asztely M, Olsson R. Dominant strictures in patients with primary sclerosing cholangitis. Am J Gastroenterol. 2004; 99(3):502–508

[34] Boberg KM, Jebsen P, Clausen OP, et al. Diagnostic benefit of biliary brush cytology in cholangiocarcinoma in primary sclerosing cholangitis. J Hepatol. 2006; 45(4):568–574

[35] Kaya M, Petersen BT, Angulo P, et al. Balloon dilation compared to stenting of dominant strictures in primary sclerosing cholangitis. Am J Gastroenterol. 2001; 96(4):1059–1066

[36] Ahrendt SA, Pitt HA, Kalloo AN, et al. Primary sclerosing cholangitis: resect, dilate, or transplant? Ann Surg. 1998; 227(3):412–423

[37] Linder S, Söderlund C. Endoscopic therapy in primary sclerosing cholangitis: outcome of treatment and risk of cancer. Hepatogastroenterology. 2001; 48(38):387–392

[38] Al Mamari S, Djordjevic J, Halliday JS, Chapman RW. Improvement of serum alkaline phosphatase to <1.5 upper limit of normal predicts better outcome and reduced risk of cholangiocarcinoma in primary sclerosing cholangitis. J Hepatol. 2013; 58(2):329–334

[39] Stanich PP, Björnsson E, Gossard AA, et al. Alkaline phosphatase normalization is associated with better prognosis in primary sclerosing cholangitis. Dig Liver Dis. 2011; 43(4):309–313

[40] Lindström L, Hultcrantz R, Boberg KM, et al. Association between reduced levels of alkaline phosphatase and survival times of patients with primary sclerosing cholangitis. Clin Gastroenterol Hepatol. 2013; 11(7):841–846

[41] Chapman MH, Webster GJ, Bannoo S, et al. Cholangiocarcinoma and dominant strictures in patients with primary sclerosing cholangitis: a 25-year single-centre experience. Eur J Gastroenterol Hepatol. 2012; 24(9):1051–1058

[42] Novotný I, Dítě P, Trna J, et al, Immunoglobulin G4-related cholangitis: a variant of IgG4-related systemic disease. Dig Dis. 2012; 30(2):216–219

[43] Al-Kawas FH. Endoscopic management of primary sclerosing cholangitis: less is better! Am J Gastroenterol. 1999; 94(9):2235–2236

[44] Bjorkman DJ, Carr-Locke DL, Lichtenstein DR, et al. Postsurgical bile leaks: endoscopic obliteration of the transpapillary pressure gradient is enough. Am J Gastroenterol. 1995; 90(12):2128–2133

[45] Pinkas H, Brady PG. Biliary leaks after laparoscopic cholecystectomy: time to stent or time to drain. Hepatobiliary Pancreat Dis Int. 2008; 7(6):628–632

[46] Agarwal N, Sharma BC, Garg S, et al. Endoscopic management of postoperative bile leaks. Hepatobiliary Pancreat Dis Int. 2006; 5(2):273–277

[47] Kaffes AJ, Hourigan L, De Luca N, et al. Impact of endoscopic intervention in 100 patients with suspected postcholecystectomy bile leak. Gastrointest Endosc. 2005; 61(2):269–275

[48] Mavrogiannis C, Liatsos C, Papanikolaou IS, et al. Biliary stenting alone versus biliary stenting plus sphincterotomy for the treatment of post- laparoscopic cholecystectomy biliary leaks: a prospective randomized study. Eur J Gastroenterol Hepatol. 2006; 18(4):405–409

[49] Katsinelos P, Kountouras J, Paroutoglou G, et al. The role of endoscopic treatment in postoperative bile leaks. Hepatogastroenterology. 2006; 53(68):166–170

[50] Katsinelos P, Kountouras J, Paroutoglou G, et al. A comparative study of 10-Fr vs. 7-Fr straight plastic stents in the treatment of postcholecystectomy bile leak. Surg Endosc. 2008; 22(1):101–106

[51] Shah JN. Endoscopic treatment of bile leaks: current standards and recent innovations. Gastrointest Endosc. 2007; 65(7):1069–1072

42 Malignant Biliary Disease

Ming-Ming Xu, Nikhil A. Kumta, Michel Kahaleh

42.1 Introduction

Cholangiocarcinoma (CCA) is a heterogeneous group of epithelial tumors arising within the biliary tract. These are conventionally divided into distal, hilar, and intrahepatic cancers by their longitudinal extent along the biliary tract and also demonstrate differences in their pathogenesis, molecular signatures, and treatment. They share a dismal prognosis due to their aggressive natural history and often late-stage disease at diagnosis. Surgical resection and in select cases, liver transplantation, offer the only durable chance of cure when CCA is diagnosed at an early stage. We will review the evolution of imaging and endoscopic tools for the diagnosis of malignant biliary disease and the available treatment options from surgery, liver transplantation, and endoscopic palliation to advances in locoregional and adjuvant therapy.

42.2 Diagnostic Approach

The early diagnosis of cholangiocarcinoma (CCA) is the most essential determinate of prognosis as curative surgical resection and liver transplantation are only possible in the small subset of patients who have resectable disease. The majority of patients present at late stage when they develop clinical symptoms due to biliary obstruction, pain, or weight loss. One of the challenges in the diagnosis of malignant biliary disease is that these symptoms can also be seen in benign causes of biliary strictures and the differentiation between malignant and benign disease can often be challenging despite the obvious difference in their clinical consequence (▶Table 42.1). Laboratory tests often show an obstructive pattern of liver chemistries, and although tumor markers such as CA 19–9 and carcinoembryonic antigen (CEA) are often used to aid in the diagnosis, current data do not support their use to independently make the diagnosis of CCA. Serum CA 19–9 cutoff values of greater than 37 U/mL has been shown have a sensitivity and specificity for malignant stricture of 73 and 63%, respectively, but can also be elevated in benign causes of cholestasis.[1]

Table 42.1 Differential diagnosis of indeterminate biliary stricture

Benign causes of biliary stricture	Malignant causes of biliary stricture
Choledocholithiasis	Cholangiocarcinoma
Postsurgical stricture	Hepatocellular carcinoma
Post liver transplant stricture	Pancreatic adenocarcinoma
Radiation-induced stricture	Ampullary adenocarcinoma
Primary sclerosing cholangitis	Gallbladder cancer
IgG4 cholangiopathy	Metastatic disease or lymphadenopathy
Benign fibrostenotic stricture	
HIV cholangiopathy	

HIV, Human Immunodeficiency Virus; IgG4, immunoglobulin G4.

42.2.1 Radiologic Imaging

Cross-sectional imaging with computed tomography (CT) or magnetic resonance imaging (MRI)/magnetic resonance cholangiopancreatography (MRCP) have become the standard imaging tools in the evaluation of suspected malignant biliary obstruction.[2] Multidetector CT (MDCT) classically shows a mass or hypoattenuating ductal thickening in the portovenous phase with or without proximal biliary ductal dilation[2] (▶Fig. 42.1). CT imaging has been shown to have high accuracy in detecting vascular involvement and distant metastases but is less accurate in the evaluation of the longitudinal extent of the tumor and local lymph node invasion.[3] The overall accuracy of CT in assessing resectability of CCA has been reported to be 60 to 88% compared to the accuracy of MRI/MRCP in assessing tumor extent and resectability of 95%.[4,5,6] MRCP has the advantage of avoiding intravenous contrast and radiation while providing similar sensitivity and specificity to endoscopic retrograde cholangiopancreatography (ERCP) for determining the level or location of obstruction and a sensitivity of 88%, specificity of 95% for determining malignancy in one large meta-analysis.[7]

42.2.2 Endoscopic Retrograde Cholangiopancreatography

Despite the high accuracy of MRCP in delineating the level of biliary obstruction and a suspected cause of biliary stricture, it ultimately cannot provide definitive tissue diagnosis. ERCP with brush cytology and endobiliary biopsy is the initial standard approach for tissue sampling in suspected biliary malignancy. The limitation of ERCP is the known poor sensitivity of brush cytology for malignancy of between 23 and 56% despite high specificity of nearly 100%.[8,9,10,11] This is likely the result of multiple factors including the desmoplastic

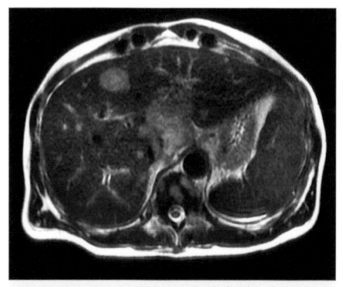

Fig. 42.1 Magnetic resonance imaging (MRI) of a hilar cholangiocarcinoma.

reaction caused by the tumor, the anatomical location of the stricture, and cellular loss during specimen processing.[12] Attempts at stricture dilation prior to brushing increase sensitivity to only 34 from 27%.[12] When endobiliary biopsy is combined with brushing, the sensitivity increases to 70%.[13] The use of a protocolized method for repeated tissue sampling with on-site cytopathology and careful specimen processing, the "smash protocol," achieved a 72% on-site pathologic diagnosis for biliary malignancy.[14]

42.2.3 Fluorescence In-Situ Hybridization

A newer, adjunctive technique to increase the diagnostic yield from brushing cytology is fluorescence in situ hybridization (FISH), which uses fluorescently labeled DNA probes to detect chromosomal aneuploidy or polysomy, which has been seen in up to 80% of CCA[15] (▶Fig. 42.2). The commercially available probes target chromosomes 3, 7, 17, and the 9p21 locus of chromosome 9. When all four probes are used in indeterminate biliary strictures, the sensitivity of FISH for malignancy is 84% with specificity of 97%.[16] FISH can significantly improve the diagnostic yield of routine cytology from ERCP without the need for additional procedures with high specificity. However, in patients with primary sclerosing cholangitis (PSC), FISH is less reliable with sensitivity for CCA of only 47%, specificity of 100%, positive predictive value of 100%, and negative predictive value of 88%.[17]

42.2.4 Cholangioscopy

The single-operator cholangioscopy (SOC) system, commonly known as the Spyglass Direct Visualization System (Boston Scientific, Natick, Massachusetts, United States) allows both direct visualization of the biliary tract and directed tissue sampling with a mini biopsy forceps (SpyBite). The system consists of a 10-F access and delivery catheter (SpyScope) through which the fiber optic probe is inserted, providing 6,000-pixel images with four-way tip maneuverability and a 30-degree view in each direction. The entire system is introduced into the biliary tree with guidewire assistance after traditional ERCP-based biliary access and fits through the working channel of the duodenoscope. A disposable 3-F SpyBite forceps can be inserted into the SpyScope working channel for visually directed biopsies. Direct cholangioscopy offers both the ability to visually characterize an indeterminate stricture as benign or malignant and to perform visually targeted biopsies of suspicious lesions (▶Fig. 42.3). Chen et al published

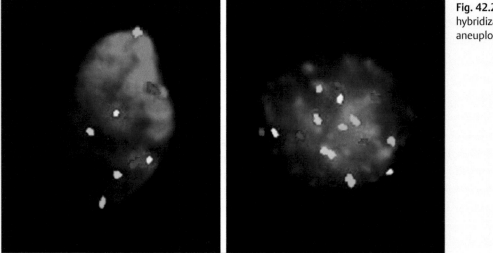

Fig. 42.2 Fluorescence in situ hybridization (FISH) showing chromosomal aneuploidy of malignant cells.

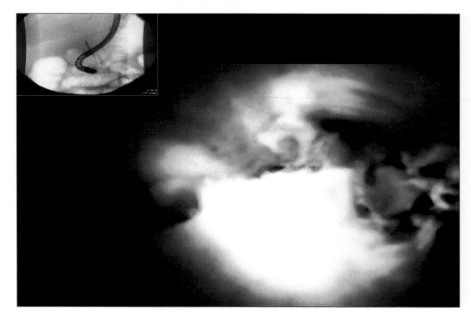

Fig. 42.3 Single-operator cholangioscopy of malignant biliary stricture.

the largest prospective, multicentered, observational study of the operating characteristics of the SOC system with 226 patients and reported a sensitivity of 78%, specificity of 82% for the visual impression of malignancy using SOC.[18] Visual impression had a higher sensitivity compared to SpyBite biopsy, which had a sensitivity of 47% and specificity of 98% for malignancy.[18] The main limitation of using cholangioscopy-based visual impression for diagnosing malignant strictures is the lack of interobserver agreement on the criteria that should be used. The tumor vessel sign has been shown to be a specific feature of malignancy but has low sensitivity of 61%.[19] One retrospective study involving multiple blinded expert endoscopists evaluating cholangioscopy videos of undifferentiated biliary strictures showed only fair agreement on the ultimate diagnosis of benign versus malignant etiology.[20] Significant complications of SOC includes a higher rate of cholangitis compared to ERCP alone (7 vs. 3%).[21] A new digital system was recently commercialized (Digital Spyglass, Boston Scientific) and provide better intraductal imaging. We, however, need further data to confirm early finding regarding its accuracy.[22]

42.2.5 Endoscopic Ultrasound-Fine Needle Aspiration

Endoscopic ultrasound (EUS) has an important complementary role to ERCP in the evaluation and staging of CCA. In the absence of a visible mass on cross-sectional imaging, EUS can identify suspicious bile duct thickening and assess for local lymphovascular invasion of the lesion[23] (▶ Fig. 42.4). The sensitivity of EUS-FNA for CCA is reported to be 53 to 89% across studies with better performance in distal CCA compared to proximal tumors.[24,25,26,27,28] EUS-FNA sensitivity is also lower in patients with previously placed biliary stents, which can cause acoustic shadowing.[23] Lastly, there is a theoretical risk of peritoneal seeding of malignant cells via the needle tract during FNA of proximal CCA, which has prompted some liver transplant centers to consider this technique a contraindication for transplantation.[29] Thus, it is important to consider resectability and transplant potential of the patient prior to any attempt at EUS-FNA of a proximal CCA.

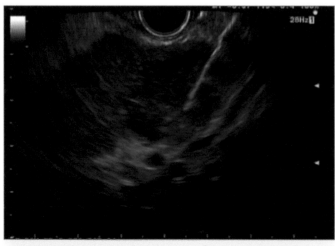

Fig. 42.4 Endoscopic ultrasound images of cholangiocarcinoma during fine-needle aspiration.

Table 42.2 Intraductal ultrasound criteria suggestive of malignant biliary stricture

Disruption of normal three-layer pattern bile duct wall

Hypoechoic mass with irregular margins

Heterogenous echo pattern

Invasion of mass into adjacent structures

Malignant lymphadenopathy (large, hypoechoic, round)

Reproduced with permission from Farrell RJ, Agarwal B, Brandwein SL, Underhill J, Chuttani R, Pleskow DK. Intraductal US is a useful adjunct to ERCP for distinguishing malignant from benign biliary strictures. Gastrointest Endosc 2002;56(5):681–687.

42.2.6 Intraductal Ultrasound

Along with EUS, intraductal ultrasound (IDUS) was developed to further enhance endobiliary imaging with a high-frequency probe that is guided directly into the biliary tree during ERCP. IDUS criteria have been developed to help with the differentiation of benign from malignant strictures (▶ Table 42.2).[30] Use of IDUS can improve the diagnostic accuracy of ERCP from 58 to 83% with improved sensitivity of 80 to 90% and specificity of 83% in diagnosing a malignant stricture.[31,32] In addition, IDUS can improve the accuracy of locoregional staging of hilar CCA compared to standard EUS because of the maneuverability of the probe to be in close proximity to the targeted tumor.[33,34]

42.2.7 Probe-based Confocal Laser Endomicroscopy

Probe-based confocal laser endomicroscopy (pCLE, Cellvizio; Mauna Kea Technologies, Paris, France) is another advanced imaging technology which uses laser light to provide in vivo microscopic-level images of the biliary epithelium in real time during ERCP. A confocal miniprobe is passed into the working channel of the duodenoscope and applied directly onto the biliary tissue. Recently the criteria to differentiate between benign and malignant strictures were refined to improve its specificity for malignancy and provide better descriptions of benign inflammatory changes in strictures (Paris classification) (▶ Fig. 42.5).[35,36] A prospective, multi-centered validation study of the Paris classification showed the combination of pCLE with ERCP had 89% sensitivity, 71% specificity, and 82% diagnostic accuracy for on-site diagnosis of malignant strictures.[36] A major limitation of pCLE is the lack of interobserver agreement in applying the criteria even among expert users of pCLE.[37]

42.3 Classification Systems

Cholangiocarcinomas are classified as extrahepatic and intrahepatic based on their anatomical location. Extrahepatic CCA include both hilar and distal common bile duct tumors. Hilar tumors are further subcategorized into types I to IV based on the Bismuth classification, which describes tumors according to their longitudinal extension along the biliary tree (▶ Fig. 42.6).[38,39] Type I refers to tumors limited to the common bile duct before the confluence, type II tumors involve the biliary confluence, type III cancers involve both the confluence and either the right (IIIa) or left (IIIb) hepatic ducts, and type IV

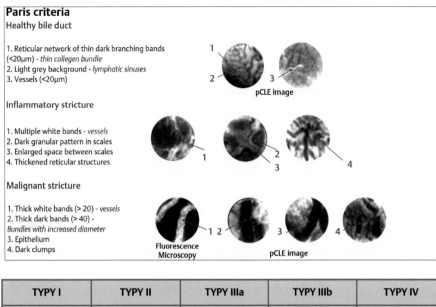

Paris criteria

Healthy bile duct

1. Reticular network of thin dark branching bands (<20μm) - *thin collegen bundle*
2. Light grey background - *lymphatic sinuses*
3. Vessels (<20μm)

pCLE image

Inflammatory stricture

1. Multiple white bands - *vessels*
2. Dark granular pattern in scales
3. Enlarged space between scales
4. Thickened reticular structures

Malignant stricture

1. Thick white bands (> 20) - *vessels*
2. Thick dark bands (> 40) - *Bundles with increased diameter*
3. Epithelium
4. Dark clumps

Fluorescence Microscopy

pCLE image

Fig. 42.5 Paris classification of probe-based confocal laser endomicroscopy findings in benign and malignant strictures.

TYPY I	TYPY II	TYPY IIIa	TYPY IIIb	TYPY IV

Fig. 42.6 Bismuth's classification of hilar cholangiocarcinoma.

refers to multifocal tumors involving both the confluence and both branches of the hepatic ducts. It is important to note that the Bismuth classification is an anatomical system of describing hilar CCA and is not a prognostic staging system. Clinical staging of CCA is based on the tumor nodal metastasis (TNM) system. Histologically, adenocarcinoma is the most common pathologic type of CCA, other rarer pathologic subtypes include papillary adenocarcinoma, intestinal type adenocarcinoma, clear cell adenocarcinoma, signet-ring cell carcinoma, and squamous cell carcinoma.[40]

42.4 Guidelines and Systematic Reviews

In 2013, the American Society of Gastrointestinal Endoscopy (ASGE) published guidelines on the evaluation of biliary neoplasm.[41] All of the modalities discussed above were reviewed and cited in the guidelines as complementary tools in the diagnostic work-up of an indeterminate biliary stricture. No algorithmic flowchart for the order or preference of use was specifically noted in the ASGE guidelines. The British Society of Gastroenterology also published updated guidelines for diagnosing CCA in 2012, which are summarized in ▶Table 42.3.[42] Our suggested algorithm for the stepwise use of these modalities in the work-up of suspected biliary malignancy is shown in ▶Fig. 42.7.

Table 42.3 British Society Guideline (2012) on the diagnosis of cholangiocarcinoma

Tumor markers

- CA 19–9 and CA 125 have low sensitivity and specificity, should only be used in conjunction with other diagnostic modalities (grade B)
- CA 19–9 should only be measured after relief of obstruction (grade B)

IgG4 cholangiopathy should be excluded prior to diagnosis of CCA

Imaging

- Contrast-enhanced high-resolution CT and/or MRI/MRCP are preferred imaging modalities in CCA (grade B)
- Contrast CT of the abdomen, chest, and pelvis should be obtained in all patients to rule out metastatic disease (grade B)

Endoscopic methods

- Invasive cholangiography should be reserved for histologic diagnosis and biliary decompression (grade B)
- FISH can enhance the diagnostic yield of routine cytology or biopsy (grade B)
- Cholangioscopy may be useful in expert centers
- EUS-guided FNA for tissue diagnosis should only be performed after surgical assessment of resectability due to risk of tumor seeding (grade B)

CA, cancer antigen; CCA, cholangiocarcinoma; CT, computed tomography; EUS, endoscopic ultrasound; FISH, fluorescence in situ hybridization; FNA, fine-needle aspiration; IgG4, immunoglobulin G4; MRCP, magnetic resonance cholangiopancreatography; MRI, magnetic resonance imaging.

Reproduced with permission from Khan SA, Davidson BR, Goldin RD, et al; British Society of Gastroenterology. Guidelines for the diagnosis and treatment of cholangiocarcinoma: an update. Gut 2012;61(12):1657–1669.

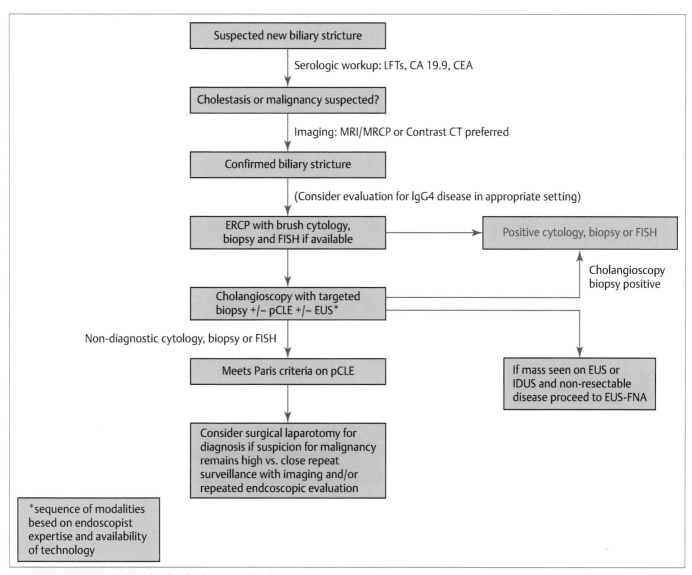

Fig. 42.7 A suggested algorithm for the diagnosis of malignant biliary stricture. CA, cancer antigen; CEA, carcinoembryonic antigen; CT, computed tomography; ERCP, endoscopic retrograde cholangiopancreatography; EUS, endoscopic ultrasound; FISH, fluorescence in situ hybridization; FNA, fine-needle aspiration; IgG4, immunoglobulin G4; LFTs, liver function tests; MRCP, magnetic resonance cholangiopancreatography; MRI, magnetic resonance imaging; pCLE, probe-based confocal laser endomicroscopy.

42.5 Therapeutic Approaches

42.5.1 Standard Techniques

Surgery

Surgical resection with negative margins, or R0 resection, is the only curative treatment for early-stage CCA. Intrahepatic CCA is treated with segmental resection or lobectomy alone with 3-year survival of 60% and 5-year survival rates of up to 22 to 44%.[43,44,45] Extrahepatic CCA in the absence of PSC is also treated with curative surgical resection. Distal extrahepatic CCA and ampullary cancers can be resected with pancreaticoduodenectomy. Types I and II Bismuth tumors are treated with en bloc resection of the extrahepatic ducts, gallbladder, and regional lymph nodes with Roux-en-Y hepaticojejunostomy.[38,46] Additional hepatic lobe resection may be needed in type III Bismuth tumors. Local lymph node involvement (N1) is not considered an absolute contraindication for resection in hilar CCA, as survival rates appear to be similar in those with and without regional lymph node involvement.[47] The absolute contraindications for surgical resection are listed in ▶ Table 42.4.[48] Five-year survival rates after R0 resection for hilar CCA are 30 to 41%, and 27 to 37% for extrahepatic tumors.[49,50,51,52] Perioperative mortality is between 5 and 10% with the primary cause being infection.[47]

42.5.2 Liver Transplantation

Liver transplantation as a curative treatment for extrahepatic CCA has been well studied, initially with dismal results, until the development by the Mayo Clinic in 2000 of a neoadjuvant protocol of chemoradiation prior to liver transplantation, which showed promising results for select patients with unresectable hilar CCA[53] (▶ Table 42.5). It has now been adopted by other expertise transplant centers as a curative treatment for hilar CCA. This protocol uses neoadjuvant external beam radiation and concurrent 5-fluorouracil (5-FU) chemotherapy, followed by brachytherapy and chemotherapy with capecitabine in multiple cycles until date of transplantation. An explorative laparotomy is performed 2 to 6 weeks after irradiation to assess for peritoneal and extrahepatic metastases, which would exclude transplant. Using their

Table 42.4 Contraindications for surgical resection of extrahepatic CCA

Bilateral lobar involvement

Unilobar involvement with contralateral portal vein or hepatic artery involvement

Bilateral portal vein or main portal vein involvement

Hepatic artery encasement

Distant lymph node metastasis

Intrahepatic metastasis (of extrahepatic CCA)

Distant metastasis

Primary sclerosing cholangitis

CCA, cholangiocarcinoma.

Adapted with permission.[48]

strict patient selection criteria (▶Table 42.4), the Mayo Clinic's single-center 1-year and 5-year disease-free survival rate under this protocol were 91 and 76%, respectively.[54,55] Later, a multicenter study using this protocol at other experienced transplant centers showed reproducible results with 5-year recurrence-free survival of 65%.[56] Liver transplantation, however, is not recommended for intrahepatic CCA due to poor outcomes with 5-year survival of less than 30%.[57]

Systemic Chemotherapy

Systemic chemotherapy in biliary tract cancers has shown modest benefit in overall survival. Many different agents have been investigated with the most commonly used chemotherapeutic agents being 5-FU and gemcitabine. 5-FU monotherapy and in combination with other chemotherapeutic agents has never been shown to significantly impact tumor growth or prolong survival.[58,59,60] The current standard chemotherapy regimen for biliary tract cancer is gemcitabine in combination with cisplatin based on a large randomized-controlled trial of 410 patients with locally advanced or metastatic biliary, ampullary, or gallbladder cancer randomized to gemcitabine monotherapy or combination therapy with cisplatin.[61] Median overall survival in the combination group was 11.7 months compared to 8.1 months in the monotherapy group.[61] The most serious adverse events of this regimen includes hematologic toxicities of neutropenia, anemia, thrombocytopenia, nonhematologic toxicities of gastrointestinal upset, rash, elevated liver function tests, and hyponatremia.[61,62]

Locoregional Therapy

Percutaneous Radiotherapy

Radiotherapy is a local ablative treatment that has been studied in the neoadjuvant, adjuvant, and palliative settings in biliary tract cancers.[63,64,65] Radiotherapy can be applied either as external beam radiation or transcatheter brachytherapy and can be used in combination with systemic chemotherapy such as 5-FU. Uncontrolled studies have shown conflicting results with some reporting prolonged survival after radiotherapy of up to 6 months compared to surgery and palliative stenting, while others failed to show any survival benefit.[65,66,67,68] There are significant adverse effects of radiotherapy including duodenal ulceration with

Table 42.5 Mayo Clinic criteria for liver transplantation of extrahepatic cholangiocarcinoma

Inclusion criteria:
- Positive cytology or biopsy
- Or CA 19–9 greater than 100 U/mL with malignant-appearing stricture without cholangitis
- Or positive FISH polysomy
- Candidate for orthotopic liver transplantation
- Hilar tumor above the cystic duct and deem unresectable by experienced surgeon

Exclusion criteria:
- Extrahepatic disease (including regional lymph node involvement)
- Discreet mass with radial diameter > 3 cm on cross-sectional imaging
- Conventionally resectable tumor
- Prior operative biopsy or attempted resection of tumor
- Prior chemotherapy or radiotherapy
- Previous malignancy within 5 y
- Uncontrolled infection
- Comorbidities precluding chemoirradiation or liver transplantation

CA, cancer antigen; FISH, fluorescence in situ hybridization.

Adapted from Heimbach JK, Gores GJ, Haddock MG, et al. Predictors of disease recurrence following neoadjuvant chemoradiotherapy and liver transplantation for unresectable perihilar cholangiocarcinoma. Transplantation 2006;82(12):1703–1707.

bleeding, gastric or duodenal obstruction, biliary stricture formation, and cholangitis related to catheter placement.[64]

Photodynamic Therapy

For unresectable CCA photodynamic therapy (PDT) is a method of palliation with supportive data of a modest survival benefit. PDT involves the intravenous infusion of a photosensitizer, most commonly a hematoporphyrin derivative, which is later photoactivated by application of a laser light that produces the specific wavelength of light at which the photosensitizing agent is activated. The laser is applied endoscopically via an intraluminal catheter during ERCP[69] (**Video 42.1**). The mechanism of cancer cell death is through the production of reactive oxygen species during the photodynamic reaction with resultant tumor cell apoptosis and vascular ischemia of tumor supplying vessels.[70,71] Multiple studies, including one randomized-controlled trial, have shown that when PDT is combined with palliative stenting, there is a significant survival benefit and improvement in quality of life.[69,72,73,74,75,76,77] A 2012 meta-analysis reported a statistically significant weighted survival advantage of 265 days in patients who underwent PDT with stenting compared to stenting alone.[78] The advantage of PDT is its relative ease of application during ERCP and the comparatively lower rate of side effects, with photosensitivity being the most common, compared to the adverse effects of systemic chemoradiation. However, other significant adverse events associated with PDT include hepatic abscess, cholangitis, facial burns, and skin rash.[79]

Biliary Stenting

Palliative biliary decompression is often necessary during the treatment course to provide relief of symptoms of biliary obstruction such as pruritus, jaundice, and cholangitis. Endoscopic biliary drainage is preferred over surgical hepaticojejunostomy or choledochojejunostomy due to its less invasive approach, fewer complications, and similar or even higher success rates that have been demonstrated in multiple high-quality randomized-controlled trials.[80,81] The first biliary stents used for palliation were plastic stents, but these had significant limitations of stent occlusion, migration, and need for exchange or replacement every 2 to 3 months. The advent of uncovered self-expanding metal stents (SEMS) in the 1990s presented an attractive alternative method of biliary decompression with lower rates of stent occlusion, cholangitis, longer complication-free survival, and lower overall cost for unresectable patients.[82,83,84,85,86] In malignant hilar tumors there remains controversy in the need for unilateral versus bilateral stenting with one randomized trial showing higher rates of success with unilateral drainage (87 vs. 77%, $p = 0.041$) and lower complication rates including lower rates of cholangitis (9 vs. 17%, $p = 0.013$).[87] Other retrospective studies showed superior long-term patency and median survival with bilateral stenting of hilar tumors.[88,89] In Bismuth I type tumors, uncovered metal stents have lower rates of migration compared to covered metal stents but higher rates of tumor ingrowth and the choice between the two is another area of ongoing controversy.[90]

42.5.3 Variation of Standard Techniques

Portal Vein Embolization

Portal vein embolization (PVE) is a technique to augment the remnant liver volume prior to surgical resection of CCA in patients who are otherwise marginal candidates for an extended hepatic resection due to a low native liver volume and concern of hepatic decompensation postoperatively.[91] Compensatory hypertrophy of the nonembolized lobe prior to surgery provides the "cushion" for maintaining adequate hepatic function postoperatively. An anticipated postresection "future liver volume" of less than 25% of the initial total liver volume has been shown to have more complications and poorer surgical outcomes.[92] When preoperative PVE is used to augment small volume livers prior to an extended hepatectomy (≥ five segments), patients who would otherwise have been excluded from potentially curative resection can become resection candidate and achieve similar survival rates as those with larger liver volumes.[92,93] Three- and 5-year survival rates after PVE of 41 and 26% were reported, similar to the 5-year survival rates for those who did not require PVE before resection.[93]

Radiofrequency Ablation

Endoscopic radiofrequency ablation (RFA) became available in 2009 after the development of the endobiliary catheter system, Habib EndoHPB, (EMcision Ltd, London) for delivery of radiotherapy directly into the bile ducts as a method of locoregional therapy for unresectable CCA. It consists of an 8-F catheter that is inserted into the biliary system after guidewire cannulation. The catheter delivers thermal energy via the bipolar probe causing local coagulative necrosis (▶Fig. 42.8). Initial studies of RFA demonstrated its safety but were aimed at prolonging stent patency and prevention of tumor ingrowth in patients who received palliative stenting.[94] In 2014, a retrospective study of patients treated with RFA and PDT was published showing similar overall survival between the two groups, but the study was limited by its retrospective,

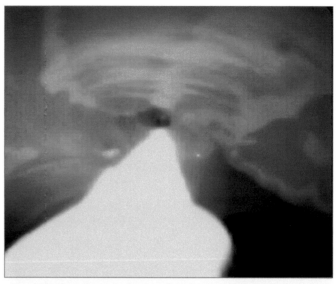

Fig. 42.8 Photodynamic therapy of cholangiocarcinoma.

nonrandomized design, small size, and unequal distribution of hilar CCA in the two treatment arms.[95] RFA provides the distinct advantage of avoiding the systemic photosensitivity associated with PDT but longer-term, multicentered, randomized head-to-head studies comparing PDT and RFA are still needed to determine the survival benefit and cost-effectiveness of these novel endoscopic therapies. Complications of RFA include cholangitis, hemobilia, and hepatic infarct.[96]

42.6 Guidelines and Reviews

Cholangiocarcinomas represent a heterogeneous group of tumors and treatment guidelines vary across societies, but any approach to the treatment of CCA should be multidisciplinary and individualized to the tumor subtype and the patient's clinical status. The British Society of Gastroenterology published a comprehensive guideline on the diagnosis and treatment of CCA in 2012 and the 2014 European Association for the Study of the Liver (EASL) guideline for intrahepatic CCA are summarized below.[42,97]

Hilar and distal cholangiocarcinoma (2012 British Society of Gastroenterology Guidelines)

- In resectable candidates, curative resection with R0 or negative margins is recommended, with or without PVE for augmentation of liver volume.
- Surgical bypass of biliary obstruction is not routinely recommended, as biliary stenting is the preferred method for palliation of obstruction.
- Liver transplantation with neoadjuvant chemoradiation can be considered for highly selected patients with hilar CCA but should not be considered for intrahepatic CCA.
- Preoperative biliary stenting in resectable disease remains controversial with conflicting data on clinical outcome.
- Initial stent insertion for biliary obstruction should be plastic until a determination of resectability is made. In those with unresectable disease a metal stent is preferred for palliation of obstruction in those with a life expectancy more than 4 months, but the choice of covered and uncovered metal stent remains controversial.
- At the time of the publication of the 2012 British Society guidelines newer endoscopic therapies for locoregional ablation were still being investigated and no recommendations can be made for their routine use.

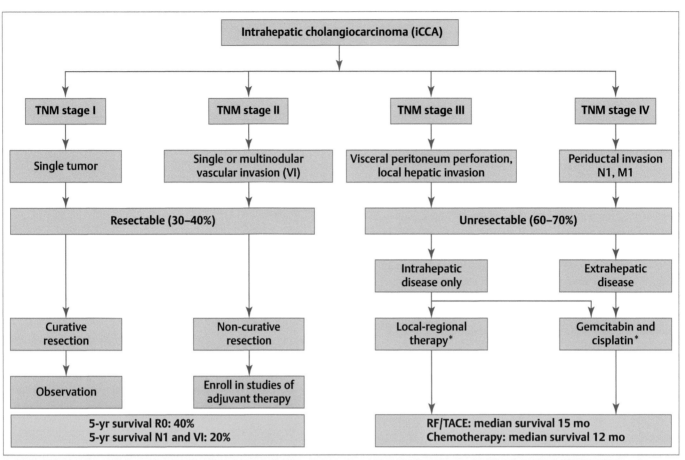

Fig. 42.9 Treatment algorithm for intrahepatic cholangiocarcinoma. RF, radiofrequency; TACE, transarterial chemoembolization; TNM, tumor node metastasis.

- Gemcitabine and cisplatin combination chemotherapy is recommended for locally advanced or unresectable CCA.
- Locoregional therapies including RFA, PDT, and transcatheter arterial embolization need to be studied in prospective randomized trials before recommendation for their routine use can be made.

Intrahepatic cholangiocarcinoma (ICCA) (2014 EASL guidelines) (▶Fig. 42.9)

- Surgical resection with goal of negative microscopic margins, R0 resection, is the treatment of choice for appropriate candidates with intrahepatic CCA (ICCA).
- Patients with obvious lymph node metastases, intrahepatic metastases, and vascular invasion should not undergo resection. Five-year survival after resection ranges from 15 to 40% in most series, with shorter survival seen in resection attempted for N1 disease.[98,99,100,101,102]
- There is no established role for adjuvant therapy postcurative resection.
- Liver transplantation is not recommended for ICCA.
- Gemcitabine and cisplatin combination chemotherapy is the practice standard regimen for unresectable CCA, including ICCA.
- There are no established first-line locoregional therapies for ICCA as most of these modalities have not been specifically investigated in ICCA and all data would be extrapolated from their use on other tumor types.

42.7 Areas of Uncertainty

There are multiple areas of uncertainty worthy of investigation in both the evaluation and management of biliary malignancy. From a diagnostic standpoint there is no standardized, sequential approach to the evaluation of a suspicious biliary stricture and the modalities used vary across institutions depending on the availabe technology and local expertise. The cost-effectiveness of each diagnostic modality individually and in combination has never been well studied. Despite the obvious clinical consequence of missing CCA we need to reconcile the cost of repeated, negative, or nondiagnostic testing of an indeterminate biliary stricture with the possibility of missing a cancer. From a therapeutic standpoint, the use of locoregional therapies such as RFA and PDT need to be better studied in large, prospective studies with head-to-head comparison to clarify their efficacy and respective roles in the treatment of CCA. The questions of covered versus uncovered SEMS and the need for bilateral biliary drainage in hilar obstruction remain controversial. As we have more conclusive data on the roles of newer endoscopic therapies for CCA, we will be able to better design multidisciplinary approaches to improve the treatment of this heterogeneous group of biliary neoplasm.

References

[1] Kim H-J, Kim M-H, Myung S-J, et al. A new strategy for the application of CA19-9 in the differentiation of pancreaticobiliary cancer: analysis using a receiver operating characteristic curve. Am J Gastroenterol. 1999; 94(7):1941–1946

[2] Zech CJ, Schoenberg SO, Reiser M, Helmberger T. Cross-sectional imaging of biliary tumors: current clinical status and future developments. Eur Radiol. 2004; 14(7):1174–1187

[3] Seo H, Lee JM, Kim IH, et al. Evaluation of the gross type and longitudinal extent of extrahepatic cholangiocarcinomas on contrast-enhanced multidetector row computed tomography. J Comput Assist Tomogr. 2009; 33(3):376–382

[4] Rösch T, Meining A, Frühmorgen S, et al. A prospective comparison of the diagnostic accuracy of ERCP, MRCP, CT, and EUS in biliary strictures. Gastrointest Endosc. 2002; 55(7):870–876

[5] Tillich M, Mischinger HJ, Preisegger KH, et al. Multiphasic helical CT in diagnosis and staging of hilar cholangiocarcinoma. AJR Am J Roentgenol. 1998; 171(3):651–658

[6] Aloia TA, Charnsangavej C, Faria S, et al. High-resolution computed tomography accurately predicts resectability in hilar cholangiocarcinoma. Am J Surg. 2007; 193(6):702–706

[7] Romagnuolo J, Bardou M, Rahme E, et al. Magnetic resonance cholangiopancreatography: a meta-analysis of test performance in suspected biliary disease. Ann Intern Med. 2003; 139(7):547–557

[8] Burnett AS, Calvert TJ, Chokshi RJ. Sensitivity of endoscopic retrograde cholangiopancreatography standard cytology: 10-y review of the literature. J Surg Res. 2013; 184(1):304–311

[9] Ponchon T, Gagnon P, Berger F, et al. Value of endobiliary brush cytology and biopsies for the diagnosis of malignant bile duct stenosis: results of a prospective study. Gastrointest Endosc. 1995; 42(6):565–572

[10] Glasbrenner B, Ardan M, Boeck W, et al. Prospective evaluation of brush cytology of biliary strictures during endoscopic retrograde cholangiopancreatography. Endoscopy. 1999; 31(9):712–717

[11] Jailwala J, Fogel EL, Sherman S, et al. Triple-tissue sampling at ERCP in malignant biliary obstruction. Gastrointest Endosc. 2000; 51(4 pt 1):383–390

[12] de Bellis M, Fogel EL, Sherman S, et al. Influence of stricture dilation and repeat brushing on the cancer detection rate of brush cytology in the evaluation of malignant biliary obstruction. Gastrointest Endosc. 2003; 58(2):176–182

[13] Schoefl R, Haefner M, Wrba F, et al. Forceps biopsy and brush cytology during endoscopic retrograde cholangiopancreatography for the diagnosis of biliary stenoses. Scand J Gastroenterol. 1997; 32(4):363–368

[14] Wright ER, Bakis G, Srinivasan R, et al. Intraprocedural tissue diagnosis during ERCP employing a new cytology preparation of forceps biopsy (Smash protocol). Am J Gastroenterol. 2011; 106(2):294–299

[15] Levy MJ, Baron TH, Clayton AC, et al. Prospective evaluation of advanced molecular markers and imaging techniques in patients with indeterminate bile duct strictures. Am J Gastroenterol. 2008; 103(5):1263–1273

[16] Gonda TA, Glick MP, Sethi A, et al. Polysomy and p16 deletion by fluorescence in situ hybridization in the diagnosis of indeterminate biliary strictures. Gastrointest Endosc. 2012; 75(1):74–79

[17] Moreno Luna LE, Kipp B, Halling KC, et al. Advanced cytologic techniques for the detection of malignant pancreatobiliary strictures. Gastroenterology. 2006; 131(4):1064–1072

[18] Chen YK, Parsi MA, Binmoeller KF, et al. Single-operator cholangioscopy in patients requiring evaluation of bile duct disease or therapy of biliary stones (with videos). Gastrointest Endosc. 2011; 74(4):805–814

[19] Kim HJ, Kim MH, Lee SK, et al. Tumor vessel: a valuable cholangioscopic clue of malignant biliary stricture. Gastrointest Endosc. 2000; 52(5):635–638

[20] Sethi A, Widmer J, Shah NL, et al. Interobserver agreement for evaluation of imaging with single operator choledochoscopy: what are we looking at? Dig Liver Dis. 2014; 46(6):518–522

[21] Sethi A, Chen YK, Austin GL, et al. ERCP with cholangiopancreatoscopy may be associated with higher rates of complications than ERCP alone: a single-center experience. Gastrointest Endosc. 2011; 73(2):251–256

[22] Amrita Sethi, Amy Tyberg, Adam Slivka, et al. Digital Single-Operator Cholangioscopy (Dsoc) Improves Interobserver Agreement (IOA) and Accuracy for Evaluation of Indeterminate Biliary Strictures Gastrointestinal Endoscopy, Vol. 83, Issue 5, AB600

[23] Mohamadnejad M, DeWitt JM, Sherman S, et al. Role of EUS for preoperative evaluation of cholangiocarcinoma: a large single-center experience. Gastrointest Endosc. 2011; 73(1):71–78

[24] Fritscher-Ravens A, Broering DC, Knoefel WT, et al. EUS-guided fine-needle aspiration of suspected hilar cholangiocarcinoma in potentially operable patients with negative brush cytology. Am J Gastroenterol. 2004; 99(1):45–51

[25] Lee JH, Salem R, Aslanian H, et al. Endoscopic ultrasound and fine-needle aspiration of unexplained bile duct strictures. Am J Gastroenterol. 2004; 99(6):1069–1073

[26] Rösch T, Hofrichter K, Frimberger E, et al. ERCP or EUS for tissue diagnosis of biliary strictures? A prospective comparative study. Gastrointest Endosc. 2004; 60(3):390–396

[27] Fritscher-Ravens A, Broering DC, Sriram PV, et al. EUS-guided fine-needle aspiration cytodiagnosis of hilar cholangiocarcinoma: a case series. Gastrointest Endosc. 2000; 52(4):534–540

[28] Eloubeidi MA, Chen VK, Jhala NC, et al. Endoscopic ultrasound-guided fine needle aspiration biopsy of suspected cholangiocarcinoma. Clin Gastroenterol Hepatol. 2004; 2(3):209–213

[29] Heimbach JK, Sanchez W, Rosen CB, Gores GJ. Trans-peritoneal fine needle aspiration biopsy of hilar cholangiocarcinoma is associated with disease dissemination. HPB (Oxford). 2011; 13(5):356–360

[30] Farrell RJ, Agarwal B, Brandwein SL, et al. Intraductal US is a useful adjunct to ERCP for distinguishing malignant from benign biliary strictures. Gastrointest Endosc. 2002; 56(5):681–687

[31] Stavropoulos S, Larghi A, Verna E, et al. Intraductal ultrasound for the evaluation of patients with biliary strictures and no abdominal mass on computed tomography. Endoscopy. 2005; 37(8):715–721

[32] Vazquez-Sequeiros E, Baron TH, Clain JE, et al. Evaluation of indeterminate bile duct strictures by intraductal US. Gastrointest Endosc. 2002; 56(3):372–379

[33] Menzel J, Poremba C, Dietl KH, Domschke W. Preoperative diagnosis of bile duct strictures—comparison of intraductal ultrasonography with conventional endosonography. Scand J Gastroenterol. 2000; 35(1):77–82

[34] Kim HM, Park JY, Kim KS, et al. Intraductal ultrasonography combined with percutaneous transhepatic cholangioscopy for the preoperative evaluation of longitudinal tumor extent in hilar cholangiocarcinoma. J Gastroenterol Hepatol. 2010; 25(2):286–292

[35] Caillol F, Filoche B, Gaidhane M, Kahaleh M. Refined probe-based confocal laser endomicroscopy classification for biliary strictures: the Paris classification. Dig Dis Sci. 2013; 58(6):1784–1789

[36] Slivka A, Gan I, Jamidar P, et al. Validation of the diagnostic accuracy of probe-based confocal laser endomicroscopy for the characterization of indeterminate biliary strictures: results of a prospective multicenter international study. Gastrointest Endosc. 2015; 81(2):282–290

[37] Talreja JP, Sethi A, Jamidar PA, et al. Interpretation of probe-based confocal laser endomicroscopy of indeterminate biliary strictures: is there any interobserver agreement? Dig Dis Sci. 2012; 57(12):3299–3302

[38] de Groen PC, Gores GJ, LaRusso NF, et al. Biliary tract cancers. N Engl J Med. 1999; 341(18):1368–1378

[39] Cheng JL, Bruno MJ, Bergman JJ, et al. Endoscopic palliation of patients with biliary obstruction caused by nonresectable hilar cholangiocarcinoma: efficacy of self-expandable metallic Wallstents. Gastrointest Endosc. 2002; 56(1):33–39

[40] Olnes MJ, Erlich R. A review and update on cholangiocarcinoma. Oncology. 2004; 66(3):167–179

[41] Anderson MA, Appalaneni V, Ben-Menachem T, et al; American Society for Gastrointestinal Endoscopy (ASGE) Standards of Practice Committee. The role of endoscopy in the evaluation and treatment of patients with biliary neoplasia. Gastrointest Endosc. 2013; 77(2):167–174

[42] Khan SA, Davidson BR, Goldin RD, et al; British Society of Gastroenterology. Guidelines for the diagnosis and treatment of cholangiocarcinoma: an update. Gut. 2012; 61(12):1657–1669

[43] Lieser MJ, Barry MK, Rowland C, et al. Surgical management of intrahepatic cholangiocarcinoma: a 31-year experience. J Hepatobiliary Pancreat Surg. 1998; 5(1):41–47

[44] Casavilla FA, Marsh JW, Iwatsuki S, et al. Hepatic resection and transplantation for peripheral cholangiocarcinoma. J Am Coll Surg. 1997; 185(5):429–436

[45] Ohtsuka M, Ito H, Kimura F, et al. Results of surgical treatment for intrahepatic cholangiocarcinoma and clinicopathological factors influencing survival. Br J Surg. 2002; 89(12):1525–1531

[46] Washburn WK, Lewis WD, Jenkins RL. Aggressive surgical resection for cholangiocarcinoma. Arch Surg. 1995; 130(3):270–276

[47] Jarnagin WR, Fong Y, DeMatteo RP, et al. Staging, resectability, and outcome in 225 patients with hilar cholangiocarcinoma. Ann Surg. 2001; 234(4):507–517, discussion 517–519

[48] Blechacz B, Gores GJ. Cholangiocarcinoma: advances in pathogenesis, diagnosis, and treatment. Hepatology. 2008; 48(1):308–321

[49] DeOliveira ML, Cunningham SC, Cameron JL, et al. Cholangiocarcinoma: thirty-one-year experience with 564 patients at a single institution. Ann Surg. 2007; 245(5):755–762

[50] Neuhaus P, Jonas S, Bechstein WO, et al. Extended resections for hilar cholangiocarcinoma. Ann Surg. 1999; 230(6):808–818, discussion 819

[51] Silva MA, Tekin K, Aytekin F, et al. Surgery for hilar cholangiocarcinoma; a 10 year experience of a tertiary referral centre in the UK. Eur J Surg Oncol. 2005; 31(5):533–539

[52] Pichlmayr R, Weimann A, Klempnauer J, et al. Surgical treatment in proximal bile duct cancer. A single-center experience. Ann Surg. 1996; 224(5):628–638

[53] De Vreede I, Steers JL, Burch PA, et al. Prolonged disease-free survival after orthotopic liver transplantation plus adjuvant chemoirradiation for cholangiocarcinoma. Liver Transpl. 2000; 6(3):309–316

[54] Heimbach JK, Gores GJ, Haddock MG, et al. Predictors of disease recurrence following neoadjuvant chemoradiotherapy and liver transplantation for unresectable perihilar cholangiocarcinoma. Transplantation. 2006; 82(12):1703–1707

[55] Gores GJ, Nagorney DM, Rosen CB. Cholangiocarcinoma: is transplantation an option? For whom? J Hepatol. 2007; 47(4):455–459

[56] Darwish Murad S, Kim WR, Harnois DM, et al. Efficacy of neoadjuvant chemoradiation, followed by liver transplantation, for perihilar cholangiocarcinoma at 12 US centers. Gastroenterology. 2012; 143(1):88–98.e3, quiz e14

[57] Pascher A, Jonas S, Neuhaus P. Intrahepatic cholangiocarcinoma: indication for transplantation. J Hepatobiliary Pancreat Surg. 2003; 10(4):282–287

[58] Takada T, Kato H, Matsushiro T, et al. Comparison of 5-fluorouracil, doxorubicin and mitomycin C with 5-fluorouracil alone in the treatment of pancreatic-biliary carcinomas. Oncology. 1994; 51(5):396–400

[59] Choi CW, Choi IK, Seo JH, et al. Effects of 5-fluorouracil and leucovorin in the treatment of pancreatic-biliary tract adenocarcinomas. Am J Clin Oncol. 2000; 23(4):425–428

[60] Patt YZ, Jones DV, Jr, Hoque A, et al. Phase II trial of intravenous flourouracil and subcutaneous interferon alfa-2b for biliary tract cancer. J Clin Oncol. 1996; 14(8):2311–2315

[61] Valle J, Wasan H, Palmer DH, et al; ABC-02 Trial Investigators. Cisplatin plus gemcitabine versus gemcitabine for biliary tract cancer. N Engl J Med. 2010; 362(14):1273–1281

[62] Suzuki E, Furuse J, Ikeda M, et al. Treatment efficacy/safety and prognostic factors in patients with advanced biliary tract cancer receiving gemcitabine monotherapy: an analysis of 100 cases. Oncology. 2010; 79(1–2):39–45

[63] Czito BG, Anscher MS, Willett CG. Radiation therapy in the treatment of cholangiocarcinoma. Oncology (Williston Park). 2006; 20(8):873–884, discussion 886–888, 893–895

[64] Foo ML, Gunderson LL, Bender CE, Buskirk SJ. External radiation therapy and transcatheter iridium in the treatment of extrahepatic bile duct carcinoma. Int J Radiat Oncol Biol Phys. 1997; 39(4):929–935

[65] Pitt HA, Nakeeb A, Abrams RA, et al. Perihilar cholangiocarcinoma. Postoperative radiotherapy does not improve survival. Ann Surg. 1995; 221(6):788–797, discussion 797–798

[66] Alden ME, Mohiuddin M. The impact of radiation dose in combined external beam and intraluminal Ir-192 brachytherapy for bile duct cancer. Int J Radiat Oncol Biol Phys. 1994; 28(4):945–951

[67] Kuvshinoff BW, Armstrong JG, Fong Y, et al. Palliation of irresectable hilar cholangiocarcinoma with biliary drainage and radiotherapy. Br J Surg. 1995; 82(11):1522–1525

[68] González González D, Gerard JP, Maners AW, et al. Results of radiation therapy in carcinoma of the proximal bile duct (Klatskin tumor). Semin Liver Dis. 1990; 10(2):131–141

[69] Ortner ME, Caca K, Berr F, et al. Successful photodynamic therapy for nonresectable cholangiocarcinoma: a randomized prospective study. Gastroenterology. 2003; 125(5):1355–1363

[70] Abels C. Targeting of the vascular system of solid tumours by photodynamic therapy (PDT). Photochem Photobiol Sci. 2004; 3(8):765–771

[71] Krammer B. Vascular effects of photodynamic therapy. Anticancer Res. 2001; 21(6B):4271–4277

[72] Berr F, Wiedmann M, Tannapfel A, et al. Photodynamic therapy for advanced bile duct cancer: evidence for improved palliation and extended survival. Hepatology. 2000; 31(2):291–298

[73] Shim CS, Cheon YK, Cha SW, et al. Prospective study of the effectiveness of percutaneous transhepatic photodynamic therapy for advanced bile duct cancer and the role of intraductal ultrasonography in response assessment. Endoscopy. 2005; 37(5):425–433

[74] Harewood GC, Baron TH, Rumalla A, et al. Pilot study to assess patient outcomes following endoscopic application of photodynamic therapy for advanced cholangiocarcinoma. J Gastroenterol Hepatol. 2005; 20(3):415–420

[75] Dumoulin FL, Gerhardt T, Fuchs S, et al. Phase II study of photodynamic therapy and metal stent as palliative treatment for nonresectable hilar cholangiocarcinoma. Gastrointest Endosc. 2003; 57(7):860–867

[76] Zoepf T, Jakobs R, Arnold JC, Apel D, Riemann JF. Palliation of nonresectable bile duct cancer: improved survival after photodynamic therapy. Am J Gastroenterol. 2005; 100(11):2426–2430

[77] Kahaleh M, Mishra R, Shami VM, et al. Unresectable cholangiocarcinoma: comparison of survival in biliary stenting alone versus stenting with photodynamic therapy. Clin Gastroenterol Hepatol. 2008; 6(3):290–297

[78] Leggett CL, Gorospe EC, Murad MH, Montori VM, Baron TH, Wang KK. Photodynamic therapy for unresectable cholangiocarcinoma: a comparative effectiveness systematic review and meta-analyses. Photodiagn Photodyn Ther. 2012; 9(3):189–195

[79] Talreja JP, Degaetani M, Ellen K, Schmitt T, Gaidhane M, Kahaleh M. Photodynamic therapy in unresectable cholangiocarcinoma: not for the uncommitted. Clin Endosc. 2013; 46(4):390–394

[80] Andersen JR, Sørensen SM, Kruse A, Rokkjaer M, Matzen P. Randomised trial of endoscopic endoprosthesis versus operative bypass in malignant obstructive jaundice. Gut. 1989; 30(8):1132–1135

[81] Smith AC, Dowsett JF, Russell RC, Hatfield AR, Cotton PB. Randomised trial of endoscopic stenting versus surgical bypass in malignant low bileduct obstruction. Lancet. 1994; 344(8938):1655–1660

[82] Moss AC, Morris E, Leyden J, MacMathuna P. Do the benefits of metal stents justify the costs? A systematic review and meta-analysis of trials comparing endoscopic stents for malignant biliary obstruction. Eur J Gastroenterol Hepatol. 2007; 19(12):1119–1124

[83] Knyrim K, Wagner HJ, Pausch J, Vakil N. A prospective, randomized, controlled trial of metal stents for malignant obstruction of the common bile duct. Endoscopy. 1993; 25(3):207–212

[84] Prat F, Chapat O, Ducot B, et al. A randomized trial of endoscopic drainage methods for inoperable malignant strictures of the common bile duct. Gastrointest Endosc. 1998; 47(1):1–7

[85] Kaassis M, Boyer J, Dumas R, et al. Plastic or metal stents for malignant stricture of the common bile duct? Results of a randomized prospective study. Gastrointest Endosc. 2003; 57(2):178–182

[86] Katsinelos P, Paikos D, Kountouras J, et al. Tannenbaum and metal stents in the palliative treatment of malignant distal bile duct obstruction: a comparative study of patency and cost effectiveness. Surg Endosc. 2006; 20(10):1587–1593

[87] De Palma GD, Galloro G, Siciliano S, Iovino P, Catanzano C. Unilateral versus bilateral endoscopic hepatic duct drainage in patients with malignant hilar biliary obstruction: results of a prospective, randomized, and controlled study. Gastrointest Endosc. 2001; 53(6):547–553

[88] Liberato MJA, Canena JMT. Endoscopic stenting for hilar cholangiocarcinoma: efficacy of unilateral and bilateral placement of plastic and metal stents in a retrospective review of 480 patients. BMC Gastroenterol. 2012; 12:103

[89] Vienne A, Hobeika E, Gouya H, et al. Prediction of drainage effectiveness during endoscopic stenting of malignant hilar strictures: the role of liver volume assessment. Gastrointest Endosc. 2010; 72(4):728–735

[90] Kullman E, Frozanpor F, Söderlund C, et al. Covered versus uncovered self-expandable nitinol stents in the palliative treatment of malignant distal biliary obstruction: results from a randomized, multicenter study. Gastrointest Endosc. 2010; 72(5):915–923

[91] Abdalla EK, Barnett CC, Doherty D, Curley SA, Vauthey JN. Extended hepatectomy in patients with hepatobiliary malignancies with and without preoperative portal vein embolization. Arch Surg. 2002; 137(6):675–680, discussion 680–681

[92] Vauthey JN, Chaoui A, Do KA, et al. Standardized measurement of the future liver remnant prior to extended liver resection: methodology and clinical associations. Surgery. 2000; 127(5):512–519

[93] Nagino M, Kamiya J, Nishio H, Ebata T, Arai T, Nimura Y. Two hundred forty consecutive portal vein embolizations before extended hepatectomy for biliary cancer: surgical outcome and long-term follow-up. Ann Surg. 2006; 243(3):364–372

[94] Steel AW, Postgate AJ, Khorsandi S, et al. Endoscopically applied radiofrequency ablation appears to be safe in the treatment of malignant biliary obstruction. Gastrointest Endosc. 2011; 73(1):149–153

[95] Strand DS, Cosgrove ND, Patrie JT, et al. ERCP-directed radiofrequency ablation and photodynamic therapy are associated with comparable survival in the treatment of unresectable cholangiocarcinoma. Gastrointest Endosc. 2014; 80(5):794–804

[96] Dolak W, Schreiber F, Schwaighofer H, et al; Austrian Biliary RFA Study Group. Endoscopic radiofrequency ablation for malignant biliary obstruction: a nationwide retrospective study of 84 consecutive applications. Surg Endosc. 2014; 28(3):854–860

[97] Bridgewater J, Galle PR, Khan SA, et al. Guidelines for the diagnosis and management of intrahepatic cholangiocarcinoma. J Hepatol. 2014; 60(6):1268–1289

[98] Tamandl D, Herberger B, Gruenberger B, Puhalla H, Klinger M, Gruenberger T. Influence of hepatic resection margin on recurrence and survival in intrahepatic cholangiocarcinoma. Ann Surg Oncol. 2008; 15(10):2787–2794

[99] Nakagohri T, Kinoshita T, Konishi M, Takahashi S, Gotohda N. Surgical outcome and prognostic factors in intrahepatic cholangiocarcinoma. World J Surg. 2008; 32(12):2675–2680

[100] Shimada K, Sano T, Nara S, et al. Therapeutic value of lymph node dissection during hepatectomy in patients with intrahepatic cholangiocellular carcinoma with negative lymph node involvement. Surgery. 2009; 145(4):411–416

[101] Nakagawa T, Kamiyama T, Kurauchi N, et al. Number of lymph node metastases is a significant prognostic factor in intrahepatic cholangiocarcinoma. World J Surg. 2005; 29(6):728–733

[102] Choi SB, Kim KS, Choi JY, et al. The prognosis and survival outcome of intrahepatic cholangiocarcinoma following surgical resection: association of lymph node metastasis and lymph node dissection with survival. Ann Surg Oncol. 2009; 16(11):3048–3056

43 Acute and Chronic Pancreatitis

Marianna Arvanitakis

43.1 Introduction

Acute pancreatitis (AP) is defined as an acute inflammation of the pancreas with involvement of various adjacent tissues and organ systems, and may be due to gallstone, alcohol, and other causes.[1] Chronic pancreatitis (CP) is an irreversible inflammatory process characterized by the destruction of pancreatic parenchyma and ductal structures associated with fibrosis.[2] It is characterized by the presence of main pancreatic duct (MPD) strictures and/or stones and may lead to pain, exocrine, and endocrine pancreatic failure. Endoscopy plays an important role in the management of acute and chronic pancreatitis. Endoscopic ultrasound (EUS) and endoscopic retrograde cholangiopancreatography (ERCP) are the two most common procedures performed in this setting. EUS is the cornerstone of diagnostic procedures, ranging from determining etiology of AP to confirming diagnosis of CP. ERCP should be considered as a therapeutic procedure only, and has been shown to be the basis of endoscopic therapy for CP, along with extracorporeal shock wave lithotripsy (ESWL). EUS-guided drainage of pancreatic collections has been applied extensively up to now for pseudocysts with mostly liquid contents, and recently developed endoscopic necrosectomy techniques have extended endoscopic management to walled-off necrosis containing solid debris. However, further studies are still required to standardize certain techniques and to investigate other alternatives. This chapter deals with diagnostic and therapeutic endoscopic procedures applied in patients with AP or CP explaining the technical modalities, and discussing indications and complications.

43.2 Diagnostic Approaches

43.2.1 Overview

EUS has largely surpassed ERCP with regard to diagnostic endoscopic procedures involving the pancreas, because of its relative limited invasiveness and low complication rates compared to ERCP (▶Table 43.1).[3,4] The most common applications include determination of AP etiology and diagnosis of CP.

43.2.2 Equipment and Techniques

EUS

EUS combines endoscopic visualization with two-dimensional ultrasound and allows high-resolution imaging of the pancreatic parenchyma and ductal structures. Both linear and radial endoscopes may be used for diagnostic procedures, but image characteristics differ. However, solely a linear endoscope can be used for therapeutic procedures, including fine-needle aspiration (FNA) and drainage.

43.2.3 Guidelines and Systematic Reviews

EUS and Diagnosis of Acute Pancreatitis Etiology

EUS may help in determining etiology in patients with unexplained AP. In a prospective study of 201 patients with a single episode of unexplained AP, EUS identified a cause in 31%, including choledocholithiasis, biliary sludge, and CP.[5] Another prospective comparative study showed that the diagnostic yield of EUS was higher than that of magnetic resonance cholangiopancreatography (MRCP) in patients with unexplained AP (51 vs. 20%, $p = 0.001$).[6] Indeed, MRCP may fail to detect small stones (< 4 mm) or stones distally situated near the papilla of Vater.[7] Regarding patients with suspected biliary AP and choledocholithiasis and given the higher morbidity of ERCP compared to EUS, sequential EUS and ERCP were assessed in two series in an effort to better triage patients in need of treatment. EUS showed high

Table 43.1 Complications of endoscopic procedures frequently utilized in the management of acute and chronic pancreatitis, according to published series

Procedure	Type of complication	Rates
EUS-FNA	Infection	0.4–1%
	Pancreatitis	0–2%
	Bleeding	0.13%
	Perforation	0.06%
ERCP	Pancreatitis[a]	1.6–15%
	Bleeding	1.3%
	Infection	1%
	Perforation	0.1–0.6%
ESWL	Pancreatitis	4.4%
	Infection	1.4%
	Steinstrasse[b]	0.4%
	Bleeding	0.3%
	Perforation	0.3%
EUS-guided drainage	Bleeding	0–9%
	Infection	0–8%
	Retroperitoneal perforation	0–5%

EUS-FNA, endoscopic ultrasound with fine-needle aspiration; ERCP, endoscopic retrograde cholangiopancreatography; ESWL, extracorporeal shock wave lithotripsy.

[a]Risk varies according to patient and procedure-related factors.

[b]Acute stone incarceration in the papilla leading to poor pancreatic juice drainage and pain, requiring emergency ERCP or ESWL.

Adapted from Early DS, Acosta RD, Chandrasekhara V, et al; ASGE Standards of Practice Committee. Adverse events associated with EUS and EUS with FNA. Gastrointest Endosc 2013;77: 839–843[3] Anderson MA, Fisher L, Jain R, Evans JA, et al; ASGE Standards of Practice Committee. Complications of ERCP. Gastrointest Endosc 2012;75:467–473[4] and Ge PS, Weizmann M, Watson RR. Pancreatic pseudocysts: advances in endoscopic management. Gastroenterol Clin North Am 2016;45:9–27.[62]

accuracy (97–98%) for choledocholithiasis detection, similar or better to ERCP.[8,9] A systematic review of all seven studies assessing the EUS-based strategy showed that ERCP was avoided in 71.2% of cases. No complications were related to EUS, whereas sphincterotomy was associated with bleeding in up to 22% of patients undergoing ERCP.[10] Regarding cost-effectiveness, a Monte Carlo decision analysis reported that the EUS-first strategy was preferable for severe biliary AP, with reduced costs, fewer therapeutic ERCPs, and fewer complications.[11] Finally, pancreatic cancer should be excluded in patients above 40 years of age with unexplained AP. The American Society of Gastrointestinal Endoscopy (ASGE) guidelines suggest EUS for the evaluation of idiopathic AP for patients older than 40 years if history, physical examination, laboratory testing, and abdominal imaging with MRCP or computed tomography (CT) are unrevealing.[2]

EUS and Diagnosis of Chronic Pancreatitis

EUS parenchymal and ductal features of CP are summarized in ▶Table 43.2. Each of these features was initially counted as 1 point (on a scale of 0–9) with higher scores increasing the probability of disease. Five or more features were consistent with CP, whereas absence of all features excluded CP.[12] However, uncertainty remained and a new consensus based on expert opinion assigned different weight to each feature to increase diagnostic accuracy[13] (▶Table 43.2). Nevertheless, this modified classification system failed to increase interobserver agreement for the diagnosis of CP compared to the initial scoring system.[14] This underscores the need to combine EUS findings with clinical, structural, and functional analyses and to be aware of the possible overdiagnosis of CP in case of recent AP, aging, male gender, tobacco or alcohol use, and obesity.[15]

43.3 Therapeutic Approaches

43.3.1 Standard Techniques

ERCP

ERCP allows therapeutic interventions of the pancreatic duct and it is the cornerstone of endoscopic therapy for pancreatic diseases. This procedure requires fluoroscopy and a fixed undercouch system to limit radiation exposure to the staff.[16] The team requires an endoscopist, an anesthesiologist, a radiology technician, and at least one nurse. The patient is in supine or prone position, for better anatomical view of the ducts. ERCP is performed with a side-viewing endoscope (duodenoscope) with a large operating channel (4.2 mm), which is introduced into the descending duodenum at a stable position en face to the papilla, as well as introduction of accessories in the bile or pancreatic duct. Necessary devices include a standard ball-tip catheter, a sphincterotome (short nose with a 20-mm wire), angulated hydrophilic-tip guidewires (0.025 and 0.035 in), balloon dilators (4–6 mm), bougies (7–10 F), Soehendra's retrievers (8.5 and 10 F) for stricture dilation, a balloon stone extractor, a small Dormia basket, and plastic straight stents (from 3- to 12-cm length and 5 to 10 F).[17] Biliary or pancreatic duct cannulation is attempted, according to the indication of ERCP.

Table 43.2 EUS criteria for diagnosis of CP (Rosemont's criteria)

Criteria	Parenchymal changes	Ductal changes	Histologic correlation
Major A	Hyperechoic foci with shadowing	MPD stones	Focal fibrosis Calcified stones
Major B	Lobularity with honeycombing		Interlobular fibrosis
Minor	Lobularity without honeycombing Hyperechoic foci without shadowing Hyperechoic strands Cysts	Irregular/dilated MPD Duct irregularity Hyperechoic MPD margins Visible side branches	Interlobular fibrosis Focal fibrosis Bridging fibrosis Cyst/pseudocyst > 3-mm head, > 2-mm body, > 1-mm tail Focal dilation, narrowing Periductal fibrosis Dilated side branches

Consistent with chronic pancreatitis: 1 major A feature and ≥ 3 minor features, 1 major A and major B features, 2 major A features. Suggestive of chronic pancreatitis: 1 major A feature and ≤ 3 minor features, 1 major B feature and ≥ 3 minor features, ≥ 5 minor features. Indeterminate for chronic pancreatitis: 3 or 4 minor features, major B feature alone or with < 3 minor features. Normal: ≤ 2 minor features without major features.

CP, chronic pancreatitis; EUS, endoscopic ultrasound; honeycombing: ≥ 3 contiguous lobules measuring at least 5 mm in length; MPD, main pancreatic duct.

Adapted from Catalano MF, Sahai A, Levy M, et al. EUS-based criteria for the diagnosis of chronic pancreatitis: the Rosemont classification. Gastrointest Endosc 2009;69:1251–1261[13] and Gardner TB, Levy MJ. EUS diagnosis of chronic pancreatitis. Gastrointest Endosc 2010;71:1280–1289.[15]

Pancreatic Sphincterotomy of the Major Papilla

Pancreatic duct cannulation is performed by placing the endoscope in front of the papilla and directing the ball-tip catheter or the sphincterotome, perpendicularly, toward the 1 o'clock direction. The guidewire technique or contrast injection may be used. Both techniques require extreme caution, especially in patients who do not have mild or moderate chronic pancreatitis, because of the high risk of post-ERCP pancreatitis, which is increased in case of multiple guidewire passes or high-volume injections.[18] Using the sphincterotome, a 5- to 10-mm incision is performed toward the 1 o'clock direction, with pure cutting current, to limit the possible future development of fibrosis and papillary stricture.[19] A pancreatic stent is usually inserted after pancreatic sphincterotomy to reduce the incidence of post-ERCP acute pancreatitis.[18]

An alternative method to pancreatic sphincterotomy utilizes an endoscopic needle knife instead of a standard pull-type sphincterotome. In this case, the pancreatic stent is inserted beforehand. The tip of the needle knife is placed at the most proximal portion of pancreatic sphincter tissue that is overlying the stent. While using the stent as a guide to direct the cut along the plane of the pancreatic duct, the needle-knife tip is advanced over the top of the stent and down its longitudinal axis thereby "unroofing" the intraduodenal portion of the major papilla.[20]

Pancreatic Sphincterotomy of the Minor Papilla

Sphincterotomy of the minor papilla might be indicated in case of pancreas divisum morphology, when pancreatic duct drainage is required. Similarly, to sphincterotomy of the major papilla, it can be performed with a standard or ultrataper pull-type sphincterotome, or with a needle-knife cut over a plastic stent. A retrospective comparative study demonstrated that overall complication as well as reintervention rates for papillary stricture were similar in those undergoing needle knife and pull-type sphincterotome minor papilla sphincterotomy.[21] The cutting wire of the sphincterotome or the needle knife is directed toward 11 o' clock and pure cutting current is used.[20]

Managing MPD Strictures

After access into the MPD and sphincterotomy, stent insertion may be performed in case of pancreatic strictures. This is achieved by first introducing the guidewire through the stricture, as far as possible, preferably with a loop at the proximal end. The second step consists of dilating, either by using a balloon, a boogie, or a Soehendra's retriever for very tight, fibrotic strictures.[22,23] Polyethylene 8.5- to 10-F pancreatic stents tailored to the shape of the pancreatic duct and length of the stricture are most commonly used[23] (▶ Fig. 43.1). Thinner stents (≤ 8.5 F) are related to more frequent hospitalizations for pain due to stent occlusion.[24]

Extracorporeal Shock Wave Lithotripsy

ESWL allows fragmentation of radio-opaque pancreatic stones before ERCP, to facilitate their extraction. The technique of ESWL requires four components, namely a shock wave generator, a focusing system, a coupling mechanism, and a localizing unit, all of which are packed in the same apparatus.[25] Best results are obtained by the third-generation lithotripters, which are equipped with bidimensional fluoroscopic and ultrasonic targeting systems. The procedure should be performed on a slightly lateral decubitus position, under general anesthesia, with a maximum of 5,000 shocks per session delivered with increasing intensity at a rate of 90 shocks per minute.[26] Successful stone fragmentation following ESWL has been defined as stones broken into fragments less than or equal to 2 or 3 mm, or by the demonstration of a decreased stone density at X-ray, an increased stone surface, and heterogeneity of the stone, which may fill the MPD and adjacent side branches.[23] ERCP may follow during the same session (**Video 43.1**).

EUS-Guided Transmural Drainage

Pancreatic collection drainage is preferably performed under combined EUS and fluoroscopy guidance, unless the collection is bulging when only fluoroscopy may be used. Nevertheless, EUS-guided drainage has higher rates of technical success.[23,27,28,29,30,31,32,33,34,35,36] Therapeutic linear EUS endoscopes should be used.

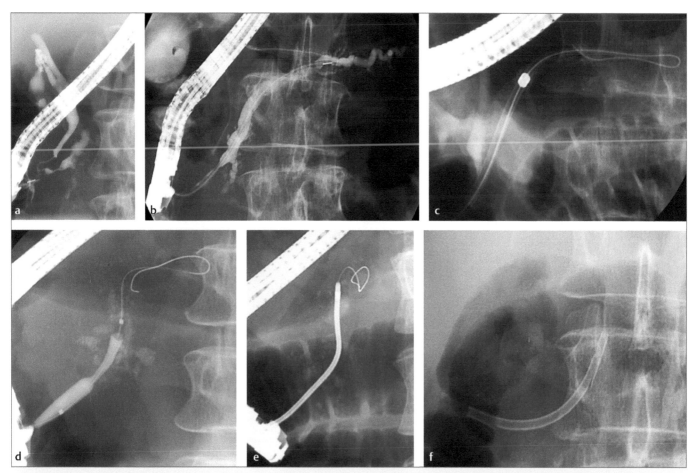

Fig. 43.1 Fluoroscopic images showing endoscopic management of patients with painful chronic pancreatitis. (**a**) Contrast injection reveals a distal main pancreatic duct stricture with upstream dilation. (**b**) Deep cannulation is achieved with a sphincterotome. (**c**) After sphincterotomy, the stricture is dilated with a plastic bougie. (**d**) Other alternative devices for dilation include the pneumatic balloon. (**e**) A Soehendra's retriever can be used for very tight strictures or in case of stones. (**f**) A straight plastic stent is inserted after dilation.

The procedure is performed with the patient under general anesthesia and endotracheal intubation, especially in case of large collections. Antibiotic prophylaxis is recommended for sterile pancreatic fluid collections Access can be gained through the stomach (cystogastrostomy), or the bulb (cystoduodenostomy). Puncture is performed by the electrosurgical needle of a 10-F cystenterostome. Then, a 0.035-in guidewire is inserted and the tract is enlarged by passing the cystenterostome into the collection, followed by the positioning of a double-pigtail stent and/ or a nasocystic catheter. For the placement of multiple stents, further dilation of the transmural path is achieved by a balloon catheter. At least two double plastic pigtail stents should be inserted[29] (**Video 43.2**).

Endoscopic Necrosectomy

Endoscopic management of necrotic pancreatic collections (walled-off necrosis) containing solid debris requires a more aggressive approach. Necrosectomy includes a first step involving transmural drainage to gain access, followed by debridement of the necrotic cavity. After initial access is established, the tract is dilated up to 15 to 20 mm, followed by placement of multiple large-bore double-pigtail stents or of a single large-diameter fully covered metallic stent.[36,37] Debridement is achieved with a forward-viewing endoscope and various devices (nets snares, baskets), preferably with at least one double-pigtail stent or catheter left in place to maintain access. Debridement is combined with irrigation and repeated if necessary.

43.3.2 Guidelines and Systemic Reviews

Biliary Acute Pancreatitis

The role and timing of ERCP in biliary AP has been the subject of numerous trial, meta-analyses, and recommendations during the last 20 years. Concerning early ERCP, the latest study from the Cochrane Collaboration included seven randomized-controlled trials and concluded that in patients with biliary AP, there is no evidence that early routine ERCP significantly affects mortality and local or systemic complications, regardless of predicted severity. However, early ERCP with biliary sphincterotomy may be beneficial in patients with co-existing cholangitis or biliary obstruction.[38] Furthermore, a recent randomized-controlled trial showed that same-admission cholecystectomy reduced the rate of recurrent gallstone-related complications in patients with mild biliary AP, with a very low risk of cholecystectomy-related complications. This study underlines the indication of same-admission cholecystectomy in patients with mild AP instead of ERCP with biliary sphincterotomy, because ERCP with sphincterotomy may reduce the risk of recurrent biliary AP but will have no effect on other biliary events such as cholecystitis.[39] However, in patients with severe biliary AP and local complications requiring interval cholecystectomy, preoperative ERCP with biliary sphincterotomy may offer some protection against recurrent biliary-related complications[40] (▶Fig. 43.2).

Sphincter of Oddi Dysfunction

Pancreatic sphincter of Oddi (SOD) can be classified in three types: type 1 with pain, more than twofold elevated pancreatic enzymes on two occasions, and dilated MPD; type 2 with pain and either elevated enzymes or dilated MPD; and type 3 with only pain[41]. Types 1 and 2 patients may present with recurrent AP. Endoscopic approach varies according to centers; some advocate biliary and/ or pancreatic sphincterotomy and others perform biliary sphincterotomy only, followed by pancreatic sphincterotomy if symptoms persist. A recent randomized trial of patients with recurrent AP demonstrated that patients with pancreatic SOD responded similarly to biliary sphincterotomy alone (51.5%) compared to combined biliary and pancreatic sphincterotomies (52.8%; $p = 1$) for the prevention of recurrent episodes of AP.[42] Furthermore, a multicenter, randomized, controlled trial failed to show any benefit of endoscopic therapy for SOD type 3 patients.[43]

Chronic Pancreatitis

Strictures

According to published series, pancreatic stenting for strictures has a technical success rate of 85 to 98% and leads to immediate pain relief in 65 to 95% of patients. During follow-up (14–58 months), persistent pain relief has been described in 32 to 68% of patients.[23] Because short periods of stenting have shown to be disappointing, MPD stenting is performed for at least a 12 months.[44] Criteria used for definitely removing stents include adequate pancreaticoduodenal outflow of contrast medium after ductal filling upstream from the stricture, and easy passage of a 6-F catheter through the stricture.[45] After prolonged MPD stenting, recurrent pain was observed in 36 to 48% of patients after "definitive" stent removal and restenting was indicated in 20 to 30% of patients.[45,46,47]

Stones

Endoscopic removal of pancreatic stones without prior ESWL has very low success rates (9%), high complication rates, and therefore should be avoided.[23,48] On the other hand, a systemic review including 11 series and 1,149 patients showed that ESWL is very effective for fragmenting radio-opaque pancreatic stones with success rates up to 89%.[49] Complication rates are low with pancreatitis occurring at 4.4%.[50] ESWL may be used alone or in combination with ERCP. A randomized-controlled trial compared ESWL alone versus ESWL followed by ERCP in 55 patients.[51] The only significant differences were longer hospital stay and higher treatment cost in the group combining ESWL with ERCP.

Regarding endoscopic therapy for CP, including ESWL and/or ERCP, many independent studies including 1,890 patients have shown its efficacy, with up to 83% of patients avoiding surgery[26,45,46,52,53,54,55,56,57] (▶Table 43.3). Two randomized trials compared endoscopic to surgical therapy for pain in CP[58,59,60] (▶Table 43.4). Although both trials showed better results in the surgery group, endoscopic therapy was suboptimal in both studies (no ESWL in the study from Dite et al, very short stenting periods in both studies). Taking into consideration the substantial morbidity and mortality (up to 4%) for surgical MPD drainage, the European Society of Gastrointestinal Endoscopy (ESGE) recommends

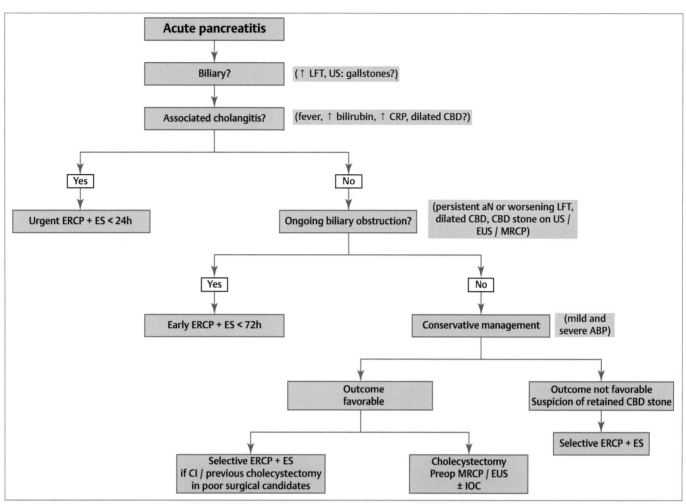

Fig. 43.2 Proposed algorithm for management of acute biliary pancreatitis. ABP, acute biliary pancreatitis; aN, abnormal; CBD, common bile duct; CI, contraindication; CRP, C-reactive protein; ES, endoscopic biliary sphincterotomy; ERCP, endoscopic retrograde cholangiopancreatography; EUS, endoscopic ultrasound; IOC, intraoperative cholangiography; LFT, liver function test; MRCP, magnetic resonance cholangiopancreatography; Preop, preoperative; US, abdominal ultrasound;

endoscopic therapy as first-line therapy for patients with painful uncomplicated CP[23] (▶Fig. 43.3, ▶Fig. 43.4).

Pancreatic Fluid Collections

Pancreatic fluid collections in AP are classified according to their contents and duration since the onset of the disease.[61] Pancreatic pseudocysts and walled-off necrosis (WON) should be differentiated from acute peripancreatic fluid collections and acute necrotic collections, both of which occur in the acute phase of pancreatitis or necrotizing pancreatitis (▶Fig. 43.5). These collections lack an encapsulated, well-defined wall. These are not candidates to endoscopic drainage and often resolve with expectant management.[62] Indications for drainage of pancreatic fluid collections include pain, infection, and compression of adjacent organs with gastric outlet syndrome or jaundice.[1,23]

Pseudocyst Drainage

A pseudocyst is defined as a fluid collection in the peripancreatic tissues, surrounded by a well-defined wall and containing essentially no solid material.[61] It can occur in both AP and CP.

Endoscopic therapy of pseudocysts may be obtained with transpapillary (through the papilla and the MPD) or transmural

drainage. Overall, endoscopic drainage is an excellent first-line therapy for the drainage of pancreatic pseudocysts, with complete resolution of pseudocysts in 71 to 95% of cases, complication rates of 0 to 37%, and procedure-related mortality of 0 to 1%.[62] Transpapillary drainage may be performed in case of a small (< 50 mm) pseudocyst communicating with the MPD. Three nonrandomized studies compared transpapillary to transmural drainage; transpapillary drainage was associated with lower morbidity (1/56 [1.8%] vs. 18/117 [15.4%] patients; p = `0.008) and similar long-term success (53/56 [94.6%] vs. 105/117 [89.7%] patients; p = 0.391) than transmural drainage.[63,64,65] EUS-guided transmural drainage is indicated for large, noncommunicating pseudocysts, which constitutes the majority of pseudocysts[27,28,29,30,31,32,33,34,35,36] (▶Table 43.5). In these cases, combining EUS-guided transmural with transpapillary drainage does not seem to improve outcome.[66] After transmural drainage and pseudocyst resolution, early stent removal (< 8 weeks) was associated with recurrences compared with stent maintenance in a randomized-controlled trial of 28 patients.[29]

Endoscopic Necrosectomy for WON

WON consists of necrotic tissue contained within the wall of reactive tissue. It is a mature, encapsulated collection of pancreatic

Table 43.3 Long-term outcome of largest series focused on endoscopic therapy for pain in patients with chronic pancreatitis

First author Year, reference	Number	ESWL (%)	Follow-up (months)	Surgery (%)	Ongoing endoscopic therapy (%)	Complete or partial pain relief (%)
Binmoeller 1995[46]	93	36	58	26	13	64
Rösch 2002[52]	1,018	50	58	24	16	85
Delhaye 2004[26]	56	100	173	21	18	65
Eleftherladis 2005[45]	100	51	69	4	38	62
Tadenuma 2005[53]	70/117[a]	100	75	1	20	70
Inui 2005[55]	504/555[a]	100	44	4	ND	ND
Farnbacher 2006[54]	98	ND	46	23	18	64
Seven 2012[56]	58/120[a]	100	52	16	8	86
Tandan 2013[57]	272/636[a]	100	> 60	9	ND	94%

ESWL, extracorporeal shock wave lithotripsy; ND, no data.

[a]Only a part of the study population had long-term follow-up.

Table 43.4 Randomized-controlled trials involving endoscopic therapy for pain in patients with chronic pancreatitis (excluding celiac plexus block trials)

	Díte et al 2003[58]		Cahen et al 2007[59]		Dumonceau et al 2007[51]	
	ERCP	Surgery	ESWL and ERCP	Surgery (LLPJ)	ESWL	ESWL and ERCP
Number	36	36	19	20	26	29
Pain relief (%) Complete Partial	15 46	34[a] 52	16 16	40 35	58 ND	55 ND
Complications (%)	8	8	58	35	0	3
Need for surgery (%)	0	3	21	5	4	10
Follow-up	5 y		6 y		4 y	

ERCP, endoscopic retrograde cholangiopancreatography; ESWL; extracorporeal shock wave lithotripsy; LLPJ, laterolateral pancreaticojejunostomy; ND, no data.

[a]p < 0.05.

and/or peripancreatic necrosis and has a well-defined inflammatory wall; usually this maturation occurs more than or equal to 4 weeks after the onset of necrotizing AP.[61] An initial retrospective comparison of endoscopic necrosectomy with conventional transmural endoscopic drainage for WON demonstrated that successful resolution was greater in the necrosectomy group (88 vs. 45%, p = 0.01) with similar complication rates.[67] The largest series focused on endoscopic necrosectomy in 197 patients and showed an overall success rate of 81 to 91% and a mortality rate of 1.9 to 7.5%.[68,69]

EUS-Guided Celiac Block

Celiac block consists of an injection of a mixture of corticoids with a local anesthetic into celiac plexus nerves to disrupt the signaling of painful stimuli through pancreatic afferent nerves.[23] EUS was superior to CT guidance in two randomized-controlled

trials.[70,71] Two meta-analyses have reported pain relief, albeit transient, in 51 to 59% of patients with painful CP.[72,73] Therefore, the ESGE guidelines recommend EUS-guided celiac block only as a second-line treatment for pain in CP.[23]

43.4 Areas of Uncertainty, Experimental Techniques, and Research

43.4.1 Diagnostic Procedures

EUS elastography is a method to assess tissue stiffness and has been shown to be highly accurate for the differential diagnosis of solid masses of the pancreas.[74] Recently, EUS elastography was also shown to be a useful tool for the diagnosis of CP by assessing the degree of fibrosis by measurement of the strain ratio. A

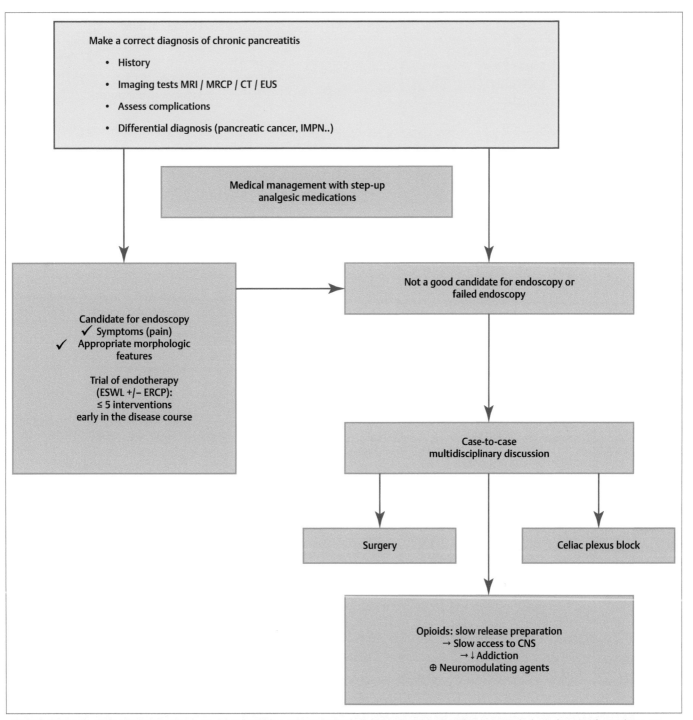

Fig. 43.3 Proposed algorithm for step-up management for patients with chronic pancreatitis. Appropriate morphologic features for endoscopic therapy are stones and/or strictures located in the head of the pancreas, with upstream main pancreatic duct dilation. CT, computed tomography; ERCP, endoscopic retrograde cholangiopancreatography; ESWL, extracorporeal shock wave lithotripsy; EUS, endoscopic ultrasound; IPMN, intraductal papillary mucinous neoplasm; MRCP, magnetic resonance cholangiopancreatography; MRI, magnetic resonance imaging.

prospective study included 191 patients with suspected or known CP and a highly significant linear correlation was found between the number of EUS criteria for CP and the strain ratio.[75] The same group also demonstrated a direct relationship between the strain ratio and the probability of pancreatic exocrine failure.[76] Therefore, this technique may have further clinical implications in the future.

Despite advanced imaging techniques, in some cases, pancreatic duct strictures remain indeterminate. Lately, intraductal imaging devices have been developed and tested in this setting. These include peroral pancreatoscopy (such as the dual- or single-operator mother–baby scope), intraductal ultrasound, and probe-based

confocal laser endomicroscopy.[77] Although these modalities offer constantly improved images with increased resolution, their diagnostic accuracy for differentiating indeterminate pancreatic strictures has still to be determined. Furthermore, issues such as learning curves, reproducibility, and cost-effectiveness have to be addressed to.

43.4.2 Therapeutic Procedures

ESGE recommends treating MPD strictures in CP patients by inserting a single, 10-F plastic stent, with stent removal planned

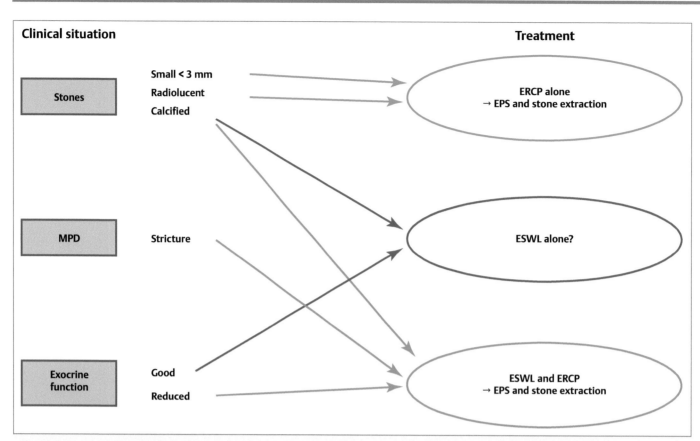

Fig. 43.5 Proposed algorithm for tailoring endoscopic treatment for patients with painful chronic pancreatitis: ESWL alone, ESWL followed by ERCP, and ERCP without previous ESWL. Determinant factors are type and size of stones, the presence or absence of main pancreatic duct strictures, and the status of exocrine function. EPS, endoscopic pancreatic sphincterotomy; ERCP, endoscopic retrograde cholangiopancreatography; ESWL, extracorporeal shock wave lithotripsy; MPD, main pancreatic duct.

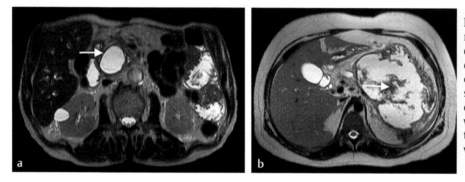

Fig. 43.5 Axial T2-weighted magnetic resonance imaging sequences depicting two different types of pancreatic fluid collections, occurring usually late (> 4 weeks) during the course of acute pancreatitis. **(a)** A pseudocyst is surrounded by a well-defined wall and contains essentially no solid material (*arrow*); **(b)** A walled-off necrosis (WON) consists of necrotic tissue contained within a well-defined wall with various degrees of solid contents (*arrow*).

within 12 months.[23] Simultaneous placement of multiple, side-by-side plastic stents has already been tested and could be applied more extensively.[78] Moreover, temporary insertion of fully covered metal stents has been reported to be safe and efficient regarding short-term pain relief after stent removal[79] (▶Fig. 43.6). Finally, in patients with strictures and an upstream MPD dilation, in whom conventional transpapillary drainage has failed and who are considered high-risk surgical candidates, EUS-guided access and drainage of the MPD may be considered.[23,80,81] In published retrospective series, pain relief has been described in 50 to 75% of patients and symptom recurrence in up to 25%. Furthermore, complication rate is high (up to 50%),

therefore these interventions should be considered only in selected patients and performed in referral centers.[82] Further studies are required to determine the place of these therapeutic modalities in the management of CP.

Self-expandable metal stents have already been introduced for transmural drainage of pancreatic collections.[83] These have a much larger luminal diameter than plastic stents and therefore may facilitate drainage. Particularly, a novel metal stent has round flared ends that may prevent stent migration and tissue injury.[62,83] It has also been proposed as the first step for endoscopic necrosectomy for WON.[62] However, high complication rates and costs might hinder generalized use of the stent.

Table 43.5 Selected large studies (n > 45) regarding EUS-guided transmural drainage of pancreatic fluid collections

First author Year, reference	N	Stents	Endoscopic necrosectomy (%)	Technical success (%)	Clinical success (%)	Complications (%)	Recurrence (%)
Kahaleh 2006[30]	46	Plastic	-	100	93	19	ND
Arvanitakis 2007[29]	46	Plastic	-	100	94	20	11
Lopes 2007[31]	51	Plastic	-	94	84	25	17
Ardengh 2008[32]	77	Plastic	-	94	91	6	11
Varadarajulu 2008[33]	60	Plastic	-	95	93	2	4
Ahn 2010[34]	47	Plastic	-	89	87	12	11
Will 2011[35]	132	Plastic	26	97	96	29	15
Seewald 2012[36]	80	Plastic	61	97	83	26	11
Lee 2014[82]	50	Plastic n = 25[a] FCSEMS n = 25	-	100	80	4	2
Walter 2015[83]	61	LAFCSEMS	24	97	79	9	ND

EUS, endoscopic ultrasound; FCSEMS, fully covered self-expandable metal stent; LAFCSEMS, Lumen-apposing fully covered self-expandable metal stent

[a]Randomized-controlled trial showing no difference between the two groups.

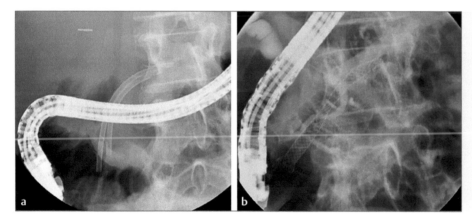

Fig. 43.6 Alternative modalities for pancreatic stenting: **(a)** with multiple plastic stents inserted side-by-side, **(b)** with a fully covered metal stent.

43.5 Conclusion

Endoscopy plays a very significant role in the diagnostic and therapeutic management of acute and chronic pancreatitis. EUS is the cornerstone of diagnostic procedures, ranging from determining etiology of AP to confirming diagnosis of CP. ERCP should be considered as a therapeutic procedure only, and has been shown to be the basis of endoscopic therapy for CP, along with ESWL. EUS-guided drainage of pancreatic collections has been applied considerably up to now for pseudocysts with liquid contents. Necrosectomy, up to now a surgical procedure, can also be tackled by endoscopic techniques, in case of WON. Further studies are still required to standardize certain techniques and to investigate other alternatives. Nevertheless, global management of pancreatic diseases still remains challenging and requires a multimodal effort, involving many disciplines such as endoscopy, radiology, surgery, and pathology.

References

[1] Working Group IAP/APA Acute Pancreatitis Guidelines. IAP/APA evidence-based guidelines for the management of acute pancreatitis. Pancreatology. 2013; 13(4, Suppl 2):e1–e15

[2] Chandrasekhara V, Chathadi KV, Acosta RD, et al; ASGE Standards of Practice Committee. The role of endoscopy in benign pancreatic disease. Gastrointest Endosc. 2015; 82(2):203–214

[3] Early DS, Acosta RD, Chandrasekhara V, et al; ASGE Standards of Practice Committee. Adverse events associated with EUS and EUS with FNA. Gastrointest Endosc. 2013; 77(6):839–843

[4] Anderson MA, Fisher L, Jain R, et al; ASGE Standards of Practice Committee. Complications of ERCP. Gastrointest Endosc. 2012; 75(3):467–473

[5] Yusoff IF, Raymond G, Sahai AV. A prospective comparison of the yield of EUS in primary vs. recurrent idiopathic acute pancreatitis. Gastrointest Endosc. 2004; 60(5):673–678

[6] Ortega AR, Gómez-Rodríguez R, Romero M, et al. Prospective comparison of endoscopic ultrasonography and magnetic resonance cholangiopancreatography in the etiological diagnosis of "idiopathic" acute pancreatitis. Pancreas. 2011; 40(2):289–294

[7] Srinivasa S, Sammour T, McEntee B, et al. Selective use of magnetic resonance cholangiopancreatography in clinical practice may miss choledocholithiasis in gallstone pancreatitis. Can J Surg. 2010; 53(6):403–407

[8] Chak A, Hawes RH, Cooper GS, et al. Prospective assessment of the utility of EUS in the evaluation of gallstone pancreatitis. Gastrointest Endosc. 1999; 49(5):599–604

[9] Liu CL, Lo CM, Chan JK, et al. Detection of choledocholithiasis by EUS in acute pancreatitis: a prospective evaluation in 100 consecutive patients. Gastrointest Endosc. 2001; 54(3):325–330

[10] De Lisi S, Leandro G, Buscarini E. Endoscopic ultrasonography versus endoscopic retrograde cholangiopancreatography in acute biliary pancreatitis: a systematic review. Eur J Gastroenterol Hepatol. 2011; 23(5):367–374

[11] Romagnuolo J, Currie G; Calgary Advanced Therapeutic Endoscopy Center study group. Noninvasive vs. selective invasive biliary imaging for acute biliary pancreatitis: an economic evaluation by using decision tree analysis. Gastrointest Endosc. 2005; 61(1):86–97

[12] Conwell DL, Zuccaro G, Purich E, et al. Comparison of endoscopic ultrasound chronic pancreatitis criteria to the endoscopic secretin-stimulated pancreatic function test. Dig Dis Sci. 2007; 52(5):1206–1210

[13] Catalano MF, Sahai A, Levy M, et al. EUS-based criteria for the diagnosis of chronic pancreatitis: the Rosemont classification. Gastrointest Endosc. 2009; 69(7):1251–1261

[14] Stevens T, Lopez R, Adler DG, et al. Multicenter comparison of the interobserver agreement of standard EUS scoring and Rosemont classification scoring for diagnosis of chronic pancreatitis. Gastrointest Endosc. 2010; 71(3):519–526

[15] Gardner TB, Levy MJ. EUS diagnosis of chronic pancreatitis. Gastrointest Endosc. 2010; 71(7):1280–1289

[16] Dumonceau JM, Garcia-Fernandez FJ, Verdun FR, et al; European Society of Digestive Endoscopy. Radiation protection in digestive endoscopy: European Society of Digestive Endoscopy (ESGE) guideline. Endoscopy. 2012; 44(4):408–421

[17] Albert J, ed. Endoscopic Retrograde Cholangiopancreatography (ERCP): Current Practice and fFture Perspectives. Bremen, Germany; Uni-Med Verlag AG: 2015

[18] Dumonceau JM, Andriulli A, Elmunzer BJ, et al; European Society of Gastrointestinal Endoscopy. Prophylaxis of post-ERCP pancreatitis: European Society of Gastrointestinal Endoscopy (ESGE) Guideline—updated June 2014. Endoscopy. 2014; 46(9):799–815

[19] Delhaye M, Matos C, Devière J. Endoscopic management of chronic pancreatitis. Gastrointest Endosc Clin N Am. 2003; 13(4):717–742

[20] Buscaglia JM, Kalloo AN. Pancreatic sphincterotomy: technique, indications, and complications. World J Gastroenterol. 2007; 13(30):4064–4071

[21] Attwell A, Borak G, Hawes R, et al. Endoscopic pancreatic sphincterotomy for pancreas divisum by using a needle-knife or standard pull-type technique: safety and reintervention rates. Gastrointest Endosc. 2006; 64(5):705–711

[22] Ziebert JJ, DiSario JA. Dilation of refractory pancreatic duct strictures: the turn of the screw. Gastrointest Endosc. 1999; 49(5):632–635

[23] Dumonceau JM, Delhaye M, Tringali A, et al. Endoscopic treatment of chronic pancreatitis: European Society of Gastrointestinal Endoscopy (ESGE) Clinical Guideline. Endoscopy. 2012; 44(8):784–800

[24] Sauer BG, Gurka MJ, Ellen K, et al. Effect of pancreatic duct stent diameter on hospitalization in chronic pancreatitis: does size matter? Pancreas. 2009; 38(7):728–731

[25] Talukdar R, Reddy DN. Pancreatic endotherapy for chronic pancreatitis. Gastrointest Endosc Clin N Am. 2015; 25(4):765–777

[26] Delhaye M, Arvanitakis M, Verset G, et al. Long-term clinical outcome after endoscopic pancreatic ductal drainage for patients with painful chronic pancreatitis. Clin Gastroenterol Hepatol. 2004; 2(12):1096–1106

[27] Varadarajulu S, Christein JD, Tamhane A, et al. Prospective randomized trial comparing EUS and EGD for transmural drainage of pancreatic pseudocysts (with videos). Gastrointest Endosc. 2008; 68(6):1102–1111

[28] Park DH, Lee SS, Moon SH, et al. Endoscopic ultrasound-guided versus conventional transmural drainage for pancreatic pseudocysts: a prospective randomized trial. Endoscopy. 2009; 41(10):842–848

[29] Arvanitakis M, Delhaye M, Bali MA, et al. Pancreatic-fluid collections: a randomized controlled trial regarding stent removal after endoscopic transmural drainage. Gastrointest Endosc. 2007; 65(4):609–619

[30] Kahaleh M, Shami VM, Conaway MR, et al. Endoscopic ultrasound drainage of pancreatic pseudocyst: a prospective comparison with conventional endoscopic drainage. Endoscopy. 2006; 38(4):355–359

[31] Lopes CV, Pesenti C, Bories E, et al. Endoscopic-ultrasound-guided endoscopic transmural drainage of pancreatic pseudocysts and abscesses. Scand J Gastroenterol. 2007; 42(4):524–529

[32] Ardengh JC, Coelho DE, Coelho JF, et al. Single-step EUS-guided endoscopic treatment for sterile pancreatic collections: a single-center experience. Dig Dis. 2008; 26(4):370–376

[33] Varadarajulu S, Tamhane A, Blakely J. Graded dilation technique for EUS-guided drainage of peripancreatic fluid collections: an assessment of outcomes and complications and technical proficiency (with video). Gastrointest Endosc. 2008; 68(4):656–666

[34] Ahn JY, Seo DW, Eum J, et al. Single-step EUS-guided transmural drainage of pancreatic pseudocysts: analysis of technical feasibility, efficacy, and safety. Gut Liver. 2010; 4(4):524–529

[35] Will U, Wanzar C, Gerlach R, Meyer F. Interventional ultrasound-guided procedures in pancreatic pseudocysts, abscesses and infected necroses—treatment algorithm in a large single-center study. Ultraschall Med. 2011; 32(2):176–183

[36] Seewald S, Ang TL, Richter H, et al. Long-term results after endoscopic drainage and necrosectomy of symptomatic pancreatic fluid collections. Dig Endosc. 2012; 24(1):36–41

[37] Trikudanathan G, Attam R, Arain MA, et al. Endoscopic interventions for necrotizing pancreatitis. Am J Gastroenterol. 2014; 109(7):969–981, quiz 982

[38] Tse F, Yuan Y. Early routine endoscopic retrograde cholangiopancreatography strategy versus early conservative management strategy in acute gallstone pancreatitis. Cochrane Database Syst Rev. 2012(5):CD009779

[39] da Costa DW, Bouwense SA, Schepers NJ, et al; Dutch Pancreatitis Study Group. Same-admission versus interval cholecystectomy for mild gallstone pancreatitis (PONCHO): a multicentre randomised controlled trial. Lancet. 2015; 386(10000):1261–1268

[40] Sanjay P, Yeeting S, Whigham C, et al. Endoscopic sphincterotomy and interval cholecystectomy are reasonable alternatives to index cholecystectomy in severe acute gallstone pancreatitis (GSP). Surg Endosc. 2008; 22(8):1832–1837

[41] Petersen BT. Sphincter of Oddi dysfunction, part 2: evidence-based review of the presentations, with "objective" pancreatic findings (types I and II) and of presumptive type III. Gastrointest Endosc. 2004; 59(6):670–687

[42] Coté GA, Imperiale TF, Schmidt SE, et al. Similar efficacies of biliary, with or without pancreatic, sphincterotomy in treatment of idiopathic recurrent acute pancreatitis. Gastroenterology. 2012; 143(6):1502–1509.e1

[43] Cotton PB, Durkalski V, Romagnuolo J, et al. Effect of endoscopic sphincterotomy for suspected sphincter of Oddi dysfunction on pain-related disability following cholecystectomy: the EPISOD randomized clinical trial. JAMA. 2014; 311(20):2101–2109

[44] Ponchon T, Bory RM, Hedelius F, et al. Endoscopic stenting for pain relief in chronic pancreatitis: results of a standardized protocol. Gastrointest Endosc. 1995; 42(5):452–456

[45] Eleftheriadis N, Dinu F, Delhaye M, et al. Long-term outcome after pancreatic stenting in severe chronic pancreatitis. Endoscopy. 2005; 37(3):223–230

[46] Binmoeller KF, Jue P, Seifert H, et al. Endoscopic pancreatic stent drainage in chronic pancreatitis and a dominant stricture: long-term results. Endoscopy. 1995; 27(9):638–644

[47] Smits ME, Badiga SM, Rauws EA, et al. Long-term results of pancreatic stents in chronic pancreatitis. Gastrointest Endosc. 1995; 42(5):461–467

[48] Farnbacher MJ, Schoen C, Rabenstein T, et al. Pancreatic duct stones in chronic pancreatitis: criteria for treatment intensity and success. Gastrointest Endosc. 2002; 56(4):501–506

[49] Nguyen-Tang T, Dumonceau JM. Endoscopic treatment in chronic pancreatitis, timing, duration and type of intervention. Best Pract Res Clin Gastroenterol. 2010; 24(3):281–298

[50] Li BR, Liao Z, Du TT, et al. Risk factors for complications of pancreatic extracorporeal shock wave lithotripsy. Endoscopy. 2014; 46(12):1092–1100

[51] Dumonceau JM, Costamagna G, Tringali A, et al. Treatment for painful calcified chronic pancreatitis: extracorporeal shock wave lithotripsy versus endoscopic treatment: a randomised controlled trial. Gut. 2007; 56(4):545–552

[52] Rösch T, Daniel S, Scholz M, et al; European Society of Gastrointestinal Endoscopy Research Group. Endoscopic treatment of chronic pancreatitis: a multicenter study of 1000 patients with long-term follow-up. Endoscopy. 2002; 34(10):765–771

[53] Tadenuma H, Ishihara T, Yamaguchi T, et al. Long-term results of extracorporeal shockwave lithotripsy and endoscopic therapy for pancreatic stones. Clin Gastroenterol Hepatol. 2005; 3(11):1128–1135

[54] Farnbacher MJ, Mühldorfer S, Wehler M, et al. Interventional endoscopic therapy in chronic pancreatitis including temporary stenting: a definitive treatment? Scand J Gastroenterol. 2006; 41(1):111–117

[55] Inui K, Tazuma S, Yamaguchi T, et al. Treatment of pancreatic stones with extracorporeal shock wave lithotripsy: results of a multicenter survey. Pancreas. 2005; 30(1):26–30

[56] Seven G, Schreiner MA, Ross AS, et al. Long-term outcomes associated with pancreatic extracorporeal shock wave lithotripsy for chronic calcific pancreatitis. Gastrointest Endosc. 2012; 75(5):997–1004.e1

[57] Tandan M, Reddy DN, Talukdar R, et al. Long-term clinical outcomes of extracorporeal shockwave lithotripsy in painful chronic calcific pancreatitis. Gastrointest Endosc. 2013; 78(5):726–733

[58] Díte P, Ruzicka M, Zboril V, Novotný I. A prospective, randomized trial comparing endoscopic and surgical therapy for chronic pancreatitis. Endoscopy. 2003; 35(7):553–558

[59] Cahen DL, Gouma DJ, Nio Y, et al. Endoscopic versus surgical drainage of the pancreatic duct in chronic pancreatitis. N Engl J Med. 2007; 356(7):676–684

[60] Cahen DL, Gouma DJ, Laramée P, et al. Long-term outcomes of endoscopic vs surgical drainage of the pancreatic duct in patients with chronic pancreatitis. Gastroenterology. 2011; 141(5):1690–1695

[61] Banks PA, Bollen TL, Dervenis C, et al; Acute Pancreatitis Classification Working Group. Classification of acute pancreatitis—2012: revision of the Atlanta classification and definitions by international consensus. Gut. 2013; 62(1):102–111

[62] Ge PS, Weizmann M, Watson RR. Pancreatic pseudocysts: advances in endoscopic management. Gastroenterol Clin North Am. 2016; 45(1):9–27

[63] Binmoeller KF, Seifert H, Walter A, Soehendra N. Transpapillary and transmural drainage of pancreatic pseudocysts. Gastrointest Endosc. 1995; 42(3):219–224

[64] Hookey LC, Debroux S, Delhaye M, et al. Endoscopic drainage of pancreatic-fluid collections in 116 patients: a comparison of etiologies, drainage techniques, and outcomes. Gastrointest Endosc. 2006; 63(4):635–643

[65] Barthet M, Lamblin G, Gasmi M, et al. Clinical usefulness of a treatment algorithm for pancreatic pseudocysts. Gastrointest Endosc. 2008; 67(2):245–252

[66] Muthusamy VR, Chandrasekhara V, Acosta RD, et al; ASGE Standards of Practice Committee. The role of endoscopy in the diagnosis and treatment of inflammatory pancreatic fluid collections. Gastrointest Endosc. 2016; 83(3):481–488

[67] Gardner TB, Chahal P, Papachristou GI, et al. A comparison of direct endoscopic necrosectomy with transmural endoscopic drainage for the treatment of walled-off pancreatic necrosis. Gastrointest Endosc. 2009; 69(6):1085–1094

[68] Seifert H, Biermer M, Schmitt W, et al. Transluminal endoscopic necrosectomy after acute pancreatitis: a multicentre study with long-term follow-up (the GE-PARD Study). Gut. 2009; 58(9):1260–1266

[69] Gardner TB, Coelho-Prabhu N, Gordon SR, et al. Direct endoscopic necrosectomy for the treatment of walled-off pancreatic necrosis: results from a multicenter U.S. series. Gastrointest Endosc. 2011; 73(4):718–726

[70] Gress F, Schmitt C, Sherman S, et al. A prospective randomized comparison of endoscopic ultrasound- and computed tomography-guided celiac plexus block for managing chronic pancreatitis pain. Am J Gastroenterol. 1999; 94(4):900–905

[71] Santosh D, Lakhtakia S, Gupta R, et al. Clinical trial: a randomized trial comparing fluoroscopy guided percutaneous technique vs. endoscopic ultrasound guided technique of coeliac plexus block for treatment of pain in chronic pancreatitis. Aliment Pharmacol Ther. 2009; 29(9):979–984

[72] Puli SR, Reddy JB, Bechtold ML, et al. EUS-guided celiac plexus neurolysis for pain due to chronic pancreatitis or pancreatic cancer pain: a meta-analysis and systematic review. Dig Dis Sci. 2009; 54(11):2330–2337

[73] Kaufman M, Singh G, Das S, et al. Efficacy of endoscopic ultrasound-guided celiac plexus block and celiac plexus neurolysis for managing abdominal pain associated with chronic pancreatitis and pancreatic cancer. J Clin Gastroenterol. 2010; 44(2):127–134

[74] Pei Q, Zou X, Zhang X, et al. Diagnostic value of EUS elastography in differentiation of benign and malignant solid pancreatic masses: a meta-analysis. Pancreatology. 2012; 12(5):402–408

[75] Iglesias-Garcia J, Domínguez-Muñoz JE, Castiñeira-Alvariño M, et al. Quantitative elastography associated with endoscopic ultrasound for the diagnosis of chronic pancreatitis. Endoscopy. 2013; 45(10):781–788

[76] Dominguez-Muñoz JE, Iglesias-Garcia J, Castiñeira Alvariño M, et al. EUS elastography to predict pancreatic exocrine insufficiency in patients with chronic pancreatitis. Gastrointest Endosc. 2015; 81(1):136–142

[77] Tringali A, Lemmers A, Meves V, et al. Intraductal biliopancreatic imaging: European Society of Gastrointestinal Endoscopy (ESGE) technology review. Endoscopy. 2015; 47(8):739–753

[78] Costamagna G, Bulajic M, Tringali A, et al. Multiple stenting of refractory pancreatic duct strictures in severe chronic pancreatitis: long-term results. Endoscopy. 2006; 38(3):254–259

[79] Shen Y, Liu M, Chen M, et al. Covered metal stent or multiple plastic stents for refractory pancreatic ductal strictures in chronic pancreatitis: a systematic review. Pancreatology. 2014; 14(2):87–90

[80] Tessier G, Bories E, Arvanitakis M, et al. EUS-guided pancreatogastrostomy and pancreatobulbostomy for the treatment of pain in patients with pancreatic ductal dilatation inaccessible for transpapillary endoscopic therapy. Gastrointest Endosc. 2007; 65(2):233–241

[81] Widmer J, Sharaiha RZ, Kahaleh M. Endoscopic ultrasonography-guided drainage of the pancreatic duct. Gastrointest Endosc Clin N Am. 2013; 23(4):847–861

[82] Lee BU, Song TJ, Lee SS, et al. Newly designed, fully covered metal stents for endoscopic ultrasound (EUS)-guided transmural drainage of peripancreatic fluid collections: a prospective randomized study. Endoscopy. 2014; 46(12):1078–1084

[83] Walter D, Will U, Sanchez-Yague A, et al. A novel lumen-apposing metal stent for endoscopic ultrasound-guided drainage of pancreatic fluid collections: a prospective cohort study. Endoscopy. 2015; 47(1):63–67

44 Pancreatic Cancers and Cystic Neoplasms

Omer Basar and William R. Brugge

44.1 Introduction

Most pancreatic cancers are ductal adenocarcinomas arising from the exocrine pancreas. Pancreatic ductal adenocarcinoma (PDAC) has a poor prognosis and age, male gender, tobacco consumption, chronic pancreatitis, and some hereditary syndromes are risk factors. Most patients are diagnosed with advanced disease usually by cross-sectional imaging. Currently endoscopic ultrasound–guided fine-needle aspiration (EUS-FNA) is the standard approach for tissue sampling of a mass lesion. Surgery is the only curative therapy. In contrast, pancreatic neuroendocrine tumors (pNETs) are less common and have a better prognosis.

Pancreatic cystic lesions (PCLs) are increasingly recognized as premalignant precursor lesions and offer the opportunity to intervene early in pancreatic cancer. Computed tomography/magnetic resonance imaging (CT/MRI) is frequently used for the initial evaluation; however, EUS-FNA is the preferred imaging tool for tissue sampling and clinical guidance. Biochemical, cytological, and DNA analysis of aspirated cyst fluid aids in the differentiation between benign, premalignant, and malignant lesions. Options for treatment include surgery and endoscopic ablation therapies. Some lesions should also be followed up conservatively.

Although pancreatic malignancies may arise from exocrine and endocrine pancreas, most cancers originate from the ductal epithelium and are termed PDACs)[1] (▶ Table 44.1). Because of its aggressive behavior, PDAC is one of the most common cancer-related deaths in United States. Screening, early diagnosis, and treatment strategies are challenging.

pNETs were formerly named islet cell tumors and are mostly indolent, with a small percentage demonstrating malignant behavior.[2] pNETs are usually an incidental finding on cross-sectional imaging.

PCLs are mostly recognized coincidentally[3,4] with a prevalence of 1.2 to 19% in different studies.[3,4,5,6] Nowadays the term, pancreatic cystic neoplasms (PCNs), is more preferred instead of PCL and these lesions are usually classified as either neoplastic or nonneoplastic (▶ Table 44.2). Most PCLs are nonneoplastic and account for 80% of the pancreatic cysts.[3,4,7] PCNs are composed of cysts with either a mucinous or serous epithelial lining. Mucinous cysts have a malignant potential whereas serous cystic neoplasm (SCN) are typically benign.

This chapter reviews the major advances in the diagnosis and management of pancreatic cancers and PCNs.

Table 44.1 2010 WHO classification of primary pancreatic malignant tumors

Epithelial tumors	
Ductal adeno CA	Adenosquamous CA
Mucinous adeno CA	Hepatoid CA
Medullary CA	Signet-ring cell CA
Undifferentiated CA	Undifferentiated CA with osteoclast-like cells
Acinar cell CA	Acinar cell cystadeno CA
IPMN with an associated invasive CA	Mixed acinar-ductal CA
Mixed acinar-neuroendocrine CA	Mixed acinar-neuroendocrine -ductal CA
Mixed ductal-neuroendocrine CA	MCN with an associated invasive CA
Pancreatoblastoma	Serous cystadeno CA
Solid pseudopapillary neoplasm	
Mesenchymal tumors	
Lymphangioma	Lipoma
Solitary fibrous tumor	Ewing's sarcoma
Desmoplastic small round cell tumor	Perivascular epithelioid cell neoplasm
Neuroendocrine neoplasms	
Pancreatic neuroendocrine microadenoma	NET G1/carcinoid
NET G2	Neuroendocrine CA
Large-cell neuroendocrine CA	Small-cell neuroendocrine CA
Enterochromaffin cell, serotonin-producing NET	Gastrinoma, malignant
Glucagonoma, malignant	Insulin-producing CA (insulinoma)
Somatostatinoma, malignant	VIPoma, malignant
Lymphomas	
Diffuse large B-cell lymphoma	

CA, carcinoma; MCN, mucinous cystic neoplasm; NET, neuroendocrine tumor.

Table 44.2 Cystic lesions of pancreas

Feature	Cyst type	Related cysts
Nonneoplastic cysts	*Epithelial*	Mucinous nonneoplastic cysts
		Endometrial cyst
		Lymphoepithelial cyst
		Enterogenous cysts
		Squamoid cysts
		Para-ampullary duodenal wall cyst
	Nonepithelial	Pseudocyst
		Simple cyst
		Retention cyst
		Infection-related cyst
Neoplastic cysts (pancreatic cystic neoplasms)	*Mucinous cystic lesions*	Intraductal papillary mucinous neoplasm
		Mucinous cystic neoplasm
	Nonmucinous cystic lesions	Serous cystic neoplasm
		Solid pseudopapillary neoplasm
		Cystic pancreatic endocrine neoplasm
		Acinar-cell cystic neoplasm
	Other neoplastic cystic lesions	Ductal adenocarcinoma with cystic degeneration

44.2 Pancreatic Cancers

44.2.1 Ductal Adenocarcinoma of the Pancreas

PDAC risk increases with age (age at median diagnosis is 71)[8] and men are slightly more affected.[9] About 80% of cases have advanced disease at diagnosis and the 5-year survival rate is only 4% in these patients.[10] The risk factors for PDAC include advanced age, male gender, "non-O" blood group, and obesity. External risk factors include exposure to high-fat diets, smoking, occupational exposure to nickel, petroleum, and wood pulp. Medical risk factors include a history of partial gastrectomy and chronic pancreatitis, or diabetes. Inherited genetic predispositions to PDAC include familial adenomatous polyposis syndrome, Lynch's syndrome, Peutz–Jeghers syndrome, hereditary pancreatitis, hereditary breast–ovarian cancer syndromes, ataxia telangiectasia, Li–Fraumeni syndrome, familial atypical multiple mole melanoma syndrome (FAMMMS).[1,11,12,13]

PDAC has a progressive cancer development pathway, which is similar to the adenoma–carcinoma sequence. Pancreatic intraepithelial neoplasias (PanIn) are the initiating precursor lesions and the degree of dysplasia increases from PanIn 1 to 3. Most of these lesions contain *KRAS* mutations, moreover PanIn 2 and 3 lesions are found to contain *p53*, *SMAD4*, and *CDKN2A* mutations.[14] Intraductal papillary mucinous neoplasms (IPMNs) and mucinous cystic neoplasm (MCN) may also initiate the tumorigenesis process, and almost half of IPMN cases contain a *KRAS* mutation (40–65% of cases).[13]

Two-thirds of PDACs are located in the head of the pancreas and present at an earlier stage than malignancies located in the body or tail. Jaundice due to biliary obstruction is the most common presenting symptom and in one-third of patients, Courvoisier's sign (a palpable gallbladder) is present. Pancreatic body and tail lesions remain asymptomatic until advanced disease progresses. Abdominal (predominantly epigastric) or midback pain, pruritus, asthenia, weight loss, and depression are the most common symptoms.[15] Pancreatic exocrine insufficiency present with steatorrhea and malabsorption, and new-onset diabetes exists in about half of the patients.[16] Migratory thrombophlebitis is another common presentation.[17]

Genetic predisposition is present in 5% of patients with PDAC and 95% are sporadic. Although screening programs in high-risk patients are not widely established in the United States, candidates listed in ▶ Table 44.3 could be candidates for screening as recommended by the International Cancer of the Pancreas Screening Consortium.[18,19]

Blood tests usually reveal a mild anemia. Cholestatic enzymes and bilirubin levels are elevated in cases with biliary obstruction. Although having a poor sensitivity in diagnosis, CA 19–9 levels are predictive for recurrent malignancy after surgery.[20]

Patients with jaundice are initially evaluated with ultrasonography (US), which has limited access to the pancreas. A hypoechoic mass in the pancreas is typical for PDAC and a "double duct sign" (dilation of both common bile duct and pancreatic duct) is also a common feature. Computed tomography (CT) and magnetic resonance imaging (MRI) are commonly used tools for the diagnosis of PDAC (▶ Fig. 44.1). A pancreatic-protocol triphasic CT is one of the best tools for staging. Unnecessary staging laparoscopies and laparotomies are 80% avoided with this protocol.[21] MRI does not usually add extra information over CT.[22] Fluorodeoxyglucose–positron emission tomography (FDG-PET) has a similar accuracy with CT/MRI; on the other hand, it may demonstrate small local and distant metastasis.[23] Nowadays, EUS-FNA is one of the best method for tissue sampling and staging (**Video 44.1**). Having a low complication rate,[24] EUS is better at detecting small lesions compared to CT/MRI[25,26] (▶ Fig. 44.2). Along with its usage in cyst fluid sampling, it has a therapeutic role in advanced PDAC (celiac ganglion blockage in cancer pain relief and biliary drainage when endoscopic retrograde cholangiopancreatography [ERCP] is not possible).

Preoperatively, PDAC is staged based on American Joint Committee on Cancer tumor, node, metastasis (TNM) system.[27] Both T1 and T2 lesions are limited to the pancreas, with a tumor dimension less than or equal to 2 cm in T1 and greater than 2 cm in T2. Superior mesenteric vein, portal vein, and splenic vein invasion is considered T3, and superior mesenteric

Table 44.3 Screening candidates for PDAC suggested by International Cancer of the Pancreas Screening Consortium

Screening candidates for PDAC	↑ Risk of PDAC
Two FDR with PDAC, with at least one affected FDR	Sixfold
Three of more blood relatives with PDAC and at least one FDR	14- to 32-fold
Peutz–Jeghers syndrome regardless of family history of PDAC	132-fold
Hereditary breast and ovarian cancer syndrome (BRCA2 mutation carriers) with either one FDR with PDAC or at least two affected family members	3.5- to 10-fold
PALB2 mutation carriers with at least one FDR with PDAC	N/A
FAMMMS (p16 mutation) carriers with at least one FDR with PDAC	9- to 47-fold
Lynch's syndrome (mismatch repair gene mutation carriers) and one FDR with PDAC	N/A

FDR, first-degree relatives; FAMMMS, familial atypical multiple mole melanoma syndrome; PDAC, pancreatic ductal adenocarcinoma.

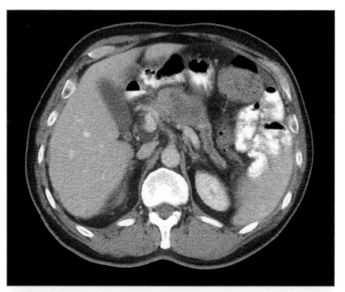

Fig. 44.1 A heterogeneous 45 × 27 mm malignant mass in the body of pancreas on computed tomography (CT).

artery and celiac axis invasion are considered T4 tumors. N1 staging describes lymph node metastasis and M1 staging indicates metastatic disease. Potentially resectable tumors are T1, T2, and T3, and T4 lesions are unresectable. Furthermore, National Comprehensive Cancer Network (NCCN) classified PDAC clinically[28] (▶Table 44.4).

A multidisciplinary approach is needed for the treatment of PDAC patients. Radical R0 resection is the only curative treatment and this takes place in less than 20% of patients. In cases with unresectable tumor or when neoadjuvant chemotherapy is planned, a histologic or cytological diagnosis is necessary. **Surgically resectable PDAC (stages I–II)** patients should undergo a Whipple procedure or distal pancreatectomy depending on the localization of PDAC. Today, laparoscopic distal pancreatectomy is the preferred technique for distal tumors.[13] The recommended therapy for **borderline resectable PDAC** is neoadjuvant chemoradiation.[13] As an adjuvant therapy, both gemcitabine and 5-fluorouracil (5-FU) were found to improve survival after R0/R1 resection.[29,30,31] On the other hand, adjuvant radiotherapy is not routinely advised.[29,30] Neoadjuvant chemotherapy has a limited efficacy and although no definite

optimal treatment is present, nab-paclitaxel (gemcitabine plus albumin-bound paclitaxel particles) and 5-FU, irinotecan, oxaliplatin, and leucovorin combination are commonly used. **Locally advanced, unresectable PDAC (stage III)** patients should receive folfirinox or gemcitabine–nab-paclitaxel as studies report similar response rates with metastatic tumors.[32] **Metastatic PDAC (stage IV)** patients should also receive the same regimen as in stage III, resulting in 10% 2-year survival rate.[33,34] Endoscopic biliary drainage, expandable metallic stent placement for duodenal obstruction, opioids, and EUS-guided celiac plexus blocks are palliative treatments for advanced PDAC (▶Fig. 44.3).

44.2.2 Pancreatic Neuroendocrine Tumors

pNETs are indolent tumors arising from cells of the endocrine and nervous system with variable malignant potential. About 1 to 2% of pancreatic tumors are pNETs[35] and their incidence increases with age. Two-thirds of pNETs are nonfunctional but secrete chromogranin, neuron-specific enolase, neurotensin, ghrelin, and human chorionic gonadotropin subunits. The symptomatic pNETs include insulinomas, gastrinomas, glucagonomas, VIPomas, and somatostatinomas.[36,37,38] Although frequently sporadic, pNETs can be a part of endocrine tumor syndromes such as multiple endocrine neoplasia type 1, von Hippel–Lindau syndrome, neurofibromatosis type 1, and tuberous sclerosis.

A combination of biochemistry and endocrine tests, imaging, endoscopic techniques, and biopsies are usually needed for diagnosis. A hormonally inactive hypervascular pancreatic mass on cross-sectional imaging is suggestive of a nonfunctional

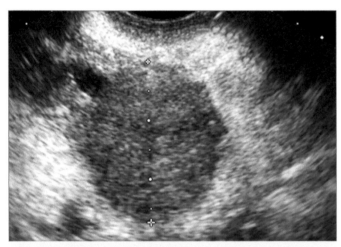

Fig. 44.2 A heterogeneous, irregular 27-mm malignant mass on endoscopic ultrasound (EUS).

Table 44.4 Clinical staging for PDAC suggested by National Comprehensive Cancer Network (NCCN)

Stage	Involvement
Local or resectable	Absence of extrapancreatic disease, no invasion of superior mesenteric artery and celiac axis, SMA and splenic vein are patent
Borderline resectable	Absence of extrapancreatic disease, SMA encasement < 180°, celiac encasement < 180° (tail), short-segment SMV occlusion, SMV/portal impingement, abutment/encasement of hepatic artery
Locally advanced or unresectable	Absence of extrapancreatic disease, SMA encasement > 180°, any celiac abutment (head) or celiac encasement > 180° (body/tail), unreconstructable SMV/portal vein occlusion; aortic invasion or encasement, lymph node metastases beyond field of resection
Metastatic disease	Extrapancreatic disease

PDAC, pancreatic ductal adenocarcinoma; SMA, superior mesenteric artery; SMV, superior mesenteric vein.

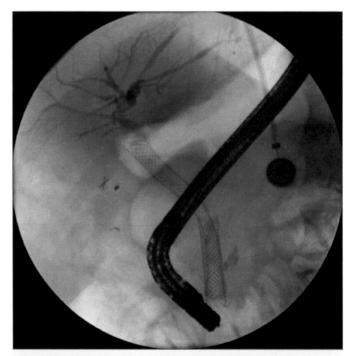

Fig. 44.3 An 82-year-old man with a history of pancreatic cancer and a metal stent placement presented with hemobilia. A 10 × 8 cm covered metal stent was placed through the previously placed 4-cm metal stent by endoscopic retrograde cholangiopancreatography (ERCP).

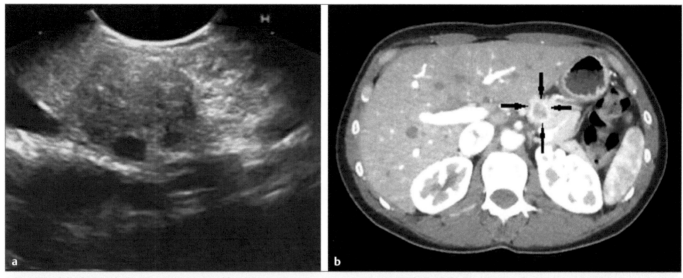

Fig. 44.4 (a) A hypoechoic, 20 × 22 mm round homogenous mass on EUS in pancreatic body consistent with pancreatic neuroendocrine tumors (pNET). (b) CT showing the same lesion.

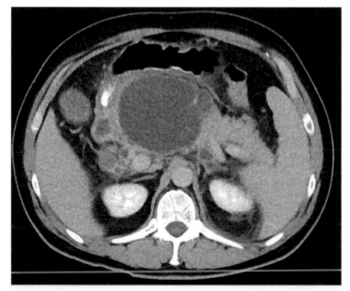

Fig. 44.5 CT showing an 11.1 × 9.1 × 17.8 cm bilobed pseudocyst.

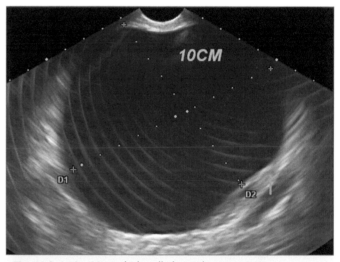

Fig. 44.6 A 10 × 10 cm thick-walled pseudocyst on EUS.

pNET, which are commonly large lesions at diagnosis with high metastasis rates.[39,40] Today, scintigraphy and EUS-guided FNA are the mostly used imaging tools to discriminate a pNET from PDAC (▶ Fig. 44.4).

The only curative treatment for pNETs is surgery. Locoregional therapy for liver metastasis, systemic chemotherapy for residual disease, and somatostatin analogs for functional pNETs are recommended.[41] The prognosis of pNETs is better, compared to PDAC, and is dependent on surgical outcomes.[42]

44.3 Cystic Lesions of Pancreas

44.3.1 Nonneoplastic Cysts

Pancreatic Pseudocysts

The most common PCLs are pancreatic pseudocysts (PPs) which are inflammatory fluid collections in the course of acute or chronic pancreatitis.[43] Pseudocysts occur in 10 to 20% of patients with acute pancreatitis with a slight male predominance.[44] After

4 weeks of acute pancreatitis, an enhancing capsule forms and may delineate a focal fluid collection, or a pseudocyst. The capsule does not contain an "epithelial lining."[45] The fluid within PPs is usually dark, opaque, and low viscosity, but may contain necrotic tissue. PPs are usually single (90%), unilocular lesions containing fluid with high amylase and lipase activity in a size ranging from 2 to 20 cm.[43,45,46]

Symptoms of PPs are abdominal pain, early satiety, and weight loss. Usually there are no specific findings on physical examination.[47] Medical history of pancreatitis, continuous abdominal pain, and consistently elevated amylase levels after clinical resolution of pancreatitis may be clues for a PP.

Initial imaging for a pseudocyst is transabdominal US, which shows an anechoic cystic lesion arising from the pancreas. Abdominal CT, which is usually superior to US, shows a well-circumscribed, thick-walled, round, or oval cystic lesion[43] (▶ Fig. 44.5). CT reveals additional information about pancreatic tissue, where there could be signs of acute or chronic pancreatitis. MRI, magnetic resonance cholangiopancreatography (MRCP), and ERCP do not contribute much to the diagnosis. With FNA capability, EUS is one of the best imaging modality to detect a PP (▶ Fig. 44.6), demonstrating an anechoic cystic lesion that is surrounded by a thick rim. Cystic fluid analysis reveals high amylase and low carcinoembryonic antigen (CEA) levels.[48] Cytology shows inflammatory cells and histiocytes; on the other hand, epithelial cells are highly suspicious for PCN and granulocytes indicate an active infection.[49]

PPs, smaller than 4 cm, frequently resolve without any treatment.[50,51,52] Either percutaneous or endoscopic drainage is the choice of treatment for large and symptomatic PPs. EUS-guided transduodenal and transgastric drainage, with a 90% success and low complication rate, is the preferred technique today.[48] In some cases, necrotic material should also be removed via a cystogastrostomy or cystoduodenostomy (**Video 44.2**). Surgical drainage is generally reserved for cases, when endoscopic drainage has failed.[53]

44.3.2 Pancreatic Cystic Neoplasms

PCNs are mainly classified as IPMN, MCN, SCN, or solid pseudopapillary neoplasm (SPN) (▶ Table 44.1). Although different frequencies are reported in the literature, in a Korean study, IPMN accounts for 41%, MCN for 25.2%, SPN for 18.3%, SCN for 15.2%.[3] General features of PCL are summarized in ▶ Table 44.5.

Intraductal Papillary Mucinous Neoplasms

IPMN is defined by intraductal proliferation of neoplastic mucin-producing columnar epithelium originating from the pancreatic duct. Papillary projections of this epithelium may rise from main duct, branch ducts, or both. It is commonly seen in older men (at 60–80s) and is classically a solitary lesion in the head of pancreas, but is multifocal sometimes (up to 30%). Approximately 20 to 50% of PCNs are believed to be IPMN.[3,54,55] When the main duct is diffusely or segmentally involved, it is termed main duct IPMN (MD-IPMN) and has a high premalignant potential.[56,57,58,59] In cases when side branches are involved, it is termed branch duct IPMN (BD-IPMN) and the annual malignancy rate is reported to be only 2 to 3%.[60,61,62] Mixed IPMN is classified when both main and side branch ducts are affected with a malignancy rate reported to be between those of MD-IPMN and BD-IPMN.

Histologically, dysplasia in IPMNs is classified as low, moderate, or high grade.[63,64] Further histologic assessments determine the subtypes of IPMN: gastric foveolar type (predominant in BD-IPMN) usually represents low-grade dysplasia.[65,66,67] Intestinal type (predominant in MD-IPMN) represents intermediate- to high-grade dysplasia and colloid type adenocarcinoma frequently develops in association with it.[68] Invasive cancers are frequently tubular-type adenocarcinomas, which have a worse

Table 44.5 General features of some pancreatic cystic lesions

Parameters	Pseudocyst	IPMN	MCN	SCN
Demographics	Adult ♂, pancreatitis history, alcohol consumption	♂ 60–70 years old	♀ 40–50 years old	♀ 60–80 years old
Descriptions	Mostly pancreatic tale localization, solitary, small to very large size, fibrous-thick capsule	Mostly pancreatic head localization, incidental and solitary. Rarely multifocal and multilocular	Mostly pancreatic body and tail localization, incidental, solitary and large, thick wall	Entire pancreas localization oligo/macrocystic or many small cysts
Cross-sectional imaging (CT/MRI)	Mostly unilocular cyst, inflammatory parenchymal findings of pancreatitis	MD: MPD is diffusely or partially involved, BD: pancreatic duct communicated solitary or cluster of cysts, sometimes multifocal	Thickly septated macrocysts, thickened wall, peripheral "eggshell calcification"	Multiple microcysts, central fibrous scar with calcification, rarely oligocystic
Endoscopic ultrasonography	Unilocular, anechoic, thick-walled cyst, chronic pancreatitis parenchymal features	MD: MPD dilation, hyperechoic nodules arising from ductal wall, BD: small, "cluster of grape-like" dilations of BD, mural nodules	Few septated big cyst, not dilated pancreatic duct, peripheral calcifications, sometimes atypical papillary projections	Multiple-anechoic, small cystic areas, "honeycomb appearance," occasionally central calcification or fibrosis
Cytology	No epithelial lining, inflammatory cells and histiocytes, degenerative debris	Papillary mucin-producing epithelium, ± atypia in various degree, staining positive with mucin, colloid-like mucin	Mucin-producing tall columnar epithelium, ± atypia in various degree, staining positive with mucin, "ovarian-like mucosa," colloid-like mucin	Mostly acellular and nondiagnostic, cluster of small cells in bland cuboidal morphology, staining positive with glycogen and negative with mucin
EUS-FNA fluid analysis	↓ Viscosity, nonmucinous, clear (brown-green in color sometimes), may be hemorrhagic, amylase ↑, lipase ↑, CEA↓↓	↑ Viscosity, viscous mucus, amylase ↑ (60%) CEA usually ↑ KRAS mutation (+) (60–80%)	↑ Viscosity, viscous mucus, amylase ↓, CEA usually ↑, KRAS mutation (+) (14%), GNAS mutation (−)	↓ viscosity, Clear fluid, May be hemorrhagic Amylase ↓↓ CEA ↓↓

BD, branch duct; CEA, carcinoembryonic antigen; CT, computed tomography; EUS-FNA, endoscopic ultrasound–guided fine-needle aspiration; IPMN, intraductal papillary mucinous neoplasm; MCN, mucinous cystic neoplasm; MD, main duct; MPD, main pancreatic duct; MRI, magnetic resonance imaging; SCN, serous cystic **neoplasm**; ♂: Men; ♀: Women; ↓: Low; ↑: High; ↓↓: Very Low.

prognosis compared to the colloid type. Intraductal oncocytic papillary cancers are infrequent and have a prognosis similar to ductal adenocarcinoma.[69,70] Gastric-type IPMN demonstrates the best prognosis, on the other hand, pancreatobiliary and intestinal type demonstrate the worse prognosis.[71]

Although abdominal pain, malaise, nausea, and vomiting may be seen in patients with IPMN, it is usually diagnosed unintentionally.[54] Serum laboratory analysis and tumor markers are generally not of diagnostic value.[3] Imaging tools not only help to diagnose an IPMN, but also help for the differential diagnosis and the evaluation for resectability. Today, upper gastrointestinal (GI) endoscopy and ERCP are not commonly used for the diagnosis.[72] Although most cystic lesions are detected by conventional imaging (US, CT, and MRI) incidentally (▶ Fig. 44.7), multidetector CT (MDCT) is currently the preferred method for evaluation. Additionally, the combination of MDCT with MRI is reported to be superior to each imaging alone.[73] Nowadays, EUS is the favored procedure, especially in patients who are prior to surgery. Papillary projections, cyst wall thickening, internal septations, mural nodule, and debris in the cyst can be visualized.[3,51,54,74] EUS can differentiate a benign cyst from malignant IPMN with an accuracy of 40 to 90%, which is superior to US, ERCP, CT, and MRI.[75]

Highly viscous cystic fluid with high CEA levels indicates a mucinous cyst (IPMN or MCN), which reflects a mucinous epithelium. A CEA cutoff value of 192 ng/mL is found to be the best predictor for a mucinous cyst, in contrast to amylase activity that does not discriminate a mucinous from nonmucinous cyst.[76] Malignant

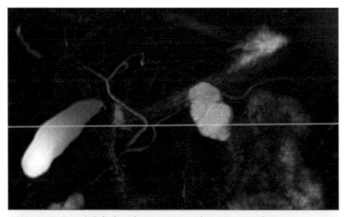

Fig. 44.7 A multilobulated, 45 × 27 mm hyperintense lesion adjacent to the body of the pancreas on magnetic resonance cholangiopancreatography (MRCP) without connection to main pancreatic duct, representing a side branch intraductal papillary mucinous neoplasm (IPMN).

cells by FNA are highly predictive of a malignant IPMN.[77] Although a *KRAS* mutation is highly specific for mucinous neoplasms,[78] it is ineffective in discriminating malignant cyst from benign cysts. Moreover, *GNAS* mutations cannot predict malignancy but may be specific for IPMN.[79]

Having a high malignancy potential, international consensus guidelines recommend a surgical resection in patients with MD-IPMN.[56,57,58,59] Given a low-risk potential, asymptomatic BD-IPMN patients without risk factors should be monitored with MRCP. Potential indications for surgical resection include the presence of a mural nodule, increase in size, and high-grade dysplasia in cytology. EUS-guided cyst ablation with alcohol or alcohol combination with paclitaxel is an alternative choice of treatment[80,81] (**Video 44.3**).

Mucinous Cystic Neoplasms

The second type of mucinous cyst is MCN, which is reported to account for 23% of resected PCN.[82] Common features of MCN include a solitary cyst in body or tail of the pancreas affecting mostly females at an age of less than 50. Commonly, it does not communicate with the pancreatic duct. An ovarian-type stroma underlies the mucin-producing columnar ductal epithelium in MCN, which stain positively for human chorionic gonadotropin, estrogen and progesterone receptors. There are three types of MCN: mucinous cystadenoma exhibiting benign features, mucinous cystic tumor with borderline features, and mucinous cystadenocarcinoma demonstrating malignant features.[83,84]

The symptoms of MCN include abdominal pain, weight loss, and fatigue in 70% of patients. Jaundice and a palpable mass could be the findings on physical examination. Laboratory tests are commonly in normal limits.[85]

A thinly septated, large solitary cyst with peripheral calcification are typical findings in CT.[86] The calcifications are lamellated and these contrast the central stellate calcifications of SCN. On MRI, peripheral calcifications, thickened wall, and septations were found to predict a malignancy in 95% of patients. Similar findings can be shown in EUS (▶ Fig. 44.8), but the FNA material provides powerful diagnostic tools. MCNs contain a thick mucin in the aspirated fluid (**Video 44.4**), which is rich in CEA, but low in amylase. The cyst fluid is often positive for *KRAS*, however, negative for GNAS.[87,88,89]

Because of having a high premalignant potential, current consensus guidelines recommend surgery for MCN.[60] Laparoscopic distal pancreatectomy with splenic preservation is the preferred surgery for lesions in the pancreatic tail. EUS-guided

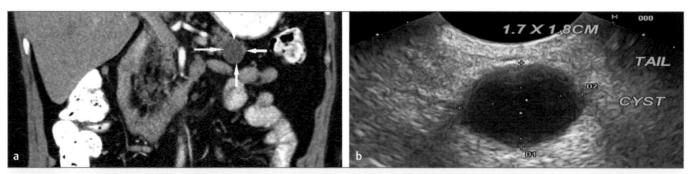

Fig. 44.8 (a) CT showing an 18-mm cystic lesion in the pancreatic tail (*white arrows*). (b) The appearance of the same lesion on EUS. Surgical histology revealed a benign mucinous cystic neoplasm (MCN).

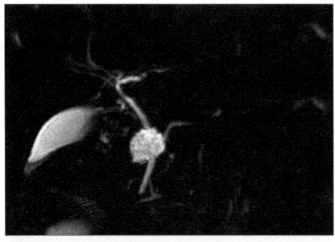

Fig. 44.9 A 28-mm, multiseptated, microcystic serous cystadenoma within the head of the pancreas on MRCP.

cyst ablation should be a choice in patients who refuse or cannot tolerate surgery.

Serous Cystic Neoplasms

SCNs are typically benign cysts in women at age less than 60, which can be located anywhere in the pancreas. These are most commonly classified as benign and serous cystadenocarcinomas are very rare. SCN contains a thin, bloody fluid, surrounded by a thin wall consisting of cuboidal epithelial cells, which stain periodic acid–Schiff (PAS) positive. These grow slowly and take a long time to reach large dimensions.[90] About 90% of von Hippel–Lindau patients develop SCN.[91]

Patients with SCN are frequently asymptomatic and CT/MRI reveals the common findings of a microcystic morphology. In the center of the lesion is a stellate-shaped central scar surrounded by multiple tiny cysts. Having similar morphology, CT/MRI sometimes fails to differentiate unilocular (oligocystic) SCN from MCN or BD-IPMN. Unilocular lesions are lobulated, thin-walled cysts usually in the pancreas (▶Fig. 44.9). The EUS findings include multiple small, anechoic thinly septated cysts. EUS-guided FNA aspiration reveals low amylase and CEA levels and infrequently PAS-positive cuboidal cells.[92]

SCN has an excellent prognosis and surgery is suggested for symptomatic patients with a large cyst (> 4 cm) and when the diagnosis is indefinite.[90,91,93]

Solid Pseudopapillary Neoplasms

SPN consists of two components: solid (solid pseudopapillary), which is formed by monomorphic epithelial cells, and cystic (hemorrhagic–necrotic pseudocystic). SPNs are large, single, round, and well-demarcated lesions that are often cystic with areas of hemorrhagic degeneration.[94] These account for about 5% of all PCNs. SPNs are most commonly found in women at their 20s or 30s. Abdominal pain, discomfort, vomiting, and weight loss associated with mass effect may be observed. SPNs are considered as low-grade malignant neoplasms.[95]

CT demonstrates a mass consisting of varying areas of nonseptated soft tissue and necrotic foci, surrounded by a thick, well-circumscribed capsule. Similarly, SPNs are well-demarcated lesions

on MRI.[96] EUS shows a well-defined hypoechoic mass with cystic and solid parts inside. The cyst fluid is highly cellular and the CEA level is low.[97]

Surgery is curative and the rate of recurrence after surgery is very low.[3]

References

[1] Muniraj T, Jamidar PA, Aslanian HR. Pancreatic cancer: a comprehensive review and update. Dis Mon. 2013; 59(11):368–402

[2] Ro C, Chai W, Yu VE, Yu R. Pancreatic neuroendocrine tumors: biology, diagnosis, and treatment. Chin J Cancer. 2013; 32(6):312–324

[3] Yoon WJ, Brugge WR. Pancreatic cystic neoplasms: diagnosis and management. Gastroenterol Clin North Am. 2012; 41(1):103–118

[4] Brugge WR. Diagnosis and management of cystic lesions of the pancreas. J Gastrointest Oncol. 2015; 6(4):375–388

[5] Laffan TA, Horton KM, Klein AP, et al. Prevalence of unsuspected pancreatic cysts on MDCT. AJR Am J Roentgenol. 2008; 191(3):802–807

[6] Moparty B, Brugge WR. Approach to pancreatic cystic lesions. Curr Gastroenterol Rep. 2007; 9(2):130–135

[7] Spinelli KS, Fromwiller TE, Daniel RA, et al. Cystic pancreatic neoplasms: observe or operate. Ann Surg. 2004; 239(5):651–657, discussion 657–659

[8] Partensky C. Toward a better understanding of pancreatic ductal adenocarcinoma: glimmers of hope? Pancreas. 2013; 42(5):729–739

[9] Howlader N, Noone AM, Krapcho M, et al. SEER Cancer Statistics Review, 1975–2010, National Cancer Institute. http://seer.cancer.gov/csr/1975_2010

[10] Vincent A, Herman J, Schulick R, et al.. Pancreatic cancer. Lancet. 2011; 378(9791):607–620. Epub 2011 May 26.

[11] Kloppel G, Hruban RH, Longnecker DS, et al. Tumours of the exocrine pancreas. In: Ham- ilton SR, Aaltonen LA, eds. World Health Organization Classification of Tumours. Pathology and Genetics of Tumours of the Digestive System. Lyon, France: IARC Press; 2000:219–251

[12] Raimondi S, Maisonneuve P, Lowenfels AB. Epidemiology of pancreatic cancer: an overview. Nat Rev Gastroenterol Hepatol. 2009; 6(12):699–708

[13] Ryan DP, Hong TS, Bardeesy N. Pancreatic adenocarcinoma. N Engl J Med. 2014; 371(11):1039–1049

[14] McCleary-Wheeler AL, McWilliams R, Fernandez-Zapico ME. Aberrant signaling pathways in pancreatic cancer: a two compartment view. Mol Carcinog. 2012; 51(1):25–39

[15] Porta M, Fabregat X, Malats N, et al. Exocrine pancreatic cancer: symptoms at presentation and their relation to tumour site and stage. Clin Transl Oncol. 2005; 7(5):189–197

[16] Chari ST, Leibson CL, Rabe KG, et al.. Probability of pancreatic cancer following diabetes: a population-based study. Gastroenterology. 2005; 129(2):504–511

[17] Khorana AA, Fine RL. Pancreatic cancer and thromboembolic disease. Lancet Oncol. 2004; 5(11):655–663

[18] Canto MI, Harinck F, Hruban RH, et al; International Cancer of Pancreas Screening (CAPS) Consortium. International Cancer of the Pancreas Screening (CAPS) Consortium summit on the management of patients with increased risk for familial pancreatic cancer. Gut. 2013; 62(3):339–347

[19] Hruban RH, Canto MI, Goggins M, et al. Update on familial pancreatic cancer. Adv Surg. 2010; 44:293–311

[20] Hernandez JM, Cowgill SM, Al-Saadi S, et al. CA 19–9 velocity predicts disease-free survival and overall survival after pancreatectomy of curative intent. J Gastrointest Surg. 2009; 13(2):349–353

[21] Kaneko OF, Lee DM, Wong J, et al. Performance of multidetector computed tomographic angiography in determining surgical resectability of pancreatic head adenocarcinoma. J Comput Assist Tomogr. 2010; 34(5):732–738

[22] Takakura K, Sumiyama K, Munakata K, et al. Clinical usefulness of diffusion-weighted MR imaging for detection of pancreatic cancer: comparison with enhanced multidetector-row CT. Abdom Imaging. 2011; 36(4):457–462

[23] Kauhanen SP, Komar G, Seppänen MP, et al. A prospective diagnostic accuracy study of 18F-fluorodeoxyglucose positron emission tomography/computed tomography, multidetector row computed tomography, and magnetic resonance imaging in primary diagnosis and staging of pancreatic cancer. Ann Surg. 2009; 250(6):957–963

[24] Eloubeidi MA, Tamhane A. Prospective assessment of diagnostic utility and complications of endoscopic ultrasound-guided fine needle aspiration. Results from a newly developed academic endoscopic ultrasound program. Dig Dis. 2008; 26(4):356–363

[25] Gress F, Savides T, Cummings O, et al. Radial scanning and linear array endosonography for staging pancreatic cancer: a prospective randomized comparison. Gastrointest Endosc. 1997; 45(2):138–142

[26] Owens DJ, Savides TJ. Endoscopic ultrasound staging and novel therapeutics for pancreatic cancer. Surg Oncol Clin N Am. 2010; 19(2):255–266

[27] Katz MH, Hwang R, Fleming JB, Evans DB. Tumor-node-metastasis staging of pancreatic adenocarcinoma. CA Cancer J Clin. 2008; 58(2):111–125

[28] Tempero MA, Malafa MP, Behrman SW, et al. Pancreatic adenocarcinoma, version 2.2014: featured updates to the NCCN guidelines. J Natl Compr Canc Netw. 2014; 12(8):1083–1093

[29] Neoptolemos JP, Stocken DD, Friess H, et al; European Study Group for Pancreatic Cancer. A randomized trial of chemoradiotherapy and chemotherapy after resection of pancreatic cancer. N Engl J Med. 2004; 350(12):1200–1210

[30] Neoptolemos JP, Stocken DD, Bassi C, et al; European Study Group for Pancreatic Cancer. Adjuvant chemotherapy with fluorouracil plus folinic acid vs gemcitabine following pancreatic cancer resection: a randomized controlled trial. JAMA. 2010; 304(10):1073–1081

[31] Oettle H, Post S, Neuhaus P, et al. Adjuvant chemotherapy with gemcitabine vs observation in patients undergoing curative-intent resection of pancreatic cancer: a randomized controlled trial. JAMA. 2007; 297(3):267–277

[32] Faris JE, Blaszkowsky LS, McDermott S, et al. FOLFIRINOX in locally advanced pancreatic cancer: the Massachusetts General Hospital Cancer Center experience. Oncologist. 2013; 18(5):543–548

[33] Conroy T, Desseigne F, Ychou M, et al; Groupe Tumeurs Digestives of Unicancer. PRODIGE Intergroup. FOLFIRINOX versus gemcitabine for metastatic pancreatic cancer. N Engl J Med. 2011; 364(19):1817–1825

[34] Von Hoff DD, Ervin T, Arena FP, et al. Increased survival in pancreatic cancer with nab-paclitaxel plus gemcitabine. N Engl J Med. 2013; 369(18):1691–1703

[35] Halfdanarson TR, Rabe KG, Rubin J, Petersen GM. Pancreatic neuroendocrine tumors (PNETs): incidence, prognosis and recent trend toward improved survival. Ann Oncol. 2008; 19(10):1727–1733

[36] Metz DC, Jensen RT. Gastrointestinal neuroendocrine tumors: pancreatic endocrine tumors. Gastroenterology. 2008; 135(5):1469–1492

[37] Klöppel G, Anlauf M. Epidemiology, tumour biology and histopathological classification of neuroendocrine tumours of the gastrointestinal tract. Best Pract Res Clin Gastroenterol. 2005; 19(4):507–517

[38] Oberg K, Eriksson B. Endocrine tumours of the pancreas. Best Pract Res Clin Gastroenterol. 2005; 19(5):753–781

[39] Falconi M, Plockinger U, Kwekkeboom DJ, et al; Frascati Consensus Conference. European . Neuroendocrine Tumor Society. Well-differentiated pancreatic nonfunctioning tumors/carcinoma. Neuroendocrinology. 2006; 84(3):196–211

[40] Plöckinger U, Wiedenmann B. Diagnosis of non-functioning neuro-endocrine gastro-enteropancreatic tumours. Neuroendocrinology. 2004; 80(suppl 1):35–38

[41] Dimou AT, Syrigos KN, Saif MW. Neuroendocrine tumors of the pancreas: what's new. Highlights from the "2010 ASCO Gastrointestinal Cancers Symposium". Orlando, FL, USA. January 22–24, 2010. Journal of the pancreas 2010;11:135–138

[42] Ehehalt F, Saeger HD, Schmidt CM, Grützmann R. Neuroendocrine tumors of the pancreas. Oncologist. 2009; 14(5):456–467

[43] Habashi S, Draganov PV. Pancreatic pseudocyst. World J Gastroenterol. 2009; 15(1):38–47

[44] Memiş A, Parildar M. Interventional radiological treatment in complications of pancreatitis. Eur J Radiol. 2002; 43(3):219–228

[45] Brun A, Agarwal N, Pitchumoni CS. Fluid collections in and around the pancreas in acute pancreatitis. J Clin Gastroenterol. 2011; 45(7):614–625

[46] Aghdassi A, Mayerle J, Kraft M, et al.. Diagnosis and treatment of pancreatic pseudocysts in chronic pancreatitis. Pancreas. 2008; 36(2):105–112

[47] Cannon JW, Callery MP, Vollmer CM, Jr. Diagnosis and management of pancreatic pseudocysts: what is the evidence? J Am Coll Surg. 2009; 209(3):385–393

[48] Brugge WR. Approaches to the drainage of pancreatic pseudocysts. Curr Opin Gastroenterol. 2004; 20(5):488–492

[49] Pitman MB, Lewandrowski K, Shen J, et al.. Pancreatic cysts: preoperative diagnosis and clinical management. Cancer Cytopathol. 2010; 118(1):1–13

[50] Balthazar EJ, Freeny PC, vanSonnenberg E. Imaging and intervention in acute pancreatitis. Radiology. 1994; 193(2):297–306

[51] Brugge WR. The use of EUS to diagnose cystic neoplasms of the pancreas. Gastrointest Endosc. 2009; 69(suppl 2):S203–S209

[52] Johnson MD, Walsh RM, Henderson JM, et al. Surgical versus nonsurgical management of pancreatic pseudocysts. J Clin Gastroenterol. 2009; 43(6):586–590

[53] Lerch MM, Stier A, Wahnschaffe U, Mayerle J. Pancreatic pseudocysts: observation, endoscopic drainage, or resection? Dtsch Arztebl Int. 2009; 106(38):614–621

[54] Farrell JJ, Brugge WR. Intraductal papillary mucinous tumor of the pancreas. Gastrointest Endosc. 2002; 55(6):701–714

[55] Sahani DV, Lin DJ, Venkatesan AM, et al. Multidisciplinary approach to diagnosis and management of intraductal papillary mucinous neoplasms of the pancreas. Clin Gastroenterol Hepatol. 2009; 7(3):259–269

[56] Salvia R, Fernández-del Castillo C, Bassi C, et al. Main-duct intraductal papillary mucinous neoplasms of the pancreas: clinical predictors of malignancy and long-term survival following resection. Ann Surg. 2004; 239(5):678–685, discussion 685–687

[57] Crippa S, Fernández-Del Castillo C, Salvia R, et al. Mucin-producing neoplasms of the pancreas: an analysis of distinguishing clinical and epidemiologic characteristics. Clin Gastroenterol Hepatol. 2010; 8(2):213–219

[58] Lafemina J, Katabi N, Klimstra D, et al. Malignant progression in IPMN: a cohort analysis of patients initially selected for resection or observation. Ann Surg Oncol. 2013; 20(2):440–447

[59] Schmidt CM, White PB, Waters JA, et al. Intraductal papillary mucinous neoplasms: predictors of malignant and invasive pathology. Ann Surg. 2007; 246(4):644–651, discussion 651–654

[60] Tanaka M, Fernández-del Castillo C, Adsay V, et al; International Association of Pancreatology. International consensus guidelines 2012 for the management of IPMN and MCN of the pancreas. Pancreatology. 2012; 12(3):183–197

[61] Kang MJ, Jang JY, Kim SJ, et al. Cyst growth rate predicts malignancy in patients with branch duct intraductal papillary mucinous neoplasms. Clin Gastroenterol Hepatol. 2011; 9(1):87–93

[62] Lévy P, Jouannaud V, O'Toole D, et al. Natural history of intraductal papillary mucinous tumors of the pancreas: actuarial risk of malignancy. Clin Gastroenterol Hepatol. 2006; 4(4):460–468

[63] Kang MJ, Lee KB, Jang JY, et al. Disease spectrum of intraductal papillary mucinous neoplasm with an associated invasive carcinoma invasive IPMN versus pancreatic ductal adenocarcinoma-associated IPMN. Pancreas. 2013; 42(8):1267–1274

[64] Sakorafas GH, Smyrniotis V, Reid-Lombardo KM, Sarr MG. Primary pancreatic cystic neoplasms revisited. Part III. Intraductal papillary mucinous neoplasms. Surg Oncol. 2011; 20(2):e109–e118

[65] Sadakari Y, Ohuchida K, Nakata K, et al. Invasive carcinoma derived from the nonintestinal type intraductal papillary mucinous neoplasm of the pancreas has a poorer prognosis than that derived from the intestinal type. Surgery. 2010; 147(6):812–817

[66] Adsay NV, Merati K, Andea A, et al. The dichotomy in the preinvasive neoplasia to invasive carcinoma sequence in the pancreas: differential expression of MUC1 and MUC2 supports the existence of two separate pathways of carcinogenesis. Mod Pathol. 2002; 15(10):1087–1095

[67] Andrejevic-Blant S, Kosmahl M, Sipos B, Klöppel G. Pancreatic intraductal papillary-mucinous neoplasms: a new and evolving entity. Virchows Arch. 2007; 451(5):863–869

[68] Yopp AC, Katabi N, Janakos M, et al. Invasive carcinoma arising in intraductal papillary mucinous neoplasms of the pancreas: a matched control study with conventional pancreatic ductal adenocarcinoma. Ann Surg. 2011; 253(5):968–974

[69] Furukawa T, Hatori T, Fujita I, et al. Prognostic relevance of morphological types of intraductal papillary mucinous neoplasms of the pancreas. Gut. 2011; 60(4):509–516

[70] Liszka L, Pajak J, Zielińska-Pajak E, et al. Intraductal oncocytic papillary neoplasms of the pancreas and bile ducts: a description of five new cases and review based on a systematic survey of the literature. J Hepatobiliary Pancreat Sci. 2010; 17(3):246–261

[71] Machado NO, Al Qadhi H, Al Wahibi K. Intraductal papillary mucinous neoplasm of pancreas. N Am J Med Sci. 2015; 7(5):160–175

[72] Konstantinou F, Syrigos KN, Saif MW. Intraductal papillary mucinous neoplasms of the pancreas (IPMNs): epidemiology, diagnosis and future aspects. JOP. 2013; 14(2):141–144

[73] Del Chiaro M, Verbeke C, Salvia R, et al; European Study Group on Cystic Tumours of the Pancreas. European experts consensus statement on cystic tumours of the pancreas. Dig Liver Dis. 2013; 45(9):703–711

[74] Brugge WR. Endoscopic approach to the diagnosis and treatment of pancreatic disease. Curr Opin Gastroenterol. 2013; 29(5):559–565

[75] Grützmann R, Niedergethmann M, Pilarsky C, Klöppel G, Saeger HD. Intraductal papillary mucinous tumors of the pancreas: biology, diagnosis, and treatment. Oncologist. 2010; 15(12):1294–1309

[76] Brugge WR, Lewandrowski K, Lee-Lewandrowski E, et al. Diagnosis of pancreatic cystic neoplasms: a report of the cooperative pancreatic cyst study. Gastroenterology. 2004; 126(5):1330–1336

[77] Michaels PJ, Brachtel EF, Bounds BC, et al.. Intraductal papillary mucinous neoplasm of the pancreas: cytologic features predict histologic grade. Cancer. 2006; 108(3):163–173

[78] Sawhney MS, Devarajan S, O'Farrel P, et al. Comparison of carcinoembryonic antigen and molecular analysis in pancreatic cyst fluid. Gastrointest Endosc. 2009; 69(6):1106–1110

[79] Dal Molin M, Matthaei H, Wu J, et al. Clinicopathological correlates of activating GNAS mutations in intraductal papillary mucinous neoplasm (IPMN) of the pancreas. Ann Surg Oncol. 2013; 20(12):3802–3808

[80] Brugge WR. Management and outcomes of pancreatic cystic lesions. Dig Liver Dis. 2008; 40(11):854–859

[81] Matthes K, Mino-Kenudson M, Sahani DV, et al. EUS-guided injection of paclitaxel (OncoGel) provides therapeutic drug concentrations in the porcine pancreas (with video). Gastrointest Endosc. 2007; 65(3):448–453

[82] Valsangkar NP, Morales-Oyarvide V, Thayer SP, et al. 851 resected cystic tumors of the pancreas: a 33-year experience at the Massachusetts General Hospital. Surgery. 2012; 152(3, suppl 1):S4–S12

[83] Sakorafas GH, Smyrniotis V, Reid-Lombardo KM, Sarr MG. Primary pancreatic cystic neoplasms revisited: part II. Mucinous cystic neoplasms. Surg Oncol. 2011; 20(2):e93–e101

[84] Bai XL, Zhang Q, Masood N, et al.. Pancreatic cystic neoplasms: a review of preoperative diagnosis and management. J Zhejiang Univ Sci B. 2013; 14(3):185–194

[85] Crippa S, Salvia R, Warshaw AL, et al. Mucinous cystic neoplasm of the pancreas is not an aggressive entity: lessons from 163 resected patients. Ann Surg. 2008; 247(4):571–579

[86] Procacci C, Carbognin G, Accordini S, et al. CT features of malignant mucinous cystic tumors of the pancreas. Eur Radiol. 2001; 11(9):1626–1630

[87] Kadayifci A, Brugge WR. Endoscopic ultrasound-guided fine-needle aspiration for the differential diagnosis of intraductal papillary mucinous neoplasms and size stratification for surveillance. Endoscopy. 2014; 46(4):357

[88] Jimenez RE, Warshaw AL, Z'graggen K, et al. Sequential accumulation of K-ras mutations and p53 overexpression in the progression of pancreatic mucinous cystic neoplasms to malignancy. Ann Surg. 1999; 230(4):501–509, discussion 509–511

[89] Iacobuzio-Donahue CA, Wilentz RE, Argani P, et al. Dpc4 protein in mucinous cystic neoplasms of the pancreas: frequent loss of expression in invasive carcinomas suggests a role in genetic progression. Am J Surg Pathol. 2000; 24(11):1544–1548

[90] Sakorafas GH, Smyrniotis V, Reid-Lombardo KM, Sarr MG. Primary pancreatic cystic neoplasms revisited. Part I: serous cystic neoplasms. Surg Oncol. 2011; 20(2):e84–e92

[91] Moore PS, Zamboni G, Brighenti A, et al. Molecular characterization of pancreatic serous microcystic adenomas: evidence for a tumor suppressor gene on chromosome 10q. Am J Pathol. 2001; 158(1):317–321

[92] Belsley NA, Pitman MB, Lauwers GY, et al.Serous cystadenoma of the pancreas: limitations and pitfalls of endoscopic ultrasound-guided fine-needle aspiration biopsy. Cancer. 2008; 114(2):102–110

[93] Farrell JJ, Fernández-del Castillo C. Pancreatic cystic neoplasms: management and unanswered questions. Gastroenterology. 2013; 144(6):1303–1315

[94] Papavramidis T, Papavramidis S. Solid pseudopapillary tumors of the pancreas: review of 718 patients reported in English literature. J Am Coll Surg. 2005; 200(6):965–972

[95] Tipton SG, Smyrk TC, Sarr MG, Thompson GB. Malignant potential of solid pseudopapillary neoplasm of the pancreas. Br J Surg. 2006; 93(6):733–737

[96] Choi JY, Kim MJ, Kim JH, et al. Solid pseudopapillary tumor of the pancreas: typical and atypical manifestations. AJR Am J Roentgenol. 2006; 187(2):W178–W186

[97] Jani N, Dewitt J, Eloubeidi M, et al. Endoscopic ultrasound-guided fine-needle aspiration for diagnosis of solid pseudopapillary tumors of the pancreas: a multicenter experience. Endoscopy. 2008; 40(3):200–203

45 Subepithelial Tumors of the Gastrointestinal Tract

Jennifer Maranki and Stavros N. Stavropoulos

45.1 Introduction

Subepithelial tumors (SETs) of the gastrointestinal (GI) tract are frequently encountered lesions and a common cause of referral for endoscopic ultrasound. While the overall prevalence is unknown, these lesions are often discovered during routine endoscopy or cross-sectional imaging performed for other reasons. On endoscopy, these are most frequently encountered in the stomach. These are often incorrectly referred to as "submucosal" tumors. The term "subepithelial" is more accurate as these tumors can be located in and/or arise from any of the layers deep to the epithelial layer of the mucosa (including the muscularis mucosae, submucosa, and muscularis propria).

SETs typically appear as a bulge within the GI lumen with normal overlying mucosa. Most of the tumors cause no symptoms, but can cause bleeding, obstruction, dysphagia, or, if in close proximity to the ampulla, jaundice, and pancreatitis. These lesions can be benign or malignant, and endoscopic ultrasound (EUS) with fine-needle aspiration (FNA) is an important modality in the diagnostic evaluation of these lesions. EUS is also useful for differentiating between mural tumors and extramural (or extrinsic) lesions. Up to 30% of suspected subepithelial mural tumors identified on routine endoscopy are found to be either extramural lesions or extrinsic compression by adjacent organs of vascular structures when evaluated with EUS.[1]

A variety of subepithelial lesions present in the GI tract, including gastrointestinal stromal tumors (GISTs), leiomyomas, carcinoids, lipomas, pancreatic rests (ectopic pancreatic tissue), duplication cysts, schwannomas, or metastatic disease. Abnormal vasculature, such as pseudoaneurysms or varices, may also present as subepithelial lesions.

In this chapter, the types of SETs as well as their endoscopic and endosonographic characteristics are discussed. Histologic and immunohistochemical features are noted, as well as high-risk features. Methods of tissue acquisition, including EUS with FNA and core biopsy are compared and contrasted. Endoscopic approaches to tumor resection are reviewed, with advantages and disadvantages of each technique.

45.2 Types of SETs

Understanding of the histologic layers of the GI wall is essential in characterizing SETs. The wall is comprised of five layers identified using EUS imaging with frequencies of 5 to 12 MHz. The innermost (first) layer, characterized by a very thin hyperechoic band, represents the superficial mucosa/interface with the lumen. Below this, a thin hypoechoic band represents deep mucosa including the muscularis mucosae (second layer). The submucosa (third layer) appears as a hyperechoic band, and deep to this, the muscularis propria (fourth layer) appears as a thick hypoechoic band. The serosa/ adventitia (fifth layer) is thin and hyperechoic, and often unable to be differentiated from surrounding structures. ▶ Table 45.1 summarizes the most common types of SETs and their corresponding wall layers.

45.2.1 Gastrointestinal Stromal Tumors

GISTs are the most frequently encountered SET of the upper GI tract.[2] These tumors are believed to arise from the interstitial cells of Cajal, and 10 to 30% are malignant at the time of diagnosis.[3] Annually, over 5,000 cases of GISTs are diagnosed.[4] Small GISTs (< 10 mm) are common in the adult population, with autopsy data from Germany reporting gross detection in 22.5% of adults over the age of 50.[5] These data suggest that most small GISTs do not progress into large macroscopic tumors despite the presence of the c-kit and *PDGFRA* mutations.[6]

Table 45.1 EUS characteristics of subepithelial tumors of the GI tract

Lesion	Echogenicity	EUS layers 2nd	3rd	4th	Other features
GIST	Hypoechoic			x	Rarely from 2nd or 3rd, may have internal anechoic echoes
Leiomyoma	Hypoechoic	x	x	x	
Carcinoid	Hypoechoic	x	x		
Duplication cyst	Anechoic	x	x	x	
Lipoma	Hyperechoic		x		Diffusely, strongly hyperechoic
Lymphoma	Hypoechoic	x	x	x	
Varices	Anechoic	x	x		Flow with Doppler, serpiginous
Neural tumors	Hypoechoic		x	x	
Pancreatic rest	Hypoechoic	x	x	x	Heterogeneous, may have anechoic ductal structures
Metastasis	Hypoechoic	x	x	x	
Granular cell tumor	Hypoechoic	x	x		

EUS, endoscopic ultrasound; GIST, gastrointestinal stromal tumor.

[a]First layer is luminal interface and mucosa, second layer is muscularis mucosa, third layer is submucosa, fourth layer is muscularis propria, fifth layer is serosa or adventitia.

Endoscopically, the lesions are most commonly encountered in the stomach. These vary is shape and size, and may have an overlying ulcer. On EUS, GISTs appear as hypoechoic masses arising from the muscularis propria (fourth layer) (▶ Fig. 45.1) or muscularis mucosa (between second and third layer). These are similar in appearance to leiomyomas, and differentiating between the two requires immunohistochemical evaluation of specimens.[7] GISTs are described as c-kit (CD117)-positive mesenchymal spindle cell or epithelioid lesions. Over 95% are positive for c-kit (CD117).[8,9] The majority of GISTs are positive for CD34, whereas a minority (20–30%) is positive for spinal muscular atrophy (SMA), and the expression of the two may be reciprocal. Even fewer express the S100 protein, and fewer than 5% are positive for desmin.[10,11,12] A newer marker for GISTs, DOG1, has shown high sensitivity and specificity for GISTs, and is particularly useful for diagnosing GISTs that are c-kit negative.[6,13,14,15,16,17] GISTs typically are found in older individuals, with the stomach being the most common site (60–70%), followed by the small intestine (20–25%), colon and rectum (5%), and esophagus (< 5%).[12]

45.2.2 Leiomyomas

Leiomyomas are benign smooth muscle tumors and appear endoscopically and endosonographically similar to GISTs, but are often smaller in size (typically < 2 cm). Occasionally, the tumors may become large. These are frequently encountered in the esophagus but can occur throughout the GI tract (▶ Fig. 45.2). These are characterized by normal overlying mucosa that can easily be tented with biopsy forceps. Similar to GISTs, these may also have a denuded or necrotic central area, particularly with large lesions. On EUS, these appear as a hypoechoic lesion arising from either the second layer (muscularis mucosa) or fourth layer (muscularis propria). Because these are unable to be differentiated from GISTs without immunochemical staining, biopsy is often required to exclude a lesion that may require endoscopic or surgical resection. Unlike GISTs, leiomyomas do not stain positive for c-kit or DOG1.

45.2.3 Carcinoids

Carcinoid tumors (▶ Fig. 45.3, ▶ Fig. 45.4) originate from neuroendocrine cells and are most frequently encountered in the small bowel. The ileum is the most common site, followed by the jejunum and duodenum.[18] Carcinoid tumors also occur in the stomach, and account for nearly 10% of all carcinoid tumors. In a retrospective, 50-year analysis of over 500 carcinoids, the male–female ratio has steadily decreased to 0.54.[19] Gastric carcinoids are classified into three types, depending on malignant potential. Type I gastric carcinoids are associated with chronic atrophic gastritis, hypergastrinemia,

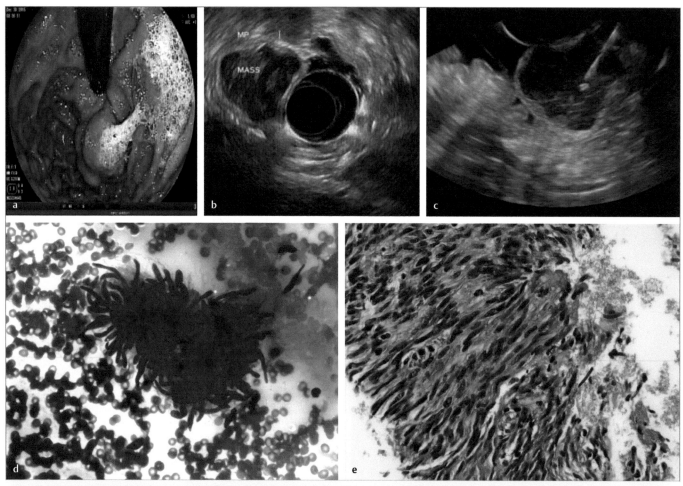

Fig. 45.1 Gastrointestinal stromal tumor (GIST) arising from the fourth wall layer. Immunohistochemistry was positive for CD-117. **(a)** Endoscopic image showing a medium-sized submucosal nodule in the cardia, best seen on retroflexion. **(b)** Radial EUS imaging of a 25-mm hypoechoic lesion arising from the muscularis propria. **(c)** Linear EUS imaging demonstrating a core needle during fine-needle biopsy within the lesion. **(d)** Diff-Quik staining revealing an abundance of spindle-shaped cells (40× magnification). **(e)** Hematoxylin and eosin staining show the lesion is composed of predominantly spindle-shaped cells with oval nuclei and eosinophilic cytoplasm (40× magnification). (Images are provided ▶ courtesy of Kaveh Sharzehi, MD, Temple University School of Medicine.)

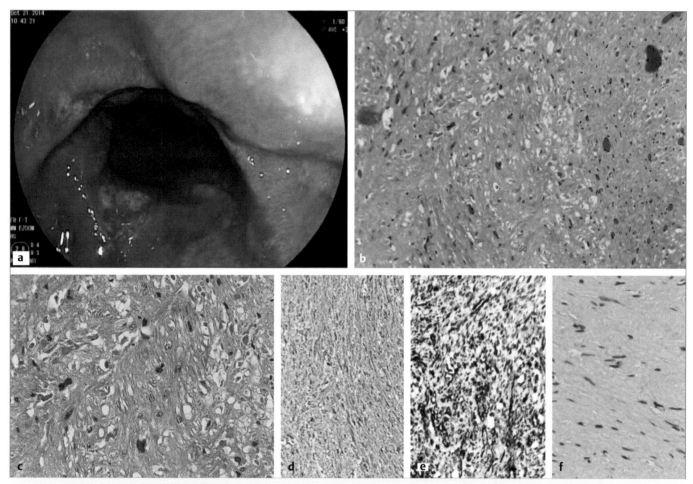

Fig. 45.2 Leiomyoma. **(a)** Endoscopic image showing a large, submucosal lesion in the distal esophagus. **(b)** Low-power H&E stain revealing a spindle cell neoplasm. **(c)** High power H&E stain. **(d)** Immunohistochemistry stains positive for Smooth Muscle Actin (SMA) and Desmin. **(e)** confirming a leiomyoma, and negative for C-Kit (CD117). **(f)** excluding a GIST.

and pernicious anemia (▶Fig. 45.3). These occur most commonly in elderly female patients and have very low malignant potential.[20] Type II gastric carcinoids are associated with hypergastrinemia due to Zollinger–Ellison syndrome and multiple endocrine neoplasia type 1 (MEN 1). These have intermediate malignant potential. Type III gastric carcinoids are sporadic, not associated with hypergastrinemia, and have the highest risk of malignant transformation.[20]

Endoscopically, carcinoids appear as sessile or semipedunculated lesions with normal overlying mucosa.[21] Carcinoid tumors may originate in the mucosal layer and penetrate into the submucosal layer, so they can often be diagnosed by mucosal biopsies.[22] On EUS examination, carcinoids appear as oval-shaped or round, hypoechoic, homogeneous tumors, most often arising from the submucosal layer (▶Fig. 45.3, ▶Fig. 45.4).[23]

45.2.4 Other Subepithelial Lesions of the Gastrointestinal Tract

Other subepithelial lesions include lipomas, pancreatic rests, duplication cysts, schwannomas, and aberrant vasculature. Metastatic lesions may also present as subepithelial lesions.

Lipomas are usually asymptomatic and can occur anywhere within the GI tract. Rarely, they can cause bowel obstruction, bleeding, or intussusception.[8] These have a smooth mucosal surface and often have a yellowish hue to the mucosa. These may

show a "pillow sign" when probed with closed biopsy forceps. On EUS, these appear as well-demarcated, oval, hyperechoic lesions arising from the submucosal layer (▶Fig. 45.5).

Pancreatic rests, or ectopic pancreatic tissue, are most frequently encountered in the stomach, most notably the antrum, but can occur throughout the GI tract. These do not typically cause symptoms, but can lead to ulceration and hemorrhage, esophageal or intestinal obstruction and intussusception, and biliary obstruction.[24] On standard endoscopy, pancreatic rests may have an umbilicated surface, sometimes described as "volcano like."[25] Endoscopic ultrasound images reveal well-circumscribed, mixed echogenicity lesions in the submucosa that can involve the muscularis as well that may contain anechoic, serpiginous ductal structures (▶Fig. 45.6).

Duplication cysts are uncommon congenital anomalies of the foregut that are often asymptomatic.[26] These are typically incidentally found on standard endoscopy or cross-sectional imaging. These appear endoscopically as round bulges that may be compressible with normal or somewhat translucent overlying mucosa. On EUS, these are smooth, spherical or tubular in shape, anechoic, with a well-defined wall, and located in the submucosa, muscularis propria, or serosal layers.[27] In the mediastinum, FNA is avoided due to the risk of infection.[28,29]

Schwannomas are benign nerve sheath tumors that can present with a variety of symptoms, including GI bleeding, abdominal pain, dysphagia, obstruction, and weight loss.[8] Histologically, they consist of spindle cells and epithelioid cells with peripheral

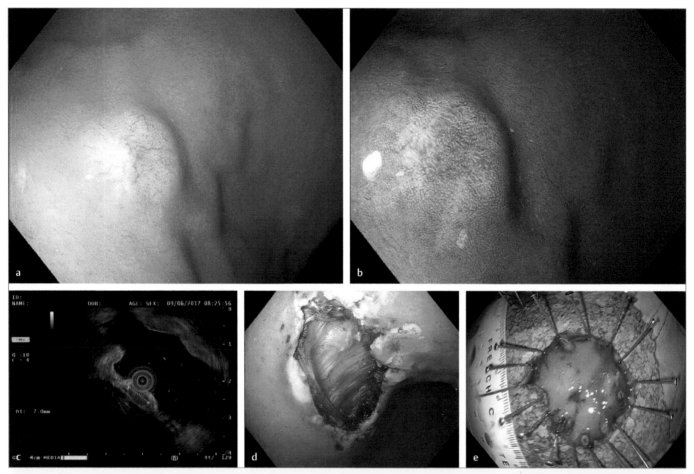

Fig. 45.3 Type I gastric carcinoid. (a) Endoscopic view of a 12 mm gastric carcinoid in the proximal stomach. (b) NBI view better defining the borders of this relatively flat lesion. (c) EUS imaging using a high frequency 20MHz mini-probe demonstrates that the lesion extends deep into the submucosa of the stomach (hyerperechoic layer 3) which is usually the case even for small carcinoids. (d) Deep resection crater with exposed muscularis propria after endoscopic submucosal dissection (ESD). Due to the deep submucosal extension of carcinoids, ESD is preferred to snare resection or endoscopic mucosal resection (EMR) which may result in a positive deep resection margin (i.e. incomplete resection). (e) Pinned ESD specimen prior to submission to pathology.

lymphoid cuffing, and stain positive for S100 and vimentin.[30,31] Endoscopically, schwannomas may have a slightly yellowish hue that can result in misidentification as lipomas. Unlike lipomas, however, endosonographically, these tumors are very low echogenicity lesions arising from the fourth layer (muscularis propria). These typically do not have internal echogenic foci but may have a marginal hypoechoic halo.[32]

Granular cell tumors are rare lesions occurring throughout the entire GI tract, with approximately one-third occurring in the esophagus.[33] These generally occur in the fourth, fifth, and sixth decades of life.[34,35] Granular cell tumors are usually solitary, but may be multifocal. These are usually incidentally found, but may cause symptoms of dysphagia, nausea, and regurgitation with lesions greater than 1 cm.[33,34] On EUS, lesions are typically less than 2 cm in size, with a homogeneous, hypoechoic lesion arising from the muscularis mucosae or submucosa.[36] Most esophageal granular cell tumors have a benign course, but cases of malignancy have been reported. It is generally accepted that tumors causing symptoms and those greater than 1 cm in size should be removed (endoscopically if possible).[33,37]

Vascular abnormalities, such as varices or pseudoaneurysm, may also appear as subepithelial lesions.[38] Gastric varies often appear as a submucosal bulge, often in the cardia and fundus, or an enlarged gastric fold. Unlike esophageal varices, gastric varices often do not have a bluish hue because these sit deeper in the gastric wall. Gastric varices should be suspected not only in patients with portal hypertension due to advanced liver disease, portal vein thrombosis, and Budd–Chiari syndrome, but also in patients with pancreatic disease causing splenic vein thrombosis. On endoscopy, other clues to the presence of portal hypertension may be seen, such as portal hypertensive gastropathy or esophageal varices. On EUS, varices appear as anechoic tubular structures in the submucosa that exhibit flow on Doppler examination.

While metastatic spread to the wall of the GI tract is rare, a variety of malignancies have been shown to spread to the gastric wall. These include melanoma and carcinomas of the lung, breast, ovaries, and kidney.[2,39,40] These appear as hypoechoic lesions in any of the layers, can have an umbilicated "volcano-like" appearance, and can be diagnosed by EUS-guided FNA (EUS-FNA) or deep biopsies depending on their depth within the wall of the GI tract.

45.3 Risk Stratification of Subepithelial Tumors

While most SETs are benign, several are malignant or have malignant potential, including GISTs, carcinoids, and lymphoma.

While all GISTs are thought to have some degree of malignant potential, GIST lesions within the small bowel are higher risk than those in the stomach or rectum.[41] Several factors, including those

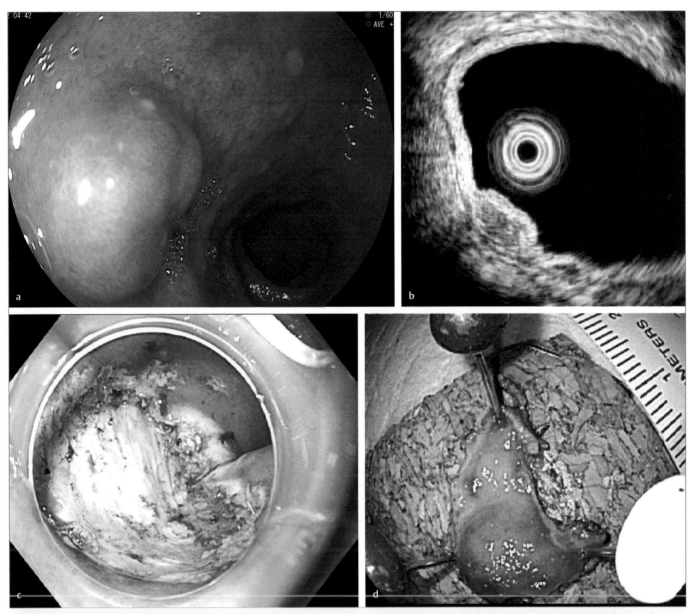

Fig. 45.4 Duodenal carcinoid. **(a)** Endoscopic view of subepithelial lesion in the proximal duodenal bulb. **(b)** EUS with miniprobe evaluation demonstrating the lesion in the submucosal layer. **(c)** Site following endoscopic submucosal dissection. **(d)** Pinning of the resection specimen onto cork.

based on overall size and mitotic rate, have been used to stratify the risk of malignancy (▶ Table 45.2).[22] Endosonographic features that have been reported to be associated with increased risk of malignancy include lesions with cystic spaces (▶ Fig. 45.7), an inhomogeneous echotexture, irregular borders, and the presence of enlarged lymph nodes.[42,43,44,45] Risk stratification is important in formulating an appropriate management strategy for GISTs.[46]

For carcinoids, risk of metastasis appears to be related to the site of the primary lesion. The rate of distant metastasis is higher in patients with small bowel carcinoids than in patients with neuroendocrine tumors (NETs) in other locations. Jejunoileal lesions are associated with a high rate of transmural invasion and aggressive behavior.[47] Further, lung and rectal carcinoids tend to remain local.[48,49]

45.4 Methods for Tissue Acquisition

Pathologic diagnosis of SETs may be helpful in clinical decision making. A variety of techniques have been applied to obtain adequate tissue for histologic analysis, and include bite-on-bite mucosal biopsies with forceps, biopsy after mucosal incision, endoscopic submucosal resection, EUS-FNA, and EUS-guided core biopsy (EUS-FNB). Several large-bore needles and core biopsy needles are currently in use for tissue acquisition (▶ Fig. 45.8).

45.4.1 Endoscopic Ultrasound-Guided Fine-Needle Aspiration

EUS-FNA is the most widely used method for tissue sampling, and is safe and effective.[2,6] Several studies have demonstrated the utility of EUS-FNA for diagnosing subepithelial lesions, and in particular, differentiating GISTs from leiomyomas.[50,51,52,53,54,55] This is especially true when on-site cytopathologic analysis of sample adequacy is undertaken.[56] In a retrospective study of 112 patients undergoing EUS-FNA of lesions arising from the fourth endosonographic layer, Hoda and colleagues reported that EUS-FNA was diagnostic in 61.6%, suspicious (spindle cells

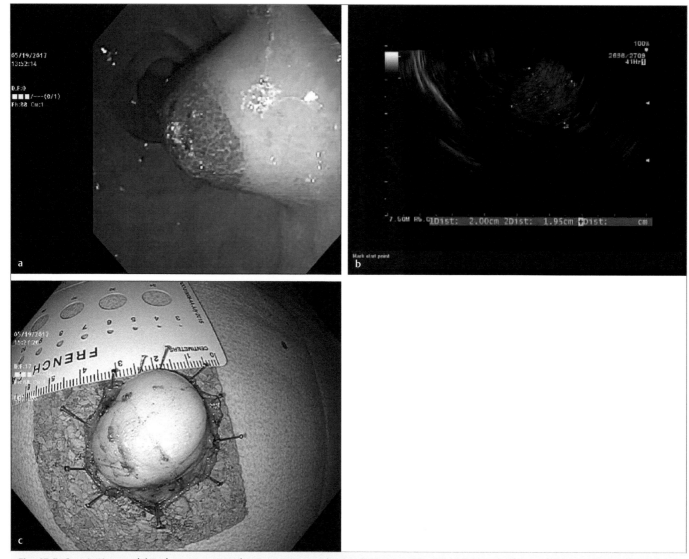

Fig. 45.5 Gastric Lipoma. **(a)** Endoscopic image showing a 3.5 cm subepithelial lesion with yellowish hue. Erythema of the mucosa overlying the lesion. **(b)** EUS imaging with a linear echoendoscope at 7.5 MHz demonstrates the typical appearance of a lipoma consisting of an oval, smooth, hyperechoic lesion arising from the submucosa. **(c)** Due to the relatively large size of the lesion with recurrent ulceration of the surface mucosa that was felt to possibly contribute to the patient's iron deficiency anemia, the lesion was resected via ESD. The image demonstrates complete enucleation of the lesion which was pinned with the mucosa overlying the lesion facing the cork.

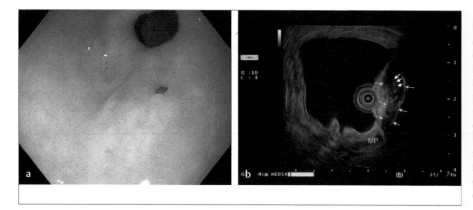

Fig. 45.6 Pancreatic rest in the gastric antrum. **(a)** Classic endoscopic appearance of a pancreatic rest: small submucosal lesion in the gastric antrum with central umbilication. **(b)** 20 MHz high frequency mini-probe EUS imaging demonstrating pancreatic parenchyma consisting of heterogeneous echotexture (hyperechoic foci in a mildly hypoechoic backround) and pancreatic ductal structures consisting of anechoic tubular structures (white arrows). Pancratic rests often extend into the muscularis propria (MP) causing thickening of the MP (blue arrows).

identified) in 22.3%, and nondiagnostic in 16.1%.[57] Mekky et al retrospectively analyzed 141 consecutive patients with gastric SETs who underwent EUS-FNA.[58] Results of the FNA were diagnostic or suggestive in over 82%, with adequate specimens being obtained in 83% of cases. Overall 49% had a definite final diagnosis, of which 60% were GISTs. EUS-FNA results were concordant with the final diagnosis in 66 of 69 lesions (accuracy rate

95.6%). Further, EUS-FNA demonstrated a sensitivity of 92.4% and specificity of 100% in differentiating benign from malignant lesions. Other studies have shown diagnostic yields ranging from 75 to 100% and sensitivities of EUS-FNA of greater than 80%.[59,60,61,62,63] Ando and colleagues reported on 49 patients with SETs originating from the muscularis propria, and found that for the diagnosis of malignant GIST, the accuracy, sensitivity, and

Table 45.2 Stratification of malignancy risk of GISTs by tumor size, mitotic count, and location

Size	Mitotic count	Risk of progressive disease (%)			
		Gastric	Jejunal/Ileal	Duodenal	Rectal
≤ 2 cm	≤ 5 per 50 HPFs	None (0)	None (0)	None (0)	None (0)
> 2 cm, ≤ 5 cm	≤ 5 per 50 HPFs	Very low (1.9)	Low (4.3)	Low (8.3)	Low (8.5)
> 5 cm, ≤ 10 cm	≤ 5 per 50 HPFs	Low (3.6)	Moderate (24)	Insufficient data	Insufficient data
> 10 cm	≤ 5 per 50 HPFs	Moderate (12)	High (52)	High (34)	High (57)
≤ 2 cm	≤ 5 per 50 HPFs	None (0)	High (50)	Insufficient data	High (54)
> 2 cm, ≤ 5 cm	≤ 5 per 50 HPFs	Moderate (16)	High (73)	High (50)	High (52)
> 5 cm, ≤ 10 cm	≤ 5 per 50 HPFs	High (55)	High (85)	Insufficient data	Insufficient data
> 10 cm	≤ 5 per 50 HPFs	High (86)	High (90)	High (86)	High (71)

HPFs, microscopic high-power field in tissue sections.

[a]Defined as metastasis or tumor-related deaths.

[b]Denotes tumor categories with very few patients.

Source: Data from Miettinen M, Lasota J. Semin Diagn Pathol 2006;23:70–83.

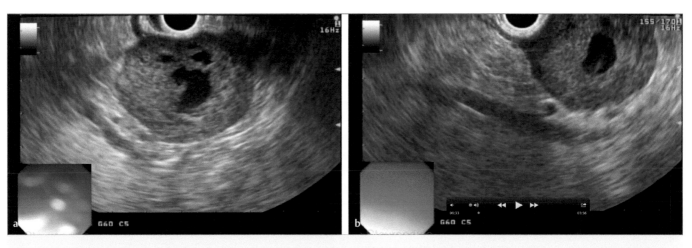

Fig. 45.7 (a, b) Gastric GIST with high-risk endosonographic appearance. This 3 × 4 cm gastric GIST had anechoic cystic spaces on EUS, a high-risk EUS feature. After en bloc endoscopic full-thickness R0 resection of the tumor, histologic analysis revealed a mitotic rate of 8/50 high-power field (HPF), consistent with a higher-risk GIST despite its gastric location and relatively small size.

specificity of EUS-FNA with the addition of immunohistochemical staining was 100%.[51] These data provide support to the use of EUS-FNA with immunohistochemical staining for the diagnosis of GISTs.[6]

Based on the data reviewed, the overall rate of definitive histologic diagnosis with EUS/FNA is relatively modest at 60 to 80%, and the amount of tissue obtained, even if adequate for definitive histologic diagnosis, may be too limited for histologic risk stratification. One approach to further optimizing tissue acquisition has been to use a larger-bore needle. Disadvantages of this approach are that the 19-gauge needle can be difficult to advance through the scope and into the lesion, resulting in a technical failure, particularly in the setting of an angulated scope. Additionally, more bleeding may occur with a larger needle. Conversely, use of a smaller-gauge (25-gauge) needle has also been explored, with the thought that it is easy to maneuver and may cause less trauma to the sampled area. While the 22-gauge needle is most commonly used, several studies have assessed the use of both 19- or 25-gauge needles.[64,65,66,67,68,69]

Other sampling techniques have also been studied. EUS-FNA using a forward-viewing echoendoscope is a modification that

has been applied in hopes of increasing the diagnostic yield. Larghi et al reported on the use of a forward-viewing EUS scope in 121 consecutive patients undergoing EUS-FNA of SETs.[70] Full histologic assessment, including immunohistochemistry, was successful in 93.4%. In terms of neoplastic versus nonneoplastic disease, the sensitivity and specificity were 92.8 and 100%, respectively. Matsuzaki et al conducted a randomized crossover study comparing forward-viewing versus oblique-viewing echoendoscopes in 41 patients with subepithelial GI lesions.[71] There was no difference in diagnostic yield between the two groups, but the forward-viewing group had shorter procedure times (21 minutes versus 27 minutes, $p = 0.009$), and superior tissue sample areas (2.46 vs. 1 mm², $p = 0.046$). ▶ Table 45.3 summarizes the yield of EUS-guided sampling.

45.4.2 Endoscopic Ultrasound-Guided Fine-Needle Biopsy and Trucut Biopsy

EUS-FNB has been proposed to overcome some of the limitations of EUS-FNA, namely inadequate tissue yield and inability to detect

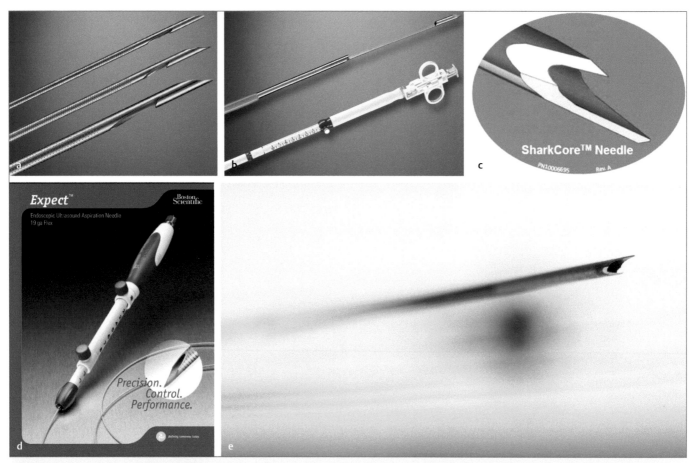

Fig. 45.8 A sample of currently available core and large-bore needles. **(a)** Cook ProCore needles. **(b)** Cook Quick-Core needle. **(c)** Boston Scientific 19-gauge flex needle. **(d)** Covidien SharkCore needle schematic. **(e)** Covidien SharkCore needle. (Cook images used with permission of Cook Medical Incorporated, Bloomington, Indiana; Boston Scientific images used with permission of Boston Scientific Corporation, Natick, Massachusetts; Covidien images used with permission of Covidien Incorporated, Mansfield, Massachusetts.)

malignant potential on cytology specimens[7] (**Video 45.1**). Levy and colleagues reported on their preliminary experience with the EUS-guided Trucut needle biopsy (EUS-TCB), suggesting adequate safety and a trend toward improved accuracy and fewer passes in 19 patients, when compared to EUS-FNA.[72] Other studies have shown modest diagnostic rates with EUS-TCB, ranging from 55 to 78%.[73,74,75,76] Diagnostic rates for EUS-FNB range from 74 to 82%.[69,77]

In a 2015 meta-analysis specifically assessing diagnostic efficacy in sampling of upper GI SETs, Zhang and colleagues reported that neither choice of FNA, TCB, or FNB, nor size of the needle appears to impact overall diagnostic rate.[78]

45.4.3 Other Tissue Acquisition Techniques

A variety of other endoscopic, non-EUS–based techniques have been reported to attempt to increase the amount of tissue obtained from SETs (▶Table 45.4). One method involves the use of forceps biopsies to take deep "well biopsies," also termed "bite-on-bite" technique. In one study of 37 subepithelial lesions found on standard endoscopy, the diagnostic yield of this technique was modest at 38%.[80] In a larger, multicenter study involving 129 patients with subepithelial lesions, definitive diagnosis with deep forceps biopsies was obtained in 59%.[81] However, 35% experienced significant bleeding following biopsy that required endoscopic hemostasis. Bite-on-bite forceps biopsy may be a reasonable first

approach in areas where EUS-FNA is not readily accessible, but it has modest yield and can be complicated by bleeding.

Another approach is to "unroof" the lesion via snare resection or needle knife incision of the mucosa/submucosa overlying a SET, followed by deep forceps biopsies or partial resection of the lesion (**Video 45.2**).[82,83,84,85,86,87]

Such techniques may result in severe delayed bleeding and chronic ulceration with bleeding of the residual SET that may convert a small asymptomatic SET into a symptomatic one requiring resection.

45.5 Management of Subepithelial Lesions

Management of SETs depends on the etiology and histology of the tumor. Many lesions, such as lipomas, pancreatic rests, duplication cysts, and varices, require no additional evaluation. Overtly malignant lesions require surgical resection if feasible. GISTs and carcinoid tumors carry significant potential for malignancy, and the management is often controversial.[2]

Sepe and Brugge proposed an algorithm for managing localized GISTs that has been adopted by the NCCN Task Force Report.[7,46] For GISTs that are symptomatic, greater than 4 or equal to 2 cm in size, or with suspicious EUS features (irregular borders, cystic spaces, ulceration, echogenic foci, and heterogeneity), resection is recommended. Otherwise, EUS surveillance should be

Table 45.3 Diagnostic yield of various EUS-guided sampling techniques in patients with GI SETs

Author	Year	Sampling technique	Needle size (G)	Number of Patients	Diagnostic (%)	Adequate for IHC	Non-diagnostic
Akahoshi	2007	FNA	22	53	79	100	21
Yoshida	2009	FNA	22	49	82	100	18
Hoda	2009	FNA	22	112	62	78	16
Hoda	2009	TCB	19	15	47	87	40
Polkowski	2009	TCB	19	49	63	86	22
Sepe	2009	FNA	19, 22, 25	37	78	35	22
Fernández-Esparrach	2010	FNA	22	40	53	82	30
Fernández-Esparrach	2010	TCB	19	40	55	95	40
Fernández-Esparrach	2010	FNA + TCB	22/19	40	78	n.r.	n.r.
Mekky	2010	FNA	22	141	62	79	17
Philipper[79]	2010	FNA	19, 22	47	34	46	26
Turhan	2010	FNA	19, 22	50	90	100	10
Dewitt	2011	TCB	19	37	79	97	21
Lee	2011	TCB	19	65	57	89	43
Suzuki	2011	FNA	22	47	75	n.r.	25
Watson	2011	FNA	19,22	65	68	n.r.	32
Eckardt	2012	FNA	19	46	52	91	48
Akahoshi	2014	FNA	22,25	90	62	n.r.	38
Larghi	2014	FNA	19	121	93	100	7
Matsuzaki	2015	FNA	19, 22, 25	41	85	n.r.	15

FNA, fine-needle aspiration; G, gauge; IHC, immunohistochemistry staining; TCB, Trucut biopsy; n.r., not reported

Table 45.4 Options for endoscopic resection of SETs

Technique	Indications	Contraindications	Advantages	Disadvantages	Complications
EMR (C, L)	SETs < 1.5 cm limited to the submucosa	SETs > 1.5 cm; SETs originating in the MP	Easy, quick technique with high success rate	Can only be applied to small endoluminal, superficial SETs	Minor hemorrhage, which is rare
Endoscopic ligation	SETs up to 2–3 cm arising from the MP with mainly intraluminal growth	SETs with extraluminal component	Easy to perform; short procedure times	Only applied to small, intraluminal SETs; unable to obtain complete pathologic evaluation, leaves tumor residua in muscularis propria	Perforation, major delayed hemorrhage
ESD	SETs limited to the submucosa (e.g., carcinoids)	Tumors with MP involvement	Allows for en bloc resection, precise histologic evaluation	Requires highly skilled manipulation by specially trained endoscopists; longer procedure times	Perforation, hemorrhage
ESE	SETs in the MP	SETs not meeting indications, SETs with extraluminal component	Not limited by size, shape, or involvement of the MP, en block resection	Similar to ESD (technically difficult, longer procedure time). May leave microscopic tumor residua in MP	Perforation, minor hemorrhage
EFTR	SETs up to 4–5 cm, involving the MP, including SETs with extraluminal component	SETs larger than 4–5 cm that may not be retrievable via luminal orifices, high-risk SETs at high risk of rupture	Allows for en bloc, full-thickness, R0 resection, precise histologic evaluation	Requires highly skilled manipulation by specially trained endoscopists; longer procedure times	Perforation, hemorrhage
STER	SETs up to 4–5 cm arising from the MP of esophagus, GEJ, and cardia, including SETs with extraluminal component	SETs larger than 4–5 cm that may not be retrievable via the tunnel and/or luminal orifices, high-risk SETs at high risk of rupture, SETs at locations where tunneling is not feasible (e.g., gastric fundus, lesser curvature etc.)	Allows for en bloc, full-thickness, R0 resection, maintains GI tract mucosal integrity facilitating secure closure	Requires highly skilled manipulation by specially trained endoscopists; longer procedure times	Perforations, hemorrhage, and for esophageal STER chest complications such as pneumothorax, infected pleural effusion/empyema

EFTR, endoscopic full-thickness resection; EMR (C, L), endoscopic mucosal tumor resection with a transparent cap (C) or ligation device (L); ESD, endoscopic submucosal dissection; ESE: endoscopic submucosal enucleation or excavation; GEJ, gastroesophageal junction; GI, gastrointestinal; MP, muscularis propria; SETs, subepithelial tumors; STER, submucosal tunneling endoscopic resection.

considered after a discussion with the patient about the risks and benefits. Of note, the NCCN guidelines initially recommended EUS surveillance at 6- to 12-month intervals, but this interval recommendation has been removed from the current version of the NCCN guidelines.[7,46]

The clinical behavior of carcinoids varies substantially based on type and location. Types I and type II gastric carcinoids tend to have a favorable prognosis.[19] Five-year survival for type I lesions is greater than 95%.[83] For types I and II lesions, endoscopic removal of small lesions (< 2 cm) is recommended (if feasible), with subsequent endoscopic surveillance (▶Fig. 45.3).[2] Type III (sporadic) carcinoids, however, have a higher malignant potential, and half will become locally invasive or metastatic. As a result, all type III gastric carcinoids, regardless of size, should be resected via partial or total gastrectomy with lymph node resection.[2,87]

Small duodenal carcinoids (less than 2 cm in size) located in the duodenal bulb can be treated with endoscopic resection (▶Fig. 45.4). Small bowel carcinoids have the potential to metastasize, regardless of size. As a result, resection of the involved segment and surrounding mesentery is recommended.[84] As these may be multifocal, evaluation of the rest of the small bowel at the time of resection is indicated.

Rectal carcinoids are often small, confined to the mucosa and submucosa, and localized at the time of diagnosis. As a result, these are frequently amenable to endoscopic resection with standard endoscopic mucosal resection (EMR) or endoscopic submucosal dissection (ESD) techniques. If they are less than 1 cm in size, standard EMR is indicated. For lesions greater than 2 cm in size, or extending into the muscularis propria, radical surgical resection is warranted. For intermediate-size lesions (1–2 cm), a transanal excision or advanced endoscopic excision technique (e.g., endoscopic submucosal dissection) is indicated.[88,89,90] Lesions arising from the colon that have not spread should be treated with partial colectomy and lymph node dissection.[91]

45.6 Endoscopic Resection of Subepithelial Tumors

Most neoplastic SETs are GISTs, the management of which hinges on risk stratification based on size and mitotic rate. However, as already reviewed, customary endoscopic sampling techniques such as EUS/FNA/FNB fail to achieve definitive histologic diagnosis in up to 30 to 40% of SETs and rarely offer adequate tissue for accurate mitotic rate assessment. Therefore, as reviewed, resection is recommended for all known or suspected GISTs that are symptomatic, have high-risk EUS features, or are ≥ 2 cm in size while lifelong surveillance at 1-year intervals is generally pursued for low-risk GISTs that are smaller than 2 cm.[46] This algorithm is often also applied to indeterminate lesions or other rare mesenchymal tumors of poorly understood malignant

potential (e.g., schwannomas, glomus tumors, granular cell tumors, etc.) for which little data exist to guide evidence-based management. This approach creates a large burden of surgery and endoscopy for small SETs less than 5 cm the majority of which are low-risk lesions. For most of these, surgery represents overtreatment driven by preoperative uncertainty and anxiety regarding risk. Furthermore, limited surgical "wedge resection" is not always possible particularly in challenging areas such as the gastroesophageal (GE) junction, esophagus, and cardia.

This situation has motivated expert endoscopists to attempt endoscopic resection of SETs smaller than 5 cm. These tumors represent an excellent target for endoscopic rather than surgical resection for the following reasons: (1) Their location in the wall of the GI tract and their frequent intraluminal growth pattern, often make them much easier to locate and remove from within the lumen of the GI tract with no need for resection of any uninvolved healthy tissue. (2) Lymph node resection is not necessary as the tumors do not metastasize via lymphatic pathways. (3) There is no need for a large margin of healthy tissue around the tumor since these tumors do not have the propensity for local recurrence seen with carcinomas; in fact, some studies show similar outcomes after R0 and R1 (macroscopically complete resection with microscopically positive margins) surgical resection of GISTs.[92,93,94] Initial attempts at endoscopic resection have included collaborative approaches with combined endoscopic and laparoscopic resection. Various techniques have been described ranging from the endoscopist providing minor assistance limited to visualization or mucosal margination of the lesion all the way to the endoscopist performing most of the resection with the surgeon providing assistance in the final stage of the resection and/or closure. Examples of such techniques include laparoscopic endoscopic combined surgery (LECS)[95] and laparoscopy-assisted endoscopic full-thickness resection (LAEFR).[95] On a recent review, these techniques were found to have 100% complete resection rates with no severe AEs with mean procedure times of approximately 3 hours and ranging up to 5 hours.[96] These approaches clearly lack the minimal invasiveness of a purely endoscopic approach since full laparoscopic access is employed. Another more recently reported purely endoscopic resection approach that we can refer to as "device-assisted endoscopic full-thickness resection" involves use of tissue apposition devices (such as devices developed for endoscopic antireflux therapies or over-the-scope clip [OTSC] devices) to achieve seromuscular layer apposition prior to full-thickness endoscopic resection.[98] Such techniques are limited to small, purely intraluminal SETs that can allow inversion of the GI wall (in the antireflux device technique) or suction of the tumor into a distal cap attachment at the tip of the endoscope (in the OTSC method). Furthermore, these devices are bulky limiting their applicability in difficult locations such as the fundus, esophagus, etc. Of more interest are techniques that have been developed as offshoots of ESD to allow "freehand" endoscopic resection of SETs. These techniques use the same devices as ESD for mucosal neoplasms, but take the resection to deeper layers including the deep submucosa, muscularis propria, or even the serosa. The first such technique that has been variably termed ESD for enucleation of SETs, endoscopic muscular dissection (EMD) or endoscopic submucosal enucleation or excavation (ESE) was developed in Asia by endoscopists experienced in ESD for mucosal neoplasms. It targets small SETs 2 to 3 cm in size with intraluminal growth and using ESD technique excavates them en bloc from the submucosa and muscularis propria. Tumors arising from the muscularis propria (e.g., GISTs) are removed by maintaining a plane of resection on the surface of the muscularis propria or the inner muscular layer. The intent is to avoid perforation (and thus also full-thickness resection)[99,100,101,102,103,104,105,106,107,108] (**Video 45.3**). In these ESE series, SETs with mean size 2 to 3 cm, arising from the submucosa or muscularis propria have been targeted with complete resection rates of 65 to 100% (lowest for tumors arising from muscularis propria) and with relatively low perforation rates of 0 to 13% and very low adverse event (AE) rates. With ESE, however, microscopic tumor residua may remain in the muscularis propria and/or serosa since full-thickness resection of the GI wall is not performed. Furthermore, ESE can only target tumors with intraluminal

growth (without any growth directed from the muscularis toward the peritoneal thoracic cavity or mediastinum). Recently, two techniques have been reported that overcome these ESE shortcomings by performing full-thickness resection of SETs. These techniques most commonly referred to as endoscopic full-thickness resection (EFTR) and submucosal tunnel endoscopic resection (STER) represent true natural orifice transluminal endoscopic surgery (NOTES) procedures that aim at en bloc, full-thickness R0 resection of SETs. EFTR was first reported in 2011 by Chinese endoscopists for gastric GISTs.[109,110] It involves full-thickness direct removal of a SET creating an intentional perforation, usually 1 to 3 cm in size which is then closed endoscopically with endoclip and endoloop techniques.[111] Our center is pioneering full-thickness resection in the United States (▶Fig. 45.9),[112] where, unlike Asia, availability of an endoscopic suturing device (Overstitch, Apollo Endosurgery, Austin, Texas, United States) allows easier and more secure closure of full-thickness defects[113] (**Video 45.4**). STER was first reported in 2012[114,115,116] not surprisingly by Asian POEM pioneers as this technique represents a direct offshoot of POEM in as much as it is mainly used for full-thickness resection of esophageal and GE junction SETs and uses a submucosal tunnel to access

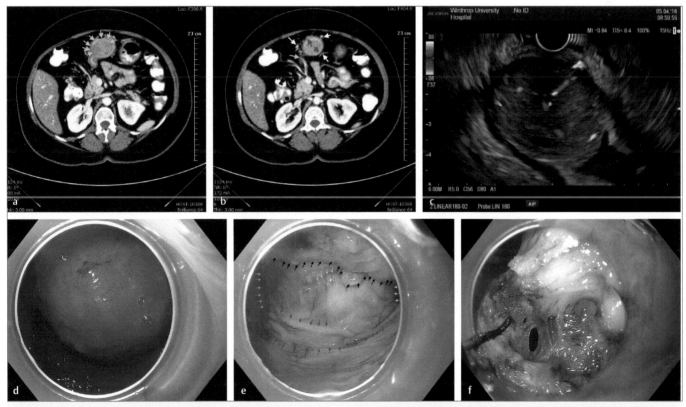

Fig. 45.9 (a) CT image intraluminal portion of GIST. (b) CT image of extraluminal portion of GIST. (c) GIST EUS with Doppler. (d) Endoscopic view of GIST. (e) EFTR submucosal dissection. (f) Initiation of full thickness resection with incision through the serosa.

(continued)

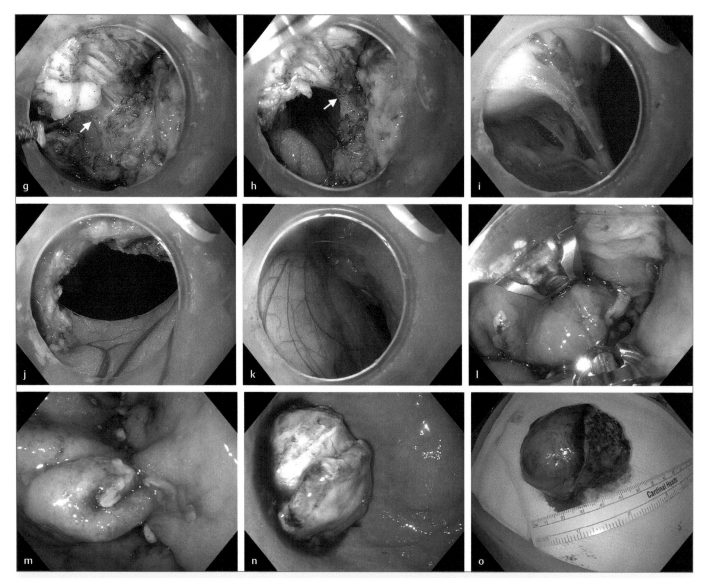

Fig. 45.9 *(continued)* **(g)** Progression of EFTR with incision of the mp initiated. **(h)** full thickness resection incision of muscularis propria circumferentially around the tumor. **(i)** Dissection of the serosal attachments to the capsule of the extralumial portion of the GIST. **(j)** EFTR completed with fat protruding through the defect. **(k)** Peritoneoscopy through the defect. **(l)** Defect closure with Overstitch.**(m)** Completed sutured closure of the defect. **(n)** Resected GIST within the gastric lumen. **(o)** Extracted GIST 5 x 6 cm.

the tumor and remove it along with the full-thickness of the GI wall from which it arises taking advantage of the tunnel concept to achieve secure closure of the perforation by simply closing the small tunnel orifice with clips (or suturing) very similarly to POEM (▶ Fig. 45.10). We summarize the Asian series (Chinese in their majority) reporting on EFTR and STER in ▶ Table 45.5 and ▶ Table 45.6, respectively. Our center has reported similar results in the only Western series to date, currently at 48 EFTRs and 14 STERs completed between 4/2012 and 11/2015.[117] (**Video 45.4** for EFTR and **Video 45.5** for STER). In the hands of expert operators, EFTR and STER provide high complete resection rates for SETs in

the 2- to 4-cm range with procedure times and adverse event rates that are similar or superior to those of surgery and with the additional advantage of minimally invasive organ-sparing resection, particularly for tumors difficult to target surgically (e.g., difficult locations and intraluminal growth pattern). EFTR and STER permit removal of lesions that have either intraluminal or extraluminal growth, but there is a size limitation of approximately 3 to 4 cm for the tumor's smallest diameter (since a larger diameter would hinder removal of the intact tumor from the tunnel and/or the mouth).

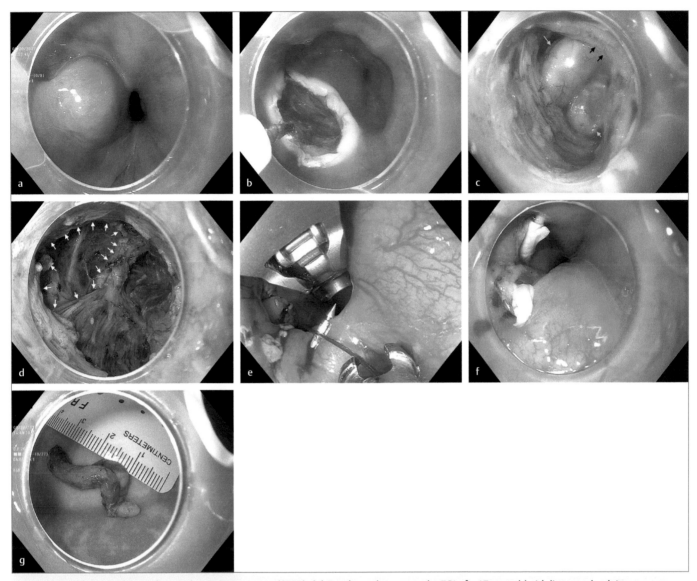

Fig. 45.10 Submucosal Tunneling Endoscopic Resection (STER). **(a)** Esophageal tumor at the EGJ of a 17 year old girl diagnosed as leiomyoma on prior EUS FNA. Due to the patient's young age the patient and her parents opted for resection rather than surveillance. **(b)** Initiation of the STER tunnel. Injection of saline in the submucosa approximately 3 cm proximal to the tumor followed by a 10-15 mm mucosal incision that will form the tunnel entry orifice. **(c)** Dissection of the tunnel and the mucosa surrounding the tumor achieves exposure of the irregularly shaped tumor (blue arrows). The tunnel can be clearly seen with the mucosa forming the ceiling of the tunnel (black arrows) and the muscularis propria with its circular muscle fibers forming the floor of the tunnel (white arrows). **(d)** Completion of the resection. A full thickness defect is seen (white arrows). The muscularis propria has been removed to achieve complete margin negative resection of the tumor exposing the mediastinal pleura, which appears as a thin transparent membrane at the bottom of the defect. **(e)** Closure of the tunnel entry using endoscopic suturing. **(f)** Completed closure of the tunnel entry sealing the tunnel and the full thickness defect under the overlying mucosa. **(g)** Ex vivo picture of the resected tumor with its intact capsule (white capsule with small vessels). The tumor has an irregular serpiginous tubular shape with dimensions of 1 x 3 cm.

Table 45.5 Selected series of endoscopic full-thickness resection (EFTR) (UGI tract except for one series by Xu et al that involved colonic SETs)

Study	Year	N	Size (mm)	Complete resection (%)	Time (min)	LOS (days)	Significant adverse events
Zhou, Surg Endosc	2011	26	28 (12–45)	100	105 (60–145)	5.5 (3–8)	None
Wang, Surg Endosc	2011	31/66 FTR	15 (8–17)	97	54	8	14% drains for peritonitis
Feng, J LEASt	2014	48	16 (5–48)	100	60 (30–270)	4–7	None
Ye, Surg Endosc	2014	51	24 (12–35)	98 1 conversion	52 (30–125)	5.9 (3–9)	None
Huang, WJG	2014	35	28 (20–45)	100	90 (60–155)	6 (4–10)	None
Guo, Surg Endosc	2015	23	12 (6–20)	100	40 (16–104)	3 (2–5)	2 peritonitis, conserve tx
Yang, Surg Endosc	2015	41	16	100	79	-	None
Xu, Endoscopy	2013	19 Colon series	18 (12–30)	84; 2 lap assist closure, 1 conversion	67 (45–130)	-	2 localized peritonitis, 1 bleeding

Table 45.6 Selected series of STER studies

Study	Year	N	Size (mm)	Complete resection (%)	Time (min)	LOS (days)	Significant adverse events
Esophageal STER series							
Inoue, *Endoscopy*	2012	11	12–30	82 (aborted 2, large [> 5 cm])	84–365	4–16	None
Gong, *Endoscopy*	2012	12	19 (10–40)	83% en bloc	48	-	2 pneumothorax (PTX)
Xu, *GIE*	2012	15 (8 FTR)	19 (12–30)	100	79 (25–130)	3.8 (3–5)	1 PTX (drain)
Lee, *Surg Endosc*	2013	5	21 (16–24)	100	35	2.8	None
Liu, *Surg Endosc*	2013	12 (7 FTR)	18 (10–30)	100	78 (130–150)	-	4 PTX/1 drain, 2 pleural effusion
Wang, *Surg Endosc*	2013	18	33	-	67	2.3	3 bleeding, 1 PTX/drain
Ye, *Surg Endosc*	2014	85 (10 FTR)	19 (10–30)	100	57 (30–115)	5.9	6 PTX
Lu, *Surg Endosc*	2014	45	12	98	84	-	None
Zhou, *WJG*	2015	21 (9 FTR)	23 (10–40)	86% en bloc 100% complete	63 (45–90)	4.3 (3–7)	1 pleural effusion/drain
Nonesophageal STER series							
Study	Year	N	Size (mm)	Complete resection (%)	Time (min)	LOS (days)	Significant adverse events
Wang, *Surg Endosc*	2014	57 (17 FTR) GE junction lesions	21.5 (6–35)	100	47 (15–120)	-	2 effusions/drained; 5 PTX/2 drained
Li, *Surg Endosc*	2015	32 Gastric lesions	23 (10–50)	100	52 (25–125)	3.9 (2–9)	1 500-cc bleed, 3 PTX/1 drain, 4 eff/1 drain, 1 abscess/drain
Lu, *PLOS one*	2015	45 Gastric lesions	19 (12–30)	93 (2 conversions)	79 (45–150)	-	7 pain, fever, no drainage
Hu, *Cancer Res Ther*	2014	12 Rectal lesions	14 (10–30)	100	49 (40–70)	3.1 (2–8)	5 fever, 1 leg swelling, emphysema

References

[1] Hwang JH, Rulyak SD, Kimmey MB; American Gastroenterological Association Institute. American Gastroenterological Association Institute technical review on the management of gastric subepithelial masses. Gastroenterology. 2006; 130(7):2217–2228

[2] Hwang JH, Kimmey MB. The incidental upper gastrointestinal subepithelial mass. Gastroenterology. 2004; 126(1):301–307

[3] Miettinen M, El-Rifai W, H L Sobin L, Lasota J. Evaluation of malignancy and prognosis of gastrointestinal stromal tumors: a review. Hum Pathol. 2002; 33(5):478–483

[4] Miettinen M, Sarlomo-Rikala M, Lasota J. Gastrointestinal stromal tumors: recent advances in understanding of their biology. Hum Pathol. 1999; 30(10):1213–1220

[5] Agaimy A, Wünsch PH, Hofstaedter F, et al. Minute gastric sclerosing stromal tumors (GIST tumorlets) are common in adults and frequently show c-KIT mutations. Am J Surg Pathol. 2007; 31(1):113–120

[6] Demetri GD, von Mehren M, Antonescu CR, et al. NCCN Task Force report: update on the management of patients with gastrointestinal stromal tumors. J Natl Compr Canc Netw. 2010; 8(Suppl 2):S1–S41, quiz S42–S44

[7] Sepe PS, Brugge WR. A guide for the diagnosis and management of gastrointestinal stromal cell tumors. Nat Rev Gastroenterol Hepatol. 2009; 6(6):363–371

[8] Salah W, Faigel DO. When to puncture, when not to puncture: submucosal tumors. Endosc Ultrasound. 2014; 3(2):98–108

[9] Stamatakos M, Douzinas E, Stefanaki C, et al. Gastrointestinal stromal tumor. World J Surg Oncol. 2009; 7:61

[10] Fletcher CD, Berman JJ, Corless C, et al. Diagnosis of gastrointestinal stromal tumors: a consensus approach. Hum Pathol. 2002; 33(5):459–465

[11] Miettinen M, Sobin LH, Lasota J. Gastrointestinal stromal tumors of the stomach: a clinicopathologic, immunohistochemical, and molecular genetic study of 1765 cases with long-term follow-up. Am J Surg Pathol. 2005; 29(1):52–68

[12] Miettinen M, Lasota J. Gastrointestinal stromal tumors—definition, clinical, histological, immunohistochemical, and molecular genetic features and differential diagnosis. Virchows Arch. 2001; 438(1):1–12

[13] West RB, Corless CL, Chen X, et al. The novel marker, DOG1, is expressed ubiquitously in gastrointestinal stromal tumors irrespective of KIT or PDGFRA mutation status. Am J Pathol. 2004; 165(1):107–113

[14] Miettinen M, Wang ZF, Lasota J. DOG1 antibody in the differential diagnosis of gastrointestinal stromal tumors: a study of 1840 cases. Am J Surg Pathol. 2009; 33(9):1401–1408

[15] Novelli M, Rossi S, Rodriguez-Justo M, et al. DOG1 and CD117 are the antibodies of choice in the diagnosis of gastrointestinal stromal tumours. Histopathology. 2010; 57(2):259–270

[16] Kara T, Serinsoz E, Arpaci RB, et al. Contribution of DOG1 expression to the diagnosis of gastrointestinal stromal tumors. Pathol Res Pract. 2013; 209(7):413–417

[17] Ho MY, Blanke CD. Gastrointestinal stromal tumors: disease and treatment update. Gastroenterology. 2011; 140(5):1372–6.e2

[18] Hemminki K, Li X. Incidence trends and risk factors of carcinoid tumors: a nationwide epidemiologic study from Sweden. Cancer. 2001; 92(8):2204–2210

[19] Modlin IM, Lye KD, Kidd M. A 50-year analysis of 562 gastric carcinoids: small tumor or larger problem? Am J Gastroenterol. 2004; 99(1):23–32

[20] Rindi G, Bordi C, Rappel S, et al. Gastric carcinoids and neuroendocrine carcinomas: pathogenesis, pathology, and behavior. World J Surg. 1996; 20(2):168–172

[21] Hirakawa K, Iida M, Matsui T, et al. Endoscopic findings in carcinoid tumor of the duodenum. Am J Gastroenterol. 1991; 86(5):603–605

[22] Menon L, Buscaglia JM. Endoscopic approach to subepithelial lesions. Therap Adv Gastroenterol. 2014; 7(3):123–130

[23] Matsumoto T, Iida M, Suekane H, et al. Endoscopic ultrasonography in rectal carcinoid tumors: contribution to selection of therapy. Gastrointest Endosc. 1991; 37(5):539–542

[24] Lai EC, Tompkins RK. Heterotopic pancreas. Review of a 26 year experience. Am J Surg. 1986; 151(6):697–700

[25] Eckardt AJ, Wassef W. Diagnosis of subepithelial tumors in the GI tract. Endoscopy, EUS, and histology: bronze, silver, and gold standard? Gastrointest Endosc. 2005; 62(2):209–212

[26] Faigel DO, Burke A, Ginsberg GG, et al. The role of endoscopic ultrasound in the evaluation and management of foregut duplications. Gastrointest Endosc. 1997; 45(1):99–103

[27] Geller A, Wang KK, DiMagno EP. Diagnosis of foregut duplication cysts by endoscopic ultrasonography. Gastroenterology. 1995; 109(3):838–842

[28] Ryan AG, Zamvar V, Roberts SA. Iatrogenic candidal infection of a mediastinal foregut cyst following endoscopic ultrasound-guided fine-needle aspiration. Endoscopy. 2002; 34(10):838–839

[29] Wildi SM, Hoda RS, Fickling W, et al. Diagnosis of benign cysts of the mediastinum: the role and risks of EUS and FNA. Gastrointest Endosc. 2003; 58(3):362–368

[30] Hou YY, Tan YS, Xu JF, et al. Schwannoma of the gastrointestinal tract: a clinicopathological, immunohistochemical and ultrastructural study of 33 cases. Histopathology. 2006; 48(5):536–545

[31] Daimaru Y, Kido H, Hashimoto H, Enjoji M. Benign schwannoma of the gastrointestinal tract: a clinicopathologic and immunohistochemical study. Hum Pathol. 1988; 19(3):257–264

[32] Jung MK, Jeon SW, Cho CM, et al. Gastric schwannomas: endosonographic characteristics. Abdom Imaging. 2008; 33(4):388–390

[33] Perçinel S, Savaş B, Yilmaz G, et al. Granular cell tumor of the esophagus: three case reports and review of the literature. Turk J Gastroenterol. 2008; 19(3):184–188

[34] Orlowska J, Pachlewski J, Gugulski A, Butruk E. A conservative approach to granular cell tumors of the esophagus: four case reports and literature review. Am J Gastroenterol. 1993; 88(2):311–315

[35] Goldblum JR, Rice TW, Zuccaro G, Richter JE. Granular cell tumors of the esophagus: a clinical and pathologic study of 13 cases. Ann Thorac Surg. 1996; 62(3):860–865

[36] Palazzo L, Landi B, Cellier C, et al. Endosonographic features of esophageal granular cell tumors. Endoscopy. 1997; 29(9):850–853

[37] Yasuda I, Tomita E, Nagura K, et al. Endoscopic removal of granular cell tumors. Gastrointest Endosc. 1995; 41(2):163–167

[38] Seicean A. Endoscopic ultrasound in the diagnosis and treatment of upper digestive bleeding: a useful tool. J Gastrointestin Liver Dis. 2013; 22(4):465–469

[39] Kadakia SC, Parker A, Canales L. Metastatic tumors to the upper gastrointestinal tract: endoscopic experience. Am J Gastroenterol. 1992; 87(10):1418–1423

[40] Sangha S, Gergeos F, Freter R, et al. Diagnosis of ovarian cancer metastatic to the stomach by EUS-guided FNA. Gastrointest Endosc. 2003; 58(6):933–935

[41] Grotz TE, Donohue JH. Surveillance strategies for gastrointestinal stromal tumors. J Surg Oncol. 2011; 104(8):921–927

[42] Chak A, Canto MI, Rösch T, et al. Endosonographic differentiation of benign and malignant stromal cell tumors. Gastrointest Endosc. 1997; 45(6):468–473

[43] Rösch T, Kapfer B, Will U, et al; German EUS Club. Endoscopic ultrasonography. Accuracy of endoscopic ultrasonography in upper gastrointestinal submucosal lesions: a prospective multicenter study. Scand J Gastroenterol. 2002; 37(7):856–862

[44] Lamba G, Gupta R, Lee B, et al. Current management and prognostic features for gastrointestinal stromal tumor (GIST). Exp Hematol Oncol. 2012; 1(1):14

[45] Palazzo L, Landi B, Cellier C, et al. Endosonographic features predictive of benign and malignant gastrointestinal stromal cell tumours. Gut. 2000; 46(1):88–92

[46] von Mehren M, Randall RL, Benjamin RS, et al. Gastrointestinal stromal tumors, version 2.2014. J Natl Compr Canc Netw. 2014; 12(6):853–862

[47] Burke AP, Thomas RM, Elsayed AM, Sobin LH. Carcinoids of the jejunum and ileum: an immunohistochemical and clinicopathologic study of 167 cases. Cancer. 1997; 79(6):1086–1093

[48] Hassan MM, Phan A, Li D, et al. Risk factors associated with neuroendocrine tumors: a U.S.-based case-control study. Int J Cancer. 2008; 123(4):867–873

[49] Wang AY, Ahmad NA. Rectal carcinoids. Curr Opin Gastroenterol. 2006; 22(5):529–535

[50] Sasaki Y, Niwa Y, Hirooka Y, et al. The use of endoscopic ultrasound-guided fine-needle aspiration for investigation of submucosal and extrinsic masses of the colon and rectum. Endoscopy. 2005; 37(2):154–160

[51] Ando N, Goto H, Niwa Y, et al. The diagnosis of GI stromal tumors with EUS-guided fine needle aspiration with immunohistochemical analysis. Gastrointest Endosc. 2002; 55(1):37–43

[52] Wiersema MJ, Vilmann P, Giovannini M, et al. Endosonography-guided fine-needle aspiration biopsy: diagnostic accuracy and complication assessment. Gastroenterology. 1997; 112(4):1087–1095

[53] Giovannini M, Seitz JF, Monges G, et al. Fine-needle aspiration cytology guided by endoscopic ultrasonography: results in 141 patients. Endoscopy. 1995; 27(2):171–177

[54] Shin HJ, Lahoti S, Sneige N. Endoscopic ultrasound-guided fine-needle aspiration in 179 cases: the M. D. Anderson Cancer Center experience. Cancer. 2002; 96(3):174–180

[55] Wiersema MJ, Wiersema LM, Khusro Q, et al. Combined endosonography and fine-needle aspiration cytology in the evaluation of gastrointestinal lesions. Gastrointest Endosc. 1994; 40(2 pt 1):199–206

[56] Klapman JB, Logrono R, Dye CE, Waxman I. Clinical impact of on-site cytopathology interpretation on endoscopic ultrasound-guided fine needle aspiration. Am J Gastroenterol. 2003; 98(6):1289–1294

[57] Hoda KM, Rodriguez SA, Faigel DO. EUS-guided sampling of suspected GI stromal tumors. Gastrointest Endosc. 2009; 69(7):1218–1223

[58] Mekky MA, Yamao K, Sawaki A, et al. Diagnostic utility of EUS-guided FNA in patients with gastric submucosal tumors. Gastrointest Endosc. 2010; 71(6):913–919

[59] Yoshida S, Yamashita K, Yokozawa M, et al. Diagnostic findings of ultrasound-guided fine-needle aspiration cytology for gastrointestinal stromal tumors: proposal of a combined cytology with newly defined features and histology diagnosis. Pathol Int. 2009; 59(10):712–719

[60] Akahoshi K, Sumida Y, Matsui N, et al. Preoperative diagnosis of gastrointestinal stromal tumor by endoscopic ultrasound-guided fine needle aspiration. World J Gastroenterol. 2007; 13(14):2077–2082

[61] Vander Noot MR, III, Eloubeidi MA, Chen VK, et al. Diagnosis of gastrointestinal tract lesions by endoscopic ultrasound-guided fine-needle aspiration biopsy. Cancer. 2004; 102(3):157–163

[62] Sepe PS, Moparty B, Pitman MB, et al. EUS-guided FNA for the diagnosis of GI stromal cell tumors: sensitivity and cytologic yield. Gastrointest Endosc. 2009; 70(2):254–261

[63] Chatzipantelis P, Salla C, Karoumpalis I, et al. Endoscopic ultrasound-guided fine needle aspiration biopsy in the diagnosis of gastrointestinal stromal tumors of the stomach. A study of 17 cases. J Gastrointestin Liver Dis. 2008; 17(1):15–20

[64] Larghi A, Verna EC, Ricci R, et al. EUS-guided fine-needle tissue acquisition by using a 19-gauge needle in a selected patient population: a prospective study. Gastrointest Endosc. 2011; 74(3):504–510

[65] Camellini L, Carlinfante G, Azzolini F, et al. A randomized clinical trial comparing 22G and 25G needles in endoscopic ultrasound-guided fine-needle aspiration of solid lesions. Endoscopy. 2011; 43(8):709–715

[66] Watson RR, Binmoeller KF, Hamerski CM, et al. Yield and performance characteristics of endoscopic ultrasound-guided fine needle aspiration for diagnosing upper GI tract stromal tumors. Dig Dis Sci. 2011; 56(6):1757–1762

[67] Eckardt AJ, Adler A, Gomes EM, et al. Endosonographic large-bore biopsy of gastric subepithelial tumors: a prospective multicenter study. Eur J Gastroenterol Hepatol. 2012; 24(10):1135–1144

[68] Akahoshi K, Oya M, Koga T, et al. Clinical usefulness of endoscopic ultrasound-guided fine needle aspiration for gastric subepithelial lesions smaller than 2 cm. J Gastrointestin Liver Dis. 2014; 23(4):405–412

[69] Kim GH, Cho YK, Kim EY, et al; Korean EUS Study Group. Comparison of 22-gauge aspiration needle with 22-gauge biopsy needle in endoscopic ultrasonography-guided subepithelial tumor sampling. Scand J Gastroenterol. 2014; 49(3):347–354

[70] Larghi A, Fuccio L, Chiarello G, et al. Fine-needle tissue acquisition from subepithelial lesions using a forward-viewing linear echoendoscope. Endoscopy. 2014; 46(1):39–45

[71] Matsuzaki I, Miyahara R, Hirooka Y, et al. Forward-viewing versus oblique-viewing echoendoscopes in the diagnosis of upper GI subepithelial lesions with EUS-guided FNA: a prospective, randomized, crossover study. Gastrointest Endosc. 2015; 82(2):287–295

[72] Levy MJ, Jondal ML, Clain J, Wiersema MJ. Preliminary experience with an EUS-guided trucut biopsy needle compared with EUS-guided FNA. Gastrointest Endosc. 2003; 57(1):101–106

[73] Fernández-Esparrach G, Sendino O, Solé M, et al. Endoscopic ultrasound-guided fine-needle aspiration and trucut biopsy in the diagnosis of gastric stromal tumors: a randomized crossover study. Endoscopy. 2010; 42(4):292–299

[74] Lee JH, Choi KD, Kim MY, et al. Clinical impact of EUS-guided Trucut biopsy results on decision making for patients with gastric subepithelial tumors ≥ 2 cm in diameter. Gastrointest Endosc. 2011; 74(5):1010–1018

[75] Dewitt J, McGreevy K, Cummings O, et al. Initial experience with EUS-guided Trucut biopsy of benign liver disease. Gastrointest Endosc. 2009; 69(3 pt 1):535–542

[76] Polkowski M, Gerke W, Jarosz D, et al. Diagnostic yield and safety of endoscopic ultrasound-guided trucut [corrected] biopsy in patients with gastric submucosal tumors: a prospective study. Endoscopy. 2009; 41(4):329–334

[77] Iglesias-Garcia J, Poley JW, Larghi A, et al. Feasibility and yield of a new EUS histology needle: results from a multicenter, pooled, cohort study. Gastrointest Endosc. 2011; 73(6):1189–1196

[78] Zhang XC, Li QL, Yu YF, et al. Diagnostic efficacy of endoscopic ultrasound-guided needle sampling for upper gastrointestinal subepithelial lesions: a meta-analysis. Surg Endosc. 2016; 30(6):2431–2441

[79] Philipper M, Hollerbach S, Gabbert HE, et al. Prosepctive comparison of endoscopic ultrasound-guided fine-needle aspiration and surgical histology in upper gastrointestinal submucosal tumors. Endoscopy. 2010 Apr; 42(4):300–5

[80] Ji JS, Lee BI, Choi KY, et al. Diagnostic yield of tissue sampling using a bite-on-bite technique for incidental subepithelial lesions. Korean J Intern Med. 2009; 24(2):101–105

[81] Buscaglia JM, Nagula S, Jayaraman V, et al. Diagnostic yield and safety of jumbo biopsy forceps in patients with subepithelial lesions of the upper and lower GI tract. Gastrointest Endosc. 2012; 75(6):1147–1152

[82] de la Serna-Higuera C, Pérez-Miranda M, Díez-Redondo P, et al. EUS-guided single-incision needle-knife biopsy: description and results of a new method for tissue sampling of subepithelial GI tumors (with video). Gastrointest Endosc. 2011; 74(3):672–676

[83] Modlin IM, Kidd M, Latich I, et al. Current status of gastrointestinal carcinoids. Gastroenterology. 2005; 128(6):1717–1751

[84] Pape UF, Perren A, Niederle B, et al; Barcelona Consensus Conference participants. ENETS Consensus Guidelines for the management of patients with neuroendocrine neoplasms from the jejuno-ileum and the appendix including goblet cell carcinomas. Neuroendocrinology. 2012; 95(2):135–156

[85] Lee HL, Kwon OW, Lee KN, et al. Endoscopic histologic diagnosis of gastric GI submucosal tumors via the endoscopic submucosal dissection technique. Gastrointest Endosc. 2011; 74(3):693–695

[86] Grubel P. Keyhole biopsy: an easy and better alternative to fine-needle aspiration or Tru-cut biopsy of submucosal gastrointestinal tumors. Endoscopy. 2010; 42(8):685–, author reply 685

[87] Thomas D, Tsolakis AV, Grozinsky-Glasberg S, et al. Long-term follow-up of a large series of patients with type 1 gastric carcinoid tumors: data from a multicenter study. Eur J Endocrinol. 2013; 168(2):185–193

[88] de Mestier L, Brixi H, Gincul R, et al. Updating the management of patients with rectal neuroendocrine tumors. Endoscopy. 2013; 45(12):1039–1046

[89] Smith JD, Reidy DL, Goodman KA, et al. A retrospective review of 126 high-grade neuroendocrine carcinomas of the colon and rectum. Ann Surg Oncol. 2014; 21(9):2956–2962

[90] Fahy BN, Tang LH, Klimstra D, et al. Carcinoid of the rectum risk stratification (CaRRs): a strategy for preoperative outcome assessment. Ann Surg Oncol. 2007; 14(5):1735–1743

[91] Caplin M, Sundin A, Nillson O, et al; Barcelona Consensus Conference participants. ENETS Consensus Guidelines for the management of patients with digestive neuroendocrine neoplasms: colorectal neuroendocrine neoplasms. Neuroendocrinology. 2012; 95(2):88–97

[92] DeMatteo RP, Lewis JJ, Leung D, et al. Two hundred gastrointestinal stromal tumors: recurrence patterns and prognostic factors for survival. Ann Surg. 2000; 231(1):51–58

[93] Pierie JP, Choudry U, Muzikansky A, et al. The effect of surgery and grade on outcome of gastrointestinal stromal tumors. Arch Surg. 2001; 136(4):383–389

[94] McCarter MD, Antonescu CR, Ballman KV, et al; American College of Surgeons Oncology Group (ACOSOG) Intergroup Adjuvant Gist Study Team. Microscopically positive margins for primary gastrointestinal stromal tumors: analysis of risk factors and tumor recurrence. J Am Coll Surg. 2012; 215(1):53–59, discussion 59–60

[95] Hiki N, Yamamoto Y, Fukunaga T, et al. Laparoscopic and endoscopic cooperative surgery for gastrointestinal stromal tumor dissection. Surg Endosc. 2008; 22(7):1729–1735

[96] Abe N, Takeuchi H, Yanagida O, et al. Endoscopic full-thickness resection with laparoscopic assistance as hybrid NOTES for gastric submucosal tumor. Surg Endosc. 2009; 23(8):1908–1913

[97] Kim HH. Endoscopic treatment for gastrointestinal stromal tumor: Advantages and hurdles. World J Gastrointest Endosc. 2015; 7(3):192–205

[98] Bauder M, Schmidt A, Caca K. Non-exposure, device-assisted endoscopic full-thickness resection. Gastrointest Endosc Clin N Am. 2016; 26(2):297–312

[99] Hyun JH, Jeen YT, Chun HJ, et al. Endoscopic resection of submucosal tumor of the esophagus: results in 62 patients. Endoscopy. 1997; 29(3):165–170

[100] Park YS, Park SW, Kim TI, et al. Endoscopic enucleation of upper-GI submucosal tumors by using an insulated-tip electrosurgical knife. Gastrointest Endosc. 2004; 59(3):409–415

[101] Rösch T, Sarbia M, Schumacher B, et al. Attempted endoscopic en bloc resection of mucosal and submucosal tumors using insulated-tip knives: a pilot series. Endoscopy. 2004; 36(9):788–801

[102] Lee IL, Lin PY, Tung SY, et al. Endoscopic submucosal dissection for the treatment of intraluminal gastric subepithelial tumors originating from the muscularis propria layer. Endoscopy. 2006; 38(10):1024–1028

[103] Probst A, Messmann H. Endoscopic therapy for early gastric cancers—from EMR to ESD, from guideline criteria to expanded criteria. Digestion. 2009; 80(3):170–172

[104] Hwang JC, Kim JH, Kim JH, et al. Endoscopic resection for the treatment of gastric subepithelial tumors originated from the muscularis propria layer. Hepatogastroenterology. 2009; 56(94–95):1281–1286

[105] Shi Q, Zhong YS, Yao LQ, et al. Endoscopic submucosal dissection for treatment of esophageal submucosal tumors originating from the muscularis propria layer. Gastrointest Endosc. 2011; 74(6):1194–1200

[106] Jeong ID, Jung SW, Bang SJ, et al. Endoscopic enucleation for gastric subepithelial tumors originating in the muscularis propria layer. Surg Endosc. 2011; 25(2):468–474

[107] Białek A, Wiechowska-Kozłowska A, Pertkiewicz J, et al. Endoscopic submucosal dissection for treatment of gastric subepithelial tumors (with video). Gastrointest Endosc. 2012; 75(2):276–286

[108] Li QL, Yao LQ, Zhou PH, et al. Submucosal tumors of the esophagogastric junction originating from the muscularis propria layer: a large study of endoscopic submucosal dissection (with video). Gastrointest Endosc. 2012; 75(6):1153–1158

[109] Wang L, Ren W, Fan CQ, et al. Full-thickness endoscopic resection of nonintracavitary gastric stromal tumors: a novel approach. Surg Endosc. 2011; 25(2):641–647

[110] Zhou PH, Yao LQ, Qin XY, et al. Endoscopic full-thickness resection without laparoscopic assistance for gastric submucosal tumors originated from the muscularis propria. Surg Endosc. 2011; 25(9):2926–2931

[111] Ye LP, Yu Z, Mao XL, et al. Endoscopic full-thickness resection with defect closure using clips and an endoloop for gastric subepithelial tumors arising from the muscularis propria. Surg Endosc. 2014; 28(6):1978–1983

[112] Stavropoulos SN, Modayil R, Friedel D, Brathwaite CE. Endoscopic full-thickness resection for GI stromal tumors. Gastrointest Endosc. 2014; 80(2):334–335

[113] Stavropoulos SN, Modayil R, Friedel D. Current applications of endoscopic suturing. World J Gastrointest Endosc. 2015; 7(8):777–789

[114] Inoue H, Ikeda H, Hosoya T, et al. Submucosal endoscopic tumor resection for subepithelial tumors in the esophagus and cardia. Endoscopy. 2012; 44(3):225–230

[115] Xu MD, Cai MY, Zhou PH, et al. Submucosal tunneling endoscopic resection: a new technique for treating upper GI submucosal tumors originating from the muscularis propria layer (with videos). Gastrointest Endosc. 2012; 75(1):195–199

[116] Gong W, Xiong Y, Zhi F, et al. Preliminary experience of endoscopic submucosal tunnel dissection for upper gastrointestinal submucosal tumors. Endoscopy. 2012; 44(3):231–235

[117] Modayil R, Stavropoulos SN. A Western perspective on "new NOTES" from POEM to full-thickness resection and beyond. Gastrointest Endosc Clin N Am. 2016; 26(2):413–432

46 Gastrointestinal Foreign Bodies

James H. Tabibian and Gregory G. Ginsberg

46.1 Introduction

Foreign bodies of the digestive (gastrointestinal [GI]) tract include nonfood objects that are intentionally or unintentionally ingested or inserted in the body, food impactions, and bezoars. Although the precise incidence of foreign bodies of the GI tract has not been well studied, this clinical scenario is frequently encountered in practice.[1,2,3,4,5,6,7,8] Given the frequency of the problem and its potential for morbidity and mortality, it is important to understand the proper methods of diagnosis and management.

46.2 Clinical Epidemiology

Esophageal food impaction is the most common foreign body type in the GI tract, with an estimated annual incidence of 16 episodes per 100,000 adults.[9] The majority of esophageal food impactions occur in patients with preexisting esophageal pathology, including benign peptic strictures, rings, eosinophilic esophagitis, surgical anastomoses, motility disorders, and (rarely) esophageal malignancy, as shown in ▶Table 46.1.[10,11,12] Types of food impaction differ by geographical region. In the United States, beef, chicken, and pork are common, whereas fish bones are more frequent in Asia and coastal areas.

True foreign body (i.e., nonfood body) ingestion occurs most frequently in the pediatric population, ages 6 months to 3 years,

Table 46.1 Underlying disorders in esophageal foreign body and food impaction

Eosinophilic esophagitis

Schatzki's ring

Schatzki's ring

Radiation-induced stricture

Zenker's (or other) diverticulum

Postsurgical (e.g., fundoplication)

Esophageal carcinoma

Achalasia

Other dysmotility condition

accounting for 80% of all true foreign body. This is attributable to children's natural oral curiosity and naiveté.[13] Typical foreign objects in this population include coins, marbles, pins, and small toys.[3,7] Adult patients at highest risk of true foreign body ingestion include those with dentures, who may accidentally ingest their own prostheses (▶Fig. 46.1) and other foreign bodies because of decreased oral tactile sensation and swallowing control, and those with altered judgment, including patients who have dementia or are intoxicated. Intentional ingestion occurs most commonly in prisoners or persons with psychiatric problems who may swallow objects for secondary gain. These patients frequently are multiple/recurrent ingestors of complex and/or hazardous foreign bodies (▶Fig. 46.2a, b). Finally, certain occupations

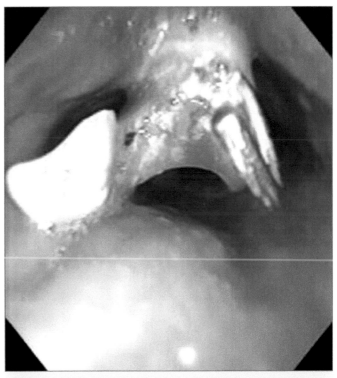

Fig. 46.1 Endoscopic view of a denture fragment in the esophagus at the level of the aortic arch.

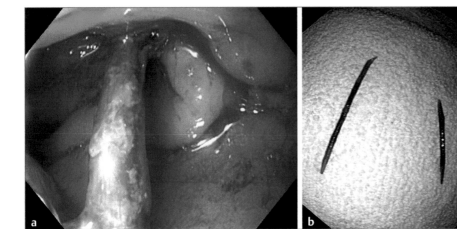

Fig. 46.2 Intentional toothpick ingestion by a prison inmate for secondary gain. The patient was transferred from the prison for therapeutic intervention. **(a)** Polypoid inflammatory changes seen in the colon in association with the embedded toothpick. **(b)** Using standard, through-the-scope biopsy forceps, the toothpick was grasped and removed in two pieces.

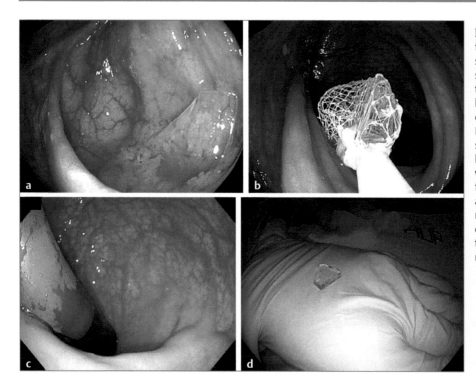

Fig. 46.3 Endoscopic removal of a glass fragment ingested while working on a skylight. (**a**) A sharp fragment of glass was seen in the right lower quadrant on computed tomography (not on plain film) and shown here in the cecum during therapeutic colonoscopy. (**b**) A Roth retrieval net (US Endoscopy, Mentor, Ohio) was used to secure the glass fragment, taking care to keep it centered in the colonic lumen during withdrawal. (**c**) Once in the rectum, the glass fragment was carefully removed through the anal canal with simultaneous manual anal retraction performed by an assistant; the colonoscope was reintroduced and confirmed the absence of trauma to the colon and rectum. (**d**) Glass fragment ex vivo.

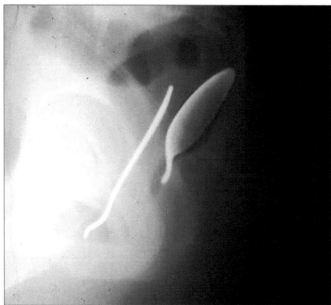

Fig. 46.4 Foreign body (broken spoon) is inserted retrograde into the rectum.

such as roofers, carpenters, tailors, and glassworkers are at risk of accidental ingestion during work with objects such as pins, nails, or glass fragments (▶Fig. 46.3a–d) that they may temporarily hold in their teeth.

Retrograde insertion of foreign objects *per ano* is usually related to sexual activity and sexual assault (▶Fig. 46.4). Rectal foreign objects can also be seen in patients with psychiatric disorders, individuals who inadvertently lose an object when trying to relieve constipation (e.g., performing mechanical disimpaction), and in cases of illicit drug smuggling.

Bezoars can form in a variety of settings and are more common in individuals with impaired gastric or transit, be it due to congenital or acquired (e.g., postoperative) motility or mechanical abnormalities. The most common types of bezoars are phytobezoars (composed of vegetable matter), trichobezoars (composed of hair), and pharmacobezoars (composed of medication), as discussed further below.

46.2.1 Overview of Pathophysiology

The majority of foreign bodies pass through the GI tract without causing symptoms or complications.[14] However, 10 to 20% cause symptoms that require intervention, in some cases surgical. Perforation and obstruction are the most serious complications of foreign objects and occur most frequently at anatomical sphincters and areas of angulation (▶Fig. 46.5). Foreign bodies can also impact and lead to complications at sites of acquired stenosis, in particular, surgical anastomoses, be these due to stricture formation, edema, or retained anastomotic sutures or staples (▶Fig. 46.6a, b).

Esophageal foreign bodies, including both esophageal food impactions and true foreign bodies, generally result in the most substantial morbidity. Esophageal foreign bodies can cause chest pain and pulmonary aspiration and can result in esophageal perforation, mediastinitis, and/or thoracic fistulization. The complication rate is directly proportional to the time the object remains in the esophagus beyond 24 hours. The esophagus has four areas of anatomical narrowing: the upper esophageal sphincter, the impression of the aortic arch, the crossing of the left main stem bronchus, and the lower esophageal sphincter. Foreign body impaction occurs preferentially in these areas of physiologic narrowing as well as in individuals with underlying esophageal pathology (structural and/or motor), as mentioned earlier.[15] Such pathology is often unrecognized or undiagnosed up until an index episode of foreign body impaction.

Once reaching the stomach, most foreign objects will pass through the GI tract within 1 to 2 weeks. Exceptions to this are sharp, large, and long objects: sharp/pointed objects have an associated perforation rate of up to approximately 35%; large objects (> 2 cm in diameter) have difficulty passing through the

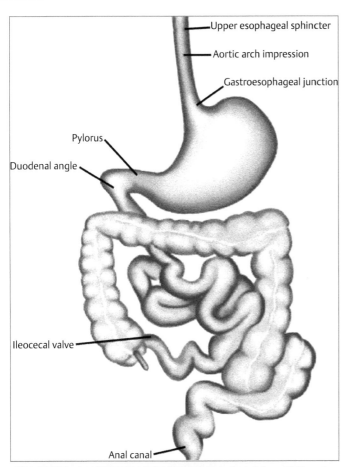

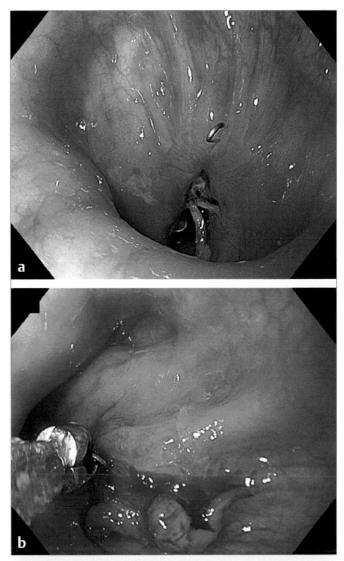

Fig. 46.5 Areas of gastrointestinal tract narrowing and angulation that predispose to foreign body impaction and obstruction.

pylorus; and objects longer than 5 cm have difficulty negotiating the pylorus and the superior and inferior duodenal angles.[16,17] The fixed angulation of the ligament of Treitz and the ileocecal valve are sites of small bowel impaction for objects that have traversed the gastric and duodenal lumen.

With respect to bezoars, phytobezoars develop with the ingestion of fibrous, poorly digestible foods such as persimmon, celery, or potato peel, etc. Trichobezoars develop classically in younger females with a psychiatric disorder that leads to ingestion of a large amount of hair. Pharmacobezoars are often the result of polypharmacy or ingestion of large, fibrous capsules/tablets.

Colorectal foreign bodies can result from anterograde passage of ingested objects or from direct retrograde insertion. The latter can cause similar complications to those that are ingested. The valves of Houston (i.e., *plicae transversae recti*) impede spontaneous passage after forceful insertion. Moreover, the internal and external anal sphincters can become spasmodic and the anal canal mucosa edematous after foreign body insertion, posing further impediment.

46.3 Patient Presentation

Clinical presentation of foreign objects in children may be subtle. Symptoms may include drooling, poor feeding, failure to thrive, or stridor/aspiration. In approximately 40% of cases, the patient is asymptomatic, and there is no report of foreign body ingestion from the patient or caregiver.[18]

Fig. 46.6 Postesophagectomy dysphagia secondary to anastomotic stricture and residual surgical material. (**a**) Staple and suture material seen at site of Ivor Lewis anastomosis. (**b**) Staples removed using staple removal forceps (Olympus, Center Valley, Pennsylvania) after performing balloon dilation at the anastomosis.

In adults, esophageal obstruction is nearly always symptomatic, with partial obstruction causing substernal chest pain, dysphagia, gagging, or a sense of choking. More complete obstruction leads to additional symptoms, namely drooling, sialorrhea, and inability to handle secretions. Small sharp objects may cause a persistent sensation of something "being stuck" in addition to chest or (referred) throat pain. Foreign bodies that have passed into the stomach infrequently cause symptoms, as mentioned above, and when they do, they are typically the direct result of a complication such as perforation, obstruction, or bleeding.

Gastric bezoars may be asymptomatic or may present with abdominal discomfort, nausea, vomiting, early satiety, or weight loss.[19] Small bowel bezoars are usually symptomatic, with obstructive symptoms.

Patients with colorectal foreign objects may be asymptomatic or present with GI bleeding, obstruction, peritonitis, or perforation. Cases of retrograde insertion generally have a distinct history, if provided.[16,17]

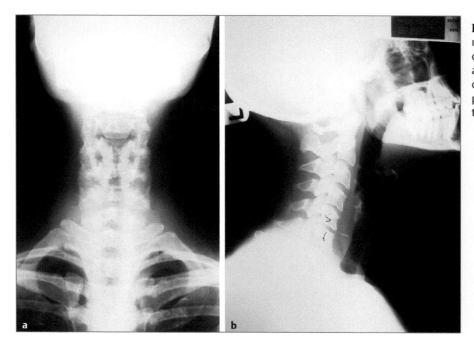

Fig. 46.7 Accidental ingestion of a metal wire fragment. While the object is obscured by the cervical vertebrae on the anteroposterior film (**a**), it is recognizable on the lateral neck film (**b**) and seen having penetrated into the soft tissue at the level of the cervical 5 to 6 intervertebral space.

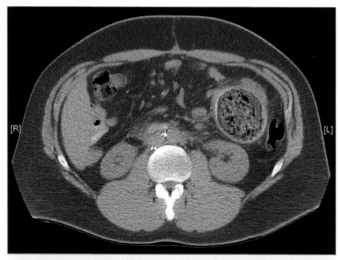

Fig. 46.8 Computerized tomography localizes a retained cloth object in the proximal jejunum not seen on plain film radiography.

46.4 Diagnosis

Obtaining a careful history is vital in the diagnosis and management of GI foreign bodies, as the majority of adults can accurately identify the timing and type of foreign body ingestion. Past medicosurgical history is important for identifying individuals at increased risk of sustaining GI tract foreign bodies as well as documenting dysphagia, previous food impaction or foreign body ingestion, and congenital or acquired anatomical abnormalities. Physical examination is generally unhelpful for determining the presence or absence of a foreign object, but it can identify complications related to a foreign object. For example, the neck and chest should be auscultated for wheezing or signs of aspiration or esophageal perforation and inspected for the presence of crepitus. Similarly, the abdomen should be examined for signs of perforation or obstruction.

Imaging of the suspected region of involvement should be considered as part of foreign object evaluation. Radiography can aid in identifying the presence, type, location, and number of foreign objects as well as complications such as perforation, subcutaneous emphysema, and obstruction.[3] Plain films have obvious diagnostic limitations in patients with esophageal food impaction and ingested foreign bodies that are not radiopaque (notably most fish bones)[20]; false-negative and false-positive rates with plain films are as high as 47 and 20%, respectively. If there is any suspicion of radio-opacity with respect to ingested foreign bodies, anteroposterior and lateral chest and neck films should be considered (▶Fig. 46.7a,b). As many foreign objects are not readily visible by plain film radiography, computed tomography (CT) imaging may be considered in lieu of simple radiographs and may be more cost-effective (▶Fig. 46.8).[21,22,23,24,25] The sensitivity and accuracy of CT are superior to plain films and can be further improved with three-dimensional reconstruction.[21,22,23,25,26] Additional details regarding initial and follow-up imaging modalities are provided in recent Radiology Society clinical guidelines.[27] Of note, barium contrast should be avoided because of the risk of aspiration with esophageal obstruction and its interference with subsequent therapeutic endoscopy (▶Fig. 46.9).

In the pediatric population, mouth-to-anus radiologic evaluation has been advocated because of the difficulty of obtaining an adequate history, especially in young children. Alternatively, and to avoid radiation, handheld metal detectors may be considered and have been shown to have a greater than 90% sensitivity and specificity in identifying the presence and location of metallic foreign bodies.[28,29,30]

Endoscopy is the most accurate diagnostic modality for food impactions, true foreign bodies, and bezoars, with an accuracy of approximately 100%. Endoscopy also offers identification of concomitant pathology such as esophageal strictures, esophagitis (reflux or eosinophilic), and mucosal trauma caused by the foreign body. Of note, foreign bodies impacted at or above the cricopharyngeus should be removed by laryngoscopy, while those below this level can be managed by flexible upper GI endoscopy.[31,32,33]

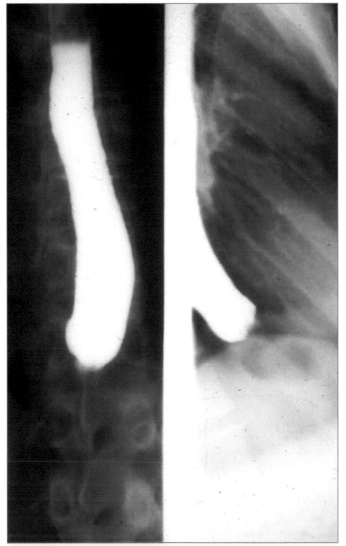

Fig. 46.9 Inadvertent contrast radiography performed in this patient with esophageal obstruction due to food bolus impaction resulted in increased risk for aspiration and complicated endoscopic management.

46.4.1 Treatment

Foreign bodies should be treated with the knowledge that 80 to 90% will pass spontaneously without complication.[2] The need to intervene is thus predicated on the individual patient, in particular symptoms, size, type, and location of the foreign body in the GI tract. While endoscopy is generally the preferred modality of intervention, other options do exist, as discussed below.

46.4.2 Pharmacologic therapies

Glucagon, a smooth muscle relaxant that reduces lower esophageal sphincter pressure, has long been employed in the management of esophageal food impaction and is indeed one of the only interventions that has been studied in a randomized-controlled trial.[34] However, the use of glucagon, typically in doses of 0.5 to 2 mg intravenously, is associated with success rates ranging only from 12 to 58% in treating esophageal food impactions.[35] Glucagon is a reasonable consideration while awaiting endoscopic therapy. However, it may cause nausea and vomiting and is not effective when there is a fixed esophageal obstruction. Moreover, it should

not delay planning for endoscopy. Other smooth muscle relaxants, such as nifedipine and nitroglycerin, are not recommended due to hypotension and other adverse effects these may cause.[36]

Effervescent agents such as carbonated soda have been described alone or in combination with other pharmacologic agents (e.g., glucagon).[37,38,39,40] The evidence for their use includes one prospective study [41] and several case series, and the collective results and anecdotal experience. There is insufficient evidence to support the use of effervescent agents in the management of esophageal food impactions or ingested foreign bodies.[40]

The use of other pharmacologic agents, such as proteolytic enzymes (including papain) should be avoided because of lack of efficacy and higher complication rates.[2,16,34,42] Pharmacologic treatment, for example, with a prokinetic agent plus a low-residue or liquid diet, may be considered for small gastric bezoars in the absence of acute obstructive symptoms, but most will require endoscopic therapy.

46.4.3 Endoscopic accessories and interventions

Foley balloon catheters, baskets, suction catheters, or magnetic catheters have been used under fluoroscopic guidance to extract esophageal foreign objects. Despite favorable published success rates, a major limitation of these methods remains lack of control during extraction of the foreign body. Complications occur particularly at the level of the upper esophageal sphincter and hypopharynx, including epistaxis, laryngospasm, and occasionally airway obstruction. The use of these methods should be limited to situations where endoscopy is not available or cannot be performed within 24 hours.

Flexible endoscopy has become the treatment of choice for esophageal food impactions and true esophageal foreign bodies based on multiple large reports of successful treatment with success rates of 95 to 100% and minimal to no complications.[36,43] Intervention is recommended for all esophageal foreign bodies ideally within 12 to 24 hours. Once ingested, nonfood foreign objects have passed distal to the esophagus, retrieval from the stomach and proximal small intestine is only generally indicated for sharp objects (because of the increased risk of perforation) and objects longer than 5 cm or with diameters greater than 2 cm (which are unlikely to negotiate around the duodenal sweep or through the pylorus, respectively). While endoscopy has an extremely high success rate in treating foreign bodies, variables that decrease the chance of successful endoscopic treatment are poor patient cooperation and ingestion of multiple complex objects. Endoscopic intervention should be avoided in cases of illicit drug "body packing," where packets of contraband are internally concealed (by ingestion or retrograde insertion), except in highly selected and individualized circumstances (▶ Fig. 46.10a, b). Attempt at endoscopic removal poses a high risk of packet rupture, which can lead to fatal drug overdose. Therefore, such cases should be managed conservatively with serial noninvasive imaging and monitoring toxicology levels, and by surgical intervention when removal is necessary.[2]

Availability of and familiarity with multiple endoscopic accessories and retrieval devices (▶ Table 46.2) are valuable for successful endoscopic management of foreign objects. Choice of equipment depends largely on foreign object type and location as

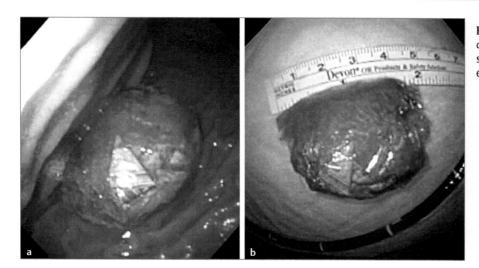

Fig. 46.10 Ingested wad of marijuana and cash. (**a**) Endoscopic view of ingesta in the stomach. (**b**) Wad ex vivo after successful endoscopic removal.

well as endoscopist experience and preference.[44,45,46] Regardless of the technique and equipment used, ex vivo practice (i.e., a "dry run") using the planned technique and equipment and an object similar to that which is in need of retrieval is often beneficial; this can serve to help determine, a priori, the suitability of the proposed method of treatment.[2]

Intravenous conscious sedation is sufficient sedation for many adult patients undergoing endoscopic management of foreign objects. However, monitored anesthesia care with propofol sedation has become increasingly common. It is important to recognize the loss of airway protective reflexes when using propofol and to ensure that risk of aspiration can be mitigated; an oroesophageal overtube may be considered as an adjunctive means to do so. Endotracheal intubation should be considered when the risk of aspiration is deemed sufficiently increased. Endotracheal intubation should also be considered in the majority of pediatric patients, in uncooperative adult patients, and for removing multiple or complex foreign objects that entail a prolonged procedural time.

46.4.4 Esophageal food impaction

Esophageal food impactions should be treated endoscopically on an urgent basis when there are signs of obstruction. The primary endoscopic technique to treat food boluses is the "push technique," which has success rates as high as 95% and low complication rates.[47] Here, the endoscope is first maneuvered around the food bolus and into the stomach to assess for distally obstructing lesions. The endoscope is then pulled back, and the food bolus is advanced carefully into the stomach. Even if the scope cannot be passed around the impacted food bolus, a trial of gently pushing the food bolus can be attempted. Forceful pushing should not be attempted as this may increase the risk of procedure-related complication.[1]

If an esophageal food impaction cannot be successfully pushed into the stomach, retrograde removal of the bolus may be performed en bloc[48] or after breaking apart the bolus with forceps, snares, or other accessories. This permits pushing the fragments into the stomach or retrograde endoscopic retrieval per os. An overtube should be considered for foods that break apart easily and/or require multiple endoscopic passes, particularly if airway protection (e.g., via endotracheal tube) has not been secured. The choice of overtube, esophageal (25 cm) versus gastric (50 cm), depends on the nature and location of the esophageal food/foreign object impaction (▶Fig. 46.11a, b). After removal (via pus

Table 46.2 Equipment for treatment and removal of gastrointestinal tract foreign bodies and food impactions

Through-the-scope retrieval accessories	Other accessory equipment
• Roth retrieval net • Rat-tooth and alligator forceps • Polypectomy snare • Three- or four-prong grasper • Dormia basket	• Overtube (esophageal or gastric) • Latex protector hood • Variceal ligator cap • Kelly's or McGill's forceps • Extractor magnet

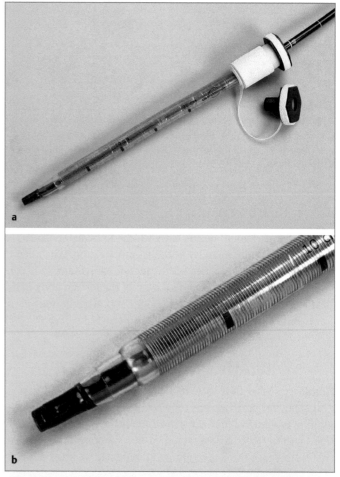

Fig. 46.11 (**a**) Commercially available oroesophageal overtube, which should be part of the readily available inventory for food impaction and ingested foreign object management. (**b**) Close-up imaging showing endoscope inside overtube with tip projecting beyond the end of the overtube.

technique or retrograde extraction), it is generally safe to perform endoscopic dilation if an esophageal stenosis is seen, unless extensive esophageal edema, erythema, or tears are present; in such scenarios, the patient should be placed on acid suppression medication, instructed on proper diet, and scheduled for esophageal dilation within approximately 4 to 6 weeks, depending on the nature of the esophageal injury and stenosis.

46.4.5 Sharp foreign bodies

All sharp foreign bodies within the reach of an endoscope should be removed if possible. Attempts should be made to remove sharp objects with the sharp end trailing distally (i.e., blunt end coming out first) to lessen the chance of perforation or mucosal tear. If a sharp object points proximally in the esophagus, it should be pushed into the stomach, rotated, and removed per os with its blunt end leading. Snares and rat tooth or alligator forceps allow the most control in removing sharp objects, and overtubes or protector hoods should be employed to protect the esophagus and oropharynx, especially if the object cannot be oriented with its sharp end trailing (▶ Fig. 46.12a–d). Sharp objects that are beyond the reach of the endoscope or cannot be removed may be observed with serial clinical examinations and radiographs. Surgery should be considered if the object does not progress in transit over approximately 3 days and clearly if there are clinical signs of perforation, obstruction, or bleeding.[49]

Long foreign bodies such as pens, toothbrushes, or silverware may not pass through the duodenal sweep, as mentioned previously, and can be difficult to remove retrograde through the lower and upper esophageal sphincters. Such objects should be grasped with a basket or snare at the tip of the object and mobilized while maintaining the object in a vertical (i.e., cephalocaudal) plane. Grasping the object closer to the center will cause the object to shift to a transverse plane, prohibiting endoscopic removal. Long foreign bodies should be endoscopically drawn into an esophageal or gastric length overtube; the object, overtube, and endoscope can then be removed as a collective unit (▶ Fig. 46.13).

46.4.6 Coins and button batteries

Coins and button batteries lodged in the esophagus can lead to pressure necrosis and perforation, with the added risk of liquefactive necrosis in the case of the latter.[2] With the development of through-the-scope retrieval nets, removal of coins and batteries has become technically facile, with the net used to snare around the object and secure control of it during removal. Once in the stomach, all but the largest coins (e.g., silver or half U.S. dollars; approximately 38 and 30 mm, respectively) will pass without complication, and batteries rarely cause problems, with the majority passing through the GI tract within 72 hours.[50]

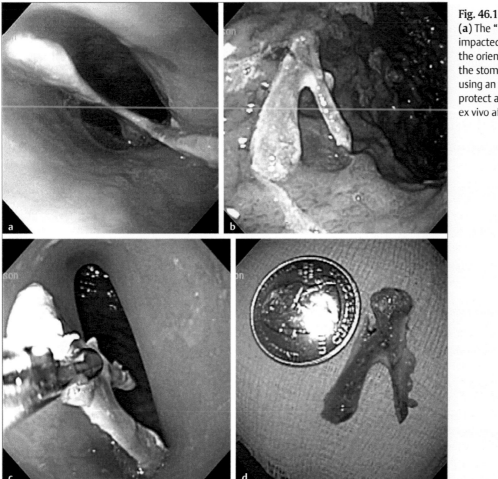

Fig. 46.12 Ingested chicken breast bone. **(a)** The "V"-shaped chicken breast bone is seen impacted in this patient's esophagus. Owing to the orientation of the bone, it was pushed into the stomach **(b)**, reoriented, and withdrawn using an over-the-scope latex hood **(c)** to protect against mucosal laceration. **(d)** Bone ex vivo after successful endoscopic removal.

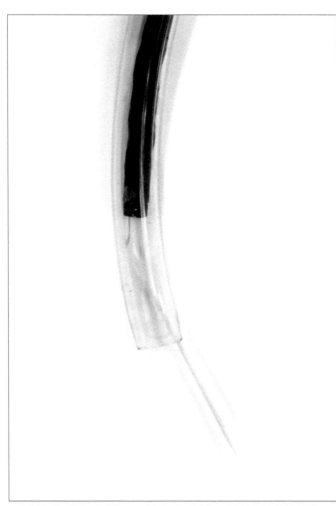

Fig. 46.13 Long and sharp, pointed objects can be safely removed by drawing the object into an overtube and withdrawing the entire assembly in unison.

46.4.7 Bezoars

With respect to bezoars, approximately 90% can be successfully treated with mechanical disruption using various endoscopic accessories. Trichobezors are an exception and typically require operative resection. After the bezoar is broken into smaller pieces, it can be retrieved retrograde per os (preferably with an overtube if multiple passes are anticipated or become needed) or allowed to pass through the GI tract. More complex endoscopic techniques such as mechanical, electrohydraulic, or neodymium-doped yttrium aluminum garnet (i.e., Nd:YAG) laser bezoar tripsy can employed for difficult-to-treat bezoars. In the rare instances of endoscopic treatment failure, surgical intervention is required. Importantly, after removal of a bezoar, patient counseling to avoid the offending ingesta (e.g., hair, high-residue foods) is critical to prevent recurrence.

46.4.8 Rectal foreign bodies

Most rectal foreign bodies can be removed manually or with the aid of an endoscope under sedation. As with upper GI foreign objects, a latex protector hood attached to the end of the scope or an overtube can be used when removing sharp objects to reduce trauma. Use of an overtube has the added advantage of overcoming the anal sphincter contraction during foreign body removal.

Larger or more complex objects may require extraction under general anesthesia with or without anal sphincter dilation or surgical intervention.[51]

46.5 Complications

The complication rate in managing all comers with foreign bodies ranges from 0 to 2% in the majority of larger studies. Complications occur more commonly when esophageal food impaction persists greater than 24 hours, with sharp and pointed objects, and in patients with a history of prior ingestions or ingestion of multiple objects. Perforation is the most notable direct complication associated with attempted removal of a foreign object. Risk factors for perforation at time of endoscopic treatment include the uncooperative (or inadequately sedated) patient, the psychiatric patient, and removal of sharp/pointed or complex objects. Cardiopulmonary complications and GI bleeding have also been described in the endoscopic removal of foreign objects but at a rate similar to that encountered with standard upper and lower endoscopy.

46.6 Conclusion and Future Trends

Gastrointestinal endoscopists will frequently encounter patients with esophageal food impaction and ingested foreign bodies. Flexible endoscopy has become the primary diagnostic and therapeutic modality for most GI tract foreign bodies. Endoscopy can provide treatment success in the majority of cases with low complication rates. Familiarity with the tools and techniques for endoscopic management enhances the likelihood for successful management.

References

[1] Eisen GM, Baron TH, Dominitz JA, et al; American Society for Gastrointestinal Endoscopy. Guideline for the management of ingested foreign bodies. Gastrointest Endosc. 2002; 55(7):802–806

[2] Webb WA. Management of foreign bodies of the upper gastrointestinal tract: update. Gastrointest Endosc. 1995; 41(1):39–51

[3] Cheng W, Tam PK. Foreign-body ingestion in children: experience with 1,265 cases. J Pediatr Surg. 1999; 34(10):1472–1476

[4] Chu KM, Choi HK, Tuen HH, et al. A prospective randomized trial comparing the use of the flexible gastroscope versus the bronchoscope in the management of foreign body ingestion. Gastrointest Endosc. 1998; 47(1):23–27

[5] Velitchkov NG, Grigorov GI, Losanoff JE, Kjossev KT. Ingested foreign bodies of the gastrointestinal tract: retrospective analysis of 542 cases. World J Surg. 1996; 20(8):1001–1005

[6] Kim JK, Kim SS, Kim JI, et al. Management of foreign bodies in the gastrointestinal tract: an analysis of 104 cases in children. Endoscopy. 1999; 31(4):302–304

[7] Hachimi-Idrissi S, Corne L, Vandenplas Y. Management of ingested foreign bodies in childhood: our experience and review of the literature. Eur J Emerg Med. 1998; 5(3):319–323

[8] Panieri E, Bass DH. The management of ingested foreign bodies in children—a review of 663 cases. Eur J Emerg Med. 1995; 2(2):83–87

[9] Longstreth GF, Longstreth KJ, Yao JF. Esophageal food impaction: epidemiology and therapy. A retrospective, observational study. Gastrointest Endosc. 2001; 53(2):193–198

[10] Sperry SL, Crockett SD, Miller CB, et al. Esophageal foreign-body impactions: epidemiology, time trends, and the impact of the increasing prevalence of eosinophilic esophagitis. Gastrointest Endosc. 2011; 74(5):985–991

[11] Desai TK, Stecevic V, Chang CH, et al. Association of eosinophilic inflammation with esophageal food impaction in adults. Gastrointest Endosc. 2005; 61(7):795–801

[12] Kerlin P, Jones D, Remedios M, Campbell C. Prevalence of eosinophilic esophagitis in adults with food bolus obstruction of the esophagus. J Clin Gastroenterol. 2007; 41(4):356–361

[13] Webb WA. Management of foreign bodies of the upper gastrointestinal tract. Gastroenterology. 1988; 94(1):204–216

[14] Schwartz GF, Polsky HS. Ingested foreign bodies of the gastrointestinal tract. Am Surg. 1976; 42(4):236–238

[15] Bloom RR, Nakano PH, Gray SW, Skandalakis JE. Foreign bodies of the gastrointestinal tract. Am Surg. 1986; 52(11):618–621

[16] Ginsberg GG. Management of ingested foreign objects and food bolus impactions. Gastrointest Endosc. 1995; 41(1):33–38

[17] Chaves DM, Ishioka S, Félix VN, et al. Removal of a foreign body from the upper gastrointestinal tract with a flexible endoscope: a prospective study. Endoscopy. 2004; 36(10):887–892

[18] Muñiz AE, Joffe MD. Foreign bodies, ingested and inhaled. JAAPA. 1999; 12(6):22–24, 27–28, 31–34 passim

[19] Diettrich NA, Gau FC. Postgastrectomy phytobezoars—endoscopic diagnosis and treatment. Arch Surg. 1985; 120(4):432–435

[20] Shaffer HA, Jr, de Lange EE. Gastrointestinal foreign bodies and strictures: radiologic interventions. Curr Probl Diagn Radiol. 1994; 23(6):205–249

[21] Zhu Z, Li W, Zhang L, et al. The predictive role of dual source CT for esophageal foreign bodies. Am J Otolaryngol. 2014; 35(2):215–218

[22] Eliashar R, Dano I, Dangoor E, et al. Computed tomography diagnosis of esophageal bone impaction: a prospective study. Ann Otol Rhinol Laryngol. 1999; 108(7 pt 1):708–710

[23] Marco De Lucas E, Sádaba P, Lastra García-Barón P, et al. Value of helical computed tomography in the management of upper esophageal foreign bodies. Acta Radiol. 2004; 45(4):369–374

[24] Shrime MG, Johnson PE, Stewart MG. Cost-effective diagnosis of ingested foreign bodies. Laryngoscope. 2007; 117(5):785–793

[25] Ma J, Kang DK, Bae JI, et al. Value of MDCT in diagnosis and management of esophageal sharp or pointed foreign bodies according to level of esophagus. AJR Am J Roentgenol. 2013; 201(5):W707–11

[26] Takada M, Kashiwagi R, Sakane M, et al. 3D-CT diagnosis for ingested foreign bodies. Am J Emerg Med. 2000; 18(2):192–193

[27] Guelfguat M, Kaplinskiy V, Reddy SH, DiPoce J. Clinical guidelines for imaging and reporting ingested foreign bodies. AJR Am J Roentgenol. 2014; 203(1):37–53

[28] Bassett KE, Schunk JE, Logan L. Localizing ingested coins with a metal detector. Am J Emerg Med. 1999; 17(4):338–341

[29] Doraiswamy NV, Baig H, Hallam L. Metal detector and swallowed metal foreign bodies in children. J Accid Emerg Med. 1999; 16(2):123–125

[30] Seikel K, Primm PA, Elizondo BJ, Remley KL. Handheld metal detector localization of ingested metallic foreign bodies: accurate in any hands? Arch Pediatr Adolesc Med. 1999; 153(8):853–857

[31] Russell R, Lucas A, Johnson J, et al. Extraction of esophageal foreign bodies in children: rigid versus flexible endoscopy. Pediatr Surg Int. 2014; 30(4):417–422

[32] Hodge D, III, Tecklenburg F, Fleisher G. Coin ingestion: does every child need a radiograph? Ann Emerg Med. 1985; 14(5):443–446

[33] Yalçin S, Karnak I, Ciftci AO, et al. Foreign body ingestion in children: an analysis of pediatric surgical practice. Pediatr Surg Int. 2007; 23(8):755–761

[34] Tibbling L, Bjorkhoel A, Jansson E, Stenkvist M. Effect of spasmolytic drugs on esophageal foreign bodies. Dysphagia. 1995; 10(2):126–127

[35] Trenkner SW, Maglinte DD, Lehman GA, et al. Esophageal food impaction: treatment with glucagon. Radiology. 1983; 149(2):401–403

[36] Ikenberry SO, Jue TL, Anderson MA, et al; ASGE Standards of Practice Committee. Management of ingested foreign bodies and food impactions. Gastrointest Endosc. 2011; 73(6):1085–1091

[37] Rice BT, Spiegel PK, Dombrowski PJ. Acute esophageal food impaction treated by gas-forming agents. Radiology. 1983; 146(2):299–301

[38] Karanjia ND, Rees M. The use of Coca-Cola in the management of bolus obstruction in benign oesophageal stricture. Ann R Coll Surg Engl. 1993; 75(2):94–95

[39] Smith JC, Janower ML, Geiger AH. Use of glucagon and gas-forming agents in acute esophageal food impaction. Radiology. 1986; 159(2):567–568

[40] Lee J, Anderson R. Best evidence topic report. Effervescent agents for oesophageal food bolus impaction. Emerg Med J. 2005; 22(2):123–124

[41] Robbins MI, Shortsleeve MJ. Treatment of acute esophageal food impaction with glucagon, an effervescent agent, and water. AJR Am J Roentgenol. 1994; 162(2):325–328

[42] Andersen HA, Bernatz PE, Grindlay JH. Perforation of the esophagus after use of a digestant agent: report of case and experimental study. Ann Otol Rhinol Laryngol. 1959; 68:890–896

[43] Ciriza C, García L, Suárez P, et al. What predictive parameters best indicate the need for emergent gastrointestinal endoscopy after foreign body ingestion? J Clin Gastroenterol. 2000; 31(1):23–28

[44] Faigel DO, Stotland BR, Kochman ML, et al. Device choice and experience level in endoscopic foreign object retrieval: an in vivo study. Gastrointest Endosc. 1997; 45(6):490–492

[45] Nelson DB, Bosco JJ, Curtis WD, et al; American Society for Gastrointestinal Endoscopy. ASGE technology status evaluation report. Endoscopic retrieval devices. February 1999. Gastrointest Endosc. 1999; 50(6):932–934

[46] Kirchner GI, Zuber-Jerger I, Endlicher E, et al. Causes of bolus impaction in the esophagus. Surg Endosc. 2011; 25(10):3170–3174

[47] Vicari JJ, Johanson JF, Frakes JT. Outcomes of acute esophageal food impaction: success of the push technique. Gastrointest Endosc. 2001; 53(2):178–181

[48] Saffouri GB, Gomez V, Tabibian JH, et al. Burn and anchor: a novel food impaction retrieval technique. Gastrointest Endosc. 2016;83(5):1029–1030

[49] Devanesan J, Pisani A, Sharma P. et al. Metallic foreign bodies in the stomach. Arch Surg. 1977; 112(5):664–665

[50] Litovitz TL. Battery ingestions: product accessibility and clinical course. Pediatrics. 1985; 75(3):469–476

[51] Kouraklis G, Misiakos E, Dovas N, et al. Management of foreign bodies of the rectum: report of 21 cases. J R Coll Surg Edinb. 1997; 42(4):246–247

Index